MORTON'S MEDICAL BIBLIOGRAPHY

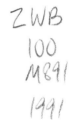

Morton's Medical Bibliography

An Annotated Check-list of Texts
Illustrating the History of Medicine
(Garrison and Morton)

Edited by Jeremy M. Norman

FIFTH EDITION

Scolar Press

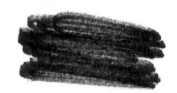

Fifth edition copyright © Jeremy M. Norman, 1991

First published 1943
Second edition 1954
Copyright L.T. Morton, 1943, 1954
Reprinted 1961 by André Deutsch
Second edition revised 1965
Third edition completely reset and printed 1970 by André Deutsch Limited
Second impression of third edition September 1976
Copyright ©1970 by Leslie T. Morton
Fourth edition completely reset and published by Gower Publishing Company Ltd
Copyright ©1983 by L.T. Morton
Fifth edition published by
Scolar Press
Gower House
Croft Road
Aldershot
Hants GU11 3HR
England

Gower Publishing Company
Old Post Road
Brookfield
Vermont 05036
USA

British Library and Library of Congress CIP data are available

ISBN 0-85967-897-0

Printed in Great Britain at the University Press, Cambridge

INTRODUCTION TO THE FIFTH EDITION

BY

LESLIE T. MORTON

In May 1960 I had the privilege of delivering a Woodward Lecture at Yale University Medical Library. The theme suggested and adopted for the lecture was an outline of events leading to the preparation and publication of *A Medical Bibliography*. The lecture was published in Lee Ash's *Serial Publications Containing Medical Classics*,[1] an index to citations to papers included in the *Bibliography*. It seemed appropriate that the introduction to this fifth edition should be prefaced by a revised and updated account of the conception, birth and development of the Bibliography to the point where it is passed on to a new compiler.

According to Garrison[2] it was Sir William Osler who suggested to Lieut.-Col. Walter D. McCaw, Librarian of the Surgeon General's Office, Washington (now the National Library of Medicine) the advantages of segregating the more valuable historic items in that library for safe keeping under glass. The task of drawing up a suitable list was entrusted to Fielding Hudson Garrison (1870-1935), Assistant Librarian. However, Wyndham D. Miles[3] records that the list was a by-product of an exhibit, initiated by McCaw, of books, pamphlets and articles that were milestones in the development of medicine from ancient times to the twentieth century and that Garrison carried out the research necessary to identify the classics. The exhibit was completed in 1910 and Garrison then wrote a 15,000-word account of the advance of medicine as illustrated by the items. Part of this article was published in the *Journal of the American Medical Association*.[4] The list itself was published in the *Index- Catalogue of the Library of the Surgeon General's Office*.[5] It contains over 2,000 items.

In 1928 Garrison was offered the post of Librarian and Lecturer on the History of Medicine at the Welch Medical Library, Johns Hopkins Hospital, by William H. Welch and in 1930 he moved to Baltimore and began working full-time at Johns Hopkins. In 1933 publication began of the *Bulletin of the Institute of the History of Medicine*, with Henry E. Sigerist as Editor. In the first volume Garrison[2] published an expanded revision of the 1912 list and recorded that the original had been used by him "as a convenient scaffolding for a book on the history of medicine". This revised list contains over 4,000 items.

I first became interested in the history of medicine in the late 1920s while working in the Medical Sciences Library at University College, London. William Sharpey, a former Professor of Physiology in the College, had bequeathed to it his fine library which contained many medical classics, including works of Vesalius, Harvey, Aselli, Boerhaave, Haller, etc. At that time they had no significance to me although I listened with interest when my seniors had them out of the safe or stacks and expounded on them.

It was Professor Charles Singer who first implanted in me an interest in medical history. His room, close to the main library, was lined with what may be regarded as the minor classics of medicine. From time to time he would ask me in to show me some treasure open on his desk – perhaps a book borrowed from the Royal College of Physicians of London or something he had just bought. He would explain its importance, and if he had bought it for his own collection he might tell me how much he had paid for it.

Although I became more interested in the subject my knowledge of it grew very slowly. I began to browse through medico-historical journals and to read books in the field. I was interested to see the *Bulletin of the Institute of the History of Medicine* when it first appeared in 1933. Garrison's Revised Check-List appeared in the November issue of that year and immediately struck me as a valuable piece of work although I had no idea at that time how important a part it was to play in my life.

At the beginning of 1933 I had moved to the library of the Royal Society of Medicine and here I was able to see much more historical material. Some requests for bibliographical information brought my mind back more than once to the Check-List but I found it difficult to consult owing to the lack of an index. In 1938 I made a more careful examination of it. I considered making author and subject indexes to it but accepted that unless they were published with a re-issued Check-List they would be of limited use. I discussed the idea with my friend the late W. J. Bishop and we concluded that if the list could be revised, expanded and annotated to provide a chronological bibliography of the most important contributions to the literature on medicine and related subjects it could be a useful reference work for medical writers and historians, research workers, librarians and others.

I next approached Grafton and Company, which specialized in the publication of library manuals and bibliographies and also carried a large stock of secondhand books in its shop opposite the British Museum. Grafton's was owned by Miss Frank Hamel, herself a distinguished author, who seemed to spend all her life at the back of the shop and was never seen without a hat. Miss Hamel was interested and agreed to undertake publication.

Garrison had died in 1935 so the next step was to ask Claudius F. Mayer and Henry Sigerist for permission to publish material that had originally appeared in the Index-Catalogue and Bulletin. Both readily gave their consent and subsequently took a keen interest in the project. I then copied out the items in the Check-List on individual slips. I decided to rearrange the entries under the main headings used in the Universal Decimal Classification system. I discarded some items dealing with botany, zoology and entomology. One laborious task was checking each name with the *Index-Catalogue* or other source and adding dates of birth and death where necessary. At a later stage and in subsequent editions finding the dates of persons whose work I myself had added proved one of the most time-consuming parts of the work.

The whole project had to be carried out in my leisure time; for this reason it took much longer than I had anticipated. My usual routine was to take a history of some particular subject and, with Garrison's *History*, and Osler's *Bibliotheca* and other aids at hand, to go thorough it with the slips making appropriate annotations and additional slips where necessary, and putting aside for further consideration items in Garrison's list that did not appear to qualify for inclusion.

Just as I was getting deeply involved in this work, war came and threatened to put an end to it. I was at first in a reserved occupation, not liable to be called for national service, but had to spend several nights each week as an air-raid warden. For a time life continued uneventfully, but our nights were soon disturbed. We would sleep fully clad and it was common practice for neighbours to come in for the evening for mutual support. I mention this only because the circumstances were not conducive to work on the project.

The situation deteriorated further. At that time I was Librarian at St. Thomas's Hospital Medical School, not far from the Houses of Parliament, a prime target. The

Hospital was severely damaged by enemy action and it was decided to evacuate part of it, together with the Medical School, out to Surrey. The School moved to Guildford, about 30 miles south-west of London. Living accommodation was hard to find but after some weeks of discomfort I was able to rent an apartment for my family over a ladies' gown shop at the junction of the High Street and the London Road. This had three rooms, so small that with our household furniture in them there was hardly room to move. The material for the bibliography, now growing and housed in shoe boxes, stood on the dining table, to be moved underneath at meal times.

In fact, this upheaval was a blessing in disguise because during the long winter evenings there was nothing else to do but work on the bibliography. Two shops, a hundred yards from our home, were taken over by the School authorities and one of them was used to house a part of the library that we had evacuated from London. Of course this included the *Index-Catalogue*! There was always the danger, though now much reduced, that a bomb might put an end to the project, so I began as soon as possible to have completed entries typed out in duplicate and to store one copy in another place. This meant that the list was being built up in rather haphazard fashion.

As work proceeded it became necessary to fill gaps both in the subject coverage and concerning individuals. I found that Garrison sometimes showed some bias towards the work of his fellow-countrymen and was not always in agreement with other writers in assigning priority. This determination of priority, however, is one of the difficulties met in compiling a work such as "Garrison-Morton". Comparatively few discoveries are clear-cut. After a "new" disease entity has been described and accepted it is not difficult for the enthusiastic specialist or historian to read into an earlier writing a description of that particular condition. The same applies to "first" descriptions of anatomical structures or physiological functions. By the time I reached that stage of the proceedings I realized how essential it was that the book should be expanded into a comprehensive annotated bibliography if it was to be of real value. I believe it was Ernest Starling who wrote: "Every discovery, however important and apparently epoch-making, is but the natural and inevitable outcome of a vast mass of work, involving many failures, by a host of different workers".

Fortunately at this time I was asked to visit the Hospital in London each Saturday to look after the literary needs of the doctors remaining on duty there. In fact this visit took up comparatively little time, and I was able to spend part of the day in the library of the Royal Society of Medicine. Much of its stock was still available in the basement stacks, and I began to check references and consult works. Each Saturday I took home a volume of the *Annals of Medical History* or some similar journal, or perhaps a history such as one of the *Clio Medica* series.

Another change occurred at this time (1941). The Medical School was moved from Guildford to Godalming, seven miles away, where part of the Hospital had been evacuated earlier. There was more accommodation for the Library and I was able to bring out more books and journals from London. It was also a more convenient place for my duplicate manuscript as I continued to live in Guildford and travelled to Godalming each day.

However, I was still hampered by the inaccessibility of some of the literature I needed. Holidays during these years were out of the question; visits to libraries in London had to be made during my Saturday trip there. I mention this only as an excuse for the shortcomings of the first edition of the book, which were not entirely due to incompetence but in some measure to the difficulty in consulting original material. I might have been considered selfish of me to persist with the work at such a time but now the book was becoming an obsession, besides providing an escape from the realities of the moment.

At that time and since, a number of people were kind enough to give their advice and criticism. I was particularly indebted to the late Dr. Bernard Samet, a refugee who came from Vienna in 1938. He had come over to requalify in order to practise in Britain. He spent many hours with me going over the material. He introduced me to Isidor Fischer, also from Vienna, who in 1932-33 had published a supplement to Hirsch's *Biographisches Lexikon der hervorragenden Ärzte* and a number of works on the history of medicine. Fischer gave me a copy of his *Eigennamen in der Krankheitsterminologie,* 1931, a comprehensive bibliography of medical eponyms. This was a most useful source book.

Correspondence with friends in the U. S. A. provided additional help. As the work progressed I became more and more absorbed in it. I decided not to plan a date for completion but to go on revising, adding and checking until such time as pressure from the publishers became too great to resist. As time went by the task of reference checking at original sources became more formidable and it was necessary to enlist outside help. Much of the time during my Saturday visits to London was spent on this dull job although by now some libraries there were closed or dispersed. Slips were sent to libraries elsewhere in the country, where staff were kind enough to help, but some items could not be checked with the originals. By 1942 most of the older material belonging to the Royal Society of Medicine had been moved to a house in St. Albans, some 23 miles north of London. My friend W. J. Bishop, who was Sub-Librarian of the Society, had recently suffered the loss of his house by bombing and was living with his family in the St. Albans premises, coming to London each day to work. He was kind enough to allow me to visit his temporary home to check references, and I recall several excursions from Guildford to St. Albans, a round journey of some 110 miles that began about 7 a.m. and ended near midnight. Although the house was quite large, books were in almost every room. The bedroom of Mr. Bishop's daughter, then 12 or 13 years old, was no exception, being lined with runs of obstetrical and gynaecological journals, which may in fact have helped her education because she eventually qualified as a physician!

By the end of 1942 sufficient material had been assembled. The slips and their duplicates were numbered and one set was sent off to the publisher early in 1943. At this point I received notice to attend a medical examination preparatory to being called up into the Armed Forces. However, it was discovered that I had a minor heart irregularity that made me unsuitable for military service, otherwise it would have been a disastrous blow to the project as I would not have been able to prepare the indexes and read the proofs. Proof reading was a pleasure after the long period of preparation, and production of the indexes was a simple but tedious matter of manipulating the duplicate set of slips.

The book at last appeared later in 1943. Considering the difficulties of the time I had reason to be very grateful to the publishers for honouring their part of the contract and for the reasonably good standard of production achieved in wartime. I learned a great deal during the preparation of the bibliography, having began it with no previous experience of such work. I put away the manuscript, determined not to look at it again for a long time.

Sources for the Bibliography. Garrison's Check-List of 1933 of course provided a good foundation as it contained about 4,200 items of which I retained 3,826. I added 1,680 items, making a total of 5,506. The most important contributions to individual subjects were found by consultation of a general history of medicine and confirmation in a history of that particular subject. The latter usually helped to fill in the relevant subject section in greater detail. In the case of the ancient writers (Hippocrates, Galen, Celsus, Aretaeus, etc.) I included the first published edition of their collected works and a good modern edition if available. The best place for them was in the Collected Works section; additionally any of their outstanding contributions to specific subjects of diseases were placed appropriately. Review articles and such publication as the *Recent Advances* series were examined for modern work.

Anyone who had contributed an important advance or who had fitted into position a small but vital piece of the puzzle qualified for inclusion. Those whose names were attached to conditions, techniques or apparatus usually deserved a place and for that reason eponymous terms were carefully examined; the eponym usually indicates priority or prominence in the field. As far as possible the first traceable description of a disease was found and included. Some early accounts, although not first, were so well written, with such complete detail and accurate description, that they deserved a place. Some surgical and other failures also deserved inclusion as pioneer work that led to later successful procedures. Nobel laureates were considered and work leading to their awards was included.

The *Bibliotheca Osleriana*, with its scholarly annotations and personal notes, was an invaluable source. The contributions to medical history of such writers as Humphry Rolleston, John Fulton and D'Arcy Power were equally valuable. Although many scholarly works on the history of special subjects have been published by British writers, a larger volume has come from the United States, where also journals on the subject have been maintained for a number of years, sometimes with the support of private individuals. (The British journal *Medical History* was begun only in 1957.) From the United States have also come reproductions of medical classics, sometimes with translations to make them even more accessible. Emerson C. Kelly's volumes of *Medical Classics* proved most useful to me and it is unfortunate that so few were published.

Some of the most valuable writings are those of the professional historians – Karl Sudhoff, Max Neuberger, Sigerist and Singer. The distinguished physician or surgeon who turns to the writing of medical history does not always do so with outstanding success, although there are notable exceptions – the Rollestons, Fulton, Guthrie, Allbutt, for example. A successful combination has sometimes been formed between the medical man and the medical librarian, as for example Willius and Keys, Bailey and Bishop. Any publication of Garrison is worth examination; he combined the knowledge of the physician with the training of the librarian. Care had to be exercised in considering items suggested by others. A specialist who has studied a subject over a number of years is liable to attach importance to some contributions out of proportion to their real significance. In attempting to review these in their proper perspective I may have overweighted some sections and covered others inadequately.

An interesting matter for consideration is the means used to communicate new discoveries. At first it had to be through the medium of books, and generally continued so for some time after journals were established. But as the tempo of discovery quickened, more and more appeared in journals and today virtually no vital work makes its first appearance in a book. The great majority of classic papers appearing in serials were published in important journals, comparatively few in unimportant or obscure journals, and very few indeed in journals of such obscurity that their contents tended to be overlooked – one thinks of Jánsky's work on blood groups and Mendel's paper on heredity. In this connexion Lee Ash's analysis[1] has proved most interesting and revealing.

In 1946 I joined the staff of the *British Medical Journal*. By 1949 the first edition of Garrison-Morton was sold out, having had a kinder reception than I could have expected. In the meantime it had made me a number of pen friends who were sending corrections and suggestions. In 1950 I began work on a second edition. Some good histories had appeared in the meantime. The Wellcome Historical Medical Library and other sources were again available. I had the opportunity to expand sections where necessary and considerably enlarged the sections on histories of medicine. The second edition appeared in 1954, containing 6,808 entries. It was reprinted in 1961 under the imprint of Andre Deutsch (who had by then taken over from Grafton responsibility for publication). It was again reprinted, with some revision, in 1965. Meanwhile in 1959 I had become Librarian at the National Institute for Medical Research, the principal research establishment of the Medical Research Council.

When the third edition was in preparation I would have liked to have taken the opportunity to alter the subject arrangement to cope with the changing face of medicine but this would have made a change of numbering necessary and I felt unable to do this because librarians and booksellers had taken to citing "Garrison-Morton" numbers in their catalogues. Instead, the numbering used in the second edition was retained, new entries were accommodated by the use of decimal points, and numbers for deleted items were not used for new works except in the case of new histories of medicine that replaced outdated works. The third edition of the bibliography appeared in 1970, the centenary year of Garrison's birth, and contained 7,534 entries.

Subsequent to the appearance of the third edition the Gower Publishing Company Limited took over responsibility for the publication of the Grafton series. The fourth edition of the *Bibliography* appeared in 1983 and contained 7,830 entries. It was extremely well produced by Gower and their printers.

During the many years I have been associated with "Garrison-Morton" I have received advice and help from many people, too numerous to mention here; the names of some are recorded in the introductions to the four editions. I would, however, record my indebtedness to the Wellcome Trust, which provided financial help towards the cost of preparing the last edition. A number of libraries, particularly those of the Wellcome Institute for the History of Medicine and the Royal Society of Medicine, have played an essential part in the task of keeping the book up to date. Most helpful of all has been my wife, who bore with patience my long absences from home during the difficult years of the war and who gave many hours to the tedious work of indexing and other routine tasks.

In conclusion I would like to refer to the oration delivered by Sir Humphry Rolleston,[6] Emeritus Regius Professor of Physic in the University of Cambridge, during the centennial celebration of the Army Medical Library (as it then was) in Washington in 1936. After outlining the development of the Library and paying a tribute to librarians in general, Sir Humphry concluded:

> The number of medical men who have been whole-time librarians of medical libraries is small; but in the United States what may have been lacking in quantity had been more than made good by quality. To three great bibliographer-librarians of the Army Medical Library tribute is justly due – Billings, Fletcher, and Garrison; for like the history of the world, that of this great library is the biography of its great men.

I personally am especially indebted to Garrison, whose pioneer work on the Check-List provided me with a hobby and an anchor for fifty years. I am confident that in the expert and enthusiastic hands of Jeremy Norman and his colleagues the *Medical Bibliography* is assured of a long and useful life. I wish him all success.

(1) Ash, L. *Serial Publications Containing Medical Classics. An Index to Citations in Garrison-Morton.* Compiled by Lee Ash, New Haven, *The Antiquarium*, 1961 (Second edition, Bethany, C.T., *The Antiquarium*, 1979).

(2) Garrison, Fielding H. A revised students' check-list of texts illustrating the history

of medicine. *Bulletin of the Institute of the History of Medicine*, 1933, **1**, 333-434.

(3) Miles, Wyndham D. *A History of the National Library of Medicine.* Washington, D. C., *U. S. Govt. Printing Office*, 1982, p. 196.

(4) Garrison, Fielding H. The historical collection of medical classics in the Library of the Surgeon General's Office. *Journal of the American Medical Association*, 1911, **56**, 1785-92.

(5) Texts illustrating the history of medicine in the Library of the Surgeon General's Office, U. S. Army. Arranged in chronological order. *Index-Catalogue of the Library of the Surgeon General's Office.* Washington, *Govt. Printing Office*, 1912, Second series, Vol. XVII, pp. 89–178 (also offprinted).

(6) Rolleston, Sir Humphry. Medical libraries. *Lancet*, 1936, **2**, 1286-9.

PREFACE AND ACKNOWLEDGEMENTS

BY

JEREMY M. NORMAN

Leslie T. Morton published the first edition of this book in London, 1943, having written much of it during the uncertain atmosphere of the Second World War. He based it on an outline of sources for the history of medicine published in 1933 by Fielding H. Garrison. Morton started on the project in 1938. Garrison had died in 1935 so the two never met and never actively collaborated on the book. However, Morton credited Garrison as the original compiler of the work on the title page and binding of the first edition. This caused the book to be referred to as "Garrison and Morton" or "Garrison-Morton" ever since the first edition, and has given many readers the false impression that Garrison was an active participant in its writing. Although Garrison was responsible for the original concept, with every new edition the book became more and more the work of Morton. To clarify this issue of authorship the title has now been changed from *A Medical Bibliography* to *Morton's Medical Bibliography.*

In his introduction to the present edition, Leslie Morton has detailed the history of this book and the important role it played in his life. Long before I undertook the editorship of this work it also had a significant place in my life. To no small extent I grew up with this book. I was introduced to it as a boy by my father, Haskell F. Norman, a physician and life-long collector of medical and scientific books, who still keeps well-thumbed copies of "Garrison-Morton" at home and at the office. I used the work for reference in my history of biological science courses during my undergraduate years at the University of California at Berkeley. As an antiquarian bookselling apprentice at John Howell Books in San Francisco from 1964 to 1969 I learned its value for identifying classics in the history of medicine and the life sciences. When I started my own antiquarian bookselling firm in 1971, specializing in the history of the sciences, I relied on the third edition as a key to medical and biological literature, and the beginning of many catalogue descriptions. Over the years the staff at Jeremy Norman & Co., Inc. and I have literally worn out several copies of the third and fourth editions in our research and cataloguing efforts.

Having used the work intensively for the past twenty-five years, it has given me great satisfaction to prepare the fifth edition. The project has involved revision of the work from literally the first entry all the way through to the end. Certain sections are extensively revised, expanded and updated; others are only slightly corrected. Virtually every section has been changed in some way. A few old entries have been moved to new locations. Sometimes this involved value judgements. For example certain works on the use of hypnosis in surgery have been moved from the category of Hypnosis under Psychiatry to the field of Anaesthesia. Certain old entries such as Celsus now have additional citations reflecting their significance in additional subjects. There are completely new sections for Ecology, Paleoanthropology: Human Prehistory, Teratology, Medical Education and the Medical Profession, Resuscitation, Aviation Medicine, Paleopathology, Sports Medicine, Paediatric Surgery, and Alternative Medicine: Acupuncture (Western References). The bibliography for Dentistry: Orthodontics: Oral Surgery has been sufficiently expanded as to warrant a completely new section. References to Geriatrics have been significantly expanded within the section on State Medicine: Public Health: Geriatrics: Hygiene. The sections on Anatomy and Medicine in Art, have been extensively rewritten and expanded. In all I have added 1,061 entries, revised or rewritten the annotations for 2,313, and deleted 119. From the approximately

7,800 entries in the fourth edition the work has been expanded to a total of 8,927. The indices to personal names and subjects are completely new for this edition.

For new entries the most difficult problems of selection remain those of recent scientific contributions. Few histories of medical specialties cover the period after 1950 in depth. With sufficient supporting documentation I did not hesitate to include contributions up to 1980, and I included a few after that date. Monographs which were instrumental in the compilation of new entries have been cited as secondary sources. Journal articles particularly useful for this purpose are cited in annotations. Coverage of secondary sources has been extended through 1990. When in doubt I have erred on the side of caution. The strength of this bibliography has always been and will remain in its selectivity.

Even though there are 8,927 entries in the bibliography, readers will note that the final entry is numbered 6810. By the third edition in 1970 it was felt that in spite of certain limitations in the organizational scheme of this book the "Garrison-Morton numbers" were already sufficiently entrenched in the library records of the world that to change them would create more harm than good. Therefore entries were added by the use of decimals. In the fifth edition there are as many as 43 decimal extensions after a few entries. To prevent confusion it has been necessary to renumber many of these decimal series.

The range of subjects covered by this work is so wide and its detail so great that this edition would not have been possible without the assistance of many collaborators. From the beginning Leslie Morton was most supportive of the project, turning over the addenda and corrigenda he had been accumulating since the fourth edition published in 1983. He was always available as a source of advice and guidance. Martha N. Steele, editor at Norman Publishing, supervised the input of the entire text of the fourth edition into word processing files. When this was done in late 1988 the multiplicity of type sizes and diversity of foreign language characters in the book prevented successful optical character recognition scanning. It required hundreds of hours of manual keystroking. I then accomplished the entire revision using the "revision marks" feature of the word processing program, which enabled me to keep track of all changes. The final manuscript was turned over to the publishers as word processing files.

The following people contributed to the fifth edition: J. Bruce Beckwith selected most of the books and wrote nearly all of the annotations for the new section on Teratology. Webb Dordick offered wide-ranging suggestions for new entries. M. Felix Freshwater provided citations for recent classics in Plastic and Reconstructive Surgery. W. Bruce Fye helped to update Cardiology and Cardiac Surgery. Carl W. Gottschalk helped revise the sections on the Kidney. K. Garth Huston, Jr. helped to compile the new section on Resuscitation. Margaret Kaiser at the History of Medicine Division of the National Library of Medicine provided key references for In-vitro Fertilization. Ralph H. Kellogg helped to revise the section on Respiratory Physiology. Joan Ecktenkamp Klein and her staff at the Claude Moore Health Sciences Library at the University of Virginia checked hundreds of periodical citations in the fourth edition and prepared a lengthy list of corrections which were incorporated into the fifth edition. Malcolm Jay Kottler suggested many changes and was the co-author of the revisions to the sections on Biology, and Evolution: Genetics: Molecular Biology. Arthur E. Lyons helped to update the sections on Neurology and Neurological Surgery. Nigel Phillips sent some useful revisions to entries in various subjects. Paul Potter was kind enough to read over all the entries on Greek and Roman Medicine, to revise a great many of these, and to suggest numerous useful new entries. Davida Rubin, chief cataloguer and my long-time collaborator at Jeremy Norman & Co., offered frequent advice and counsel. Many entries were revised from annotations previously published in her catalogues. Roy Rubin collaborated on the extensive revisions to Orthopaedics and the new Sports

Medicine section. Ira M. Rutkow updated the section on Hernia and helped to improve all of the surgical sections with his research on the history of surgery in the United States. R. Ted Steinbock provided references for the new section on Paleopathology. George Wantz collaborated with Ira Rutkow on the hernia revisions. Richard J. Wolfe of the Francis A. Countway Library at Harvard provided invaluable assistance in enabling me to use the rich collections of that library for research and reference checking. Nancy W. Zinn of the University of California, San Francisco, offered me convenient access to the historical collections in that library. My thanks to you all.

Over the nearly fifty years of its existence this work has benefited much from the constructive suggestions of readers. Your revisions and suggestions will be much appreciated, and will be considered for the eventual sixth edition.

To Susan McNaughton, Senior Editor at Scolar Press, and her staff, my thanks for professional management of this complex production. To my father, Haskell F. Norman, thanks for introducing me to this book in the first place and for encouraging me to undertake this revision. To my wife, Jane Morrissey Norman, thanks for tolerating the seemingly endless hours of my writing this book throughout our engagement. Your cheerful co-operation, and your single requirement that I could not work on the book after dinner, made this book possible.

CONTENTS

COLLECTED WORKS: OPERA OMNIA

See also 2189-2238, Medicine, general works; 5547-5632, Surgery, general works.

1   HAMMURABI, *King of Babylon. fl.* 1792-1750 B.C.
The code of Hammurabi, King of Babylon about 2000 B.C. Autographed text, transliteration, translation, glossary, index of subjects, lists of proper names, signs, numerals, corrections, and erasures, with map, frontispiece, and photograph of text, by Robert Francis Harper. Chicago, *Callaghan & Co.,* 1904.
    The Code of Hammurabi was found among the clay tablets of the library of Ashurbanipal. It is now in the Louvre. It was first published in Scheil: *Mémoires de la Délégation en Perse,* Paris, 1902, **4,** 4-162. The Code mentions the fees payable to a physician following successful treatment; these varied according to the station of the patient. Similarly, the punishment for the failure of an operation is set out. At least this shows that in Babylon 4,000 years ago the medical profession had advanced far enough in public esteem to warrant the payment of adequate fees.

2   EBERS PAPYRUS.
Papyros Ebers. Das älteste Buch über Heilkunde. Aus dem Aegyptischen zum erstenmal vollständig übersetzt von H. Joachim. Berlin, *G. Reimer,* 1890.
    The Ebers Papyrus dates from about 1552 B.C. The original, now at Leipzig, was discovered about 1862 and was purchased by Georg Ebers in 1873. The papyrus measures 20.23 m. in length and 30 cm. in height. It is the most important medical papyrus yet recovered; it is written in hieratic script and contains the most complete record of Egyptian medicine known. Ebers published a facsimile of the papyrus, with a partial translation, in 1875.

3   ———. The papyrus Ebers. The greatest Egyptian medical document. Translated by B. Ebbell. Copenhagen, *Levin & Munksgaard,* 1937.
    Best English translation so far published.

4   WRESZINSKI, Walter. 1880-
Der grosse medizinische Papyrus des Berliner Museums (Pap. Berl. 3038) in Facsimile und Umschrift mit Uebersetzung, Kommentar und Glossar. Herausg. von W. Wreszinski. Leipzig, *J. C. Hinrichs,* 1909.
    The Greater German Papyrus (Brugsch Papyrus) dates from about 1300 B.C. The above facsimile reproduction and translation forms vol. 1 of the *Medizin der alten Aegypter* series.

5   CHESTER BEATTY PAPYRUS.
Le papyrus médical Chester Beatty. Par le Dr. Frans Jonckheere. Bruxelles, *Fondation Egyptologique Reine Elisabeth,* 1947. *La Médicine Egyptienne,* No. 2.
    A hieratic papyrus of the 13th-12th century B.C. It is a fragment of a monograph on diseases of the anus. It was reproduced with hieroglyphic transcription by A. H. Gardiner in 1935.

6   KÜCHLER, FRIEDRICH.
Beiträge zur Kenntnis der assyrisch-babylonischen Medizin. Texte mit
Umschrift, Uebersetzung und Kommentar. Leipzig, *J. C. Hinrich, 1904.*
      Medical texts from the library of Ashurbanipal, together with German
translations. A valuable paper on this subject is M. Jastrow's "The medicine
of the Babylonians and Assyrians", *Proc. roy. Soc. Med.* 1913-14, **7,** Sect.
Hist. Med., 109-76.

7   THOMPSON, REGINALD CAMPBELL. 1876-1941
Assyrian medical texts. From the originals in the British Museum. London,
Oxford Univ. Press, 1923.
      Facsimiles of the texts of 660 cuneiform medical tablets, many of which
were hitherto unpublished, from the library of Ashurbanipal. The tablets
date back to the seventh century B.C. No translations are included, but
Thompson has interpreted and systematized many of the texts in a later
work (*Proc. roy. Soc. Med.,* 1924, **17,** Sect. Hist. Med., 1-34; 1926, **19,** Sect.
Hist. Med., 29-78).

8   AYURVEDA
The Ayurvedic system of medicine. By NAGENDRA NATH SEN GUPTA. 3 vols.
Calcutta, *K. R. Chatterjee,* 1901-07.
      Ayurveda is the most ancient system of Hindu medicine; only fragments
of the original remain. The early Hindus believed it to be of divine origin
and ascribed it to Brahma. It dates from *circa* 1400-1200 B.C. Reprinted Delhi,
Indian Book Centre, 1984.

9   CHARAKA SAMHITA.
[Charaka Samhita. Edited by JIBANANDA VIDYASAGARA.] Calcutta, *Sarasvati Press,*
1877.
      Sanskrit text. Authorities vary as to the date of Charaka. He is said to
have lived at times varying between 800 B.C. and A.D. 78. The Samhita, or
Sanhita, is one of the most ancient and complete systems of Hindu
medicine to have survived. It is arranged in the form of dialogues between
master and pupil and is divided into eight books. Charaka's writing is
superior to that of Susruta in the accuracy of his descriptions. What Susruta
is to surgery, Charaka is to medicine.

10   ———. The Charaka Samhita. Edited and published with translations in
Hindi, Gujerati and English, *Shree Gulabkunverba Ayurvedic Society.* 6 vols.
Jamnagar, 1949.

11   SUŚRUTA SAMHITA.
[Suśruta Samhita. The system of Hindu medicine taught by Dhanwantari.
Compiled by Suśruta. Edited and published by PANDIT-KULAPATI JIBANANDA
VIDYASAGARA.] 5th ed. Calcutta, 1909.
      Sanskrit text. The Suśruta Samhita required a good educational foun-
dation of a student of medicine. Suśruta is said to have lived in the 6th or
5th centuries, B.C. The writings of Suśruta and Charaka formed the
groundwork of all the Hindu medical and surgical systems which followed.
The Suśruta Samhita is divided into six books and contains a fairly accurate
description of the human body, besides some surgery. This work was first
published in the West in the Latin translation of Franz Hessler (1799-1890),
5 vols., Erlangen, 1844-55.

12 ———. An English translation of the Suśruta Samhita...translated and edited by K. K. BHISHAGRATNA. 2nd ed. Varanasi, *Chowkhamba Sanskrit Series Office,* 1963.

13 HIPPOCRATES. 460-375 B.C.
Oeuvres complètes d'Hippocrate. Traduction nouvelle avec le texte grec en regard...Par E. LITTRÉ. 10 vols. Paris, *J. B. Baillière,* 1839-61.

Although none of the seventy odd works in this collection can be attributed with certainty to Hippocrates, the writings retain their historical significance as the earliest extant sources of Western medical thought and practice. The first complete edition in Latin was issued from Rome by Fabius Calvus in 1525, and the Greek *editio princeps* was published by the Aldine Press a year later in Venice. Important Greek editions to follow were those of Janus Cornarius, Basel, 1538, Anuce Foes [Foesius], Frankfurt, 1595, and Littré. The above bilingual edition was the result of 22 years of continuous labour. Reprinted Amsterdam, 1961. For a detailed bibliography of modern editions and translations *see* P. Potter, *Short handbook of Hippocratic medicine*, Quebec, 1988.

14 ———. The genuine works of Hippocrates. Translated from the Greek, with a preliminary discourse and annotations by FRANCIS ADAMS. 2 vols. London, *Sydenham Society,* 1849.

Francis Adams, surgeon of Banchory, Scotland, prepared this partial translation to acquaint his contemporaries with "the opinions of an author, whom I verily believe to be the highest exemplar of professional excellence which the world has ever seen". It is the last English edition of the Hippocratic writings intended to serve as actual medical instruction. Several reprints have been published.

15 ———. Opera. Recensuit H. KUEHLEWEIN. 2 vols. Lipsiae, *B. G. Teubner,* 1894-1902.

This Greek edition, originally planned to include the whole collection in seven volumes, was abandoned in 1907 with the founding of the *Corpus Medicorum Graecorum* series, which to date includes about one fifth of the corpus in seven volumes. Both editions employ manuscripts and methods unknown to Littré to achieve a decisive improvement on his text.

16 ———. [Works] with an English translation by W. H. S. JONES, E. T. WITHINGTON, and PAUL POTTER. 6 vols. London, *W, Heinemann,* 1923-88.

Greek–English edition in the *Loeb Classical Library*. Contains something over half of the Hippocratic corpus.

16.1 ———. The medical works of Hippocrates. A new translation by J. CHADWICK and W. N. MANN. Oxford, *Blackwell,* [1950].

This collection of translations is partly reprinted with an introduction by G.E.R. Lloyd and the addition of three new translations by I.M. Lonie as Hippocratic Writings, Harmondsworth, *Penguin Classics,* 1978.

16.2 DIOCLES *of Carystus. fl.* 360 B.C.
Die Fragmente der sikelischen Ärzte Akron, Philistion und des Diokles von Karystos. Herausgegeben von M. WELLMANN. Berlin, *Weidmann,* 1901.

16.3   PRAXAGORAS *of Cos. fl.* 340 B.C.
The fragments of Praxagoras of Cos and his school. Collected, edited and translated by FRITZ STECKERL. Leiden, *E.J. Brill,* 1958.

17   ARISTOTLE. 384-322 B.C.
Opera. Edidit Academia Regia Borussica. 5 vols. Berolini, *Reimer,* 1831-70.
Greek–Latin bilingual text. Aristotle, at one time tutor to Alexander the Great, was, among other things, the first observational biologist, and the founder of comparative anatomy. His views had a profound influence in determining the direction of medical and biological thought; perhaps no other man has so dominated and advanced science as a whole than Aristotle. There were numerous Latin editions of Aristotle's collected works printed in the 15th century. The first edition of the Greek text was published by Aldus Manutius of Venice (6 vols., 1495-98).

18   ——. The works of Aristotle translated into English. Edited by J. A. SMITH and W. D. ROSS. 12 vols. Oxford, *Clarendon Press,* 1908-52.
The *Loeb Classical Library* has published 23 vols. of Aristotle's works (Greek and English text), 1926-70.

18.1   HEROPHILUS. *fl.* 290 B.C.
Herophilus: The art of medicine in early Alexandria. Edition, translation and essays by H. VON STADEN. Cambridge, *Cambridge University Press,* 1989.
The first comprehensive presentation of the ancient evidence for the achievements of Herophilus and his school, including edited versions of all original Greek and Latin texts plus English translations, with in-depth commentaries. In most cases these are the first English translations of the texts concerned.

18.2   HERACLIDES *of Tarentum. fl.* 75 B.C.
Die griechische Empirikerschule. Sammlung der Fragmente und Darstellung der Lehre von Karl Deichgräber. Berlin, *Weidmann,* 1930.

19   ASCLEPIADES *of Bithynia.* 124-56 B.C.
Fragmenta. Digessit et curavit C. G. GUMPERT. Vinariae, *Industrie-Comptoir,* 1794.
After the fall of Corinth (146 B.C.), Greek physicians migrated to Rome. There, before the advent of Asclepiades, the Greek physicians were despised and distrusted. Asclepiades may be said to have established Greek medicine in Rome on a respectable footing. Gumpert has preserved what is left of his writings in the above Greek edition. See R. M. Green, *Asclepiades, his life and writings,* New Haven, 1955, which includes a translation of Gumpert's *Fragmenta. See* No. 1984.

20   CELSUS, AULUS AURELIUS CORNELIUS. 25 B.C.-A.D. 50
De medicina. Florentiae, *Nicolaus [Laurentius],* 1478.
The *De Medicina* is the oldest medical document after the Hippocratic writings. Written about A.D. 30, it remains the greatest medical treatise from ancient Rome, and the first Western history of medicine. Celsus's superb literary style won him the title of *Cicero medicorum. De medicina* deals with diseases treated by diet and regimen and with those amenable to drugs and surgery. The manuscript of *De Medicina* was lost during the Middle Ages and re-discovered in Milan in 1443. The above work, edited by Bartholomaeus Fontius, was one of the first medical books to be

printed. *See* Osler, *Incunabula medica,* 147. First English translation by J. Grieve, London, 1756. *See* Nos. 3666.8, 5548.1, 5733.50, & 6375.

21 ——. De medicina. With an English translation by W. G. SPENCER. 3 vols. London, *W. Heinemann,* 1935-38.
   Loeb Classical Library. Text in Latin and English. This edition is based on the scholarly text of F. Marx published as *Corpus Medicorum Latinorum I,* Leipzig, 1915.

22 ARETAEUS *the Cappadocian.* A.D. 81-?138
   Τα Σωζομενα. The extant works of Aretaeus, the Cappadocian. Edited and translated by FRANCIS ADAMS. London, Sydenham Society, 1856.
   Aretaeus left many fine descriptions of disease; in fact Garrison ranks him second only to Hippocrates in this respect. His works were first published in Latin translation by Junius Paulus Crassus at Venice in 1552, with the Greek *editio princeps* following two years later in Paris. The first English translation by J. Moffat was published in London, 1785. The valuable edition by Adams includes the Greek text with an English translation. Reprinted Boston, *Milford House,* 1972. The standard modern edition is that of C. Hude, *Corpus Medicorum Graecorum II,* Berlin, 1958.

23 RUFUS *of Ephesus.* fl. A.D. 100
   De vesicae remumque morbis. De purgantibus medicamentis. De partibus corporis humani...Parisiis, *A. Turnebus,* 1554.
   Greek *editio princeps* edited by Jacques Goupyl. In his day Rufus stood out among his contemporaries as a great surgeon. He is particularly remembered for his work on haemostasis; he also wrote a treatise on gout. Rufus is mentioned by Chaucer's doctor.

24 ——. Œuvres, texte collationné sur les manuscrits, traduit pour la première fois en français avec une introduction. Publication commencée par CH. DAREMBERG, continuée et terminée par CH. EMILE RUELLE. Paris, *J.B. Baillière,* 1879.
   Greek–French edition containing all the extant works of Rufus, as well as fragments collected from a wide range of ancient and medieval sources. Reprinted Amsterdam, 1963. The treatise *On the interrogation of the patient* was published as *Corpus Medicorum Graecorum Supplement IV,* Berlin, 1962, and *Diseases of the Kidney and Bladder* as *CMG III,* 1, Berlin, 1977.

25 ANONYMUS LONDINENSIS.
   Anonymus Londinensis. Auszüge eines unbekannten aus Aristoteles-Menons Handbuch der Medizin und aus Werken anderer älterer Aerzte. Berlin, *G. Reimer,* 1896.
   The important B. M. Papyrus 137, found in 1891, was deciphered by Sir Frederick Kenyon; a Greek text edited by Hermann Diels was published in 1893, and the above German translation (by H. Beckh and F. Spät) appeared in 1896. The work is a treatise on medicine, written about A.D. 150. It contains extracts from a lost collection of the opinions of the earlier Greek physicians, and throws some light on early Greek medicine.

26 ——. The medical writings of Anonymus Londinensis. By W. H. S. JONES. Cambridge, *University Press,* 1947.
   Greek and English text on facing pages.

27   GALEN. A.D. 130-200
Librorum pars prima [-quinta]...5 vols. [Venetiis, *in aedibus Aldi, et Andreae Asulani soceri,* 1525].

Greek *editio princeps* of the complete works, edited by Andrea Torresani [Asulanus] and G.B. Oppizzoni [Opizo]. A two-volume Latin edition appeared in 1490 in Venice. Galen stands second only to Hippocrates in importance in ancient Greek medicine. His writings dominated Byzantine, Arabic, and medieval medicine for over a millenium, being superseded in anatomy only with Vesalius, in physiology with Harvey, and in pathology with Boerhaave.

28   ——. Opera omnia. Editionem curavit C. G. KÜHN. 20 vols. [in 22]. Lipsiae, *C. Cnobloch,* 1821-33.

This Greek–Latin edition is reprinted from much earlier editions, and owes its frequent citation only to the fact that no other complete edition has succeeded it: both text and translation leave much to be desired. Reprinted with an epilogue by K. Schubring, Hildesheim, *G. Olms,* 1965.

29   ——. [Opera omnia]. Corpus Medicorum Graecorum V... (Lipsiae et) Berolini, *B. G. Teubner/Akademie-Verlag,* 1914-.

As of 1990 about twenty volumes containing perhaps a fifth of the Corpus have been published. Although the principles of the edition have varied somewhat over the 75 year course of the project, all volumes represent a decisive advance over Kühn (No. 28). Important treatises accompanied by English translations are: *Galen on the Doctrines of Hippocrates and Plato,* edited and translated by Phillip De Lacy, C.M.G. V, 4, 1,2, 3 vols., 1978-84. *Galen on Prognosis,* edited and translated by Vivian Nutton, C.M.G. V, 8, 1, 1979. *Galen on examinations by which the best physicians are recognized,* edited in Arabic and translated by Albert Iskandar, C.M.G. Supplementum Orientale IV, 1988.

30   ANTYLLUS. *fl.* A.D. 250
Antylli veteris chirurgi quae apud Oribasium libro xliv, xlv et 1 leguntur fragmenta. Dissertatio...publice defendet F. C. F. WOLZ. Jenae, *typ. Schreiberi* [1842].

One of the most daring and accomplished of surgeons, Antyllus is particularly remembered for his work on the surgery of aneurysm. He was first to recognize two forms of aneurysm – one caused by dilatation and the other following wounding of an artery. Much of his writing is available to us only through the industry of Oribasius who included it in his compilations. A German version of Antyllus is in *Janus,* 1847, **2,** 298-329, 744-71; 1848, **3,** 166-84.

31   ORIBASIUS. A.D. 325-403
Œuvres d'Oribase, texte grec, en grande partie inédit...traduit pour la première fois en français; par les DRS. BUSSEMAKER et DAREMBERG. 6 vols. Paris, *Imp. nationale,* 1851-76.

Oribasius was a compiler of existing knowledge rather than an original writer. His output was immense; he compiled the *Synagoge,* an encyclopaedic digest of medicine, hygiene, therapeutics, and surgery from Hippocrates to his own times, in 70 volumes. The unwieldiness of the work was probably the reason why he also wrote a synopsis of it. Only 17 volumes have survived.

32 ——. Collectionum medicarum reliquiae. Synopsis ad Eustathium. Libri ad Eunapium. Corpus Medicorum Graecorum VI, 1-3. 5 vols. Lipsiae et Berolini, *B.G. Teubner,* 1926-31.

Contains selections from the writings of medical men, the originals of some of whose works no longer exist, and who would have been forgotten but for the compilations of Oribasius. Writers included are Agathinus, Antyllus, Apollonius, Archigenes, Athenaeus, Ctesias, Dieuches, Diocles, Dioscorides, Herodotus, Justus, Lycus, Menemachus, Mnesitheus Atheniensis, Mnesitheus Cyzicenus, Oribasius, Philagrius, Philotimus, Philumenus, Sabinus, Xenocrates, Zopyrus. Reprinted Amsterdam, 1964.

33 AETIUS *of Amida.* A.D. 502-575
Βιβλίων ἰατρικῶν τομος ά. Librorum medicinalium tomus primus, primi scilicet libri octo nunc primum in lucem editi. [Venetiis, *in aedibus haeredum Aldi Manutii et Andreae Asulani*], 1534.

Greek *editio princeps* of the first half of the *Tetrabiblion,* the second half of which has never been published. Complete Latin translations of the four volumes, each containing four parts or books, were provided by J.B. Montanus and Janus Cornarius, Basel, 1533-35, etc. The standard Greek edition of books 1-8 is now A. Olivieri, *Corpus Medicorum Graecorum VIII,* 1-2, Berlin, 1935-50. In the *Tetrabiblion* Aetius collected together works of other men which might have been forgotten but for him. Among them may be mentioned Rufus of Ephesus, Antyllus, Leonides, Soranus, Philumenus. In this work is also to be found Aetius's own original work on the treatment of aneurysm by ligation of the brachial artery above the sac. *See* Nos. 5814 and 6136.

34 ALEXANDER *of Tralles.* A.D. 525-605
Practica. [Lugduni, *per F. Fradin,* 1504].

Incomplete medieval Latin translation of the main medical work of Alexander. The complete Greek text was first published in Paris by Robert Estienne [Stephanus] in 1548.

35 ——. Alexander von Tralles. Original-Text und Uebersetzung...von THEODOR PUSCHMANN. 2 vols. Wien, *W. Braumüller,* 1878-79.

In the main Alexander Trallianus was a compiler, but some of the work in his writings appears to be his own. His original description of worms and vermifuges make him the first parasitologist. The above Greek–German text is the best so far published, and includes a biography. Reprinted, Amsterdam, 1963.

35.1 ——. Œuvres médicales d'Alexander de Tralles, le dernier auteur classique des grands médecins grecs de l'antiquité. Ed. F. BRUNET. 4 vols. Paris, *Geuthner,* 1933-37.

36 PAUL *of Aegina.* A.D. 625-690
The seven books of Paulus Aegineta. Translated from the Greek...by FRANCIS ADAMS. 3 vols. London, *Sydenham Society,* 1844-47.

Paulus Aegineta was the most important physician of his day and a skilful surgeon. He gave original descriptions of lithotomy, trephining, tonsillectomy, paracentesis and amputation of the breast; the first clear description of the effects of lead poisoning also comes from him. His work first appeared in Greek from the famous Aldine Press in Venice in 1528, edited by F. Torresani [Asulanus]. Three Latin translations were published in 1532. The first, entitled *Opus divinum* was translated from the Aldine edition by A. Torinus, and published by A. Cratander. It included books 1-5 and 7. The second, entitled *De medica materia...* published in Venice by L. Giunta, included the sixth book on surgery. The third, entitled *Opus de re medica*, published in Paris by S. de Colines, was based on a new, improved text and included all seven books in the translation of J. Winter of Andernach. This first English translation of the complete work by Adams is accompanied by a very extensive commentary "embracing a complete view of the knowledge possessed by the Greeks, Romans, and Arabians on all subjects connected with medicine and surgery".

37   ———. [Opera] ed. J. L. HEIBERG. Corpus Medicorum Graecorum IX. 2 vols. Lipsiae et Berolini, *B.G. Teubner,* 1921-24.
       Standard Greek text.

38   BUDGE, *Sir* ERNEST ALFRED THOMPSON WALLIS. 1857-1934
       Syrian anatomy, pathology and therapeutics or "The Book of Medicines". The Syriac text...with an English translation, *etc.* 2 vols. London, *H. Milford,* 1913.
       Text and translation of a Syrian manuscript which throws some light on Syrian medicine.

39   RHAZES [ABU BAKR MUHAMMAD IBN ZAKARIYA AL-RAZI]. *circa* 854-925 or 935
       Liber nonus ad Almansorem, cum commentario SILLANI DE NIGRIS. [Padua, *B. Valdezochius*], 1476.
       The *Almansor,* so named after the prince to whom it was addressed, was a popular textbook and one of the first to be printed. Rhazes ranks with Hippocrates and Galen as one of the founders of clinical medicine. Only one copy of the above edition of his work is known to exist; it was bought by Sir William Osler in 1915 and bequeathed by him to the British Museum. For its full collation see the *Bibliotheca Osleriana,* No. 451.

39.1 ———. Liber ad Almansorem. [Translated from the Arabic by Gerard of Cremona, with 22 other medical tracts by Rhazes, Maimonides, Hippocrates, Avenzoar, etc.] [Venice: *Bonetus Locatellus, for Octavianus Scotus,* 1497].
       The best edition of the opuscula of Rhazes, containing the second printing of the celebrated *Liber ad Almansorem,* not to be confused with *Liber nonus ad Almansorem* (No. 39), as well as *De aegritudine puerorum* (No. 6313), and other works by Rhazes. This edition also contains the first edition of Rhazes' *De proprietatibus membrorum et nocumentis sexaginta animalium.* The *Liber ad Almansorem* first appeared in its entirety in 1481 with 14 other titles. When republished in 1497, additional works by Rhazes, Maimonides and Avenzoar were included for a total of 23 separate titles. (Works by Hippocrates, Mesuë, and Maimonides also included here were previously cited in a later separate collected edition as No. 53.)

40   ———. Liber Elhavi seu totum continentis Bubikir Zacharie Errasis filii, traducti ex arabice in latinum per MAG. FERRAGIUM. [Brescia, *J. Britannicus*], 1486.
       The *Al-Hawi,* or *Continens.* It is a great encyclopaedia of medicine. The above first Latin translation by Ferragut is the largest and heaviest of the medical incunabula. The original manuscript was in Arabic.

42   HALY ABBAS ['ALI IBN-AL-'ABBAS AL MAJUSI]. 930-994.
Liber artis medicine, qui dicitur regalis. Venetiis, *B. Ricius*, 1492.

The *Almaleki*, or *Liber regius*, of Haly Ben Abbas was the leading treatise of medicine for a hundred years, when it was displaced by Avicenna's *Canon* (*see* No. 43).

43   AVICENNA [ABU-'ALI AL-HUSAYN IBN ADALLAH IBN-SINA]. 980-1037
Liber canonis. Mediolani, *P. de Lavagna*, 1473.

Avicenna is said to have written more than 100 books, most of which have perished. He was an experienced physician; he wrote on the aetiology of epilepsy and described diabetes, noticing the sweetish taste of the urine. His *Canon* is one of the most famous medical texts ever written, a complete exposition of Galenism. Neuburger says: "It stands for the epitome of all precedent development, the final codification of all Graeco-Arabic medicine". It dominated the medical schools of Europe and Asia for five centuries. The above is a Latin translation by Gerard of Cremona. Choulant mentions two other undated, and probably earlier, editions.

44   ——. Kitāb al-Qānūn fi al-ṭibb. [Libri V Canonis medicinae.] Romae, *in typ. Medicea*, 1593.

Title transliterated. Text and title page (except imprint) are in Arabic. First printing of the text in Arabic. See also S. M. Afnan, *Avicenna, his life and works*. London, 1958.

45   ——. A treatise on the Canon of Medicine incorporating a translation of the First Book. By O.C. GRUNER. London, *Luzac & Co.*, 1930.

This translation of Book I of the *Canon* is accompanied by a large number of valuable notes and comments on the text, which bring out the close connection between Arabic and Chinese medicine, and the influence which Avicenna had upon many medieval scholars. A translation direct from Arabic into English by H. A. Hameed *et al.* was published in New Delhi, 1970.

46   CONSTANTINE *of Africa*. 1015-1087
Opera. 2 vols. Basileae, *H. Petrus.* 1536-39.

Many of the writings of Constantine were merely translations into Latin of Greek, Arabic and Jewish writers. His importance lies in the fact that by such Latinizing he placed Mohammedan thought and culture at the disposal of European medicine from the 12th to 17th centuries. For a time he taught at the School of Salerno.

47   AVENZOAR [ABUMERON]. ?1092-1162
Liber Teisir, sive rectificatio medicationis et regiminis. Venetiis, *J. & G. de Gregoriis*, 1490.

This is a Latin translation from the Hebrew version of 1280. Avenzoar, the greatest Moslem physician of the Western Caliphate, described the itch-mite, *Sarcoptes scabiei*, serous pericarditis, mediastinal abscess, pharyngeal paralysis and otitis media. He was the first to attempt total extirpation of the uterus. He anticipated the modern stomach tube and advocated rectal feeding. He carefully described, but did not perform, lithotomy, and is apparently the first to mention a lithotrite.

48   AVERROËS [ABU'L WALID MUHAMMAD IBN AHMAD IBN MUHAMMAD IBN RUSHD].
1126-1198
Colliget. Ferrarae, *L. deValentia de Rubeis,* 1482.

The *Kitab-al-Kullyat* or *Colliget* (Book of Universals) was an "attempt to found a system of medicine upon the neo-Platonic modification of Aristotle's philosophy" (Garrison, p. 132). Averroës was the best commentator upon Aristotle, and scholars still turn to him for the interpretation of obscure passages in the great philosopher's writings. He was the last of the great Arab physicians.

49   SCHOOL OF SALERNO
Collectio Salernitana...raccolti ed illustrati da G.E.T. [i.e. A.W.E.T. HENSCHEL., C. DAREMBERG ed E. S. DE RENZI. 5 vols. Napoli, *Filiatre-Sebezio,* 1852-59.

The School of Medicine at Salerno dispelled the stagnation of medicine which had persisted throughout the Dark Ages. Its masters were the first medieval physicians to cultivate medicine as an independent science. Many of the documents compiled at the School are included in the above work, having been found in the Breslau Codex of the mid 12th century, discovered in 1837. The *Regimen Sanitatis Salernitanum* was among the earlier medical works printed, its first edition appearing in Cologne, about 1480. It underwent at least 25 editions in the 15th century. The School at Salerno was eclipsed by the rise of Montpellier and Bologna to the front rank; it was suppressed by Napoleon in 1811. Reprinted, Bologna, *Forni,* 1967.

50   ——. Magistri Salernitani nondum editi. Ed. PIERO GIACOSA. 1 vol. and atlas. Torino, *frat. Bocca,* 1901.

Reproduction of some of the texts produced at the School of Salerno. In all, it is believed that the total output from the School numbered 100 texts, including the famous poem *Regimen Sanitatis Salernitanum,* or *Flos Medicae.*

51   ——. The school of Salernum. Regimen sanitatis Salernitanum, the English version by Sir JOHN HARINGTON. History of the School of Salernum by FRANCIS R. PACKARD, and a note on the prehistory of the Regimen Sanitatis by FIELDING H. GARRISON. New York, *Hoeber,* 1920. Reprinted New York, 1970.

52   ARTICELLA
Articella. [Padua, *N. Petri, circa* 1476.]

A collection of classical texts on medicine, written in Latin. Includes works of Hippocrates, Galen, Theophilus, and Johannitius. As a medical library in one volume, which underwent six editions in the 15th century and many other editions in the first half of the 16th century, the work reflects changing attitudes to various ancient texts and translations through the constant evolution of its contents.

53   MAIMON, MOSHE BEN [MAIMONIDES]. 1135-1204
Hoc in volumine hec continentur Aphorismi Rabi Moysi. Aphorismi Jo. Damasceni [i.e. the elder Mesue] Liber secretorum Hypocratis...[Venice, Hammon, 1500.]

An edition of the Latin translation of Maimonides' Aphorismi (first published, Venice, 1489), together with a compilation of the works of Mesue, Avenzoar, Galen, etc. Page for page reprint, Venice, 1508. *See* No. 6495.90.

54   MEDICI ANTIQUI OMNES.
Medici antiqui omnes, qui latinis literis diversorum morborum genera et
remedia persecuti sunt. Venetiis, *apud Aldi filios,* 1547.
Contains selections from the writings of Celsus, Plinius Secundus,
Soranus, Apuleius, Barbarus, Musa, Priscianus, Trotula, Macer, Caelius
Aurelianus, Marcellus Empiricus, Scribonius Largus, Serenus Samonicus,
Strabus Gallus.

55   MEDICAE ARTIS PRINCIPES.
Medicae artis principes post Hippocratum et Galenum. Graeci Latinitate
donati. Excudebat H. STEPHANUS. 2 vols. [Genevae], *typ. H. Stephanus,* 1567.
Contains work of Aretaeus, Rufus of Ephesus, Alexander of Tralles, Paul
of Aegina, Oribasius, Sextus Philosophicus, Aetius, Philaretius, Theophilus,
Actuarius Zach. fil., Nicholaus Myrepsus Alexandrinus, Celsus, Scribonius
Largus, Marcellus Empiricus, Quintus Serenus Samonicus.

56   GRASSI, GIUNIO PAOLO. ?-1574
Medici antique Graeci: Aretaeus, Palladius, Ruffus, Theophilus: physici &
chirurgi...Omnes a Junio Paulo Crasso...Latio donati. Basileae, *ex officina
Petri Pernae,* 1581.

57   PARACELSUS THEOPHRASTUS PHILIPPUS AUREOLOUS BOMBASTUS VON HOHENHEIM.
1493-1541.
Sämtliche Werke...Herausg. von K. SUDHOFF und W. MATHIESSEN. 14 vols.
München, Berlin, *O. W. Barth, R. Oldenbourg,* 1922-33.
Paracelsus, a much-travelled man, was one of the most remarkable
figures in medicine. He was first to write on miners' diseases, to establish
the relationship between cretinism and endemic goitre and to note the
geographic differences in diseases. Sudhoff studied Paracelsus exhaustively. The first definitive collection of his works, edited by J. Huser, 10
vols., Basel, 1589-91, was reprinted, Hildesheim, *G. Olms,* 1971-74. A
selection of the writings of Paracelsus was edited by J. Jacobi and translated
by N. Guterman, 1951. J. Hargrave published a biography in 1951. See also
W. Pagel's *Paracelsus,* Basel & New York, *Karger,* 1958.

58   ———. Theophrastus Paracelsus Werke. Besorgt von W.E. PEUCKERT. Bd. 1-
5. Basel, *Schwabe,* 1965-69.
Osler said that Paracelsus was "the Luther of medicine, for when
authority was paramount he stood out for independent study".

59   PARÉ, AMBROISE. 1510-1590
Œuvres complètes d'Ambroise Paré. 3 vols. Paris, *Baillière,* 1840-41.
The best edition of Paré's works, edited by J. F. Malgaigne. An English
translation by Thomas Johnson appeared as early as 1634. *See also* No. 5565.
Janet Doe published *A bibliography of the works of Ambroise Paré,*
Chicago, 1943 and F. R. Packard published *Life and times of Ambroise
Paré.,.* New York, 1921. The comprehensive historical introduction to
Malgaigne's edition was translated by Wallace Hamby as *Surgery and
Ambroise Paré* Oklahoma, *Norman,* 1965.

60   BAILLOU, GUILLAUME DE [BALLONIUS]. 1538-1616
Opera medica omnia. 4 vols. Venetiis, *apud A. Jeremiam,* 1734-36.
De Baillou, "the first epidemiologist of modern times", foreshadowed
much that was afterwards taught by Sydenham. He first described

whooping-cough and introduced the term "rheumatism". He was Court physician during the reign of Henri IV of France. See the article on Baillou by E. W. Goodall in *Ann. med. Hist.,* 1935, **7,** 409-27.

60.1   FABRY VON HILDEN, WILHELM. 1560-1624
Opera quae extant omnia...partim nunc recens in lucem edita. Francofurti ad Moenum, *Sumptibus Johannis Beyeri,* 1646.
The collected works of the "father of German surgery". German translation, Frankfurt, 1652.

61   SENNERT, DANIEL. 1572-1637
Opera. 6 vols. Lugduni, *J. A. Huguetan,* 1676.
Besides giving early accounts of scarlatina and rubella, Sennert added to the knowledge of scurvy, dysentery and alcoholism. He was an able clinician but a believer in witchcraft. His *Opera* was first published in 1641; the edition given above is regarded as the best.

61.1   HARVEY, WILLIAM. 1578-1657
The works of William Harvey. Translated from the Latin, with a life of the author, by ROBERT WILLIS. London, *Sydenham Society,* 1847.
See Sir Geoffrey Keynes's *Life of William Harvey,* Oxford, 1966, (2nd printing, with corrections, 1978) and his *Bibliography of the writings of William Harvey,* 3rd ed., revised by Gweneth Whitteridge and Christine English, Winchester, *St. Paul's Bibliographies,* 1988.

61.2   SPIEGHEL, ADRIAAN VAN DER [SPIGELIUS]. 1578-1625
Opera quae extant omnia. Ex recension Joh. Antonidae vander Linden. Amsterdam, *Blaeu,* 1645.
Spieghel succeeded Casseri in the chair of anatomy at Padua. This edition of his collected writings contains the second printing of the 97 copperplates first printed in Casseri's *Tabulae anatomicae* (No. 381) plus 9 exquisite plates also by Valesio and Fialetti from Casseri's treatise, *De formatu foetu,* and a tenth plate representing the hymen. This splendid volume contains the second edition of No. 5229, and, in addition to Spigelius's writings, contains the 4th edition of Aselli (No. 1094), and the 5th edition of Harvey (No. 759).

62   WILLIS, THOMAS. 1621-1675
Opera omnia. 2 vols. Genevae, *apud Samuelem de Tournes,* 1676-80.
Willis was remarkable for his careful clinical observation. He was second only to Sydenham in his day. To him we owe the original descriptions of several conditions.

63   SYDENHAM, THOMAS. 1624-1689
Opera omnia. Ed. GULIELMUS ALEXANDER GREENHILL. London, *Sydenham Society,* 1844.
Sydenham is one of the greatest figures in internal medicine, and has been called the "Father of English Medicine". His reputation rests on his first-hand accounts of such conditions as the malarial fevers of his times, gout, scarlatina, measles, etc. A better edition of the above (editio altera) appeared in 1846. The original work, printed in 1685, is called *editio altera;* although no earlier edition is known to exist. An edition of Sydenham's Opuscula was published in Amsterdam, 1683. See K. Dewhurst's *Dr Thomas Sydenham, his life and original writings.,* London, *Wellcome Institute,* 1966.

64   ———. The works of Thomas Sydenham. Translated from the Latin edition of Dr. GREENHILL with a life of the author by R. G. LATHAM. 2 vols. London, *Sydenham Society*, 1848-50.

Best English translation of Sydenham's works.

65   REDI, FRANCESCO. 1626-1697
Opere. 7 vols. Venezia, *Remondini*, 1762.

Redi was a leading physician in Italy. He is best remembered for his experiments discrediting the theory of spontaneous generation and for his pioneer work in the field of parasitology (*see* No. 2448.1); see also the article on Redi by R. Cole in *Ann. med. Hist.*, 1926, **8**, 347-59.

66   MALPIGHI, MARCELLO. 1628-1694
Opera omnia. 2 vols. Londini, *R. Scott*, 1686.

Malpighi was the founder of histology and the greatest of the microscopists. In 1660 he was the first to see the capillary anastomosis between the arteries and the veins, thus helping the completion of Harvey's work on the circulation. He was a great embryologist; his name is perpetuated in the "Malpighian bodies", "Malpighi's layer" of the epidermis, "Malpighi's (splenic) corpuscles". Malpighi was an excellent draughtsman but a poor writer. *See* No. 534.1 *Marcello Malpighi and the evolution of embryology*, by H. B. Adelmann.

67   LEEUWENHOEK, ANTONJ VAN. 1632-1723
Ontledingen en ontdekkingen. 6 vols. Leiden, 1693-1718.

Leeuwenhoek was one of the first and greatest of the microbiologists. Many of his discoveries were communicated by him to the Royal Society in London. He discovered protozoa and bacteria. He is said to have had 250 microscopes and 419 lenses, many of them ground by himself. (*See also* Nos. 98, 265, 860.) An English translation of his works omitting all references to spermatozoa appeared in 2 vols. in 1798-1807. Clifford Dobell's study, *Antony van Leeuwenhoek and his 'little animals"*, London, 1932, reveals many new facts about the man, and includes the best bibliography. 10 vols. of his collected letters have been published in Dutch and English. (Lisse, *Swets & Zeitlinger*, 1939-1979.)

68   BAGLIVI, GIORGIO. 1668-1707
Opera omnia medico-practica et anatomica. Lugduni, *Anisson & J. Posuel*, 1704.

Baglivi, Professor of Anatomy at Rome, had a short but brilliant career. He wrote *Praxis medica* and *De fibra motrice*, and originated the so-called "solidar" pathology; he also devoted much time to experimental physiology. Baglivi was a strong advocate of specialism.

69   STAHL, GEORG ERNST. 1660-1734
Theoria medica vera. Halae, *lit. Orphanotrophiei*, 1708 [1707].

See No. 70. A three-volume German translation of the above was published in Berlin in 1831-33.

70   ———. Œuvres médico-philosophiques et pratiques. 6 vols. Paris, *J. B. Baillière*, 1859-64.

Stahl was responsible for the re-introduction of the idea of a "sensitive soul", propounded by van Helmont. The Stahlian "animism" considered the body to be composed of passive or "dead" substance, which became animated by the soul during life, returning to passivity or "death" on the departure of the soul from the body.

71   LANCISI, GIOVANNI MARIA. 1654-1720
Opera quae hactenus prodierunt omnia. 2 vols. Genevae, *J. A. Cramer et fil.*, 1718.
      Lancisi, great Italian clinician, was the first to describe cardiac syphilis; he was also notable as an epidemiologist, with a clear insight into the theory of contagion. He was physician to Pope Clement XI, who turned over to him the forgotten copper plates executed by Eustachius in 1552. Lancisi published these with his own notes in 1714. (*See* No. 391.) Note that Lancisi's posthumous *De aneurysmatibus* published in 1728 (No. 2973) appears only in later collected editions.

72   HOFFMANN, FRIEDRICH. 1660-1742
Opera omnia physico-medica. (Supplementum, *etc.*) 9 vols. Genevae, *fratres de Tournes,* 1740-53.
      Hoffmann of Halle was the most important of the Iatromechanists. He believed an ether-like "vital fluid" to be present in the nervous system and to act upon the muscles, giving them "tonus".

73   BOERHAAVE, HERMAN. 1668-1738
Opera omnia medica. Venetiis, *apud L. Basilium,* 1742.
      Boerhaave had a great reputation as a clinician; he was, in fact, the creator of the modern method of clinical teaching. His writings had an enormous influence during his lifetime. Haller, Cullen, Pringle, van Swieten and de Haen were among his pupils. His greatest work was his *Elementa chemiae,* published in 2 vols. at Leiden, 1732. The definitive bibliography is G.A. Lindeboom, *Bibliographia Boerhaaviana,* Leiden, *E.J. Brill,* 1959. See also Lindeboom's *Herman Boerhaave, the man and his work,* London, *Methuen,* 1968.

74   HUXHAM, JOHN. 1692-1768
Opera physico-medica. Lipsiae, *J. P. Kraus,* 1764.
      Huxham, a Devonshire man, was a pupil of Boerhaave. His most important contributions to medicine were in connection with fevers and infectious diseases.

75   WERLHOF, PAUL GOTTLIEB. 1699-1767
Opera medica. 3 vols. Hannoverae, *imp. frat. Helwingiorum,* 1775-76.
      Werlhof, a contemporary and friend of Haller, is remembered for his classic description of purpura haemorrhagica (*see* No. 3052). He was Court physician at Hanover.

76   CULLEN, WILLIAM. 1710-1790
The works. 2 vols. Edinburgh, *W. Blackwood,* 1827.
      Cullen was the most conspicuous figure in the history of the Edinburgh Medical School during the 18th century. He was an inspiring teacher and was instrumental in founding the Glasgow Medical School in 1744. His clinical lectures were notable as being the first given in the vernacular instead of in Latin.

77   CAMPER, PIETER. 1722-1789
Sämmtliche kleinere Schriften. 3 vols. Leipzig, *S. L. Crusius,* 1784-90.

Camper, an artist of skill, made his mark as an anthropologist and craniologist. He discovered the processus vaginalis of the peritoneum and the fibrous structure of the eye, and made several other important contributions to medical science. English translation, 1794.

78   HUNTER, JOHN. 1728-1793
The works of John Hunter. With notes. Edited by J. F. PALMER. 4 vols. and atlas. London. *Longman*, [1835]-37.

Hunter gave a great impetus to the study of morbid anatomy; he was the veritable founder of experimental and surgical pathology and one of the three greatest surgeons of all time. He was responsible for the commencement of some of the greatest medical museums; the Hunterian museum of the Royal College of Surgeons of England was based on his own private collection; much of it was destroyed during an air raid in World War II. Vol. I of the above work includes Drewry Ottley's Life of Hunter. A list of the books written by Hunter, and their location in British libraries, was published by W. R. LeFanu in 1946. The biography by Jessie Dobson, Edinburgh, 1969, includes a chronological list of Hunter's writings. For a detailed analysis of his scientific works within the context of his life see *John Hunter...*by George Qvist, London, [1981].

79   HEWSON, WILLIAM. 1739-1774
The works. Edited with an introduction and notes by G. GULLIVER. London, *Sydenham Society,* 1846.

Hewson was a pupil of the Hunters. In 1769 his memoir on the lymphatics in fishes won for him the Copley Medal of the Royal Society. His most important work is probably his "Experimental inquiry into the properties of the blood", 1771. *See also* Nos. 863, 1102.

80   RUSH, BENJAMIN. 1745-1813
Medical inquiries and observations. 5 vols. Philadelphia, *Prichard & Hall,* 1789-98.

Rush was considered the ablest American clinician of his time. He was a friend of Benjamin Franklin and one of the signatories of the Declaration of Independence. His many writings are distinguished for their classical style; several are dealt with elsewhere in this bibliography.

82   PURKYNĚ, JAN EVANGELISTA [PURKINJE]. 1787-1869
Sebrané spisy. Opera omnia. Tom. 1-12. v Praze, *Purkyňova Spolestnost,* 1918-73.

Purkyně was Professor of Physiology at Breslau and Prague. Eminent as physiologist and microscopist, he was first to use the microtome. *See* Kruta, V. *J.E. Purkyně, Physiologist. A short account of his contributions...with a bibliography of his works.* (Prague, *Academia Publishing House,* 1969).

82.1   SEMMELWEIS, IGNAZ PHILIPP. 1818 - 65
Semmelweis' gesammelte Werke. [Edited by] DR. TIBERIUS VON GYORY. Jena, *Gustav Fischer,* 1905.

An annotated edition, reprinting the texts of Semmelweis's works on puereral fever as a septicaemia (No. 6275) and on the aetiology of puerperal sepsis (No. 6277) as well as other gynaecological papers and articles on Semmelweis by Hebra and Skoda, among others.

83   PASTEUR, LOUIS. 1822-1895
Œuvres de Pasteur, réunies par Pasteur VALLERY-RADOT. 7 vols. Paris, *Masson,*
1922-39.
      One of the founders of bacteriology, Pasteur is at the same time one of
the greatest figures in the history of medicine. His work on fermentation,
the doctrine of spontaneous generation (which he exploded), virus diseases and preventive vaccinations, was fundamental. The standard biography is René Vallery-Radot, *La Vie de Pasteur,* Paris, 1900. English translation, 2 vols., 1901. See also E. Duclaux, *Pasteur: Histoire d'un esprit,* (Paris,
1896). English translation, Philadelphia, 1920.

84   CHARCOT, JEAN MARTIN. 1825-1893
Œuvres complètes. 9 vols. Paris, *Bureaux de Progrès Médical [and other
publishers],* 1886-91.
      Charcot, famous teacher at La Salpêtrière, created there the greatest
neurological clinic of modern times. He was a pioneer of psychotherapy
and left many memorable descriptions of nervous disorders. Pierre Marie,
who died in 1940, was a pupil of Charcot.

85   LISTER, JOSEPH, 1*st Baron Lister.* 1827-1912
Collected papers. 2 vols. Oxford, *Clarendon Press,* 1909.
      Lister, a pupil of Sharpey, became Professor of Surgery successively at
Glasgow, Edinburgh and King's College, London. He was the first medical
man in Britain to be raised to the peerage. The founder of the antiseptic
principle, his work had a profound effect upon modern surgery and
obstetrics. It is to be remembered that Oliver Wendell Holmes and Ignaz
Semmelweis had both, before Lister, striven without success to obtain the
adoption of antisepsis in obstetrics. Because Lister never wrote any books,
his *Collected papers* remain his lasting monument. Sir Rickman Godlee's
biography of Lister appeared (2nd ed.) in 1918. A shorter biography was
published by H. C. Cameron in 1948, and another by D. Guthrie in 1949.
See also R. Fisher, *Joseph Lister,* New York, *Stein & Day,* 1977.

86   KOCH, ROBERT. 1843-1910
Gesammelte Werke. 2 vols. [in 3]. Leipzig, *G. Thieme,* 1912.
      By his demonstration of the life-cycle of the anthrax bacillus, Koch in
1877 was the first to show a specific micro-organism to be the cause of a
definite disease. For his work on tuberculosis, he received the Nobel Prize
in 1905. See T.D. Brock, *Robert Koch: a life in medicine and bacteriology,*
Madison, *Science-Tech Publishers,* 1988.

86.1   PAVLOV, IVAN PETROVITCH. 1849-1936
Sämtliche Werke. 6 vols. Berlin, *Akademie-Verlag,* 1956.

86.2   WELCH, WILLIAM HENRY. 1850-1934
Papers and addresses. 3 vols., Baltimore, *Johns Hopkins Press,* 1920.
      Reprints Welch's papers with an introduction by Simon Flexner and a
chronological bibliography.

86.3   HALSTED, WILLIAM STEWART. 1852-1922
Surgical papers. 2 vols. Baltimore, *Johns Hopkins Press,* 1924.
      In spite of an addiction to cocaine hydrochlorate from experimentation
with it as a surgical anaesthetic in 1884 until his death, Halsted was among
the greatest of all surgical innovators and teachers. While pioneering

important new procedures, he developed the modern system of residency training and was the first to use rubber gloves in surgery. Like Lister, he never wrote any books, and his collected papers remain his lasting monument.

86.4   EHRLICH, PAUL. 1854-1915

Collected papers of Paul Ehrlich. Compiled and edited by F. HIMMELWEIT. 3 vols. London, *Pergamon Press,* 1956-60.

Vol. I: *Histology, biochemistry, and pathology;* Vol. 2: *Immunology and cancer research;* Vol. 3: *Chemotherapy.* Most texts are in German. English translations are also published when available. The set includes new English translations of a few items. Volume 4, intended to contain Ehrlich's collected letters and a complete bibliography, was never published. See M. M. Marquardt's *Paul Ehrlich,* 1949, and E. Bäumler's, *Paul Ehrlich, scientist for life,* G. Edwards transl., [1984].

86.5   CORPUS MEDICORUM GRAECORUM.

Ediderunt Academiae Berolinensis Hauniensis Lipsiensis, Lipsiae et Berolini, *B. G. Teubner* until 1945, thereafter Berlin, *Akademie-Verlag,* 1908-

This series sets as its goal the scholarly edition of all extant ancient Greek medical texts, including those lost in the original language but preserved in medieval translations. To date about fifty volumes have appeared. These are numbered as follows: I. Hippocrates, II. Aretaeus, III. Rufus, IV. Soranus, V. Galen, VI. Oribasius, VII. Alexander of Tralles, VIII. Aetius of Amida, IX. Paulus of Aegina, X. Minor Writers, XI. Minor commentators on Hippocrates and Galen. Miscellaneous works are included in Supplementa and Supplementa Orientalia.

86.6   CORPUS MEDICORUM LATINORUM.

Editum consilio et auctoritate Instituti Puschmanniani Lipsiensis. Lipsiae et Berolini, *B. G. Teubner* until 1945, thereafter, Berlin, *Akademie-Verlag,* 1915-.

As of 1990 eight volumes have been published (*). The completed series would include: I. Celsus*; II. Scribonius Largus, Quintus Serenus* etc.: III. Plinius Secundus Iunior*; IV. Antonius Musa, Pseudo-Apuleius, Sextus Placitus, etc.*; V. Marcellus*; VI. Cassius Felix, Theodorus Priscianus; VII. Caelius Aurelianus*; VIII. Anthimus*, Mustio, etc.

86.7   FREUD, SIGMUND. 1856-1939

The collected edition of the psychological works of Sigmund Freud. Translated from the German under the general editorship of JAMES STRACHEY. 24 vols. London, *Hogarth Press,* 1966-74.

For biography see E. Jones, *Sigmund Freud, life and work,* 3 vols., London, 1953-57; and P. Gay, *Sigmund Freud: a life for our time,* New York, 1988. For iconography see E. Freud, L. Freud, & I. Grubrich-Simitis, *Sigmund Freud: his life in pictures and words,* New York, [1978].

BIOLOGY

87   EMPEDOCLES. *circa* 490-430 B.C.
The fragments of Empedocles. Translated by W. E. LEONARD. *Monist,* 1907, **17,** 451-74.
Empedocles was a Greek philosopher, statesman, physician and reformer. His poem on Nature originally ran to 5,000 lines, of which only 400 are now left. He believed in four ultimate elements—fire, air, water and earth, these being brought into union and parted by the two powers, love and hate.

87.1   THEOPHRASTUS *of Eresos. circa* 371- *circa* 287 B.C.
[De historia et causis plantarum]. [Treviso, *Bartholomaeus Confalonerius,* 1483].
    The earliest work of scientific botany. Theophrastus, a student of Aristotle, succeeded his teacher as head of the Athens Peripatetic School. His system of botanical classification, analogous to the zoological system in Aristotle's *Historia animalium,* maintained its authority until the advent of the microscope in the mid 17th century. First edition in Greek in Aristotle, *[Opera omnia],* Venice, Aldus Manutius, 1495-98. Greek–English bilingual edition edited by Sir A. Hort, in *Loeb Classics,* 2 vols., 1916. *See No.* 1783.

88   LUCRETIUS *Carus,* TITUS. *fl.* 98-55 B.C.
De rerum natura. [Brescia,] Thomas Ferrandus, [1473].
    The work is a reasoned system of philosophy written in verse. Book V attempts an explanation of the origin of the universe and life, and the gradual advance of man from the savage state. All these topics are treated from the viewpoint that the world is not itself divine nor directed by a divine agency. Definitive edition with translation, commentary, *apparatus criticus* and prolegomena by Cyril Bailey, 3 vols., London, *Oxford University Press,* 1947.

89   PLINIUS *Secundus,* CAIUS. A.D. 23-79
    Historia naturalis, libri XXXVII. Venice, *Johann von Speier,* 1469. The most ancient Western encyclopaedia extant, Pliny's *Historia* contained all that was known in his time of geography, mineralogy, anthropology, botany, zoology and meteorology. Books XX-XXXII deal with medicine. This was the one work of classical antiquity which, despite the low quality of its material, was read steadily throughout the Dark Ages. The botanical errors were not corrected until 1492 (Leoniceno, *see* No. 1798). Pliny's work was one of the very first scientific texts to be printed. The first English translation by Philemon Holland appeared in 1601. The modern English translation of the *Natural history* with parallel Latin text is that of W.H.S. Jones, H. Rackham, and D.E. Eichholz in the *Loeb Classical Library,* 10 vols., London, *W. Heinemann,* 1948-63.

91   BARTHOLOMEW *Anglicus* [DE GLANVILLA (BARTHOLOMAEUS)] *fl.* 1250
De proprietatibus rerum. [Bazel, *B. Ruppel, circa* 1470.]
    A condensed encyclopaedia of what was then understood by natural science. The work was probably written about the middle of the 13th century. It was one of the most widely read scientific works of the Middle Ages. Caxton is said to have learned to print from this book.

92 ——. De proprietatibus rerum. [London, *Wynkyn de Worde*, 1495.]

This English translation of Bartholomaeus Anglicus was made by John of Trevisa in 1398. Bibliographically it is of interest as being one of the earliest books printed in London, one of the finest of the 15th century, and the first book printed on paper made in England. See also *On the properties of things. John Trevisa's translation of Bartholomaeus Anglicus' De proprietatibus rerum. A critical text edited by M. C. Seymour*, 2 vols., London, 1975.

93 LEONARDO DA VINCI. 1452-1519

Codice sul volo degli uccelli. Pubblicato da T. Sabachnikoff; transcrizione e note di G. Piumati, con traduzione francese di C. Ravaisson-Mollien. Paris, *E. Rouveyre*, 1893.

The scientific study of the mechanics of flight begins with Leonardo's investigations on birds, undertaken during his attempts to build a flying machine. The original manuscript of this work is now in Rome.

94 ——. The notebooks of Leonardo da Vinci. Arranged, rendered into English and introduced by Edward MacCurdy. 2 vols. London, *Cape*, 1938.

2nd edition, 1956 (reprinted London, *Cape*, 1977).

95 HERBAL

Herbarius Mainz, *P. Schoeffer*, [14]84.

One of the earliest illustrated books on plants, which also contains some fanciful pictures of animals. It was probably compiled by Johann von Kaub from the works of earlier writers. Facsimile reprints 1924 and 1968. *See* No. 1796.

96 ——. Ortus sanitatis. Moguntiae, *J. Meydenbach*, 1491.

First edition of a herbal and general treatise on natural history which became very popular. Despite its quaint and often fanciful woodcuts of animals and plants, it stimulated other more scientific treatises on botany and zoology. Available in facsimile in W. L. Schreiber's *Die Krauterbücher des XV und XVI Jahrhunderts*, Munich, 1924. An English translation of *circa* 1521 (S.T.C. 22367) was reprinted London, *Quaritch*, 1954, edited by N. Hudson. *See* No. 1797.

97 REDI, Francesco. 1626-1697

Esperienze intorno alla generazione degl'insetti. Firenze, *all'Insegna della Stella*, 1668.

The first scientific study of the question of spontaneous generation. Redi's experiments dealt the first real blow to the doctrine of spontaneous generation. In these experiments Redi made use of what we now term "controls". English translation, 1909.

98 CAMERER, Rudolph Jakob [Camerarius]. 1685-1721

De sexu plantarum epistola. Tübingen, *Vidua Rommeii*, 1694.

First experimental demonstration of the sexuality of plants. Camerer showed that in flowering plants the anthers are male organs, and that the ovary with style and stigma are female, and that pollen is required for the production of viable seeds. Until his work, the continuity of reproductive processes in plants and animals had been a matter of speculation; after it, the scientific study of fertilization and hybridization became possible.

99   LINNÉ, CARL VON [LINNAEUS]. 1707-1778
Systema naturae. Lugduni Batavorum, *apud Theodorum Haak,* 1735.

In this work Linnaeus developed the first logical and modern classifications of plants, animals and minerals. Its most valuable feature, the binomial nomenclature (genus and species) was probably devised in the first place by Joachim Jung, about 1640. The most important edition of the *Systema naturae* is the tenth, published in 2 vols., 1758-59.

99.1   ——. Species plantarum...2 vols. Stockholm, *Salvius,* 1753.

The first full-dress appearance of Linnaeus's binomial system. Describing about 8,000 plant species from all over the world in the binomial system, the book demonstrated the value of a binomial system of nomenclature for biology generally, and was the stimulus to the development of this type of classification throughout the field. English translation, 2 vols., Lichfield, 1787.

100   SPALLANZANI, LAZZARO. 1729-1799
Saggio di osservazioni microscopiche concernenti il sistema della generazione dei Signori de Needham e Buffon. *In his:* Dissertazione due...Modena, 1765.

Spallanzani, a believer in preformation theory, found that he could prevent contamination by microorganisms in strongly heated infusions protected from aerial contamination, but he observed that as soon as air was allowed to enter the flask, microorganisms proliferated. He was one of the first to dispute the doctrine of spontaneous generation.

101   ——. Prodromo di un opera da imprimersi sopra le riproduzione animali. Modena, *Giovanni Montanari,* 1768.

In this preliminary to a larger work on regeneration which was never published, Spallanzani described regenerative capacities of remarkable complexity and repetitiveness in the land snail, salamander and toad and frog, establishing the general law that an inverse ratio obtains between the regenerative capacity and age of the individual. English translation, London, 1769.

102   ——. Opusculi di fisica animale e vegetabile. 2 vols. Modena, *Soc. tipografica,* 1776.

Later confutation of the theory of spontaneous generation. Spallanzani's conclusions were similar to those expressed by Pasteur nearly a century later. His collected works were published in Milan, 2 vols., 1932-33. English translation, 2 vols., London, 1784.

103   INGEN-HOUSZ, JAN. 1730-1799
Experiments on vegetables, discovering their great power of purifying the common air in the sun-shine, and of injuring it in the shade at night. To which is joined, a new method of examining the accurate degree of salubrity of the atmosphere. London, *P. Elmsley and H. Payne,* 1779.

Ingen-Housz showed that the green parts of plants, when exposed to light, fix the free carbon dioxide of the atmosphere, but that in darkness plants have no such power. Thus he proved that animal life is dependent ultimately on plant life, a discovery of fundamental importance in the economy of the world of living things. Reprinted, with biography, by H. S. Reed in *Chronica Botanica,* Waltham, Mass., 1949, **11,** nos. 5-6.

104   BLUMENBACH, Johann Friedrich. 1752-1840
Ueber den Bildungstrieb und das Zeugungsgeschäft. Göttingen, *J. C. Dieterich,* 1781.
     Blumenbach, Professor of Medicine at Göttingen, was the founder of modern anthropology. In the above work he rejected the "preformation" theory and advanced the theory of epigenesis as the true explanation of the phenomenon of embryological development. English translation, London, [1792?].

104.1   SPRENGEL, Christian Konrad. 1750-1816
Das entdeckte Geheimnis der Natur im Bau und in der Befruchtung der Blumen. Berlin, *Friedrich Vieweg,* 1793.
     Sprengel demonstrated for the first time that the whole structure of nectar-bearing flowers is adapted for fertilization by insects. In his study of the Rose-bay Sprengel discovered dichogamy – that in some plants the two sexes (stigmas and anthers) while occurring in one blossom, mature at different times. This prevents the flowers from being fertilized by their own pollen, and necessitates fertilization by the pollen carried to them by insects.

105   DARWIN, Erasmus. 1731-1802
Zoonomia; or the laws of organic life. 2 vols. London, *J. Johnson,* 1794-96.
     Grandfather of Charles Darwin and Francis Galton, Erasmus Darwin provided in *Zoonomia,* his major work in medicine and natural science, the first consistent all-embracing hypothesis of evolution. Nevertheless, his grandson, Charles, said Erasmus's theory had no effect on his *On the origin of species.*

105.1   TREVIRANUS, Gottfried Reinhold. 1776-1837
Biologie...6 vols. Gottingen, *Röwer,* 1802-22.
     Simultaneously with Lamarck, Treviranus coined the term "biology" for the study of living things, and he was the first to use it in a book title. This massive work was a summary of all basic knowledge about the structure and function of living matter. Treviranus wrote that any living creature has the ability to adapt its organization to changing external conditions. Thus both Haeckel and Weismann considered Treviranus to be a precurser of evolution theory, even though Treviranus never explained how changes in organic structures occurred nor how they could become hereditary.

106   OKEN, Lorenz. 1779-1851
Die Zeugung. Bamberg, Würzburg, *J. A. Goebhardt,* 1805.
     Oken maintained that all organic beings originate from, and consist of, cells, and that organisms are produced by an agglomeration of these cells.

107   ISIS.
Isis, oder encyclopädische Zeitung (verzüglich für Naturgeschichte, vergleichende Anatomie und Physiologie), von Oken. 41 vols. Jena, *etc.,* 1817-48.
     Oken, a leading light in the Nature–Philosophical School in Germany, produced important work in the field of biology. He founded the journal *Isis,* which published articles of great value; its incursion into the field of German politics led to a demand for the resignation of Oken from his professorship or the suppression of his journal. Oken resigned and continued to publish *Isis.*

108   DUTROCHET, René Joachim Henri. 1776-1847
        Recherches anatomiques et physiologiques sur la structure intime des
        animaux et des végétaux. Paris, *J. B. Baillière,* 1824.

109   BROWN, Robert. 1773-1858
        Observations on the organs and mode of fecundation in Orchideae and
        Asclepiadeae. *Trans. Linn. Soc.,* 1829-32, **16,** 685-746.
        Discovery, in 1831, of the cell nucleus.

109.1   WAGNER, Rudolph. 1805-1864
        Einige Bemerkungen und Fragen über das Keimbläschen (vesicula
        germinativa). *Arch. Anat. Physiol. wiss. Med.,* 1835, 373-7.
        Wagner saw and described the nucleolus.

110   DUTROCHET René Joachim Henri. 1776-1847
        Mémoires pour servir à l'histoire anatomique et physiologique des végétaux
        et des animaux. 2 vols. and atlas. Paris, *J. B. Baillière,* 1837.
            Dutrochet asserted that respiration follows the same pattern in both
        animals and plants, showing that the minute openings on the surface of
        leaves (the stomata) communicate with lacunae in deeper tissue. He also
        demonstrated that only the green parts of the plant can absorb carbon
        dioxide, thereby transforming light energy into chemical energy. The
        Mémoires are a collection of all his more important biological papers.

111   EHRENBERG, Christian Gottfried. 1795-1876
        Die Infusionsthierchen als vollkommene Organismen. 1 vol. and atlas.
        Leipzig, *L. Voss,* 1838.
            In this monumental work Ehrenberg extended Müller's bacteriological
        classification.(*See* No. 2466.) Like Müller, he made no distinction between
        protozoa and bacteria, classing them both as infusoria. His classification
        included *Vibrio, Spirillum* and *Spirochaeta.* The fine plates in this book
        were drawn by Ehrenberg himself.

112   SCHLEIDEN, Matthias Jakob. 1804-1881
        Beiträge zur Phytogenesis. *Arch. Anat. Physiol. wiss. Med.,* 1838, 137-76.
            Schleiden demonstrated that plant tissues are made up of and devel-
        oped from groups of cells, of which he recognized the "cytoblast" or cell-
        nucleus. He observed with great accuracy certain other activities of the cell,
        and is an important figure in the development of the cell theory. Unfortu-
        nately he held that young cells develop spontaneously from the cytoblast,
        an acceptance of the theory of spontaneous generation. English translation
        (Sydenham Society) 1847.

112.1   SCHWANN, Theodor. 1810-1882
        Ueber die Analogie in der Structur und dem Wachsthum der Thiere und
        Pflanzen. *Neue Not. Geb. Nat. Heil.,* Jan. 1838, 33-36; Feb. 1838, 225-29;
        April 1838, 21-23.
            Schwann's three-part preliminary application of Schleiden's "watch-
        glass" cell theory to the genesis of animal cells. Schleiden communicated
        the theory to him verbally. This paper actually pre-dates Schleiden's first
        publication (No. 112) but Schwann gives Schleiden full credit for the
        Uhrglastheorie. English translation with commentary in L.J. Rather, P.
        Rather, and J.B. Frerichs, *Johannes Müller and the nineteeth century
        origins of tumor cell theory,* Canton, Mass., [1986].

113 ——. Mikroskopische Untersuchungen über die Uebereinstimmung in der Struktur und dem Wachsthum der Thiere und Pflanzen. Berlin, *Sander,* 1839.

Mainly devoted to the investigation of the elementary structure of animal tissues, Schwann's *Untersuchungen* had an important bearing on the development of the doctrine of the cell structure of animal tissue. In this work Schwann discarded Schleiden's *Uhrglastheorie* and put forward a theory of his own. In the same work he described the neurilemma, the "sheath of Schwann". Schwann was Professor of Anatomy and Physiology at Liège. English translation (Sydenham Society), 1847. See M. Florkin, *Naissance et déviation de la théorie cellulaire dans l'œuvre de Theodore Schwann.* Paris, *Hermann,* 1960.

114 MOHL, Hugo von. 1805-1872
Grundzüge der Anatomie und Physiologie der vegetabilischen Zelle. *In:* Rudolph Wagner's Handwörterbuch der Physiologie. Braunschweig, *F. Vieweg und Sohn,* 1851.

Von Mohl saw and described cell division. English translation, London, 1852.

115 MOLESCHOTT, Jacob. 1822-1893
Der Kreislauf des Lebens. Mainz, *V. von Zabern,* 1852.

This work attacked Liebig's theories, although courteously. Moleschott, a Dutch physiologist, evolved a purely materialistic conception of the world. He considered life a magnificent metabolic process, and thought a product of the activities of the brain.

116 REMAK, Robert. 1815-1865
Ueber extracelluläre Entstehung thierischer Zellen und über die Vermehrung derselben durch Theilung. *Arch. Anat. Physiol. wiss. Med.,* 1852, 47-57.

Remak was the first to point out that growth of new tissues was accomplished by the division of pre-existing cells.

117 SCHULTZE, Maximilian Johann Sigismund. 1825-1874
Ueber Muskelkörperchen und das, was man eine Zelle zu nennen habe. *Arch. Anat. Physiol. wiss. Med.,* 1861, 1-27.

Schultze showed the cell to be a clump of nucleated protoplasm, stating that each muscle fibre or primitive muscle bundle was developed from a single myoblast by successive divisions of its cell or nucleus. His work settled the controversy with regard to the place of the cell in muscle tissue and stimulated the histologists to investigate the nature of intercellular tissue. Partial English translation in No. 143.1.

118 ——. Das Protoplasma der Rhizopoden und der Pflanzenzellen. Leipzig, *Engelmann,* 1863.

Schultze showed that protoplasm is practically identical in all living cells.

119 SPENCER, Herbert. 1820-1903
The principles of biology. 2 vols. London, *Williams & Norgate,* 1864-67.

Spencer conceived that every species is endowed with its own type of physiological unit, each unit being capable, under certain circumstances, of reproducing the whole organism. Spencer set forth doctrines of evolution some years before the appearance of the *Origin of species.*

120   HAECKEL, Ernst Heinrich Philipp August. 1834-1919
        Die Gastraea-Theorie, die phylogenetische Classification des Thierreichs
        und die Homologie der Keimblätter. *Jena. Z. Naturw.,* 1874, **8,** 1-55.
            Haeckel's gastraea theory, which considers the two-layered gastrula as
        the ancestral form of multicellular animals.

122   FLEMMING, Walther. 1843-1905
        Beiträge zur Kenntniss der Zelle und ihrer Lebenserscheinungen. *Arch. mikr.
        Anat.,* 1879, **16,** 302-436; 1880, **18,** 151-259.
            Classic account of cell division and karyokinesis. Flemming named the
        nuclear substance "chromatin" and gave the name "mitosis" to cell division.
        Translation of Part II in *J. Cell Biol.,* 1965, **25,** No. 1, pt. 2, 3-69. See also
        Flemming's book on the subject, *Zellsubstanz, Kern und Zellteilung,*
        Leipzig, 1882.

123   STRASBURGER, Eduard Adolf. 1844-1912
        Ueber Zellbildung und Zelltheilung. 3te. Aufl. Jena, *G. Fischer,* 1880.
            A pioneer work on the formation and division of cells. In this third
        edition Strasburger established one of the principles of modern cytology,
        i.e., that independent cell formation does not occur but that fresh nuclei
        invariably arise through the division of older ones. The first edition of this
        book appeared in 1875.

125   LOEB, Jacques. 1859-1924
        Der Heliotropismus der Thiere und seine Uebereinstimmung mit dem
        Heliotropismus der Pflanzen. Würzburg, *G. Hertz,* 1890.
            Loeb founded the theory of "tropisms" as the basis of the psychology of
        the lower forms of life. English translation in Loeb's *Studies in general
        physiology,* Vol. 1, 1-88. Chicago, 1905.

126   ALTMANN, Richard. 1852-1900
        Die Elementarorganismen und ihre Beziehungen zu den Zellen. Leipzig,
        Veit & Comp., 1890.
            Mitochondria described, p. 145.

127   DAVENPORT, Charles Benedict. 1866-1944
        Experimental morphology. 2 pts. New York, *Macmillan,* 1897-99.
            Reprinted, 1908.

128   MORGAN, Thomas Hunt. 1866-1945
        Regeneration. New York, *Macmillan,* 1901.

129   DRIESCH, Hans Adolf Eduard. 1867-1941
        Die organischen Regulationen. Leipzig, *W. Engelmann,* 1901.

132   MINOT, Charles Sedgwick. 1852-1914
        The problem of age, growth and death. New York, *G. P. Putnam,* 1908.
            Minot's theory of ageing, based on cytomorphosis and the rate of
        growth. This work first appeared as a paper in vol. 7 of the *Popular Science
        Monthly,* 1907.

134   KEEBLE, *Sir* Frederick William. 1870-1952
        Plant animals. Cambridge, *University Press,* 1910.

135   LOEB, JACQUES. 1859-1924
       The mechanistic conception of life. Chicago, *University Press* (1912).

136   ABDERHALDEN, EMIL. 1877-1950
       Handbuch der biologischen Arbeitsmethoden. Herausgegeben von E.
       ABDERHALDEN. Vol. 1-107. Berlin, Wien, *Urban & Schwarzenburg,* 1920-39.

137   PEARL, RAYMOND. 1879-1940
       The biology of death. Philadelphia, *Lippincott Co.,* 1922.
       Raymond Pearl did important work on the subject of vital statistics.

138   ROBERTSON, THORBURN BRAILSFORD. 1884-1930
       The chemical basis of growth and senescence. Philadelphia, *J. B. Lippincott*
       (1923).

139   LOEB, JACQUES. 1859-1924
       Regeneration from a physico-chemical viewpoint. New York, *McGraw Hill
       Book Co.,* 1924.

139.1 BAKER, JOHN RANDAL. 1900-1984
       The cell-theory: a restatement, history, and critique. *Q. J. micr. Sci.,* 1948,
       89, 103-25, **90,** 87-108; 1952, **93,**157-90.

139.2 LEWIS, WARREN HARMON. 1870-1964
       Pinocytosis. *Bull. Johns Hopk. Hosp.,* 1931, **49**, 17-27.
       Discovery of pinocytosis.

History of General Biology

141   RADL, EMMANUEL. 1873-1942
       Geschichte der biologischen Theorien seit dem Ende des siebzehnten
       Jahrhunderts. 2 pts. Leipzig, *Engelmann,* 1905-09.
       Second edition, extensively revised as *Geschichte der biologischen
       Theorien in der Neuzeit,* pt.1., Leipzig-Berlin, 1913. English translation of
       pt 2. as *The history of biological theories,* London, 1930.

142   NORDENSKIÖLD, NILS ERIK. 1872-1933
       The history of biology: a survey. Translated by L. B. EYRE. New York, *Knopf,*
       1928.
       Previously published in Swedish and German editions. Many reprints
       were published.

143   KROGMAN, WILTON MARION. 1903-
       A bibliography of human morphology, 1914-1939. Chicago, *University Press,*
       1941.

143.1 HALL, THOMAS S.
       A source book in animal biology. New York, *McGraw-Hill,* 1951.

144   SINGER, CHARLES JOSEPH. 1876-1960
       A history of biology to about the year 1900. A general introduction to the
       study of living things. 3rd ed. London & New York, *Abelard-Schuman,* 1959.

145 BODENHEIMER, FREDERICK SIMON. 1897-1959
The history of biology. London, *Dawsons* [1958].

145.1 HUGHES. ARTHUR. 1908-
A history of cytology. New York, *Abelard-Schuman*, 1959.

145.2 LENOIR, TIMOTHY.
The strategy of life: teleology and mechanics in nineteenth century German biology. Dordrecht, *D. Reidel*, 1982.

ECOLOGY

See also DEMOGRAPHY; STATISTICS

145.50 EVELYN, JOHN. 1620-1706
Fumifugium: or the inconveniencie of the aer and smoak of London dissipated. Together with some remedies humbly proposed. London, *Gabriel Bedel*, 1661.
  A pioneering attack on air pollution caused by "the hellish and dismall cloud of sea-coal" which perpetually enveloped London. Of course, the problems Evelyn wrote about did not go away, and the work continued to be reprinted, with at least four editions published in the 20th century, including one in 1961 by the National Society for Clean Air.

145.51 ———. Sylva, or a discourse of forest- trees, and the preservation of timber in His Majesty's dominions. London, *Jo. Martyn and Ja. Allestry*, 1664.
  A protest against the careless destruction of England's forests to fuel the furnaces of the glass and iron industries. The work was influential in establishing a much-needed programme of reforestation that had a lasting effect on the British economy. This was the first official publication of the newly established Royal Society.

145.52 INGEN-HOUSZ, JAN. 1730-1799
Experiments on vegetables, discovering their great power of purifying the common air in the sun-shine, and of injuring it in the shade at night. To which is joined, a new method of examining the accurate degree of salubrity of the atmosphere. London, *P. Elmsley and H. Payne,* 1779.
  Ingen-Housz showed that the green parts of plants, when exposed to light, fix the free carbon dioxide of the atmosphere, but that in darkness plants have no such power. Thus he proved that animal life is dependent ultimately on plant life, a discovery of fundamental importance in ecology.

145.53 ZIMMERMAN, EBERHARD AUGUST WILHELM VON. 1743-1815
Specimen zoologiae geographicae, quardupem domicilia et migrationes sistens. Leiden, *Theodor Haak*, 1777.
  The first textbook of zoogeography, containing the first world map showing the distribution of mammals.

145.54 SAUSSURE, NICOLAS-THÉODORE DE. 1767-1845
Recherches chimiques sur la végétation. Paris, *Nyon*, An XII [1804].
  In this foundation work on phytochemistry, Saussure analysed the chief active components of plants, their synthesis and decomposition. He specified the relationships between vegetation and the environment. He

showed that plants grown in closed vessels took their entire carbon content from the enclosed gas, and thus demolished the old theory that plants derive carbon from the so-called "humus" of the soil.

145.55   HUMBOLDT, Friedrich Wilhelm Heinrich Alexander von. 1769-1859 & BONPLAND, Aimé J.A. 1773-1858.
Essai sur la géographie des plantes; accompagné d'un tableau physique des régions équinoxales. Paris, *Levrault, Schoell*, 1805.
One of the first works on the geographical distribution of plants. Humboldt was a pioneer student of geographical– ecological plant associations.

145.56   EDWARDS, William Frédéric. 1776-1842
De l'influence des agens physiques sur la vie. Paris, *Crochard*, 1824.
Edwards studied the influence of environmental factors on animal life, concluding that vital processes depend on external physical and chemical forces but are not entirely controlled by them. English translation by Thomas Hodgkin, with important additional material by Hodgkin and others, London, 1832. *See* No. 1991.

145.57   VERHULST, Pierre François. 1804-1849
Notice sur la loi que la population suit dans son accroissement. *Corresp. Math. et Phys.*, 1838, **10**, 113-21.
Verhulst constructed the simplest mathematical model of a continously growing population with an upper limit to its size.

145.58   ——. Recherches mathématiques sur la loi d'accroissement de la population. *Mem. Acad. Roy. Belg.*, 1845, **18**, 1-38.
In his second paper on population growth Verhulst introduced the term, *logistic*. He modified his equation so its early part is exponential and becomes logistic only after a definite length of time. Verhulst published a second paper on this subject: Deuxième mémoire sur la loi d'accroissement de la population. *Mem. Acad. Roy. Belg.*, 1847, **20**, 1-32.

145.59   MARSH, George Perkins. 1801-1882
Man and nature; or, physical geography as modified by human action. New York, *Charles Scribner*, 1864.
"The fountainhead of the conservation movement" (Mumford). This is a comprehensive scientific account of man's enormous and often destructive impact on the physical world. Marsh warned of the dangers of the reckless misuse of land then endemic in the United States, using the ruined lands of the Mediterranean region as an example of America's probable future, and called for a scientific programme to restore the land.

145.60   WALLACE, Alfred Russel. 1823-1913
The geographical distribution of animals. 2 vols. London, *Macmillan*, 1876.
Wallace studied the fauna of the Malay peninsula and was struck both with its resemblances to and differences from that of South America. His studies resulted in the above world-wide study, which pioneered the science of zoogeography.

145.61   MÖBIUS, Karl August. 1825-1908
Die Auster und die Austernwirtschaft. Berlin, *Verlag von Wiegandt*, 1877.

In this study of oyster culture precipitated by the impoverishment of natural oyster beds, Möbius provided the earliest description of a marine animal community maintained in a state of equilibrium by limitations of resources.

145.62　FORBES, Stephen Alfred. 1844-1930
The lake as a microcosm. *Bull. Sci. Assoc. Peoria, Ill.,* 1887, 77-87.
　　Forbes was the first to apply ecological principles to limnology. He emphasized population regulation and the dynamic nature of the community.

145.63　LOTKA, Alfred James. 1880-1949
Elements of physical biology. Baltimore, *Williams & Wilkins,* 1925.
　　In this landmark of theoretical population ecology Lotka attempted to provide for parts of biology a basis comparable to that given by theoretical physics to experimental physics. This was the first great exposition and elaboration of Verhulst's logistic. (No. 145.56). Reprinted, New York, 1956 as *Elements of mathematical biology.*

145.64　VOLTERRA, Vito. 1860-1940
Variazioni e fluttuazioni del numero d'individui in specie animali conviventi. *Mem. R. Acad. Naz. dei Lincei* (ser.6), 1926, **2**, 31-113.
　　The mathematician Volterra created the basic equations for two species interactions. Abridged English translation as appendix to R. Chapman, *Animal ecology,* New York, 1931.

145.65　ELTON, Charles Sutherland. 1900-
Animal ecology. London, *Sidgwick and Jackson,* 1927.
　　Elton integrated the concepts of food chains, pyramids of numbers, and the "niche" into a useful framework for ecology.

145.66　GAUSE, George Francis. 1910-
The struggle for existence. Baltimore, *Williams & Wilkins,* 1934.
　　Gause developed the concept of competitive exclusion as formulated by Volterra.

145.67　LINDEMAN, Raymond L.
The trophic-dynamic aspect of ecology. *Ecology,* 1942, **23**, 399-418.
　　"The birth of ecosystem ecology" (McIntosh). Lindeman described energy flow in ecosystems in a form amenable to productive abstract analysis.

History of Ecology

145.90　HUTCHINSON, George Evelyn. 1903-
An introduction to population ecology. New Haven, *Yale University Press,* [1978].
　　This elegantly written textbook by a pioneering authority is based on a carefully documented historical approach to the subject.

145.91　McINTOSH, Robert Patrick.
The background of ecology: concept and theory. Cambridge, *Cambridge University Press,* [1985].

See also 198-215, CRANIOLOGY

146   HERODOTUS. *circa* 484-425 B.C.
       The History of Herodotus of Halicarnassus. The translation of G. RAWLINSON revised & annotated by A.W. LAWRENCE...To which is added a life of Herodotus. London, *The Nonesuch Press*, 1935.
       George Rawlinson's edition of Herodotus is probably the most useful, the notes being of particular value. For this superbly produced edition Rawlinson's work was revised by A.W. Lawrence, the brother of the more widely celebrated T.E. Lawrence.

147   ——. Works of Herodotus. Translated by A. D. GODLEY. 4 vols. London, *Heinemann,* 1920-24.
       Greek and English text, *Loeb Classics* series. Herodotus travelled much in Greece, Asia Minor and North Africa, before settling in Italy. His *History* includes careful observations on the nature and habits of various peoples, and may be regarded as the first work on anthropology.

148   GALEN. A.D. 130-200
       De temperamentis libri III recensuit G. HELREICH.Lipsiae, *B.G. Teubner,* 1904.
       Reprinted Stuttgart, 1969.

149   DÜRER, ALBRECHT. 1471-1528
       Vier Bücher von menschlicher Proportion. (Nürnberg, *J. Formschneyder),* 1528.
       Written, designed, and illustrated by Dürer, this work is notable for its extraordinary series of anthropometrical woodcuts. The first two books deal with the proper proportions of the human form; the third changes the proportions according to mathematical rules, giving examples of extremely fat and thin figures, while the last book depicts the human figure in motion and treats of foreshortenings. Dürer's work is the first attempt to apply anthropometry to aesthetics. The woodcuts represent the first attempt to employ cross-hatching to depict shades and shadows in wood engraving. Facsimile edition with commentary volume by M. Steck, Zurich, *J.S. Dietikon,* [1969]. Dürer's manuscript prepared for the printer for the first part of the above work is preserved at Dresden along with many other anatomical studies by him. See *The human figure by Albrecht Dürer. The complete "Dresden Sketchbook"* edited with introduction, translation and commentary by W. L. Strauss. New York, 1972.

150   PORTA, GIOVANNI BATTISTA DELLA. 1536-1615
       De humana physiognomonia libri IIII. Vici Æquensis, *apud I. Cacchium,* 1586.
       Della Porta preceded Lavater in attempting to estimate human character by the features. This is one of the first works on the ancient "science" of physiognomy to be extensively illustrated.

151   ELSHOLTZ, JOHANN SIGMUND. 1623-1688
       Anthropometria. Patavii, *typ. M. Cadorini,* 1654.
       Elsholtz was the first physician to study anthropometry and human proportion.

152   CARDANO, GIROLAMO [CARDANUS]. 1501-1576
Metoposcopia libris tredecim et octingentis faciei humanae eiconibus complexa. Paris, *T. Jolly,* 1658.
Contains 800 illustrations of the human face. Cardan, Professor of Medicine at Padua as well as a celebrated mathematician and scientist, claimed to be able to draw horoscopes from the appearance of the face. A French translation was also published in 1658.

153   TYSON, EDWARD. 1650-1708
Orang-outang, sive homo sylvestris: or, the anatomy of a pygmie compared with that of a monkey, an ape, and a man. London, *T. Bennet & D. Brown,* 1699.
The first really important work on comparative morphology. Tyson originated the "missing link" idea in this study of the anatomy of a chimpanzee which he called a "pygmie". Facsimile reprint, 1966. Biography of Tyson by Ashley Montagu, Philadelphia, 1943.

154   LAVATER, JOHANN CASPAR. 1741-1801
Von der Physiognomik. Leipzig, *Weidmanns Erben,* 1772.
Lavater was the last of the descriptive physiognomists. He expanded the above work into *Physiognomische Fragmente zur Beförderung der Menschenkenntnis und Menschenliebe,* 1775-78. This was translated into English by H. Hunter as *Essays on physiognomy,* 3 vols. in 5, London, 1789-98 [i.e.1788-99] and other editions. His work was very influential on portraiture.

155   RUBENS, PIERRE PAUL. 1577-1640
Théorie de la figure humaine. Paris, *C. A. Jombert,* 1773.
This work on the human figure, published more than 100 years after the death of Rubens, is one of a handful of anatomical treatises illustrated by an artist of the first magnitude.

156   BLUMENBACH, JOHANN FRIEDRICH. 1752-1840
De generis humani varietate nativa. Gottingae, *A. Vandenhoeck,* 1775.
Blumenbach was the founder of anthropology. In this, his doctoral dissertation, he classified mankind into four races, based on selected combinations of head shape, skin colour and hair form. In the second edition (1781) he found it necessary to expand this division into five races, but his famous terms "Caucasian, Mongolian, Ethiopian, American, and Malayan" were not used until the third edition of 1795. English translation in Blumenbach, *The anthropological treatises...,* translated by T. Bendyshe, London, 1865.

156.1   SMITH, SAMUEL STANHOPE. 1750-1819
An essay on the causes of the variety of complexion and figure in the human species. Philadelphia, *Robert Aitken,* 1787.
In the first significant anthropological work produced in America, Smith argued that racial differences were produced by environment, contradicting the prevalent theories of separate creations of discrete and different races. Reprint of 2nd., enlarged edition, 1810, Cambridge, Mass., *Harvard University Press,* 1965.

157   BLUMENBACH, JOHANN FRIEDRICH. 1752-1840
Beyträge zur Naturgeschichte. 2 pts. Göttingen, 1790-1811
English translation, London, 1865.

158   CAMPER, PIETER. 1722-1789
        Ueber den natürlichen Unterschied der Gesichtszüge in Menschen
        verschiedener Gegenden und verschiedenen Alters. Berlin, *Vossische
        Buchhandlung,* 1792.
            This work on physiognomy includes Camper's description of his
        craniometrical methods. Camper is chiefly remembered for the "facial
        angle" of his own invention. The book first appeared in Dutch in 1791.
        English translation in Camper, *The works...on the connexion
        between...anatomy and the arts,* London, 1794. *See* No. 6604.90.

159   PRICHARD, JAMES COWLES. 1786-1848
        Researches into the physical history of man. London, *J. & A. Arch,* 1813.
            Prichard, a Bristol physician, classified and systematized facts relating
        to the races of men better than any previous writer. The second edition of
        his book, 1826, contains a remarkable anticipation of modern views on
        evolution, views which were suppressed in later editions. Facsimile edited
        with an introductory essay [and bibliography] by G. W. Stocking, Jr.,
        Chicago, *University Press,* 1973. The one-volume first edition was unillus-
        trated. By the 3rd edition the work was expanded to 5 vols.(1836-47) and
        contained many colour plates. In that form it synthesized all then known
        information about the various races of mankind, forming a basis for
        modern ethnological research.

160   PURKYNĚ, JAN EVANGELISTA [PURKINJE]. 1787-1869
        Commentatio de examine physiologico organi visus et systematis cutanei.
        Vratislavae, *typis Universitatis* [1823].
            Purkyně was the first to classify fingerprints. Reprinted in his *Opera omnia*
        (No. 82), vol. 1, pp. 163-94, 1918. English translation in John, *Jan Evangelista
        Purkyně,* Philadelphia, 1959.

161   KNOX, ROBERT. 1791-1862
        The races of men. London, *H. Renshaw,* 1850.
            Knox, anatomist at Edinburgh, and notorious for his association with
        the resurrectionists, made important researches in the field of ethnology
        while serving as an army surgeon at the Cape of Good Hope.

164   QUATREFAGES DE BRÉAU, JEAN ARMAND DE. 1810-1892
        Unité de l'espèce humaine. Paris, *L. Hachette,* 1861.
            De Quatrefages was one of the most eminent French anthropologists.

165   HUXLEY, THOMAS HENRY. 1825-1895
        Evidence as to man's place in nature. London, *Williams & Norgate,* 1863.
            Huxley showed that in the visible characters man differs less from the
        higher apes than do the latter from lower members of the same order of
        primates. He also provided the first thorough and detailed comparative
        description of the Neanderthal remains. *See* No. 204.

167   ——. On the methods and results of ethnology. *Proc. Roy. Inst. Gr. Brit.,*
        1862-66, **4**, 461-63.
            Includes Huxley's classification of mankind by means of the hair.

168   PRUNER-BEY, FRANZ. 1808-1882
        De la chevelure comme caractéristique des races humaines. *Mém. Soc.
        Anthrop. Paris,* 1865, **2**, 1-35; 1872, **3**, 77-92.

Pruner-Bey did the first important work on the classification of races according to texture and shape in section of hair.

169   BROCA, Pierre Paul. 1824-1880.
Mémoires d'anthropologie. 3 vols. Paris, *C. Reinwald,* 1871-77.
Most often remembered for his contributions to neurology, Broca was among the greatest of the French anthropologists. He originated modern craniometry and in that connection devised many craniometric and cranioscopic instruments. *See also* No. 344 *et al.*

170   DARWIN, Charles Robert. 1809-1882
The descent of man, and selection in relation to sex. 2 vols. London, *J. Murray,* 1871.
This is really two works. The first demolished the theory that the universe was created for Man, while in the second Darwin presented a mass of evidence in support of his earlier hypothesis regarding sexual selection. Edited reprint, *Princeton Univ. Press,* 1981.

171   QUETELET, Lambert Adolphe Jacques. 1796-1874
Anthropométrie, ou mesure des différentes facultés de l'homme. Bruxelles, *C. Muquardt,* 1870.
In his classification of various populations, Quetelet adopted the plan of determining the standard or typical "mean man" as a basis, using stature, weight, or complexion, etc., as a measure in each particular race or population.

172   TYLOR, *Sir* Edward Burnett. 1832-1917
Primitive culture...2 vols., London, *John Murray,* 1871.
The standard work on primitive religion for many years. Tylor approached his subject from the point of view of psychology, exploring the nature of belief in spirits, omens, magic, etc. His work has important ties with the analytical psychology of Jung.

173   SPENCER, Herbert. 1820-1903
Descriptive sociology: a cyclopaedia of facts; representing the constitution of every type and grade of human society, *etc.* London, 1873-
Spencer founded and edited this great series, which still continues to be published.

174   LOMBROSO, Cesare. 1836-1909
L'uomo delinquente, studiato in rapporto alla antropologia, alla medicina legale ed alle discipline carcerarie. Milano, *U. Hoepli,* 1876.
Lombroso inaugurated the doctrine of a "criminal type". His systematic studies showed that in general the criminal population exhibits a higher percentage of physical, nervous and mental anomalies than the normal population; this he attributed partly to degeneration and partly to atavism.

175   TOPINARD, Paul. 1830-1912
L'anthropologie. Paris, *C. Reinwald,* 1876.
Topinard was curator of the museum of the Société d'Anthropologie de Paris. "Topinard's angle" and "line", both described in this book, are landmarks employed in anthropometry. English translations 1878 and 1894.

176   VIRCHOW, RUDOLF LUDWIG KARL. 1821-1902
Beiträge zur physischen Anthropologie der Deutschen. *Abh. k. preuss. Akad. Wiss. Berl.* 1876, Phys.-math. Klasse, Abt. 1, 1-390.
     Virchow made an important survey of the physical characters of the German people. Outside pathology of which he was the Master, Virchow's greatest scientific interest was anthropology.

177   FAULDS, HENRY. 1844-1930
On the skin-furrows of the hand. *Nature (Lond.),* 1880, **22,** 605.
     Faulds's fingerprint method of identification.

179   PLOSS, HERMANN HEINRICH. 1819-1885
Das Weib in der Natur- und Völkerkunde. 2 vols. Leipzig, *T. Grieben,* 1885.
     A vast amount of data concerning every aspect of woman is collected into these volumes. Anthropology, psychology, aesthetics, physiology are all treated at length in what has become a standard and authoritative work. Subsequent editions were edited by Max and Paul Bartels and by von Reitzenstein. An English translation by E. J. Dingwall was published in London in 1935 (3 volumes); the translator added much to the value of both text and plates.

180   RATZEL, FRIEDRICH. 1844-1904
Völkerkunde. 2 vols. Leipzig, Wien, *Bibliographisches Inst.,* 1885-88.
     One of the greatest books on ethnology. Ratzel emphasized the importance of the investigation of the history of primitive peoples in the study of ethnology.

181   BERTILLON, ALPHONSE. 1853-1914
Les signalements anthropométriques. Paris, *G. Masson,* 1886.
     Bertillon invented a method ("Bertillonage") of identifying persons by means of selected measurements, the five following measurements being used as the basis of his system: head length, head breadth, length of middle finger, length of left foot, and length of forearm from elbow to extremity of middle finger. His method was used particularly for the identification of criminals.

182   QUATREFAGES DE BRÉAU, JEAN LOUIS ARMAND DE. 1810-1892
Les pygmées. Paris, *J. B. Baillière,* 1887.
     De Quatrefages showed that pygmies are descended from ancient races and are not, as was believed by many, a retrograde or degenerate type of negro of comparatively recent growth. English translation, 1895.

183   WIEDERSHEIM, ROBERT ERNST EDUARD. 1848-1923
Der Bau des Menschen als Zeugniss für seine Vergangenheit. Freiburg, *J. C. B. Mohr,* 1887.
     English translation, London, 1893.

184   FRAZER, *Sir* JAMES GEORGE. 1854-1941
The golden bough. 2 vols. London, *Macmillan & Co.,* 1890.
     Although Frazer's theoretical evolutionary sequence of magical, religious, and scientific thought is no longer accepted, and though his broad general psychological theory has proved unsatisfactory, it enabled him to compare and synthesize (in the 3rd edition, 12 vols., 1911-15) a wider

range of information and religious and magical practices than has been achieved by any other single anthropologist. New abridgement, 1959.

185 BRÜCKE, Ernst Wilhelm von, *Ritter*. 1819-1892
Schönheit und Fehler der menschlichen Gestalt. Wien, *W. Braumüller,* 1891.

186 GALTON, *Sir* Francis. 1822-1911
Finger prints. London, *Macmillan,* 1892.
The use of fingerprints as identification marks was known to the Chinese, but Galton was among the first to explain their possibilities in the identification of criminals. "Galton's delta" is a triangular area of papillary ridges on the distal pads of the digits.

187 ELLIS, Henry Havelock. 1859-1939
Man and woman. London, *W. Scott,* 1894.
A study of the constitutional differences between man and woman.

188 STRATZ, Carl Heinrich. 1858-1924
Die Schönheit des weiblichen Körpers. Stuttgart, *F. Enke,* 1899.

189 HENRY, *Sir* Edward Richard, *Bart*. 1850-1931
Classification and uses of finger prints. London, *Routledge*, 1900.
The Henry system of fingerprint classification which he developed as Inspector-General of Police in Bengal, is the basis for the system presently in use throughout the world.

190 MARTIN, Rudolf. 1864-1925
Lehrbuch der Anthropologie. Jena, *G. Fischer,* 1914.
Exhaustive bibliography. 2nd ed., 1928.

194.1 HOLLANDER, Eugen. 1867-1932.
Äskulap und Venus. Eine Kultur- und Sittengeschichte im Spiegel des Ärztes. Berlin, *Popylaen-Verlag,* 1928.
An exhaustive and well-illustrated survey of medical anthropology with emphasis on sexuality.

195 MOURANT, Arthur Ernest. 1904-
The use of blood groups in anthropology. *J. roy. anthrop. Inst.,* 1947, **77,** 139-44.

History of Anthropology

196 HADDON, Alfred Cort. 1855-1940
History of anthropology. With the help of A. Hingston Quiggin. London, *Watts & Co.,* 1910.
Revised edition, 1934.

197 PENNIMAN, Thomas Kenneth. *d.* 1977
A hundred years of anthropology. 3rd ed. London, *Duckworth,* 1965.
Includes a useful chronological table and a valuable bibliography. First published 1935.

197.1   TANNER, JAMES MOURILYAN
A history of the study of human growth. Cambridge, *Cambridge University Press*, [1981].

197.2   BARSANTI, GUILIO, *et al.*
Misur d'uomo. Strumenti, teorie e pratiche dell'antropometria e della psicologia sperimentale tra '800 e '900. Firenze, [*Istituto e Museo di Storia della Scienza*,] 1986.
Extensively annotated and illustrated catalogue of an exhibition of books and instruments documenting the history of measuring techniques in physical anthropology and experimental psychology in the 18th and 19th centuries. With S. Gori-Savellini, P. Guarnieri, and C. Pogliano.

197.3   STOCKING, GEORGE W., JR.
Victorian anthropology. New York, *Free Press*, 1987.

CRANIOLOGY

198   BLUMENBACH, JOHANN FRIEDRICH. 1752-1840
Decas collectionis suae craniorum diversarum gentium illustrata. 6 pts. plus supplement. Gottingae, *J. C. (H.) Dieterich*, 1790-1828.
Blumenbach was the founder of craniology, and his craniological collection served as the principal foundation for his investigations into the natural history of mankind. He used the *norma verticalis*, the shape of the skull as seen from above, as the means of distinguishing three types: Mongols, Negroes, and Caucasians. The above work includes a description of the uncinate ("Blumenbach's") process. *See* No. 156.

199   OKEN, LORENZ. 1779-1851
Ueber die Bedeutung der Schädelknochen. Jena, *J. C. G. Göpferdt*, 1807.
Oken's vertebral theory of the skull.

200   GOETHE, JOHANN WOLFGANG VON. 1749-1832
Ueber den Zwischenkiefer des Menschen und der Thiere. *Nova Acta Acad. Leopold.-Carol. (Halle)*, 1831, **15**, 1-48.
Goethe discovered the intermaxillary bone; he was one of the pioneers of evolution and the first to use the term "morphology".

201   MORTON, SAMUEL GEORGE. 1799-1851
Crania Americana. Philadelphia, *J. Dobson*, 1839.
In his day Morton was the most eminent craniologist in the United States. He had a collection of nearly 1,000 skulls.

202   RETZIUS, ANDERS ADOLF. 1796-1860
Om formen af nordboernes cranier. *Förhandl. skand. Naturforsch.*, 1842, **3**, 157-201.
Retzius introduced the method of classifying races according to the cranial or cephalic index. A German translation of his paper is available in the *Arch. Anat. Physiol. wiss. Med.*, 1845, 84-129.

203   DAVIS, JOSEPH BARNARD. 1801-1881, & THURNHAM, JOHN. 1810-1873.
Crania Britannica. 6 pts. London, *printed for the subscribers*, 1856-65.

203.1 RÜTIMEYER, Ludwig. 1825-1895, & HIS, Wilhelm, Snr. 1831-1904.
Crania Helvetica. Basel, Genf. *H. Georg,* 1864.

203.2 QUATREFAGES DE BRÉAU, Jean Louis Armand de. 1810-1892, & HAMY,
Ernest Theodore Jules. 1842-1908.
Crania ethnica. 2 pts. Paris, *J. B. Baillière,* 1872-82.

203.3 RETZIUS, Magnus Gustaf. 1842-1919
Finska kranier. Stockholm, *Central-Tryckeriet,* 1878.

203.4 TÖRÖK, Aurel von.
Grundzüge einer systematischen Kraniometrie. Stuttgart, *F. Enke,* 1890.
Török made an exhaustive study of craniometry and proposed 5,000
different measurements of a single skull.

203.5 VIRCHOW, Rudolf Ludwig Karl. 1821-1902
Crania ethnica Americana. Berlin, *A. Asker,* 1892.
Virchow was an expert craniologist.

203.6 BUXTON, L. H. Dudley, & MORANT, Geoffrey McKay.
The essential craniological technique. *J. roy. anthrop. Inst.,* 1933, **63,** 19-
47.

PALEOANTHROPOLOGY: HUMAN PREHISTORY

203.7 ESPER, Johann Friedrich. 1732-1781
Ausfürliche Nachricht von neuentdeckten Zoolithen, unbekannter
vierfüsiger Thiere...Nuremberg, *Georg Knorrs,* 1774.
Esper was the first to record the finding, in Gailenreuth Cave, of human
bones alongside the remains of unknown and probably extinct animals.
The implications of this dramatic observation published in a colour plate
book about unusual fossil animal bones seem to have been unnoticed by
the scientific establishment. Also French translation, Nuremberg, *Knorrs,*
1774. *See* No. 2312.1.

203.8 SCHMERLING, Phillipe-Charles. 1791-1836
Recherches sur les ossemens fossiles découvertes dans les cavernes de la
province de Liège. 2 vols. and atlas. Liège, *Collardin,* 1833-34.
A physician from Delft, Schmerling found extensive human remains
and artifacts associated with the remains of extinct animals in the caverns
around Liège. He concluded that these findings were evidence for human
antiquity. Although Schmerling's findings were widely acknowledged, the
scientific establishment was not yet ready to accept the idea of the antiquity
of man.

203.9 BOUCHER DE PERTHES, Jacques. 1788-1868
Antiquités celtiques et antédiluviennes. 3 vols. Paris, *Treuttel & Würtz,* 1847-
64.
Customs inspector at Abbéville and a prolific writer on diverse subjects,
Boucher de Perthes found extensive deposits of flint implements in
association with the bones of mammoths and other fossil animals. His
work presented the first convincing proof that man had been a contem-

porary of the mammoth. A portion of the first volume of this work was first published in Paris, 1846 as *De l'industrie primitive ou des arts a leur origine.*

204 SCHAAFHAUSEN, HERMANN. 1816-1893
Zur Kenntniss der ältesten Rassenschädel. *Arch. Anat. Physiol. wiss. Med.,* 1858, 453-78.

First description of the Neanderthal skull, the first human fossil skull morphologically distinct from the skulls of modern *Homo sapiens,* discovered in 1856 in Neanderthal Cave in the Neander Valley, near Düsseldorf. English translation, with comments, by G. Busk entitled "On the crania of the most ancient races of man" in *Nat. Hist. Rev.,* 1861, **1**, 155-76. Huxley (No. 165) made much of this discovery; however, because the skull was not unearthed from demonstrably ancient strata, its age was disputed until a more rigorously unearthed find occurred in 1886.

204.1 LYELL, *Sir* CHARLES. 1797-1875
The geological evidences of the antiquity of man with remarks on theories of the origin of species by variation. London, *John Murray,* 1863.

Lyell's summary discussion of the evidence for human antiquity "introduced a wide readership to the new view and to the facts that supported it, thus laying the synthetic foundation for future work" (Grayson). This work also contained Lyell's first published statements about Darwin's theory of evolution by natural selection.

210 DUBOIS, EUGÈNE. 1858-1940
Pithecanthropus erectus. Eine menschenähnliche Uebergangsform aus Java. Batavia, *Landesdruckerei,* 1894.

Discovery of *Homo erectus,* the oldest type of *Homo.* The skull-cap of *Pithecanthropus erectus* (Java man), the earliest type of ape-like man known, was discovered by Dubois at Trinil, Java, in 1891. It is here described for the first time.

211 DAWSON, CHARLES. 1864-1916, and WOODWARD, ARTHUR SMITH. 1864-1944
On the discovery of a palaeolithic skull and mandible in a flint-bearing gravel overlying the Wealden (Hastings Beds) at Piltdown, Fletching (Sussex). With an appendix by GRAFTON ELLIOT SMITH. *Quart. J. Geol. Soc.,* 1913, **69**, 117-151.

The first scientific report on "Piltdown man" (Eoanthropus dawsoni,) one of the longest-lasting and most influential hoaxes ever perpetrated. Smith Woodward wrote the report but gave primary authorship to Dawson who had "discovered" the fossil. It was not completely debunked until 1953. See J.S. Weiner, K.P. Oakley, and W.E. Le Gros Clark, The solution of the Piltdown problem. *Bull. B.M. (Nat.Hist.) Geol.,* 1953, **2**, 139-146, and J.S. Weiner, *The Piltdown forgery,* 1955.

211.1 DART, RAYMOND ARTHUR. 1893-1988
Australopithecus africanus: The man-ape of South Africa. *Nature (Lond.),*1925, **115**, 195-99.

Discovery in 1924 of the first member of the genus *Australopithecus,* the first "fossil man" found in Africa.

212   SMITH, *Sir* GRAFTON ELLIOT. 1871-1937
The Rhodesian skull. *Brit. med. J.*, 1922, **1,** 197-8.
Description of the skull found at Broken Hill, Rhodesia, in 1921.

213   ——. Sinanthropus – Peking Man; its discovery and significance. *Sci. Monthly,* 1931, **33,** 193-212.
Elliot Smith visited Peking to view the skull of *Sinanthropus pekinensis,* discovered by W. C. Pei on December 2, 1929. A preliminary description by Pei is to be found in *Bull. geol. Soc. China,* 1929, **8,** 3.

214   WEIDENREICH, FRANZ. 1873-1948
The skull of Sinanthropus pekinensis. *Geological Survey of China,* New series D, No. 10, 1943.

214.1   BROOM, ROBERT. 1866-1951
Pretoria: The South African fossil ape-men. The Australopithecinae. Part I. The occurrence and general structure of the South African ape-men. *Transvaal Mus. Mem.,* 1946, **2,** 7-144.
With this comprehensive report Broom presented his case to the scientific establishment that Australopithecus probably represented the stock from which mankind had evolved. With G.W.H. Schepers.

214.2   LEAKEY, LOUIS SEYMOUR BAZETT. 1903-1972 *et al.*
Age of Bed I, Olduvai Gorge, Tanganyika, *Nature,* 1961, **191,** 478-79.
Introduction of the potassium-argon dating method to palaeoanthropology, proving that fossils, *Australopithecus (Zinjanthropus) boisei,* found in Olduvai Gorge were 1.75 million years old. With J.F. Evernden and G.H. Curtis.

214.3   JOHANSON, DONALD C. 1943- , and TAIEB, MAURICE.
London: Plio-pleistocene hominid discoveries in Hadar, Ethiopia. *Nature,* 1976, **260,** 293-97.
Report on the Afar fossils representing a minimum of 35 and a maximum of 65 individuals, all about 3,000,000 years old. The most famous of these is called "Lucy". Another large collection of bones is sometimes called "The Family".

History of Human Prehistory

214.9   READER, JOHN.
Missing links: The hunt for earliest man. Boston, *Little, Brown,* [1981].
An entertaining and superbly illustrated, but carefully documented account of the major fossil finds from Neanderthal to Australopithecus Afarensis.

214.91   GRAYSON, DONALD K.
The establishment of human antiquity. New York: *Academic Press,* 1983.
The most complete historical treatment of the pre-1900 literature.

EVOLUTION: GENETICS: MOLECULAR BIOLOGY

215 HALE, *Sir* Matthew. 1609-1676
The primitive organization of mankind considered and examined according to the light of nature. London, *William Shrowsbery*, 1677.

Hale, Chief Justice of the King's Bench, "seems to have been the first to use the expression 'Geometrical Proportion' for the growth of a population from a single family" (Hutchinson). In this he anticipated Malthus (No. 215.4). He believed that in animals, especially insects, various natural calamities reduce the numbers to low levels intermittently, so maintaining a balance of nature.

215.1 MAUPERTUIS, Pierre Louis Moreau de. 1698-1759.
Dissertation physique à l'occasion du nègre blanc. Leiden, *[publisher not identified]*, 1744.

Stimulated by the much talked about appearance of an albino negro in Paris, Maupertuis expressed theories of biparental heredity and epigenesis which substantially anticipated those of Darwin, Mendel, and De Vries nearly a century and a half later.

215.2 ———.Vénus physique, contenant deux dissertations, l'une, sur l'origine des hommes et des animaux, et l'autre, sur l'origine des noirs. [The Hague?], 1745.

English translation, *The earthly Venus,* was published in New York, 1966. Includes a reprint of No. 215.1.

215.3 HERDER, Johann Gottfried von. 1744-1803
Ideen zur Philosophie der Geschichte der Menschheit. 4 vols., Riga & Leipzig, *Hartknoch*, 1784-91.

Herder's history has long been regarded as a very strong statement of Darwinian evolution before Darwin: many single passages come close to the evolution theory. Among the passages most often regarded as anticipating Darwin are those on the temporal sequence of forms from simpler to more highly organized, and on the overabundance of nature with the ensuing struggle for existence between species and individuals.

215.4 MALTHUS, Thomas Robert. 1766-1834
An essay on the principle of population, as it affects the future improvement of society. London, *J. Johnson,* 1798.

Malthus laid down the principle that populations increase in geometrical ratio, but that subsistence increases only in arithmetical ratio. His work was an important influence on both Darwin and Wallace in their formulation of the concept of natural selection. *See* No. 1693.

215.5 LAMARCK, Jean Baptiste Pierre Antoine de Monet de. 1744-1829
Système des animaux sans vertèbres. Paris, *Chez l'auteur*, [1801].

The "Discours d'ouverture" contains Lamarck's first published statement of the theory of the inheritance of acquired characteristics. *See* No. 316.

216 ———.Philosophie zoologique. 2 vols. Paris, *J. B. Baillière,* 1809.
Lamarck was one of the greatest of the comparative anatomists. This work is considered the greatest exposition of his argument that evolution occurred by the inheritance of characteristics acquired by animals as a

result of the use or disuse of organs in response to external stimuli. English translation by H. Elliot, 1914.

216.1   ADAMS, JOSEPH. 1756-1818
A treatise on the supposed hereditary properties of diseases. London, *J. Callow,* 1814.
    Adams was a pioneer in medical genetics. He distinguished between familial and hereditary diseases, saw that an increase in hereditary disease frequency in isolated areas could be caused by inbreeding, and suggested the establishment of hereditary disease registers.

216.2   WELLS, WILLIAM CHARLES. 1757-1817
Two essays: upon single vision with two eyes; the other on dew...An account of a female of the white race of mankind, part of whose skin resembles that of a negro...London, *Archibald Constable,* 1818.
    First statement of the theory of natural selection. Wells's paper on a white woman with patchy brown discoloration of the skin contains an almost complete anticipation of Darwin's theory of natural selection, although it was completely ignored until it was resurrected by a correspondent of Darwin in the 1860s. The volume also contains Wells's autobiography. *See* no. 1604.

216.3   MATTHEW, PATRICK. 1790-1874
On naval timber and arboriculture. London, *Longman...,* 1831.
    The "first clear and complete" anticipation of the Darwinian theory of evolution by natural selection. The appendix to Matthew's work actually uses the expression, "natural process of selection". See W.J. Dempster, *Patrick Matthew and natural selection: A nineteenth century gentleman-farmer, naturalist and writer,* Edinburgh, *Paul Harris,* 1983.

217   STEENSTRUP, JOHANNES JAPETUS SMITH. 1813-1897
Om Fortplantning og Udvikling gjennem vexlende Generations-raekker. Kjøbenhavn, *C. A. Reitzel,* 1842.
    Steenstrup is responsible for the theory of the "alternation of generation". He showed that certain animals produce offspring which never resemble them but which, on the other hand, bring forth progeny which return in form and nature to their grandparents or more distant ancestors. An English translation of the book was published by the Ray Society of London in 1845.

218   CHAMBERS, ROBERT. 1802-1871
Vestiges of the natural history of creation *and* Explanations: a sequel to "Vestiges..." 2 vols. London, *J. Churchill,* 1844-45.
    This outspoken statement of a belief in evolution, published anonymously to protect Chambers's reputation as a publisher, anticipated Darwin's *Origin* by 16 years and generally prepared the public for Darwin's theories. For a scientific book in the Victorian era, it became a sensational best seller. Authorship was not revealed until the 12th edition (1884) 13 years after Chambers's death. Facsimile reprint, Leicester, *Univ. Press,* 1969. See M. Millhauser, *Just before Darwin: Robert Chambers and 'Vestiges',* Middletown, *Wesleyan University Press,* [1959].

219   DARWIN, CHARLES ROBERT 1809-1882, & WALLACE, ALFRED RUSSEL. 1823-1913
On the tendency of species to form varieties: and on the perpetuation of varieties and species by natural means of selection. *J. Proc. Linn. Soc.* (1858), 1859, **3,** Zool., 45-62.

The first printed exposition of the "Darwinian" theory of evolution by natural selection. Had not Wallace independently discovered the theory of natural selection, it is possible that the extremely cautious Darwin might never have published his evolutionary theories during his lifetime. However, Wallace conceived the theory during an attack of malarial fever in Ternate in the Mollucas (February, 1858) and sent a manuscript summary to Darwin, who feared that his discovery would be pre-empted. In the interest of justice Hooker and Lyell suggested joint publication of Wallace's paper, *On the tendency of varieties to depart indefinitely from the original type*, prefaced by a section of a manuscript of a work on species written by Darwin in 1844, when it was read by Hooker, plus an abstract of a letter by Darwin to Asa Gray, dated 1857, to show that Darwin's views on the subject had not changed between 1844 and 1857.

220   DARWIN, CHARLES ROBERT. 1809-1882
On the origin of species by means of natural selection. London, *J. Murray,* 1859.

Prepared under the advice of Lyell and Hooker, and brought to press soon after publication of the joint paper by Darwin and Wallace (No.219), this was Darwin's greatest work and one of the most important books ever published. The whole edition of 1250 copies was sold on the day of publication. Although the theory of evolution can be traced to the ancient Greek belief in the "great chain of being", Darwin's greatest achievement was to make this centuries-old "underground" concept acceptable to the scientific community by cogently arguing for the existence of a viable mechanism – natural selection – by which new species evolve over vast periods of time. Darwin's influence on biology was fundamental, and continues to be felt today. He remains one of the best-known scientists of all time. Facsimile reproduction, with introduction by E. Mayr, Cambridge, Mass., 1964. *See* R.B. Freeman, *The works of Charles Darwin: an annotated bibliographical handlist.* 2nd ed. Folkestone, Kent, *Dawson,* 1977.

220.1   BATES, HENRY WALTER. 1825-1892
Contributions to an insect fauna of the Amazon valley: Lepidoptera: Heliconidae. *Trans. Linn. Soc.,* 1862, **23**, 495-566.

Bates spent eleven years in the Amazon and there collected 8,000 species of insects new to science. In the above paper he clearly stated and solved the problem of "mimicry", known today as "Batesian mimicry". The superficial resemblance of a palatable species (mimic) to an unpalatable species (model) is a form of protective colouration that has evolved by natural selection. (*See also* No. 228.1).

220.2   HUXLEY, THOMAS HENRY. 1825-1895
On our knowledge of the causes of the phenomenon of organic nature. London, *Robert Hardwicke,* 1862.

This series of six lectures delivered to "working men" in November and December, 1862 includes Huxley's first book-form exposition of Darwin's theories, of which he was probably the greatest popular exponent. A prolific essayist as well as author of hundreds of scientific papers, Huxley was one of the most eloquent of all English writers on the natural sciences. *See also* No. 165.

221   MÜLLER, JOHANN FRIEDRICH THEODOR. 1821-1897
Für Darwin. Leipzig, *Engelmann,* 1864.

Müller, the first German to support Darwin, studied the development of the Crustacea in Brazil and published some of his results in the above little book, which contains much original information. He realized the bearing of individual development on the theory of evolution. English translation as *Facts and arguments for Darwin*, London, 1869. Repr., 1968.

222   MENDEL, GREGOR JOHANN. 1822-1884
Versuche über Pflanzen-Hybriden. *Verh. naturf. Vereins Brünn* (1865), 1866, **4**, 3-47.

Discovery of the Mendelian ratios, the most significant single achievement in the history of genetics. The story of how Mendel published his paper in this relatively obscure journal only to have his discovery ignored during his lifetime has been frequently retold. In 1900 Correns and de Vries (Nos. 239.01 and 239.1) rediscovered the Mendelian ratios almost simultaneously. William Bateson first translated the above work into English in *J. Roy. Hort. Soc.*, 1901, **26**, 1-32. The following year he published his first monograph on Mendel (No. 241).

223   HAECKEL, ERNST HEINRICH PHILIPP AUGUST. 1834-1919
Generelle Morphologie der Organismen. 2 vols. Berlin, *G. Reimer,* 1866.

Haeckel, one of the greatest morphologists of the 19th century, accepted the general principles of Darwinism, disagreeing on some points. He was the first to promote Darwin's theories in Germany. This work contains the first statement of his theory that "ontogeny recapitulates phylogeny". *See* No. 224.

224   ———. Natürliche Schöpfungsgeschichte. Berlin, *G. Reimer,* 1868.

In the above work Haeckel constructed the first of the now commonplace ancestral trees, depicting the evolution of life from the simplest organisms through 21 stages of development to modern man – the 22nd and final stage. Within this general scheme he created the concept of the *Phylum* (i.e. stem) to accommodate all organisms descended from a common form, and created the word *Phylogeny* to describe their evolutionary development from common form to distinct species. He suggested that within each species the term *Ontogeny* should describe the development of the individual from conception to maturity. From this he proposed his famous biogenetic law, "Ontogeny recapitulated Phylogeny". His Phyletic Museum at Jena is probably the finest collection of serial illustrations of evolution and development in the world. English translation, 2 vols., London, 1876. Darwin wrote in *The Descent of man* (No. 227) "if [the English translation of] this work had appeared before my essay [*Descent...*] had been written, I should probably never have completed it. Almost all the conclusions at which I have arrived I find confirmed by this naturalist, whose knowledge on many points is much fuller than mine". *See* No. 223.

224.1   DARWIN, CHARLES ROBERT. 1809-1882
The variation of animals and plants under domestication. 2 vols. London, *J. Murray,* 1868.

Darwin carried out numerous investigations with pigeons and various plants. He recognized continuous and discontinuous variation; he concluded that crossing tends to keep populations uniform.

226   GALTON, *Sir* FRANCIS. 1822-1911
Hereditary genius. London, *Macmillan & Co.,* 1869.

Galton investigated the families of great men and suggested that genius was hereditary, and thus founded the science of Eugenics, although he did not coin the word until 1883 (*see* No. 230). Karl Pearson's, *The life, letters and labours of Francis Galton*, 3 vols. in 4, Cambridge, 1914-30, is one of the most remarkable biographies ever published on a scientist.

227   DARWIN, CHARLES ROBERT. 1809-1882
The descent of man, and selection in relation to sex. 2 vols. London, *J. Murray,* 1871.
This is really two works. The first demolished the theory that the universe was created for Man, while in the second Darwin presented a mass of evidence in support of his earlier hypothesis regarding sexual selection. Edited reprint, *Princeton Univ. Press,* 1981.

228   WALLACE, ALFRED RUSSEL. 1823–1913
Contributions to the theory of natural selection. London, *Macmillan,* 1870.
Reprints, with important revisions and additions, nine important papers concerning natural selection, which had previously appeared in journals, and publishes for the first time a major paper on *The limits of natural selection as applied to man.* Unlike Darwin, Wallace believed that at some point during man's history man had partially escaped natural selection, and that a "higher intelligence" had a part in the development of the human race.

228.1   MÜLLER, JOHANN FRIEDRICH THEODOR. 1821-1897
Ueber die Vortheile der Mimicry bei Schmetterlingen. *Zool. Anz.* 1878, **1,** 54-5.
Bates's theory of mimicry (No. 220.1) did not account for the superficial resemblances between two or more unpalatable species. Müller explained such mimicry, known today as "Müllerian mimicry". A predator must learn which potential prey are palatable. The colouration of an unpalatable species serves as warning colouration to predators. When warning colouration is shared by two or more unpalatable species, the warning colours are recognized more quickly by the predator and the number of individuals destroyed in each species is reduced while the predator learns.

229   ROUX, WILHELM. 1850-1924
Über die Bedeutung der Kerntheilungsfiguren. Leipzig, *F. Engelmann,* 1883.
Roux investigated why the nucleus undergoes the precise division of mitosis while the rest of the cell undergoes a rather crude division when one cell splits into two. He argued that mitosis ensures a precise halving of the nucleus, suggesting that the nucleus contains the material basis of heredity.

229.1   STRASBURGER, EDUARD ADOLF. 1844-1912
Neue Untersuchungen über den Befruchtungsvorgang bei den Phanerogamen als Gründlage für eine Theorie der Zeugung. Jena, *Gustav Fischer,* 1884.
Like Roux (No. 229), Strasburger hypothesized that the cell nucleus contained the material basis of heredity, and developed the idea with evidence from microscopical observations.

230 GALTON, *Sir* Francis. 1822-1911
Inquiries into human faculty and its development. London, *Macmillan & Co.*, 1883.
Galton, cousin of Charles Darwin, founded the science of Eugenics. In his important *Inquiries* he showed mathematically "the results of his experiments on the relations between the powers of visual imagery and of abstract thought, of the associations between the elements of different sense departments, of the correlation of mental traits, the associations of words, and the times taken in making the associations" (T. K. Penniman). The word "eugenics" first appears in the above book.

231 KÖLLIKER, Rudolph Albert von. 1817-1905
Die Bedeutung der Zellenkerne für die Vorgänge der Vererbung. *Z. Wiss. Zool.*, 1885, **42,** 1-46.
Along with Roux, Kölliker stated that hereditary characters were transmitted by the cell nucleus.

231.1 BOVERI, Theodor. 1862-1915
Zellen-Studien. *Jena Z. Naturw.*, 1888, **22,** 685-882.
Boveri gave decisive proof of the maintenance of chromosomal individuality.

233 GALTON, *Sir* Francis. 1822-1911
Natural inheritance. London, *Macmillan & Co.*, 1889.
By the employment of statistical methods Galton propounded a "law of filial regression". This book represents the first statistical study of biological variation and inheritance.

234 WEISMANN, August Friedrich Leopold. 1834-1914
Amphimixis, oder die Vermischung der Individuen. Jena, *G. Fischer,* 1891.
By "amphimixis" Weismann meant the union of the two parent germs, which he considered the principal source of heritable variation in evolution by natural selection. English translation in Weismann's *Essays upon Heredity*, Vol. 2, Oxford, 1892.

235 ——. Aufsätze über Vererbung und verwandte biologische Fragen. Jena, *G. Fischer,* 1892.
Weismann produced experimental evidence that acquired characters are not transmitted.

236 ——. Das Keimplasma. Jena, *G. Fischer,* 1892.
Weismann elaborated the theory of the continuity of the germ plasm. English edition, 1893.

237 BATESON, William. 1861-1926
Materials for the study of variation treated with especial regard to discontinuity in the origin of species. London, *Macmillan & Co.*, 1894.
Bateson was convinced that discontinuity was the more important type of variation among animals and plants "in some unknown way a part of their nature and not directly dependent upon natural selection at all". He showed that Darwin's concept of variation needed modification.

238   WILSON, EDMUND BEECHER. 1856-1939
       The cell in development and inheritance. New York, *Macmillan & Co.,*
       1896.
       Wilson emphasized the function of cytology in the study of embryol-
       ogy, heredity, evolution and general physiology. The above work has
       been called the single most influential treatise on cytology of the 20th
       century. The third edition was extensively revised and enlarged as *The cell
       in development and heredity*, 1925. 1st ed. reprinted, New York, 1966.

239   GALTON, *Sir* FRANCIS. 1822-1911
       The average contribution of each several ancestor to the total heritage of
       the offspring. *Proc. roy. Soc. Lond.,* 1897, **61,** 401-13.
       Galton's "law of ancestral heredity".

239.01 VRIES, HUGO MARIE DE. 1848-1935
       Das Spaltungsgesetz der Bastarde. *Ber. dtsch. bot. Ges.,* 1900, **18,** 83-90.
       De Vries and Correns independently rediscovered and confirmed
       Mendel's laws. This is De Vries's most important paper on the subject. De
       Vries's first published paper on the topic is "Sur la loi de disjonction des
       hybrides", *C.R. Acad. Sci. (Paris),* 1900, **130,** 845-47. Reading of this paper
       led Correns to write his own paper (No. 239.1), although Correns claimed
       he had previously and independently arrrived at the same conclusions.
       English translation in No. 258.4.

239.1 CORRENS, CARL FRANZ JOSEPH ERICH. 1864-1933
       G. Mendel's Regel über das Verhalten der Nachkommenschaft der
       Rassenbastarde. *Ber. dtsch. botanisch. Ges.,* 1900, **18,** 158-67.
       Correns had come to the same conclusions as Mendel before seeing the
       latter's 1865 paper. Of the three "rediscoverers" of Mendel's laws, Correns
       showed the greatest understanding of them. English translation in No.
       258.4.

239.2 TSCHERMAK VON SEYSENEGG, ERICH. 1871-1962
       Über küntsliche Kreuzung von *Pisum sativum. Z. landwirtsch. Versuchsw.
       in Österreich,* 1900, **3,** 465-555.
       With Correns and de Vries, Tschermak brought Mendel's work into
       prominence and confirmed it, although Tschermak may not have fully
       understood the Mendelian laws before he had read Mendel's work. See
       also Tschermak's first paper on the subject: "Über künstliche Kreuzung bei
       Pisum Sativum", *Ber. dtsch. bot. Ges.,* 1900, **18,** 232-39.

240   VRIES, HUGO MARIE DE. 1848-1935
       Die Mutationstheorie. 2 vols. Leipzig, *Veit & Co.,* 1901-3.
       The theory of mutation was first advanced by de Vries. Abridged
       English translation, Chicago, 1909.

241   BATESON, WILLIAM. 1861-1926
       Mendel's principles of heredity: a defence. Cambridge, *Cambridge Univ.
       Press,* 1902.
       The first book on Mendelism in English, and the first English textbook
       of genetics. It contains a reprint of the first English translation of Mendel's
       "Versuch über Pflanzen-Hybriden" from the *J. Roy. Horticult. Soc.,* which
       Bateson had published the previous year together with the first edition in
       English of Mendel's second paper on Hieracium (1869). Bateson named

the science, "genetics" in 1905-6. He published a much-expanded second edition as *Mendel's principles of Heredity*, Cambridge, *Cambridge University Press*, 1909.

241.1   BOVERI, THEODOR. 1862-1915
Über mehrpolige Mitosen als Mittel zur Analyse des Zellkerns. *Verh. phys.-med. Ges. Wurzburg*, 1903, **35,** 67-90.
Boveri's experiments, involving multipolar mitoses in sea urchin eggs fertilized by two sperm, demonstrated that different chromosomes perform different functions in development. English translation in No. 534.3.

242   JOHANNSEN, WILHELM LUDVIG. 1857-1927
Ueber Erblichkeit in Populationen und in reinen Linien. Jena, *G. Fischer,* 1903.
More support for the Mendelian law of inheritance was provided by Johannsen, a Danish botanist, who showed that in certain self-fertilizing plants a pure line of descendants can be maintained indefinitely, in which case natural selection is not effective, selection depending upon genetic variability. He introduced the term "gene" in 1909.

242.1   SUTTON, WALTER STANBOROUGH. 1877-1916
The chromosomes in heredity. *Biol. Bull.,* 1903, **4,** 231-51.
Sutton advanced the theory that Mendel's factors were hereditary particles borne by the chromosomes and that Mendel's laws for his factors were the direct result of the behaviour of chromosomes in meiosis. Boveri independently proposed a similar view (No. 242.2), which became known as the "Sutton–Boveri hypothesis".

242.2   BOVERI, THEODOR. 1862-1915
Ergebnisse über die Konstitution der chromatischen Substanz des Zellkerns. Jena, *G. Fischer,* 1904.
   See No. 242.1.

242.3   BATESON, WILLIAM. 1861-1926, *et al.*
Further experiments on inheritance in sweet peas and stocks; preliminary account. *Proc. roy. Soc. B,* 1906, **77,** 236-8.
W. Bateson, E. R. Saunders and R. C. Punnett noted the phenomena of linkage of genes.

243   HARDY, GODFREY HAROLD. 1877-1947
Mendelian proportions in a mixed population. *Science*, 1908, **28**, 49-50.
   Hardy–Weinberg equilibrium.

244   WEINBERG, WILHELM. 1836-1937
Über den Nachweis der Vererbung beim Menschen. *Jahr. Ver. f. Vaterländ. Nat. Würt.*, 1908, **64**, 369-82.
Weinberg, a general practitioner and obstetrician in Stuttgart, was also a founder of population genetics. He discovered the Hardy–Weinberg equilibrium.

244.1   GARROD, *Sir* ARCHIBALD EDWARD. 1857-1936
Inborn errors of metabolism. London, *H. Frowde,* 1909.
Garrod established chemical individuality as the paradigm of Mendelian variation. *See* Nos. 253.2 and 3921.

245   NILSSON-EHLE, NILS HERMAN. 1873-1949
   Kreuzungsuntersuchungen an Hafer und Weizen. *Lunds Univ. Arsskr.,*
   1909, N.F. Afd.2, **5,** Nr. 2, 1-122; 1911, N.F. Afd.2, **7,** Nr. 6, 1-84.
    The "multiple factor" theory advanced by Nilsson-Ehle brought under
   the Mendelian law cases which, by their extreme variability of inheritance,
   might be considered exceptions to it.

245.1   EAST, EDWARD MURRAY. 1879-1938
   A Mendelian interpretation of variation that is apparently continuous.
   American naturalist, 1910, **44,** 65-82.
    East published simultaneously and independently a theory essentially
   identical to Nilsson-Ehle (No. 245).

245.2   MORGAN, THOMAS HUNT. 1866-1945
   Sex-linked inheritance in *Drosophila. Science,* 1910, **32,** 120-22.
    Demonstration of sex-linked inheritance.

245.3   ——. Random segregation versus coupling in Mendelian inheritance.
   Science, 1911, **34,** 384.
    Morgan proposed that the Mendelian factors (genes) are arranged in a
   linear series on chromosomes and that the degree of linkage between two
   genes on the same chromosome depends upon the distance between
   them. This fundamental idea enabled his student Sturtevant to map genes
   on chromosomes. (*See* No. 245.2).

245.4   STURTEVANT, ALFRED HENRY. 1891-1970
   The linear arrangement of six sex-linked factors in *Drosophila,* as shown
   by their mode of association. *J. exp. Zool.,* 1913, **14,** 43-59.
    Proof that the genes are arranged in a linear sequence along the
   chromosome. The work paved the way for the construction of chromosome maps for other species besides *Drosophila.*

245.5   BRIDGES, COLIN BLACKMAN. 1889-1938
   Non-disjunction of the sex chromosome of *Drosophila. J. Exp. Zool.,* 1913,
   15, 587-606.
    Bridges discovered non-disjunction, failure of chromosome pairs to
   segregate regularly during meiosis.

246   MORGAN, THOMAS HUNT. 1866-1945, *et al.*
   The mechanism.of Mendelian heredity. New York, *H. Holt,* 1915.
    With A.H. Sturtevant, H.J. Muller, and C.B. Bridges. Summarizes the
   major early findings of Morgan's *Drosophila* research group, which based
   its research on the rapidly reproducing small vinegar fly, *Drosophila*
   melanogaster, often called the fruit fly. This epoch-making book presented evidence showing that genes were arranged linearly on chromosomes and that the Mendelian laws could be shown to be based on
   observable events occurring in cells. The group also showed that heredity
   could be studied rigorously and quantitatively. Morgan was awarded the
   Nobel Prize for physiology in 1933.

248   FISHER, Sir RONALD AYLMER. 1890-1962
   The correlation between relatives on the supposition of Mendelian inheritance. *Trans. Roy. Soc. Edin.,* 1918, **52,** 399-433.

Fisher reconciled Mendelian genetics with the biometric observations of Karl Pearson and Francis Galton. Reprinted, with extended commentary in *Eugen. Lab. Mem., Univ. Coll. Lond.,* 1966, **41**.

251   MORGAN, THOMAS HUNT. 1866-1945
The theory of the gene. New Haven, *Yale Univ. Press,* 1926.

251.1   MULLER, HERMANN JOSEPH. 1890-1967
Artificial transmutation of the gene. *Science,* 1927, **66**, 84-7.

Muller was awarded the Nobel Prize in 1946 for his work on the genetic effects of radiation. His paper records the first successful attempt at inducing genetic mutation.

251.2   GRIFFITH, FREDERICK. ?1879-1941
The significance of pneumococcal types. *J. Hyg. (Camb.),* 1928, **27**, 113-59.

Griffith's experiments on transforming type II pneumococci into type III were repeated by Avery who was able sixteen years later (No. 255.3) to demonstrate that DNA was the transforming material.

253   FISHER, *Sir* RONALD AYLMER. 1890-1962
The genetical theory of natural selection. Oxford, *Clarendon Press,* 1930.

The first coherent general algebraic analysis of Mendelian population behaviour. The work contains Fisher's rigorous development of his "fundamental theorem of natural selection"–"the rate of increase in fitness of any organism at any time is equal to its genetic variance in fitness at that time". Along with Wright (No. 253.1) and Haldane (No. 254), Fisher established mathematical population genetics.

253.1   WRIGHT, SEWALL. 1889-1988
Evolution in Mendelian populations. *Genetics,* 1931, **16**, 97-159.

First detailed presentation of Wright's quantitative theory of the effects of mutation, migration, selection, and population size on changes in gene frequencies in populations.

253.2   GARROD, *Sir* ARCHIBALD EDWARD. 1857-1936
The inborn factors in disease. Oxford, *Clarendon Press,* 1931.

Garrod argued that chemical individuality could result in individuals having a predisposition to certain diseases. This view has become particularly significant in light of the establishment of recombinant DNA methods to identify inherited genetic defects. Reprint with epilogue by C.R. Scriver and B. Childs, and bibliography of Garrod's writings, Oxford, *Oxford University Press,* 1989.

254   HALDANE, JOHN BURDON SANDERSON. 1892-1964
The causes of evolution. London, *Longmans, Green & Co.,* 1932.

Haldane's summary of his mathematical theory of natural selection. The detailed mathematical theory appeared as *Mathematical theory of natural and artificial selection,* first published (Pt. I) in *Trans. Camb. philos. Soc.,* 1924, **23**, 19-41, and (Pts. II-IX) in *Proc. Camb. philos. Soc.,* vol. 1, 23, 26, 27, 28. Pt. X appeared in *Genetics,* 1934, **19**, 412-29.

254.1   TIMOFEEFF-RESSOVSKY, NIKOLAI VLADIMIROVICH. 1900- , *et al.*
•   Ueber die Natur der Genmutation und der Genstruktur. *Nachr. Ges. Wiss. Göttingen, math.-fis. Kl.,* Fachgr. 6, 1935, **1,** 189-245.

     X-ray mutagenesis of *Drosophila.* A paper of fundamental importance in molecular biology; the "target theory". This has been called the "green paper", referring to the colour of the paper cover of the *Nachrichten,* and also the *Dreimännerwerk,* for the three writers, Timoféeff-Ressovsky, K. G. Zimmer, and Max Delbrück.

254.2   DOBZHANSKY, THEODOSIUS. 1900-1975
     Genetics and the origin of species. New York, *Columbia Univ. Press,* 1937.

254.3   BEADLE, GEORGE WELLS. 1903- , & TATUM, EDWARD LAWRIE. 1909-1975
     Genetic control of biochemical reactions in *Neurospora. Proc. nat. Acad. Sci. (Wash.),* 1941, **27,** 499-506.

     The work of Beadle and Tatum on mutations induced with *Neurospora crassa* opened up a new field, biochemical genetics. They shared the Nobel Prize in 1958 with J. Lederberg (No. 255.4) for their researches on the mechanism by which the chromosomes in the cell nucleus transmit inherited characters.

255   HUXLEY, *Sir* JULIAN SORELL. 1887-1975
     Evolution: the modern synthesis. London, *Allen & Unwin,* 1942.

255.1   MAYR, Ernst. 1904-
     Systematics and the origin of species. New York, *Columbia Univ. Press,* 1942.

255.2   SIMPSON, GEORGE GAYLORD. 1902-1984
     Tempo and mode in evolution. New York, *Columbia Univ. Press,* 1944.

255.3   AVERY, OSWALD THEODORE. 1877-1955, *et al.*
     Studies on the chemical nature of the substance inducing transformation of pneumococcal types. Induction of transformation by a deoxyribonucleic acid fraction isolated from pneumococcus type III. *J. exp. Med.,* 1944, **79,** 137-58.

     Demonstration that deoxyribonucleic acid (DNA) is the basic material responsible for genetic transformation. With C. M. MacLeod and M. McCarty.

255.4   LEDERBERG, JOSHUA. 1925- , & TATUM, EDWARD LAWRIE. 1909-1975
     Gene recombination in *Escherichia coli. Nature (Lond.),* 1946, **158,** 558.

     Discovery of sexual processes in the reproduction of bacteria. Lederberg shared the Nobel Prize with Tatum and Beadle (No. 254.3) in 1958.

255.5   BARR, MURRAY LLEWELLYN. 1908- , & BERTRAM, EWART GEORGE. 1923-
     A morphological distinction between neurones of the male and female, and the behaviour of the nucleolar satellite during accelerated nucleoprotein synthesis. *Nature (Lond.),* 1949, **163,** 676-7.

     Barr and Bertram showed that it is possible to determine the genetic sex of an individual according as to whether there is a chromatin mass present on the inner surface of the nuclear membrane of cells with resting or intermittent nuclei (sex chromatin). See also *Anat. Rec.,* 1952, **112,** 709-12, and *Surg. Gynec. Obstet.,* 1953, **96,** 641-8.

255.6   CHARGAFF, ERWIN. 1905-
Chemical specificity of nucleic acids and the mechanism of their enzymatic degradation. *Experientia (Basel)*, 1950, **6**, 201-9.
Between 1946 and 1950 Chargaff carried out chemical studies that revolutionized attitudes towards DNA.

255.7   GEDDA, LUIGI.
Studio dei gemelli. Roma, *Edizioni Orizzonto Medico*, 1951.
The first truly comprehensive work on the scientific study of twins. (1381pp., 547 illustrations, 161 tables). English translation of the first half of the work, with some revisions: *Twins in history and science*, Springfield, C.C. Thomas, [1961].

256   HERSHEY, ALFRED DAY. 1908-   , & CHASE, MARTHA COWLES. 1927-
Independent functions of viral protein and nucleic acid in growth of bacteriophage. *J. gen. Physiol.*, 1952, **36**, 39-56.
DNA shown to be the carrier of genetic information in virus reproduction. Hershey shared the Nobel Prize in 1969 with S. E. Luria and M. Delbrück.

256.1   ZINDER, NORTON DAVID. 1928-   , & LEDERBERG, JOSHUA. 1925-
Genetic exchange in Salmonella. *J. Bact.*, 1952, **64**, 679-99.
Description of a new mechanism ("transduction") for the transfer of genetic characters from one bacterial strain to another.

256.2   MOORE, KEITH LEON. 1925- , *et al*
The detection of chromosomal sex in hermaphrodites from a skin biopsy. *Surg. Gynec. Obstet.*, 1953, **96**, 641-48.
Sex chromatin demonstrated in humans. With M. A. Graham and M. L. Barr.

256.3   WATSON, JAMES DEWEY. 1928-   , & CRICK, FRANCIS HARRY COMPTON. 1916-
Molecular structure of nucleic acids. A structure for deoxyribose nucleic acid. *Nature (Lond.)*, 1953, **171**, 737-38.
Watson and Crick shared the Nobel Prize with M. H. F. Wilkins (No. 256.4) for the discovery of the molecular structure of DNA. Later they proposed how DNA might explain the chemical mechanism by which cells passed on their character accurately. (Genetical implications of the structure of deoxyribonucleic acid, *Nature, (Lond.)*, 1953, **171**, 964-7.)

256.4   WILKINS, MAURICE HUGH FREDERICK. 1916-   , *et al.*
Helical structure of crystalline deoxypentose nucleic acid. *Nature (Lond.)*, 1953, **172**, 759-62.
With W. E. Seeds, A. R. Stokes, and H. R. Wilson. Wilkins discovered the double helix structure of DNA. He shared the Nobel Prize with Crick and Watson in 1962.

256.5   TJIO, JOE HIN, & LEVAN, ALBERT. 1905-
The chromosome number in man. *Hereditas (Lund)*, 1956, **42**, 1-6.
Proof that the normal chromosome number in man is 46.

256.6   MESELSON, MATTHEW STANLEY. 1930- & STAHL, FRANKLIN WILLIAM. 1929-
The replication of DNA in Escherichia coli. *Proc. Nat. Acad. Sci.*,1958, **44**, 671-82.
First proof of semi-conservative replication of DNA.

256.7   LYON, MARY FRANCES.
Gene action in the *X*-chromosome of the mouse (*Mus musculus* L). *Nature (Lond.)*, 1961, **190**, 372-73.
Theory of differential inactivation of the *X*-chromosome. See also *Amer. J. hum. Genet.*, 1962, **14,** 135-48.

256.8   CRICK, FRANCIS HARRY COMPTON. 1916- , *et al.*
General nature of the genetic code for proteins. *Nature (Lond.)*, 1961, **192,** 1227-32.
The codons in DNA specifying amino acids in proteins. With L. Barnett, S. Brenner, and R. J. Watts-Tobin.

256.9   JACOB, FRANÇOIS. 1920- , & MONOD, JACQUES. 1910-1976.
Genetic regulatory mechanisms in the synthesis of proteins. *J. molec. Biol.,* 1961, **3,** 318-56.
Jacob, Monod, and André Lwoff shared the Nobel Prize in 1965 for their discovery of a gene whose function is to regulate the activity of other genes.

256.10   BRENNER, SYDNEY. 1927- , *et al.*
An unstable intermediate carrying information from genes to ribosomes for protein synthesis. *Nature (Lond.)* 1961, **190,** 576-80.
Demonstration of the existence of "messenger" RNA. With F. Jacob and M. Meselson. The following paper (pp. 581-85) by F. Gros *et al.* is also relevant.

256.11   MATTHAEI, J. HEINRICH, & NIRENBERG, MARSHALL WARREN. 1927-
Characteristics and stabilization of DNAase-sensitive protein synthesis in *E. coli* extracts. *Proc. nat. Acad. Sci. (Wash.)* 1961, **47,** 1580-88.
Nirenberg shared the Nobel Prize in 1968 with H. G. Khorana and R. W. Holley for his work on DNA. With Matthaei he demonstrated that messenger RNA is required for protein synthesis and that synthetic messenger RNA preparations can be used to decipher various aspects of the genetic code.

256.12   GURDON, JOHN BERTRAND. 1933-
Adult frogs derived from the nuclei of single somatic cells. *Develop. Biol.,* 1962, **4,** 256-73.
Demonstration that somatic and germinal nuclei are genetically equivalent. Gurdon transplanted cell nuclei from tadpoles into enucleated eggs and developed normal tadpoles.

257   NISHIMURA, S. *et al.*
Synthetic deoxyribopolynucleotides as templates for ribonucleic acid polymerase: the formation and characterization of a ribopolynucleotide with a repeating trinucleotide sequence. *Proc. nat. Acad. Sci. (Wash.),* 1964, **52,** 1494-1501.

257.1   HAMILTON, WILLIAM DONALD. 1936-
The genetical evolution of social behaviour I, II. *J. Theoret. Biol.,* 1964, **7,** 1-52.
Hamilton's mathematical theory of kin selection as an explanation for the evolution of social behaviour (including supposedly altruistic behaviour), is the foundation of sociobiology.

257.2   HOLLEY, ROBERT WILLIAM. 1922- , *et al.*
Structure of a ribonucleic acid. *Science*, 1965, **147,** 1462-65.
The complete sequence of an alanine transfer RNA determined – the first nucleic acid structure to be determined. With seven co-authors. Holley was a Nobel laureate in 1968 for his work on transfer RNA.

257.3   JACKSON, DAVID ARCHER. 1942- , SYMONS, ROBERT, & BERG, PAUL. 1926-
Biochemical method for inserting new genetic information into DNA of simina virus 40: circular SV40 DNA molecules containg Lambda phage genes and the galactose operon of *Escherichia coli. Proc. nat. Acad. Sci.* (Wash.), 1972, **69,** 2904-2909.
First recombinant DNA molecules generated.

257.4   LOBBAN, PETER & KAISER, ARMIN DALE. 1927-
Enzymatic end-to-end joining of DNA molecules. *J. molec. Biol.*, 1973, **78,** 453-471.

257.5   COHEN, STANLEY NORMAN. 1935- , CHANG, A.C.Y., BOYER, HERBERT WAYNE. 1936- , & HELLING, ROBERT BRUCE. 1936- .
Construction of biologically functional bacterial plasmids *in vitro. Proc. nat. Acad. Sci., (Wash.)*, 1973, **70,** 3240-3244.
First practical method for cloning genes, by the formation of recombinant plasmids which can be used to infect plasmid-free bacteria.

257.6   WILSON, EDWARD OSBORNE. 1929-
Sociobiology: the new synthesis. Cambridge, Mass., *Harvard University Press,* 1975.
Integration of biological and evolutionary theory with the study of social behaviour and social organization of animal populations.

History of Evolution: Genetics: Molecular Biology

258   LOVEJOY, ARTHUR ONCKEN. 1873-1962
The great chain of being: a study of the history of an idea. Cambridge, Mass., *Harvard University Press,* 1936.

258.1   LESKY, ERNA
Die Zeugungs- und Vererbungslehren der Antike und ihr Nachwirken. Wiesbaden, *Franz Steiner,* 1950.
A study of the earliest "scientific" theories of heredity and genetics.

258.2   PETERS, JAMES ARTHUR. 1922-
Classic papers in genetics. Edited by JAMES A. PETERS. Englewood Cliffs, N.J., *Prentice-Hall Inc.,* 1959.

258.3   STURTEVANT, ALFRED HENRY. 1891-1970
A history of genetics. New York, *Harper & Row,* 1965.

258.4   DUNN, LESLIE CLARENCE. 1893-1974
A short history of genetics. The development of the main lines of thought: 1864-1939. New York, *McGraw-Hill,* 1965.

258.5   CARLSON, Elof Axel. 1931-
The gene: a critical history. Philadelphia, *W. B. Saunders,* 1966.

258.6   STERN, Curt. 1902-1981, & SHERWOOD, Eva R.
The origins of genetics. A Mendel source book. San Francisco, *Freeman,*
1967.

258.7   PROVINE, William B.
The origins of theoretical population genetics. Chicago, *University of
Chicago Press,* 1971.

258.8   STUBBE, Hans, 1902-
Kurze Geschichte der Genetik bis zur Wiederentdeckung der
Vererbungsregeln Gregor Mendels. Zweite Ausgabe. Jena, *VEB Gustav
Fischer Verlag,* 1965.
> Revised and enlarged English translation, Cambridge, Mass., *Massachusetts Institute of Technology Press,* 1972.

258.9   OLBY, Robert. 1933-
The path to the double helix. London, *Macmillan,* 1974.
> A well-documented history of molecular biology.

258.10   PORTUGAL, Franklin H. & COHEN, Jack S.
A century of DNA: a history of the discovery of the structure and function
of the genetic substance. Cambridge, Mass., *MIT Press,* 1977.

258.11   JUDSON, Horace Freeland.
The eighth day of creation. Makers of the revolution in biology. New York,
Simon & Schuster, 1979.

258.12   MAYR, Ernst. 1904-
The growth of biological thought. Diversity, evolution, and inheritance.
Cambridge, Mass., *Harvard University Press,* 1982.
> An interpretive history of what Mayr calls "ultimate" explanations in
biology, reflecting Mayr's expertise in systematics, evolution, and genetics.

258.13   BOWLER, Peter.
Evolution: the history of an idea. Berkeley, *University of California Press,*
1984.

259   STELLUTI, Francesco. 1577-1653
Persio tradotto. Roma, *G. Mascardi,* 1630.
> First book to contain illustrations of natural objects as seen through the
microscope, specifically an engraving of the exterior surface of bees. The
work includes the Latin text of the Satyrae VI of Aulus Persius Flaccus
together with an Italian translation and notes by Stelluti.

259.1   ODIERNA, Giovan Battista. 1569-1660
l'Occhio della mosca *In his:* Opusculi...Palermo, *Cirillo,* 1644.
     The first microscopical section in biology is discussed and illustrated in Odierna's study of the fly's eye, which is also the first description of the faceted eye of an arthropod.

260   BOREL, Pierre [Borellus.] 1620-1689
Historiarum, et observationum medico-physicarum, centuria. Castris, *apud A. Colomerium,* 1653.
     The first work to apply microscopy to medicine. Borel probably saw the blood corpuscles and *Sarcoptes scabiei.*

261   ———. De vero telescopii inventore. Hagae-Comitum, *A. Vlacq,* 1655.
     Borel collected evidence to show that Zacharias (sometimes called Zacharias Janssen) invented the compound microscope about 1590. Zacharias was a spectacle-maker of Middelburg, Holland.

262   HOOKE, Robert. 1635-1703
Micrographia, or some physiological descriptions of minute bodies made by magnifying glasses; with observations and inquiries thereupon. London, *J. Martyn & J. Allestry,* 1665.
     Hooke, at one time research assistant to Robert Boyle, was one of the greatest inventive geniuses of all time. He constructed one of the most famous of the early compound microscopes. His *Micrographia* is the earliest work devoted entirely to an account of microscopical observations and is probably the most influential book in the entire history of microscopy. It is also the first book on the subject in English. Containing 38 copperplate engravings mostly after drawings by Hooke, with some probably after drawings by the architect and occasional scientist, Sir Christopher Wren (1632-1723), *Micrographia* is one of the most dramatically illustrated books of the 17th century. Among itsm any innovations, it includes the coinage of the modern biological usage of the word "cell" to describe the microscopic structure of tissue. Numerous facsimile reprints have been published.

263   ZAHN, Johann. 1641-1707
Oculus artificialis teledioptricus sive telescopium. 3 pts. Herbipoli, *Q. Heyl,* 1685-86.
     Includes the first complete history of early microscopes.

264   BONANNI, Filippo [Buonanni.] 1638-1725
Observationes circa viventia...cum micrographia curiosa. Romae, *typ. D. A. Herculis,* 1691.
     Illustrates several early microscopes, including the famous microscopes of the Bolognese Joseph Campani.

265   LEEUWENHOEK, Antonj van. 1632-1723
Ontledingen en ontdekkingen, *etc.* 6 vols. Leiden, Delft, 1693-1718.
     A collection in Dutch of many contributions sent by van Leeuwenhoek to the Royal Society of London, and first published in English translation in *Philosophical Transactions.* He is one of the greatest figures in the history of microscopy. He was first to describe spermatozoa, and the red blood corpuscles, discovered the crystalline lens, and was the first to see protozoa under the microscope. He introduced staining in histology in 1719 (saffron for muscle fibres). *See* No. 67.

265.1   DEIJL, Harmanus van. 1738-1809
Kort bericht der trapsgewijze verbeteringen aan achromatische verrekijkers.
Natuurk. Verh. Maatsch. Wetensch. Haarlem, 1807, **3,** 133-52.
Van Deijl introduced an achromatic objective.

266   AMICI, Giovanni Battista. 1784-1863
De microscopi catadiottrici memoria. Modena, 1818.
Amici constructed the first microscope with achromatic lenses and
suggested water-immersion for improved achromatic lenses of the com-
pound microscope. A translation in French of the above appears in *Ann.
Chim. Phys. (Paris),* 1820, **13,** 384-410.

266.1   GORING, C. R. 1792-1840
On Mr. Tulley's thick aplanatic object-glasses, for diverging rays; with an
account of a few microscopic test objects. *Quart. J. Sci.,* 1827, **22,** 265-84.
Goring was an Edinburgh medical practitioner. He commissioned
Tulley and others to make various modifications to the microscope. The
above paper reports the first effective achromatic object-glass.

267   LISTER, Joseph Jackson. 1786-1869
On some properties in achromatic object-glasses applicable to the improvement of the microscope. *Phil. Trans.,* 1830, **120,** 187-200.
The principle of the modern microscope was worked out by J. J. Lister,
father of Lord Lister. His important improvements in achromatic lenses
make him one of the most prominent figures in the history of modern
microscopy.

267.1   DONNÉ, Alfred. 1801-1878
Cours de microscopie. 1 vol. and atlas. Paris, *J. B. Baillière,* 1844-45.
The atlas includes the first engravings from photomicrographs, in this
case, daguerreotypes. One is reproduced by A. Hughes, *J. roy. micr. Soc.,*
1955, **75,** 1-22 (pl. IV).

268   HIS, Wilhelm, *Sr.* 1831-1904
Beschreibung eines Mikrotoms. *Arch. mikr. Anat.,* 1870 **6,** 229-32.
His was, more than any other man, responsible for the introduction of
the microtome, although Ranvier and other Frenchmen had earlier employed
microtomes of simpler types.

268.1   STEPHENSON, John Ware.
On a large-angled immersion objective, without adjustment collar; with
some observations on "numerical aperture". *J. roy. micr. Soc.,* 1878, **1,** 51-
6.
Stephenson suggested the oil immersion lens system to Abbe, who
developed it.

269   ABBE, Ernst. 1840-1905
Ueber neue Mikroskope. *S. B. Jena. Ges. Med.,* 1886, **2,** 107-28 (suppl. to
Jena Z. Naturw. 1887, **20**).
Fundamental improvements in the microscope were made by Abbe,
who was a mathematician. In 1878 he introduced the oil immersion lens;
in 1886 he made an apochromatic objective corrected for three colours in
which the secondary spectrum was not noticeable, while he is also

remembered for the sub-stage condenser which bears his name. A translation of the above article is in *J. roy. micr. Soc.*, 1887, 20-34.

269.1   KÖHLER, AUGUST. 1866-1948
Mikrophotographische Untersuchungen mit ultraviolettem Licht. *Z. wiss. Mikr.*, 1904, **21**, 129-65, 273-304.
The ultraviolet light microscope was conceived and designed by Köhler.

269.2   HEIMSTÄDT, OSKAR. 1879-1944
Das Fluoreszenzmikroskop. *Z. wiss. Mikr.*, 1911, **28**, 330-37.
Fluorescence microscopy.

269.3   KNOLL, MAX.1879-1969 & RUSKA, ERNST. 1906-
Beitrag zur geometrischen Elektronenoptik. *Ann. Physik*, 1932, **12**, 607-61.
Electron microscope. See also their later paper in *Z. Physik.* 1932, **78**, 318.

269.4   HAITINGER, MAX. 1868-1946
Die Methoden der Fluoreszenzmikroskopie. In E. ABDERHALDEN: *Handbuch der biologischen Arbeitsmethoden,* Berlin, Abt. II, Teil 3, pp. 3307-37, 1934.
Modern methods of fluorescence microscopy were developed by Haitinger.

269.5   ZERNIKE, FRITS. 1888-1966
Das Phasenkontrastverfahren b.d. mikroskopischen Beobachtung. *Phys. Z.*, 1935, **36**, 848-51.
Phase contrast microscopy was invented by Zernike. He was awarded the Nobel Prize for physics in 1953.

269.6   BARNARD, JOSEPH EDWIN. 1869-1949, & WELCH, FRANK V.
Microscopy with ultra-violet light. A simplification of method. *J. roy. micr. Soc.*, 1936, **56**, 365-71.

269.7   COSSLETT, VERNON ELLIS. 1908- , & NIXON, W. C.
X-ray shadow microscope. *Nature (Lond.)*, 1951, **168**, 24-5.

269.8   EHRENBERG, WERNER. 1901- , & SPEAR, W.E.
An electrostatic focusing system and its application to a fine focus x-ray tube. *Proc. phys. Soc. (Lond.) B*, 1951, **64**, 67-75.
X-ray microscopy.

History of Microscopy

270   HARTING, PIETER. 1812-1885
Het mikroskoop. 4 vols. Utrecht, 1848-54.
Exhaustive history of the microscope. The work was translated into German, appearing (second edition) in 1866; this last was reprinted Amsterdam, 3 vols., 1970.

271   CLAY, REGINALD STANLEY, & COURT, THOMAS H.
The history of the microscope. London, *Griffin,* 1932.
The best history of microscopes up to 1800. Reprinted London, 1971.

272   CONN, HAROLD JOEL. 1886-1975, *et al.*
History of staining. 2nd ed. Geneve, N.Y., *Biotech Publications*, 1948. 3rd. by George C. Lusk & Frederick H. Kasten. Baltimore, *Williams & Wilkins*, 1983.

273   FREUND, HUGO, & BERG, ALEXANDER.
Geschichte der Mikroskopie. 3 vols. Frankfurt, *Umschau*, 1963-66.
A biographical history.

273.1   BRADBURY, SAVILE.
The evolution of the microscope. Oxford, *Pergamon Press*, 1967.

273.2   MARTON, LADISLAUS LASZLO. 1901-1979
Early history of the electron microscope. San Francisco, *San Francisco Press*, 1968.

ZOOLOGY AND COMPARATIVE ANATOMY

274   ARISTOTLE. 384-322 B.C.
De historia animalium *in his* [De animalibus] Translated by THEODORE GAZA; edited by LUDOVICUS PODOCATHARUS. [Venice: *Johann de Colonia & Johannes Manthen*, 1476]
Aristotle was the first scientist to gather empirical evidence about the biological world through observation. By his careful observations and excellent accounts of the natural history of those living creatures which he was able to investigate, Aristotle may be considered the first scientific naturalist. English trans. *in his* Works...edited by J.A. Smith and W.D. Ross, Oxford, 1910, **4**, 486a-633a. For an evaluation of the biological work of Aristotle, see Singer's *History of biology,* 1950, pp. 9-44.

275   ——. De partibus animalium. *In his* [De animalibus] Translated by THEODORE GAZA; edited by LUDOVICUS PODOCATHARUS. [Venice: *Johann de Colonia & Johannes Manthen*, 1476]
The first animal physiology. English trans. *in his* Works...edited by J. A. Smith and W. D. Ross, Oxford, 1912, **5**, 639a-697b. This edition excluded annotations by the translator, W. Ogle, which were published in the edition of London, 1882.

276   ALBERTUS MAGNUS [ALBERT VON BOLLSTADT.] ?1193-1280
De animalibus. Rome, *Simon Nicolai Chardella, de Lucca*, 1478.
Albertus slavishly followed Aristotle, although sometimes criticizing him. He was a Dominican monk and the most eminent naturalist of the 13th century; his work on animals contained a good deal of personal observation. See also *De animalibus libri xxxi. Nach der Cölner Urschrift herausgegeben* von H. Stadler. 2 vols. Münster, 1916-1921.

276.1   CONRAD VON MEGENBERG. *circa* 1309-1374
Buch der Natur. Augsburg, *Johann Bämler*, [14]75.
The first printed book to contain illustrations of animals, and the first notable scientific book in German. It discusses animals, birds, fish, anatomy, physiology, plagues, the medicinal value of plants and stones, etc.

277   TURNER, WILLIAM. 1510-1568
        Avium praecipuarum...historia. Coloniae, *J. Gymnicus,* 1544.
        The first book on birds with clear descriptions of the appearance of individual birds based on the author's own experiences and observations. Turner attempted to determine those birds named by Aristotle and Pliny; he added notes from his own observations on birds, identifying numerous northern European and English species for the first time. Annotated English translation with Latin text, Cambridge, 1903.

278   BELON, PIERRE [BELLONIUS]. 1517-1564
        L'histoire naturelle des estranges poissons marins. Paris, *R. Chaudière,* 1551.
        This, Belon's first biological work, is regarded as the earliest modern scientific work in the field of comparative anatomy.

279   ——. De aquatilibus. Parisiis, *C. Stephanus,* 1553.

280   GESNER, CONRAD. 1516-1565
        Historia animalium. 5 vols. Tiguri, *apud C. Froschouerum,* 1551-1587.
        Gesner was a man of great industry. His *Historia animalium* is considered one of the starting points of modern zoology; it contains 4,500 pages and nearly 1,000 woodcuts, some being by Albrecht Dürer. It includes the names of all the known animals in the ancient and modern languages, together with a mass of information regarding them. Portions of this work were translated by Edward Topsel as *The historie of four-footed beasts.* London, 1658.

281   WOTTON, EDWARD. 1492-1555
        De differentiis animalium. Lutetiae Parisiorum *M. Vascosanus,* 1552.
        Wotton is considered the founder of modern zoology. Basing his work on Aristotle, he rejected the fantastic additions which had accrued to the writings of the latter during the Middle Ages. His book is beautifully printed but not illustrated.

282   RONDELET, GUILLAUME [RONDELETIUS]. 1507-1566
        Libri de piscibus marinis. (Universae aquatilium pars altera.) 2 vols. Lugduni, *apud Matthiam Bonhomme,* 1554-55.
        Rondelet wrote this book with the idea of verifying Aristotle, but in it he described many forms of fishes for the first time. The book is an accurate account of his investigation of Mediterranean fishes and marine animals, and Singer says that Fig. 51, illustrating the structure of a sea urchin, is the earliest figure we have of a dissected vertebrate. Rondelet also observed the relationship between embryo and mother in the placental dogfish.

283   BELON, PIERRE [BELLONIUS]. 1517-1564
        L'histoire de la nature des oyseaux. Paris, *B. Preuost, G. Cauellat,* 1555.
        Belon's book on birds is well illustrated, including plates of the skeletons of man and bird side by side and in the same posture, to compare them bone for bone.

284   COITER, VOLCHER. 1534-1576
        Lectiones Gabrielis Falloppi...Diversorum animalium sceletorum explicationes. Noribergae, *in off. T. Gerlachii,* 1575.
        Coiter was a pupil of Fallopius and Eustachius, and became town physician of Nuremburg. His book on comparative osteology, contained

in his edition of the lectures of Fallopius, extended his studies begun in his work of 1572-73, (No. 1539). Coiter's study of the skeleton of the foetus and of a child six months old was the first study of developmental osteology and showed where ossification begins. The copperplate engravings are after drawings by Coiter. Biography and English translation by B. T. W. Nuyens and A. Schierbeck, Haarlem, 1956.

285   RUINI, Carlo. ?1530-1598
Dell'anotomia, et dell'infermità del cavallo. Bologna, *G. Rossi,* 1598.

First book devoted exclusively to the structure of a single species other than man. Besides being one of the foundation-stones of modern veterinary medicine, it contains a description of the lesser circulation. The admirable woodcuts were inspired by those in Vesalius's *De humani corporis fabrica* (1543) .

286   CASSERI, Giulio [Julius Casserius *Placentinus*]. ?1561-1616
De vocis auditusque organis historia anatomica. 2 pts. Ferrariae, *exc. V. Baldinus, typ. Cameralis,* 1600-01.

Casseri, originally a servant to Fabrizio, was personally trained by his employer and eventually succeeded to Fabrizio's chair of anatomy. He investigated the structure of the auditory and vocal organs in most of the domestic animals. The book includes a description of the larynx more accurate than that of any previous author, and is also notable for its fine copperplate engravings. Translation of chap. I-VIII (the section on the larynx) in *Acta otol. (Stockh.),* 1969, Suppl. 261.

287   JONSTON, John [Johnstone]. 1603-1675
Thaumatographia naturalis. Amsterdami, *G. Blaeu,* 1632.

A compilation of all the contemporary zoological knowledge. Jonston, born in Scotland, spent most of his life on the mainland of Europe.

288   MOFFET, Thomas [Moufet, Muffetus]. 1553-1604
Insectorum sive minimorum animalium theatrum. Londoni, *ex. off. typ. Thom. Cotes,* 1634.

Moffet travelled extensively in Europe and kept copious notes of his observations on insects. These he published in the above folio, together with many excellent woodcut illustrations. To date, this was the best work of its kind and it set a new standard of accuracy in the study of the invertebrates. An English translation, *Theater of Insects,* appeared in 1658.

289   SEVERINO, Marco Aurelio [Severinus]. 1580-1656
Zootomia Democritaea: id est, anatome generalis totius animantium opificii. Noribergae, *lit. Endterianis,* 1645.

One of the most important of the early works on comparative anatomy. It includes the *Anatomia porci,* attributed to Copho of Salerno. Severinus dissected many animals and was convinced that the microscope would throw light on comparative anatomy.

290   ALDROVANDI, Ulisse [Aldrovandus]. 1522-1605
Opera omnia. 13 vols. Bononiae, *J. B. Bellagamba (and others),* 1599-1667.

Aldrovandi, first director of the botanical garden at Bologna, was a prolific writer. Some of his writings made their first appearance in print after his death. He designed them as a whole to form an enormous illustrated encyclopaedia of biology.

291   GOEDAERT, JAN [GOEDARTIUS]. 1620-1668
        Metamorphosis et historia naturalis insectorum. 3 pts. Medioburgi, *Jacobum Fierensium*, 1662-67.
        English translation, London, 1682.

292   CHARLETON, WALTER. 1619-1707
        Onomasticon zoicon, plerorumque animalium differentias et nomina propria pluribus linguis exponens. Cui accedunt mantissa anatomica, et quaedam de variis fossilium generibus. Londoni, *apud. J. Allestry*, 1668.
        Gives a list of the English, Latin, and Greek names of all the then known animals.

292.1   PRIVATE COLLEGE OF AMSTERDAM
        Observationes anatomicae selectiores. [Part II: Observationum anatomicarum... pars altera]. Amsterdam, *Caspar Commelin*, 1667-1673.
        The only publications of one of the earliest scientific societies, active from 1664 to 1672. Founded by Gerard Blaes, and numbering Jan Swammerdam among its members, the college devoted itself to comparative anatomical and physiological investigations of the lower vertebrates, concentrating primarily on fishes and mammals. The above works contain the first publication of Swammerdam's early experiments with neuro-muscular physiology. Other portions of the works were probably written by Blaes. Facsimile edition edited by F.J. Cole, Berkshire, *University of Reading*, 1938.

293   MALPIGHI, MARCELLO. 1628-1694
        Dissertatio epistolica de bombyce. Londini, *J. Martyn & J. Allestry*, 1669.
        Malpighi's work on the silkworm represents the first monograph on an invertebrate and records one of the most striking pieces of research work on his part. He dissected the silkworm under the microscope with great skill and observed its intricate structure; before the appearance of this work the silkworm was believed to have no internal organs.

294   SWAMMERDAM, JAN. 1637-1680
        Historia insectorum generalis. 2 pts. Utrrecht [*sic*], *M. van Dreunen*, 1669.
        Swammerdam, one of the greatest of the early microscopists, spent much time on the study of insects, and mapped out a natural classification of them.

294.1   REDI, FRANCESCO. 1626-1697.
        Esperienze intorno a diverse cose naturali...Firenze, *All' Insegno della Nave*, 1671.
        Includes the first scientific study of an electric fish. While the torpedo's peculiar properties had provoked scientific speculation since at least the time of Aristotle, Redi was the first to perform an actual dissection of the fish for scientific purposes. He was the first to locate and examine the torpedo's electric organs.

295   PERRAULT, CLAUDE. 1613-1688
        Mémoires pour servir à l'histoire des animaux. 2 vols., Paris, *Imprimerie Royale*, 1671-76.
        The early biological work of the French Académie des Sciences was issued chiefly as anatomical descriptions of various animals. It was conducted by a team of comparative anatomists led by Perrault that included G.J. Duverney, J. Pecquet, M. Charas and P. de la Hire. Issued in large folio

format and intended for presentation by Louis XIV, this important text is one of the most sumptuously produced of all early biological works. English translation, London, 1678.

296   BLAES, GERARD [BLASIUS]. 1626-1682
Anatome animalium. Amstelodami, *J. a Someren,* 1681.
    "The first comprehensive manual of comparative anatomy based on the original and literary researches of a working anatomist" (Cole). Blaes anticipated Cowper in finding the Cowper's glands, which he illustrated in his plate of the genitalia and os penis of the rat. The 85 pages devoted to the anatomy of the dog was the first comprehensive and original treatise on a vertebrate since Ruini (No. 285).

297   GREW, NEHEMIAH. 1641-1712
Musaeum Regalis Societatis, or a catalogue and description of the natural and artificial rarities belonging to the Royal Society and preserved at Gresham College. Whereunto is subjoyned the comparative anatomy of stomachs and guts. London, *H. Newman,* 1681.
    Grew, secretary to the Royal Society, compiled this great illustrated catalogue of its museum, then housed at Gresham College. Published with the catalogue is Grew's study of the stomach organs, which is the first zoological book to have the term "comparative anatomy" on the title page, and also the first attempt to deal with one system of organs only by the comparative method.

298   SNAPE, ANDREW, *Jnr.*
The anatomy of an horse. London, *M. Flesher,* 1683.
    First book in English on equine anatomy, largely a translation of Ruini (No. 285).

299   RAY, JOHN. 1628-1705
Synopsis methodica animalium quadrupedum et serpentini generis. Londini, *S. Smith, & B. Walford,* 1693.
    This work contains the first really systematic classification of animals. Much of its general arrangement of animals survives in modern systems of classification.

300   TYSON, EDWARD. 1650-1708
Orang-outang, sive homo sylvestris: or, the anatomy of a pygmie compared with that of a monkey, an ape, and a man. London, *T. Bennet & D. Brown,* 1699.
    The earliest work of importance in comparative morphology. Tyson compared the anatomy of man and monkeys and between the two he placed the chimpanzee, which he regarded as the typical pygmy. This was the origin of the idea of a "missing link" in the ascent of man from the apes. *See also* No. 153.

301   RÉAUMUR, RENÉ ANTOINE FERCHAULT DE. 1683-1757
Sur les diverses reproductions qui se font dans les écrevisses, les omars, les crabes, etc. *Mém. Acad. roy. Sci (Paris),* 1712, 226-45.
    Réaumur showed that crustaceans replace their lost limbs, a fact until then disputed.

302   VALLISNIERI, ANTONIO [VALLISNERI]. 1661-1730
Istoria del camaleonte Affricano e di varj animali d'Italia. Venezia, *G. G. Ertz,* 1715.

303   VALENTINI, MICHAEL BERNHARD. 1657-1729
Amphitheatrum zootomicum. Francofurti ad Moenum, *sumpt. haered. Zunnerianorum,* 1720.
     "First extensive work on the comparative anatomy of vertebrates" (Casey Wood).

304   RÉAUMUR, RENÉ ANTOINE FERCHAULT DE. 1683-1757
Mémoires pour servir à l'histoire des insectes. 6 vols. Paris, *Mortier,* 1734-42.
     Réaumur's greatest work. It describes the appearance, habits and locality of all the known insects except the beetles, and includes 267 plates.

305   LYONET, PIETER. 1707-1789
Traité anatomique de la chénille. La Haye, 1762.
     Lyonet's great monograph on the goat moth caterpillar remains today among the greatest examples of anatomical examination.

306   BAKER, HENRY. 1698-1774
An attempt towards a natural history of the polype. London, *R. Dodsley,* 1743.

307   TREMBLEY, ABRAHAM. 1710-1784
Mémoires, pour servir à l'histoire d'un genre de polypes d'eau douce, à bras en forme de cornes. Leyden, *J. & H. Verbeek,* 1744.
     Trembley discovered the hydra and was the first to observe in it asexual reproduction, regeneration, and photosensitivity in an animal without eyes. His experiments were of great importance in the study of regeneration of lost parts. He was the first to make permanent grafts and to witness cell-division. A biography of Trembley was published by J. R. Baker, London, 1952. English translation in S.G. and H.M. Lenhoff, *Hydra and the birth of experimental biology,* Pacific Grove, CA, 1986.

308   BONNET, CHARLES. 1720-1793
Traité d'insectologie. 2 pts. Paris, *Durand,* 1745.
     This pioneering work on experimental entomology incorporates Bonnet's most important discovery – parthenogenetic reproduction – based on his study of aphids. Bonnet used the result of this and other discoveries as a basis for speculation about life on earth. This work presents in tabular form his version of the "great chain of being". Bonnet's concept of the essential continuity of life, a consequence of his discovery and preformationist interpretation of parthenogenesis, was a major force in the shaping of later evolutionary opinion. *See* No. 472.

308.1   STUBBS, GEORGE. 1724-1806
The anatomy of the horse. London, *J. Purser for the author,* 1766.
     The first original work on equine anatomy after Ruini (No. 285). Stubbs, the great painter of animals, prepared his own dissections of horse carcasses, and personally engraved the 24 double folio plates for this work, a task that took him seven or eight years to complete. Besides the first issue of this work, copies with text leaves identical to the first edition exist with

the plates printed on paper watermarked 1798, 1813, and 1815. *See* No. 6610.54.

309   HUNTER, John. 1728-1793
Observations on certain parts of the animal oeconomy. London, 1786.
Includes John Hunter's observations on the secondary sexual characteristics in birds, on the descent of the testis, on the air sac in birds, on the structure of the placenta, etc., together with the original description of the olfactory nerves.

310   RUSSELL, Patrick. 1727-1805
An account of Indian serpents. 4 vols. London, *G. Nicol,* 1796-1809.
First attempt at a description of Indian serpents and serpent venoms. Includes the original description of Russell's viper, *Daboia russellii.*

311   CUVIER, Georges Léopold Chrétien Frédéric Dagobert, *Baron.* 1769-1832
Leçons d'anatomie comparée. 5 vols. Paris, *Baudouin,* an VIII [1800]-1805.
Cuvier ranks with von Baer as one of the founders of modern morphology. Vols. 1-2 ed. by C. Duméril, and vols. 3-5 ed. by G.L. Duvernoy, but Cuvier took full responsibility for the contents of this work.

312   BLUMENBACH, Johann Friedrich. 1752-1840
Handbuch der vergleichenden Anatomie. Göttingen, *H. Dieterich,* 1805.
Blumenbach, physiologist and anthropologist, was Professor of Medicine at Göttingen. He was the first to show the value of comparative anatomy in the study of anthropology; his classic text went through many editions; it was translated into English in 1807.

313   VICQ D'AZYR, Félix. 1748-1794
Œuvres recueillies... par Jacques L. Moreau [de la Sarthe]. 6 vols. and atlas. Paris, *L. Duprat-Duverger,* 1805.
Vicq d'Azyr has been called the greatest comparative anatomist of the 18th century. The mammillo-thalamic tract is named the "bundle of Vicq d'Azyr". *See* No. 401.2.

314   MECKEL, Johann Friedrich, *the younger.* 1781-1833
Beyträge zur vergleichenden Anatomie. 2 vols. Leipzig, *C. H. Reclam,* 1808-11.
See No. 318.

315   HOME, *Sir* Everard. 1756-1832
Lectures on comparative anatomy, in which are explained the preparations in the Hunterian collection. 6 vols. London, *G & W. Nicol, etc.,* 1814-28.
Plagiarized from the manuscripts of John Hunter, Home's father-in-law, and of immense importance for publication of Hunter's researches. Home destroyed the original manuscripts on which his work was based after he corrected the page proofs. See Qvist, *John Hunter* (1981).

316   LAMARCK, Jean Baptiste Pierre Antoine de Monet de. 1744-1829
Histoire naturelle des animaux sans vertèbres. 7 vols. Paris, *Verdière,* 1815-22.
An elaborate expansion of Lamarck's one-volume work with the same title published in Paris, 1801 (No.215.5). As a systematist Lamarck made

important contributions to biology. He separated spiders and crustaceans from insects, made advances in the classification of worms and echinoderms, and introduced the classification of animals into vertebrates and invertebrates. The introduction to this work includes Lamarck's summary of his four laws of evolution.

317 CHAMISSO, LUDWIG ADALBERT VON. 1781-1838
De salpa. Berolini, *apud F. Dümmlerum,* 1819.
 In this monograph on certain *Vermes* is included the first description of several of the Tunicates and the earliest use of the expression "alternation of generations".

318 MECKEL, JOHANN FRIEDRICH, *the younger.* 1781-1833
System der vergleichenden Anatomie. 5 vols. [in 6]. Halle, *Renger,* 1821-31.
 Meckel is considered the greatest comparative anatomist before Johannes Müller.

319 GEOFFROY SAINT-HILAIRE, ÉTIENNE. 1772-1844, & CUVIER, FRE;DE;RIC. 1773-1838
Histoire naturelle des mammifères. 4 vols. Paris, *Belin & Blaise,* 1824-42.

322 AUDUBON, JOHN JAMES LAFOREST. 1785-1851
The birds of America. 4 vols. London, *The Author,* 1827-38.
 Contains 435 hand-coloured plates in double elephant folio format. This is widely regarded as the greatest illustrated ornithological work ever published. With the assistance of William Macgillivray, Audubon wrote a five-volume text for this atlas, entitled *Ornithological biography,* Edinburgh, 1831-39. Numerous reproductions of these famous plates have been published, as well as two complete full-size facsimile editions of this massive work.

324 BUFFON, GEORGES LOUIS LECLERC, *Comte.* 1707-1788
Histoire naturelle générale et particulière...44 vols. plus atlas. Paris, *Imprimerie Royale* [etc.], 1749- "An XII" [1803/04].
 This vast work is divided into seven parts. I: Histoire naturelle générale et particulière...15 vols., by Buffon and L.J.M. Daubenton (1749-67). II: Histoire naturelle des oiseaux. 9 vols., by Buffon, P. Guéneau de Montbeillard and G.L.C.A. Bexon (1770-1783). III: Histoire naturelle des mineraux. 5 vols., by Buffon (1783-88). IV: Supplement. 7 vols., by Buffon, the last volume finished by La Cépède after Buffon's death (1774-1789). V: Histoire naturelle des quadrupèdes ovipare et des serpents. 2 vols., by Le Compte de la Cépède (1788-89). VI: Histoire naturelle des poissons. 5 vols., by La Cépède (1798- "An XI" [1802/03]). Histoire naturelle des cétacées. 1 vol., by La Cépède. (An XII [1803/04]). "Natural history, prior to Buffon, had all the earmarks of an avocation, a hobby. Buffon is the one who raised it to the status of a science" (Mayr). Buffon is also regarded as an important early contributor to the history of evolutionary thought as he introduced a large number of evolutionary problems, such as common descent, extinction, and reproductive isolation of species, into the realm of scientific investigation.

325 OWEN, *Sir* RICHARD. 1804-1892
Memoir on the pearly nautilus (Nautilus pompilius, Linn.). London, *W. Wood,* 1832.

326 ROYAL COLLEGE OF SURGEONS OF ENGLAND.
Descriptive and illustrated catalogue of the physiological series of comparative anatomy contained in the Museum [by RICHARD OWEN]. 5 vols. [in 6]. London, *R & J. E. Taylor*, 1833-40.

When Hunter died his museum was cared for by his faithful assistant and amanuensis, the artist and anatomist, William Clift, who persuaded the Government to purchase it. Owen later became curator and his monumental catalogue is still of value today. A history of the museum from its foundation to its destruction by a high-explosive bomb in May 1941, is given in G. Grey Turner's *Hunterian Museum,* 1946.

326.1 HOLBROOK, JOHN EDWARDS. 1794-1871
North American herpetology; or, a description of the reptiles inhabiting the United States. 4 vols., Philadelphia, *J. Dobson,* 1836-38.

The greatest American book on herpetology, and one of the finest American colour plate books on natural history. The fourth volume is particularly rare.

327 CUVIER, GEORGES LÉOPOLD CHRÉTIEN FRÉDÉRIC DAGOBERT, *Baron*. 1769-1832
Le règne animal. 3me édition. 20 vols. Paris, *Fortin, Masson & Cie.,* 1836-49.

Cuvier's most comprehensive work represented the fruits of a lifetime's study of living and fossil animals. In his day Cuvier exerted an enormous influence on science. He played a leading part in the development of the science of palaeontology and stimulated the study of comparative anatomy. First edition, 4 vols., Paris, *Deterville,* 1817. Several English translations are available. See Coleman, *Georges Cuvier zoologist,* Cambridge, *Harvard University Press,* 1964.

328 MÜLLER, JOHANNES. 1801-1858
Ueber die Lymphherzen der Schildkröten. Berlin, *Druckerei d. k. Akad.,* 1840.

329 OWEN, *Sir* RICHARD. 1804-1892
Odontography, or, a treatise on the comparative anatomy of the teeth. 2 vols. London, *H. Baillière,* 1840-45.

Owen's comprehensive investigation of the morphology of mammalian teeth led him into palaeontology, of which he soon became one of the masters. Owen, son-in-law of William Clift, was from 1836-56 Hunterian professor at the Royal College of Surgeons. During the 1860s he was one of the most virulent opponents of Darwinism.

329.1 SAVAGE, THOMAS S. 1804-1880 & WYMAN, JEFFRIES. 1814-1874.
A description of the characters and habits of troglodytes gorilla, and of the osteology of the same. *Boston J. Nat. Hist.,* 1847, **5**, 417-27, 429-30, 432-33, 435, 436-441.

First description of the gorilla. Savage, an American physician/clergyman, worked extensively as a missionary physician in Africa.

330 OWEN, *Sir* RICHARD. 1804-1892
On the archetype and homologies of the vertebrate skeleton. London, *J. Van Voorst,* 1848.

Owen's vertebral theory of the origin of the skull, later refuted by Huxley and others.

331 SIEBOLD, CARL THEODOR ERNST VON. 1804-1885, & STANNIUS, HERMANN FRIEDRICH. 1808-1883.
Lehrbuch der vergleichenden Anatomie. 2 vols. Berlin, *Veit & Co.,* 1846-48.
English translation of vol. 1, Boston, 1854.

333 AGASSIZ, LOUIS JEAN RODOLPHE. 1807-1873
Contributions to the natural history of the United States. 4 vols. Boston, *Little, Brown & Co.,* 1857-62.
Agassiz was the leading comparative anatomist in America and a virulent opponent of Darwinism. Ten volumes of this set were planned but only four appeared. Volume one contains his theoretical work, *Essay on Classification.* The remainder of the set is valuable for its descriptions of American turtles.

334 BRONN, HEINRICH GEORG. 1800-1862
Die Klassen und Ordnungen des Thier-Reichs. Vol. 1-. Leipzig, *C. F. Winter,* 1859-
This great systematic work, begun by Bronn, is being continued by other naturalists. It deals with both recent and fossil zoology.

335 COUCH, JONATHAN. 1789-1870
A history of the fishes of the British Isles. 4 vols. London, *Groombridge and Sons,* [1860]-1865.
Couch, a general practitioner at Polperro, Cornwall, became one of the greatest authorities on British fishes. The work, a monument of industry and patience, includes some fine plates, also by Couch.

336 OWEN, *Sir* RICHARD. 1804-1892
On the anatomy and physiology of the vertebrates. 3 vols. London, *Longmans, Green,* 1866-68.
1. Fishes and reptiles; 2. Birds; 3. Mammals. The most important work on the subject since Cuvier. It is based entirely on personal observations.

337 GEGENBAUR, CARL. 1826-1903
Grundzüge der vergleichenden Anatomie der Wirbelthiere. 2te. Aufl. Leipzig, *W. Engelmann,* 1870.
Gegenbaur's best work. He stressed the value of comparative anatomy as the basis of the study of descent, considering that knowledge of the relations of corresponding parts in different animals was more important even than comparative embryology in this respect.

338 HUXLEY, THOMAS HENRY. 1825-1895
A manual of the anatomy of vertebrated animals. London, *J. & A. Churchill,* 1871.
Huxley was among those who refuted Owen's theory of the vertebral skull.

339 DOHRN, ANTON. 1840-1909
Der Ursprung der Wirbelthiere und das Princip des Functionswechsels. Leipzig, *W. Engelmann,* 1875.

Dohrn's theory of change of function as the origin of evolutionary novelties.

343   WIEDERSHEIM, ROBERT ERNST EDUARD. 1848-1923
Lehrbuch der vergleichenden Anatomie der Wirbelthiere. 2 vols., Jena, *G. Fischer,* 1882-83.
    English translation, London, 1886.

344   BROCA, PIERRE PAUL. 1824-1880
Mémoires sur le cerveau de l'homme et des primates. Paris, *C. Reinwald,* 1888.

345   LANKESTER, *Sir* EDWIN RAY. 1847-1929
A treatise on zoology. Edited by E. RAY LANKESTER. 9 vols. London, *Black,* 1900-09.

346   THEOBALD, FREDERICK VINCENT. 1868-1930
A monograph of the Culicidae, or mosquitoes. 4 vols. and atlas. London, *Longmans & Co.,* 1901-10.

347   DUCKWORTH, WYNFRID LAURENCE HENRY. 1870-1956
Morphology and anthropology. Cambridge, *Univ. Press,* 1904.

348   MORGAN, THOMAS HUNT. 1866-1945
Experimental zoology. New York, *Macmillan & Co.,* 1907.

349   PATTON, WALTER SCOTT. 1876-1960, & CRAGG, FRANCIS WILLIAM. 1882-1924
A textbook of medical entomology. London, Madras, and Calcutta, *Christian Literature Society for India,* 1913.

350   TILNEY, FREDERICK. 1875-1938
The brain from ape to man. With chapters on the reconstruction of the grey matter in the primate brainstem by HENRY ALSOP RILEY. 2 vols. New York, *P. B. Hoeber,* 1928.
    Classic study of the evolution of the central nervous system in the higher mammals.

351   ZUCKERMAN, SOLLY, *Baron Zuckerman of Burnham Thorpe,* 1904-
The social life of monkeys and apes. London, *Kegan Paul,* 1932.
    A study of the relationship of Man to the other primates, from the physiological and biochemical standpoint. Zuckerman's work is considered the first adequate interpretation of simian society. 2nd ed., 1980.

352   CLARK, *Sir* WILFRID EDWARD LE GROS. 1895-1971
History of the primates. London, *British Museum (Natural History),* 1949

History of Zoology

353   CARUS, JULIUS VICTOR. 1823-1903
Geschichte der Zoologie. München, *R. Oldenbourg,* 1872.
    French edition, 1880.

353.1   RUSSELL, EDWARD STUART. 1887-1954
Form and function: a contribution to the history of animal morphology.
London, *John Murray*, 1916.

354   WOOD, CASEY ALBERT. 1856-1942
An introduction to the literature of vertebrate zoology. London, *Oxford Univ. Press*, 1931.
A comprehensive summary and bibliography of the literature on vertebrate zoology. Reprint, 1979.

355   HASSALL, ALBERT. 1862-1942, *et al.*
Index-catalogue of medical and veterinary zoology. Pt. 1-. Washington, *Govt. Printing Off.*, 1932-
In progress.

356   COLE, FRANCIS JOSEPH. 1872-1959
A history of comparative anatomy. From Aristotle to the eighteenth century. London, *Macmillan & Co.*, 1944.
Reprinted, *Dover Publications*, 1978.

356.1   RAVEN, CHARLES E.
English naturalists from Neckham to Ray. Cambridge, *University Press*, 1947.

356.2   STRESEMAN, ERWIN. 1889-1972.
Die Entwicklung Der Ornithologie von Aristoteles bis zur Gegenwart. Berlin, *F.W. Peters*, 1951.
Revised English translation by H. and C. Epstein, ed. by G. Cottrell, with a foreword and an epilogue on American ornithology by E. Mayr. Cambridge, Mass., *Harvard University Press*, 1975.

357   PETIT, GEORGES.1892-1973, & THEODORIDES, JEAN. 1926-
Histoire de la zoologie des origines à Linné. Paris, *Hermann*, 1962.

358   NISSEN, CLAUS. 1901-1975
Die zoologische Buchillustration. Ihre Bibliographie und Geschichte. 2 vols., Stuttgart, *Hiersemann*, 1966-78.
The most comprehensive history and historical bibliography of zoological illustration.

358.1   SERVICE, MICHAEL WILLIAM.
A short history of medical entomology. *J. med. Entomol.*, 1978, **14,** 603-26.

ANATOMY AND PHYSIOLOGY

ANATOMY

359   GALEN. A.D. 130-200
De anatomicis administrationibus, libri i-ix. *In his* Opera omnia ed. cur. C. G. KÜHN, Lipsiae, *C. Cnobloch*, 1821, **2,** 215-731.
Galen's anatomical writings are a repository of all contemporary knowledge, together with some of his own views and discoveries. He had

a good knowledge of osteology and myology, some knowledge of angiology and less of zoology. Although not to be regarded as the founder of the science of anatomy, he is nevertheless its first important witness. English translation by C. Singer (1956).

360 ——. Sieben Bücher Anatomie des Galen. 2 vols. Leipzig, *J. C. Hinrichs,* 1906.

Books 9, 5-15 are lost in the Greek original, but preserved in a ninth century Arabic version, which M. Simon here edits and translates into German. An English translation of Simon's Arabic text was published by W.L.H. Duckworth, M.C. Lyons and B. Towers, Cambridge, 1962.

361 MONDINO DE'LUZZI [MUNDINUS]. ?1275-1326
Anothomia. Papiae, *Antonio De Carcano,* 1478.

The first modern book devoted solely to anatomy; written for his students in 1316. Mundinus re-introduced human dissection, which had been neglected for 1500 years before him; he was the most noted dissector of his period. The medieval anatomical vocabulary, well set forth by Mundinus, was derived mainly from Arabic; Singer, in his translation of the work, 1925, has added an ample glossary of terms of Arabic origin. Facsimile reproduction, in E. Wickersheimer's *Anatomies de Mondino dei Luzzi et de Guido de Vigevano,* Paris, 1926.

362 MONDEVILLE, HENRI DE. ?1260-1320
Die Anatomie des Heinrich von Mondeville. Nach einer Handschrift der Königlichen Bibliothek zu Berlin von Jahre 1304 zum ersten Male herausgegeben von J. PAGEL. Berlin, *G. Reimer,* 1889.

Mondeville was the first teacher known to have lectured with the aid of illustrations, using 13 charts of human anatomy. He lectured at Montpellier.

363 KETHAM, JOHANNES DE. *d. circa* 1490
Fasciculus medicinae. Venetiis, *per Johannem & Gregorius fratres de Forlivio,* 1491.

A collection of short medical treatises which circulated widely in manuscript, some as early as the 13th century, and was perhaps attributed by the printers to its former owner, Johannes von Kirchheim, a professor of medicine in Vienna about 1460. His name was probably corrupted by the printers to Ketham. The great importance of this book is that it includes the first printed anatomic illustrations of any kind. Singer's edition, which includes his translation of the commentary by Karl Sudhoff, was published at Milan, 1924. The first English translation of Ketham's text by Luke Demaitre, republishing Singer's translation of Sudhoff's commentary, was published at Birmingham by *The Classics of Medicine Library,* 1988. This edition reproduces the woodcuts in colour from an original hand-coloured copy at Yale's Cushing/Whitney Medical Library, together with selected illustrations from the Italian 1493 edition with Singer's commentary.

363.1 ——. Fasciculo di medicina. Venice: *Johannes & Gregorius de Gregoriis, de Forlivio,* 1493/4.

This Italian translation contains an entirely new and more extensive series of woodcuts and additional text. The dramatically improved and more realistic illustrations, which were reproduced in the numerous later editions, are by an unknown artist, about whom there has been much speculation. He was certainly close to the school of Bellini. The dissection scene appears in colour only in this edition and is one of the first three known examples of colour printing, its four colours having been applied by means of stencils. Facsimile edition with extensive commentary by Charles Singer, 2 vols., Milan, 1925. Facsimile edition, Munich, 1979.

363.2 PEYLIGK, JOHANNES. 1474-1522
Philosophia naturalis compendium. Leipzig, *Melchior Lotter*, 1499.
The last section of this commentary on Aristotle is an illustrated summary of anatomy, the text of which was derived, with some modifications, from medieval manuscripts. The series of eleven woodcuts has been called "the first series of anatomical figures specially prepared for a printed book".

363.3 HUNDT, MAGNUS, *the Elder.* 1449-1519
Antropologium de ho[min]is dignitate, natura, et p[ro]prietatibus. [Leipzig, *Wolfgang Stöcklin*, 1501].
Includes the first illustrations of the viscera in a printed book. The four woodcuts are derived with modifications from Peyligk (No. 363.2).

363.4 ZERBI, GABRIELE. 1445-1505
Liber anathomie corporis humani & singulorum membrorum illius. [Venice, *Locatello for the heirs of Scoto*, 1502].
"The first systematic and sufficiently detailed examination of the human body since Mundinus, far outstripping the latter in scientific accuracy" (Lind, *Pre-Vesalian anatomy*, 10, also 141-56). *See also* Nos. 1589.1 and 1758.1.

364 LEONARDO DA VINCI. 1452-1519
I manoscritti de Leonardo da Vinci della Reale Biblioteca di Windsor. Pubblicata da TEODORO SABACHNIKOFF. Transcritti e annotati da GIOVANNI PIUMATI. 2 vols. Parigi, *E. Rouveyre*, 1898-1901.
Includes ff. A-B of his anatomical MSS. Text in French and Italian.

365 ——. Quaderni d'anatomia I-VI. Fogli della Royal Library di Windsor, pubblicati da C. L. VANGENSTEN, A.FONAHN, H. HOPSTOCK. 6 vols. Christiania, *J.Dybwad*, 1911-16.
Leonardo, "the greatest artist and scientist of the Italian Renaissance, was the founder of iconographic and physiologic anatomy" (Garrison). He made over 750 sketches of all the principal organs of the body, drawings which were adequately reproduced only in recent times. His notes accompanying the drawings are in mirror-writing. Text in Italian, English, and German.

366 ——. Leonardo da Vinci on the human body. The anatomical, physiological, and embryological drawings of Leonardo da Vinci. With translations, emendations, and biographical introduction by CHARLES D. O'MALLEY and J. B. DE C. M. SAUNDERS. New York, *Henry Schuman*, 1952.
Includes 215 plates.

366.1 ——. Corpus of the anatomical studies in the collection...at Windsor Castle. Edited by K. D.KEELE AND C. PEDRETTI. 3 vols. New York, *Johnson Reprint Corporation*, 1980.

Splendid edition reproducing all of the drawings in colour, and with the original chronology and integrity of the drawings restored. Text provides transliteration of Leonardo's notes in the original Italian plus English translation, commentary, etc. Combines material previously published less elegantly and accurately in Nos. 364 & 365. For a scientific analysis of Leonardo's medical writings see K.D. Keele's *Leonardo da Vinci's elements of the science of man*, New York, *Academic Press*, 1983. For Leonardo's contributions to neuroanatomy see E.M. Todd, *The neuroanatomy of Leonardo da Vinci*, Santa Barbara, *Capra Press*, [1983]. For his work on vision see D.S. Strong, *Leonardo on the eye, An English translation and critical commentary on Ms. D. in the Bibliothèque Nationale...* New York, *Garland*, 1979.

367   BERENGARIO DA CARPI, Giacomo. *circa* 1460-1530[?]
Commentaria cum amplissimis additionibus super anatomia Mundini una cum textu ejusdem in pristinum et verum nitorem redacto. Bononiae, *imp. per H. de Benedictis,* 1521.

Berengario introduced iconography and independent anatomical observation into the teaching of anatomy. His *Commentaria* was the first work since the time of Galen to display any considerable amount of anatomical information based upon personal investigation and observation. The *Commentaria* contains the first mention of the vermiform appendix, as well as the first good account of the thymus. The description of the male and female reproductive organs, of reproduction itself, and of the foetus, is more extensive than any earlier account. *See* No. 6010.

368   ——. Isagogae breves perlucide ac uberime in anatomiam humani corporis a communi medicorum academia usitatam. Bononiae, *B. Hectoris,* 1522.

A revised and condensed version of the *Commentaria* (No.367). This is the work by which Berengario is best known. Includes a description of the valves of the heart. English translation by L. R. Lind, Chicago, 1959. The second edition (1523) contains 3 more anatomical woodcuts depicting the heart and brain.

368.01   BRUNSCHWIG, Hieronymus. 1450-*circa* 1512
The noble experyence of the vertuous handywarke of surgeri. London, *Peter Treveris,* 1525.

This translation of Brunschwig's surgery (No. 5559) includes the first anatomical text to be printed in English, a 13-page section with 4 woodcuts. Facsimile, Amsterdam, 1973.

368.1   EDWARDES, David. 1502-1542
De indiciis et praecognitionibus, opus apprime utile medicis. Eiusdem in anatomicen introductio luculenta et brevis. Londini, *R. Redmanus,* 1532.

First anatomical text by an Englishman. The only known copy is in the British Museum. Edwardes made the first recorded dissection in England (1531). Reproduced in facsimile with an English translation by C. D. O'Malley and K. F. Russell, London, 1961. See biographical note by A. Rook and M. Newbold, *Med. Hist.,* 1975, **19,** 389.

369   LAGUNA, Andrés [Lacuna]. 1499-1560
Anatomica methodus, seu de sectione humani corporis contemplatio. Parisiis, *apud J. Kerver,* 1535.

Includes the first description of the ileo-caecal valve. Laguna, a Spanish anatomist, travelled much in Europe and became physician to Charles V. English translation in No. 461.3.

370   DRYANDER, JOHANN [EICHMANN]. 1500-1560
Anatomia capitis humani, Marpurgi, *E. Cervicorni,* 1536.
The first work on the anatomy of the head. Illustrated with 11 woodcuts. English translation in No. 461.3.

371   ——. Anatomiae, hoc est, corporis humani dissectionis pars prior. Marpurgi, *apud E. Cervicornum,* 1537.
Dryander was among the first to make illustrations after his own dissections. His unfinished *Anatomiae,* expanded from the *Anatomia* published the previous year, is one of the most important of the pre-Vesalian atlases. Choulant ascribes the woodcuts to the school of Hans Brosamer (Frankfurt) while Herrlinger suggests that they may come from the Basel school. This book includes the first printing of Gabriele de Zerbis's *Anatomia infantis* and Copho's *Anatomia porci.*

372   VESALIUS, ANDREAS. 1514-1564
Tabulae anatomicae sex. Venetiis, *sumpt. J. S. Calcarensis,* 1538.
Vesalius' first anatomical publication, consisting of six oversized anatomical charts, resembling fugitive sheets. The three skeletal woodcuts are signed by the artist, Jan Stephan van Calcar, who also acted as the publisher. The other woodcuts were engraved after drawings by Vesalius. Only two complete sets of the original edition exist – one in the Bibliotheca Nazionale Marciana, Venice, and the other in the Hunterian Collection at the University of Glasgow Library, donated by Sir William Stirling-Maxwell, who published a limited edition facsimile of his copy for private distribution (London, 1874). Singer and Rabin, *A prelude to modern science,* Cambridge, 1946, reproduces the sheets half-size with commentary. A full-size facsimile appears in Vesalius, *Tabulae Anatomicae,* Munich, *Bremer Press,* 1934. The woodcuts also appear with commentary in Saunders and O'Malley, *The illustrations from the works of Andreas Vesalius,* Cleveland, *World Publishing,* 1950.

372.1   ——. Andreas VESALIUS's first public anatomy at Bologna, 1540. An eyewitness report by BALDASAR HESELER together with his notes on MATTHAEUS CURTIUS's lectures on anatomia. MUNDINI edited, with an introduction, translation into English and notes by RUBEN ERIKSSON. Uppsala, *Almqvist & Wiksells,* 1959.
A unique manuscript discovery helping us to bridge the gap in the development of Vesalius's ideas between the *Tabulae anatomicae sex* (1538) and the *Fabrica* (1543).

373   CANANO, GIOVANNI BATTISTA. 1515-1579
Musculorum humani corporis picturata dissectio. [Ferrara, 1541?].
Contains copper-plates of the bones and muscles of the upper limb, from drawings by Girolamo da Carpi, which "in realism and exactitude surpassed anything between Leonardo and Vesalius; but having seen the woodcuts of [Vesalius's] *Fabrica,* the high-minded Ferrarese deliberately suppressed his own book, and only 11 copies are now extant" (A. C. Klebs). The first book in which each muscle was illustrated separately. This fine work was reprinted in facsimile in Florence, 1925, edited by Harvey Cushing and E. C. Streeter. English translation in No. 461.3.

373.1   RYFF, WALTHER HERMANN. (d. before 1562)
Des aller fürtrefflichsten...erschaffen. Das is des menchen...warhafftige
beschreibung oder Anatomi...[Strasbourg, *Balthassar Beck*], 1541.

This plagiarism of Vesalius's *Tabulae anatomicae sex* contains 25
woodcuts by Hans Baldung Grien (1484/1485-1545), and represents the
artist's only contribution to medical illustration. The woodcuts include the
best illustrations of brain dissection techniques published before Vesalius's
Fabrica.

374   LOBERA DE AVILA, LUIS. *fl.* 1551
Libro de anatomia *In:* Remedio de cuerpos humanos y silva de experiencias
y otras cosas utilissimas: nuevamente compuesto... [Alcalá de Henares,
Juan de Brocar, 1542?].

Text in Spanish and Latin.

375   VESALIUS, ANDREAS. 1514-1564
De humani corporis fabrica libri septem. Basileae, *ex off. Ioannis Oporini,*
1543.

Published when the author was only 29 years old, the *Fabrica* revolutionized not only the science of anatomy but how it was taught.
Throughout this encylopaedic work on the structure and workings of the
human body, Vesalius provided a fuller and more detailed description of
the human anatomy than any of his predecessors, correcting errors in the
traditional anatomical teachings of Galen. Even more epochal than his
criticism of Galen and other medieval authorities was Vesalius's assertion
that the dissection of cadavers must be performed by the physician himself.

As revolutionary as the contents of the *Fabrica* and the anatomical
discoveries which it published, was its unprecedented blending of scientific exposition, art and typography. The title page and series of woodcut
musclemen remain the most famous anatomical illustrations of all time.
The artist or artists responsible for these masterworks has been the source
of continuing scholarly speculation for centuries, but any definite attribu-
tion remains unproven.   In *The illustrations from the works of Andreas
Vesalius* (1950) Saunders and O'Malley published reduced versions of all
the illustrations from Vesalius's writings, with a commentary and biographical sketch. The standard biography is C.D. O'Malley, *Andreas Vesalius
of Brussels*, Berkeley, 1964. Harvey Cushing's classic *Biobibliography of
Andreas Vesalius* (1943) appeared in a second edition, Hamden, Conn.,
1962, and the third edition is in preparation. See also the dated but classic
work, M. Roth, *Andreas Vesalius Bruxellensis,* Berlin, *Reimer,* 1892;
reprinted Amsterdam, *Asher,* 1965.

376   ——. Suorum de humani corporis fabrica librorum epitome. Basileae (*ex
off. J. Oporini,* 1543).

The *Epitome,* which Vesalius viewed as a sort of outline guide to the
encycyclopaedic *Fabrica*, falls in the tradition of anatomical fugitive sheets
and the *Tabulae Anatomicae sex.* Published in a larger format than the
folio *Fabrica*, it contains a series of wall charts illustrated with woodcuts,
in which seven oversize figures appear for the first time. Planned by
Vesalius along with the *Fabrica*, the *Epitome* was probably published almost simultaneously, making the *Fabrica* one of very few epochal publications to be issued together with a "précis" by the author.   Reduced size
facsimile reproduction, with translation, New York, 1949.

376.1   GEMINUS, THOMAS. circa 1510-1562.
          Compendiosa totius anatomie delineatio, aere exarata. London, [John
          Herford, 1545.]
              Although by tradition and Vesalius's own comments this work has been
          considered the first of the many plagiarisms of Vesalius's *Fabrica and
          Epitome,* Geminus gave full credit to Vesalius in a bold headline on the first
          leaf of text. He did, however, redraw Vesalius's woodcuts without permis-
          sion. This is the second work printed in England with engraved plates. The
          new medium of copperplate engraving used by Geminus allowed a
          sharpness of line impossible for the wood engravers employed by Vesalius.
          The title page was called by Hind, "the first engraving of any artistic
          importance produced in England". The book provided a summary view
          of Vesalius's discoveries more complete than the *Epitome* but without the
          size and expense of the *Fabrica.* English translation by the pioneer English
          playwright, Nicholas Udall, 1553. Facsimile edition of the translation with
          introduction by C.D. O'Malley, London, 1959. *See* No. 6139.

377   ——. De humani corporis fabrica libri septem. Basileae, *J. Oporinus,* 1555.
              Containing Vesalius's final revisions of the text, this edition is also
          superior for its enlarged format, improved typography and printing, better
          paper, larger woodcut initials, and changes to the lettering of the anatomi-
          cal woodcuts. Most of the original woodblocks from the second edition
          along with the anatomical captions were splendidly reprinted as *Icones
          Anatomicae* by the Bremer Press for the New York Academy of Medicine
          and the University of Munich, 1934. The woodblocks had been preserved
          in the University of Munich but were destroyed in World War II.

378   ESTIENNE, CHARLES [STEPHANUS]. 1504-1564
          De dissectione partium corporis humani. Parisiis, *apud S. Colinaeum,* 1545.
              First published work to include illustrations of the whole external
          venous and nervous systems. A French translation appeared from the same
          press in 1546. The physician author was the son of Henri Estienne, the
          founder of the Estienne dynasty of scholar-printers, and the son-in-law of
          the printer of this book, Simon de Colines. The magnificent woodcuts in
          this work were by Jean ("Mercure") Jollat and the surgeon/artist and
          collaborator on the work, Estienne de la Rivière, possibly after designs by
          the Florentine artist/architect Giovanni Battista Rosso. The cuts were
          begun as early as 1530 by Jollat, and Estienne and Rivière collaborated on
          the book as early as 1539. However publication of this manual of
          dissection was delayed because of a lawsuit brought against Estienne by
          Rivière. Had the book appeared prior to 1543 as planned it would have
          eclipsed some of the innovation of Vesalius's *Fabrica.* Reprint of French
          translation, Paris, *Azoulay,* 1972.

378.01   MONTAÑA DE MONTSERRATE, BERNARDINO. circa 1480-?
          Libro de la anathomia del hombre. Valladolid, *Sebastian Martinez,* 1551.
              The first Spanish anatomy book in the Spanish language, the second
          anatomy book ever published in Spain, and the work that introduced
          Vesalian illustrations to Spain. The text is a version of Henri de Mondeville's
          medieval anatomy. The 12 anatomical woodcuts may have been executed
          by the printer, Sebastian Martinez.

378.02   VALVERDE, JUAN DE HAMUSCO. *fl.* 1550
          Historia de la composicion del cuerpo humano...Rome, *Antonio Sala-
          manca,* 1556.

The first great original medical book in Spanish and the most original of the "plagiarisms" from Vesalius, although Valverde freely acknowledged that he took his illustrations from Vesalius, providing only four entirely new plates in his 42 engravings from the Vesalian woodcuts. The plates were engraved by Nicolas Beatrizet probably after Gaspar Becerra, a pupil of Michelangelo. The book contains numerous revisions to Vesalius and other discoveries by Valverde.

378.1   COLOMBO, MATTEO REALDO [COLUMBUS]. *circa* 1510-1559
De re anatomica libri xv. Venetiis, *ex typ. Nicolai Beuilacquae,* 1559.
Colombo was a pupil of Vesalius and succeeded him in the chair of anatomy at Padua before proceeding to chairs first at Pisa and later at Rome. His book, published just after his death, rectified a number of anatomical errors, but he plagiarized and disparaged his predecessors. He described the pulmonary circulation but may have read the account of Servetus published six years previously. He gave a clear description of the mode of action of the pulmonary, cardiac, and aortic valves. The only illustration in this work is the fine woodcut title page influenced by the title page of the *Fabrica* and suggesting the relief by Donatello entitled *Miser's Heart.* Colombo met Michelangelo in 1547 and supposedly he attempted to commission Michelangelo to illustrate this book. Unfortunately that project never transpired. English translation of the section on pulmonary circulation in John Banister, *The historie of man sucked from the sappe of the most approved anathomistes...*London, *John Daye,* 1578. English translation of book XV by R.J. Moes and C.D. O'Malley, *Realdo Colombo: "On those things rarely found in anatomy", Bull. Hist. Med.,* 1960, **34**, 508-28.

378.2   FALLOPPIO, GABRIELE [FALLOPIUS]. 1523-1562
Observationes anatomicae. Venetiis, *apud M. A. Ulmum,* 1561.
Fallopius studied under Vesalius and became professor of anatomy at Ferrara (1547), Pisa (1548) and Padua (1551). He was a careful dissector, a great observer, and an accurate recorder. He discovered and first described the chorda tympani and semicircular canals, correctly described the structure and course of the cerebral vessels, knew the circular folds of the small intestines. He enumerated all the nerves of the eye, and introduced a number of anatomical names. He is eponymously remembered by the Fallopian tube and the Fallopian aqueduct.

379   BAUHIN, CASPAR [BAUHINUS]. 1560-1624
Theatrum anatomicum infinitis locis auctum, ad morbos accommodatum, *etc.* Basileae, *S. Henric Petri,* 1592.
Includes historical data. Bauhin was professor of anatomy at Basle.

380   GUIDI, GUIDO [VIDIUS]. 1508-1569
De anatome corporis humani libri vii. Venetiis, *apud Juntas,* 1611.
Guidi, professor of philosophy and medicine at Pisa, discovered the Vidian nerve, the Vidian canal, and the Vidian artery. The above was edited by his nephew.

381   CASSERI, GUILIO [JULIUS CASSERIUS *Placentinus*]. 1561?-1616
Tabulae anatomicae lxxiix. Venetiis, *apud E. Deuchinum,* 1627.
First publication of the very beautiful copperplates engraved by Francesco Valesio after Odoardo Fialetti, a pupil of Titian. Casseri commis-

sioned these plates covering the whole field of human anatomy for his unfinished masterwork entitled *Theatrum anatomicum*. For this publication, the editor, Daniel Rindfleisch (Bucretius) added another 20 plates by the same artist/engraver team. *See* No. 61.2.

381.1   GRACHT, Jacob van der. 1593-1652
Anatomie der uuterlicke deelen van het menschelick lichaem...Graven Hagae, *den Auteur*, 1634.
    The earliest of all independent works on anatomy for graphic or plastic artists.

382   HIGHMORE, Nathaniel. 1613-1685
Corporis humani disquisitio anatomica. Hagai-Comitis, *S. Broun*, 1651.
    Highmore is remembered for his description of the "antrum of Highmore" (already noticed by Casserius and figured by Leonardo da Vinci), the seminal ducts and the epididymis. This was also the first English work to accept Harvey's ideas on the circulation. The interesting engraved title page compares the body allegorically to a garden.

383   KERCKRING, Thomas Theodor. 1640-1693
Spicilegium anatomicum. Amstelodami, *sumpt. A. Frisii*, 1670.
    Kerckring made important investigations on the development of the foetal bones. He was the first to describe the large ossicle sometimes present at the lambdoidal suture; his name is remembered in the *valvulae conniventes* of the small intestine, previously described by Fallopius.

384   GENGA, Bernardino. 1665-1734
Anatomia chirurgica. Roma, *A. Ercole*, 1672.
    First book devoted entirely to surgical anatomy.

385   BIDLOO, Govert. 1649-1713
Anatomia humani corporis, centum et quinque tabulis, per artificiosiss. G. de Lairesse ad vivum delineatis. Amstelodami, *vid. J. à Someren*, 1685.
    The value of Bidloo's *Anatomia* lies chiefly in the 105 fine copperplate engravings drawn by Gérard de Lairesse, and engraved by Pieter van Gunst. These are masterpieces of Dutch baroque art. When William of Orange came to England in 1688, Bidloo was chosen to accompany him as his physician. Facsimile reprint, Paris, 1972. See P. Dumaître, *La curieuse destinée des planches anatomiques de Gérard de Lairesse*, Amsterdam, *Rodopi*, 1982.

385.1   COWPER, William. 1666-1709
The anatomy of humane bodies, with figures drawn after the life by some of the best masters in Europe. Oxford, *Sam. Smith*, 1698.
    The most elaborate and beautiful of all 17th century English treatises on anatomy and also one of the most extraordinary plagiarisms in the entire history of medicine. Cowper purchased sets of the van Gunst copperplates used to illustrate Bidloo's book, and issued them under his own name with an English text and a new illustrated appendix. For the frontispiece Cowper had a small printed flap with his own name pasted over Bidloo's title and name. Naturally Bidloo accused Cowper of plagiarism and published the record of the case in the following polemic: *Gulielmus Cowper, criminis literarii citatus, coram tribunali nobiliss., ampliss: Societatis Britanno-Regiae*, Leiden, 1700.

386   GENGA, BERNARDINO. 1655-1734
Anatomia per uso et intelligenza del disegno ricercata non solo su gl'ossi,
e muscoli del corpo humano. Roma, *G. J. de Rossi,* 1691.
     Contains 56 copper-plates, excellent anatomically and artistically, with
commentary by Giovanni Maria Lancisi. This is one of the finest of all books
on anatomy for artists. English translation with plates re-engraved, London, *Senex,* [1723].

387   HAVERS, CLOPTON. *d.*1702
Osteologia nova, or some new observations of the bones. London, *S. Smith,*
1691.
     Havers discovered the Haversian canals and made important observa-
tions of the physiology of bone growth and repair. The Haversian lamellae,
glands, and folds, are also named after him. The Haversian canals were
observed by van Leeuwenhoek in 1686.

388   VERHEYEN, PHILIPPE. 1648-1710
Anatomia corporis humani. Lovanii, 1693.
     This work was widely used for some years after publication, supersed-
ing Bartholin in popularity. Second edition, with supplement, 2 vols.,
Louvain, 1706-12.

389   RUYSCH, FREDERIK. 1638-1731
Thesaurus anatomicus. i-x. Amstelaedami, *J. Wolters,* 1701-16.
     Ruysch, professor of anatomy at Leyden and Amsterdam, is notable for
his method of injecting the vessels. The recipe for the material used by
Ruysch has remained a secret. He gave the first description of bronchial
blood vessels and vascular plexuses of the heart, demonstrated the valves
of the lymphatics, and made a great number of other important discoveries
in anatomy.

390   CHESELDEN, WILLIAM. 1688-1752
The anatomy of the humane body. London, *N. Cliff & D. Jackson,* 1713.
     Although Cheselden is best known for his accomplishments in the field
of surgery, he wrote two important books on anatomy. The above was for
many years a textbook of the English medical schools and ran through 13
editions.

391   EUSTACHI, BARTOLOMEO [EUSTACHIUS]. *circa* 1510/1520-1574
Tabulae anatomicae. Romae, *ex off. F. Gonzagae,* 1714.
     A romantic history attaches to this fine collection of plates, drawn by
Eustachius himself and completed in 1552. They remained unprinted and
forgotten in the Vatican Library until discovered in the early 18th century,
and were then presented by Pope Clement XI to his physician, Giovanni
Maria Lancisi. The latter published them in 1714 together with his own
notes. These copperplates are more accurate than the work of Vesalius.
Singer was of the opinion that had they appeared in 1552 Eustachius would
have ranked with Vesalius as one of the founders of modern anatomy. He
discovered the Eustachian tube, the thoracic duct, the adrenals and the
abducens nerve, and gave the first accurate description of the uterus. He
also described the cochlea, the muscles of the throat and the origin of the
optic nerves.

392   SANTORINI, GIOVANNI DOMENICO. 1681-1737
       Observationes anatomicae. Venetiis, *apud J. B. Recurti,* 1724.
          Santorini was one of the ablest dissectors of his day. In the above work
       many new discoveries of anatomical details are set forth, together with
       corrections of some of the errors of earlier anatomists. The work describes
       the four major discoveries for which Santorini is known eponymically:
       Santorini's cartilage, Santorini's vein, Santorini's duct, and Santorini's
       caruncula.

392.1 COWPER, WILLIAM. 1666-1709
       Myotomia reformata. London, *Robert Knaplock,* 1724.
          This work made a modest first appearance in 1694 as an octavo, but
       Cowper worked until his death on a new edition which was finally
       published posthumously under the supervision and at the expense of
       Richard Mead (1673-1754). This sumptuous folio with engravings after
       Rubens and Raphael and an ingenious set of historiated initials ranks
       among the most artistic anatomical atlases of the period.

393   CHOVET, ABRAHAM. 1704-1799
       A syllabus or index, of all the parts that enter the composition of the human
       body...For the use of those that go through courses of anatomy. London,
       1732.
          Chovet was born in England and died in Philadelphia. He made many
       beautiful wax models to illustrate his lectures, and was among the first to
       popularize the use of wax and natural preparations in the teaching of
       anatomy, devices which he advocated in his *Syllabus.* The book gives an
       interesting picture of the methods employed in the teaching of anatomy in
       the mid 18th century. Chovet's famous collection of models went to
       Pennsylvania University, where it later perished in a fire.

394   WINSLOW, JACQUES BÉNIGNE. 1669-1760
       Exposition anatomique de la structure du corps humain. Paris, *G. Desprez
       et J. Dessesartz,* 1732.
          The foramen between the greater and lesser sacs of the peritoneum
       (described on pages 352-65), is named after Winslow. His *Exposition* is
       distinguished as being the first book on descriptive anatomy to discard
       physiological details and hypothetical explanations foreign to the subject.
       He did much to condense and systematize the anatomical knowledge of
       his time. Includes a reprint of the text of Stensen, *Discours sur l'anatomie
       du cerveau,* Paris, 1669. English translation, 2 vols., 1733-34. *See* No. 1314.

395   CHESELDEN, WILLIAM. 1688-1752
       Osteographia, or the anatomy of the bones. London, 1733.
          This splendidly designed and illustrated work contained full and
       accurate descriptions of all the human bones, as well as many of animals.
       Cheselden is the first person to have used the camera obscura to gain
       precision in his illustrations, and the vignette on the title page shows him
       using this instrument. The engravings are beautifully executed by Van der
       Gucht. In 1720 Cheselden inaugurated lectures on anatomy and surgery at
       St. Thomas's Hospital. See the paper by K. F. Russell, *Bull. Hist. Med.,* 1954,
       28, 32-49, which mentions a trial issue of the book, dated 1728. See also
       Russell, *British Anatomy 1525-1800,* 2nd ed., 1987. Facsimile reprint of
       the undated remainder issue printed without text, Philadelphia, 1968.

395.1   NESBITT, ROBERT. 1700-1761
Human osteogeny explained in two lectures. London, W. Innys, 1736.
Nesbitt pointed out that bones may develop in membrane as well as cartilage, an observation which was ignored until the 19th century. He left an outstanding description of bone growth.

395.2   CORTONA, PIETRO DA [BERRETINI]. 1596-1669
Tabulae anatomicae. Rome, *Fausti Amidei,* 1741.
27 anatomical copperplates after drawings by the most influential painter of the Italian Baroque movement, who also excelled as an architect. The editor, Cajetano Petrioli, supplied the text and small numbered anatomical "figures" in the margins of the plates. The original drawings for the plates are preserved in the Hunterian Collection at the University of Glasgow Library. See J.M. Norman (ed.), *The anatomical plates of Pietro da Cortona,* New York, *Dover,* 1986.

396   LIEUTAUD, JOSEPH. 1703-1780
Essais anatomiques. Paris, *P. M. Huart,* 1742.
Lieutaud rectified many anatomical errors, described carefully the structure and relations of the heart and its cavities, and added to the contemporary knowledge concerning the bladder. The trigonum vesicae is named "Lieutaud's trigone".

396.1   WEITBRECHT, JOSIAS. 1702-1747
Syndesmologia sive historia ligamentorum corporis humani, St. Petersburg, *Academy of Sciences,* 1742.
Weitbrecht is known for "Weitbrecht's ligament" (of the elbow), "Weitbrecht's foramen ovale" (gap in the capusle of the shoulder joint between the glenal-humeral ligaments), and "Weitbrecht's fibres" (retinacular fibres of the neck of the femur). English translation by E. B. Kaplan, Philadelphia, *Saunders,* 1969.

397   HALLER, ALBRECHT VON. 1708-1777
Icones anatomicae. 8 pts. Gottingae, *A. Vandenhoeck,* [1743]-56.
Accurate and beautiful engravings of the diaphragm, uterus, ovaries, vagina, arteries, with explanatory observations.

398   GAUTIER D'AGOTY, JACQUES FABIAN. 1717-1786
Essai d'anatomie en tableaux imprimés. Paris, *chez Gautier,* 1745.
Remarkable for its striking mezzotints printed in colour.

399   ALBINUS, BERNHARD SIEGFRIED. 1697-1770
Tabulae sceleti et musculorum corporis humani. Lugduni Batavorum, *J. & H. Verbeek,* [1737-] 1747.
The splendid series of 40 large copperplates of the bones and muscles in this work were drawn and engraved by Jan Wandelaar (1690-1759). They established a new standard in anatomical illustration, and remain unsurpassed for their artistic beauty and scientific accuracy. English translation with new engravings of the plates, London, *Knapton,* 1749.   The first extensive biography of Albinus, Punt, *Bernard Siegfried Albinus...on "human nature",* Amsterdam, *B.M. Israël,* 1983, publishes the original plans, designs and drawings for his anatomy.

399.1   SANTORINI, GIOVANNI DOMENICO. 1681-1737
         Septemdecim tabulae...Parma, *Typographia Regia,* 1775.
         Santorini died before the completion of these anatomical plates which
         he intended to be his *chef d'œuvre.* This elegantly printed volume is the
         only significant medical book printed by the celebrated Giambattista
         Bodoni for the Duke of Parma.

399.2   MONRO, ALEXANDER *Secundus.* 1733-1817.
         A description of all the bursae mucosae of the human body. Edinburgh, *C.
         Elliot,* 1788.
         The first serious study of this subject and the most original anatomical
         work by the greatest of the Monro dynasty. *See* No. 1385.

400   SOEMMERRING, SAMUEL THOMAS. 1755-1830
         Vom Baue des menschlichen Körpers. 5 pts. Frankfurt a. M., *Varrentrapp
         u. Wenner,* 1791-96.
         Soemmerring's text-book contained only facts actually observed by
         him. He departed from the usual practice of including physiology with
         anatomy. The book was very popular in German medical schools, and
         Meckel considered it Soemmerring's best work. It includes a very full list
         of what Soemmerring considered his anatomical discoveries.

401   ——. Tabula sceleti feminini juncta descriptione. Trajecti ad Moenum,
         Varrentrapp undWenner, 1797.
         Soemmerring was noted for his accuracy in anatomical illustration, and
         the above work is a fine example of his artistic sense. For it he selected the
         skeleton of a well-built girl of 20 years. Great care was taken in selecting
         the most appropriate posture and the contour of an ideally perfect female
         body in which the skeleton might be drawn in order properly to observe
         its proportions.

401.1   GAMELIN, JACQUES. 1738-1803
         Nouveau recueil d'ostéologie et de myologie...Toulouse, *J.F. Desclassan,*
         1779.
         "Without contest the most beautiful of all anatomies for the artist and
         one of the most remarkable books of its time" (Hahn & Dumaitre). The
         plates in this work are more fantastic than any other anatomy, suggesting
         the work of Goya, who may have known or studied with Gamelin since
         Gamelin taught in Rome during the time Goya was there.

401.2   VICQ D'AZYR, FÉLIX. 1748-1794.
         Traité d'anatomie et de physiologie avec des planches coloriées réprésentant
         au naturel les divers organes de l'homme et des animaux. Tome premier
         [all published]. Paris, *François Ambroise Didot l'aîné,* 1786.
         The most accurate neuroanatomical work produced before the advent
         of microscopic staining techniques. Vicq d'Azyr identified accurately for
         the first time many of the cerebral convolutions, along with various internal
         structures of the brain. This was the first volume of an ambitious study of
         anatomy and physiology which remained unfinished at Vicq d'Azyr's
         premature death.

401.3   BELL, JOHN. 1763-1820 & BELL, *Sir* CHARLES. 1774-1842
         The anatomy of the human body. 4 vols. Edinburgh, *Cadell & Davies,* 1797-
         1804.

"The first great textbook contributed by the British school to modern anatomy"(Russell, No. 461).

402   BELL, *Sir* CHARLES. 1774-1842
        A system of dissections. 2 vols. Edinburgh, *Mundell & Son,* 1798-1803.
        Published in 7 fascicules and appendix while Bell was still a student, this was Bell's first independent venture as an author. The anatomical work of Charles Bell and his brother John was the most important in the British Isles during the early part of the 19th century.

403   BICHAT, MARIE FRANÇOIS XAVIER. 1771-1802
        Anatomie générale, appliquée à la physiologie et à la médicine. 4 vols. [in 2]. Paris, *Brosson, Gabon & Cie.,* an X [1802].
        Bichat revolutionized descriptive anatomy. Where Morgagni and others had conceived of whole organs being diseased, Bichat showed how individual tissues could be separately affected. He covered tissue pathology, system by system in the *Anatomie générale,* showing that tissues from different organs are similar and subject to the same diseases, and identifying 21 different types of tissues. This was done essentially without a microscope, but marks the beginning of modern histology. The above work and No. 404 are remarkable in their total reliance on verbal description to convey anatomical detail, since neither work contains a single illustration. English translation, 3 vols., Boston, 1822.

404   ———. Traité d'anatomie descriptive. 5 vols. Paris, *Gabon & Cie.,* an X-XII [1801-03].
        Bichat's last work, unfinished at his death. Vol. 4 was prepared by Mathieu-François Buisson and vol. 5 by Philibert-Joseph Roux. See No. 1315.

405   BURNS, ALLAN. 1781-1813
        Observations on the surgical anatomy of the head and neck. Edinburgh, *T. Bryce,* 1811.
        See also Nos. 2889, 3055. Burns was the first to suggest (p. 31) ligature of the innominate artery. His book describes "Burns's space", the fascial space at the suprasternal notch.

406   MEDICO, GIUSEPPE DEL.
        Anatomia per uso de'pittori e scultori. Roma, *V. Poggioli,* 1811.
        This anatomy for artists and sculptors contains 38 good copperplates in black and red.

407   MECKEL, JOHANN FRIEDRICH, *the younger.* 1781-1833
        Handbuch der menschlichen Anatomie. 4 vols. *Halle & Berlin,* 1815-20.

408   RIEMER, PIETER DE. 1760-1831
        Afbeeldingen van de juiste plaatsing der inwendige deelen van het menschelijk ligchaam. 's-Gravenhage, *J. Allart,* 1818.
        First use of frozen sections for anatomical illustration. De Riemer appears to have been the first to freeze tissues in order to permit fine sectioning.

409   CLOQUET, JULES GERMAIN. 1790-1883
        Anatomie de l'homme. 5 vol. Paris, *C. de Lasteyrie,* 1821-31.
        The first anatomical atlas illustrated by lithography, containing 300 plates in folio format. This was probably the most elaborate of the

lithographic "incunabula" produced by de Lasteyrie, one of the pioneer lithographers in France. Cloquet was professor of clinical surgery, Paris. Second edition in reduced format, Paris, 1825-[36].

409.1   MASCAGNI, PAOLO. 1752-1815
Anatomia universa...2 vols. Pisa, *Niccolo Capurro,* [1822], 1823-30, [1832].
    The largest of all medical books from the standpoint of format. The 44 life size engraved plates are reproduced in double elephant folio size measuring 950 x 635 mm., and include an almost incredible level of detail. Published posthumously in fascicules over ten years, very few sets were issued. Those with the plates hand-coloured by the artist, Antonio Serrantoni, are among the most breathtakingly beautiful of all anatomical studies. Three plates placed end-to-end illustrate the entire figure life-size. Incomplete piracy by Antommarchi (1823-26). Small folio authorized edition with more conveniently sized versions of the dramatic colour plates, 2 vols., Firenze, *Batelli,* 1833. *See also* no. 1104.

410   QUAIN, JONES. 1796-1865
Elements of descriptive and practical anatomy. London, *W. Simpkin & R. Marshall,* 1828.
    Among the most important of the English textbooks on anatomy. An eleventh edition was published in 1908-29.

411   FLAXMAN, JOHN. 1755-1826
Anatomical studies of the bones and muscles, for the use of artists. London, *M. A. Nattali,* 1833.
    Plates engraved by Henry Landseer from Flaxman's drawings.

411.1   BELL, CHARLES. 1774-1842
The hand: Its mechanism and vital endowments as evincing design. London, *William Pickering,* 1833.
    Classic work on the anatomy, physiology, bio-mechanics, comparative anatomy, and adaptive importance of the hand. The first edition has 288pp. An enlarged second edition with 314pp. was also published in 1833, without notice on the title page.

412   HUXLEY, THOMAS HENRY. 1825-1895
On a hitherto undescribed structure in the human hair sheath. *Lond. med. Gaz.,* 1845, **36,** 1340-41.
    "Huxley's layer" and "membrane" of the root sheath of hair follicles.

413   HYRTL, JOSZEF. 1810-1894
Lehrbuch der Anatomie des Menschen. Prag, *F. Ehrlich,* 1846.
    Hyrtl's *Lehrbuch* passed through 22 editions and was translated into the principal modern languages.

414   ———. Handbuch der topographischen Anatomie. 2 vols. Wien, *W. Braumüller,* 1847.
    Hyrtl, professor of anatomy at Vienna, published the first text on topographical anatomy in German. He was for 30 years the most popular lecturer on the subject in Europe, and ranks as one of the greatest of medical scholars.

415   KNOX, ROBERT. 1791-1862
A manual of artistic anatomy. London, *H. Renshaw,* 1852.

Knox, remembered because of his indiscreet association with the Edinburgh "resurrectionists", was one of the best teachers of anatomy during the 19th century.

416   PIROGOV, NIKOLAI IVANOVICH. 1810-1881
Anatome topographica sectionibus per corpus humanum congelatum triplici directione ductis illustrata. 8 pts. Petropoli, *J. Trey,* 1852-59.
     Pirogov was the greatest of all Russian surgeons. In Russian medicine he is approached only by Pavlov. He introduced the teaching of applied topographical anatomy in Russia. His great atlas of 220 plates represents the first use on a grand scale of frozen sections in anatomical illustration, an idea first carried out by de Riemer (No. 408).

417   HENLE, FRIEDRICH GUSTAV JAKOB. 1809-1885
Handbuch der systematischen Anatomie des Menschen. 3 vols. Braunschweig, *F. Vieweg u. Sohn,* 1855-71.
     Considered by many authorities to be the greatest of the modern systems of anatomy. Many structures are named after Henle, including the looped portion of the uriniferous tubules of the kidney, the layer of cells in the root sheath of a hair, and the ampulla of the uterine tube.

418   GRAY, HENRY. 1825-1861
Anatomy, descriptive and surgical. London, *J. W. Parker & Son,* 1858.
     Gray's textbook of anatomy remains today a standard work on the subject in the English-speaking world. The 37th edition appeared in 1989; the first American edition was published at Philadelphia, 1859.

419   HUMPHRY, *Sir* GEORGE MURRAY. 1820-1896
A treatise on the human skeleton, including the joints. Cambridge, *Macmillan & Co.,* 1858.
     Humphry was professor of anatomy at Cambridge and became the first professor of surgery there. He founded the *Journal of Anatomy and Physiology* in 1867. "Humphry's ligament" of the knee-joint is described on p. 546 of the above book and pictured on plate 53, fig. 1.

420   OLLIER, LOUIS ZAVIER EDOUARD LÉOPOLD. 1830-1900
Des moyens chirurgicaux de favoriser la reproduction des os après les résections *Gaz. hebd. Méd. Chir.* 1858, **5,** 572-7, 651-3, 733-6, 769-70, 853-7, 890, 899-905.
     "Ollier's layer", the osteogenetic layer of the periosteum.

421   LEIDY, JOSEPH. 1823-1891
An elementary treatise on human anatomy. Philadelphia, *J. B. Lippincott,* 1861.
     Leidy himself illustrated this book. He was professor of anatomy at Philadelphia and the leading American anatomist of his time.

422   SIBSON, FRANCIS. 1814-1876
Medical anatomy: or, illustrations of the relative position and movements of the internal organs. 7 pts. London, *J. Churchill,* [1855]-69.
     Sibson was professor of medicine at St. Mary's Hospital. "Sibson's fascia" and "muscle" are named after him. Plates 19-21 show movements, structure and sounds of the heart.

423   HEITZMANN, CARL. 1836-1896
Die descriptive und topographische Anatomie des Menschen. Wien, *W. Braumüller,* 1870.

424   BRAUNE, CHRISTIAN WILHELM. 1831-1892
        Topographisch-anatomischer Atlas. Nach Durchschnitten angefrornen
        Cadavern. Leipzig, *Veit & Co.,* 1872.
            Fine illustrations of frozen sections.

425   HYRTL, JOSZEF. 1810-1894
        Die Corrosions-Anatomie und ihre Ergebnisse. Wien, *W. Braumüller,* 1873.
            Hyrtl, skilled in making anatomical preparations, built up a collection
        which was unsurpassed in Europe. In the above work he described a
        method of his own invention, in which he injected the blood supplies of
        the different organs, the adjacent parts being eaten away by acids, in order
        to show the finest ramifications. The technique of wax impregnation and
        later corrosion was of course known to the Hunters.

426   REID, ROBERT WILLIAM. 1851-1939
        Observations on the relation of the principal fissures and convolutions of
        the cerebrum to the outer surface of the scalp. *Lancet,* 1884, **2,** 539-40.
            Reid's base line – the anthropometric base line on the skull.

427   KOLLMANN, JULIUS KONSTANTIN ERNST. 1834-1918
        Plastische Anatomie des menschlichen Körpers. Leipzig, *Veit & Co.,* 1886.
            "Illustrated with lithographs from hand-drawings, photographs from
        the nude, ethnic studies of facial features...The text...is of unusual historic
        interest, and includes special chapters on the anatomy of the infant, human
        proportions, and ethnic morphology" (Choulant, transl. Frank).

428   TESTUT, JEAN LEO. 1849-1925
        Traité d'anatomie humaine. 3 vols. Paris, *O. Doin,* 1889-92.
            7th edition, 1921-23.

429   BRODIE, CHARLES GORDON. 1860-1933
        Dissections illustrated. London, *Whittaker & Co.,* 1892-95.
            "Brodie's ligament", the transverse humoral ligament, described.

430   SPALTEHOLZ, KARL WERNER. 1861-1940
        Handatlas der Anatomie des Menschen. 3 vols. Leipzig, *S. Hirzel,* 1895-1903.
            16th edition in English, 1967.

431   MACEWEN, *Sir* WILLIAM. 1848-1924
        Atlas of head sections. Glasgow, *J. Maclehose,* 1893.
            Intended to supplement and illustrate Macewen's neurosurgical text-
        book published the same year (No.4872).

432   HIS, WILHELM, *Snr.* 1831-1904
        Die anatomische Nomenclatur. Leipzig, *Veit & Co.,* 1895.
            His was largely responsible for the Basle Nomina Anatomica, the first
        attempt to produce a standard anatomical nomenclature. English transla-
        tion by L. F. Barker, 1907.

433   BARDELEBEN, KARL VON. 1849-1918
        Handbuch der Anatomie des Menschen. Herausgegeben von K. VON
        BARDELEBEN. 32 parts. Jena, *G. Fischer,* 1896-1934.
            An important collective work.

434 ———. Lehrbuch der systematischen Anatomie des Menschen. Berlin, Wien, *Urban & Schwarzenberg,* 1906.

435 MERKEL, Friedrich Sigmund. 1845-1919
Die Anatomie des Menschen. 3 pts. Wiesbaden, *J. F. Bergmann,* 1913-14.

436 WOERDEMANN, Martinus Willem. 1892–
Nomina anatomica Parisiensia (1955) and B.N.A. (1895). Utrecht, *Oostboek,* 1957.
Includes historical sketch of the systems of anatomical nomenclature.

436.1 NETTER, Frank Henry. 1906-
Atlas of human anatomy. Summit, N.J., *Ciba-Geigy Corporation,* [1989].
The culmination of the life work of the greatest anatomical illustrator of the 20th century. Includes 514 full-colour plates, many of which were created for this atlas. Reproduction of previously published plates was enhanced in this superbly produced work. With S. Colacino, consulting editor.

History of Anatomy

See also ART AND MEDICINE

437 BAUHIN, Caspar [Bauhinus]. 1560-1624
Anatomica corporis virilis et muliebris historia. Lugduni, *J. le Preux,* 1597.

437.1 PORTAL, Antoine. 1742-1832
Histoire de l'anatomie et de la chirurgie. 6 vols. [in 7]. Paris, P.F. *Didot le jeune,* 1770-73.
A biobibliographical survey to 1755.

438 HALLER, Albrecht von. 1708-1777
Bibliotheca anatomica. 2 vols. Tiguri, *apud Orell, Gessner,* etc., 1774-77.
Haller is one of the greatest names in medical bibliography. While pursuing his monumental scientific career he found time to compile bibliographies of botany, anatomy, medicine and surgery which together form the most exhaustive summary of previous writings on these subjects. Reprinted, Hildesheim, *G. Olms,* 1969.

439 HYRTL, Joszef. 1810-1894
Antiquitates anatomicae rariores. Vindobonae, *typ. Congregationis Mechitaristicae,* 1835.

440 CHOULANT, Johann Ludwig. 1791-1861
Geschichte und Bibliographie der anatomischen Abbildung. Leipzig, *R. Weigel,* 1852.
In this classic work Choulant traced the evolution of anatomical illustration from the early schematic plates up to his own time, including a valuable bibliography. Reprinted, Wiesbaden, 1974. An English translation of the work by Mortimer Frank appeared in 1920 (Chicago, *University Press*) and this is enriched by a chapter on anatomical illustration since Choulant, written by F. H. Garrison. A reprint of the translation appeared in 1945 with additional essays by Garrison *et al,* plus a new historical essay by Charles Singer. This was reprinted in 1962 (New York, *Hafner.*)

442   KEEN, WILLIAM WILLIAMS. 1837-1932
       A sketch of the early history of practical anatomy. Philadelphia, *J. B. Lippincott,* 1874.
           Reprinted in Keen's *Addresses and other papers,* Philadelphia, 1905.

443   HYRTL, JOSZEF. 1810-1894
       Das Arabische un Hebräische in der Anatomie. Wien, *W. Braumüller,* 1879.
           Hyrtl, professor of anatomy at Prague and Vienna, retired in 1874 and devoted his leisure to the writing of this and the following work. He ranks with Littré as one of the greatest medical scholars.

444   ———. Onomatologia anatomica Geschichte und Kritik der anatomischen Sprache der Gegenwart. Wien, *W. Braumüller,* 1880.
           A classic work on anatomical terminology. Reprinted, Hildesheim, *G. Olms,* 1970.

444.1 BAILEY, JAMES BALKE.
       The diary of a resurrectionist 1811-1812, to which are added an account of the resurrection men in London and a short history of the passing of the Anatomy Act. London, *Swan Sonnenschein,* 1896.
           First-hand account of the activities of the so-called "sack-em-up" men who flourished in England and Scotland until passage in 1832 of the Anatomy Act provided legal means for physicians to obtain cadavers for dissection.

446   DUVAL, MATHIAS MARIE. 1844-1907, & CUYER, EDOUARD. 1852-?
       Histoire d'anatomie plastique. Paris, *Picard & Kann,* 1898.

447   TÖPLY, ROBERT, *Ritter,* VON. 1856-1947
       Studien zur Geschichte der Anatomie im Mittelalter. Leipzig, Wien, *F. Deuticke,* 1898.

448   ———. Geschichte der Anatomie. In Puschmann's *Handbuch der Geschichte der Medizin,* Jena, 1903, **2**, 155-326.

449   HOPF, LUDWIG. 1838-
       Die Anfänge der Anatomie bei den alten Kulturvölkern. Breslau, *J. U. Kern,* 1904.
           Abhandlungen zur Geschichte der Medizin, Breslau, Heft 9.

450   BARDEEN, CHARLES RUSSELL. 1871-1935
       Anatomy in America. *Bull. Univ. Wisconsin,* 1905, No. 115, 85-208.

451   SUDHOFF, KARL FRIEDRICH JAKOB. 1853-1938
       Tradition und Naturbeobachtung in den Illustrationen medicinischer Handschriften und Frühdrucke vornehmlich des 15. Jahrhunderts. Leipzig, *J. A. Barth,* 1907.

452   ———. Ein Beitrag zur Geschichte der Anatomie im Mittelalter, speziell der anatomischen Graphik nach Handschriften des 9. bis 15. Jahrhunderts. Leipzig, *J. A. Barth,* 1908.
           Studien zur Geschichte der Medizin, Leipzig, Heft 4. Reprinted Hildesheim, 1964.

454   SINGER, CHARLES JOSEPH. 1876-1960
The evolution of anatomy. A short history of anatomical and physiological discovery to Harvey. London, *Kegan Paul,* 1925.

     This invaluable reference book was reprinted under the title *A short history of anatomy and physiology from the Greeks to Harvey*, Dover, 1957.

456   CORNER, GEORGE WASHINGTON. 1889-1981
Anatomical texts of the earlier Middle Ages. Washington, 1927. *Carnegie Inst. Publication No. 364.*

     A valuable study of the history of medieval anatomy.

459   WEGNER, RICHARD NIKOLAUS. 1884-
Das Anatomenbildnis. Seine Entwicklung im Zusammenhang mit der anatomischen Abbildung. Basel, *Schwabe,* 1939.

460   DOBSON, JESSIE. 1906-1984
Anatomical eponyms: being a biographical dictionary of those anatomists whose names have become incorporated into anatomical nomenclature, with definitions of the structures to which their names have been attached and references to the works in which they are described. 2nd ed. Edinburgh, *E. & S. Livingstone,* 1962.

461   RUSSELL, KENNETH FITZPATRICK. 1911-1987
British anatomy 1525-1800; a bibliography of works published in Britain, America, and on the Continent. 2nd edition. Winchester, England, *St. Paul's Bibliographies,* 1987.

     Full descriptions, frequently annotated, of 901 items.

461.1   WOLF-HEIDEGGER, GERHARD, & CETTO, ANNA MARIA.
Die anatomische Sektion in bildlicher Darstellung. Basel, *Karger,* 1967.

461.2   HERRLINGER, ROBERT. 1914-1968.
Geschichte der medizinische Abbildung. 2nd ed. 2 vols. München, *Moos,* 1967-72.

     A history of medical illustration, but primarily covering the history of anatomy. English transl. of Vol.1 (to 1600), London, *Pitman,* 1970. Vol. 2 edited by Marielene Putscher extends the work to recent times.

461.3   LIND, LEVI ROBERT. 1906-
Studies in pre-Vesalian anatomy. Biography, translation, documents. Philadelphia, *American Philosophical Soc.,* 1975.

     Includes Alessandro Achillini, Alessandro Benedetti, Berengario da Carpi, Gabriele Zerbi, Niccolo Massa, Andrés de Laguna, J. Dryander and G. B. Canano.

461.4   PERSAUD, T. V. N.
Early history of human anatomy, from antiquity to the beginning of the modern era. Springfield, Il., *Charles C. Thomas,* 1984.

EMBRYOLOGY

462   ARISTOTLE. 384-322 B.C.
De generatione animalium *In his* [De animalibus] Translated by Theodore Gaza; edited by Ludovicus Podcatharus. Venice, *Johann de Colonia & Johannes Manthen,* 1476.

The first textbook of embryology. Aristotle classified animals according to their embryological characters, wrote at length on generation and the theories concerning it which were current in his day, and dealt exhaustively with the whole subject of embryology. "The depth of Aristotle's insight into the generation of animals has not been surpassed" (Needham). English translation *in his* Works...edited by J. A. Smith and W. D. Ross. Oxford, 1912, **5,** 715a-789b. Also translated by A. L. Peck, *Loeb Classics,* 1953.

463   RUEFF, JACOB [RUFF; RUOFF]. 1500-1558
Ein schön lustig Trosbüchle... Zurich, *C. Froschauer,* 1554.

This is an improved version of Rösslin's *Der swangern frawen.* Its importance to the embryologist lies in Rueff's illustrations, which show contemporary ideas about mammalian embryology. A Latin translation was issued simultaneously by the same publisher.

464   ARANZI, GIULIO CESARE [ARANZIO; ARANTIUS]. 1530-1589
De humano foetu. Bononiae, *J. Rubrius,* 1564.

Aranzi believed the maternal and foetal circulations to be separate. He described the ductus arteriosus and ductus venosus of the foetus, and the corpora Arantii in the heart valves. Incidentally, he was the first to record a pelvic deformity.

464.1   COITER, VOLCHER. 1534-1576
Externarum et internarum principalium humani corporis partium tabulae. Noribergae, *T. Gerlatzeni,* 1572.

Includes epochal, although unillustrated, studies of the anatomy of the chick, describing observations made on 20 successive days. These presented the first systematic study since the three-period description of Aristotle.

465   FABRIZIO, GIROLAMO [FABRICIUS AB AQUAPENDENTE]. 1533-1619
De formato foetu. Venetiis, *per F. Bolzettam,* 1600. [Colophon: *Laurentius Pasquatus,* 1604].

Fabricius wrote at great length on embryology, inventing many theories, some of which were false. His illustrations marked a great advance on previous work. Fabricius recorded for the first time the dissection of several embryos. Facsimile reprint with translation by H. B. Adelmann, 1942.

466   ——. De formatione ovi et pulli. Patavii, *ex. off. A. Bencÿ,* 1621.

467   HARVEY, WILLIAM. 1578-1657
Exercitationes de generatione animalium. Londini, *O Pulleyn,* 1651.

Harvey was among the first to disbelieve the erroneous doctrine of the "preformation" of the foetus; he maintained that the organism derives from the ovum by the gradual building up and aggregation of its parts. The chapter on midwifery in this book is the first work on that subject to be written by an Englishman. This book also demonstrates Harvey's intimate knowledge of the existing literature on the subject. He corrected many of the errors of Fabricius. Harvey considered this to be the culminating work of his life, and more significant than *De motu cordis.* See *The analysis of the De generatione animalium of William Harvey* by A. W. Meyer, Stanford Univ. Press, 1936. First English translation, London, 1653. New translation, with introduction and notes by G. Whitteridge, Oxford, *Blackwell,* 1980.

467.1   HIGHMORE, NATHANIEL. 1613-1685.
The history of generation...London, *John Martin,* 1651.
Highmore's account of the development of the chick is the first embryological study based on microscopical examination, predating Malpighi (No. 468) by more than twenty years. This is also the first book in English to refer to the microscope. It was published within weeks of Harvey's book (No. 467). Harvey and Highmore had collaborated on embryological research at Oxford since the 1640s.

467.2   NEEDHAM, WALTER. 1631?-1691?
Disquisitio anatomica de formatu foetu. London, *Radulph Needham,* 1667.
Founding work of developmental chemical embryology, the first book to report chemical experiments on the developing mammalian embryo, and the first to give practical instructions on dissection of embryos. Needham was also the first to describe the solid bodies in the amniotic fluid, and to give a comparative account of the secondary apparatus of generation.

468   MALPIGHI, MARCELLO. 1628-1694
De ovo incubato observationes. Londini, *J. Martyn,* 1673.
First accurate description, from the microscopical point of view, of the chick embryo. *See* No. 467.1. English translation in No. 534.1

469   ——. Dissertatio epistolica de formatione pulli in ovo. Londini, *J. Martyn,* 1673.
This and the *De ovo incubato* (No. 468) placed the study of embryology on a sound basis, surpassing in accuracy all other contemporary work on the subject and foreshadowing some of the more important general lines of research in embryology. English translation in No. 534.1.

469.1   CASSEBOHM, JOHANN FRIEDRICH. 1699?-1743
Tractatus quatuor anatomici de aure humana. Tractatus quintus anatomicus de aure humana. Cui accedit tractatus sextus de aure monstri humani. Halae Magdeburgi, *sumtibus Orphanotrophei,* 1734-35.
Cassebohm's studies of the embryonic ear far surpassed his predecessors, including Valsalva and Morgagni, and were not themselves surpassed until the work of Huschke and von Baer. See No. 1547.

469.2   HALLER, ALBRECHT VON. 1708-1777
Sur la formation du coeur dans le poulet...2 vols. Lausanne, *Bousquet,* 1758.
Haller devised a numerical method to demonstrate the rate of growth of the foetus, showing that the rate of growth is relatively rapid in the earlier stages but that the tempo gradually decreases. He calculated the rate of growth of the chick and of the human embryo.

470   WOLFF, CASPAR FRIEDRICH. 1733-1794
Theoria generationis. Halae ad Salam, *lit. Hendelianis,* 1759.
Wolff observed in great detail the early processes of embryonic differentiation. He disposed of the "preformation" theory, substituting his view that the organs are formed from leaf-like (blastodermic) layers. He thus laid

the foundation of the "germ-layer" theory of Baer and Pander. His book includes descriptions of the "Wolffian bodies" and "ducts". Reprinted 1966.

471 ——. De formatione intestinorum praecipue. *Novi Comment. Acad. Sci. Petropol.,* 1768, **12**, 43-7, 403-507; 1769, **13**, 478-530.

One of the acknowledged classics of embryology. Wolff's description of the formation of the chick's intestine by the rolling inwards of a leaf-like layer of the blastoderm was important as proving his theory of epigenesis. A German translation by J. F. Meckel was published in 1812.

472 BONNET, CHARLES. 1720-1793
Considérations sur les corps organisés. 2 vols. Amsterdam, *M. M. Rey,* 1762.

Bonnet's theory of generation offered the best synthesis of 18th century ideas of development and remained a leading authority until von Baer. Bonnet believed in the preformation of the embryo. He used many of Haller's arguments to support his own opinions. J. Needham (No.533) calls him an organicistic preformationist, for his objection to epigenesis lay in the fact that it apparently did not allow for the integration of the organism as a whole.

473 SOEMMERRING, SAMUEL THOMAS. 1755-1830
Icones embryonum humanorum. Francofurti ad Moenum, *Varrentrapp u. Wenner,* 1799.

Soemmerring met William Hunter during a visit to London in 1778. The latter's classic work on the pregnant uterus (No. 6157) dealt only with the latter half of pregnancy. Soemmerring therefore decided, in a supplementary volume, to deal with the appearance of the embryo during the first half of pregnancy. This book is one of the best illustrated of Soemmerring's works.

474 PANDER, HEINRICH CHRISTIAN. 1794-1865
Dissertatio sistens historiam metamorphoseos, quam ovum incubatum prioribus quinque diebus subit. Wirceburgi, *T. E. Nitribitt,* 1817.

Pander's doctoral thesis in which he announced his discovery of the trilaminar structure of the chick blastoderm, which term he also coined. This discovery stimulated von Baer's research. Pander later paid for the publication of an illustrated German-language edition of the thesis. The original Latin edition has no illustrations.

474.1 PRÉVOST, JEAN LOUIS. 1790-1850, & DUMAS, JEAN BAPTISTE ANDRÉ. 1800-1884
Deuxième mémoire sur la génération. Rapports de l'œuf avec la liqueur fécondante. Phénomènes appréciables, résultant de leur action mutuelle. Développement de l'œuf des Batraciens. *Ann. Sci. nat. (Paris),* 1824, **2,** 100-120, 129-49.

Prévost and Dumas proved that the frog egg is fertilized by the entry of spermatozoa.

475 MÜLLER, JOHANNES. 1801-1858
Ueber die Entwickelung der Eier im Eierstock bei den Gespenstheuschrecken. *Nove Acta phys.-med. Acad. Caes. Leopold nat. curios.,* Bonn, 1825, **12,** 553-672.

Discovery of the Müllerian duct.

476   PURKYNĚ, JAN EVANGELISTA [PURKINJE]. 1787-1869
Symbolae ad ovi ovium historiam ante incubationem. Vratislaviae, *typ. Universitatis,* 1825.

First description of the germinal vesicle in the embryo, "Purkyně's vesicle". This is located on the spot of the yolk where the embryo develops. Later identified with the cell nucleus, this formed a bridge between the large avian egg and the small ova of other animals, stimulating the researches of von Baer (No. 477). Reprinted in his *Opera selecta,* Prague, 1948, pp. 1-25; 2nd ed. Leipzig, *L. Voss,* 1830, reprinted in his *Opera omnia,* vol. 1, pp. 195-218. English translation of 2nd ed., in *Essays in biology in honor of Herbert M. Evans* (1943).

477   BAER, CARL ERNST VON. 1792-1876
De ovi mammalium et hominis genesi, Lipsiae, *L. Vossius,* 1827.

Announces Baer's discovery of the mammalian ovum, the culmination of a search begun by scientists at least as early as the work of de Graaf in the 17th century (No.1209). The pamphlet was reprinted in facsimile in *Isis,* 1931, **16,** 315-30. English translation by C. D. O'Malley, *Isis,* 1956, **47,** 117-53.

478   PRÉVOST, JEAN LOUIS. 1790-1850, & DUMAS, JEAN BAPTISTE ANDRÉ. 1800-1894
Mémoire sur le développement du poulet dans l'œuf. *Ann. Sci. nat. (Paris),* 1827, **12,** 415-43.

First description of the segmentation of the frog's egg.

479   BAER, CARL ERNST VON. 1792-1876
Ueber Entwicklungsgeschichte der Thiere. 2 vols. in 3. Königsberg, *Bornträger,* 1828-88.

Baer, the father of modern embryology, definitely established the "germ-layer theory", discovered the notochord and the human ovum, and postulated the law of corresponding stages in embryonic development. With Cuvier he is the founder of modern morphology. Later in his life he devoted much time to the study of anthropology. Part of vol. 1 was published in No. 599. In response to demands by subscribers to the treatise, the publishers issued vol. 2 in incomplete form in 1837. The conclusion to vol. 2, sometimes called volume 3, was edited by Ludwig Stieda and published 12 years after von Baer's death.

480   RATHKE, MARTIN HEINRICH. 1793-1860
Abhandlungen zur Bildungs- und Entwicklungs-Geschichte der Menschen und der Thiere. 2 pts. Leipzig, *F. C. W. Vogel,* 1832-33.

Rathke's most notable discovery was of structures homologous with gill slits in bird and mammalian embryos. He discredited the vertebral theory of the skull.

481   SCHWANN, THEODOR. 1810-1882
De necessitate aëris atmosphaerici ad evolutionem pulli in ovo incubito. Berolini, *typ. Nietackianis,* 1834.

Proof that air is necessary in the development of the embryo.

482   REICHERT, KARL BOGISLAUS. 1811-1883
Ueber die Visceralbogen der Wirbelthiere. Berlin, *Sittenfeld,* 1837.

First description of the visceral arches in vertebrates.

483   RATHKE, MARTIN HEINRICH. 1793-1860
        Entwicklungsgeschichte der Natter (Coluber natrix). Koenigsberg,
        Börntrager, 1839.
        "Rathke's pouch", a diverticulum from the embryonic buccal cavity.

484   BISCHOFF, THEODOR LUDWIG WILHELM. 1807-1882
        Entwickelungsgeschichte des Kaninchen-Eies. Braunschweig, *F. Vieweg
        u. Sohn,* 1842.
        Bischoff contributed important original work on the development of
        the rabbit.

484.1   BARRY, MARTIN. 1802-1855
        Spermatozoa observed within the mammiferous ovum. *Phil. Trans,* 1843, 33.
        Barry was the first to observe the spermatozoon within the ovum.

485   REMAK, ROBERT. 1815-1865
        Untersuchungen über die Entwickelung der Wirbelthiere. Berlin, *G. Reimer,* 1855.
        Simplification of von Baer's classification of the germ-layers.

486   GEGENBAUR, CARL. 1826-1903
        Ueber den Bau und die Entwickelung der Wirbelthier-Eier mit partieller
        Dottertheilung. *Arch. Anat. Physiol wiss. Med.,* 1861, 491-529.
        Proof that the ovum is unicellular in all vertebrates.

487   KÖLLIKER, RUDOLPH ALBERT VON. 1871-1905
        Entwicklungsgeschichte des Menschen und der höheren Thiere. Leipzig,
        W. Engelmann, 1861.
        First book on comparative embryology.

488   SCHULTZE, MAXIMILIAN JOHANN SIGISMUND. 1825-1874
        Observationes nonnulae de ovorum ranarum segmentatione, quae
        "Furchungsprocess" dicitur. Bonnae, *Formis C. Georgi,* 1863.
        Best contemporary description of the segmentation furrowing of the egg.

489   HIS, WILHELM, *Snr.* 1831-1904
        Beobachtungen über den Bau des Säugethier-Eierstockes. *Arch mikr. Anat.,*
        1865, **1,** 151-202.
        His was the greatest of the 19th-century embryologists.

490   ———. Die Häute und Höhlen des Körpers. Basel, *Schwighauser,* 1865.
        A new classification of tissues based on histogenesis.

491   LANGHANS, THEODOR. 1839-1915
        Zur Kenntnis der menschlichen Placenta. *Arch Gynäk.,* 1870, **1,** 317-34.
        "Langhans's layer"—the cytotrophoblast, the individual cells of which
        are termed "Langhans's cells".

492   WALDEYER-HARTZ, HEINRICH WILHELM GOTTFRIED. 1836-1921
        Eierstock und Ei. Leipzig, *W. Engelmann,* 1870.
        Waldeyer discovered the germinal epithelium.

493   HAECKEL, ERNST HEINRICH PHILIPP AUGUST. 1834-1919
        Anthropogenie oder Entwicklungsgeschichte des Menschen. Leipzig, *W.
        Engelmann,* 1874.

494   HIS, Wilhelm, *Snr.* 1831-1904
Unsere Körperform und das physiologische Problem ihrer Entstehung.
Leipzig, *F. C. W. Vogel,* 1874.

      In this work His compared the various layers and organs of the embryo
to a series of elastic tubes and plates. He thought that the local inequalities
of growth and the differences in the consistency of the tissues might
account for the various organs and structures. This work led to the idea of
"developmental mechanics".

495   HERTWIG, Wilhelm August Oscar. 1849-1922
Beiträge zur Kenntnis der Bildung, Befruchtung und Theilung des
thierischen Eies. *Morph. Jb.,* 1876, **1,** 347-434.

      Demonstration of the fact that the spermatozoon enters the ovum and
that fertilization occurs by the union of the nuclei of the male and female
sex cells. Hertwig also established that the transfer of hereditary material
is part of the same nuclear process. Hertwig was professor of anatomy at
Jena and Berlin.

496   BENEDEN, Edouard van. 1846-1910
Le maturation de l'œuf, la fécondation et les premières phases du
développement embryonnaire des mammifères. *Bull Acad. roy. Sci. Belg.,*
1875, 2 sér., **40,** 686-736.

      First detailed description of the segmentation of the mammalian ovum.

497   ——. Contributions à l'histoire de la vésicule germinative et du premier
noyau embryonnaire. *Bull. Acad. Roy. Sci. Belg.,* 1876, 2 sér., **41,** 38-85.

      Independently of Flemming, van Beneden discovered the centrosome.

498   FLEMMING, Walther. 1843-1905
Beobachtungen über die Beschaffenheit des Zellkerns. *Arch. mikr. Anat.,*
1877, **13,** 693-717.

      Discovery of the centrosome.

499   WHITMAN, Charles Otis. 1842-1910
The embryology of *Clepsine. Quart. J. micr. Sci.,* 1878, **18,** 215-315.

      The study of cell-lineage was initiated by Whitman's paper on *Clepsine.*

500   BALFOUR, Francis Maitland. 1851-1882
A treatise on comparative embryology. 2 vols. London, *Macmillan & Co.,*
1880-81.

      This classic work sums up all the previous knowledge on the subject
and includes Balfour's own important contributions. Balfour, a pupil of
Michael Foster, became professor of animal morphology in 1882; in the
same year he met his death in a mountaineering accident.

501   HIS, Wilhelm, *Snr.* 1831-1904
Anatomie menschlicher Embryonen. 3 pts. and atlas. Leipzig, *F. C. W. Vogel,*
1880-85.

      A systematic account of early human embryology that stimulated
further investigation in a field in which His stood highest among his
contemporaries. He was the first to study the human embryo as a whole.

502   HERTWIG, Wilhelm August Oscar. 1849-1922, & HERTWIG, Karl Wilhelm Theodor Richard. 1850-1937
Die Coelomtheorie; Versuch einer Erklärung des mittleren Keimblattes. Jena, *G. Fischer,* 1881.
The "coelom" theory formulated to account for the classification and phylogeny of metazoan animals.

502.1   BENEDEN, Edouard van. 1846-1910
Récherches sur la maturation de l'œuf, la fécondation et la division cellulaire. *Arch. de Biol.,* 1883, **4**, 265-640.
This work extended Hertwig's work on fertilization (No. 495) down to the level of chromosomes, which were clearly visible in *Ascaris* after the sperm and egg united.

503   PFLÜGER, Eduard Friedrich Wilhelm. 1829-1910, & SMITH, William J.
Untersuchungen über Bastardirung der anuren Batrachier und die Principien der Zeugung. *Pflüg. Arch. ges. Physiol.,* 1883, **32**, 519-41.
Pflüger was one of the earliest workers in the field of experimental embryology. Above, his first work on the subject, deals with the cross-fertilization of different species of frog.

504   HERTWIG, Wilhelm August Oscar. 1849-1922
Lehrbuch der Entwicklungsgeschichte des Menschen und der Wirbelthiere. Jena, *G. Fischer,* 1886.

505   ROUX, Wilhelm 1850-1924
Beiträge zur Entwickelungsmechanik des Embryo. Ueber die künstliche Hervorbringung halber Embryonen durch Zerstörung einer der beiden ersten Furchungskugeln, sowie über die Nachentwickelung (Postgeneration) der fehlenden Körperhälfte. *Virchows Arch. path. Anat.,* 1888, **114**, 113-53, 246-91.
Roux is regarded as the founder of developmental mechanics ("Entwicklungsmechanik" as he named it). His work on the production of half-embryos initiated a turning point by shifting emphasis from descriptive to experimental embryology. Roux believed that the above work showed that the nucleus of each blastomere is capable of directing a specific independent line of differentiation. He eventually concluded that the nucleus is made up of hereditary particles. Partial English translation in No. 534.3.

506   MINOT, Charles Sedgwick. 1852-1914
Uterus and embryo. *J. Morph.,* 1889, **2**, 341-462.

507   ———. A theory of the structure of the placenta. *Anat. Anz.,* 1891, **6**, 125-31.

509   DRIESCH, Hans Adolf Eduard. 1867-1941
Entwicklungsmechanische Studien. I. Der Werth der beiden ersten Furchungszellen in der Echinodermentwicklung. Experimentelle Erzeugen von Theil- und Doppelbildung. II. Ueber die Beziehungen des Lichtes zur ersten Etappe der thierischen Formbildung. *Z. wiss. Zool.,* 1892, **53**, 160-84.
In the spring of 1891 Driesch succeeded in separating the blastomeres of the cleaving sea urchin egg. English translation in No. 534.3.

510   WILSON, EDMUND BEECHER. 1856-1939
       The cell-lineage of *Nereis*. *J. Morph.*, 1892, **6**, 361-480.
       Wilson traced the development of *Nereis* in minute detail from fertilized
       egg to the free-swimming larval stage, a pioneer study of cell-lineage.

511   LOEB, JACQUES. 1859-1924
       Ueber die Grenzen der Theilbarkeit der Eisubstanz. *Pflüg. Arch. ges. Physiol*,
       1894-95, **59**, 379-94.
       English translation in Loeb's *Studies in general physiology*, Vol.1.,
       Chicago, 1905.

512   LILLIE, FRANK RATTRAY. 1870-1947
       The embryology of the Unionidae. A study in cell-lineage. *J. Morph.* 1895,
       10, 1-100.

513   KEIBEL, FRANZ KARL JULIUS. 1861-1929
       Normentafeln zur Entwicklungsgeschichte der Wirbelthiere. Hrsg. von
       FRANZ KEIBEL. 16 pts. Jena, *G. Fischer*, 1897-1938.

514   MORGAN, THOMAS HUNT. 1866-1945
       The development of the frog's egg; an introduction to experimental
       embryology. New York, *Macmillan & Co.*, 1897.
       First work in English on experimental embryology.

515   SCHAPER, ALFRED. 1863-1905
       Die frühesten Differenzirungsvorgänge in Centralnervensystem. *Wilhelm
       Roux Arch. EntwMech. Org.*, 1897, **5**, 81-132.

515.1 LOEB, JACQUES. 1859-1924
       On the nature of the process of fertilization and the artificial production of
       normal larvae (plutei) from the unfertilized eggs of the sea urchin. *Amer J.
       Physiol.*, 1899, **3**, 135-38.
       Loeb first succeeded in achieving parthenogenesis in 1899.

516   MALL, FRANKLIN PAINE. 1862-1917
       Contributions to the study of the pathology of early human embryos. 3 pts.
       Baltimore, *etc.*, 1899-1908.

516.1 PETERS, HUBERT. 1859-1934
       Ueber die Einbettung des menschlichen Eies und das früheste bisher
       bekannte menschliche Placentationsstadium. Leipzig, Wien, *F. Deuticke*,
       1899.

517   KORSCHELT, EUGEN. 1858-1946, & HEIDER, KARL. 1856-1935
       Lehrbuch der vergleichenden Entwicklungsgeschichte der wirbellosen
       Thiere. Jena, *G. Fischer*, 1902-09.

517.1 HENKING, HERMANN. 1858-1942
       Untersuchungen über den ersten Entwicklungsvorgänge in den Eiern der
       Insekten. II. Ueber Spermatogenese und deren Beziehung zur
       Eientwicklung bei *Pyrrhocoris apterus*, *L. Z. wiss. Zool.*, 1891, **51**, 685-736.
       Henking observed an element among chromosomes that showed
       peculiar behaviour during meiosis. These were the first observations on
       what were subsequently called sex chromosomes.

518   McCLUNG, CLARENCE ERWIN. 1870-1946
        The accessory chromosome; sex determination. *Biol Bull.*, 1902, **3**, 43-84.
        The accessory chromosomes were shown by McClung to be the
        determinants of sex.

519   WILSON, EDMUND BEECHER. 1856-1939
        Experimental studies on germinal localisation. *J. exp. Zool.*, 1904, **1**, 1-73.

520   HERTWIG, WILHELM AUGUST OSCAR. 1849-1922
        Handbuch der vergleichenden und experimentellen Entwicklungslehre
        der Wirbelthiere. Hrsg. von OSCAR HERTWIG. 3 vols. [in 6]. Jena, *G. Fischer,*
        1906.

521   HARRISON, ROSS GRANVILLE. 1870-1959
        Observations on the living developing nerve fiber. *Anat. Rec.*, 1907, **1**, 116-
        18.
        Harrison demonstrated the development of nerve fibres by independ-
        ent growth from cells outside the organism.

522   LEWIS, WARREN HARMON. 1870-1964
        Experiments on the origin and differentiation of the optic vesicle in
        amphibia. Amer. J. Anat., 1907-08, 7, 259-77.

523   BRYCE, THOMAN HASTIE. 1862-1946, & TEACHER, JOHN HAMMOND. 1869-1930
        Contributions to the study of the early development and imbedding of the
        human ovum. An early ovum imbedded in the decidua. Glasgow, *J.*
        Maclehose & Sons, 1908.
        The "Bryce-Teacher ovum", age estimated at 13-14 days.

524   LOEB, JACQUES. 1859-1924
        Ueber den chemischen Character des Befruchtungvorgangs. Leipzig, *W.*
        Englemann, 1908.

525   ——. Die chemische Entwicklungserregung des tierischen Eies; künstliche
        Parthenogenese. Berlin, *J. Springer,* 1909.
        Artificial parthenogenesis. For Loeb's first paper on this subject see No.
        515.1. Translated and revised in Loeb's *Artificial parthenogenesis and*
        fertilization, 1913.

526   KEIBEL, FRANZ KARL JULIUS. 1861-1929, & MALL, FRANKLIN PAINE. 1862-1917
        Manual of human embryology. Edited by F. KEIBEL and F. P. MALL. 2 vols.
        Philadelphia, *J. B. Lippincott,* 1910-12.
        The important studies on human embryos, originated by His, were
        carried on by his pupils, Keibel and Mall. This classic work written by
        American and German experts "has not yet been superceded" (D.S.B.).

527   ROUX, WILHELM. 1850-1924
        Terminologie der Entwicklungsmechanik. Leipzig, *W. Engelmann,* 1912.

527.1   LILLIE, FRANK RATTRAY. 1870-1947
        The mechanism of fertilization. *Science,* 1913, **38**, 524-8.

528   PARKER, GEORGE HOWARD. 1864-1955
The elementary nervous system. Philadelphia, *J. B. Lippincott,* 1919.
Important studies on the survival of primitive types of neuromuscular mechanism in some of the higher vertebrates.

529   GOLDSCHMIDT, RICHARD BENEDICT. 1878-1958
Geschlechtsbestimmung. Berlin, 1921.
English translation, 1923.

530   SPEMANN, HANS. 1869-1941, & MANGOLD, HILDE.
Über Induktion von Embryonalanlagen durch Implantation artfremder Organisatoren. *Wilhelm Roux Arch. EntwMech. Org.,* 1924, **100,** 599-638.
Spemann was awarded the Nobel Prize in 1935 for his discovery of "organizers" in animal development. English translation in No. 534.3.

531   NEEDHAM, JOSEPH. 1900-
Chemical embryology. 3 vols. Cambridge, *Univ. Press,* 1931.

531.1   HOLTFRETER, JOHANNES. 1901-
Gewebeaffinität, ein Mittel der embryonalen Formbildung. *Arch. exp. Zellforsch.,* 1939, **23,** 169-209.
Tissue affinity as a means of embryonic morphogenesis. English translation in No. 534.3.

532   ROCK, JOHN. 1890-1984, & HERTIG, ARTHUR TREMAIN. 1904-
Some aspects of early human development. *Amer. J. Obstet. Gynec.,* 1942, **44,** 973-83; 1943, **45,** 356.
Report of the youngest normal implanted fertilized human ovum, fertilization age about 7 1/2 days. Hertig and Rock published a more detailed study in *Contr. Embryol. Carneg. Instn,* 1945, **31,** 65-84.

532.1   ROCK, JOHN. 1890-1984, & MENKIN, MIRIAM F.
In vitro ferilization and cleavage of human ovarian eggs. *Science,* 1944, **100,** 105-07.
First *in vitro* fertilization of human eggs.

532.2   CHANG, MIN CHUEH. 1908-
Fertilizing capacity of spermatozoa deposited into the fallopian tubes. *Nature*, 1951, 168, 697-98.
Discovery that maturation of the sperm in the mammalian female tract is a necessary step in reproduction. This was co-discovered and called capacitation by Austin in the same year. See C.R. Austin, Observation on the penetration of the sperm into the mammalian eggs. *Aust. J. sci. Res.,* 1951, **B4,** 581-.

532.3   ——. Fertilization of rabbit ova in vitro. *Nature,* 1959, **184,** 466-67.
The birth of normal rabbits from *in vitro* fertilization and embryo transfer was the first proof that births resulting from this procedure are normal.

532.4   EDWARDS, ROBERT GEOFFREY. 1925- , BAVISTER, B.D., & STEPTOE, PATRICK CHRISTOPHER. 1913-1988
Early stages of fertilization *in vitro* of human oocytes. *Nature,* 1969, **221,** 632-35.
First successful in-vitro fertilization of human oocytes.

532.5   STEPTOE, Patrick Christopher. 1913-1988, & EDWARDS, Robert Geoffrey. 1925-
Birth after the reimplantation of a human embryo. (Letter to the editor). *Lancet*, 1978, **2**, 366.
First successful human birth after *in vitro* fertilization and embryo transfer.

History of Embryology

532.9   COLE, Francis Joseph. 1872-1959
Early theories of sexual generation. Oxford, *Clarendon Press*, 1930.

533   NEEDHAM, Joseph. 1900-
A history of embryology. Cambridge, *Univ. Press*, 1934.
An exhaustive history of the subject. Deals with embryology from the earliest times to the beginning of the 19th century and includes a valuable bibliography and many illustrations. Second edition, 1959.

534   MEYER, Arthur William. 1873-1966
The rise of embryology. Stanford, Calif., *Stanford Univ. Press*, 1939.
Includes a fine bibliography.

534.1   ADELMANN, Howard Bernhardt. 1898-1988
Marcello Malpighi and the evolution of embryology. 5 vols. Ithaca, N.Y., *Cornell Univ. Press*, 1966.
Vol. 1 is an exhaustive biography of Malpighi; the remaining 4 volumes provide an extensive account of the development of embryology, and annotated English translations of Nos. 468 & 469.

534.2   GASKING, Elizabeth B.
Investigations into generation, 1651-1828. Baltimore, *Johns Hopkins Press*, 1966.

534.3   OPPENHEIMER, Jane Marion. 1911-
Essays in the history of embryology and biology. Cambridge, Mass., *M.I.T. Press*, 1967.

534.4   ROGER, Jacques.
Les sciences de la vie dans la pensée française du XVIIIe siecle. Genération des animaux de Descartes à l'Encyclopédie. 2e ed. Paris, *Armand Colin*, 1971.

534.41   WILLIER, Benjamin Harris. 1890-1972, & OPPENHEIMER, Jane Marion. 1911-
Foundations of experimental embryology. Edited by Benjamin H. Willier and Jane M. Oppenheimer. 2nd ed. New York, *Hafner Press*, 1974.
14 classic contributions to embryology (in English translations where appropriate) with historical commentaries.

534.42   HORDER, T.J. *et al* (eds.)
A history of embryology. Cambridge, *Cambridge Univ. Press*, 1986.

534.50   LYCOSTHENES, Conrad Wolffhart. 1518-1561
Prodigiorum ac ostentorum chronicon. Basel, *Heinrich Petri*, 1557.
This enclyclopaedic chronology of portentious events in human history
includes many monstrous births, both human and animal. Actual cases are
uncritically mingled with mythical creatures. German translation, 1557.

534.51   PARÉ, Ambroise. 1510-1590
Deux livres de chirurgie. I. De la generation de l'homme... II. Des monstres
tant terrestres que marins avec leurs portraits. Paris, *André Wechel*, 1573.
Many reports of real malformations are intermixed with mythical
accounts. English translations, 1634, and later. Recent English translation,
Chicago, *University of Chicago Press*, 1982.

534.52   LICETI, Fortunio. 1577-1657
De monstrorum caussis, natura, & differentiis libri duo. Patavii, *Apud
Casparem Crivellarium*, 1616.
One of the earliest classifications of deformities, Liceti's work was still
under review in works on malformation in the 19th century. Includes both
real and imaginary cases. The first of many illustrated editions appeared in
Padua, 1634. This edition includes accurate descriptions of cases observed
by Liceti in the years following the first edition.

534.53   ALDROVANDI, Ulisse. 1522-1605
Monstrorum historia... Bartholomaeus Ambrosinus... volumen composuit.
Bononiae, *Nicolai Tebaldini*, 1642.
Aldrovandi assembled a large collection of specimens and notes on
monsters which were published posthumously by Bartholommeo
Ambrosini (1588-1657), who added a number of personally observed
cases. Among the latter is the first detailed description and illustration of
bladder exstrophy. Valuable case descriptions are mingled with fictitious
ones, including specimens of false chimeras apparently created to please
Aldrovandi's patrons. Some of these can still be seen in the Aldrovandi
collection at the University of Bologna.

534.54   HALLER, Albrecht von. 1708-1777
Operum anatomici argumenti minorum tomus tertius, De Monstris.
Lausanne, *François Grasset*, 1768.
Reprints and updates Haller's earlier essays on various malformations.
This work marks the beginning of scientific teratology, placing it on a
foundation of sound anatomical description.

534.55   SOEMMERRING, Samuel Thomas. 1755-1830
Abbildungen und Beschreibungen einiger Missgeburten. Mainz,
Universitazbehandlung, 1791.
Most of the plates demonstrate a progressive series of specimens with
duplication anomalies of the face and head, from midfacial cleft to
complete dicephalus. This arrangement of malformations into a continu-
ous series with definable steps anticipated the taxonomic approach of the
Geoffroy Saint-Hilaires.

534.56   MECKEL, JOHANN FRIEDRICH, *the younger.* 1781-1833
Handbuch der pathologischen Anatomie. 2 vols., Halle, *Carl Heinrich Reclam,* 1812-1816.
Meckel classified malformations systematically, on the basis of altered developmental mechanisms, basing his work on embryology. See No. 2284.

534.57   GEOFFROY SAINT-HILAIRE, ÉTIENNE. 1772-1844
Philosophie anatomique, Tome II, Des monstruosités. Paris, chez l'Auteur, 1822.
The elder Geoffroy Saint-Hilaire is credited with coining the word Teratology, and was the first seriously to attempt the experimental production of anomalies, by manipulating chick eggs. See T. Cahn, *La vie et l'œuvre d'Etienne Geoffroy Saint-Hilaire,* Paris, 1962.

534.58   GEOFFROY SAINT-HILAIRE, ISIDORE. 1805-1861
Histoire générale et particulière des anomalies de l'organisation chez l'homme et les animaux. 3 vols. and atlas. Paris, *J.-B. Baillière,* 1832-37.
Isidore, the son of Étienne (*See* No. 534.57) organized all known human and animal malformations taxonomically. Many principles governing abnormal development were enunciated for the first time in this work. It also introduced hundreds of names for specific malformations, many of which are still in use. For comprehensive coverage of rare anomalies it is still of value as a reference source.

534.59   GURLT, ERNST FRIEDRICH. 1794-1882
Handbuch der pathologischen Anatomie der Haus-Säugethiere. 2 vols. and atlas. Berlin, *G. Reimer,* 1832.
The most comprehensive treatise on malformations of domesticated animals, as well as an important contribution to general teratology. The superb atlas illustrates many rare animal terata. See also his *Über thierische Missgeburten, ein Beitrag zur pathologischen Anatomie und Entwicklungsgeschichte.* Berlin, *A. Hirschwald,* 1877.

534.60   OTTO, ADOLPH WILHELM. 1786-1845
Monstrorum sexcentorum descriptio anatomica. Vratislaviae, *F. Girt,* 1841.
Brief but accurate descriptions of 600 human and animal specimens, with 30 outstanding plates.

534.61   VROLIK, WILLEM. 1801-1863
Tabulae ad illustrandam embryogenesin hominis et mammalium tam naturalem quem abnormem. Amsterdam, *G.M.P., Londinck,* 1849.
The 100 plates of this volume contain some of the most accurate and beautiful depictions of human and animal malformations ever published. Text in Dutch and Latin.

534.62   PANUM, PETER LUDWIG. 1820-1885
Untersuchungen über die Entstehung der Missbildungen Zunächst in den Eiern der Vögel. Berlin, *Georg Reimer,* 1860.
The first monograph on experimental teratology.

534.63   FÖRSTER, AUGUST. 1822-1865
Die Missbildungen des Menschen, systematisch dargestellt. 2 vols. Jena, *Friedrich Mauke,* 1861.
An encyclopaedia of cases from the literature and from Förster's personal experience. It contains an extremely useful bibliography of

teratology which served as the basis for all subsequent bibliographies of the subject.

534.64   FISHER, George Jackson. 1825-1893
Diploteratology. *Trans. med. Soc. N.Y.*, **1865**: 232-68; **1866**: 206-96; **1867**: 396-430; **1868**: 276-306.
Includes a valuable history of teratology with a detailed bibliography. Fisher assembled one of the largest of all libraries on teratology.

534.65   DARESTE, Camille. 1822-1899
Récherches sur la production artificielle des monstruosités, ou essais de teratologénie expérimentale. Paris, Reinwald, 1877.
Dareste devoted his career to experimental teratology, and in this work established the field as a science. The second edition (1891) is greatly revised and enlarged. Contains a valuable history of experimental teratology.

534.66   AHLFELD, Friedrich. 1843-
Die Missbildungen des Menschen. 2 vols. and atlas. Leipzig, *F. W. Grunow*, 1880-82.
Reproduces plates of important specimens from otherwise inaccessible sources.

534.67   TARUFFI, Cesare. 1821-1902
Storia della teratologia. 8 vols., Bologna, *Regia Tipographia*, 1881-94.
The most extensive history and bibliography of teratology ever published, despite the fact that the section on malformations of single organs and parts was never completed. Contains excerpts and detailed abstracts of innumerable rare specimens from otherwise unobtainable sources.

534.68   HIRST, Barton Cooke. 1861-1935, & PIERSOL, George Arthur. 1856-1924
Human monstrosities. 4 vols., Philadelphia, *Lea Brothers*, 1891-93.
The first large work on the subject illustrated primarily by photographs of specimens.

534.69   BALLANTYNE, John William. 1861-1923
Manual of antenatal pathology and hygiene. Volume 2, The embryo. Edinburgh, *William Green*, 1904.
The most complete history of teratology in English, and among the best in any language. American edition, New York, 1905.

534.70   SCHWALBE, Ernst. 1871-1920
Die Morphologie der Missbildungen des Menschen und der Thiere. Jena, *Gustav Fischer*, 1906-1952.
The first volume is an important contribution to general teratology, including a good history of the topic, and enunciating Schwalbe's "teratogenic termination period", the guiding principle for estimating the timing of teratogenic events. Volume 2 (1907) covers diploteratology. Volume 3 on individual malformations appeared in 3 parts between 1909 and 1937. Posthumous volumes were edited by Georg B. Gruber beginning in 1927.

534.71   WARKANY, Josef. 1902-
Congenital malformations. Chicago, *Year Book*, 1971.
The *magnum opus* of the greatest teratologist of the 20th century, whose contributions span all aspects of the field, both clinical and experimental.

History of Teratology

534.90   GRUBER, GEORG B. 1884-1964
Studien zur Historik der Teratologie. *Zent. allg. Path.*, 1963, **105**, 219-237, 293-316.

HISTOLOGY

535   MALPIGHI, MARCELLO. 1628-1694
De viscerum structura exercitatio anatomica. Bononiae, *ex typ. J. Montj,* 1666.
Includes Malpighi's classic essay on the kidney, the "Malpighian bodies" which have perpetuated his name. The book also includes (pp. 125-26) the first description of Hodgkin's disease. Strangely enough, Malpighi gives no illustration of the kidney in this work. For a reproduction and English translation of this work, see *Ann. med. Hist.*, 1925, **7**, 245-63.

536   ———. Anatome plantarum. 2 pts. Londini, *J. Martyn,* 1675-79.
Malpighi was the founder of microscopic anatomy and a pioneer in the study of plant development. He approached the subject through the study of plant tissues.

537   BICHAT, MARIE FRANÇOIS XAVIER. 1771-1802
Traité des membranes en général et diverses membranes en particulier. Paris, *Richard, Caille & Ravier,* an VIII [1800].
Bichat conceived the idea of a science of anatomy and pathology based upon an accurate classification of the various tissues of the body, their distribution in the various organs and parts, and their particular susceptibilities to disease (Corner). He is regarded as the founder of modern histology and tissue pathology. English translation, Boston, 1813.

538   MÜLLER, JOHANNES. 1801-1858
De glandularum secernentium structura penitiori. Lipsiae, *sumpt. L. Vossii,* 1830.
Müller's most important histological work. In it he described the microscopic anatomy of a large series of secreting glands. Müller's greatest influence was not so much through his own work as through the influence he had upon his pupils at Bonn and Berlin. English translation, 1839.

539   HENLE, FRIEDRICH GUSTAV JACOB. 1809-1885
Symbolae ad anatomiam villorum intestinalium, imprimis eorum epithelii et vasorum lacteorum. Berolini. *A. Hirschwald,* 1837.
Henle first described the epithelia of the skin and intestines, and defined the structure and function of columnar and ciliated epithelium. He applied the term "epithelium": to all mucous membranes in the body. Modern knowledge of the epithelial tissues starts with Henle. English translation and commentary in L.J. Rather, P. Rather, & J.B. Frerichs, Johannes Müller and the nineteenth century origins of tumour cell theory, Canton, Mass., *Science History Publications,* 1986.

540   ———. Ueber die Ausbreitung des Epithelium im menschlichen Körper. *Arch. Anat. Physiol. wiss. Med.,* 1838, 103-28.
Henle broadened the scope of his study of epithelium (No. 539) to include the covering layers of the true body cavities.

541   ROSENTHAL, JOSEPH.
De formatione granulosa in nervis aliisque partibus organismi animalis.
Breslau, 1839.
       In 1839 Purkyně was the first to use the term *protoplasma,* by which he
described the embryonic ground substance. This fact is recorded in the
inaugural dissertation of one of his students, J. Rosenthal.

542   BOWMAN, *Sir* WILLIAM. 1816-1892
On the minute structure and movements of voluntary muscle. *Phil. Trans.,*
1840, **130,** 457-501; 1841, **131,** 69-72.
       Classical description of striated muscle.

543   HENLE, FRIEDRICH GUSTAV JACOB. 1809-1885
Allgemeine Anatomie Leipzig, *L. Voss,* 1841.
       Many of the histological discoveries of Henle are described in the
above. He classified tissues histologically.

543.1 LEBERT, HERMANN. 1813-1878
Physiologie pathologique. 2 vols. & atlas. Paris, *Baillière,* 1845.
       One of the earliest and most important atlases of pathological histology.
Lebert's work played an important role in introducing the cellular idea of
pathology, laying the groundwork for Virchow's theories.

544   HASSALL, ARTHUR HILL. 1817-1894
The microscopic anatomy of the human body, in health and disease. 2 vols.
London, *S. Highley,* [1846]-1849.
       First English textbook on microscopical anatomy. His description of the
concentric corpuscles of the thymus (p. 9) led to the term "Hassall's
corpuscles".

545   SHARPEY, WILLIAM. 1802-1880
Bone or osseous tissue. In Quain, J. *Anatomy.* 5th ed., London, 1848, cxxxii-
clxiii.
       The discovery of the "fibres of Sharpey" is reported on pp. cxlii-cxliii.

546   KÖLLIKER, RUDOLPH ALBERT VON. 1817-1905
Handbuch der Gewebelehre des Menschen. Leipzig, *W. Engelmann,* 1852.
       Isolation of smooth muscle.

548   GERLACH, JOSEPH VON. 1820-1896
Mikroskopische Studien aus dem Gebiete der menschlichen Morphologie.
Erlangen, *F. Enke,* 1858.
       Gerlach introduced several staining methods, the most important of
which (a transparent solution of ammonia carmine and gelatin) is called
"Gerlach's stain"; it was the first satisfactory histological stain.

548.1 RECKLINGHAUSEN, FRIEDRICH DANIEL VON. 1833-1910
Ueber Eiter- und Bindegewebskörperchen. *Virchows Arch. path. Anat.,*
1863, **28,** 157-97.
       Recklinghausen described granular cells in the frog mesentery, later
named "mast cells" by Ehrlich (No. 553.1).

549   KLEBS, Theodor Albrecht Edwin. 1834-1913
       Die Einschmelzungs-Methode, ein Beitrag zur mikroskopischen Technik.
       Arch. mikr. Anat., 1869, **5,** 164-6.
       Introduction of paraffin embedding.

550   STRICKER, Salomon. 1834-1898
       Handbuch der Lehre von den Geweben des Menschen und der Thiere. 2
       vols. Leipzig, *W. Engelmann,* 1869-72.
       One of the greatest of textbooks on histology. English translation, 3
       vols., 1870-73.

551   FISCHER, Ernst.
       Ueber den Bau der Meissner'schen Tastkörperchen. *Arch. mikr. Anat.,*
       1876, **12,** 364-90.
       Includes first account of demonstration of nerve endings by means of
       the gold chloride method.

552   KUPFFER, Karl Wilhelm von. 1829-1902
       Ueber Sternzellen der Leber. *Arch. mikr. Anat.,* 1876, **12,** 353-8.
       "Kupffer's cells" – stellate cells in the lining of the blood channels in the
       liver.

553   DUVAL, Mathias Marie. 1844-1907
       Technique de l'emploi du collodion humide pour la pratique des coupes
       microscopiques. *J. Anat. Physiol. (Paris),* 1879, **15,** 185-8.
       Introduction of collodion for embedding.

553.1 EHRLICH, Paul. 1854-1915
       Beiträge zur Kenntniss der granulirten Bindegewebszellen und der
       eosinophilen Leukocythen. *Arch. Anat. Physiol., Physiol. Abt.,* 1879, 166-
       69.
       Mast cells; *see* No. 548.1.

554   ——. Ueber die Methylenblaureaction der lebenden Nervensubstanz.
       Dtsch. Med. Wschr., 1886, **12,** 49-52.
       Ehrlich's method of intravital staining.

555   HERTWIG, Wilhelm August Oscar. 1849-1922, & HERTWIG, Karl Wilhelm
       Theodor Richard. 1850-1937
       Untersuchungen zur Morphologie und Physiologie der Zelle. 6pts. Jena, *G.
       Fischer,* 1884-90.

556   ——. Die Zelle und die Gewebe. 2 pts. Jena, *G. Fischer,* 1893-8.
       Part 1 was translated as *The cell: outlines of general anatomy and
       physiology,* London, 1895.

557   BLUM, F.
       Der Formaldehyd als Härtungsmittel. Vorläufige Mittheilung. *Z. wiss. Mikr.,*
       1893, **10,** 314-15.
       Formalin first used for tissue fixation.

558   HARRISON, Ross Granville. 1870-1959
       The outgrowth of the nerve fibre as a mode of protoplasmic movement. *J.
       exp. Zool,* 1910, **9,** 787-846.

The inauguration of tissue culture was made possible by Harrison's proof of the outgrowth of nerve-fibres from ganglion cells.

559   CARREL, ALEXIS. 1873-1944
Rejuvenation of cultures of tissues. *J. Amer. med. Ass.*, 1911, **57,** 1611.
    Extra-vital cultivation and rejuvenation of tissue. Carrel was awarded the Nobel Prize in 1912.

560   ——. & BURROWS, MONTROSE THOMAS. 1884-1947
Cultivation of tissues in vitro and its technique. *J. exp. Med.*, 1911, **13,** 387-96; 415-21.
    Carrel demonstrated the potential immortality of mammalian tissue. He was able to keep the excised viscera of an animal alive and functioning physiologically *in vitro.* For his later work see the same journal, 1911, **14,** 244-7; 1913, **18,** 155-61.

560.1 RAMÓN Y CAJAL, SANTIAGO. 1852-1934
Estudios sobre la degeneración y regeneración de sistema nervioso. 2 vols., Madrid, *N. Moya,* 1913-14.
    The most complete work on the subject so far written. Ramón y Cajal, great neuroanatomist and histologist, was for many years in charge of the institute bearing his name at Madrid. He gained the Nobel Prize in 1906. English translation, 2 vols., London, 1928. Reprinted 1959.

561   LEWIS, MARGARET REED. 1881- , & LEWIS, WARREN HARMON. 1870-1964
Mitochondria and other cytoplasmic structures in tissue cultures. *Amer. J. Anat.*, 1914-15, **17,** 339-401.
    Original investigations upon the visible mitochondria.

562   ASCHOFF, KARL ALBERT LUDWIG. 1866-1942
Das reticulo-endotheliale System. *Ergebn. inn Med.*, 1924, **26,** 1-118.
    In an earlier paper on this subject (*Münch. med. Wschr.*, 1922, **69,** 1352-56) Aschoff introduced the term "reticuol-endotheolial system"; as early as 1914 he grouped certain phagocytic cells into his system.

563   MÖLLENDORFF, WILHELM VON. 1887-1944
Handbuch der mikroskopischen Anatomie des Menschen. 7 vols. [in 17] Berlin, *J. Springer,* 1927-43.

566.1 FELL, *Dame* HONOR BRIDGETT. 1900-1986, & ROBISON, ROBERT. 1883-1941
The growth, development and phosphatase activity of embryonic avian femora in limb-buds cultivated *in vitro. Biochem. J.*, 1929, **23,** 767-84.
    First modern organ cultures.

566.2 SANFORD, KATHERINE KOONTZ. 1915- , *et al.*
The growth in vitro of single isolated tissue cells. *J. nat. Cancer Inst.*, 1948, **9,** 229-46.
    First successful cloning of tissue cells. With W. R. Earle and G. D. Likely.

566.3 ATERMAN, KURT.
Some local factors in the restoration of the rat's liver after partial hepatectomy. 1. Glycogin; the Golgi apparatus; sinusoidal cells; the basement membranes of the sinusoids. *Arch. Path. (Chicago)*, 1952, **53,** 197-208.
    First detailed account of lysosomes.

566.4   DUVE, Christian de. 1917- , *et al.*
Tissue fractionation studies. 6. Intracellular distribution patterns of enzymes in rat-liver tissue. *Biochem. J.,* 1955, **60,** 604-18.
      Lysosomes. With B. C. Pressman, R. Gianetto, R. Wattiaux and F. Appelmans.

567   BAKER, John Randal. 1900-1984
The discovery of the uses of colouring agents in biological micro-technique. *J. Quekett micr. Club,* 1943, ser. 4, **1**, 256-75.

567.1   MURRAY, Margaret Ransome. 1901- , & KOPECH, Gertrude. 1915-
A bibliography of the research in tissue culture 1884-1950. An index to the literature of the living cell cultivated in vitro. 2 vols. New York, *Academic Press,* 1953.

567.2   BRACEGIRDLE, Brian. 1933-
A history of microtechnique. The evolution of the microtome and the development of tissue preparation. London, *Heinemann,* 1978. Second edition, revised, Chicago, *Science Heritage Library*, 1987.

568   ARISTOTLE. 384-322 b.c.
De motu animalium. De incessu animalium. *In his* Works, edited by J. A. Smith and W. D. Ross, Oxford, 1912, **5,** 698a-714b.

569   GALEN. a.d. 130-200
On the natural faculties. With an English translation by A. J. Brock. London, *W. Heinemann,* 1916.
      Greek–English in the Loeb Classical Library. Before Harvey, Galen was the most important figure in experimental physiology.

570   ——. De usu partium libri XVII recensuit G. Helmreich. 2 vols., Lipsiae, *B.G. Teubner,* 1907-09. Reprinted Amsterdam, 1968. An English translation with a very useful introduction and notes was published by M.T. May, 2 vols., Ithaca, N.Y., 1968.

571   NEMESIUS, *Bishop of Emesa. fl.* a.d. 400
Divini Gregorii Nyssae episcopi qui fuit frater Basilii Magni libri octo: I. De homine...Strassburg, *Matthias Schurer,* 1512.
      Nemesius' *De natura hominis,* a physiological and psychological study of man, was highly esteemed during the Middle Ages. He was one of the first to propose that mental processes were localized in the cells or ventricles of the brain, and his comments on the heartbeat and pulse have been erroneously interpreted as an anticipation of Harvey's theory of the circulation. English translation, London, 1636.

572   FERNEL, Jean François. 1497-1558
De naturali parte medicinae libri septem. Parisiis, *apud Simonem Colinaeum,* 1542.
      The earliest work devoted exclusively to physiology and the first to call the subject by that name. It was re-issued in 1554 as part of Fernel's *Medicina* (No. 2271). Fernel suggested that physicians should themselves

study the human body and not accept tradition. See Sir Charles Sherrington's *The endeavour of Jean Fernel,* Cambridge, 1946.

572.1   SANTORIO, SANTORIO [SANCTORIUS]. 1561-1636
Methodi vitandorum errorum omnium, qui in arte medica... Venice, *Bariletto,* 1603.
First mention of Santorio's pulse-clock ("pulsilogium") and his scale. Through most of the 17th and 18th centuries Santorio's name was linked with that of Harvey as the greatest figure in physiology and experimental medicine because of his introduction of precision instruments for quantitative studies. He was also the founder of modern metabolic research.

572.2   ——.Commentaria in artem medicinalem Galeni. Venice, *Jocobus Antonius Somaschus,* 1612.
First printed mention of the air thermometer, an instrument that played a vital part in the creation of static medicine. This device was similar to Galileo's open-air thermoscope, of which Santorio may have known, but he was the first to transform the thermoscope into a thermometer by adding a scale with fixed reference points.

573   ——. Ars...de statica medicina aphorismorum sectionibus septem comprehensa. Venetiis, *apud N. Polum,* 1614.
This collection of aphorisms is the work by which Santorio's ideas became widely known. See also nos. 572.1 & 572.2. For description of his experiments, see No. 2668. English translations by Abdiah Cole (1663), John Davies (1676), and others.

574   DESCARTES, RENÉ. 1596-1650
De homine figuris et latinitate donatus a Florentio Schuyl. Lugduni Batavorum, *apud F. Moyardum & P. Leffen,* 1662.
Descartes considered the human body a material machine, directed by a rational soul located in the pineal body. This book was the first attempt to cover the whole field of "animal physiology". The work is really a physiological appendix to his *Discourse on method,* 1637. The first edition was translated from the French. The French text first appeared in 1664. It was translated, with commentary by T. S. Hall, and published in Cambridge, Mass., in 1972 as *Treatise of man.* See G.A. Lindeboom, *Descartes and medicine,* Amsterdam, *Rodopi,* 1979.

575   CROONE, WILLIAM. 1633-1684
De ratione motus musculorum. Londini, *excud. J. Hayes,* 1664.
Croone accumulated a large fortune from his practice; with it his widow endowed the Croonian Lectures at the Royal College of Physicians, London. He believed muscular contraction to be brought about by the action of a "spirituous liquor" passing from the nerves and interacting with substances in the muscle. Translation of an extract in J. F. Fulton's *Selected readings in the history of physiology,* 2nd ed., 1966, pp. 207-9.

576   STENSEN, NIELS [STENO, NICOLAUS]. 1638-1686
De musculis et glandulis observationum specimen. Hafniae, *lit. M. Godiechenii,* 1664.
Stensen described the structure of muscles, the *fibra motrix,* confirming that contraction actually occurs in the muscle fibres, not in the tendon as Galen had thought. He attempted a geometrical description of muscle

contraction. He described the anatomy of the heart and its function as a muscle, and described the anatomy and function of the respiratory muscles including the diaphragm. English translation of the section on the muscles and the tongue in J.E. Poulson & E. Snorrason, *Nicolaus Steno 1638-1686, A re-consideration by Danish scientists.* Gentofte, Denmark, 1986.

577 ——. Elementorum myologiae specimen. Florentiae, *ex typ. sub signo Stellae,* 1667.

In this work Stensen, in collaboration with the mathematician Vincenzio Viviani (1622-1703), a pupil of Galileo, developed a geometrical description of muscular contraction, and attempted to show theoretically that muscles did not increase in volume during contraction. The appendix contains his anatomical descriptions of the head of two sharks. In discussing the relationship of the shark teeth to similar-shaped fossil stones found in the Mediterranean, Stensen developed theories of how geological structures and fossils might be formed. This was translated by A. Garboe as *The earliest geological treatise (1667),* London, 1958.

578 MAYOW, JOHN. 1643-1679
Tractatus quinque medico-physici. Oxonii, *e theatro Sheldoniano,* 1674.

Mayow was the first to locate the seat of animal heat in the muscles; he discovered the double articulation of the ribs with the spine and came near to discovering oxygen in his suggestion that the object of breathing was to abstract from the air a definite group of life-giving "particles". He was the first to make the definite suggestion that it is only a special fraction of the air that is of use in respiration. His *Tractatus,* embodying all his brilliant conclusions, is one of the best English medical classics. English translation, Edinburgh, 1907.

579 GLISSON, FRANCIS. 1597-1677
Tractatus de ventriculo et intestinis. Londini, *H. Brome,* 1677.

Glisson introduced the idea of irritability as a specific property of all human tissue, a hypothesis which had no effect upon contemporary physiology, but which was later demonstrated experimentally by Haller (No. 587).

580 KIRCHER, ATHANASIUS. 1602-1680
Physiologia Kircheriana experimentalis. Amstelaedami, *J. Waesberg,* 1680.

Includes the first recorded experiment in hypnotism in animals.

581 BOERHAAVE, HERMAN. 1668-1738
Institutiones medicae in usus annuae exercitationis domesticos digestae. Lugduni Batavorum. *J. van der Linden,* 1708.

One of Boerhaave's best works. The first part deals with physiology, with important observations upon digestion.

582 STAHL, GEORG ERNST. 1660-1734
Theoria medica vera. Halle, *lit. Orphanotrophei,* 1708.

Stahl tried to explain vital phenomena by mystical means. He was the head of the so-called Animistic School which explained disease as caused by misdirected activities on the part of the soul.

583 HOFFMANN, FRIEDRICH. 1660-1742
Fundamenta physiologiae. Halle, 1718.

Hoffmann was a writer of extraordinary versatility, and the first to perceive pathology as an aspect of physiology. His *Fundamenta* is an outstanding treatise on physiology. English translation by L. King, London, 1971.

584   BELCHIER, JOHN. 1706-1785
An account of the bones of animals being changed to a red colour by aliment only. *Phil. Trans.* (1735-6), 1738, **39**, 287-8; 299-300.

Belchier fed animals with madder, noting that new bone formed subsequent to its ingestion was stained red. This was the earliest attempt at vital staining and is also important as making possible the study of osteogenesis.

585   HALLER, ALBRECHT VON. 1708-1777
Primae lineae physiologiae in usum praelectionum academicarum. Gottingae, *A. Vandenhoeck,* 1747.

Haller was one of the most imposing figures in the whole of medicine, besides being a superb bibliographer and the founder of medical bibliography. As a physiologist he was the greatest of his time. Many apparently "new" discoveries of later times had already been accounted for by Haller. The above work includes (p. 259) Haller's resonance theory, similar to that already propounded by Du Verney and (more than 100 years later) by Helmholtz (No. 1562). English editions 1754 and later.

586   LA METTRIE, JULIEN OFFRAY DE. 1709-1751
L'homme machine. Leyde, *E. Luzac, fils,* 1748.

La Mettrie attempted among other things to prove the materialism of the soul. Because of his blatant and aggressive atheism, all of La Mettrie's writings were placed on the Index and systematically burned. Owing to its heretical nature, this anonymous work was also ordered to be burnt by the magistrates of Leiden. An English translation appeared in 1749. See Vartanian, *L'homme machine, a study in the origins of an idea,* Princeton, 1960.

587   HALLER, ALBRECHT VON. 1708-1777
De partibus corporis humani sensibilibus et irritabilibus. *Comment. Soc. reg. sci. Gotting.* (1752), 1753, **2**, 114-58.

Glisson in 1677 had introduced the concept of "irritability" as a specific property of all tissues. Haller, in the above work, recorded his experimental proof of this, and distinguished between nerve impulse (sensibility) and muscular contraction (irritability). English translation in *Bull. Hist. Med.,* 1937, **4**, 651-99.

588   ——. Elementa physiologiae corporis humani. 8 vols. Lausanne, Berne, 1757-66.

Haller synthesized the whole physiological knowledge of his time. In the above, probably his greatest work, Haller included some anatomical descriptions which were most valuable. He is said to have written more than 1300 scientific papers.

589   WALSH, JOHN. ?1725-1795
Of the electric property of the torpedo. *Phil Trans.,* 1773, **63**, 461-77.

The first accurate study of the electrical organs of the torpedo fish were made by Walsh, who was given the Copley Medal of the Royal Society for his work on the subject. Walsh proved that the shock of the torpedo was electrical and that the fish could only send the shock through a conductor.

590   BLAGDEN, *Sir* CHARLES. 1748-1820
        Experiments and observations in an heated room. *Phil. Trans.*, 1775, **65,**
        111-23; 484-94.
        First demonstration of the importance of perspiration in the mainten-
        ance of constant body temperature.

591   CRAWFORD, ADAIR. 1748-1795
        Experiments and observations on animal heat. London, *J. Murray,* 1779.
        Earliest experiments upon animal calorimetry.

592   LAVOISIER, ANTOINE LAURENT. 1743-1794, & LA PLACE, PIERRE SIMON DE. 1749-
        1827
        Mémoire sur la chaleur. *Hist Acad. roy. Sci. (Paris),* (1780), 1784, 335-408.
        These workers invented an ice calorimeter, with it measured the
        respiratory quotient of a pig, and demonstrated the analogy between
        respiration and combustion.

593   GALVANI, LUIGI. 1737-1798
        De viribus electricitatis in motu musculari commentarius. *Bonon. Sci. Art.*
        Inst. Acad. Comment., Bologna, 1791, **7,** 363-418.
        In the course of his experiments on irritable responses caused by static
        electricity applied to frog muscles, Galvani produced electric current from
        the contact of two different metals in a moist environment. Galvani
        mistakenly believed this phenomenon (which his nephew Giovanni
        Aldini called "galvanism") to be animal electricity. *See* No. 594.1 Facsimile
        of Volta's copy, with English translation, and bibliography of editions and
        translations by J.F. Fulton and M.E. Stanton, Norwalk, Conn., *Burndy Lib-*
        rary, 1953.

594   SÉGUIN, ARMAND. 1768-1835, & LAVOISIER, ANTOINE LAURENT. 1743-1794
        Premier mémoire sur la respiration des animaux. *Hist Acad. Sci. (Paris),*
        (1789), 1793, 566-84.
        Séguin and Lavoisier measured the metabolism of a man (Séguin
        himself). They made three observations of fundamental importance in this
        respect; that the intensity of oxidation in man is dependent upon (1) food,
        (2) environmental temperature, and (3) mechanical work.

594.1   [GALVANI, LUIGI. 1737-1798]
        Dell'uso e dell'attività dell arco conduttore nelle contrazioni dei muscoli.
        Bologna, *S. Tommaso d'Aquino,* 1794.
        The first account of Galvani's electrical experiments without the pres-
        ence of metals, in which he demonstrated the presence of electrical energy
        in living tissue by showing that convulsions in frog nerve-muscle prepara-
        tions could be produced simply by touching nerve to muscle. This
        observation of the injury current of nerve or demarcation current was the
        first proof of animal electricity. The key experiment appears in a 23-page
        "Supplemento" following p. 168. Some authorities consider this a joint
        publication of Galvani and Aldini. *See* No. 593.

595   CRUIKSHANK, WILLIAM CUMBERLAND. 1745-1800
        Experiments on the insensible perspiration of the human body. London,
        G. Nicol, 1795.
        Demonstration that carbon dioxide is given off by the skin. This book
        was first privately printed in 1779; above is the corrected edition.

596   REIL, JOHANN CHRISTIAN. 1759-1813
Von der Lebenskraft. *Arch. Physiol. (Halle)*, 1796, **1**, 8-162.
Reil advanced the doctrine of the life-force as the chemical expression
of physiological function. Like Glisson and Hunter, he recognized irritability as a specific property of tissue. He founded the *Archiv für die Physiologie*,
the first journal of physiology.

597   BICHAT, MARIE FRANÇOIS XAVIER. 1771-1802
Recherches physiologiques sur la vie et la mort. Paris, *Brosson, Gabon et
Cie.*, an VIII [1800].
When Volta questioned the validity of experiments claiming to show
responsiveness of an *ex vivo* heart, devoid of blood flow and nervous
connections, Bichat obtained permission to experiment upon the freshly
killed bodies of those guillotined during the French Revolution. His trials
on both laboratory animals and human cadavers led him to conclude that
cardiac excitation by electricity would occur only when the organ was
stimulated by direct contact. English translation of second edition, Philadelphia, 1809.

597.1   MAGENDIE, FRANÇOIS. 1783-1855
Précis élémentaire de physiologie. 2 vols., Paris, *Méquignon-Marvis*, 1816-
17.
The first modern physiology textbook in which doctrine gave way to
simple, precise descriptions of experimental facts. Vol. 2 contains Magendie's
classic demonstration of the importance of nitrogenous food, or protein,
in the food supply of mammals. *See* No. 1041.1

598   ——. Mémoires sur le mécanisme de l'absorption chez les animaux à sang
rouge et chaud. *J. Physiol. exp. path.*, 1821, **1**, 1-17, 18-31.
Magendie, the pioneer of experimental physiology in France, demonstrated the absorption of fluids and semisolids to be a function of the blood-
vessels, as well as of the lymphatics. He was the founder, in 1821, of the
Journal de physiologie expérimentale.

598.1   EDWARDS, WILLIAM FREDERIC. 1776-1842
De l'influence des agens physiques sur la vie. Paris, *Crochard*, 1824.
Edwards studied the influence of environmental factors on animal life,
concluding that vital processes depend on external physical and chemical
forces but are not entirely controlled by them. His book is a pioneer work
in animal ecology. English translation by Thomas Hodgkin, with important
additional material by Hodgkin and others, London, 1832. *See* No. 1991.

599   BURDACH, KARL FRIEDRICH. 1776-1847
Die Physiologie als Erfahrungswissenschaft. 6 vols. Leipzig, Königsberg,
1826-40.
Burdach's great textbook of physiology was planned to run to 10 vols.,
but the death of his wife quenched his enthusiasm for the task. Parts of the
text were written by von Baer, Rathke, Johannes Müller, R. Wagner and
others, under the direction of Burdach. Von Baer's contribution includes
material also published the same year in *Ueber Entwicklungsgeschichte der
Thiere*. Burdach's unsatisfactory editing of it for *Die Physiologie* stimulated
von Baer to have his own separate book published. *See* No. 479.

600   SHARPEY, William. 1802-1880
On a peculiar motion excited in fluids by the surfaces of certain animals.
Edinb. med. surg. J., 1830, **34,** 113-22.

Sharpey was the first occupant of the chair of anatomy and physiology
at University College, London, this chair being the first official recognition
of physiology in any English medical school. He wrote a memorable paper
on cilia and ciliary motion. Through his students Sharpey was the founder
of the British school of physiology. Among his pupils were Michael Foster,
Burdon-Sanderson and Schäfer.

601   MÜLLER, Johannes. 1801-1858
Handbuch der Physiologie des Menschen. 2 vols. Coblenz, *J. Hölscher,* 1834-
40.

The first modern, systematic textbook on physiology, presenting an
authoritative and discerning survey of each aspect of the science. This is
also one of the best reviews of physiological literature during the first part
of the 19th century. Through an extensive series of publications and the
Arch. Anat. Physiol. wiss. Med. which he edited, Müller made fundamental
contributions to anatomy and physiology, pathological anatomy and
histology, embryology, and zoology. Vol. 1 was issued in parts, 1833-34,
and Vol. 2 was issued in parts, 1837-40. A somewhat abbreviated English
translation was published, 1838-42.

602   PURKYNĚ, Jan Evangelista. 1787-1869, & VALENTIN, Gabriel Gustav. 1810-
1883
De phaenomeno generali et fundamentali motus vibratorii contini in
membranis. Wratislaviae, *sumpt. A. Schulz et soc.,* 1835.

Classical paper on ciliary epithelial motion. Reprinted in Purkyně's *Opera
omnia* (No. 82), pp. 277-371, 1918. English translation in *Dublin J. med.
chem. Sci.,* 1835, **7,** 279-84.

603   SHARPEY, William. 1802-1880
Cilia. In Todd's *Cyclopaedia of anatomy and physiology.* London, 1835-36,
1, 606-38.

The important discoveries of Purkyně and Valentin, together with additional observations by Sharpey himself were embodied in an article
written by him for Todd's *Cyclopaedia.*

604   WEBER, Wilhelm Eduard. 1804-1891, & WEBER, Eduard Friedrich Wilhelm.
1806-1871
Mechanik der menschlichen Gehwerkzeuge. 1 vol. and atlas. Göttingen, *in
der Dieterichschen Buchhandlung,* 1836.

A pioneering study of the physiology and biomechanics of motion and
locomotion. The atlas contains illustrations that were printed directly from
actual bones embedded in the printing plates.

605   MATTEUCCI, Carlo. 1811-1868
Sur le courant électrique ou propre de la grenouille. *Ann. Chim.,* 1838, **68,**
93-106.

Matteucci established the difference of potential between injured nerve
and its muscle.

606 MAYER, JULIUS ROBERT VON. 1814-1878
Bemerkungen über die Kräfte der unbelebten Natur, *Ann. Chem. Pharm. (Lemgo)*, 1842, **42**, 233-40.
Mayer demonstrated the principle of the conservation of energy as far as physiological processes are concerned.

607 WAGNER, RUDOLPH. 1805-1864
Handwörterbuch der Physiologie ... hrsg. VON R. WAGNER. 4 vols. Braunschweig, *F. Vieweg & Sohn,* 1842-53.
Wagner was professor at Göttingen. His literary output was enormous. In the above work he contributed the sections on sympathetic nerves, nerve-ganglia, and nerve-endings. This work contained 63 extensive review articles from 30 authors.

608 MATTEUCCI, CARLO. 1811-1868, & HUMBOLDT, FRIEDRICH HEINRICH ALEXANDER VON. 1769-1859
Sur le courant électrique des muscles des animaux vivants ou récemment tués. *C. R. Acad. Sci. (Paris),* 1843, **16**, 197-200.
Matteucci's "rheoscopic frog" effect.

609 DU BOIS-REYMOND, EMIL. 1818-1896
Ueber den sogennanten Froschstrom. *Ann. Physik. (Berl.),* 1843, **58**, 1-30.
First description and definition of electrotonus.

610 ——. Untersuchungen über thierische Elektricität. 2 vols. [in 3]. Berlin, *G. Reimer,* 1848-84.
A pupil of J. Müller, Emil du Bois-Reymond was the founder of modern electrophysiology. He introduced faradic stimulation and made an exhaustive investigation of physiological tetanus. Above is a collective edition of his writings on the subject. Extracts were translated into English in H.B. Jones, *On animal electricity*...London, 1852, and more extensive portions in C.E. Morgan, *Electrophysiology and therapeutics*, New York, 1868.

611 HELMHOLTZ, HERMANN LUDWIG FERDINAND VON. 1821-1894
Ueber die Erhaltung der Kraft, eine physikalische Abhandlung. Berlin, *G. Reimer,* 1847.
An epoch-making work which led the way to the acceptance of the fundamental physical doctrine of the conservation of energy.

612 ——. Ueber die Wärmeentwickelung bei der Muskelaction. *Arch. Anat. Physiol. wiss. Med,* 1848, 144-64.
Helmholtz showed the muscles to be the principal source of animal heat.

613 MOLESCHOTT, JACOB. 1822-1893
Physiologie des Stoffwechsels in Pflanzen und Thieren. Erlangen, *F. Enke,* 1851.

614 DUCHENNE DE BOULOGNE, GUILLAUME BENJAMIN AMAND, 1806-1875
De l'électrisation localisée et de son application à la physiologie, à la pathologie et à la thérapeutique. Paris, *J. B. Baillière,* 1855.
Duchenne classified the electrophysiology of the entire muscular system and summed up his findings in the above work. The application of his results to pathological conditions marks him as the founder of electro-

therapy. An *Album de photographies pathologiques* was published in 1862 to accompany the text of the second edition, 1861. Engl. trans. of 3rd ed., Philadelphia, 1871. *See* Nos. 1995 & 4543.

615   BERNARD, CLAUDE. 1813-1878
Leçons de physiologie expérimentale appliquée à la médecine. 2 vols. Paris, *J. B. Baillière,* 1855-56.
Claude Bernard made strenuous efforts to introduce experimental methods into physiology. The above includes his classic work on the function of the liver, pancreas, and gastric glands. *See also* No. 634.

616   ——. Analyse physiologique des propriétés des systèmes musculaires et nerveux au moyen de curare. *C. R. Acad. Sci. (Paris),* 1856, **43,** 825-29.
Bernard paralysed motor nerve-endings with curare and demonstrated the independent excitability of muscle; his paper is the classic proof of Haller's doctrine of irritability.

617   FICK, ADOLPH. 1829-1901
Die medizinische Physik. Braunschweig, *F. Vieweg,* 1856.

618   KÖLLIKER, RUDOLPH ALBERT VON. 1817-1905, & MÜLLER, HEINRICH. 1820-1864
Nachweis der negativen Schwankung des Muskelstroms am natürlich sich contrahirenden Muskel. *Verh. phys.-med. Ges. Würzburg,* 1856, **6,** 528-33.
Kölliker and Müller were the first to measure action currents from cardiac muscle.

619   RAINEY, GEORGE. 1801-1884
On the formation of the skeletons of animals, and other hard structures formed in connexion with living tissues. *Brit. for. med.-chir. Rev.,* 1857, **20,** 451-76.
Includes description of "Rainey's tubes" or "corpuscles" in connexion with the process of calcification of tissues.

620   KÜHNE, WILLY. 1837-1900
Untersuchungen über Bewegungen und Veränderungen der contraktilen Substanz. *Arch. Anat. Physiol. wiss. Med.,* 1859, 564-642, 748-835.
Proof of the coagulability of muscle proteins.

621   PFLÜGER, EDUARD FRIEDRICH WILHELM. 1829-1910
Untersuchungen über die Physiologie des Electrotonus. Berlin, *A. Hirschwald,* 1859.
One of the most interesting works of its time on the physiology of nerve. In it Pflüger first stated the laws governing the make and break stimulation of nerve with the galvanic current. Pflüger was a pupil of Müller and du Bois-Reymond.

622   BERNARD, CLAUDE. 1813-1878
Du rôle des actions réflexes paralysantes dans le phénomène des sécrétions. *J. Anat. Physiol. (Paris),* 1864, **1,** 507-13.
Studies of the "paralytic secretions" occasioned by section of glandular nerves.

623 FICK, ADOLPH. 1829-1901
Untersuchungen über elektrische Nervenreizung. Braunschweig, *F. Vieweg*, 1864.

 Among the instruments introduced by Fick for the study of muscle and nerve physiology were the myotonograph, the cosine lever, and an improved thermopile.

624 DUCHENNE DE BOULOGNE, GUILLAUME BENJAMIN AMAND. 1806-1875
Physiologie des mouvements demontrée à l'aide de l'expérimentation électrique et de l'observation clinique, et applicable à l'étude des paralysies et des déformations. Paris, *J. B. Baillière*, 1867.

 A monumental work, the result of twenty years' study of electro-muscular stimulation "to determine the proper action which the muscles possess in life". The book contains an excellent record of the kinesiology of the entire muscular system. English translation by E. B. Kaplan, Philadelphia, 1949.

625 HERMANN, LUDIMAR. 1838-1914
Untersuchungen über den Stoffwechsel der Muskeln, ausgehend vom Gaswechsel derselben. Berlin, *A. Hirschwald*, 1867.

 Hermann's views on nitrogen metabolism in muscular work correctly anticipated the later conclusions of Fletcher, Hopkins, and others.

626 FLINT, AUSTIN, *Jnr.* 1836-1915
On the physiological effects of severe and protracted muscular exercise; with especial reference to the influence of exercise upon the excretion of nitrogen. *N. Y. med. J.*, 1871, **13**, 609-97.

 Flint made investigations on the nitrogen output of a long-distance walker, before, during, and after the latter's attempt to walk 400 miles in five days. The useful data in this paper are often referred to in discussions on the subject. Edition in book form, New York, *D. Appleton*, 1871.

627 PFLÜGER, EDUARD FRIEDRICH WILHELM. 1829-1910
Ueber die Diffusion des Sauerstoffs, den Ort und die Gesetze der Oxydationsprocesse im thierischen Organismus. *Pflüg. Arch. ges. Physiol.*, 1872, **6**, 43-64, 190.

628 HAUGHTON, SAMUEL. 1821-1897
Principles of animal mechanics. London, *Longmans, Green, & Co.*, 1873.

 Haughton stated that the muscular mechanism is so arranged that its work is carried out with the minimum of muscular contraction. This he called the "principle of least action". His opposition to Darwinism is especially noticed in this book.

629 STIRLING, WILLIAM. 1851-1932
Ueber die summation elektrischer Hautreize. *Arb. Physiol. Anst. Leipzig*, (1874), 1875, **9**, 223-91.

 Stirling, a pupil of Ludwig, became a great teacher of physiology. His paper on the summation of electrical stimuli to the skin was a prize thesis.

630 ECK, NIKOLAI VLADIMIROVICH. 1848-1908
K voprosu o perevyazkie vorotnoi veni. Predvaritelnoye soobshtshenize. [On the ligature of the portal vein.] *Voyenno med. J.*, 1877, **130**, No. 2, 1-2.

Eck developed the "Eck fistula" for the experimental study of diseases of the liver and the relation of the liver to metabolism. English translation in *Surg. Gynec. Obstet.*, 1953, **96,** 375.

631   FOSTER, *Sir* MICHAEL. 1836-1907
A text-book of physiology. London, *Macmillan,* 1877.
Foster was one of the greatest of the modern teachers of physiology. He became professor at Cambridge in 1883. Many great scientists are numbered among his pupils. See G.L. Geisen, Michael Foster and the Cambridge School of Physiology. Princeton, *Princeton University Press*, 1978.

632   ROMANES, GEORGE JOHN. 1848-1894
Observations on the locomotor system of Medusae. *Phil. Trans.*, (1876), 1877, **166,** 269-313; (1877), 1878, **167,** 659-752; (1880), 1881, **171,** 161-202.
Romanes' work with electro-stimulation directly influenced Gaskell in his artificial production of "heart-block", the name for which Gaskell based on an expression of Romanes. *See* No. 829.

633   PFLÜGER, EDUARD FRIEDRICH WILHELM. 1829-1910
Ueber Wärme und Oxydation der lebendigen Materie. *Pflüg. Arch. ges. Physiol.*, 1878, **18,** 247-380.

634   BERNARD, CLAUDE. 1813-1878
Leçons de physiologie opératoire. Paris, *J. B. Baillière,* 1879.
In this, his last work, Bernard showed himself "the unapproachable master in the technique of experimental procedure" (Garrison).

635   VOIT, CARL VON. 1831-1908
Handbuch der Physiologie des Gesammt-Stoffwechsels und der Fortpflanzung. Leipzig, *F. C. W. Vogel,* 1881.
Forms vol. 6, pt. 1 of Hermann's *Handbuch der Physiologie.*

636   MOSSO, ANGELO. 1846-1910
Les lois de la fatigue étudiées dans les muscles de l'homme. *Arch. ital. Biol.*, 1890, **13,** 123-86.
Mosso invented the ergograph from the study of voluntary contraction. The description of the instrument is on pages 124-41 of the above article.

637   BRAUNE, CHRISTIAN WILHELM. 1831-1892, & FISCHER, OTTO. 1861-1917
Die Bewegungen des Kniegelenkes. *Abh. math.-phys. Cl. k. sächs. Ges. Wiss. Leipzig,* 1891, **17,** 78-150.
Investigation of the mechanics of motion on mathematical lines. *See also* No. 645.

638   CHAUVEAU, JEAN BAPTISTE AUGUSTE. 1827-1917
Le travail musculaire et l'énergie qu'il représente. Paris, *Asselin & Houzeau,* 1891.
Important studies on thermodynamics of muscular work.

639   MOSSO, ANGELO. 1846-1910
La fatica. Milano, *frat. Treves,* 1891.
Mosso investigated muscular fatigue with the ergograph of his invention. He showed fatigue to be due to a toxin produced by muscular contraction. English translation, 1906.

640   NOORDEN, CARL HARKO VON. 1858-1944
        Beiträge zur Lehre von Stoffwechsel. I. Grundriss einer Methodik der
        Stoffwechsel-Untersuchungen. Berlin, *A. Hirschwald,* 1893.

641   WOLFF, JULIUS. 1836-1902
        Das Gesetz der Transformation der Knochen. Berlin, *A. Hirschwald,* 1892.
            "Wolff's law" stated that every change in form and function of a bone,
        or in its function alone, is followed by certain definite changes in its internal
        architecture and equally definite secondary alterations in its mathematical
        laws. English translation by P. Maquet and R. Furlong. Berlin, *Springer-
        Verlag,* 1986.

642   ENGELMANN, THEODOR WILHELM. 1843-1909
        Ueber den Ursprung der Muskelkraft. Leipzig, *W. Engelmann,* 1893.

643   MAREY, ÉTIENNE JULES. 1830-1904
        Le mouvement. Paris, *G. Masson,* 1894.
            Marey, like Muybridge (No. 650-51), was a pioneer in the use of serial
        pictures as a method of studying the mechanics of locomotion. English
        translation, 1895.

644   BIEDERMANN, WILHELM. 1852-1929
        Elektrophysiologie. Jena, *G. Fischer,* 1895.
            First exhaustive treatise on electrophysiology. English translation, 2
        vols., London, 1896-98.

645   BRAUNE, CHRISTIAN WILHELM. 1831-1892, & FISCHER, OTTO. 1861-1917
        Der Gang des Menschen. *Abh. math.-phys. Cl. k. sächs. Ges. Wiss. Leipzig,*
        1895, **21,** 153-322.
            Classic study of the human gait. The authors calculated the external and
        internal forces involved in walking and described the kinematics and
        kinetics of the movement. English translation by P. Maquet & R. Furlong,
        Berlin, *Springer-Verlag,* 1987.

646   RICHET, CHARLES ROBERT. 1850-1935
        Dictionnaire de physiologie. Vols. 1-10. Paris, *F. Alcan,* 1895-1928.
            Covers A–Moelle épinière only.

647   STARLING, ERNEST HENRY. 1866-1927
        On the absorption of fluids from the connective tissue spaces. *J. Physiol.
        (Lond.),* 1896, **19,** 312-26.
            Starling discovered the functional significance of the serum proteins.

648   ATWATER, WILBUR OLIN. 1844-1907, & LANGWORTHY, CHARLES FORD.
        1864-1932.
        A digest of metabolism experiments in which the balance of income and
        outgo was determined. Washington, *Govt. Printing Off.,* 1898.

649   SHARPEY-SCHAFER, *Sir* EDWARD ALBERT. 1850-1935
        Text-book of physiology. Edited by E. A. SCHÄFER. 2 vols. Edinburgh, *Y. J.
        Pentland,* 1898-1900.
            A collective work and a classic textbook of physiology. Sharpey-
        Schafer is one of the greatest names in British physiology. He was a pupil
        of Sharpey, and when that great man died without any known descendants

117

Schäfer gave the name to his son, in order to perpetuate it. When his son was killed in the war of 1914-1918, Schäfer added it to his own.

649.1   MAGNUS-LEVY, Adolf. 1865-1955, & FALK, Ernst.
Der Lungengaswechsel des Menschen in den verschiedenen. Altersstufen. *Arch. Anat. Physiol., Physiol. Abt.,* 1899, Suppl.-Bd, 314-81.
The first systematic study of the basal metabolism of normal individuals from childhood to old age.

650   MUYBRIDGE, Eadweard [James Edward Muggeridge]. 1830-1904.
Animals in motion. London, *Chapman & Hall,* 1899.

651   ——. The human figure in motion. An electro-photographic investigation of consecutive phases of muscular actions. London, *Chapman & Hall,* 1901.
Muybridge, an Englishman, made exhaustive photographic investigations of consecutive animal movements while he was in America. More than 100,000 photographs were embodied in his *Animal locomotion. An electro-photographic investigation of consecutive phases of animal movements,* 1872-85. Philadelphia, 1887. The great cost of producing this work of 11 folio volumes with 781 photo-engravings restricted its sale to a very few copies and the above two books are abridgements. This pioneer study of serial photography demonstrated the possibilities of motion pictures and foreshadowed the modern cinematograph. Reprinted New York, 1955. All 781 plates from the 1887 *Animal locomotion* were re-published New York, *Dover,* 1979, with introduction by A. Mozley.

652   LUCIANI, Luigi. 1840-1919
Fisiologia dell'uomo. 3 vols. Milan, *Società Edit. Libraria,* 1901-11.
5th edition (5 vols.), 1919-21; English translation (5 vols.), London, 1911-21. Luciani was professor of physiology successively at Siena, Florence, and Rome.

653   BERNSTEIN, Julius. 1839-1917
Untersuchungen zur Thermodynamik der bioelektrischen Ströme. *Pflüg. Arch. ges. Physiol.,* 1902, **92,** 521-62; 1908, **122,** 129-95; **124,** 462-68.
Bernstein's important studies on the nature of muscular contraction included the observation that changes in surface tension are a controlling factor in the development of the energy of muscular contraction.

654   LOEB, Jacques. 1859-1924
The dynamics of living matter. New York, *Columbia University Press,* 1906.

655   LAPICQUE, Louis. 1866-1952
Définition expérimentale de l'excitabilité. *C. R. Soc. Biol. (Paris),* 1909, **67,** 280-83.
Lapicque first defined "chronaxia", the duration of excitation of tissue. Partial translation in J. F. Fulton's *Selected readings in the history of physiology,* 2nd ed., 1966, pp. 233-34.

656   WINTERSTEIN, Hans. 1879-1963
Handbuch der vergleichenden Physiologie. Hrsg. von Hans Winterstein. 4 vols. Jena, *G. Fischer,* 1910-25.

656.1 MACEWEN, *Sir* William. 1848-1924
The growth of bone. Glasgow, *J. Maclehose,* 1912.
Throughout his life Macewen devoted much time to the study of bone growth. His researches revolutionized ideas concerning osteogenesis.

657 BENEDICT, Francis Gano. 1870-1957, & CATHCART, Edward Provan. 1877-1954
Muscular work. A metabolic study. Washington, *Carnegie Inst.,* 1913.

658 BAYLISS, *Sir* William Maddock. 1860-1924
Principles of general physiology. London, *Longmans, Green,* 1915.
Bayliss's book treats of general physiology from the physical chemical point of view. For some years it remained the most important book of its kind, and today is still of great value for its historical information and its accurate bibliography. A fifth edition, edited by L. E. Bayliss, appeared in 1959-60.

659 HILL, Archibald Vivian. 1886-1977, & HARTREE, William. 1870-1943
The four phases of heat-production of muscle. *J. Physiol. (Lond.),* 1920, **54,** 84-128.
Hill and Hartree made valuable contributions to the knowledge of the thermodynamics of muscle. Hill shared the Nobel Prize with Meyerhof in 1922 for his discovery relating to the production of heat in muscle. *See also Physiol. Rev.,* 1922, **2,** 310-41, and Hill, A. V., *Trails and trials in physiology: a bibliography 1909-1964,* 1965.

660 READ, Jay Marion. 1889-
Correlation of basal metabolic rate with pulse rate and pulse pressure. *J. Amer. med. Ass.,* 1922, **78,** 1887-89.
Read's formula for computation of basal metabolic rate.

661 MAGNUS, Rudolf. 1873-1927
Körperstellung. Berlin, *J. Springer,* 1924.
A classic work on muscle tone and posture, a subject upon which Magnus spent many years of study. He demonstrated among other things that the labyrinth is the one sense organ entirely concerned with posture and equilibrium. English translation, New Delhi, 1987.

662 BETHE, Albrecht. 1872-1954, *et al.*
Handbuch der normalen und pathologischen Physiologie. Hrsg. von. A. Bethe, G. Bergmann, *etc.* 18 vols. Berlin, *J. Springer,* 1925-32.

663 FULTON, John Farquhar. 1899-1960
Muscular contraction and the reflex control of movement. Baltimore, *Williams & Wilkins,* 1926.
A detailed study of the physiology of skeletal muscle. A valuable historical introduction will be found on pp. 3-55, and the book includes an extensive bibliography.

663.1 MAGNUS, Rudolf. 1873-1927
Cameron Prize Lectures on some results of studies in the physiology of posture. *Lancet,* 1926, **2,** 531-36, 585-88.
Magnus demonstrated the function of the otoliths and semicircular canals of the inner ear in regulating the equilibrium of the body.

119

664 CANNON, WALTER BRADFORD. 1871-1945
The wisdom of the body. New York, *Norton & Co.,* 1932.
  A discussion of the regulation of body fluids, hunger, thirst, temperature, oxygen supply, water, sugar, and proteins of the body, and the role of the sympathetic-adrenal mechanism.

For history, see Nos. 1571-1588.11

BIOCHEMISTRY

665 HELMONT, JEAN BAPTISTE VAN. 1577-1644
Ortus medicinae. Amstelodami, *apud L. Elzevirium,* 1648.
  Helmont was one of the founders of biochemistry. He was the first to realize the physiological importance of ferments and gases, and indeed invented the word "gas". He introduced the gravimetric idea in the analysis of urine. Helmont published very little during his life. The above work is a collection of his writings, issued by his son, Franz Mercurius, who also worked with the Cabalist scholar/mystic, Christian Knorr von Rosenroth (1636-89) on the expanded German language version (Sulzbach, *Endters Söhne,* 1683), considered the best edition of the text. English translation from the Latin, London, *L. Loyd,* 1662. The German edition was reprinted with notes by W. Pagel & K. Kemp, Munich, *Kösel,* 1971.

665.1 BOYLE, ROBERT. 1627-1691
Certain physiological essays. London, *Henry Herringman,* 1661.
  In this prelude to Boyle's *Sceptical chymist* Boyle describes his corpuscular view of digestion, "giving recognition to the existence of the agents now designated the 'enzymes' " (Fulton, *Bibliography of Robert Boyle* [1961] 25). The above work also contains Boyle's first published accounts of chemical experiments.

666 ——. A defence of the doctrine touching the spring and weight of the air. London, *J. G. for Thomas Robinson,* 1662.
  Boyle's law. The above pamphlet was appended to the second edition of Boyle's *The spring and weight of the air,* 1662. The relevant passage is reproduced in J. F. Fulton's *Selected readings in the history of physiology,* 2nd ed., 1966, pp. 8-10. Fulton published an annotated bibliography of Boyle's works in 1956 (2nd ed., 1961).

666.1 BOERHAAVE, HERMAN. 1668-1738
Elementa chemiae. 2 vols., Lugduni Batavorum, *Apud Isaacum Severinum,* 1732.
  Boerhaave was the first to separate out urea from urine, and to do so without adding chemical substances such as alcohol or nitric acid. He first published his method for isolating it in the above work. English translation, London, 1735.

667 ROUELLE, HILAIRE MARIE. 1718-1779
Observations sur l'urine humaine. *J. Méd. Chir Pharm.,* 1773, **40,** 451-68.
  Discovery of urea, independently of Boerhaave. Rouelle isolated urea as the alcohol-soluble substance from urine. He was the first to present proof of the high nitrogen content of urea.

668   SCHEELE, CARL WILHELM. 1742-1786
Undersökning om blasestenen. *Kongl. Vetenskaps-Acad. Handl.*, 1776, **37**, 327-32.
Discovery of uric acid. English translation in his *Chemical Essays,* London, 1786.

668.1   WOLLASTON, WILLIAM HYDE. 1766-1828
On cystic oxide, a new species of urinary calculus. *Phil. Trans.,* 1810, **100**, 223-30.
Cystine, the first amino-acid to be isolated, was prepared by Wollaston from a urinary calculus. This was also the first report of cystinuria.

668.2   CHEVREUL, MICHEL EUGÈNE. 1786-1889
Recherches chimiques sur plusieurs corps gras, et particulièrement sur leurs combinations avec les calculs. Cinquième mémoire. Des corps qu'on a appelés adipocire, c'est-à-dire, de la substance cristallisée des calculs biliaires humains, du spermacéti et de la substance grasse des cadavres. *Ann. Chim. (Paris),* 1815, **95**, 5-50.
Chevreul characterized cholesterol.

668.3   BRACONNOT, HENRI. 1780-1855
Mémoire sur la conversion de matières animales en nouvelles substances par le moyen de l'acide sulfurique. *Ann. Chim. Phys.,* 1820, Sér. 2, **13**, 113-15.
Isolation of glycine and leucine.

669   CHEVREUL, MICHEL EUGÈNE. 1786-1889
Recherches chimiques sur les corps gras d'origine animale. Paris, *F. G. Levrault,* 1823.
A classic study of animal fats. Chevreul discovered that fats are composed of fatty acids and glycerol.

670   DUTROCHET, RENÉ JOACHIM HENRI. 1776-1847
Nouvelles observations sur l'endosmose et l'exosmose. *Ann. Chim. Phys.,* 1827, **35**, 393-400; 1828, **37**, 191-201; 1832, **49**, 411-37; **51**, 159-66; 1835, **60**, 337-68.
The process by which water passes through a membrane from a solution on the one side to another solution on the other side has been known, since the classic work of Dutrochet, as "endosmosis" or "exosmosis"; the pressure due to this passage of water has naturally been called "osmotic".

671   WÖHLER, FRIEDRICH. 1800-1882
Ueber künstliche Bildung des Harnstoffs. *Ann. Phys. Chem. (Leipzig),* 1828, **12**, 253-6.
The synthetic preparation of urea was the first occasion that an organic compound was built up from inorganic materials. Wöhler's discovery led eventually to the brilliant results that have been achieved in attempts to synthesize other organic compounds. A French translation of this article appears in *Ann. Chim. (Paris),* 1828, **37**, 330-34. English translation in Leicester & Klickstein (eds.), *A source book in chemistry 1400-1900,* Cambridge, Mass., 1952.

672   CHEVREUL, MICHEL EUGÈNE. 1786-1889
Neues eigenthümliches stickstoffhaltiges Princip, in Muskelfleisch
gefunden. *J. Chem. Physik.*, 1832, **65**, 455-56.
Isolation of creatine from muscle.

673   MÜLLER, JOHANNES. 1801-1858
Ueber Knorpel und Knochen. *Ann. Pharm. (Heidelberg)*, 1837, **21**, 277-82.
Isolation of chondrin and glutin.

674   SCHWANN, THEODOR. 1810-1882
Vorlaüfige Mittheilung betreffend Versuche über die Weingährung und
Fäulniss. *Ann. Phys. Chem. (Leipzig)*, 1837, **41**, 184-93.
Proof that putrefaction is produced by living bodies. Independently of
Cagniard-Latour, Schwann discovered the yeast cell. He is regarded as the
founder of the germ theory of putrefaction and fermentation.

675   CAGNIARD-LATOUR, CHARLES, *Baron.* 1777-1859
Mémoire sur la fermentation vineuse. *Ann. Chim. Phys.*, 1838, **68**, 206-22.
The earliest demonstration of the true nature of yeast was made by
Cagniard-Latour in 1836. All his work on the subject is summed up in this
paper.

676   MULDER, GERARD JOHANN. 1802-1880
Action de l'acide hydrochlorique sur la protéine. *Bull. Sci. Phys. nat. (Leyde)*,
1838, 153.
Mulder gave the name *protéine* to a substance which he believed to be
the essential constituent of all organized bodies. Later, with Liebig, he
found there was no such definite compound, but the work remained to
designate the nitrogenous products of which it was a mixture.

677   LIEBIG, JUSTUS VON. 1803-1873
Die organische Chemie in ihrer Anwendung auf Physiologie und Pathologie.
Braunschweig, *F. Vieweg,* 1842.
First classification of the organic foodstuffs and the processes of
nutrition. With this book Liebig introduced the concept of metabolism into
physiology. English translation, London, 1842.

678   WÖHLER, FRIEDRICH. 1800-1882
Umwandlung der Benzoësäure in Hippursäure im lebenden Organismus.
Ann. Phys. Chem. (Leipzig), 1842, **56**, 638-41.
Discovery that benzoic acid taken in with food is excreted in the urine
as hippuric acid – a discovery of importance in the chemistry of metabo-
lism. (But *see* the footnote to p. 474 of Garrison's *History of medicine,* 1929.)

679   PETTENKOFER, MAX JOSEF VON. 1818-1901
Notiz über eine neue Reaction auf Galle und Zucker. *Ann. Chem. Pharm.*
1844, **52**, 90-96.
Pettenkofer's test for bile. Previously there had been no means of
recognizing the presence of the bile salts.

680   FEHLING, HERMANN CHRISTIAN VON. 1812-1885
Quantitative Bestimmung des Zuckers im Harn. *Arch. physiol. Heilk.,* 1848,
7, 64-73.
Fehling's test for sugar in the urine.

681   STRECKER, ADOLPH. 1822-1871
Untersuchung der Ochsengalle. *Ann. Chem Pharm.*, 1848, **65**, 1-37; **67**, 1-60; 1849, **70**, 149-97.

682   LUDWIG, CARL FRIEDRICH WILHELM. 1816-1895
Ueber die endosmotischen Aequivalent und die endosmotische Theorie. *Z. rat. Med.*, 1849, **8**, 1-52.
      In this development of his theory of urinary secretion (*see* No. 1232) Ludwig made important observations on endosmosis.

683   MILLON, AUGUST NICOLAS EUGÈNE. 1812-1867
Sur un réactif propre aux composés protéiques. *C. R. Acad. Sci. (Paris)*, 1849, **28**, 40-42.
      Millon discovered a special reagent for proteids.

684   FUNKE, OTTO. 1828-1879
Atlas der physiologischen Chemie. Leipzig, *W. Englemann*, 1853.

685   LIEBIG, JUSTUS VON. 1803-1873
Ueber einige Harnstoffverbindungen und eine neue Methode zur Bestimmung von Kochsalz und Harnstoff im Harn. *Ann. Pharm. (Heidelberg)*, 1853, **85**, 289-328.
      Liebig's method of estimating urea.

685.1   FRERICHS, FRIEDRICH THEODOR. 1819-1885, & STAEDELER, GEORG. 1821-1871
Ueber das Vorkommen von Leucin und Tyrosin in der menschlichen Leber. *Arch. Anat Physiol. wiss. Med.*, 1854, 382-92.
      Discovery of leucine and tyrosine in the urine.

686   GRAHAM, THOMAS. 1805-1869
On osmotic force. *Phil. Trans.*, 1854, **144**, 177-228.
      Investigation of osmotic force; provided important information for the physiologists.

687   MARCET, WILLIAM. 1829-1900
On the immediate principles of human excrements in the healthy state. *Phil. Tran.*, 1857, **147**, 403-13.
      First important publication on coprosterol as a product of excretion.

688   GRAHAM, THOMAS. 1805-1869
Liquid diffusion applied to analysis. *Phil. Trans.*, 1861, **151**, 183-224.
      Graham's method of separating animal and other fluids by dialysis introduced the distinction between colloidal and crystalloid substances.

690   COHNHEIM, JULIUS FRIEDRICH. 1839-1884
Zur Kenntnis der zuckerbildenden Fermente. *Virchows Arch. path. Anat.*, 1863, **28**, 241-53.
      Investigation of the sugar-forming ferments.

692   TRAUBE, Moritz. 1826-1894
        Experimente zur Theorie der Zellenbildung und Endosmose. *Arch. Anat. Physiol. wiss. Med.*, 1867, 87-165.
        Employing, for the first time, copper ferrocyanide as a semi-permeable membrane, Traube investigated osmosis and the permeability of membranes.

693   JAFFE, Max. 1841-1911
        Beitrag zur Kenntniss der Gallen- und Harnpigmente. *J. prakt. Chem.*, 1868, **104**, 401-06.
        Jaffe discovered urobilin in the urine.

694   ———. Ueber das Vorkommen von Urobilin im Darminhalt. *Zbl. med. Wiss.*, 1871, **9**, 465-66.
        Discovery of urobilin in the intestines.

695   MIESCHER, Johann Friedrich. 1844-1895
        Ueber die chemische Zusammensetzung der Eiterzellen. In: F. Hoppe-Seyler: *Medicinisch-chemische Untersuchungen,* Berlin, 1871, Heft 4, 441-60.
        Miescher discovered a substance which he termed nuclein (nucleoprotein), later shown to be the hereditary genetic material. He demonstrated it in pus cells. He was also first to suggest the existence of the genetic code (see *Nature (Lond.)*, 1967, **215,** 556).

696   VIERORDT, Karl. 1818-1884
        Die quantitative Spectralanalyse in ihrer Anwendung auf Physiologie, Physik, Chemie und Technologie. Tübingen, *H. Laupp,* 1876.
        Vierordt's spectral analyses of haemoglobin, bile and urine were of great value. He studied the variations in the spectrum of oxyhaemoglobin produced by different dilutions of this substance and was thus able to estimate the haemoglobin content of the blood.

697   JAFFE, Max. 1841-1911
        Ueber die Ausscheidung des Indicans unter physiologischen und pathologischen Verhältnissen. *Virchows Arch. path. Anat.*, 1877, **70,** 72-111.
        Isolation of indican in the urine.

698   PFEFFER, Wilhelm Friedrich Philipp. 1845-1920
        Osmotische Untersuchungen. Leipzig, *W. Engelmann,* 1877.
        The osmotic pressures of solutions were found by Pfeffer to be directly in proportion to the concentration of the solute and to the absolute temperature. English translation, 1895.

699   WALTER, Friedrich.
        Untersuchungen über die Wirkung der Säuren auf den thierischen Organismus. *Arch. exp. Path. Pharmak.*, 1877, **7**, 148-78.

700   BERNARD, Claude. 1813-1878
        La fermentation alcoolique. *Rev. sci. (Paris),* 1878, **16**, 49-56.
        Bernard disbelieved Pasteur's definition of a ferment as "a living form originating from a germ".

700.1   KÜHNE, WILLY. 1837-1900
Erfahrungen und Bemerkungen über Enzyme und Fermente. *Untersuch. physiol. Inst. Univ. Heidelberg,* 1878, **1**, 291-324.
Kühne introduced the term "enzyme".

701   HOPPE-SEYLER, ERNST FELIX IMMANUEL. 1825-1895
Physiologische Chemie. Berlin, *A. Hirschwald,* 1881.
Hoppe-Seyler, one of the greatest of the physiological chemists, founded the *Zeitschrift für physiologische Chemie* and wrote a classical textbook on the subject.

702   KOSSEL, ALBRECHT. 1853-1927
Zur Chemie des Zellkerns. *Hoppe-Seyl. Z. physiol. Chem.,* 1882-83, **7**, 7-22; 1886, **10**, 248-64; 1896-97, **22**, 176-87.
Among the many important contributions of Kossel was his study of the chemistry of the cell and cell-nucleus. He was professor of physiology at Marburg and Heidelberg and was awarded the Nobel Prize for Physiology in 1910.

703   KJELDAHL, JOHANN. 1849-1900
En ny Methode til kvaelstofbestemmelse i organiske Stoffer. *Medd. Carlsberg Lab. (Kbh.),* 1883, **2**, 1-27.
Kjeldahl, a Danish chemist, devised a method of determining the amount of nitrogen in an organic compound ("Kjeldahl's method"). A German translation is in *Z. anal. Chem.,* 1883, **22**, 366-82.

704   KÜLZ, RUDOLPH EDUARD. 1845-1895
Ueber eine neue linksdrehende Säure (Pseudooxybuttersäure). *Z. Biol,* 1884, **20**, 165-78; 1887, **23**, 329-39.
Isolation of ß-oxybutyric acid. (Title of second paper: Beiträge zur Kenntniss der activen ß-Oxybuttersäure).

705   BRIEGER, LUDWIG. 1849-1909
Ueber Ptomaine. 3 vols. Berlin, *A. Hirschwald,* 1885-86.
Brieger isolated and determined the composition of a number of the ptomaines.

706   VAN'T HOFF, JACOBUS HENDRICUS. 1852-1911
Lois d'équilibre chimique dans l'état dilué, gazeux ou dissous. *K. Svenska vetenskAkad. Handl.,* Stockholm, 1885, **21**, No. 17, pp. 1-41.
Van't Hoff stated that osmotic pressure is proportional to the concentration if the temperature remains invariable, and proportional to the absolute temperature if the concentration remains invariable.

707   HAY, MATTHEW. 1855-1932
Test for the bile acids. In LANDOIS and STIRLING: *Text-book of human physiology,* 2nd ed., London, 1886, **1**, 381.
Hay devised a test for the determination of bile acids in the urine.

708   JAFFE, MAX. 1841-1911
Ueber den Niederschlag, welchen Pikrinsäure in normalen Harn erzeugt und über eine neue Reaction des Kreatinins. *Hoppe-Seyl. Z. physiol. Chem.* 1886, **10**, 391-400.
Jaffe's creatinine test.

709   ARRHENIUS, Svante August. 1859-1927
        Ueber die Dissociation der in Wasser gelösten Stoffe. *Z. Physikal. Chem.*
        1887. **1,** 631-48.
        The electrolytic dissociation theory of Arrhenius.

710   BUNGE, Gustav von. 1844-1920
        Lehrbuch der physiologischen und pathologischen Chemie. Leipzig, *F. C.
        W. Vogel,* 1887.

711   Van't HOFF, Jacobus Hendricus. 1852-1911
        Die Rolle des osmotischen Druckes in der Analogie zwischen Lösungen
        und Gasen. *Z. physikal. Chem.,* 1887, **1,** 481-508.

712   VAUGHAN, Victor Clarence. 1851-1929 & NOVY, Frederick George. 1864-
        1957
        Ptomaines and leucomaines, or the putrefactive and physiological alkaloids,
        Philadelphia, *Lea Bros. & Co.,* 1888.

713   ALTMANN, Richard. 1852-1900
        Ueber Nucleinsäuren. *Arch. Anat. Physiol., Physiol. Abt.,* 1889, 524-36.

714   BERTHELOT, Pierre Eugène Marcelin. 1827-1907
        Fixation de l'azote par la terre végétale nue ou avec le concours des
        légumineuses. *Rev. sci. (Paris),* 1889, **43,** 450-54.
        Berthelot showed that bacteria acting in clay soils are able to fix
        nitrogen.

715   STADELMANN, Ernst. 1853-1941
        Ueber den Einfluss der Alkalien auf den menschlichen Stoffwechsel.
        Stuttgart, *F. Enke,* 1890.

716   DRECHSEL, Edmund. 1843-1897
        Der Abbau der Eiweissstoffe. *Arch. Anat. Physiol. Abt.,* 1891, 248-78.
        Drechsel discovered that the protein molecule contains both mono-
        and di-amino acids.

717   HARLEY, Edward Vaughan Berkeley. 1863-1923
        The behaviour of saccharine matter in the blood. *J. Physiol. (Lond.),* 1891,
        12, 391-408.
        Destruction of sugar in the blood.

718   HOPKINS, *Sir* Frederick Gowland. 1861-1947
        On the estimation of uric acid in the urine: a new process by means of
        saturation with ammonium chloride. *Proc. Roy. Soc.,* 1892, **52,** 93-98.
        Hopkins's method of estimating uric acid in urine.

719   KOSSEL, Albrecht. 1853-1927
        Ueber die Nucleinsäure. *Arch. Anat. Physiol., Physiol. Abt.,* 1893, 157-64;
        1894, 194-203.
        See No. 702.

719.1   BUCHNER, Eduard. 1860-1907
        Alkoholische Gärung ohne Hefezellen. *Ber. dtsch. chem. Ges.,* 1897, **30,**
        117-24, 1110-13, 2668-78.

Discovery of cell-free fermentation, the turning point in the study of enzymes. Buchner received the Nobel Prize for Chemistry in 1907 for this work. Third paper written with R. Rapp.

720 FISCHER, EMIL. 1852-1919
Bedeutung der Stereochemie für die Physiologie. *Hoppe-Seyl. Z. physiol. Chem.*, 1898-99, **26**, 60-87.

721 KOSSEL, ALBRECHT. 1853-1927
Ueber die Eiweissstoffe. *Dtsch. med. Wschr.*, 1898, **24**, 581-82.
Kossel forecast the polypeptide nature of the protein molecule.

722 KASTLE, JOSEPH HOEING. 1864-1916, & LOEVENHART, ARTHUR SALOMON. 1878-1929
Concerning lipase, the fat-splitting enzyme, and the reversibility of its action. *Amer. chem. J.*, 1900, **24**, 491-525.
Demonstration of the reversible action of lipase.

723 HOPKINS, *Sir* FREDERICK GOWLAND. 1861-1947, & COLE, SYDNEY WILLIAM. 1877-1952
A contribution to the chemistry of proteids. I. A preliminary study of a hitherto undescribed product of tryptic digestion. *J. Physiol. (Lond.)*, 1901, **27**, 418-28.
Isolation of tryptophan.

724 HÖBER, RUDOLF OTTO ANSELM. 1873-1953
Physikalische Chemie der Zelle und Gewebe. Leipzig, *W. Engelmann,* 1902.

725 HAMBURGER, HARTOG JAKOB. 1859-1924
Osmotischer Druck und Ionenlehre in den medicinischen Wissenschaften. 3 vols. Wiesbaden, *J. F. Bergmann,* 1902-04.
Includes an account of all the methods of determining osmotic pressure.

725.1 LEVENE, PHOEBUS AARON THEODORE. 1869-1940
Darstellung und Analyse einiger Nucleinsäuren. *Hoppe-Seyl. Z. physiol. Chem.*, 1903, **39**, 4-8, 133-35, 479-83.
Chemical distinction between DNA and RNA. Levene elucidated the fundamentals of nucleic acid chemistry. His work led to the tetranucleotide hypothesis.

726 BOHR, CHRISTIAN. 1855-1911, *et al.*
Ueber einen in biologischer Beziehung wichtigen Einfluss, den die Kohlensäurespannung des Blutes auf dessen Sauerstoffbindung übt. *Skand. Arch. Physiol,* 1904, **16**, 402-12.
Bohr, Hasselbalch, and Krogh showed, in the experimental animal, that the affinity of blood for oxygen depends upon carbon dioxide pressure. English translation in No. 1588.16.

727 ABDERHALDEN, EMIL. 1877-1950
Abbau und Aufbau der Eiweisskörper im tierischen Organismus. *Hoppe-Seyl. Z.physiol. Chem.,* 1905, **44**, 17-52.

728   KNOOP, FRANZ. 1875-1946
Die Abbau aromatischer Fettsäuren im Tierkörper. *Beitr. chem. Physiol. Path.*, 1905, **6**, 150-62.
ß-oxidation theory.

729   ZSIGMONDY, RICHARD ADOLF. 1866-1930
Zur Erkenntnis der Kolloide. Jena, *G. Fischer,* 1905.

730   FISCHER, EMIL. 1852-1919
Untersuchungen über Aminosäuren, Polypeptide und Proteine. 2 vols., Berlin, *J. Springer,* 1906-23.
In a series of papers, Fischer showed that animal and vegetable proteins are composed of a series of amino-acids united by elimination of water.

730.1   HOWELL, WILLIAM HENRY. 1860-1945
Note upon the presence of amino-acids in the blood and lymph as determined by the ß naphthalinsulphochloride reaction. *Amer. J. Physiol.,* 1906, **17**, 273-79.
Demonstration of the presence of amino-acids in the blood.

731   PAVY, FREDERICK WILLIAM. 1829-1911
On carbohydrate metabolism. London, *J. & A. Churchill,* 1906.

732   WILLCOCK, EDITH GERTRUDE, & HOPKINS, *Sir* FREDERICK GOWLAND. 1861-1947
The importance of individual amino-acids in metabolism. *J. Physiol. (Lond.),* 1906, **35**, 88-102.
Demonstration of the importance of tryptophan in diet. The pioneer work of Hopkins led eventually to the discovery of vitamins.

733   FLETCHER, *Sir* WALTER MORLEY. 1873-1933, & HOPKINS, *Sir* FREDERICK GOWLAND. 1861-1947
Lactic acid in amphibian muscle. *J. Physiol. (Lond.),* 1907, **35**, 247-309.
Explanation of the production of lactic acid in normal muscular contraction.

734   DAKIN, HENRY DRYSDALE. 1880-1952
The oxidation of butyric acid by means of hydrogen peroxide with formation of acetone, aldehydes, and other products. *J. biol. Chem.,* 1908, **4**, 77-89.
See No. 735.

735   ———. Comparative studies of the mode of oxidation of phenyl derivatives of fatty acids by the animal organism and by hydrogen peroxide. *J. biol. Chem.* 1908, **4**, 419-35; **5**, 173-85, 303-09; 1909, **6**, 203-43.
Dakin's oxidation theory.

736   GRUBE, KARL ADOLPH. 1866-
Ueber die kleinsten Moleküle, welche die Leber zur Synthese des Glykogenes verwerten kann. *Pflüg. Arch. ges. Physiol,* 1908, **121**, 636-40.

737   FREUNDLICH, HERBERT. 1880-1941
Kapillarchemie. Leipzig, *Akademische Verlagsgesellschaft,* 1909.

738   OSTWALD, Carl Wilhelm Wolfgang. 1883-1943
Grundriss der Kolloidchemie. Dresden, *Steinkopff,* 1909.

739   KASTLE, Joseph Hoeing. 1864-1916
The oxidases and other oxygen-catalysts concerned in biological oxidations. *Bull. Hyg. Lab. U.S. publ. Hlth Serv.,* No. 59, Washington, 1910.

740   TRAUBE, Isidor. 1860-1943
Die Theorie des Haftdrucks (Oberflächendrucks) und ihre Bedeutung für die Physiologie. *Pflüg. Arch. ges. Physiol.,* 1910, **132,** 511-38; 1911, **140,** 109-34.

741   DAKIN, Henry Drysdale. 1880-1952
Oxidations and reductions in the animal body. London, *Longmans,* 1912.

741.1   FOLIN, Otto Knut Olof. 1876-1934, & FARMER, Chester Jefferson. 1886-1969
A new method for the determination of total nitrogen in urine. *J. biol. Chem.,* 1912, **11,** 493-501.

        Folin introduced several micro-methods for the determination of nitrogen, urea, creatine, etc.

741.2   ABEL, John Jacob. 1857-1938, *et al.*
On the removal of diffusible substances from the circulating blood of living animals by dialysis. *J. Pharmacol.,* 1914, **5,** 275-316.

        Haemodialysis. *See also* No. 1976. Preliminary communication in *Trans Ass. Amer. Phycns.,* 1913, **28,** 51-4. With L. G. Rowntree and B. B. Turner.

742   HASSELBALCH, Karl Albert. 1874-1962
Die Berechnung der Wasserstoffzahl des Blutes aus der freien und gebundenen Kohlensäure desselben, und die Sauerstoffbindung des Blutes als Funktion der Wasserstoffzahl. *Biochem. Zeit.,* 1917, **78,** 112-144.

        Henderson–Hasselbalch equation for the determination of pH concentration in the blood. English translation in No. 1588.16.

743   JONES, Walter. 1865-1935
The action of the boiled pancreas extract on yeast nucleic acid. *Amer. J. Physiol.,* 1920, **52,** 203-7.
        Ribonuclease.

744   BELL, Richard D., & DOISY, Edward Adelbert. 1883-1986
Rapid colorimetric methods for the determination of phosphorus in urine and blood. *J. biol. Chem.,* 1920, **44,** 55-67.

745   HOPKINS, *Sir* Frederick Gowland. 1861-1947
On an autoxidisable constituent of the cell. *Biochem. J.,* 1921, **15,** 286-305.
        Isolation of glutathione.

746   ROBISON, Robert. 1883-1941
The possible significance of hexosephosphoric esters in ossification. *Biochem. J.,* 1923, **17,** 286-93.

        Records an important advance in the knowledge concerning the conversion of blood calcium into the insoluble calcium of bone.

747   JACKSON, Henry. 1892-
       Studies in nuclein metabolism. II. The isolation of a nucleotide from human
       blood. *J. biol. Chem.*, 1924, **59**, 529-34.
           Jackson demonstrated the existence of pentose nucleotides in normal
       blood.

748   MEYERHOF, Otto Fritz. 1884-1951
       Chemical dynamics of life phenomena. Philadelphia, *J. B. Lippincott,* 1924.

749   CLUTTERBUCK, Percival Walter, & RAPER, Henry Stanley, 1882-1951
       A study of the oxidation of the ammonium salts of normal saturated fatty
       acids and its biological significance. *Biochem. J.,* 1925, **19**, 385-96.

750   WARBURG, Otto Heinrich. 1883-1970
       Ueber die katalytischen Wirkungen der lebendigen Substanz. Berlin, *J.
       Springer,* 1928.

751   FISKE, Cyrus Hartwell. 1890-1978, & SUBBAROW, Yella-pragada, 1896-1948
       Phosphorus compounds of muscle and liver. *Science,* 1929, **70**, 381-382.
           Discovery of adenosine-5'-triphosphate (ATP).

751.1 KREBS, *Sir* Hans Adolf. 1900-1981, & JOHNSON, William Arthur.
       Citric acid in intermediate metabolism in animal tissues. *Enzymologia,* 1937,
       4, 148-56.
           Citric acid cycle of aerobic carbohydrate metabolism. Krebs shared the
       Nobel Prize with Fritz Lipmann (No. 751.3) in 1953.

751.2 COHN, Edward Joseph. 1895-1953, *et al.*
       Chemical, clinical, and immunological studies on the products of human
       plasma fractionation. I. The characterization of the protein fractions of
       human plasma. *J. clin. Invest.,* 1944, **23**, 417-32.
           Fractionation of plasma proteins. With J. L. Oncley, L. E. Strong, W. L.
       Hughes, and S. H. Armstrong.

751.3 LIPMANN, Fritz Albert. 1899- , & KAPLAN, Nathan Oram. 1917-1986
       A common factor in the enzymatic acetylation of sulfanilamide and of
       choline. *J. biol. Chem.,* 1946, **162**, 743-44.
           Coenzyme A.

751.4 CORI, Carl Ferdinand. 1896-1984
       Enzymatic reactions in carbohydrate metabolism. *Harvey Lect.* (1945-46),
       1947, **41**, 253-72.
           C. F. Cori and Mrs. G. T. Cori (1896-1957) shared (with Houssay) the
       Nobel Prize in 1947 for their researches on the course of the catalytic
       transformation of glycogens.

752.3 GRUNBERG-MANAGO, Marianne, & OCHOA DE ALBORNOZ, Severo.
       1905-
       Enzymatic synthesis and breakdown of polynucleotides; polynucleotide
       phosphorylase. *J. Amer. chem. Soc.,* 1955, **77**, 3165-66.
           Ochoa shared the Nobel Prize with Kornberg in 1959 for their artificial
       synthesis of nucleic acids by means of enzymes. The above paper describes
       the discovery of an enzyme able to catalyse the removal of a terminal
       phosphate group from ribonucleoside diphosphates.

752.4   KORNBERG, ARTHUR. 1918- , *et al.*
Enzymic synthesis of deoxyribonucleic acid. *Biochim. Biophys. Acta.,* 1956, **21,** 197-98.
With I. R. Lehman, M. J. Bessman, and E. S. Simms. Kornberg shared the Nobel Prize with Ochoa in 1959.

752.5   THEORELL, AXEL HUGO TEODOR. 1903-1982
The nature and mode of action of oxidation enzymes. Nobel Lecture, December 12, 1955. In *Festschrift Arthur Stoll,* Basel, Birkhäuser, 1957, pp. 35-47.
Theorell was awarded a Nobel Prize in 1955 for his discoveries relating to the nature and mode of action of oxidizing enzymes. The above paper summarizes his work in this field.

752.6   GILHAM, PETER THOMAS. 1930- , & KHORANA, HAR GOBIND. 1922-
Studies on polynucleotides. I. A new and general method for the chemical synthesis of the C_5'-C_3' internucleotide linkage. Synthesis of deoxyribo-dinucleotides. *J. Amer. chem. Soc.,* 1958, **80,** 6212-22.
Khorana shared the Nobel Prize (Physiology) with R. W. Holley and M. W. Nirenberg in 1968 for the techniques he established for the synthesis of polynucleotides.
H. G. Khorana, T. M. Jacob, and S. Nishimura were principally responsible for producing evidence confirming the genetic code.

752.7   ROBSON, GEORGE ALAN. 1934- , BUTCHER, REGINALD WILLIAM. 1930- , & SUTHERLAND, EARL WILBER. 1915-
Cyclic AMP. *Ann. Rev. Biochem.,* 1968, **37,** 149-74.
Sutherland elucidated the role of cyclic adenosine monophosphate, the second messenger mediating actions in a wide range of hormonal effects. He received the Nobel Prize in 1971.

For history, see Nos. 1581, 1588.6, 1588.9, 1588.11

CARDIOVASCULAR SYSTEM

753   IBN-AL-NAFIS [ABŪ-HASAN ALĀ-ŪD-DĪN ALI IBN ABI-AL-HAZIN]. *circa* 1210-1288
Ibn an Nafis und seine Theorie des Lungenkreislaufs. Von MAX MEYERHOF, *Quell. Stud. Gesch. Med.,* 1933, **4,** 37-88.
Ibn-al-Nafis, a Syrian physician, described the lesser circulation in his commentary on the anatomy of the *Canon* of Avicenna, 1268. This was discovered in three Arabic MSS by Mohyi el Din el Tatawi, who included a German translation in his inaugural dissertation, Freiburg, 1924. Meyerhof includes 29 pages of Arabic text in his paper. A translation of the relevant passage is in *Ann. Surg.,* 1936, **104,** 1-8, and in *Bull. med. Hist.,* 1955, **29,** 430-40.

754   SERVETUS, MICHAEL. 1511-1553
Christianismi restitutio. Vienne, *Balthasar Arnoullet,* 1553.
Contains (pp. 168-73) the first printed description of the lesser circulation. Because of the heretical nature of this book on the reform of Christianity, it was printed secretly at Vienne, France, although copies had circulated in manuscript as early as 1546. Servetus, a physician, was burnt at the stake at Champel, Geneva, by order of Calvin. Virtually the entire edition of 1000 copies was burned with him. Only three copies survive –

Richard Mead's copy in the Bibliothèque Nationale, Paris, a copy in the Imperial Library, Vienna, and a copy lacking the title page and the first 16pp., said to be Calvin's personal copy, at the University Library, Edinburgh. It was reprinted in facsimile in 1790 at Nuremberg. Servetus's passages describing the pulmonary circulation are also translated in J. F. Fulton's *Selected readings in the history of physiology,* 2nd ed., 1966, pp. 44-45. See Fulton & Stanton, *Michael Servetus, humanist and martyr. With a bibliography of his works,* New York, *Reichner,* 1953.

755   CESALPINO, ANDREA [CAESALPINUS]. 1525-1603
Peripateticarum quaestionum libri quinque. Venetiis, *apud Iuntas,* 1571.
Cesalpino preceded Harvey in the discovery of the concept of the circulation, and Harvey must have known of his ideas, but Cesalpino's idea of the circulation was not supported by convincing experimental work or quantitative evidence.

756   ——. Quaestionum peripateticum, libri V. Venetiis, *apud Juntas,* 1593.
A greatly expanded second edition. The results of tying a vein and the centripetal flow in veins were first recorded in print by Cesalpino (lib. ii, Qu. xvii, p. 234). See the English translation, with commentary, of the portions of this work relevant to the circulation by Clark, Nimis and Rochefort in *J. hist. med. & all. sci.,* 1978, **33**, 185-213.

757   FABRIZIO, GIROLAMO [FABRICIUS AB AQUAPENDENTE]. 1537-1619
De venarum ostiolis. Patavii, *ex typ. L. Pasquati,* 1603.
Fabricius, teacher of Harvey at Padua, discovered the venous valves, and illustrated them in life-size copperplates in this monograph. He failed to recognize their true function, however, considering this to be merely a delaying of the blood flow. This work must have influenced Harvey to turn his experimental efforts toward an accurate explanation for the existence of the venous valves. This line of research eventually led him to develop an accurate knowledge of how the circulation worked. Facsimile edition, with English translation, edited by K. J. Franklin, 1933.

758   HARVEY, WILLIAM. 1578-1657
Praelectiones anatomiae universalis. London, *J. Churchill,* 1886.
Facsimile reproduction with transliteration of Harvey's manuscript notes for a Lumleian Lecture, 1616. These show that at that date Harvey had already completed his demonstration of the circulation of the blood. English translation with annotations, Berkeley, 1961. Edited, with an introduction, translation, and notes by G. Whitteridge, *Edinburgh,* 1964.

759   ——. Exercitatio anatomica de motu cordis et sanguinis in animalibus. Francofurti, *sumpt. Guilielmi Fitzeri,* 1628.
Discovery and experimental proof of the circulation of the blood. Together with Vesalius's *Fabrica* (1543), Harvey's *De motu cordus* shares the honour as the greatest book in the history of medicine. By fundamentally changing our conceptions of the functions of the heart and blood vessels, Harvey pointed the way to reform of all of physiology and medicine. During the mid 17th century new mechanical and chemical systems of physiology incorporated the circulation as a basic assumption in the explanation of a wide range of vital phenomena, and while subsequent developments in physiology have led to great changes in thinking about the functions of the circulation, they have abundantly confirmed the

importance of Harvey's discovery as the cornerstone of modern physiology and medicine. The book was reprinted in facsimile in 1928 (*Monumenta medica,* Vol. 5, Florence). The Latin text, with an English translation by K. J. Franklin, was published in Oxford, 1957, and a translation with introduction and notes was published by G. Whitteridge in 1976 (Oxford, Blackwell). *See also* No. 61.1.

760   MALPIGHI, MARCELLO. 1628-1694
De pulmonibus observations anatomicae. Bononiae, *B. Ferronius,* 1661.

    Discovery of the capillary circulation. This book, which is very rare, consists of two letters to Borelli describing observations made through the microscope on the lung of a living frog. In the second letter Malpighi described small channels connecting arteries with veins, the capillaries. This was the first proof that blood circulation occurred within a closed hydraulic system. The second edition was published as an appendix to Thomas Bartholin's *De pulmonum substantia et motu diatribe,* 1663. It is republished in his *Opera omnia,* Lugduni Batavorum, 1687, ii, 331. A facsimile was published in Milan in 1958; English translation by J. Young in *Proc. roy. Soc. Med.,* 1929-30, Sect. Hist. Med., **23**, 1-11. *See* No. 915

761   LOWER, RICHARD. 1631-1691
Tractatus de corde. Londini, *J. Allestry,* 1669.

    Lower was the first to demonstrate the scroll-like structure of the cardiac muscle. He was one of the first to transfuse blood. Chapter III of the above work records how Lower injected dark venous blood into the insufflated lungs; he concluded that its subsequent bright red colour was due to its absorption of some of the air passing though the lungs. The British Museum copy of this book bears the signature of Walter Charleton, followed by the date "1668"; it is possible, therefore, that the book actually appeared in that year and not in 1669. Facsimile, with translation, London, 1932.

762   BORELLI, GIOVANNI ALFONSO. 1608-1679
De motu animalium. 2 pts. Romae, *ex typ. A. Bernabo,* 1680-81.

    Borelli originated the neurogenic theory of the heart's action and first suggested that the circulation resembled a simple hydraulic system. He was the first to insist that the heart beat was a simple muscular contraction. One of the founders of biomechanics, Borelli was a representative of the Iatro-Mathematical School, which treated all physiological happenings as rigid consequences of the laws of physics and mechanics. English translation by P. Maquet from the 1743 edition, Berlin, *Springer-Verlag,* 1989. *See* No. 3669.2.

762.1   BELLINI, LORENZO. 1643-1704
De urinis et pulsibus de missione sanguinis de febribus de morbis capitis, et pectoris. Bononiae, Ex typographia Antonii Pisarii, 1683.

    Bellini began to develop his hydraulic iatromechanics in this work, in which he considered the blood as a physical fluid with simple mechanical and mathematicizable properties. *See* No. 4162.

763   THEBESIUS, ADAM CHRISTIAN. 1686-1732
Disputatio medica inauguralis de circulo sanguinis in corde. Lugduni Batavorum, *A. Elzevier,* 1708.

    First description of the coronary valves and the venae thebesii.

764   POURFOUR DU PETIT, FRANÇOIS. 1664-1741
Mémoire dans lequel il est démontré que les nerfs intercostaux fournissent des rameaux que portent des espirits dans les yeux. *Hist. Acad. roy. Sci. (Paris) (Mém)*, 1727, 1-19.
Discovery of the vasomotor nerves (*see also* No. 1313).

765   HALES, STEPHEN. 1677-1761
Statical essays, containing haemastaticks. Vol. 2. London, *W. Innys & R. Manby*, 1733.
In this work is recorded Hales's invention of the manometer, with which he was the first to measure blood-pressure. His work is the greatest single contribution to our knowledge of the vascular system after Harvey, and led to the development of the blood-pressure measuring instruments now in universal use. Partial reprint in Willius & Keys, *Cardiac classics,* 1941, pp. 131-55.

765.1   TAUBE, HARTWIG WILHELM LUDWIG. 1706-
Dissertationem inauguralem de vera nervi intercostalis origine. Gottingae, *apud Abram Vandenhoeck,* 1743.
Taube described the carotid body and named it "ganglion minutum", See J. Pick, *J. Hist. Med.,* 1959, **14,** 61-73.

765.2   CARSON, JAMES. 1772-1843
An inquiry into the causes of the motion of the blood; with an appendix, in which the process of respiration and its connexion with the circulation of the blood are attempted to be elucidated. Liverpool, *Longman & Col,* 1815.
Carson recognized the vital effect on venous return played by the negative pressure in the pleural cavity.

766   WEBER, ERNST HEINRICH. 1795-1878 & WEBER, WILHELM EDUARD. 1804-1891
Wellenlehre auf Experimente gegründet. Leipzig, *Gerhard Fleischer,* 1825.
The first work to apply hydrodynamics to the circulation of the blood.

767   POISEUILLE, JEAN LÉONARD MARIE. 1799-1869
Recherches sur la force du coeur aortique. Paris, *Thèse No.* 166, 1828.
Poiseuille was the first after Stephen Hales to make any important addition to the knowledge of the physiology of circulation. In his graduation thesis, above, he described a "haemodynamometer" invented by himself and which he used to repeat some of Hales's blood-pressure experiments. With his haemomanometer, a mercury manometer, which was a great improvement on the long tube used by Hales, Poiseuille showed that the blood-pressure rises and falls on expiration and inspiration, and measured the degree of arterial dilatation produced by each heart beat. English translation in *Edinb. med. surg. J.,* 1829, **32,** 28-38. *See also* his paper in *J. Physiol. exp. path.,* 1828, **8,** 272-305.

768   ——. Recherches expérimentales sur le mouvement des liquides dans les tubes de très petits diamètres. *C. R. Acad. Sci. (Paris),* 1840, **11,** 961-67, 1041-48; 1841, **12,** 112-15.
Poiseuille's law of the flow of liquids in tubes — fundamental in blood viscosimetry. Abstract; complete monograph in *Mém. Acad. roy. Sci. (Paris),* 1846, **9,** 433-544.

768.1   HALL, MARSHALL. 1790-1857
A critical and experimental essay on the circulation of the blood. London,
R. B. Seeley & W. Burnside, 1831.
Marshall Hall clearly distinguished arterioles and venules from capillaries,
and he described arteriovenous shunts.

769   HENLE, FRIEDRICH GUSTAV JACOB. 1809-1885
Gefässnerven. In his *Allgemeine Anatomie,* Leipzig, 1841, p. 510, 690.
Demonstration of the presence of smooth muscle in the endothelial
coat of small arteries.

770   LUDWIG, CARL FRIEDRICH WILHELM. 1816-1895
Beiträge zur Kenntniss des Einflusses der Respirationsbewegungen auf den
Blutlauf im Aortensystem. *Arch. Anat. Physiol. wiss. Med.,* 1847, 242-302.
Ludwig changed Poiseuille's haemodynamometer into the kymograph
by the addition of a float and caused this float to write on a recording
cylinder. Abridged English translation in Ruskin (No. 3160.1).

771   VOLKMANN, ALFRED WILHELM. 1800-1887
Die Hämodynamik nach Versuchen. Leipzig, *Breitkopf & Härtel,* 1850.

772   VIERORDT, KARL. 1818-1884
Die bildliche Darstellung des menschlichen Arterienpulses. *Arch. physiol.
Heilk.,* 1854, **13,** 284-87.
Vierordt invented a sphygmograph which acted on the principle that
indirect estimation of blood-pressure could be accomplished by measuring
the counter-pressure necessary to obliterate the arterial pulsation. This was
the first instrument with which a tracing of the human pulse could be made.
The paper is the first record of a study with an instrument of precision of
the pulse in health and disease. Vierordt expanded this work into book
form: *Die Lehre von Arterienpuls,* Braunschweig, Vieweg, 1855.

773   FAIVRE, JEAN.
Études expérimentales sur les lésions organiques du coeur. *Ann. Soc. Méd.
Lyon,* 1856, 2 sér., **4,** 180-88.
Faivre made the first accurate estimation of the blood-pressure in man,
by connecting the artery with a mercury manometer and making direct
readings. These investigations were important, since they established
normal values. The paper was republished in book form in 1856. English
translation of part 2 in Ruskin (No. 3160.1).

774   BERNARD, CLAUDE. 1813-1878
De l'influence de deux ordres de nerfs qui déterminent les variations de
couleur du sang veineux dans les organes glandulaires. *C. R. Acad. Sci.,
(Paris),* 1858, **47,** 245-53; 393-400.
Discovery of the vasoconstrictor and vasodilator nerves and description of their function of regulating the blood supply to the different parts
of the body.

775   VIERORDT, KARL. 1818-1884
Die Erscheinungen und Gesetze der Stromgeschwindigkeitin des Blutes.
Frankfurt a.M., *Meidinger Sohn & Co.,* 1858.
Vierordt estimated, by means of a "haemotachometer" of his own
invention, the rate of the blood flow in various arteries, and also the
influence of the blood volume, pulse rate and respiratory rate upon it.

776   MAREY, ETIENNE JULES. 1830-1904
Recherches sur le pouls au moyen d'un nouvel appareil enregistreur le
sphygmographe. Paris, *E. Thunot et Cie.*, 1860.
    Invention of the modern sphygmograph. Also published in *C.R. Acad.
Sci. (Paris)*, 1860, **51**,281-309. Preliminary paper in same journal, 1860, **50**,
634-37.

777   POISEUILLE, JEAN LEONARD MARIE. 1799-1869
Sur la pression du sang dans le système artériel. *C. R. Acad. Sci. (Paris)*,
1860, **51**, 238-42.

778   LUDWIG, CARL FRIEDRICH WILHELM. 1816-1895
Die physiologischen Leistungen des Blutdrucks. Leipzig, *S. Hirzel*, 1865.
    Ludwig's inaugural address at Leipzig, in which he introduced the idea
of keeping alive excised portions of organs by means of artificial circulation, or perfusion. He suggested that the blood-pressure had a stimulating
effect on the vagus.

779   DOGIEL, JAN. 1830-1905
Die Ausmessung der strömenden Blutvolumina. *Arb. physiol. Anst. Lpz.*
(1867), 1868, **2**, 196-271.
    Invention of the *Stromuhr,* for measurement of the velocity of the
blood. Dogiel was a pupil of Ludwig.

780   THANHOFFER, LAJOS VON. 1843-1909
Die beiderseitige mechanische Reizung des Nv. vagus beim Menschen.
Zbl. med. Wiss., 1875, **13**, 403-06.

781   KRIES, N. VON.
Ueber den Druck in den Blutcapillaren der menschlichen Haut. *Arb. physiol.
Anst. Lpz.* (1875), 1876, **10**, 69-80.

782   STRICKER, SALOMON. 1834-1898
Untersuchungen über die Gefässernerven-Wurzeln des Ischiadicus. *S. B.
k. Akad. Wiss. Wien, math.-nat. Cl.*, 1876, 3 Abt., **74**, 173-85.
    Stricker was the first to describe vasodilatation on stimulation of the
posterior nerve roots.

782.1   ROUGET, CHARLES MARIE BENJAMIN. 1824-1904
Sur la contractilité capillaires sanguins. *C. R. Acad. Sci. (Paris)*, 1879, **88**,
916-18.
    Rouget made an important investigation of the control of capillary
circulation. He described cells ("Rouget's cells") on the outer surfaces of
capillary walls, considered to be contractile. English translation in No.
1588.3.

783   MAREY, ETIENNE JULES. 1830-1904
La circulation du sang à l'état physiologique et dans les maladies. Paris, *G.
Masson,* 1881.

784   BRAUNE, CHRISTIAN WILHELM. 1831-1892
Das Venensystem des menschlichen Körpers. 2 pts. and atlas. Leipzig, *Veit & Co.,* 1884-89.
Like Braune's other anatomical works, this is notable for its excellent illustrations.

785   MALL, FRANKLIN PAINE. 1862-1917
Der Einfluss der Systems der Vena portae auf die Vertheilung des Blutes. *Arch. Anat. Physiol. Abt.,* 1892, 409-53.

786   PORTER, WILLIAM TOWNSEND. 1862-1949
On the results of ligation of the coronary arteries. *J. Physiol. (Lond.),* 1893-94, **15,** 121-38; *J. exp. Med.,* 1896, **1,** 46-70.
"Following coronary ligation Porter noted that the procedure frequently resulted in fibrillary contractions of the heart and sudden death. However, death did not always occur and this led him to conclude that Cohnheim's (1881) consistently fatal results were due to operative trauma and that the coronary arteries were not end arteries" (Willius & Dry).

787   TIGERSTEDT, ROBERT ADOLF ARMAND. 1853-1923
Lehrbuch der Physiologie des Kreislaufes. Leipzig, *Veit & Co.,* 1893.

788   GIBSON, ALEXANDER GEORGE. 1875-1950
The significance of a hitherto undescribed wave in the jugular pulse. *Lancet,* 1907, **2,** 1380-82.
The physiological wave sometimes found in mid-diastole, when the pulse is slow, was first described by Gibson. He termed it the *b*-wave.

789   HARTMANN, HENRI. 1860-1952
Some considerations upon high amputation of the rectum. *Ann. Surg.,* 1909, **50,** 1091-94.
"Hartmann's critical point", the site on the large intestine where the lowest sigmoid artery meets the superior rectal arterial branch.

790   LOMBARD, WARREN PLIMPTON. 1855-1939
The blood-vessels in the arterioles, capillaries and small veins of the human skin. *Amer. J. Physiol,* 1911-12. **29,** 335-62.
Lombard soaked the skin in cedarwood oil, rendering transparent the superficial epidermal layers, and thus making possible many direct observations on it.

791   SOLLMANN, TORALD HERMANN. 1874-1965, & BROWN, EDGAR DEWIGHT. 1869-
The blood pressure fall produced by traction on the carotid artery. *Amer. J. Physiol.,* 1912, **30,** 88-104.
First description of the carotid sinus depressor reflex.

792   DALE, *Sir* HENRY HALLETT. 1875-1968, & RICHARDS, ALFRED NEWTON. 1876-1966
The vasodilator action of histamine and of some other substances. *J. Physiol. (Lond.),* 1918-19, **52,** 110-65.
Dale and Richards studied the effect of histamine on the control of the circulation and showed its peripheral action to be located in the capillaries and smaller arterioles.

793   KROGH, SCHACK AUGUST STEENBERG. 1874-1949
The anatomy and physiology of the capillaries. New Haven, *Yale Univ. Press,*
1922.
     Silliman Lectures. A second edition appeared in 1929. Krogh received
the Nobel Prize for Physiology in 1920. His most important work was on
the physiology of capillaries.

794   HERING, HEINRICH EWALD. 1866-1948
Der Karotisdruckversuch. *Münch med. Wschr.,* 1923, **70,** 1287-90.

795   ——. Die Aenderung der Herzschlagzahl durch Aenderung des arteriellen
Blutdruckes erfolgt aus reflektorischem Wege; gleichzeitig eine Mitteilung
über die Funktion des Sinus caroticus, beziehungsweise der Sinusnerven.
Pflüg. Arch. ges. Physiol., 1924, 206, 721-3.
     First description of the structure and function of the sinus nerve and the
reflex character of carotid pressure.

795.1   LANDIS, EUGEN MARKLEY. 1901-
The capillary pressure in frog mesentery as determined by micro-injection
methods. *Amer. J. Physiol.,* 1926, **75,** 548-70.
     Direct measurement of the blood pressure within the capillaries.

796   BLUMGART, HERRMAN LUDWIG. 1895-1977, & WEISS, SOMA. 1898-1942
Studies in the velocity of blood flow. *J. clin. Invest.,* 1927, **4,** 1-13, 15-31,
149-71, 173-97, 199-209, 389-425, 555-74.
     First practical method of measuring circulation time.

797   LEWIS, *Sir* THOMAS. 1881-1945
The blood-vessels of the human skin and their responses. London, *Shaw,*
1927.

798   REIN, FRIEDRICH HERMANN. 1898-1953
Die Thermo-Stromuhr. Ein Verfahren zur fortlaufenden Messung der
mittleren absoluten Durchfulssmengen in uneröffneten Gefässen in situ.
Z. Biol, 1928, **87,** 394-418.
     Introduction of the *Thermostromuhr,* an instrument for measuring the
velocity of the blood flow.

799   WIGGERS, CARL JOHN. 1883-1963
The pressure pulses in the cardiovascular system. London, *Longmans, Green
& Co.,* 1928.
     Wiggers, professor of physiology at the Western Reserve University,
Cleveland, contributed much to the knowledge of the circulation and
devised several instruments to promote the study of this subject.

800   STANDARDISATION of methods of measuring the arterial blood pressure.
Joint report of the committees appointed by the Cardiac Society of Great
Britain and Ireland, and the American Heart Association. *Brit. Heart J.,*
1939, **1,** 261-67.

Anatomy & Physiology of the Heart

801   EUSTACHI, BARTOLOMEO [EUSTACHIUS]. *circa* 1510/20-1574
Opuscula anatomica. Venetiis, *V. Luchinus,* 1564.
Plate VIII illustrates the "Eustachian valve", the valvula venae cavae in the right auricle.

802   PINEAU, SÉVERIN. *d.*1619.
Opusculum physiologum & anatomicum in duos libellos distinctum. In quibus primum, De integritatis & corruptionis virginum notis...Paris, *Steph. Prevosteau,* 1597.
In 1595 Pineau demonstrated the vestigial foramen ovale in the adult heart, settling the question of the perviousness of the septum of the heart. His work was first published in 1597. He published this study in a frank treatise on virginity and the ways of losing it.

802.1   BOTALLO, LEONARDO (BOTALLUS). *circa* 1519-1587/88
Opera omnia medica et chirurgica. Lugduni, *D & A., à Gassbeeck,* 1660.
"Botallo's duct", the ductus arteriosus; "Botallo's foramen", the foramen ovale interauriculare; and "Botallo's ligament", the ligamentum arteriosum, are described in this work. However two of these traditional attributions of discovery should more accurately be called independent rediscovery since Botallo's duct had been mentioned in the 2nd century by Galen. More recently Falloppio had mentioned the ductus arteriosus in 1561 and Vesalius had mentioned both the ductus arteriosus and the foramen ovale in 1561.

803   VALSALVA, ANTONIO MARIA. 1666-1723
Opera. 2 vols. Venetiis, *apud F. Pitteri,* 1740.
Valsalva described the aortic "sinus of Valsalva".

804   SKODA, JOSEF. 1805-1881
Ueber den Herzstoss und die durch die Herzbewegungen verursachten Töne. *Med. Jb. k. österr. Staates (Wien),* 1837, N.F., **13,** 227-266.
Skoda's theory of the heart beat.

805   PURKYNĚ, JAN EVANGELISTA [PURKINJE]. 1787-1869
Nowe spostrzezenia i badainia w przedmiocie fizyologii i drobnowidzowéj anatomii. *Rocz. Wydzialu lekar. Univ. Jagiel,* 1839, **2,** 44-67.
The "Purkinjě fibres"; identification of the conductor system of the heart. Reprinted in his *Opera omnia,* 1939, **3,** 52-63. German version in *Arch. Anat. Physiol. wiss. Med.,* 1845, 281-95; English translation by W. W. Gull in *Lond. med. Gaz.,* 1845, **36,** 1066-69, 1156-58. Historical note by V. Kruta in *Bull. N.Y. Acad. Med.,* 1971, **47,** 351-7.

806   REMAK, ROBERT. 1815-1865
Neurologische Erläuterungen. *Arch. Anat. Physiol. (Lpz.),* 1844, 463-72.
Remak was first to describe the intrinsic ganglia of the heart.

807   WEBER, EDUARD FRIEDRICH WILHELM. 1806-1871, & WEBER, ERNST HEINRICH. 1795-1878
Experimenta, quibus probatur nervos vagos rotatione machinae galvanomagneticae irritatos, motum cordis retardare et adeo intercipare. *Ann. univ. Med. (Milano),* 1845, 3 ser., **20,** 227-33.

The discovery of the inhibitory power of the vagus. Also published in Wagner's *Handwörterbuch der Physiologie*, 1846, **3,** 45-51. Partial translation in J. F. Fulton's *Selected readings in the history of physiology,* 2nd ed., 1966. p.296.

808   WILD, F.
Ueber die peristaltische Bewegung des Oesophagus, nebst einigen Bemerkungen über diejenigen des Darms. *Z. rat. Med.,* 1846, **5,** 76-132.
      Includes (pp. 76-77) a description of what is probably the first perfusion of the isolated heart.

809   LUDWIG, CARL FRIEDRICH WILHELM. 1816-1895
Über die Herznerven des Frosches. *Arch. Anat. Physiol wiss. Med.,* 1848, 139-43.

810   HOFFA, MORITZ, & LUDWIG, CARL FRIEDRICH WILHELM. 1816-1895
Einige neue Versuche über Herzbewegung. *Z. rat. Med.,* 1850, **9,** 107-44.
      Experimental ventricular fibrillation.

811   BIDDER, FRIEDRICH HEINRICH. 1810-1894
Ueber functionell verschiedene und räumlich getrennte Nervencentra im Froschherzen. *Arch. Anat. Physiol. wiss. Med.,* 1852, 163-177.
      Discovery of the ganglion cells at the auriculo-ventricular junction, "Bidder's ganglion".

812   STANNIUS, HERMANN FRIEDRICH. 1808-1883
Zwei Reihen physiologischer Versuche. *Arch. Anat. Physiol. wiss. Med.,* 1852, 85-100.
      Stannius initiated research on the physiology of the conduction system of the heart. He illustrated vagal inhibition of the heart beat and indicated the existence of the pacemaker of the heart. Stannius also showed that the apex of the heart ceases to beat rhythmically when separated physiologically by ligature or clamp from the rest of the heart, while the sinus remains unaffected. Partial translation in J. F. Fulton's *Selected readings in the history of physiology,* 2nd. ed., 1966, pp. 59-60.

812.1   BERNARD, CLAUDE. 1813-1878
Leçons de physiologie expérimentale appliquée à la médecine. Vol. 1. Paris, *J. B. Baillière,* 1855.
      P. 126: Catheterization of the heart of a dog (in some editions, p. 119).

812.2   GROUX, EUGÈNE ALEXANDER. 1833-78.
Fissura sterni congenita. New observations and experiments made in Amerika [sic] and Great Britain...Hamburg, *Köhler,* 1859.
      Records first use of telegraphy to record and measure the heart beat and pulse. This was done in Boston with an instrument placed against Groux's chest, the other end of which was in contact with the circuit breaker of the telegraph. Dr. J.B. Upham called his device a sphygmosphone. Includes reprint of Report of the Committee of the N.Y. Pathological Society, appointed to examine the case of Mr. E. A. Groux...*Amer. med. Month.,*1959, **11,** 35-40. with supplementary material, and new illustrations.

813 MAREY, ÉTIENNE JULES. 1830-1904
Loi qui préside à la fréquence des battements du coeur. *C. R. Acad. Sci. (Paris),* 1861, **53,** 95-8.
Marey's law of the heart. Marey was the first to realize the relationship between the blood pressure and the heart rate.

814 GOLTZ, FRIEDRICH LEOPOLD. 1834-1902
Ueber Reflexionen von und zum Herzen (Klopfversuch). *Königsb. med. Jb.,* 1862, **3,** 271-4.
Rapidly-repeated blows on the belly of a frog caused cessation of the heart-beat, which Goltz concluded was brought about by reflex inhibition through the vagus, an important contribution to the knowledge of the mechanism of shock.

815 BEZOLD, ALBERT VON. 1836-1868
Untersuchungen über die Innervation des Herzens Leipzig, *W. Engelmann,* 1863.
Discovery of the accelerator or excitatory nerve fibres of the heart (pp. 191-232), "Bezold's ganglia".

816 CHAUVEAU, JEAN BAPTISTE AUGUSTE. 1827-1917, & MAREY, ÉTIENNE JULES. 1830-1904
Appareils et expériences cardiographiques. *Mém. Acad. imp. de Méd. (Paris),* 1863, **26,** 268-319.
First direct records of the heart impulse by means of a "cardiac sound" and the sphygmograph – recording tambours, which wrote on a moving drum covered with smoked paper.

817 CZERMAK, JOHANN NEPOMUK. 1828-1873
Ueber mechanische Vagus-Reizung beim Menschen. *Jena. Z. Med., Naturw.,* 1865-66, **2,** 384-6.
"Czermak's vagus pressure". Czermak found that mechanical pressure on a spot of the carotid triangle in the neck produced lowering of the heart rate.

818 TRAUBE, LUDWIG. 1818-1876
Ueber periodische Thätigkeits-Aeusserungen des vasomotorischen und Hemmungs-Nervencentrums. *Zbl. med. Wiss.,* 1865, **3,** 881-5.
First description of the rhythmic variations in tone of the vasoconstrictor centre (Traube–Hering waves).

819 CYON, ELIE DE. 1842-1912, & LUDWIG, CARL FRIEDRICH WILHELM. 1816-1895
Die Reflexe eines der sensiblen Nerven des Herzens auf die motorischen der Blutgefässe. *Arb. physiol Anst. Leipzig,* (1866), 1867, **1,** 128-49.
Discovery of the vasomotor reflexes.

819.1 BERNSTEIN, JULIUS. 1839-1917
Über den zeitlichen Verlauf der negativen Schwankung des Nervenstroms. *Pflügers Arch. ges. Physiol.,* 1868, 1, 173-207.
Bernstein introduced the differential rheotome, and the first electrocardiograms were obtained with it by Marchand in 1877 (No. 823.1).

820   FICK, ADOLPH. 1829-1901
Ueber die Messung des Blutquantums in den Herzventrikeln. *S. B. phys.-med. Ges. Würzburg,* 1870, 16.
Fick's principle for the calculation of cardiac output based on measuring the minute volume of oxygen consumption and the arteriovenous oxygen difference.

821   SCHMIEDEBERG, JOHANN ERNST OSWALD. 1838-1921
Untersuchungen über einige Giftwirkungen am Froschherzen. *Arb. physiol. Anst. Leipzig,* (1870), 1871, **5,** 41-52.
First investigation of the effect of poisons on the frog's heart. In some cases Schmiedeberg found that stimulation of the vagus after administration of poisons produced acceleration of the heart rate.

822   BOWDITCH, HENRY PICKERING. 1840-1911
Ueber die Eigenthümlichkeiten der Reizbarkeit, welche die Muskelfasern des Herzens zeigen. *Arb. physiol. Anst. Leipzig,* (1871), 1872, **6,** 139-76.
Bowditch established the "all-or-nothing" principle of heart muscle contraction. He founded, at Harvard, the first physiological laboratory in the United States.

823   TALMA, SAPE. 1847-1918
Beiträge zur Theorie der Herz- und Arterientöne. *Dtsch. Arch. klin. Med.,* 1874, **15,** 77-98.

823.1   MARCHAND, RICHARD.
Beiträge zur Kenntniss der Reizwell und Contractionswelle des Herzmuskels. *Pflügers Arch. ges. Physiol.,* 1877, **15,** 511-36.
Marchand obtained the first electrocardiogram. Using the differential rheotome he measured the time course of the potential variations from the frog's heart.

824   BURDON-SANDERSON, *Sir* JOHN SCOTT. 1828-1905, & PAGE, FREDERICK JAMES MONTAGUE. 1848-1907
On the time-relations of the excitatory process in the ventricle of the heart of the frog. *J. Physiol. (Lond.),* 1879-80, **2,** 384-435.
These workers were among the first to study the action currents of the heart, and made the first records (with the capillary electrometer) of the minute electrical current produced by the beating of the heart. *See also* No. 831.

825   TALMA, SAPE. 1847-1918
Zur Genese der Herztöne. *Pflüg. Arch. ges. Physiol.,* 1880, **23,** 275-8.

826   RINGER, SYDNEY. 1834-1910
Regarding the action of hydrate of soda, hydrate of ammonia, and hydrate of potash on the ventricle of the frog's heart. *J. Physiol. (Lond.),* 1880-82, **3,** 195-202.
"Ringer's solution".

827   MARTIN, HENRY NEWELL. 1848-1896
On a method of isolating the mammalian heart. *Science,* 1881, **2,** 228.

Martin devised a form of perfusion of the isolated mammalian heart – one of the greatest single contributions ever to come from an American physiological laboratory. This made possible his later work on the heart.

828 ——. Observations on the direct influence of variations of arterial pressure upon the rate of beat of the mammalian heart. *Stud. Biol. Lab. Johns Hopk. Univ.*, 1882, **2**, 213-33.

829 GASKELL, WALTER HOLBROOK. 1847-1914
On the rhythm of the heart of the frog, and on the nature of the action of the vagus nerve. *Phil. Trans.*, 1882, **173**, 993-1033.
Croonian Lectures, 1881. Gaskell's classical memoir on the muscles and nerves of the heart included a description of "Gaskell's nerves", the accelerator nerves of the heart. He showed that the motor impulses from the nerve ganglia in the sinus venosus influence the heart rhythm but do not originate cardiac movements, which are due to the rhythmic contraction of the heart muscle. This led to the artificial production of "heart-block", the name for which Gaskell based on an expression of Romanes. *See* No. 632.

830 ——. On the innervation of the heart, with special reference to the heart of the tortoise. *J. Physiol. (Lond.)*, 1883-84, **4**, 43-127.
In his important investigation of the innervation of the heart, Gaskell showed that the efferent vasconstrictor fibres originated from the lateral horn of the spinal cord.

831 BURDON-SANDERSON, *Sir* JOHN SCOTT. 1828-1905, & PAGE, FREDERICK JAMES MONTAGUE. 1848-1907
On the electrical phemomena of the excitatory process in the heart of the frog and of the tortoise, as investigated photographically. *J. Physiol. (Lond.)*, 1883-84, **4**, 327-38.
See No. 824.

832 MARTIN, HENRY NEWELL. 1848-1896
The direct influence of gradual variations of temperature upon the rate of beat of the dog's heart. *Phil. Trans.*, 1883, **174**, 663-88.
Martin was among the first to study the effect of temperature changes upon the isolated heart.

833 WALLER, AUGUSTUS DÉSIRÉ. 1856-1922
A demonstration on man of electromotive changes accompanying the heart's beat. *J. Physiol. (Lond.)*, 1887, **8**, 229-34.
Waller was first to use electrodes and leads in demonstrating the action currents of the heart, avoiding the necessity of opening the chest of laboratory animals and preparing the way for present-day clinical electrocardiography. He obtained the first electrocardiogram in man.

834 MACKENZIE, *Sir* JAMES. 1853-1925
Pulsation in the veins, with the description of a method for graphically recording them. *J. Path. Bact.*, 1892, **1**, 53-89.
The phlebograph, which developed into the polygraph. With it Mackenzie obtained simultaneous tracings of the pulsations of the jugular vein and radial artery.

835 ROY, Charles Smart. 1854-1897, & ADAMI, John George. 1862-1926
Contributions to the physiology and pathology of the mammalian heart.
Phil. Trans., 1892, ser. B., **183,** 199-298.

836 HIS, Wilhelm, *Jnr.* 1863-1934
Die Thätigkeit des embryonalen Herzens und deren Bedeutung für die
Lehre von der Herzbewegung beim Erwachsenen. *Arb. med. Klin. Leipzig,*
1893, 14-50.
 His described the atrioventricular bundle which was later named after
him. English translation in F. A. Willius and T. E. Keys, *Cardiac classics,*
1941, p. 695.

837 KENT, Albert Frank Stanley. 1863-1958
Researches on the structure and function of the mammalian heart. *J. Physiol.
(Lond.),* 1893, **14,** 233-54.
 Kent also discovered the atrioventricular bundle ("bundle of Kent"), a
narrow band of muscle between the auricles and ventricles of the heart.
Its purpose is to act as a bridge for contractile impulses between the
auricles and ventricles.

838 BRAUN, Ludwig. 1867-1936
Ueber Herzbewegung und Herzstoss. Jena, *G. Fischer,* 1898.
 First employment of cinematograph to record the cardiac changes
during all phases of heart contraction.

838.1 PRÉVOST, Jean Louis. 1790-1850, & Battelli, F.
La mort par les décharges électriques. *J. Physiol. (Paris),* 1899, **1,** 1085-1100.
 "Prévost and Battelli produced ventricular fibrillation in dogs by shock-
ing with weak currents. They then shocked the fibrillating heart with a
stronger current—the second, or counter, shock. The fibrillation stopped,
and a few seconds later the heart resumed its normal beating" (Callahan *et
al., Classics of Cardiology,* Vol. 3)

839 MacCALLUM, John Bruce. 1876-1906
On the muscular architecture and growth of the ventricles of the heart. In
Contributions to the science of medicine. Dedicated . . . to W. H. Welch.
Baltimore, 1900, pp. 307-35.
 A classic account of the development and architecture of the muscular
wall of the heart.

840 EINTHOVEN, Willem. 1860-1927
Un nouveau galvanomètre. *Arch. néerl. Sci. exactes nat.,* 1901, 2 sér., **6,**
625-33.
 One of the most distinguished of modern physiologists, Einthoven
directed much of his research to the development and perfection of
recording instruments. His most famous work was in connexion with his
string galvanometer, a perfection of the instrument invented by J. S. C.
Schweigger, of Halle. Einthoven was awarded the Nobel Prize in 1924.

841 FRIEDENTHAL, Hans Wilhelm Karl. 1870-
Ueber die Entfernung der extracardialen Herznerven bei Saügethieren.
Arch. Anat. Physiol., Physiol. Abt., 1902, 135-45.

842 EINTHOVEN, WILLEM. 1860-1927
The string galvanometer and the human electro-cardiogram. *K. Akad Wet. Amst., Proc. Sect. Sci.*, 1903-04, **6**, 107-15.

Einthoven showed how his string galvanometer could portray the electrical changes occurring in the human heart. Modern electrocardiography became a reality through his work, and the string galvanometer finally displaced the capillary electrometer in the measurement of the electric current produced by the contracting heart. Also in *Ann. Physik*, 1903, **12**, 1059.

843 FRANK, OTTO. 1865-1944
Die unmittelbare Registrierung der Herztöne. *Münch. med. Wschr.*, 1904, **51**, 953-54.

Frank obtained the first perfect pulse curves with special manometers, the so-called "Frank capsules".

843.1 CREMER, MAX. 1865-1935
Über die direkte Ableitung der Aktionsströme des menschlichen Herzens vom Oesophagus und über das Elektrokardiogramm des Fötus. *Münch. med. Wschr.*, 1906, **53**, 811-13.

Fetal electrocardiogram recorded. Cremer was also the first to record an electrocardiogram with an electrode in the oesophagus.

844 KEITH, *Sir* ARTHUR. 1866-1955, & FLACK, MARTIN WILLIAM. 1882-1931
The form and nature of the muscular connections between the primary divisions of the vertebrate heart. *J. Anat. Physiol. (Lond.)*, 1906-07, **41**, 172-89.

Discovery of the sino-atrial node, the "pacemaker of the heart". Reprinted in Willius & Keys, *Cardiac classics*, 1941, pp. 747-62.

845 TAWARA, SUNAO. 1873-1952
Das Reizleitungssystem des Säugethierherzens. Jena, *G. Fischer*, 1906.

Tawara discovered and described the atrioventricular node – "node of Tawara".

846 EINTHOVEN, WILLEM. 1960-1927
Die Registrierung der menschlichen Herztone mittels des Saitengalvanometers. *Pflüg. Arch. ges. Physiol.*, 1907, **117**, 461-72.

Phonocardiography.

847 MACKENZIE, *Sir* JAMES. 1853-1925
The extra-systole. A contribution to the functional pathology of the primitive cardiac tissue. *Quart. J. Med.*, 1907-08, **1**, 131-49, 481-90.

848 EPPINGER, HANS. 1879-1946, & ROTHBERGER, CARL JULIUS. 1871-
Ueber die Folgen der Durchschneidung der Tawaraschen Schenkel der Reizleitungssystems. *Z. klin. Med.*, 1910, **70**, 1-20.

First experimental study of the electrocardiographic changes in bundle-branch block.

849 ABEL, JOHN JACOB. 1857-1938
On the action of drugs and the function of the anterior lymph hearts in cardiectomized frogs. *J. Pharmacol.*, 1913, **3**, 581-608.

Abel was one of America's most distinguished pharmacologists. See A. M. Harvey: Pharmacology's giant, *Johns Hopk. med. J.,* 1974, **135,** 245-58.

850   ——. & TURNER, Benjamin Bernard. 1871-
On the influence of the lymph hearts upon the action of convulsant drugs in cardiectomized frogs. II. *J. Pharmacol.,* 1914, **6,** 91-122.

851   BAINBRIDGE, Francis Arthur. 1874-1921
On some cardiac reflexes. *J. Physiol. (Lond.),* 1914, **48,** 332-40.
Bainbridge found that cardiac reflex action is produced by inhibition of vagus tone and excitation of the accelerator nerves.

852   SMITH, Fred M. 1888-1946
The ligation of coronary arteries with electrocardiographic study. *Arch. intern. Med.,* 1918, **22,** 8-27.

853   STARLING, Ernest Henry. 1866-1927
The Linacre lecture on the law of the heart. London, *Longmans, Green & Co.,* 1918.
Starling's "law of the heart".

854   LEWIS, *Sir* Thomas. 1881-1945
The mechanism and graphic registration of the heart beat. London, *Shaw & Sons,* 1920.
Sir Thomas Lewis was a pioneer in the application to clinical medicine of the electrocardiographic method for examination of the heart. His book is both an exhaustive treatise on the subject and a valuable bibliographical source. The above is the second edition of *The mechanism of the heart beat,* 1911; third edition, 1925.

855   GROSS, Louis. 1894-
The blood supply to the heart. New York, *P. B. Hoeber,* 1921.

856   SPALTEHOLZ, Karl Werner. 1861-1940
Die Arterien der Herwand. Leipzig, *S. Hirzel,* 1924.

856.1   DALE, *Sir* Henry Hallett. 1975-1968, & SCHUSTER, Edgar Hermann Joseph. 1899-1969
A double perfusion-pump. *J. Physiol. (Lond.),* 1928, **64,** 356-64.
Mechanical heart.

857   GROLLMAN, Arthur. 1901-1980
The determination of the cardiac output of man by the use of acetylene. *Amer. J. Physiol.,* 1929, **88,** 432-45.
Grollman introduced the acetylene method of determination of cardiac output.

858   ——. The cardiac output of man in health and disease. Springfield, *C. C. Thomas,* 1932.

858.1   LINDBERGH, Charles Augustus. 1902-1974
An apparatus for the culture of whole organs. *J. Exp. Med.,*1935, **62,** 409-31.

In 1931, the year before his son's sensational kidnapping, the celebrity aviator began working with Alexis Carrel at the Rockefeller Institute on a perfusion pump which would allow the cultivation of whole organs *in vitro*. His pump maintained a sterile, pulsating circulation of fluid through excised organs, and enabled Carrel to keep organs such as the thyroid gland and kidney alive and functioning. It is a forerunner of the modern heart pump. (*See also* No. 856.1). Reprinted in Carrel and Lindbergh, *The culture of organs*, New York, Paul Hoeber, 1938.

859   McMICHAEL, *Sir* JOHN. 1904- , & SHARPEY-SCHAFER, EDWARD PETER. 1908-1963
Cardiac output in man by a direct Fick method. *Brit. Heart J.*, 1944, **6,** 33-40.

859.1   DODRILL, FOREST DEWEY. 1902- , *et al.*
Some physiologic aspects of the artificial heart problem. *J. thorac. Surg.*, 1952, **24,** 134-50.
First successful apparatus for the complete bypass of the heart. With E. Hill and R. Gerisch.

HAEMATOLOGY

See also 2011-2028.1, BLOOD TRANSFUSION; 3048-3155.4, DISORDERS OF THE BLOOD.

860   LEEUWENHOEK, ANTONJ VAN. 1632-1723
Microscopical observations concerning blood, milk, bones, the brain, spittle, and cuticula, etc. *Phil. Trans.*, 1674, **9,** 121-28.
First really accurate description of the red blood corpuscles, which Swammerdam had noted in 1658.

861   BOYLE, ROBERT. 1627-1691
Memoirs for the natural history of humane blood, especially the spirit of that liquor. London, *S. Smith,* 1684.
The first analysis of blood, Boyle's *Memoirs* may be considered the first scientific study in physiological chemistry, exhibiting methods which have become universally adopted. This is Boyle's most important medical work.

862   MENGHINI, VINCENZO. 1704-1759
De ferrearum particularum sede in sanguine. *Bonon. Sci. Art. Inst. Acad. Comment.*, 1746, **2,** pt.2, 244-66.
Discovery of iron in the blood.

863   HEWSON, WILLIAM. 1739-1774
An experimental inquiry into the properties of the blood...Part III. A description of the red particles of the blood. London, *T. Cadell,* 1771.
Hewson established the fact that fibrinogen is responsible for the clotting of blood; he first described the lymphocyte.

863.1   WELLS, WILLIAM CHARLES. 1757-1817
Observations and experiments on the colour of blood. *Phil. Trans.*, 1797, **87,** 416-31.
Wells showed that the colouring matter in the blood was not iron but a complex organic substance subsequently identified as haematin.

864 DONNÉ, ALEXANDRE. 1801-1878
De l'origine des globules du sang, de leur mode de formation et de leur fin.
C. R. Acad. Sci. (Paris), 1842, **14,** 366-68.
Announces the discovery of the blood platelets.

865 BUCHANAN, ANDREW. 1798-1882
On the coagulation of blood and other fibriniferous liquids. *Lond. med.
Gaz.,* 1845, n.s. **1,** 617-21.
Buchanan extracted the fibrin ferment of blood. He showed that it was
capable of coagulating blood and other serous fluids not in themselves
coagulable.

865.1 REICHERT, KARL BOGISLAUS. 1811-1883
Beobachtungen über eine eiweissartige Substanz in Krystallform. *Müller's
Arch. Anat. Physiol. wiss. Med.,* 1848, 197-251.
Reichert obtained haemoglobin crystals in the guinea pig.

866 FUNKE, OTTO. 1828-1879
Ueber das Milzvenenblut. *Z. rat. Med.,* 1851, n.F. **1,** 172-218; 1852, **2,** 198-
217.
Discovery of haemoglobin. (Title of second paper: Neue Beobachtungen
über die Krystalle des Milzvenen- und Fisch-Blutes).

867 VIERORDT, KARL. 1818-1884
Neue Methode der quantitativen mikroskopischen Analyse des Blutes.
Arch. physiol Heilk., 1852, **11,** 26-46.
Vierordt was the first to devise an exact method of enumerating the red
blood corpuscles. *See also* his later paper: Zählungen der Blutkörperchen
des Menschen, in the same volume, pp. 326-31.

868 WELCKER, HERMANN. 1822-1897
Bestimmungen der Menge des Körperblutes und der Blutfärbekraft, sowie
Bestimmungen von Zahl, Maass Oberfläche und Volum des einzelnen
Blutkörperchens bei Thieren und bei Menschen. *Z. rat. Med.,* 1858, 3 R.,
4, 145-67; 1863, 3 R., **20,** 257-307.
Welcker was the first to determine the total blood volume and the
volume of the normal red blood cells. Earlier paper in *Vjschr. prakt. Heilk.,*
1854, **44,** 63.

869 SCHMIDT, ALEXANDER. 1831-1894
Ueber den Faserstoff und die Ursachen seiner Gerinnung. *Arch. Anat.
Physiol. wiss. Med.,* 1861, 545-87, 675-721; 1862, 428-69, 533-64.

870 HOPPE-SEYLER, ERNST FELIX IMMANUEL. 1825-1895
Ueber das Verhalten des Blutfarbstoffe im Spectrum des Sonnenlichtes.
Virchows Arch. path. Anat., 1862, **23,** 446-49.
See No. 873.

871 LISTER, JOSEPH, *1st Baron Lister.* 1827-1912
On the coagulation of the blood. *Proc. roy. Soc. (Lond.),* (1862), 1863, **12,**
580-611.
In his Croonian Lecture Lister exploded the theory that blood coagulation is due to ammonia and showed that, in the blood vessels, it depends
upon their injury. He further showed that by carrying out the strictest

precautions he could keep blood free from putrefaction indefinitely, thus supporting his theory that bacteria were the cause of wound suppuration.

872   STOKES, *Sir* GEORGE GABRIEL. 1819-1903
On the reduction and oxidation of the colouring matter of the blood. *Proc. roy. Soc. (Lond.)*, 1863-64, **13**, 355-64.
Discovery that oxygen can be removed from haemoglobin by reducing agents.

873   HOPPE-SEYLER, ERNST FELIX IMMANUEL. 1825-1895
Ueber den chemischen und optischen Eigenschaften des Blutfarbstoffs. *Virchows Arch. path. Anat.*, 1864, **29**, 233-35, 597-600.
Hoppe-Seyler obtained haemoglobin in crystalline form and made other important discoveries in haematology. *See also* No. 870.

873.1   BIZZOZERO, GIULIO. 1846-1901
Sulla funzione ematopoietica del midollo delle ossa. *R. C. R. Ist. Lomb. Sci. Lett.*, 1868, 2 ser., **1**, 815-18.
Bizzozero demonstrated that erythropoiesis and leucopoiesis take place in the bone marrow.

873.2   NEUMANN, ERNST. 1834-1918
Ueber die Bedeutung des Knochenmarkes für die Blutbildung. *Zbl. med. Wiss.*, 1868, **6**, 689; *Arch. Heilk.*, 1869, **10**, 68-102.
Independently of Bizzozero (No. 873.1), Neumann showed that erythropoiesis and leucopoiesis take place in the bone marrow.

874   PREYER, THIERRY WILHELM. 1841-1897
Die Blutkrystalle. Jena, *Mauke,* 1871.

875   OSLER, *Sir* WILLIAM, *Bart.* 1849-1919
An account of certain organisms occurring in the liquor sanguinis. *Proc. roy. Soc. (Lond.)*, (1873), 1874, **22**, 391-98.
One of the best early descriptions of the blood platelets was given by Osler. He noticed that white thrombi were almost entirely composed of them.

876   MALASSEZ, LOUIS CHARLES. 1842-1909
Nouvelle méthode de numération des globules rouges et des globules blancs du sang. *Arch. Physiol. norm. path.*, 1874, 2 sér., **1**, 32-52.
Malassez designed the first haemocytometer, the instrument being given that name by Gowers, who modified it in 1877.

877   HAMMARSTEN, OLOF. 1841-1932
Undersökningar af de s.k. fibringeneratorerna fibrinet samt fibrinogenets koagulation. *Upsala LäkFören. Förh.*, 1875-76, **11**, 538-79.
Investigating the mechanism of blood coagulation, Hammarsten showed it to be accomplished by the splitting up of fibrinogen into fibrin and other substances.

878   GOWERS, *Sir* WILLIAM RICHARD. 1845-1915
An apparatus for the clinical estimation of haemoglobin. *Trans. clin. Soc. Lond.*, 1879, **12**, 64-67.

Gowers introduced the colorimetric method of estimating haemo-globin and devised a haemoglobinometer for the purpose. This was modified by Haldane (*see* No. 891). Previously Hoppe-Seyler had used a haematinometer.

879   HAYEM, GEORGES. 1841-1933
Recherches sur l'évolution des hématies dans le sang de l'homme et des vertébrés. *Arch. Physiol. norm. path.*, 1878, **5**, 692-734.
First accurate counts of the blood platelets.

880   EHRLICH, PAUL. 1854-1915
Methodologische Beiträge zur Physiologie und Pathologie der verschiedenen Formen der Leukocyten. *Z. klin. Med.*, 1879-80, **1**, 553-560.
Foundation of the differential blood count technique.

881   BIZZOZERO, GIULIO. 1846-1901
Su di un nuovo elemento morfologico del sangue dei mammiferi e della sua importanza nella trombosi e nella coagulazione. *Osservatore*, 1882, **17**, 785-87; **18**, 97-99.
Bizzozero gave the blood platelets their name and found that they play a part in blood coagulation. A German translation with additions is in *Virchows Arch. path. Anat.*, 1882, **90**, 261-332.

882   GRÉHANT, NESTOR. 1838-1910, & QUINQUAUD, CHARLES EUGENE. 1841-1894
Mésure du volume de sang contenu dans l'organisme d'un mammifère vivant. *C. R. Acad. Sci. (Paris)*, 1882, **94**, 1450-53.
A method of determining blood volume with carbon monoxide.

883   HAYEM, GEORGES. 1841-1933
Du sang et de ses altérations anatomiques. Paris, *G. Masson*, 1889.

884   ARTHUS, NICOLAS MAURICE. 1862-1945, & PAGES, CALIXTE.
Nouvelle théorie chimique de la coagulation du sang. *Arch. Physiol. norm. path.*, 1890, 5 ser., **2**, 739-46.
First demonstration of the essential role of calcium in the mechanism of blood coagulation.

885   HEDIN, SVEN GUSTAF. 1859-1933
Der Hämatokrit, ein neuer Apparat zur Untersuchung des Blutes. *Skand. Arch. Physiol.*, 1890-91, **2**, 134-40.
Hedin's haematocrit. He first briefly described it in *Upsala LäkFören. Förh.*, 1889, **24**, 440. Hedin is best known for his career outside the laboratory as an explorer.

886   HOWELL, WILLIAM HENRY. 1860-1945
The life history of the formed elements of the blood, especially the red blood corpuscles. *J. Morph.*, 1890-91, **4**, 57-116.
Includes description of "Howell's bodies" seen in mature erythrocytes and called also "Howell–Jolly bodies" after the later description by J. M. J. Jolly.

887   EHRLICH, PAUL. 1854-1915
Farbenanalytische Untersuchungen zur Histologie und Klinik des Blutes. Berlin, *A. Hirschwald*, 1891.
Extension of Ehrlich's work on the differential blood count.

888   SCHMIDT, ALEXANDER. 1831-1894
       Zur Blutlehre. Leipzig, *F. C. W. Vogel,* 1892.
       Schmidt established several new facts regarding blood coagulation.

889   LANDSTEINER, KARL. 1868-1943
       Zur Kenntniss der antifermentativen, lytischen und agglutinierenden
       Wirkungen des Blutserums und der Lymphe. *Zbl. Bakt.,* 1900, **27,** 357-62.
       Landsteiner discovered that human blood contains iso-agglutinins
       capable of agglutinating other human red blood cells. He divided human
       blood into three groups. He was awarded the Nobel Prize for medicine in
       1930.

890   TALLQVIST, THEODOR WALDEMAR. 1871-1927
       Ein einfaches Verfahren zur directen Schätzung der Färbestärke des Blutes.
       Z. klin. Med., 1900, **40,** 137-41.
       Tallqvist's haemoglobin scale.

891   HALDANE, JOHN SCOTT. 1860-1936
       The colorimetric determination of haemoglobin. *J. Physiol. (Lond.),* 1901,
       26, 497-504.
       Haldane's haemoglobinometer and method for determination of hae-
       moglobin.

892   SAHLI, HERMANN. 1856-1933
       Über ein einfaches und exactes Verfahren der klinischen Hämometrie.
       Verh. dtsch. Congr. inn. Med., 1902, **20,** 230-34.
       Sahli's method for the determination of haemoglobin.

893   DECASTELLO, ALFRED VON. 1872- , & STURLI, ADRIANO. 1873-1964
       Ueber die Isoagglutinine im Serum gesunder und kranker Menschen.
       Münch. med. Wschr., 1902, **49,** 1090-95.
       Following Landsteiner's division of human blood into three groups,
       Decastello and Sturli discovered a fourth (the rarest) group.

894   MORAWITZ, PAUL OSKAR. 1879-1936
       Beiträge zur Kenntniss der Blutgerinnung. *Dtsch. Arch. klin. Med.,* 1903-
       04, **79,** 1-28, 215-33, 432-42.
       Morawitz's theory of blood coagulation.

895   VAUGHAN, VICTOR CLARENCE. 1851-1929
       On the appearance and significance of certain granules in the erythrocytes
       of man. *J. med. Res.,* 1903, **10,** 342-66.
       Reticulocytes described.

896   JANSKÝ, JAN. 1873-1921
       Haematologické studie u psychotiku. *Sborn. Klinicky,* 1906-07, **8,** 85-139.
       Janský demonstrated that blood could be classified into four groups; he
       named these O, A, B, and AB. His work, published in a little-known journal,
       was at first overlooked, and in 1910 Moss independently published work
       on exactly similar lines. A French résumé of the paper is in the above
       journal, pp. 131-33, and a German summary in *Jb. Neurol. Psychiat.,* 1907,
       1028.

897   WRIGHT, James Homer. 1871-1928
        The origin and nature of the blood plates. *Boston med. surg. J.,* 1906, **154,** 643-45.
        Discovery of the role of the megakaryocytes in the formation of the blood platelets.

898   DUNGERN, Emil von. 1876-1961, & HIRSZFELD, Ludwik. 1884-1954
        Ueber Vererbung gruppenspezifischer Strukturen des Blutes. *Z. Immun-Forsch.,* 1910, **6,** 284-92.
        Proof that blood groups are inherited according to Mendelian laws.

899   HOWELL, William Henry. 1860-1945
        The preparation and properties of thrombin, together with observations on antithrombin and prothrombin. *Amer. J. Physiol.,* 1910, **26,** 453-73.

900   MOSS, William Lorenzo. 1876-1957
        Studies on isoagglutinins and isohemolysins. *Johns Hopk. Hosp. Bull.,* 1910, **21,** 63-70.
        Moss showed that the blood of all individuals could be placed into one of four groups. His classification has been the one most commonly used until recently. The work was similar to that of Janský and completed before the writer learned of the latter's publication.

901   PRICE-JONES, Cecil. 1863-1943
        The variation in the sizes of red blood cells. *Brit. med. J.,* 1910, **2,** 1418-19.
        Price-Jones described a method for the direct measurement of red blood cells, which has led to the term, "Price-Jones curve". *See also* his book, *Red blood cell diameters,* London, 1933.

902   HOWELL, William Henry. 1860-1945
        The role of antithrombin and thromboplastin (thromboplastic substance) in the coagulation of blood. *Amer. J. Physiol.,* 1911-12, **29,** 187-209.

903   KEITH, Norman Macdonnell. 1885-1976, *et al.*
        A method for the determination of plasma and blood volume. *Arch. intern. Med.,* 1915, **16,** 547-76.
        N. M. Keith, L. G. Rowntree, and J. T. Geraghty devised a method for determination of plasma and blood volume, which includes the injection of a dye.

904   McLEAN, Jay. 1890-1957
        The thromboplastic action of cephalin. *Amer. J. Physiol.,* 1916, **41,** 250-57.
        McLean extracted from dog liver a substance which retarded blood coagulation *in vitro* and which, after further work by Howell and Holt (No. 905), was named heparin.

905   HOWELL, William Henry. 1860-1945, & HOLT, Luther Emmett. 1855-1924
        Two new factors in blood coagulation — heparin and pro-antithrombin. *Amer. J. Physiol.,* 1918-19, **47,** 328-41.
        Isolation of heparin.

906   PAPPENHEIM, Artur. 1870-1916
        Morphologische Hämatologie. Hrsg. von H. Hirschfeld. Bd. 1. Leipzig, *W. Klinkhardt,* 1919.

907   HAYEM, GEORGES. 1841-1933
L'hématoblaste, troisième élement du sang. Paris, *Presse univ. de France,* 1923.
    Hayem first named the haematoblasts in 1877 (*Mém. Soc. Biol. (Paris),* 1877, **29,** 97). His view, reiterated in 1923, was that they were the early stages of red blood cells and regenerated the blood.

907.1   BERNSTEIN, FELIX. 1878-
Ergebniss einer biostatischen zusammenfassenden Betrachtung über die erblichen Blutstrukturen des Menschen. *Klin. Wschr.,* 1924, **3,** 1495-97.
    Bernstein determined the exact method of inheritance of the ABO blood groups.

908   MAXIMOW, ALEXANDER. 1874-1928
Relation of blood cells to connective tissues and endothelium. *Physiol. Rev.,* 1924, **4,** 533-63.
    Maximow's blood regeneration theory.

909   DOAN, CHARLES AUSTIN. 1896- , CUNNINGHAM, ROBERT SYDNEY. 1891- , & SABIN, FLORENCE RENA. 1871-1953
Experimental studies on the origin and maturation of avian and mammalian red blood-cells. *Contr. Embryol. Carneg. Instn.,* 1925, **16,** 163-226.

910   LANDSTEINER, KARL. 1868-1943, & LEVINE, PHILIP. 1900-1987
A new agglutinable factor differentiating individual human bloods. *Proc. Soc. exp. Biol. (N.Y.),* 1927, **24,** 600-02.
    Discovery of M and N agglutinogens. See also the same journal, pp. 941-42.

911   BERGENHEIM, BENGT LUDVIG. 1898- , & FÅHRAEUS, ROBERT [ROBIN] SANNO. 1888-1968
Über spontane Hämolysinbildung im Blut, unter besonderer Berücksichtigung der Physiologie der Milz. *Z. ges. exp. Med.,* 1936, **97,** 555-87.
    Lysolechtin found in normal blood.

912   BOYD, WILLIAM CLOUSER. 1903-1983
Blood groups. *Tab. biol. (Amst.),* 1939, **17,** 113-240.
    Boyd showed that blood groups are inherited and not changed by environment.

912.1   LEVINE, PHILIP. 1900-1987 , & STETSON, RUFUS E.
An unusual case of intra-group agglutination. *J. Amer. med. Ass.,* 1939, **113,** 126-27.
    Discovery of the Rh antigen.

912.2   LANDSTEINER, KARL. 1868-1943, & WIENER, ALEXANDER SOLOMON. 1907-1976
An agglutinable factor in human blood recognized by immune sera for Rhesus blood. *Proc. Soc. exp. Biol. (N.Y.),* 1940, **43,** 223.
    Recognition of the Rh antigen.

912.3   MOUREAU, PAUL. 1904-
Recherches sur un nouvel hémo-agglutinogène du sang humain. *Acta biol. belg.,* 1941, **1,** 123-28.

Moureau discovered the Rh factor independently of Levine and others whose work was not known to him owing to the military occupation of Belgium. See also his paper in *Amer. J. clin. Path.*, 1946, **16,** 373-79.

912.4   COHN, EDWIN JOSEPH. 1892-1953, *et al.*
Chemical, clinical, and immunological studies on the products of human plasma fractionation. *J. clin. Invest.*, 1944, **23,** 417-606.
Discovery of the blood derivatives.

912.5   OWREN, PAUL ARNOR. 1905-
The coagulation of blood. Investigations on a new clotting factor. *Acta med. scand.*, 1947, Suppl. 194, 1-327.
Discovery of the Factor V. Preliminary account in *Proc. Norwegian Acad. Sci.*, 1941, **17,** 21.

913   WALSH, ROBERT JOHN, & MONTGOMERY, CARMEL M.
A new human *iso*-agglutinin subdividing the *MN* blood groups. *Nature (Lond.)*, 1947, **160,** 504-5.
S blood-group antigen.

For history, see 1572, 1588.2.

RESPIRATORY SYSTEM

914   BOYLE, ROBERT. 1627-1691
New experiments physico-mechanical touching the spring of the air. Oxford, *H. Hall for T. Robinson,* 1660.
Boyle showed the effects of the elasticity, compressibility, and weight of air. He investigated its function in respiration, combustion, and conveyance of sound. The importance of this work in the history of respiration is Boyle's demonstration that air is essential for life.

915   MALPIGHI, MARCELLO. 1628-1694
De pulmonibus observationes anatomicae. Bononiae, *B. Ferronius* 1661.
Malpighi demonstrated that the pulmonary tissues are vesicular in nature and showed that the trachea ends in bronchial filaments. His *De pulmonibus* includes his demonstration of the capillary anastomosis between arteries and veins. *See* No. 760.

916   HOOKE, ROBERT. 1635-1703
An account of an experiment of preserving animals alive by blowing through their lungs with bellows. *Phil. Trans.*, 1667, **2,** 539-40.
By blowing air from a bellows over the exposed lungs of a dog, Hooke proved that respiratory motion is not necessary to maintain life, but that the essential feature of respiration lies in certain blood changes in the lungs. Reprinted in J. F. Fulton's *Selected readings in the history of physiology,* 2nd ed., 1966, pp. 121-23.

917   HALLER, ALBRECHT VON. 1708-1777
De respiratione experimenta anatomica, quibus aëris inter pulmonem et pleuram absentia demonstratur et musculorum intercostalium internorum officium adseritur. 2 pts. Gottingae, *A. Vandenhoeck,* 1746-1747.
First investigation of the action of the intercostal muscles in respiration.

918   HAMBERGER, GEORG ERHARD. 1697-1755
De respirationis mechanismo et usu genuino. Jenae, *apud J. C. Croekerum,* 1748.
Hamberger disputed Haller's interpretation that both the intercostal muscles lifted the ribs and were therefore responsible for respiration.

919   BLACK, JOSEPH. 1728-1799
Dissertatio medica inauguralis de humore acido a cibis orto, et magnesia alba. Edinburgi, *G. Hamilton & J. Balfour,* 1754.
Isolation of carbon dioxide. English translation, Minneapolis, 1973.

920   PRIESTLEY, JOSEPH. 1733-1804
Observations on the different kinds of air. *Phil. Trans.,* 1772, **62,** 147-264.
The isolation of oxygen was first achieved by Priestley. He also demonstrated that plants immersed in water give off oxygen and that this gas is essential for animal life.

921   RUTHERFORD, DANIEL. 1749-1819
De aëre fixo dicto, aut mephitico. Edinburgi, *Balfour & Smellie,* 1772.
Discovery of nitrogen.

922   LAVOISIER, ANTOINE LAURENT. 1743-1794
Mémoire sur la nature du principe qui se combine avec les métaux pendant leur calcination, et qui en augmente le poids. *Hist. Acad. roy. Sci.* (1775), 1778, 520-26.
Although Priestley isolated oxygen, it was Lavoisier who discovered its real significance. He showed the true nature of the interchange of gases in the lungs and exploded Stahl's phlogiston theory. Lavoisier was guillotined during the French Revolution.

923   ———. Mémoire sur la formation de l'acide, nommé air fixe ou acide crayeux, et que je désignerai désormais sous le nom d'acid du charbon. *Hist. Acad. roy. Sci.* (1781), 1784, 448-67.

924   ———. Mémoire sur l'affinité du principe oxygine avec les différentes substances auxquelles il est susceptible de s'unir. *Hist. Acad. roy. Sci.,* (1782), 1785, 530-40.

925   CAVENDISH, HENRY. 1731-1810
Experiments on air. *Phil. Trans.,* 1784, **74,** 119-53.
Cavendish isolated hydrogen in 1766, and later demonstrated the composition of air.

926   HASSENFRATZ, JEAN HENRI. 1755-1827
Mémoire sur la combinaison de l'oxigène avec le carbone et l'hydrogène du sang, sur la dissolution de l'oxigène dans le sang, et sur la manière dont le calorique se dégage. *Ann. Chim.,* 1791, **9,** 261-74.
Hassenfratz, a pupil of Lagrange, maintained that the oxidation of carbon and hydrogen took place in the blood, and not in the lungs as taught by others.

927   REISSEISEN, Franz Daniel. 1773-1828, & SOEMMERRING, Samuel Thomas. 1755-1830
       Über den Bau der Lungen. Berlin, *in den Vossischen Buchhandlung,* 1808.
       In 1804 the Berlin Akademie der Naturwissenschaften offered a prize for the best essay on the structure and function of the lungs. The prize was won by Reisseisen, while Soemmerring received honourable mention. The texts of both works were published in one volume; Soemmerring's essay was entitled "Ueber die Structur, die Verrichtung und den Gebrauch der Lungen".

928   LEGALLOIS, Julien Jean César. 1770-1814
       Expériences sur le principe de la vie. Paris, *D'Hautel,* 1812.
       Legallois described the action of the vagus nerve on respiration. He showed that bilateral section of the vagus can produce fatal broncho-pneumonia. The above work includes (p. 37) his location of the respiratory centre in the medulla. Legallois is also remembered for his reviving, after Borelli, the neurogenic theory of the heart's action; namely that the motor power of the heart comes from the spinal cord via branches of the sympathetic nerves. English translation, Philadelphia, 1813. *See* No. 1389.2.

929   MAGNUS, Heinrich Gustav. 1802-1870
       Ueber die im Blute enthaltenen Gase, Sauerstoffe, Stickstoff, und Kohlensäure. *Ann. Phys. Chem. (Leipzig),* 1837, **12,** 583-606.
       First quantitative analysis of the blood gases. Magnus proved that the arterial blood contains a higher concentration of oxygen than venous blood and that the latter had a higher carbon dioxide content.

930   HUTCHINSON, John. 1811-1861
       On the capacity of the lungs, and on the respiratory functions, with a view of establishing a precise and easy method of detecting disease by the spirometer. *Med.-chir. Trans.,* 1846, **29,** 137-252.
       Invention of the spirometer, making possible the determination of the vital capacity of the lungs. Hutchinson's work first appeared in summary form in *Lancet,* 1844, **1,** 390-391, 567-70.

931   SCHIFF, Moritz. 1823-1896
       Die Ursache der Lungenveränderung nach Durchschneidung der pneumogastrischen Nerven. *Arch. physiol Heilk,* 1847, **6,** 690-721, 769-804.
       Study of the effect of section of the vagus on respiration. *See also* No. 933.

932   REGNAULT, Henri Victor. 1810-1878, & REISET, Jules. 1818-1896
       Recherches chimiques sur la respiration des animaux des diverses classes. *Ann. Chim. Phys.,* 1849, 3 sér. **26,** 219-519.
       First determination of the respiratory quotient.

933   SCHIFF, Moritz. 1823-1896
       Ueber den Einfluss der Vagusdurchschneidung auf das Lungengewebe. *Arch. physiol. Heilk,* 1850, **9,** 625-62.
       See No. 931.

934   MEYER, Lothar. 1830-1895
       Die Gase des Blutes. *Z. rat. Med.,* 1857, **8,** 256-316.
       Meyer showed that the oxygen in the blood was not held in simple solution but came off in quantity only when the air pressure was reduced to one fiftieth of an atmosphere.

935   MEYER, LOTHAR. 1830-1895.
De sanguine oxydo carbonico infesto. Wratislaviae, *typ. Grasii, Barthii et soc.*, 1858.
Investigation of the blood gases.

935.1   SMITH, EDWARD. ?1818-1874
Experimental inquiries into the chemical and other phenomena of respiration, and their modifications by various physical agents. *Phil. Trans.*, 1859, 149, 681-714.
Smith invented a respirometer to study changes in respiratory function under various conditions. See also the following paper (pp. 715-42) on the effects of foods on respiration. For an account of his work in this and other fields, *see* C. B. Chapman, *J. Hist. Med.*, 1967, **22**, 1-26.

935.2   JOURDANET, DENIS
Les altitudes de l'Amérique tropicale comparées au niveau des mers au point de vue de la constitution médicale. Paris, *Baillière*, 1861.
Jourdanet discovered the anoxaemia theory of high altitude sickness. *See* No. 943.1.

936   SCHULTZE, MAXIMILIAN JOHANN SIGISMUND. 1825-1874
Untersuchungen über den Bau der Nasenschleimhaut, namentlich die Structur und Endigungsweise der Geruchsnerven bei dem Menschen und den Wirbelthieren. *Abh. naturf. Ges. Halle*, 1862, **7**, 1-100.
Schultze's classic paper on the nerves to the neuro-epithelium in the special sense organs marks an epoch in histology. He describes the cells of the olfactory mucous membrane, "Schultze's cells".

937   PETTENKOFER, MAX JOSEF VON. 1818-1901
Ueber die Respiration. *Ann. Chem. Pharm (Heidelberg)*, 1862-63, Suppl. 2, 1-52.

938   ———. & VOIT, CARL VON. 1831-1908
Untersuchungen über die Respiration. *Ann. Chem. Pharm. (Heidelberg)*, 1862-63, Suppl. 2, 52-70.
The first combined feeding–respiration experiments. Pettenkofer and Voit devised an apparatus for their important experiments on respiration and metabolism. They were first to estimate the amounts of protein, fat, and carbohydrate broken down in the body.

939   PFLÜGER, EDUARD FRIEDRICH WILHELM. 1829-1910
Zur Gasometrie des Blutes. *Zbl. med. Wiss.*, 1866, **4**, 305-8.
Pflüger showed that respiratory changes take place in the tissues.

940   ———. Ueber die Ursache der Athembewegungen, sowie der Dyspnoë und Apnoë. *Pflüg. Arch. ges. Physiol.*, 1868, **1**, 61-106.
Pflüger investigated the cause of the initiation of respiration in newborn animals. English translation in No. 1588.16.

941   HERING, KARL EWALD KONSTANTIN. 1834-1918
Die Selbststeuerung der Athmung durch den *Nervus vagus. S.B.k. Akad. Wiss., math.-nat. Cl. (Wien)*, 1868, 2. Abt., **57**, 672-77.

942   BREUER, Josef. 1842-1925
        Die Selbststeuerung der Athmung durch den *Nervus vagus. S.B.k. Akad.
        Wiss., math.-nat. Cl. (Wien)*, 1868, 2. Abt., **58**, 909-37.
        "Hering–Breuer reflex"; *see also* the previous entry. English translation
        of both papers in R. Porter (ed.), Hering–Breuer Centenary Symposium,
        London, *Churchill,* 1970.

943   LUSCHKA, Hubert von. 1820-1875
        Der Kehlkopf des Menschen. Tübingen, *H. Laupp,* 1871.

943.1   JOURDANET, Denis
        Influence de la pression de l'air sur la vie de l'homme. Paris, *Masson,* 1875.
        Jourdanet's observational work in remote areas of Latin America and
        Asia produced important evidence for Bert's proof that altitude sickness is
        due to anoxaemia. In *La pression barométrique* (No. 944) Bert describes
        how Jourdanet made it possible for him to do his laboratory work on
        altitude physiology, and how the two agreed to each take half the field:
        Bert, the laboratory work; and Jourdanet, the observational. Bert also
        credits Jourdanet with the theory of anoxaemia. Extensively illustrated.
        Second edition, 2 vols., 1876. *See* No. 935.2.

944   BERT, Paul. 1833-1886
        La pression barométrique. Recherches de physiologie expérimentale.
        Paris, *G. Masson,* 1878.
        The greatest work in the history of altitude physiology, in which Bert
        proved that the principal symptoms of altitude sickness arise from reduced
        partial pressure of oxygen and not from diminution of total pressure. Bert
        introduced oxygen apparatus to avert the dangerous consequences of
        ascent to high altitudes, and was the first to study the conditions of high-
        altitude ascents in a pressure chamber. He also explained the aetiology and
        mechanism of caisson disease. English translation, 1943, reprinted Bethesda,
        Md., 1979.

945   MARTIN, Henry Newell. 1848-1896, & HARTWELL, Edward Mussey. 1850-
        1922
        On the respiratory function of the internal intercostal muscles. *J. Physiol.
        (Lond.),* 1879-80, **2**, 24-27.
        The important work of Martin and Hartwell on the intercostal muscles
        settled the controversy regarding their function.

946   ZUCKERKANDL, Emil. 1849-1910
        Normale und pathologische Anatomie der Nasenhöhle und ihrer
        pneumatischen Anhänge. 2 vols. Wien, *W. Braumüller,* 1882-92.

947   HEAD, *Sir* Henry. 1861-1940
        On the regulation of respiration. *J. Physiol. (Lond.),* 1889, **10**, 1-70, 279-90.
        Demonstration of the action of the vagus in respiration.

949   HÜFNER, Carl Gustav von. 1840-1908
        Neue Versuche zur Bestimmung der Sauerstoffcapacität des Blutfarbstoffs.
        Arch. Anat. Physiol., Physiol. Abt., 1894, 130-76.
        Hüfner showed that 1 gm. haemoglobin combines with 1.34 cc oxygen.

950   MOSSO, ANGELO. 1846-1910
Fisiologia dell'uomo sulle Alpi. Studii fatti sul Monte Rosa. Milano, *frat. Treves,* 1897.

Mosso made important investigations on respiration at high altitudes. He considered that the respiratory symptoms produced at high altitudes were due to lack of carbon dioxide. English translation, London, 1898.

951   HALDANE, JOHN SCOTT, 1860-1936
A contribution to the chemistry of haemoglobin and its immediate derivatives. *J. Physiol. (Lond.),* 1898, **22**, 298-306.

Potassium ferricyanide method for the determination of oxygen in oxyhaemoglobin.

951.1   ——. Some improved methods of gas analysis. *J. Physiol. (Lond.),* 1898, **22**, 465-80.

The Haldane apparatus for the analysis of the repiratory gases, which proved a method that could measure oxygen and carbon dioxide to 0.005%. It was the cornerstone of all respiratory gas analysis until P.F. Scholander's apparatus (No. 971.1).

951.2   FREDERICQ, LÉON. 1851-1935
Sur la cause de l'apnée. *Arch. Biol.,* 1901, **17**, 561-576.

Fredericq "established that chemical changes in the blood acting somewhere in the head were the major factor in the regulation of breathing" (Kellogg). English translation in No. 1588.16.

952   MOSSO, ANGELO. 1846-1910
La physiologie de l'apnée étudiée chez l'homme. *Arch. ital. Biol.,* 1903-04, **40,** 1-30.

First studies of the physiology of apnoea in man.

953   TISSOT, JULES.
Nouvelle méthode de mesure et d'inscription du débit et des mouvements respiratoires de l'homme et des animaux. *J. Physiol. Path. gén.,* 1904, **6,** 688-700.

Tissot spirometer.

954   HALDANE, JOHN SCOTT. 1860-1936, & PRIESTLEY, JOHN GILLIES. 1880-1941
The regulation of the lung-ventilation. *J. Physiol. (Lond.),* 1905, **32,** 225-66.

Proof of the regulation of respiration by CO_2 concentration of the alveolar air.

955   DOUGLAS, CLAUDE GORDON. 1882-1963
A method for determining the total respiratory exchange in man. *J. Physiol. (Lond.),* 1911, **42,** Proc. Physiol. Soc., xvii-xviii.

Douglas bag.

956   PETERS, *Sir* RUDOLPH ALBERT. 1889-1982
Chemical nature of specific oxygen capacity in haemoglobin. *J. Physiol. (Lond.),* 1912, **44,** 131-49.

Peters made accurate determinations of the ratio of iron to oxygen in the blood.

957   DOUGLAS, CLAUDE GORDON. 1882-1963, *et al.*
        Physiological observations made on Pike's Peak, Colorado, with special
        reference to adaptation to low barometric pressures. *Phil. Trans. B,* 1913,
        203, 185-318.
            With J. S. Haldane, Y. Henderson, and E. C. Schneider.

958   CHRISTIANSEN, JOHANNE OSTENFELD. 1882-1968, *et al.*
        The absorption and dissociation of carbon dioxide by human blood. *J.
        Physiol. (Lond.),* 1914, **48,** 244-71.
            With C. G. Douglas and J. S. Haldane. CO_2 dissociation curves. These
        workers discovered that haemoglobin indirectly greatly assists the trans-
        port of CO_2 by the blood.

959   MEYERHOF, OTTO FRITZ. 1884-1951
        Ueber das Vorkommen des Coferments des alcoholischen Hefegärung im
        Muskelgewebe und seine muttmassliche Bedeutung im Atmungs-
        mechanismus. *Hoppe-Seyl. Z. physiol. Chem.,* 1918, **101,** 165-75.
            Meyerhof shared the Nobel Prize for physiology with A. V. Hill in 1922
        for his work on the physiology of muscle.

960   JOFFE, JACK, & POULTON, EDWARD PALMER. 1883-1939
        The partition of CO_2 between plasma and corpuscles in oxygenated and
        reduced blood. *J. Physiol. (Lond.),* 1920-21, **54,** 129-51.

961   HALDANE, JOHN SCOTT. 1860-1936
        Respiration. New Haven, *Yale Univ. Press,* 1922.
            An account of the work of the Oxford School of Physiology, in particular
        the Pike's Peak expedition (No. 957). Second edition, 1935, with J. G.
        Priestley.

962   HARTRIDGE, HAMILTON. 1886-1976, & ROUGHTON, FRANCIS JOHN WORSLEY.
        1899-1972
        The velocity with which carbon monoxide displaces oxygen from com-
        bination with haemoglobin. *Proc. roy. Soc. B,* 1923, **94,** 336-67.

963   LUMSDEN, THOMAS WILLIAM.
        The regulation of respiration. *J. Physiol. (Lond.),* 1923-24, **58,** 81-91, 111-
        26.
            Lumsden introduced the concept of subsidiary respiratory centres in
        the brain stem.

963.1   VAN SLYKE, DONALD DEXTER. 1883-1971, & NEILL, JAMES M. 1894-1964
        The determination of gases in blood and other solutions by vacuum
        extraction and manometric measurement. *J. biol. Chem.,* 1924, **61,** 523-573.
            Method for the manometric analysis of gases in blood and other
        solutions.

964   BARCROFT, *Sir* JOSEPH. 1872-1947
        The respiratory function of the blood. Cambridge, *Univ. Press,* 1913.
            Barcroft's studies of the oxygen-carrying capacity of the blood are
        recorded in the above monograph. He particularly concentrated on
        elucidation of the oxygen dissociation curve. The second edition, 2 vols.,
        Cambridge, 1925-28, was greatly revised and enlarged.

965   GESELL, ROBERT. 1886-1954
          The chemical regulation of respiration. *Physiol. Rev.*, 1925, **5,** 551-95.

966   HENRIQUES, OSCAR M. 1895-1953
          Die Bindungsweise des Kohlendioxyds im Blute. *Biochem. Z.*, 1928, **200,**
          1-24.
              Carbamino reaction.

967   HEYMANS, CORNEILLE JEAN FRANÇOIS. 1892-1968
          Le sinus carotidien et la zone homologue cardio-aortique. Paris, *Presses univ.
          de France,* 1929.
              His work on the sinus–aorta mechanism in respiration gained Heymans
          the Nobel Prize in 1938.

968   KEILIN, DAVID. 1887-1963
          Cytochrome and respiratory enzymes. *Proc. roy. Soc. B,* 1929, **104,** 206-52.
              Keilin discovered cytochrome and laid the foundations of the modern
          concept of cellular respiration. *See* No. 1588.3.

969   WARBURG, OTTO HEINRICH. 1883-1970, & NEGELEIN, ERWIN.
          Ueber den Absorptionsspektrum des Atmungsferments. *Biochem. Z.,* 1929,
          214, 64-100.
              Warburg discovered the nature and function of the respiratory ferment.
          He was awarded the Nobel Prize for physiology in 1931.

970   ———. & CHRISTIAN, WALTER. 1907-1955
          Ueber ein neues Oxydationsferment und sein Absorptionsspektrum.
          Biochem. Z., 1932, **254,** 438-58.

971   MELDRUM, NORMAN URQUHART. 1907-1933, & ROUGHTON, FRANCIS JOHN
          WORSLEY. 1899-1972
          Carbonic anhydrase. Its preparation and properties. *J. Physiol. (Lond.),*
          1933, **80,** 113-42.
              Isolation of carbonic anhydrase.

971.1   SCHOLANDER, PER FREDRIK. 1905-1980
          Analyzer for accurate estimate of respiratory gases in one-half cubic
          centimeter samples. *J. biol. Chem.,* 1947, **167,** 235-50.
              An improvement on the classic Haldane method for analysing oxygen
          and carbon dioxide in respiratory gases. It provides comparable accuracy
          over a wider range of gas concentrations with a gas sample of only 0.5 ml
          instead of 25 ml.

DIGESTIVE SYSTEM

See also 665-752.13, BIOCHEMISTRY.

972   GLISSON, FRANCIS. 1597-1677
          Anatomia hepatis. Londini, *typ. Du-Gardianis,* 1654.
              First accurate description of the capsule of the liver (Glisson's capsule)
          and its blood-supply. He also described the sphincter of the bile duct
          ("Glisson's sphincter", the sphincter of Oddi). This is the first book printed

in England which gives a detailed account of a single organ based on original research. *See* No. 1098.1.

973 STENSEN, NIELS. [STENO]. 1638-1686
Observationes anatomicae, quibus varia oris, oculorum & narium vas describuntur novique salivae, lacrymarum & muci fontes deteguntur. Lugduni Batavorum, *J. Chouët,* 1662.

Includes the first account of the excretory duct of the parotid gland ("Stensen's duct"), discovered by Stensen. He first reported his discovery in a letter to his teacher, Thomas Bartholin, dated April, 22, 1661. Facsimile reproduction, with English translation, Copenhagen, 1951.

974 GRAAF, REGNIER DE. 1641-1673
De succi pancreatici natura et usu exercitatio anatomico-medica. Lugduni Batavorum, *ex. off. Hackiana,* 1664.

De Graaf was an early investigator of the pancreatic secretion. He collected the pancreatic juice of dogs by means of artificial pancreatic fistulae, commenting on the small quantity of juice secreted and on its alkaline character. The French edition, Paris, 1666, contained a revised and enlarged text. Partial translation in J. F. Fulton, *Selected readings in the history of physiology,* 2nd ed., 1966, pp. 167-68. Full English translation from 2nd ed. (1671), London, 1676.

974.1 WEPFER, JOHANN JACOB. 1620-1695
Cicutae aquaticae historia et noxae. Basileae, *J. R. König,* 1679.

Discovery of the duodenal (Brunner's) glands (*see also* No. 975). Wepfer was Brunner's father-in-law.

974.2 BARTHOLIN, CASPAR. 1655-1738
Du ductu salivati hactenus non descriptio. Hafniae, *typ. J. P. Bockenhoffer,* 1684.

"Bartholin's duct" and "gland", the sublingual salivary gland and ducts.

975 BRUNNER, JOHANN CONRAD A. 1653-1727
De glandulis in intestino duodeno hominis detectis. Heidelbergae, *C. E. Buchta,* 1687.

"Brunner's glands", earlier described by Wepfer (No. 974.1).

976 VATER, ABRAHAM. 1684-1751
Dissertatio anatomica qua novum bilis diverticulum circa orificium ductus choledochi ut et valvulosam colli vesicae felleae constructionem ad disceptandum proponit. Wittenbergae, *lit. Gerdesianus,* 1720.

Following Vater's classic description of the ampulla of the bile duct, it was named the "ampulla of Vater".

977 POUPART, FRANÇOIS. 1661-1709
[Suspenseurs de l'abdomen]. *Hist. Acad. roy. Sci.,* Paris, 1730, 51.

"Poupart's ligament", the inguinal ligament.

978 LIEBERKÜHN, JOHANN NATHANAEL. 1711-1756
De fabrica et actione villorum intestinorum tenuium hominis. Lugduni Batavorum, *C. & G. J. Wishof,* 1745.

"Lieberkühn's glands" or "crypts" described. They were discovered by Malpighi in 1688.

979   RÉAUMUR, RENÉ ANTOINE FERCHAULT DE. 1683-1757
Sur la digestion des oiseaux. *Hist. Acad. roy. Sci.,* (1752), 1756, 266-307, 461-95.
    Using a pet buzzard, de Réaumur succeeded in isolating the gastric juice and demonstrating its solvent effect on foods.

980   STEVENS, EDWARD. 1755?-1834
Dissertatio physiologica inauguralis de alimentorum concoctione. Edinburgi, *Balfour et Smellie,* 1777.
    First isolation of human gastric juice. Stevens was also the first successfully to perform an *in vitro* digestion, proving the presence in the gastric juice of the active principle necessary for the assimilation of food. An English translation is included in Spallanzani's *Dissertations relative to the natural history of animals,* 1784, vol. 1, pp. 303-16. English translation, with biography of Stevens, Montreal, 1969.

981   SPALLANZANI, LAZZARO. 1729-1799
Dissertazioni di fisica animale e vegetabile. Vol. 1. Modena, *Presso la Società Tipografica,* 1780.
    Spallanzani confirmed earlier doctrines of the solvent property of the gastric juice and discovered the action of the saliva in digestion. He stated that gastric juice can act outside the body and can prevent or inhibit putrefaction. He obtained gastric juice by tying a sponge on a piece of string, then allowing it to be swallowed. English translation, 1784.

982   YOUNG, JOHN RICHARDSON. 1782-1804
An experimental inquiry into the principles of nutrition, and the digestive process. Philadelphia, *Eaken & Mecum,* 1803.
    Young, one of the first American experimental physiologists, showed the solvent principle in the gastric juice to be an acid, but wrongly inferred that it was phosphoric acid. He also deduced the association and synchrony between gastric juice and saliva. Reprinted, Urbana, Ill., 1959.

983   HESSELBACH, FRANZ KASPAR. 1759-1816
Anatomisch-chirurgische Abhandlung ueber den Ursprung der Leistenbrüche. Würzburg, *Baumgärtner,* 1806.
    Hesselbach's "fascia", "ligament", and "triangle" described.

984   MECKEL, JOHANN FRIEDRICH, *the younger.* 1781-1833
Ueber die Divertikel am Darmkanal. *Arch. Physiol. (Halle),* 1809, **9,** 421-53.
    "Meckel's diverticulum".

985   MAGENDIE, FRANÇOIS. 1783-1855
Mémoire sur le vomissement. Paris, *Crochard,* 1813.
    Physiologists still consult Magendie's classic description of the physiology of deglutition and vomiting. Magendie proved, against the current theory of Haller, that the stomach was passive rather than active in vomiting. This was essentially correct; however Magendie did fail to observe the active role of the plyloric end of the stomach. English translation in *Ann. Phil.,* London, 1813, **1,** 429-38.

985.1   ———. Mémoire sur l'usage de l'epiglotte dans la déglutition...Paris, *Méquignon-Marvis,* 1813.

Magendie showed that the epiglottis is not necessary for swallowing, which disproved the accepted doctrine that the epiglottis was necessary to cover the glottis to prevent food from entering the trachea.

986   BRODIE, *Sir* Benjamin Collins, *Bart*. 1783-1862
Experiments and observations on the influence of the nerves of the eighth pair on the secretions of the stomach. *Phil. Trans.*, 1814, **104**, 102-06.
Before turning to surgery, Brodie did important work in physiology. Above is his study of the influence of the pneumogastric nerve on gastric secretion.

987   PROUT, William. 1785-1850
On the nature of the acid and saline matters usually existing in the stomachs of animals. *Phil. Trans.*, 1824, **114,** 45-49.
Proof that the gastric juice contains free hydrochloric acid.

987.1   BEAUMONT, William. 1785-1853
A case of wounded stomach [by Joseph Lovell]. *Medical Recorder*, 1825, **8**, 14-19, 840.
Beaumont's first report on Alexis St. Martin was accidentally published under the name of Joseph Lovell, Surgeon-General of the U.S. Army. *See* No. 989.

987.2   ——. Further experiments on the case of Alexis San Martin, who was wounded in the stomach by a load of buckshot. *Medical Recorder*, 1826, **9**, 94-97.
In this and No. 987.1 Beaumont first described his   revolutionary experiments on Alexis St. Martin. He continued these researches and published his monograph in 1833. *See* No. 989.

988   TIEDEMANN, Friedrich. 1781-1861, & GMELIN, Leopold. 1788-1853
Die Verdauung nach Versuchen. 2 vols. Heidelberg, *K. Groos,* 1826-27.
Confirmation of the work of Prout.

989   BEAUMONT, William. 1785-1853
Experiments and observations on the gastric juice, and the physiology of digestion. Plattsburgh, *F. P Allen,* 1833.
Alexis St. Martin, a Canadian half-breed who had sustained a gastric fistula, was treated and investigated by Beaumont. With his human medium, Beaumont was the first to study digestion and the movements of the stomach *in vivo.* His work on the subject was the most important before Pavlov. Edinburgh imprint, 1838. Second edition, corrected, Burlington, Vt., 1847. Facsimile reprint, Cambridge, *Harvard Univ. Press,* 1929.

990   MÜLLER, Johannes. 1801-1858, & SCHWANN, Theodor. 1810-1882
Versuche über die künstliche Verdauung des geronnenen Eiweisses. *Arch. Anat. Physiol. wiss. Med.,* 1836, 66-89.

991   SCHWANN, Theodor. 1810-1882
Ueber das Wesen des Verdauungsprocesses. *Arch. Anat. Physiol. wiss. Med.,* 1836, 90-138.
Beaumont had considered that the gastric juice contained some other active chemical substance besides hydrochloric acid. Schwann proved this to be pepsin.

992   BOUSSINGAULT, JEAN BAPTISTE, 1802-1887
Analyses comparées des alimens consommés et des produits rendus par une vache laitière. *Ann. Chim.*, 1839, **71**, 113-36.
The first analysis of foodstuffs and fertilizers. Boussingault made a balance of intake and outgo of nutrients in food and excreta.

992.1   BASSOV, VASILI. 1812-1879
Voie artificielle dans l'estomac des animaux. *Bull. Soc. imp. Naturalistes Moscou,* 1843, N.S. **16**, 315-19.
First gastric fistula established specially for the purpose of experimentation.

992.2   BLONDLOT, NICOLAS. 1810-1877
Traité analytique de la digestion considérée particulièrement dans l'homme et dans les animaux. Paris, *Fortin, Masson et Cie.,* 1843.
Gastric fistula for experimental purposes.

992.3   BERNARD, CLAUDE. 1813-1878
Du suc gastrique et de son rôle dans la nutrition. Paris, *Rignous,* 1843.
Bernard showed that if sucrose is injected directly into the blood it is eliminated by the kidneys while glucose is retained, and that gastric juice transforms sucrose into assimilable sugar. See F.J. Holmes, *Claude Bernard and animal chemistry: The emergence of a scientist,* Cambridge, Mass., 1974. This includes a history of research on digestion from 1750-1848.

993   SCHWANN, THEODOR. 1810-1882
Versuche um auszumitteln, ob die Galle im Organismus eine für das Leben wesentliche Rolle spielt. *Arch. Anat. Physiol. wiss. Med.,* 1844, 127-59.
Proof of the indispensability of bile to digestion.

994   GERLACH, JOSEPH. 1820-1896
Beobachtung einer tödlichen Peritonitis, als Folge einer Perforation des Wurmfortsatzes. *Z. rat. Med.,* 1847, **6**, 12-23.
Description of "Gerlach's valve", sometimes seen at the orifice of the appendix.

995   BERNARD, CLAUDE. 1813-1878
De l'origine du sucre dans l'économie animale. *Arch. gén. Méd.,* 1848, 4 sér., **18**, 303-19.
Bernard's first communication regarding his investigation of the glycogenic function of the liver. Reprinted, with translation, in *Med. Classics,* 1939, **3**, 552-80.

996   ——. Du suc pancréatique et de son rôle dans les phénomènes de la digestion. *Arch. gén Méd.,* 1849, **19**, 60-81.
Discovery of the digestive action of the pancreatic juice, especially its role in the digestion and absorption of fats. Reprinted, with translation, in *Med. Classics,* 1939, **3**, 581-617.

997   MOLESCHOTT, JACOB. 1822-1893
Die Physiologie der Nahrungsmittel. Darmstadt, *C. W. Leske,* 1850.

998   LUDWIG, Carl Friedrich Wilhelm. 1816-1895
        Neue Versuche über die Beihilfe der Nerven zur Speichelabsonderung. *Z. rat. Med.*, 1851, n.F. **1**, 254-77.
        The innervation of the salivary glands first elucidated.

999   BIDDER, Friedrich Heinrich. 1810-1894, & SCHMIDT, Carl. 1822-1894
        Die Verdauungssäfte und der Stoffwechsel. Mitau & Leipzig, *G. A. Reyher,* 1852.
        Even after the work of Prout and Beaumont, some physiologists thought that the free acid of the gastric juice was lactic acid; Bidder and Schmidt finally proved that normally the gastric juice always contains HCl in excess.

999.1   BERNARD, Claude. 1813-1878
        Nouvelles recherches expérimentales sur les phénomènes glycogéniques du foie. *C. R. Soc. Biol. (Mémoires),* (1857) 1858, 2 sér. **4**, 1-7.
        Discovery of glycogen. See also *C. R. Acad. Sci. (Paris),* 1857, **44,** 578-86, 1325-31.

1000   ——. Sur le mécanisme de la formation du sucre dans le foie. *C. R. Acad. Sci. (Paris),* 1855, **41,** 461-69.
        The culmination of Bernard's work on the glycogenic function of the liver. He invented the term "internal secretion" and can be said to have started the scientific investigation of the internal secretions, although for 30 years the significance of his work was not generally realized. By his research on glycogen Bernard showed that the body can not only break down, but can also build up, complex chemical substances.

1000.1 ——. Mémoire sur le pancréas et sur le rôle du suc pancréatique dans les phénomènes digestifs. *Suppl. C. R. Acad. Sci. (Paris),* 1856, 1, 379-563.
        The most beautifully illustrated of all Bernard's writings which summed up the results of his work on the role of the pancreas in digestion. English translation reproducing the colour plates in colour. London, 1985.

1001   CORVISART, François Rémy Lucien. 1824-1882
        Sur une fonction peu connue du pancréas. La digestion des aliments azotés. 10 pts. Paris, *V. Masson,* 1857-63.
        Corvisart showed that pancreatic proteolysis takes place at body temperature, in acid, alkaline, or neutral media.

1002   SAPPEY, Marie Philbert Constant. 1810-1896
        Mémoire sur un point d'anatomie pathologique relatif à l'histoire de la cirrhose. *Mém. Acad. imp. Méd. (Paris),* 1859, **23**, 269-78.
        "Sappey's veins" in the falciform ligament of the liver.

1003   BRÜCKE, Ernst Wilhelm von, *Ritter.* 1819-1892
        Beiträge zur Lehre von der Verdauung. *S.B.k. Akad. Wiss. Wien,* 1861, math.-nat.Kl., **43**, Abt.2, 601-23.

1004   DANILEVSKY, Aleksandr Yakolevich. 1838-1923
        Ueber specifisch wirkende Körper des natürlichen und künstlichen pancreatischen Saftes. *Virchows Arch. path. Anat.,* 1862, **25**, 279-307.
        Discovery of trypsin.

1005   FLINT, AUSTIN, *Jnr.* 1936-1915
Experimental researches into a new excretory function of the liver, consisting in the removal of cholesterine from the blood and its discharge from
the body in the form of stercorine. *Amer. J. med. Sci.,* 1862, n.s. **44,** 305-
65.
Discovery, in the faeces, of "stercorine" (coprosterol).

1006   AUERBACH, LEOPOLD. 1828-1897
Ueber einen Plexus gangliosus myogastricus. *Jber. schles. Ges. vaterl. Cultur,*
(1862), 1863, **40,** 103-04.
Auerbach's plexus and ganglion. See also his book *Ueber einen Plexus
myentericus,* Breslau, *Morgenstern,* 1862.

1007   THIRY, LUDWIG. 1817-1897
Ueber eine neue Methode den Dünndarm zu isolieren. *S.B. k. Akad. Wiss.
Wien,* math.-nat. Kl., 1865, Abt. I, **50,** 77-96.
Thiry-Vella fistula. *See also* No. 1014.

1008   HEIDENHAIN, RUDOLF PETER HEINRICH. 1834-1897
Beiträge zur Lehre von der Speichelsecretion. *Stud. physiol. Inst. Breslau,*
1868, **4,** 1-124.

1009   LANGERHANS, PAUL. 1847-1888
Beiträge zur mikroskopischen Anatomie der Bauchspeicheldrüse. Inaugural-Dissertation. Berlin, *Gustav Lange,* 1869.
First account of the islands of Langerhans. In 1893 E. Laguesse attached
the name of Langerhans to the structures. Langerhans did not suggest any
function for them. The book has been reprinted with an English translation
by H. Morrison, *Bull. Hist. Med.,* 1937, **5,** 259-97.

1010   PASCHUTIN, VICTOR VASILYEVICH. 1845-1901
Einige Versuche mit Fermenten, welche Stärke und Rohrzucker in
Traubenzucker verwandeln. *Arch. Anat. Physiol. wiss. Med.,* 1871, 305-84.

1011   HEIDENHAIN, RUDOLF PETER HEINRICH. 1834-1897
Ueber die Wirkung einiger Gifte auf die Nerven der glandula submaxillaris.
Pflüg. Arch. ges. Physiol., 1872, **5,** 309-18.
Study of the effect of poisons on the nerves of the submaxillary gland.

1012   KÜHNE, WILLY. 1837-1900
Ueber das Trypsin. *Verh. naturh.-med. Ver. Heidelberg,* 1874-77, n.F. **1,**
194-98.
Isolation of trypsin.

1012.1   HEIDENHAIN, RUDOLF PETER HEINRICH. 1834-1897
Ueber die Pepsinbildung in den Pylorusdrüsen. *Pflüg. Arch. ges. Physiol.,*
1878, **18,** 169-71.
Heidenhain pouch.

1013   LUCIANI, LUIGI. 1840-1919
Fisiologia del digiuni. Firenze, *Sucessori Le Monnier,* 1881.
Luciani distinguished three stages of starvation in man – hunger,
physiological inanition, and pathological inanition.

1014 VELLA, Luigi. 1825-1886
Nuovo metodo per avere il succo enterico puro, e stabilirne le proprietà fisiologiche. *Mem. r. Accad. Sci. Ist. Bologna,* 1881, **2,** 515-38.

1015 KRONECKER, Karl Hugo. 1839-1914, & MELTZER, Samuel James. 1851-1920
Der Schluckmechanismus, seine Erregung und seine Hemmung. *Arch. Anat. Physiol., Physiol. Abt.,* 1883, *Suppl.-Bd.,* 328-62.
An experimental study, by means of a balloon, of swallowing and of oesophageal contractions.

1016 KÜHNE, Willy. 1837-1900, & CHITTENDEN, Russell Henry. 1856-1943
Ueber die nächsten Spaltungsproducte der Eiweisskörper. *Z. Biol.,* 1883, **19,** 159-208.
Kühne and Chittenden isolated and named several new substances during their investigation of the products of digestion. *See also* the same journal, 1884, **20,** 11-51; 1886, **22,** 409-58; 1889, **25,** 358-67.

1017 ESCHERICH, Theodor. 1857-1911
Die Darmbakterien des Säuglings und ihre Beziehungen zur Physiologie der Verdauung. Stuttgart, *F. Enke,* 1886.
Includes the first account of *Bact. coli* infection. The organism was later renamed *Escherichia coli.*

1018 ODDI, Ruggero. 1864-1913
D'une disposition à sphincter spéciale de l'ouverture du canal cholédoque. *Arch. ital. Biol.,* 1887, **8,** 317-22.
"Sphincter of Oddi" of the bile duct, already known to Glisson in 1654. Reprinted as a pamphlet, Perugia, 1887.

1018.1 HARTMANN, Henri. 1860-1952
Quelques points de l'anatomie et de la chirurgie des voies biliaires. *Bull. Soc. anat. Paris,* 1891, 5 sér., **5,** 480-500.
"Hartmann's pouch", a dilatation of the neck of the gall-bladder.

1019 HEIDENHAIN, Rudolf Peter Heinrich. 1834-1897
Neue Versuche über die Aufsaugung im Dünndarm. *Pflüg. Arch. ges. Physiol.,* 1894, **56,** 579-631.

1020 NUTTALL, George Henry Falkiner. 1862-1937, & THIER-FELDER, Hans. 1858-1930
Thierisches Leben ohne Bakterien im Verdauungskanal. *Hoppe-Seyl. Z. physiol. Chem.,* 1895-96, **21,** 109-21; 1896-97, **22,** 62-73; 1897, **23,** 231-35.
Proof that healthy life and perfect digestion are possible without the presence of bacteria in the digestive tract.

1021 KULTSCHITZKY, Nikolai. 1856-1925
Zur Frage über den Bau des Darmkanals. *Arch. mikr. Anat.,* 1897, **49,** 7-35.
The "cells of Kultschitzky" in the epithelium of the intestine, between the cells which line the gland of Lieberkühn.

1022   PAVLOV, IVAN PETROVITCH. 1849-1936
Lektsii o rabotie glavnikh pishtshevarîtelnikh zhelyoz. [Lectures on the work of the principal digestive glands.] St. Petersburg, *I. N. Kushnereff,* 1897.

    Pavlov made perhaps the greatest contribution to our knowledge of the physiology of digestion. Especially notable was his method of producing gastric and pancreatic fistulae for the purpose of his experiments. The second published edition was a German translation by A. Walther, Wiesbaden, *J.F. Bergmann,* 1898. The work was translated into English in 1902, with a second edition appearing in 1910. A translation of Pavlov's description of the stomach pouch devised by him is in J. F. Fulton's *Selected readings in the history of physiology,* 2nd ed., 1966, pp. 192-93. He was awarded the Nobel Prize in physiology in 1904. *See also* No. 1445.

1023   ADDISON, CHRISTOPHER. *1st Viscount Addison of Stallingborough.* 1869-1951
On the topographical anatomy of abdominal viscera in man, especially the gastrointestinal canal. *J. Anat. Physiol.,* 1899, **33,** 565-86.

    "Addison's transpyloric plane". Addison was Britain's first Minister of Health (1919-21).

1024   BAYLISS, *Sir* WILLIAM MADDOCK. 1860-1924, & STARLING, ERNEST HENRY. 1866-1927
The mechanism of pancreatic secretion. *J. Physiol. (Lond.),* 1902, **28,** 325-53.

    Demonstration of the existence of secretin in the duodenal secretion. Preliminary note in *Lancet,* 1902, **1,** 813.

1025   RUBNER, MAX. 1854-1932
Die Gesetze des Energieverbrauchs bei der Ernährung. Leipzig & Wien, *F. Deuticke,* 1902.

    Rubner's classic work on the influence of foodstuffs on metabolism. In it he introduced the term "specific dynamic action of the foodstuffs".

1026   EDKINS, JOHN SYDNEY. 1863-1940
The chemical mechanism of gastric secretion. *J. Physiol. (Lond.),* 1906, **34,** 133-44.

    Gastric secretin (gastrin) was first described by Edkins. A preliminary communication is in *Proc. roy. Soc. B,* 1905, **76,** 376.

1027   BENEDICT, FRANCIS GANO. 1870-1957
The influence of inanition on metabolism. Washington, *Carnegie Inst.,* 1907.

1028   LONDON, EFIM SEMENOVICH. 1869-1939, & DOBROVOLSKAJA, N.
Studien über die spezifische Anpassung der Verdauungssäfte. *Hoppe-Seyl. Z. physiol. Chem.,* 1910, **68,** 374-77.

1029   CANNON, WALTER BRADFORD. 1871-1945
The mechanical factors of digestion. London, *E. Arnold,* 1911.
    Summarized research begun in 1896. *See* No. 3519.

1030   CARLSON, ANTON JULIUS. 1875-1956
Contributions to the physiology of the stomach. *Amer. J. Physiol.,* 1912-13, **31,** 151-68, 175-92, 212-22, 318-27; 1913, **32,** 245-63.

Carlson recorded stomach movements by means of a balloon inserted through a gastric fistula. Much of his important work on gastric physiology is summed up in his book. *See* No. 1033.

1031   GLÉNARD, ROGER. 1880-1964
Le mouvement de l'intestin en circulation artificielle. Paris, 1913.
Cinematographic studies of the movements of the intestines in animals. A thesis presented to the Faculty of Science, Paris University.

1032   BABKIN, BORIS PETROVICH. 1877-1950
Die äussere Sekretion der Verdauungsdrüsen. Berlin, *J. Springer,* 1914.

1033   CARLSON, ANTON JULIUS. 1875-1956
The control of hunger in health and disease. Chicago, *Univ. Press,* (1916).

1034   TRENDELENBURG, PAUL. 1884-1931
Physiologische und pharmakologische Versuche über die Dünndarmperistaltik. *Arch. exp. Path. Pharmak.,* 1917, **81,** 55-129.

1035   ALVAREZ, WALTER CLEMENT. 1884-
The mechanics of the digestive tract. New York, *P. H. Hoeber,* 1922.
Includes (p. 111) his smooth diet for duodenal ulcer. Fourth edition entitled *Introduction to gastro-enterology,* 1950.

1036   DuBOIS, EUGÈNE FLOYD. 1882-1959
Basal metabolism in health and disease. Philadelphia, *Lea & Febiger,* 1924.

1037   IVY, ANDREW CONWAY. 1893-1977, & FARRELL, JAMES IRVING. 1900-
Contributions to the physiology of gastric secretion. The proof of a humoral mechanism. A new procedure for the study of gastric physiology. *Amer. J. Physiol.,* 1925, **74,** 639-49.

1038   KOSAKA, T., & LIM, ROBERT KHO-SENG. 1897-1969
Demonstration of the humoral agent in fat inhibition of gastric secretion. *Proc. Soc. exp. Biol. (N.Y.),* 1930, **27,** 890-91.
The work of Kosaka and Lim led to the discovery of a hormone inhibiting gastric secretion ("enterogastrone").

1038.1   NORTHROP, JOHN HOWARD. 1891-
Crystalline pepsin. *J. gen. Physiol.,* 1930, **13,** 739-80.
Crystallization of pepsin and its identity as a protein.

1039   ÅGREN, GUNNAR. 1907-
Ueber die pharmakodynamischen Wirkungen und chemischen Eigenschaften des Secretins. *Skand. Arch. Physiol.,* 1934, **70,** 10-87.
Preparation of crystalline secretin.

1040   HAHN, PAUL FRANCIS. 1908-1967, *et al.*
Radioactive iron absorption by gastro-intestinal tract. Influence of anemia, anoxia, and antecedent feeding distribution in growing dogs. *J. exp. Med.,* 1943, **78,** 169-88.
An important contribution to the knowledge of iron absorption. With W. F. Bale, J. F. Ross, W. M. Balfour, and G. H. Whipple.

1040.1   HARPER, ALFRED ALEXANDER. 1907- , & RAPER, HENRY STANLEY. 1882-1951
Pancreozymin, a stimulant of the secretion of pancreatic enzymes in
extracts of the small intestine. *J. Physiol. (Lond.),* 1943, **102,** 115-25.

1041   WOLF, STEWART GEORGE. 1914- , & WOLFF, HAROLD GEORGE. 1898-1962
Human gastric function. An experimental study of a man and his stomach.
New York, *Oxford University Press,* 1943.
     Important experiments on gastric function, made on "Tom", a man who
had a gastric fistula from the age of 9. Second edition in 1947.

Nutrition: Vitamins

1041.1   MAGENDIE, FRANÇOIS. 1783-1855
Précis élémentaire de physiologie. 2 vols., Paris, *Méquignon-Marvis,* 1816-
17.
     Vol. 2 contains Magendie's classic demonstration of the importance of
nitrogenous food, or protein, in the food supply of mammals. In the course
of his experiments on dogs fed non-nitrogenous substances, Magendie
also induced the first experimental cases of an avitaminosis (specifically,
lack of vitamin A.) *See* No. 597.1.

1042   LUNIN, NIKOLAI IVANOVICH. 1853-1937
Ueber die Bedeutung der anorganischen Salze für die Ernährung des
Thiers. *Hoppe-Seyl. Z. physiol. Chem.,* 1881, **5,** 31-39.
     Working in Bunge's laboratory, Lunin prepared synthetic milk diets and
showed that they lacked an unknown factor necessary for animal growth,
and that animals cannot live on a chemically pure (i.e. vitamin-free) diet.
This was the starting point of modern research on vitamins.

1043   CHITTENDEN, RUSSELL HENRY. 1856-1943
Physiological economy in nutrition. New York, *F. A. Stokes Co.,* 1904.
     Chittenden, founder of the first laboratory of physiological chemistry in
the U.S.A., made many important experiments in nutrition, especially in
connexion with the low protein diet advocated by him.

1044   HOPKINS, *Sir* FREDERICK GOWLAND, 1861-1947
The analyst and the medical man. *Analyst,* 1906, **31,** 385-404.
     Hopkins predicted the existence of vitamins as early as 1906. He fed
animals a diet of zein which failed to maintain growth; however, the
animals grew at once when casein was substituted. He concluded that "in
the organs must appear special, indispensable active substances which the
tissues can only make from special precursors in the diet".

1045   LUSK, GRAHAM. 1866-1932
The elements of the science of nutrition. Philadelphia, *W. B. Saunders,*
1906.
     A classic exposition of respiratory and intermediary metabolism.
Fourth edition, 1928. Reprint of Lusk's personal annotated copy of the
fourth edition, with biography and bibliography of his writings, New York,
Johnson Reprint, 1976.

1046   STEPP, WILHELM OTTO. 1882-1963
        Versuche über Fütterung mit lipoidfreier Nahrung. *Biochem. Z.*, 1909, **22,**
        452-60.
            Stepp discovered that removal of fat from the diet greatly reduced its
        nutritive value but that substitution of pure fats did not make good the
        deficiency. He thus discovered the existence of fat-soluble vitamins,
        without fully realizing it. For his later papers, see the same journal, 1911,
        57, 135; 1913, **62,** 405.

1047   FUNK, CASIMIR. 1884-1967
        On the chemical nature of the substance which cures polyneuritis in birds
        induced by a diet of polished rice. *J. Physiol., (Lond.)*, 1911-12, **43,** 395-
        400.
            One of the earliest attempts to isolate what later became known as
        vitamin B$_1$. *See* No. 1051.

1048   HOPKINS, *Sir* FREDERICK GOWLAND. 1861-1947
        Feeding experiments illustrating the importance of accessory factors in
        normal dietaries. *J. Physiol. (Lond.)*, 1912, **44,** 425-60.
            Hopkins shared the Nobel Prize in Physiology with Eijkman in 1929 for
        his discovery of the growth-stimulating vitamins.

1049   McCOLLUM, ELMER VERNER. 1879-1967, & DAVIS, MARGUERITE. 1887-
        The necessity of certain lipids in the diet during growth. *J. biol. Chem.*,
        1913, **15,** 167-75.
            Discovery of "fat-soluble A" (vitamin A). *See also J. biol. Chem.*, 1915,
        23, 181-246, in which the same authors showed the necessity in diet for at
        least two factors – "fat-soluble A" and "water-soluble B".

1050   OSBORNE, THOMAS BURR. 1859-1929, & MENDEL, LAFAYETTE BENEDICT. 1872-
        1935
        The relation of growth to the chemical constituents of the diet. *J. biol. Chem.*,
        1913, **15,** 311-26.
            Like McCollum and Davis, Osborne and Mendel showed the necessity
        in diet of a factor which was later to be known as vitamin A.

1051   FUNK, CASIMIR. 1884-1967
        Die Vitamine. Wiesbaden, *J. F. Bergmann*, 1914.
            A pioneer work in the study of vitamins. Much of the previous literature
        is reviewed. Funk introduced the term "vitamine", later changed to "vita-
        min". In 1912 (*J. State Med.*, **20,** 341) he postulated his theory of the
        existence of unknown but essential factors in diet. *See* No. 1047.

1052   McCOLLUM, ELMER VERNER. 1879-1967
        The newer knowledge of nutrition. New York, *Macmillan Co.*, 1918.

1053   DRUMMOND, *Sir* JACK CECIL. 1891-1952
        Note on the role of the antiscorbutic factor in nutrition. *Biochem. J.*, 1919,
        13, 77-80.
            In 1920 Drummond suggested the term "vitamin".

1054   STEENBOCK, HARRY. 1886-1967, *et al.*
Fat-soluble vitamine. VII. The fat-soluble vitamine and yellow pigmentation in animal fats with some observations on its stability to saponification. *J. biol. Chem.,* 1921, **47,** 89-109.
Separation of vitamin A from vitamin D. With M. Sell and M. Van R. Buell.

1054.1   McCOLLUM, ELMER VERNER. 1879-1967, *et al.*
Studies on experimental rickets. XXI. An experimental demonstration of the existence of a vitamin which promotes calcium deposition. *J. biol. Chem.,* 1922, **53,** 293-312.
Discovery of vitamin D. with N. Simmonds, J. E. Becker, and P. G. Shipley.

1055   EVANS, HERBERT MCLEAN. 1882-1971, & BISHOP, KATHARINE SCOTT. 1889-1976
On the existence of a hitherto unrecognized dietary factor essential for reproduction. *Science,* 1922, **56,** 650-51.
Discovery of vitamin E. See also their later paper in *J. Amer. med. Ass.,* 1923, **81,** 889-92.

1056   STEENBOCK, HARRY. 1886-1967, *et al.*
Fat-soluble vitamin. XXVI. Antirachitic property of milk and its increase by direct irradiation and by irradiation of the animal. *J. biol. Chem.,* 1925, **66,** 441-49.
Demonstration that the therapeutic properties of ultra-violet light could be effectively stored in foods and later released after consumption. With E. B. Hart, C. A. Hoppert, and A. Black.

1057   GOLDBERGER, JOSEPH. 1874-1929, *et al.*
A further study of butter, fresh beef, and yeast as pellagra preventives, with consideration of the relation of factor P-P of pellagra (and black tongue of dogs) to vitamin B. *U.S. publ. Hlth Rep.,* 1926, **41,** 297-318.
Anti-pellagra vitamin (B_2, riboflavine). With G. A. Wheeler, R. D. Lillie, and L. M. Rogers.

1058   JANSEN, BAREND COENRAAD PETRUS. 1884-1962, & DONATH, WILLIAM FREDERICK. 1889-1957
Antineuritisch Vitamine. *Chem. Weekbl.,* 1926, **23,** 201-03.
Isolation of vitamin B_1 (aneurine) in crystalline form.

1058.1   ROSENHEIM, OTTO. 1871-1955, & WEBSTER, THOMAS ARTHUR.
The anti-rachitic properties of irradiated sterols. *Biochem. J.,* 1926, **20,** 537-44.
Proof that the irradiation of ergosterol formed vitamin D.

1059   SZENT-GYÖRGYI, ALBERT. 1893-1987
Observations on the function of peroxidase systems and the chemistry of the adrenal cortex. Description of a new carbohydrate derivative. *Biochem. J.,* 1928, **22,** 1387-1409.
Isolation of vitamin C, ascorbic acid. Szent-Györgyi was awarded a Nobel Prize in 1937 for his discoveries in connexion with the biological combustion process with special reference to vitamin C and the catalysis of fumaric acid.

1060   WILLIAMS, ROBERT RUNNELS. 1886-1965, & WATERMAN, ROBERT EDWARD. 1899-
The tripartite nature of vitamin B. *J. biol. Chem.,* 1928, **78,** 311-22.
Vitamin B$_3$.

1061   BOURDILLON, ROBERT BENEDICT. 1889-1971, *et al.*
The absorption spectrum of vitamin D. *Proc. roy. Soc. B,* 1929, **94,** 561-83.
See No. 1065. With C. Fischmann, R. G. C. Jenkins, and T. A. Webster.

1062   DAM, CARL PIETER HENRIK. 1895-1976
Cholesterinstoffwechsel in Hühnereiern und Hühnchen. *Biochem. Z.,* 1929, **215,** 475-92.
Discovery of the dietary anti-haemorrhagic factor, vitamin K. Dam shared the Nobel Prize with E. A. Doisy in 1943.

1063   BURR, GEORGE OSWALD. 1896- , & BURR, MILDRED M.
On the nature and rôle of the fatty acids essential in nutrition. *J. Biol. Chem.,* 1930, **86,** 587-621.
Demonstration of the need of the body for certain unsaturated fatty acids (vitamin F).

1064   CARTER, CYRIL WILLIAM. 1898- , *et al.*
Maintenance nutrition in the adult pigeon and its relation to torulin (vitamin B$_1$). *Biochem. J.,* 1930, **24,** 1832-51.
Discovery of vitamin B$_5$, probably identical with nicotinic acid. With H. W. Kinnersley and R. A. Peters.

1065   BOURDILLON, ROBERT BENEDICT. 1889-1971, *et al.*
The quantitative estimation of vitamin D by radiography. London, *H. M. Stationery Office,* 1931.
Medical Research Council Special Report No. 158. R. B. Bourdillon, H. M. Bruce, C. Fischmann, R. G. C. Jenkins, and T. A. Webster isolated from irradiated ergosterol a crystalline compound, calciferol, which, weight for weight, has 400,000 times the anti-rachitic value of cod liver oil. *See also* No. 1061.

1066   BROWNING, ETHEL.
The vitamins. London, *Baillière, Tindall & Cox,* 1931.

1067   ASKEW, FREDERIC ANDERTON, *et al.*
Crystalline vitamin D. *Proc. roy. Soc. B,* 1932, **109,** 488-506.
Written with R. B. Bourdillon, H. M. Bruce, R. K. Callow, J. St. L. Philpot, and T. A. Webster.

1068   REICHSTEIN, TADEUS. 1897- , *et al.*
Synthese der d- und l-Ascorbinsäure (C-Vitamin). *Helv. chim. Acta,* 1933, **16,** 1019-33.
T. Reichstein, A. Grüssner, and R. Oppenauer synthesized vitamin C.

1068.1 WILLIAMS, ROGER JOHN. 1893-1988, *et al.*
"Pantothenic acid", a growth determinant of universal biological occurrence. *J. Amer. chem. Soc.,* 1933, **55,** 2912-27.
Discovery of pantothenic acid (vitamin B$_3$). with C. M. Lyman, G. H. Goodyear, J. H. Truesdail, and D. Holaday.

1069   ELLINGER, PHILIPP. 1887-1952, & KOSCHARA, WALTER. 1904-1945
        The lyochromes: a new group of animal pigments. *Nature (Lond.)*, 1934,
        133, 553-56.
        Chemical formula of riboflavine (vitamin B$_2$).

1070   EVANS, HERBERT MCLEAN. 1882-1971, *et al.*
        Vital need of the body for certain unsaturated fatty acids. *J. biol. Chem.,*
        1934, **106,** 431-50.
        Isolation of vitamin F (linolenic acid). With S. Lepkovsky and E. A.
        Murphy.

1071   ——. The isolation from wheat-germ oil of an alcohol, α-tocopherol,
        having the properties of vitamin E. *J. biol. Chem.,* 1936, **113,** 319-32.
        Isolation of vitamin E. With O. H. Emerson and G. A. Emerson.

1071.1 KÖGL, FRITZ. 1897-1954, & TÖNNIS, BENNO.
        Über das Bios-Problem. Darstellung von krystallisiertem Biotin aus Eigelb.
        Hoppe-Seyl. Z. physiol. Chem., 1936, **242,** 43-73.
        Isolation of biotin.

1072   RUSZNYAK, STEPHAN, & SZENT-GYÖRGYI, ALBERT. 1893-1987
        Vitamin P: Flavonols as vitamins. *Nature (Lond.)*, 1936, **138,** 27.
        Discovery of vitamin P ("citrin").

1073   WILLIAMS, ROBERT RUNNELS. 1886-1965, & CLINE, JOSEPH KALMAN, 1908-
        Synthesis of vitamin B$_1$. *J. Amer. chem. Soc.,* 1936, **58,** 1504-05.
        Synthesis of aneurine.

1074   HOLMES, HARRY NICHOLLS. 1879-1958, & CORBET, RUTH E.
        A crystalline vitamin A concentration. *Science,* 1937, **85,** 103.

1075   TODD, ALEXANDER ROBERTUS, *Lord Todd of Trumpington.* 1907- , *et al.*
        Studies on vitamin E. The isolation of ß-tocopherol from wheat germ oil.
        Biochem. J., 1937, **31,** 2257-63.
        With F. Bergel and T. S. Work.

1076   KOEHN, CARL JAMES. 1910- , & ELVEHJEM, CONRAD ARNOLD. 1901-1962
        Further studies on the concentration of the antipellagra factor. *J. biol. Chem,*
        1937, **118,** 693-99.
        Chicken pellagra factor.

1077   ELVEHJEM, CONRAD ARNOLD. 1901-1962, *et al.*
        The isolation and identification of the anti-black tongue factor. *J. biol. Chem.,*
        1938, **123,** 137-49.
        Isolation of nicotinic acid, the pellagra-preventing factor. With R. J.
        Madden, F. N. Strong, and D. W. Woolley.

1078   HARRIS, LESLIE JULIUS. 1898-1973
        Vitamins and vitamin deficiencies. Vol. 1. London, *J. & A. Churchill,* 1938.

1079   KARRER, PAUL. 1889-1971, *et al.*
        α-Tocopherol. *Helv. chim. Acta,* 1938, **21,** 520-25.
        P. Karrer, H. Fritzsche, B. H. Ringier, and H. Salomon synthesized
        vitamin E (α-tocopherol).

1080   DAM, CARL PIETER HENRIK. 1895-1976, *et al.*
        Isolierung des Vitamins K in hochgereinigter Form. *Helv. chim. Acta,* 1939,
        22, 310-313.
            Isolation of vitamin K_1 from alfalfa. It was isolated independently by R.
        W. McKee and his co-workers, *J. Amer. chem. Soc.,* 1939, **61,** 1295.

1081   BINKLEY, STEPHEN BENNETT. 1910- , *et al.*
        The isolation of vitamin K_1. *J. biol. Chem.,* 1939, **130,** 219-34.
            With D. W. MacCorquodale, S. A. Thayer, and E. A. Doisy.

1082   ———. The constitution of vitamin K_2. *J. biol. Chem.,* 1940, **133,** 721-29.
            Structural formula of vitamin K_2. With R. W. McKee, S. A. Thayer, and
        E. A. Doisy. Dam and Doisy shared a Nobel Prize in 1943 for their work on
        vitamin K.

1083   FIESER, LOUIS FREDERICK. 1899-1977
        Synthesis of vitamin K_1. *J. Amer. chem. Soc.,* 1939, **61,** 3467-75.

1084   ANSBACHER, STEFAN. 1905-
        p-Aminobenzoic acid, a vitamin. *Science,* 1941, **93,** 164-65.
            Recognition of ß-amenobenzoic acid as a member of the vitamin-B
        complex.

1085   VIGNEAUD, VINCENT DU. 1901-1978, *et al.*
        A further note on the identity of vitamin H with biotin. *Science,* 1940, **92,** 609-
        10.
            Isolation of ß-biotin (formerly known as vitamin H). With D. B. Melville,
        P. György, and C. S. Rose.

1086   HOGAN, ALBERT GARLAND. 1884-1961, & PARROTT, ERNEST MILFORD. 1903-
        Anemia in chicks caused by a vitamin deficiency. *J. biol. Chem.,* 1940, **132,**
        507-17.
            Isolation of vitamin B_c (folic acid, pteroylglutamic acid). Preliminary
        communication in *J. biol. Chem.,* 1939, **128,** xlvi-xlvii.

1086.1 DRAGSTEDT, LESTER REYNOLD. 1893-1975, *et al.*
        Observations on a substance in pancreas (a fat metabolizing hormone)
        which permits survival and prevents liver changes in depancreatized dogs.
        Amer. J. Physiol., 1936, **117,** 175-81.
            Lipocaic. With J. Van Prohaska and H. P. Harms.

1087   WAWRA, CECIL Z., & WEBB, JOHN LEYDEN. 1914-1966
        The isolation of a new oxidation-reduction enzyme from lemon peel
        (vitamin P). *Science,* 1942, **96,** 302-03.
            Isolation of vitamin P (hesperidin chalcone).

1088   HARRIS, STANTON AVERY. 1902- , *et al.*
        Synthetic biotin. *Science,* 1943, **97,** 447-48.
            Synthesis of biotin. With D. E. Wolf, R. Mozingo, and K. Folkers.

1089   KÖGL, FRITZ. 1897-1954, & HAM, E.J. TEN.
        Zur Kenntnis des ß-Biotins. 34. Mitteilung über pflanzliche Wachstumstoffe.
        Hoppe-Seyl. Z. physiol. Chem., 1943, **279,** 140-52.
            Isolation of α-biotin.

1090   SHORB, MARY SHAW. 1907-
        Unidentified growth factors for *Lactobacillus lactis* in refined liver extract.
        J. biol. Chem., 1947, **169,** 455-56.
            Mary Shorb provided a method of biological assay of liver extracts that
        made possible the isolation of vitamin B_{12}.

1091   RICKES, EDWARD LAWRENCE. 1912- , *et al.*
        Crystalline vitamin B_{12}. *Science,* 1948, **107,** 396-97.
            With N. G. Brink, F. R. Koniuszy, T. R. Wood, and K. Folkers.

1092   SMITH, ERNEST LESTER. 1904-
        Presence of cobalt in the anti-pernicious anaemia factor. *Nature (Lond.),*
        1948, **162,** 144-45.
            Independently of Rickes *et al.,* Lester Smith isolated vitamin B_{12} in Britain.
        See also Nature (Lond.), 1948, **161,** 638.

History of Nutrition

1092.50 SALMONSEN, ELLA MAUD. 1885-1971
         Bibliographical survey of vitamins 1650-1930, with a section on patents by
         M. H. Wodlinger. Chicago, *M. H. Wodlinger,* 1932.

1092.51 DRUMMOND, *Sir* JACK CECIL. 1891-1952, & WILBRAHAM, ANNE, *Lady*
         Drummond. d.1952
         The Englishman's food. A history of five centuries of English diet. London,
         Jonathan Cape, (1939).
             Revised edition, 1958.

1092.52 McCOLLUM, ELMER VERNER. 1879-1967
         A history of nutrition. Boston, *Houghton Mifflin Co.,* 1957.

1092.53. BÖTTCHER, HELMUTH MAXIMILIAN. 1895-
          Das Vitaminbuch. Die Geschichte der Vitaminforschung. Köln, *Kiepenheuer*
          & Witsch, 1965.

1092.54 DARBY, WILLIAM J. *et al.*
         Food: The gift of Osiris. 2 vols. New York, *Academic Press,* 1977.
             Extensively illustrated history of nutrition in ancient Egypt. With P.
         Ghalioungui and L. Grivetti.

1093   EUSTACHI, BARTOLOMEO [EUSTACHIUS]. *circa* 1510/20-1574
        Opuscula anatomica. Venetiis, *V. Luchinus,* 1564.
            Eustachius recognized the thoracic duct in the horse and even detected
        some of its valves. His work on this structure was forgotten until Aselli's
        description of the lacteals.

1094   ASELLI, Caspare. 1581-1626
De lactibus sive lacteis venis. Mediolani, *apud Io. B. Bidellium,* 1627.
Records the discovery of the lacteal vessels. Aselli's book has also the distinction of including the first anatomical plates printed in colours (four chiaroscuro woodcuts, 16" x 10"). Reprinted Leipzig, 1968; Milan, 1972.

1095   PECQUET, Jean. 1622-1674
Experimenta nova anatomica, quibus incognitum chyli receptaculum, et ab eo per thoracem in ramos usque subclavis vasa lactea deteguntur. Parisiis, *Apud Sebastianum Cramoisy et Gabrielem Cramoisy,* 1651.
Pecquet discovered the thoracic duct in dogs and its relation to the lacteals. Using a dog that was digesting, he described the thoracic duct, its entry into the subclavian veins, and the receptaculum chyli or chyle reservoir. The chyle reservoir had been sought after since Aselli's discovery of the chyliferous vessels (lacteals) in the dog. English translation, London, 1653.

1096   BARTHOLIN, Thomas. 1616-1680
De lacteis thoracicis in homine brutisque. Hafniae, *M. Martzan,* 1652.
Contains Bartholin's discovery of the thoracic duct. English translation, 1653.

1097   ———. Vasa lymphatica. Hafniae, *Petrus Hakius,* 1653.
Bartholin disputed the claim of Rudbeck as to priority in the discovery of the intestinal lymphatics. Although anticipated in this by Rudbeck, there is no doubt that Bartholinus was the first to appreciate the significance of the lymphatic system as a whole. Facsimile edition, 1916.

1098   RUDBECK Olof. 1630-1702
Nova exercitatio anatomica, exhibens ductus hepaticos aquosos, et vasa glandularum serosa. Arosiae, *excud. E. Lauringerus,* 1653.
Rudbeck claimed to have discovered the intestinal lymphatics and their connexion with the thoracic duct in 1651, a claim disputed as to priority by Bartholin (Nos. 1096-97). This book was reproduced in facsimile in 1930. English translation in *Bull. Hist. Med.,* 1942, **11,** 304-39.

1098.1   GLISSON, Francis. 1597-1677
Anatomia hepatis ... subjiciuntur nonnulla de lymphae-ductibus nuper repertis. Londini, *typ. Du-Gardianis,* 1654.
Independently of Bartholin and Rudbeck, George Joyliffe (1621-58) observed the lymphatics. He communicated his discovery to Glisson early in 1652 and the latter included an account in the above work (Cap. xxxi). *See* No. 972.

1099   RUYSCH, Frederik. 1638-1731
Dilucidatio valvularum in vasis lymphaticis et lacteis. Hagae-Comitiae, *ex officina H. Gael,* 1665.
First description of the valves of the lymphatics, discovered by Ruysch. Facsimile reprint, Niewkoop, *De Graaf,* 1964.

1100   PEYER, Johann Conrad. 1653-1712
Exercitatio anatomico-medica de glandulis intestinorum, earumque usu et affectionibus. Scafhusae, *Onophrius et Waldkirch,* 1677.
Includes a description of "Peyer's patches", the lymphoid follicles in the small intestine which have an important rôle in typhoid. They were first

described by J. N. Pechlin (1644-1706) in his *De purgantium medicamentorum facultatibus exercitatio nova,* 1672.

1101   NUCK, ANTONJ. 1650-1692
De ductu salivali novo, saliva, ductibus oculorum aquosis, et humore oculi aqueo. Lugduni Batavorum, *P. vander Aa,* 1685.
Nuck's name has been attached to the glands and duct described by him.

1102   HEWSON, WILLIAM. 1739-1774
Experimental inquiries: Part the second. Containing a description of the lymphatic system in the human subject and in other animals. Together with observations on the lymph, and the changes which it undergoes in some diseases. London, *J. Johnson,* 1774.
Hewson gave the first complete account of the anatomical peculiarities of the lymphatics. He divided the lymphatics into two groups – superficial and deep. He described the leucocytes as derived from the lymphatic glands and thymus.

1103   CRUIKSHANK, WILLIAM CUMBERLAND. 1745-1800
The anatomy of the absorbing vessels of the human body. London, *G. Nicol,* 1786.
With Hunter and Hewson, Cruikshank laid the foundation of modern knowledge concerning the lymphatics. He was Dr. Johnson's physician and William Hunter's assistant.

1104   MASCAGNI, Paolo. 1752-1815
Vasorum lymphaticorum corporis humani historia et ichnographia. Senis, ex typ. *P. Carli,* 1787.
Mascagni, Professor of Anatomy at Siena, made several discoveries regarding the lymphatics. His beautiful atlas contained 41 engravings of the lymphatics and gained him lasting fame. He had previously published a *Prodrome,* in French, 1784; this contained only four plates.

1105   WEBER, ERNST HEINRICH. 1795-1878
Microscopische Beobachtungen über die sichtbare Fortbewegung der Lymphkörnchen in den Lymphgefässen der Froschlarven. *Arch. Anat. Physiol. wiss. Med.,* 1837, 267-72.

1106   NOLL, FRIEDRICH WILHELM.
De cursu lymphae in vasis lymphaticis. Marburgi Cattorum, *typ. Elwerti,* 1849.
Noll advanced the theory that lymph is formed by the diffusion of fluids from the blood through the vessel walls into the surrounding tissues.

1107   HIS, WILHELM. *Snr.* 1831-1904
Untersuchungen über den Bau der Lymphdrüsen. Leipzig, *W. Engelmann,* 1861.
Histology of the lymphatics. His himself drew the illustrations.

1108   RECKLINGHAUSEN, FRIEDRICH DANIEL VON. 1833-1910
Die Lymphgefässe und ihre Beziehung zum Bindegewebe. Berlin, *A. Hirschwald,* 1862.
"Recklinghausen's canals", the lymph canaliculi.

1109   HIS, WILHELM, *Snr.* 1831-1904
Ueber das Epithel der Lymphgefässwurzeln und über die von Recklinghausen'schen Saftcanälchen. *Z. wiss. Zool.,* 1863, **13,** 455-73.

1110   SAPPEY, MARIE PHILIBERT CONSTANT. 1810-1896
Anatomie, physiologie, pathologie des vaisseaux lymphatiques. Paris, *A. Delahaye & E. Lacrosnier,* 1874-75.
Notable for its illustrations.

1111   WALDEYER-HARTZ, HEINRICH WILHELM GOTTFRIED. 1836-1921
Ueber den lymphatischen Apparat des Pharynx. *Dtsch. med. Wschr.,* 1884, **10,** 313.
"Waldeyer's tonsillar ring", the lymphoid ring of the nasopharynx.

1112   STARLING, ERNEST HENRY. 1866-1927
The influence of mechanical factors on lymph production. *J. Physiol. (Lond.),* 1894, **16,** 224-67.

1113   SABIN, FLORENCE RENA. 1871-1953
The origin and development of the lymphatic system. Baltimore, *Johns Hopkins Press,* 1913.

1114   YOFFEY, JOSEPH MENDEL. 1902-
The quantitative study of lymphocyte production. *J. Anat. (Lond.),* 1933, **67,** 250-62; 1935-36, **70,** 507-14.

DUCTLESS GLANDS: INTERNAL SECRETION

See also 3789-3911, ENDOCRINE DISORDERS

1116   WHARTON, THOMAS. 1614-1673
Adenographia: sive, glandularum totius corporis descriptio. Londini, *typ. J. G. impens. Authoris,* 1656.
    Wharton described the duct of the submaxillary salivary gland ("Wharton's duct"). He described the thyroid more accurately than his predecessors, naming it. He also described "Wharton's jelly" of the umbilical cord (pp.243-44). Wharton explained the role of saliva in mastication and digestion, but provided erroneous explanations for the functions of the adrenals and thyroid. *Adenographia* gave the first thorough account of the glands of the human body, which Wharton classified as excretory, reductive, and nutrient. He differentiated the viscera from the glands and explained their relationship. Wharton was one of the few physicians to remain in London during the plague of 1666.

1117   BORDEU, THÉOPHILE DE. 1772-1776
Recherches sur les maladies chroniques. VI. Anlayse médicinale du sang. Paris, 1775.
    De Bordeu first conceived the idea of internal secretion by his hypothesis that every organ, tissue, and cell discharges into the blood products which influence other parts of the body.

1118   LEGALLOIS, JULIEN JEAN CÉSAR. 1770-1814
Le sang, est-il identique dans tous les vaisseaux qu'il parcourt? Paris, *l'Auteur,* An X [1801].

Like de Bordeu, and more definitely, Legallois anticipated the conception of internal secretions. He surmised from the identity in composition of all varieties of arterial blood and the diversity of venous blood in different parts of the body, that this diversity is acquired, in each case from the loss of some substance from the organ from which the vein proceeds.

1119   COOPER, *Sir* ASTLEY PASTON, *Bart.* 1768-1841
The anatomy of the thymus gland. London, *Longman,* 1832.
Cooper, the most popular surgeon in London during the early part of the 19th century, was connected with both Guy's and St. Thomas's Hospitals. Among his best works is his description of the thymus; he described the "reservoir" of the thymus as lined by smooth mucous membrane and running spirally, not straight, through the gland.

1120   HEIDENHAIN, RUDOLF PETER HEINRICH. 1834-1897
Ueber secretorische und trophische Drüsennerven. *Pflüg. Arch. ges. Physiol.,* 1878, **17,** 1-67.
Investigation of the secretory and trophic nerves of glands. Heidenhain considered all secretory phenomena to be intracellular, rather than mechanical, processes.

1121   BAYLISS, *Sir* WILLIAM MADDOCK. 1860-1924, & STARLING, ERNEST HENRY. 1866-1927
The chemical regulation of the secretory process. *Proc. roy. Soc. B,* 1904, **73,** 310-22.
Bayliss and Starling developed the theory of hormonal control of internal secretion.

1122   STARLING, ERNEST HENRY. 1866-1927
The Croonian Lectures on the chemical correlation of the functions of the body. *Lancet,* 1905, **2,** 339-41, 423-25, 501-03, 579-83.
Starling constructed a general scheme of the "hormones" as he named the internal secretions. This is the first appearance of the word, which was suggested by W. B. Hardy.

1123   BIEDL, ARTUR. 1869-1933
Innere Sekretion. Berlin, Wien, *Urban & Schwarzenburg,* 1910.
Biedl showed that the adrenal cortex is essential for life. His book (4th ed., 1922) includes an exhaustive bibliography. An English translation appeared in 1912.

1124   CANNON, WALTER BRADFORD. 1871-1945
Bodily changes in pain, hunger, fear, and rage. New York, *D. Appleton,* 1915.
Observation of the effect of strong emotions on gastrointestinal motility (No. 1029) led Cannon to examination of the sympathetic nervous system and its emergency function. Cannon showed the close connexion between the endocrine glands and the emotions.

1125   TRENDELENBURG, PAUL. 1884-1931
Die Hormone; ihre Physiologie und Pharmakilogie. 2 vols., Berlin, *J. Springer,* 1929-1934.

Thyroid: Parathyroids

1126   KING, THOMAS WILKINSON. 1809-1847
Observations on the thyroid gland, with notes on the same subject by Sir Astley Cooper. *Guy's Hosp. Rep.*, 1836, **1**, 429-56.

King, sometimes referred to as the "father of endocrinology", anticipated the endocrine action of the thyroid.

1126.1   OWEN, *Sir* RICHARD. 1804-1892
On the anatomy of the Indian rhinoceros (Rh. unicornis *L.*). *Trans. Zool. Soc. Lond.*, 1852, **4**, 31-58.

Owen was the first to describe the parathyroids.

1127   SANDSTRÖM, IVAR VICTOR. 1852-1889
Om en ny körtel hos menniskan och atskilliga däggdjur. *Upsala Läkaref. Förh.*, 1880, **15**, 441-71.

Remak, Owen, and Virchow had previously noted the presence of what may have been parathyroids; the first systematic account of them was given by Sandström. An English translation of this paper appeared in *Bull. Inst. Hist. Med.*, Baltimore, 1938, **6**, 192-222; a translation was also published in book form at Baltimore, 1938.

1128   HORSLEY, *Sir* VICTOR ALEXANDER HADEN. 1857-1916
On the function of the Thyroid gland. *Proc. roy. Soc. (Lond.)*, 1884-85, **38**, 5-7; 1886, **40**, 6-9.

From his experimental work Horsley produced evidence to support the view that myxoedema, cretinism and operative cachexia strumpriva are all due to thyroid deficiency.

1129   ——. Functional nervous disorders due to loss of thyroid gland and pituitary body. *Lancet*, 1886, **1**, 5.

First successful experimental hypophysectomy; two dogs survived five and six months respectively after this operation.

1130   GLEY, EUGÈNE. 1857-1930
Sur les fonctions du corps thyroïde. *C. R. Soc. Biol. (Paris)*, 1891, **43**, 841-47.

Gley re-discovered the parathyroids and later came across Sandström's description (*see* No. 1127). Gley seems to have been the first to understand their real significance; his work showed the necessity of the parathyroids for the maintenance of life.

1131   BAUMANN, EUGEN. 1846-1896
Ueber das normale vorkommen von Jod im Thierkörper. *Hoppe-Seyl. Z. physiol. Chem.*, 1895-96, **21**, 319-30, 481-93; **22**, 1-17.

Demonstration of the presence of iodine in organic combination in the thyroid. Baumann isolated an iodine-containing compound ("Thyrojodin"). The biochemical research stimulated by this work led eventually to the discovery of thyroxine. Second paper is written with E. Roos.

1131.1   HUTCHISON, *Sir* ROBERT. 1871-1960
The chemistry of the thyroid gland and the nature of its active constituent. *J. Physiol. (Lond.)*, 1896, **20**, 474-96.

Isolation of a globulin afterwards named thyroglobulin.

1132   HUNT, REID. 1870-1948, & SEIDELL, ATHERTON. 1878-1961
Studies on thyroid. I. The relation of iodine to the physiological activity of
thyroid preparations. *Bull. Hyg. Lab. U.S. Publ. Hlth. Serv.,* No. 47, 1909.

1133   KENDALL, EDWARD CALVIN. 1886-1972
The isolation in crystalline form of the compound containing iodine, which
occurs in the thyroid; its chemical nature and physiologic activity. *J. Amer.
med. Ass.,* 1915, **64,** 2042-43; *Trans. Ass. Amer. Physicians,* 1915, **30,** 420-
49.
    Kendall isolated in crystalline form the thyroid hormone "thyroxine" on
Christmas Day, 1914.

1134   HUNT, REID. 1870-1948
The acetonitril test for thyroid and of some alterations of metabolism. *Amer
J. Physiol.,* 1923, **63,** 257-99.
    The acetonitril test was introduced by Hunt in 1905 (*J. biol. Chem.,* **1,**
33) and later modified by him. It shows the activity of thyroid preparations
to be proportional to their iodine content.

1135   HANSON, ADOLPH MELANCTHON. 1888-1959
An elementary chemical study of the parathyroid glands of cattle. *Milit. Surg.,*
1923, **52,** 280-84.
    Hanson isolated the first really potent parathyroid extract.

1136   COLLIP, JAMES BERTRAM. 1892-1965
The extraction of a parathyroid hormone which will prevent or control
parathyroid tetany and which regulates the level of blood calcium. *J. biol.
Chem.,* 1925, **63,** 395-438.
    Isolation of parathormone, the active principle of the parathyroids.

1137   HARINGTON, *Sir* CHARLES ROBERT. 1897-1972
Chemistry of thyroxine **I.** *Biochem. J.,* 1926, **20,** 293-313.
    Harington showed that thyroxine is a derivative of tyrosine, and he gave
its formula as $C_{15}H_{11}O_4NI_4$.

1138   ——. & BARGER, GEORGE. 1878-1939
Chemistry of thyroxine. III. Constitution and synthesis of thyroxine.
Biochem. J., 1927, **21,** 169-81.
    Synthesis of thyroxine.

1138.01   LOEB, LEON. 1865-1959, and BASSETT, R.B.
Effect of hormones of anterior pituitary on thyroid gland in the guinea pig.
Proc. Soc. Exp. Biol. Med., 1929, **26,** 860-62.
    Loeb and Aron (No.1138.2) demonstrated the thyroid-stimulating
hormone (TSH) in the anterior pituitary.

1138.02   ARON, MAX. 1892-1974
Action de la préhypophyse sur le thyroïde chez le cobaye. *C.R. Soc. Biol.
Fil.,* 1929, **102,** 682-684.
    Simultaneously with Loeb (No. 1138.1) Aron demonstrated the thyroid-
stimulating hormone (TSH) in the anterior pituitary.

1138.1   GROSS, JACK. 1921- , & PITT-RIVERS, ROSALIND VENETIA. 1907-1990
          3:5:3'-Triiodothyronine. I. Isolation from thyroid gland and synthesis.
          Biochem. J., 1953, **53,** 645-50.
          Discovery of the second thyroid hormone, triiodothyronine.

1138.2   COPP, DOUGLAS HAROLD. 1915-, *et al.*
          Evidence for calcitonin – a new hormone from the parathyroid that lowers
          blood calcium. *Endocrinology,* 1962, **70,** 638-49.
          With E. C. Cameron, B. A. Cheney, A. G. F. Davidson, and K. G. Henze.

Adrenals

1139   EUSTACHI, BARTOLOMEO [EUSTACHIUS]. *circa* 1510/20-1574
          Opuscula anatomica. Venetiis, *V. Luchinus,* 1564.
          Includes first description of the adrenals.

1140   BROWN-SÉQUARD, CHARLES EDOUARD. 1817-1894
          Recherches expérimentales sur la physiologie et la pathologie des capsules
          surrénales. *C. R. Acad. Sci. (Paris),* 1856, **43,** 422-25; 542-46.
          Brown-Séquard found that excision of both adrenals in animals invariably
          proved fatal, thus determining their indispensability. He also believed that
          they had an antitoxic influence upon the blood. His experimental work
          was of great importance in the development of our knowledge of the
          internal secretions.

1141   VULPIAN, EDME FÉLIX ALFRED. 1826-1887
          Note sur quelques réactions propres à la substance des capsules surrénales.
          C. R. Acad. Sci. (Paris), 1856, **43,** 663-65.
          Vulpian discovered adrenaline in the adrenal medulla.

1143   OLIVER, GEORGE. 1841-1915, & SHARPEY-SCHAFER, *Sir* EDWARD ALBERT.
          1850-1935
          The physiological effects of extracts of the suprarenal capsules. *J. Physiol.
          (Lond.),* 1895, **18,** 230-76.
          These workers demonstrated the existence of a pressor substance
          (adrenaline) in the adrenal medulla. Preliminary communications regarding
          the above appeared in the proceedings of the Physiological Society, *J.
          Physiol.,* 1894, **16,** p. i-v; 1895, **17,** p. ix-xiv.

1144   ABEL, JOHN JACOB. 1857-1938, & CRAWFORD, ALBERT CORNELIUS. 1869-1921
          On the blood-pressure-raising constituent of the suprarenal capsule. *Johns
          Hopk. Hosp. Bull.,* 1897, **8,** 151-57.
          Abel and Crawford further investigated the pressor substance of Oliver
          and Schäfer calling it "epinephrine".

1145   ABEL, JOHN JACOB. 1857-1938
          Ueber den blutdruckerregenden Bestandtheil der Nebenniere, das
          Epinephrin. *Hoppe-Seyl. Z. physiol. Chem.,* 1899, **28,** 318-62.

1146   TAKAMINE, JOKICHI. 1854-1922
          The blood-pressure-raising principle of the suprarenal glands. *Therap. Gaz.,*
          1901, **17,** 221-24; *Amer. J. Pharm.,* **73,** 523-31.
          Isolation of adrenaline.

1147   ALDRICH, Thomas Bell. 1861-
A preliminary report on the active principle of the suprarenal gland. *Amer.
J. Physiol.,* 1901, **5,** 457-61.
      Independently of Takamine, Aldrich succeeded in isolating adrenaline
in a crystalline form. He gave it the formula $C_9H_{13}NO_3$. Adrenaline was the
first hormone to be isolated.

1147.1   STOLZ, Friedrich. 1860-1936
Ueber Adrenalin und Alkylaminoacetobrenzcatechin. *Ber. dtsch. chem.
Ges.,* 1904, **37,** 4149-54.
      Synthesis of adrenaline.

1148   ROGOFF, Julius Moses. 1883-1966, & STEWART, George Neil. 1860-1930
Further studies on adrenal insufficiency in dogs. *Science,* 1927, **66,** 327.
      Cortical hormone first obtained.

1149   PFIFFNER, Joseph John. 1903-1975, & SWINGLE, Wilbur Willis. 1891-
The preparation of an active extract of the supra-renal cortex. *Anat. Rec.,*
1929, **44,** 225.
      First practical method of preparing an extract of the active agent of the
adrenal cortical hormone. It was named cortin until it was recognized that
there are several active agents in the secretion.

1150   KENDALL, Edward Calvin. 1886-1972, *et al.*
Isolation in crystalline form of the hormone essential to life from the
suprarenal cortex; its chemical nature and physiologic properties. *Proc.
Mayo Clin.,* 1934, **9,** 245-50.
      Together with H. L. Mason, B. F. McKenzie, C. S. Myers, and G. A.
Koelsche, Kendall reported the isolation in crystalline form of cortin
$(C_{20}H_{30}O_5)$.

1151   ——. A physiologic and chemical investigation of the suprarenal cortex. *J.
biol. Chem.,* 1936, **114,** lvii-lviii.
      Isolation of nine closely related steroid hormones from adrenal cortical
extracts; one of these was Compound E $(C_{21}H_{28}O_5)$ which in 1939 was
renamed cortisone. With H. L. Mason, C. S. Myers, and W. D. Allers. See also
the same journal, 1936, **114,** 613; **116,** 267.

1152   WINTERSTEINER, Osker Paul. 1898-1971, & PFIFFNER, Joseph John. 1903-
1975
Chemical studies on the adrenal cortex. II. Isolation of several physiologically inactive crystalline compounds from active extracts. III. Isolation of two new physiologically inactive compounds. *J. biol. Chem.,* 1935,
111, 599-612; 1936, **116,** 291-305.
      Isolation of Compound F, identical with Kendall's Compund E. *See* No.
1151.

1153   REICHSTEIN, Tadeus. 1897-
Über Bestandteile der Nebennieren-Rinde. VI. Trennungsmethoden sowie
Isolierung der Substanzen Fa, H, und J. *Helv. chim. Acta,* 1936, **19,** 1107-
26.
      Isolation of Compound Fa, identical with Compounds E and F. Reichstein
shared the Nobel Prize with Kendall and Hench in 1950.

1154   FREMERY, P. DE, *et al.*
Corticosteron, a crystallized compound with the biological activity of the
adrenal-cortical hormone. *Nature (Lond.)*, 1937, **139,** 26.
     Isolation of corticosterone. With E. Laqueur, T. Reichstein, R. W.
Spanhoff, and I. E. Uyldert.

1155   BERGSTRÖM, SUNE. 1916- , *et al.*
Isolation of *nor*-adrenaline from the adrenal gland. *Acta chem. scand.,*
1949, **3,** 305-6.
     With U.S. von Euler and U. Hamberg. *See also* fuller account in *Acta
physiol. scand.,* 1950, **20,** 101-8. Noradrenaline was independently isolated by B. F. Tullar, *Science,* 1950, **109,** 536-7.

1155.1   GRUNDY, HILARY M., *et al.*
Isolation of a highly active mineralocorticoid from beef adrenal extract.
Nature (Lond.), 1952, **169,** 795-96.
     Isolation of aldosterone. With S. A. Simpson and J. F. Tait.

1155.2   WOODWARD, ROBERT BURNS. 1917- , *et al.*
The total synthesis of steroids. *J. Amer. chem. Soc.,* 1952, **74,** 4223-51.
     Synthesis of cortisone. With F. Sondheimer, D. Taub, K. Heusler, and W.
M. McLamore.

Pituitary

1156   RATHKE, MARTIN HEINRICH. 1793-1860
Ueber die Entstehung der Glandula pituitaria. *Arch. Anat. Physiol. wiss.
Med.,* 1838, 482-85.
     Important description of the pituitary.

1157   VASSALE, GUILIO. 1862-1912, & SACCHI, ERCOLE.
Sulla distruzione della ghiandola pituitaria. *Riv. sper. Freniat.,* 1892, **18,** 525-
61.
     Vassale and Sacchi showed water and mineral metabolism to be
affected by hypophysectomy.

1158   PAULESCO, NICOLAS. 1869-1931
L'hypophyse du cerveau. I. Physiologie. Paris, *Vigot Frères,* 1908.
     Paulesco found that the removal of the anterior pituitary had fatal
results, while removal of the posterior lobe had negative results.

1159   DALE, *Sir* HENRY HALLETT. 1875-1968
The action of extracts of the pituitary body. *Biochem. J.,* 1909, **4,** 427-47.
     Oxytocic action of posterior pituitary injection.

1160   CROWE, SAMUEL JAMES. 1883-1955, *et al.*
Experimental hypophysectomy. *Johns Hopk. Hosp. Bull,* 1910, **21,** 127-69.
     First experimental evidence of the relationship between the pituitary
and the reproductive system. With H. W. Cushing and J. Homans.

1161   CUSHING, HARVEY WILLIAMS. 1869-1939
The functions of the pituitary body. *Amer. J. med. Sci.,* 1910, **139,** 473-84.
     See No. 3896.

1162 ASCHNER, BERNHARD. 1883-1960
Über die Funktion der Hypophyse. *Pflüg. Arch. ges. Physiol.*, 1912, **146,** 1-146.
 Aschner was able to keep his hypophysectomized dogs alive indefinitely. He found that they developed genital hypoplasia.

1162.1 GAINES, WALTER LEE. 1881-
A contribution to the physiology of lactation. *Amer. J. Physiol.*, 1915, **38,** 285-312.
 Gaines demonstrated the action of the pituitary in lactation.

1163 EVANS, HERBERT MCLEAN. 1882-1971, & LONG, JOSEPH ABRAHAM. 1879-
The effect of the anterior lobe administered intraperitoneally upon growth, maturity and oestrus cycles of the rat. *Anat. Rec.*, 1921, **21,** 62-63.
 Evans and Long discovered the growth hormone of the anterior pituitary, showing that continued injections of an anterior pituitary extract produced an acceleration in the growth-rate of laboratory animals.

1164 ABEL, JOHN JACOB. 1857-1938, & ROUILLER, CHARLES AUGUST. 1883-
Evaluation of the hormone of the infundibulum of the pituitary gland in terms of histamine, with experiments on the action of repeated injections of the hormone on the blood pressure. *J. Pharmacol.*, 1922-23, **20,** 65-84.

1165 ABEL, JOHN JACOB. 1857-1938, *et al.*
Further investigations on the oxytocic-pressor-diuretic principle of the infundibular portion of the pituitary gland. *J. Pharmacol.*, 1923-24, **22,** 289-316.
 With C. A. Rouiller and E. M. K. Geiling.

1166 SMITH, PHILIP EDWARD. 1884-1970
The induction of precocious sexual maturity by pituitary homeotransplants. *Amer. J. Physiol.*, 1927, **80,** 114-25.
 Smith was able to induce precocious sexual maturity in mice and rats by the implantation of pituitary tissue.

1167 ——, & ENGLE, EARL THERON. 1896-1957
Experimental evidence regarding the rôle of the anterior pituitary in the development and regulation of the genital system. *Amer. J. Anat.*, 1927, **40,** 159-217.
 Pituitary tissue implanted in the immature mouse was found by these writers to cause precocious sexual maturity. Thus they showed that the activity of the gonads is maintained by the anterior lobe of the pituitary.

1168 ZONDEK, BERNHARD. 1891-1966, & ASCHHEIM, SELMAR. 1878-1965
Das Hormon des Hypophysenvorderlappens. *Klin. Wschr.*, 1927, **6,** 348-52; 1928, **7,** 831-35.
 Isolation of the gonadotrophic hormone of the anterior pituitary (Prolan A & B).

1168.1 KAMM, OLIVER. 1888-1965, *et al.*
The active principles of the posterior lobe of the pituitary gland. I. The demonstration of the presence of two active principles. II. The separation of the two principles and their concentration in the form of potent solid preparations. *J. Amer. chem. Soc.*, 1928, **50,** 573-601.
 Isolation of vasopressin and oxytocin. With T. B. Aldrich, I. W. Grote, L. W. Rowe, and E. P. Bugbee.

1168.2 STRICKER, P., & GRUETER, F.
Action du lobe antérieur de l'hypophyse sur la montée laiteuse. *C. R. Soc. Biol. (Paris),* 1929, **99,** 1978-80.
Demonstration of the existence of a pituitary lactogenic hormone (prolactin).

1169 HOUSSAY, Bernardo Alberto. 1887-1971, & BIASOTTI, Alfredo. 1903-
La diabetes pancreática de los perros hipofisoprivos. *Rev. Soc. argent. Biol.,* 1930, **6,** 251-96.
Houssay's depancreatized hypophysectomized dog. This work led to Houssay's demonstration of the importance of the anterior pituitary in sugar metabolism, for which he shared the Nobel Prize in 1947. *See also Endocrinology,* 1931, **15,** 511-23.

1170 COLLIP, James Bertram. 1892-1965, *et al.*
The adrenotropic hormone of the anterior pituitary lobe. *Lancet,* 1933, **2,** 347-48.
Isolation of an impure "adrenotropic hormone" containing adrenocorticotropic principle. With E. M. Anderson and D. L. Thomson.

1171 RIDDLE, Oscar. 1877-1968, *et al.*
The preparation, identification and assay of prolactin – a hormone of the anterior pituitary. *Amer. J. Physiol.,* 1933, **105,** 191-216.
With R. W. Bates and S. W. Dykshorn.

1172 VAN DYKE, Harry Benjamin. 1895-1971
The physiology and pharmacology of the pituitary body. 2 vols. Chicago, *Univ. Press,* 1936-39.
Includes an extensive bibliography.

1173 YOUNG, *Sir* Frank George. 1908-1988
Permanent experimental diabetes produced by pituitary (anterior lobe) injections. *Lancet,* 1937, **2,** 372-74.
Anterior pituitary diabetogenic hormone.

1173.1 LI, Choh Hao. 1913- , *et al.*
Interstitial cell stimulating hormone. II. Method of preparation and some physico-chemical studies. *Endocrinology,* 1940, **27,** 803-08.
Isolation of the interstitial cell stimulating (luteinizing) hormone. With M. E. Simpson and H. M Evans.

1174 ——. Adrenocorticotropic hormone. *J. biol. Chem.,* 1943, **149,** 413-24.
Isolation of pure adrenocorticotropic hormone (ACTH) from sheep pituitary glands. With H. M. Evans and M. E. Simpson.

1175 SAYERS, George. 1914- , *et al.*
Preparation and properties of pituitary adrenocorticotropic hormone. *J. biol. Chem.,* 1943, **149,** 425-36.
Isolation of ACTH from swine pituitaries. With A. White and C. N. H. Long.

1175.1 LI, Choh Hao. 1913- , *et al.*
Isolation and properties of the anterior hypophyseal growth hormone. *J. biol. Chem.,* 1945, **159,** 353-66.

Isolation of the anterior pituitary growth hormone. With H. M. Evans and M. E. Simpson.

1175.2 ———. Isolation of pituitary follicle-stimulating hormone (FSH). *Science*, 1949, **109**, 445-46.
With M. E. Simpson and H. M. Evans.

1175.3 VIGNEAUD, VINCENT DU. 1901-1978, *et al.*
The synthesis of an octapeptide amide with the hormonal activity of oxytocin. *J. Amer. chem. Soc.*, 1953, **75**, 4879-80.
Synthesis of oxytocin. With C. Ressler, J. M. Swan, C. W. Roberts, P. G. Katsoyannis, and S. Gordon. For his work on the synthesis of oxytocin and other posterior pituitary hormones, du Vigneaud was awarded a Nobel Prize (Chemistry) in 1955.

1175.4 ———. A synthetic preparation possessing biological properties associated with arginine-vasopressin. *J. Amer. chem. Soc.*, 1954, **76**, 4751-52.
Synthesis of vasopressin. With D. T. Gish and P. G. Katsoyannis.

Gonads: Sex Hormones

1176 BERTHOLD, ARNOLD ADOLPH. 1803-1861
Transplantation der Hoden. *Arch Anat. Physiol. wiss. Med.*, 1849, 42-46.
Berthold showed that transplantation of a cock's testes to another part of the body prevented atrophy of the comb, the usual sequel to castration. He was thus the first to prove the existence of an internal secretion. English translation in *Bull. Hist. Med.*, 1944, **16**, 399-401.

1177 BROWN-SÉQUARD, CHARLES EDOUARD. 1817-1894
Expérience démontrant la puissance dynamogénique chez l'homme d'un liquide extrait de testicules d'animaux. *Arch. Physiol. norm. path.*, 1889, 5 sér., **1**, 651-58.
Brown-Séquard injected into himself a testicular extract in order to bring about rejuvenation. He reported much benefit but his advocacy of this method evoked scepticism and criticism, although it stimulated research on internal secretion, being perhaps the first employment of "male sex hormone". Further papers on this subject were published by Brown-Séquard in the same journal, 1889, 5 sér., **1**, 739-46; 1890, **2**, 201-08, 443-57, 641-48; and 1891, **3**, 747-61.

1178 POEHL, ALEKSANDR VASSILIEVIC [VON PEL]. 1858-1898
[On spermin.] *J. Russk. fis.-chim. Obsh.*, 1891, **23**, 151-55.
Isolation of spermin from the testis.

1178.1 KNAUER, EMIL., 1867-1935
Einige Versuche über Ovarientransplantation bei Kaninchen. *Zbl. Gynäk.*, 1896, **20**, 524-28.
Knauer implanted ovaries into immature or castrated animals, producing development of sexual characteristics, thus demonstrating the existence of an ovarian hormone.

1179 SOBOTTA, ROBERT HEINRICH JOHANNES. 1869-1945
Ueber die Bildung des Corpus luteum bei der Maus. *Arch. mikr. Anat.*, 1896, **47**, 261-308.

1180   LANE-CLAYPON, Janet Elizabeth. 1877-1967, & STARLING, Ernest Henry. 1866-1927
An experimental enquiry into the factors which determine the growth and activity of the mammary glands. *Proc. roy. Soc. B,* 1905-06, **77,** 505-22.

In their classic paper on the mammary gland, these workers attributed its changes during pregnancy to the foetus.

1181   HITSCHMANN, Fritz. 1870-1926, & ADLER, Ludwig. 1876-1958
Der Bau der Uterusschleimhaut des geschlechtsreifen Weibes besonderer Berücksichtigung der Menstruation. *Mschr. Geburt. Gynäk.,* 1908, **27,** 1-82.

First definite description of the cyclical changes in the endometrium, which were shown to be a normal physiological process.

1182   STOCKARD, Charles Rupert. 1879-1939, & PAPANICOLAOU, George Nicholas. 1883-1962
The existence of a typical oestrus cycle in the guinea-pig; with a study of its histological and physiological changes. *Amer. J. Anat.,* 1917, **22,** 225-83.

The vaginal smear test for oestrus; it demonstrates the histological changes occurring in the vagina during the menstrual cycle.

1183   ALLEN, Edgar. 1892-1943, & DOISY, Edward Adelbert. 1893-1986
An ovarian hormone. *J. Amer. med. Ass.,* 1923, **81,** 819-21.

Isolation of the active principle of the ovarian hormone (oestrin). More detailed account in *J. biol. Chem.,* 1924, **61,** 711-23.

1184   ——. The induction of a sexually mature condition in immature females by injection of the ovarian follicular hormone. *Amer. J. Physiol.,* 1924, **69,** 577-88.

Test for recognition of the oestrus hormone.

1185   ——. The menstrual cycle of the monkey, *Macacus rhesus:* Observations on normal animals, the effects of removal of the ovaries and the effects of injection of ovarian and placental extracts into the spayed animals. *Contr. Embryol. Carneg. Instn.,* 1927, **19,** 1-44.

This paper marks the beginning of modern knowledge of the menstrual cycle. Allen showed that uterine bleeding occurs as a withdrawal effect when oestrogen ceases to act on the endometrium.

1186   LAQUEUR, Ernst. 1880-1947, *et al.*
Über das Vorkommen weiblichen Sexualhormons (Menformon) im Harn von Männern. *Klin. Wschr.* 1927, **6,** 1859.

Discovery of the oestrogenic activity of male urine. With E. Dingemanse, P. C. Hart, and S. E. de Jongh.

1187   McGEE, Lemuel Clyde. 1904-
The effect of the injection of a lipoid fraction of bull testicle in capons. *Proc. Inst. Med. Chicago,* 1927, **6,** 242-54.

McGee prepared the first active male hormone extract from the lipoid fraction of bull testes. His paper includes a preliminary account of the capon-comb test. *See* No. 1191.

1188   CORNER, GEORGE WASHINGTON. 1889-1981, & ALLEN, WILLARD MYRON. 1904-
        Physiology of the corpus luteum. *Amer. J. Physiol,* 1929, **88,** 326-46.
        Discovery of the corpus luteum hormone, progesterone.

1189   FUNK, CASIMIR. 1884-1967, & HARROW, BENJAMIN. 1888- 1970
        The male hormone. *Proc. Soc. exp. Biol. (N.Y.),* 1929, **26,** 325-26.
        Funk and Harrow obtained crude active male hormone extracts from
        male urine.

1190   MARRIAN, GUY FREDERIC. 1904-1981
        The chemistry of oestrin. I. Preparation from urine and separation from an
        unidentified solid alcohol. *Biochem. J.,* 1929, **23,** 1090-98.
        Isolation of pregnanediol.

1191   MOORE, CARL RICHARD. 1892-1955, *et al.*
        The effects of extracts of testis in correcting the castrated condition in the
        fowl and in the mammal. *Endocrinology,* 1929, **13,** 367-74.
        C. R. Moore, T. F. Gallagher, and F. C. Koch were the first to obtain a
        potent testicular extract containing the male sex hormone, androsterone,
        later obtained in crystalline form by Butenandt. They also gave a detailed
        account of the capon-comb test for the assay of the male hormone.

1192   COLLIP, JAMES BERTRAM. 1892-1965
        The ovary-stimulating hormone of the placenta. *Canad. med. Ass. J.,* 1930,
        22, 215-19, 761-74.
        Collip's anterior-pituitary-like (A-L-P) factor.

1193   DOISY, EDWARD ADELBERT. 1893-1986, *et al.*
        The preparation of the crystalline ovarian hormone from the urine of
        pregnant women. *J. biol. Chem.,* 1930, **86,** 499-509.
        Isolation for the first time of a pure crystalline hormone (oestrone).
        Doisy shared the Nobel Prize with Dam in 1943. Written with C. D. Veler
        and S. A. Thayer. Preliminary communication in *Amer. J. Physiol.,* 1929, **90,**
        329-30.

1194   MARRIAN, GUY FREDERIC. 1904-1981
        The chemistry of oestrin. III. An improved method of preparation and the
        isolation of active crystalline material. *Biochem. J.,* 1930, **24,** 435-45.
        Crystalline oestriol obtained.

1195   BUTENANDT, ADOLF FRIEDRICH JOHANN. 1903-
        Ueber die chemische Untersuchung der Sexualhormone. *Z. angew. Chem.,*
        1931, **44,** 905-08.
        The male sex hormone, androsterone, was isolated in crystalline form
        by Butenandt. He shared the Nobel Prize for chemistry with Ruzicka (No.
        1201) in 1939.

1196   ZONDEK, BERNHARD. 1891-1966
        Die Hormone des Ovariums und des Hypophysenvorderlappens. Berlin,
        J. Springer, 1931.
        Second edition, 1935.

1197 ALLEN, EDGAR. 1892-1943
Sex and internal secretions; a survey of recent research. Baltimore, *Williams & Wilkins,* 1932.
 Second edition, 1939, with C. H. Danforth and E. A. Doisy.

1198 BROWNE, JOHN SYMONDS LYON. 1904-
Chemical and physiological properties of crystalline oestrogenic hormones. *Canad. J. Res.,* 1933, **8,** 180-97.
 Oestriol obtained from placental tissue.

1199 KAUFMANN, CARL.
Die Behandlung der Amenorrhoë mit hohen Dosen der Ovarialhormone. *Klin. Wschr.,* 1933, **12,** 1557-62.
 First use of oestrogenic hormone in ovariectomized women, with production of the typical cyclical endometrial changes.

1200 BUTENANDT, ADOLF FRIEDRICH JOHANN. 1903-
Neuere Ergebnisse auf dem Gebiet der Sexualhormone. *Wien klin. Wschr.,* 1934, **47,** 897-901, 934-36.
 Progesterone obtained in crystalline form.

1201 RUZICKA, LEOPOLD. 1887-1976, *et al.*
Über die Synthese des Testikelhormons (Androsteron) und Stereoisomerer desselben durch Abbau hydrierter Sterine. *Helv. chim. Acta,* 1934, **17,** 1395-1406.
 First complete synthesis of a sex hormone (androsterone). With M. W. Goldberg, J. Meyer, H. Brüngger, and E. Eichenberger. Ruzicka shared the 1939 Nobel Prize for Chemistry with Butenandt (No. 1195).

1201.1 DAVID, K., *et al.*
Über krystallinisches männliches Hormon aus Hoden (Testosteron), wirksamer als aus Harn oder aus Cholesterin bereitetes Androsteron. *Hoppe-Seyl. Z. physiol. Chem.,* 1935, **233,** 281-82.
 Isolation of testosterone from the testis. With E. Dingemanse, J. Freud, and E. Laqueur.

1202 MacCORQUODALE, DONALD WILLIAM. 1898- , *et al.*
The isolation of the principal estrogenic substance of liquor folliculi. *J. biol. Chem.,* 1936, **115,** 435-48.
 Isolation of oestradiol. With S. A. Thayer and E. A. Doisy.

For history, see 1588.

Pancreas

1203 LANGERHANS, PAUL. 1847-1888
Beiträge zur mikroskopischen Anatomie der Bauchspeicheldrüse. Inaugural-Dissertation. Berlin, *Gustav Lange,* 1869.
 First account of the "islands of Langerhans". Reprinted with English translation, 1937. *See also* No. 1009.

1204 MEYER, JEAN DE. 1878-1934
Action de la sécrétion interne du pancréas sur différent organes et en particulier sur la sécrétion rénale. *Arch. Fisiol.,* 1909, **7**, 96-99.
  De Meyer was apparently the first to suggest the name "insuline" for the substance then believed to be secreted by the pancreas.

1205 BANTING, *Sir* FREDERICK GRANT. 1891-1941, & BEST, CHARLES HERBERT. 1899-1978
The internal secretion of the pancreas. *J. Lab. clin. Med.,* 1921-22, **7**, 251-66.
  Isolation of insulin. The first report on the subject was made by Banting, Best and Macleod at a meeting of the American Physiological Society, Dec. 28, 1921, and published in *Amer. J. Physiol.,* 1922, **59**, 479. Charles Best's *Selected papers,* including those cited in this bibliography, were published in Toronto, 1963.

1206 ABEL, JOHN JACOB. 1857-1938
Crystalline insulin. *Proc. nat. Acad. Sci. (Wash.),* 1926, **12**, 132-36.
  Crystalline insulin first obtained. See also *J. Pharmacol.,* 1927, **31,** 65-85.

1207 RYLE, ANDREW PETER, *et al.*
The disulphide bonds of insulin. *Biochem. J.,* 1955, **60,** 541-56.
  Structure of insulin. With F. Sanger, L. F. Smith and R. Kitai. Sanger received the Nobel Prize in Chemistry in 1958 for this work; he shared the Prize in 1980 for work on the sequencing of DNA.

1207.1 KUNG, YUEH-TING, *et al.*
Total synthesis of crystalline bovine insulin. *Scientia sin.,* 1965, **14,** 1710-16.

GENITO-URINARY SYSTEM

1208 FALLOPPIO, GABRIELE [FALLOPIUS]. 1523-1562
Observationes anatomicae. Venetiis, *apud M. A. Ulmum,* 1561.
  Fallopius is best remembered for his account of the tubes named after him. In this completely unillustrated work he also left excellent descriptions of the ovaries, hymen, clitoris, and round ligaments. He gave to the vagina and the placenta their present scientific names, and definitely proved the existence of the seminal vesicles. Photographic reproduction with annotated Italian version, 2 vols., Modena, 1964.

1209 GRAAF, REGNER DE. 1641-1673
De mulierum organis generationi inservientibus. Lugduni Batavorum, *ex. off. Hackiana,* 1672.
  De Graaf demonstrated ovulation anatomically, pathologically and experimentally. In the above work he included the first account of the "Graafian follicle". Translation of Chapter XII, dealing with the ovaries, by G. W. Corner in *Essays in biology in honor of Herbert M. Evans,* Berkeley, 1943. Complete English translation of this and No. 1210 by H.D. Jocelyn and B.P. Setchell, *J. Reprod. Fertil.,* Suppl. 17, 1972.

1210 ——. De virorum organis generationi inservientibus, de clysteribus et de usu siphonis in anatomia. Lugduni Batavorum, *ex. off. Hackiana,* 1668.

Exact and detailed account of the male reproductive system. This work and No. 1209 were translated into English and published as Suppl. 17 to *J. Reprod. Fertil,* 1972. Facsimile of originals, Nieuwkoop, *De Graaf,* 1965.

1211   SWAMMERDAM, JAN. 1637-1680
Miraculum naturae, sive uteri muliebris fabrica. Lugduni Batavorum, *apud S. Mathaei,* 1672.
After de Graaf published his work on ovulation (No. 1209), Swammerdam asserted his priority in the above work, noting that his researches had been acknowledged in 1668 by van Horne.

1212   MÉRY, JEAN. 1645-1722
Observations anatomiques. *J. Sçavans,* 1684, 129.
Includes a brief description of "Cowper's glands".

1213   NUCK, ANTONJ. 1650-1692
Adenographia curiosa et uteri foeminei anatome nova. Lugduni Batavorum, *apud Jordanum Luchtmans,* 1691.
Description of the "canal of Nuck".

1214   COWPER, WILLIAM. 1666-1709
An account of two new glands and their excretory ducts, lately discovered in human bodies. *Phil. Trans.,* (1699), 1700, **21**, 364-69.
Cowper's description of the glands which bear his name. He was forestalled in their discovery by Jean Méry.

1215   LITTRE, ALEXIS. 1658-1726
Description de l'urèthre de l'homme. *Hist. Acad. roy. Sci. (Paris),* (1700), 1719, Mém., 311-16.
"Littre's glands" described.

1216   NABOTH, MARTIN. 1675-1721
De sterilitate mulierum. Leipzig, *A. Zeidler,* 1707.
The Nabothian cysts and glands of the cervix uteri first described (sect. xv).

1217   DOUGLAS, JAMES. 1675-1742
A description of the peritonaeum, and of that part of the membrana cellularis which lies on its outside. With an account of the true situation of all the abdominal viscera, in respect of these two membranes. London, *J. Roberts,* 1730.
Douglas described the peritoneum in detail; his name is perpetuated in the "pouch", "line", and "fold of Douglas". He was a friend of John Hunter and brother of John Douglas, the lithotomist.

1218   CRUIKSHANK, WILLIAM CUMBERLAND. 1745-1800
Experiments in which, on the third day after impregnation, the ova of rabbits were found in the Fallopian tubes, and on the fourth day after impregnation in the uterus itself, with the first appearances of the foetus. *Phil. Trans.,* 1797, **87,** 197-214.
Cruikshank showed that the impregnated ovum stayed in the fallopian tube for a period before implantation in the uterus.

1219   KÖLLIKER, RUDOLPH ALBERT VON. 1817-1905
        Beiträge zur Kenntniss der Geschlechtsverhältnisse und der
        Samenflüssigkeit wirbelloser Thiere. Berlin, *W. Logier,* 1841.

1220   ———. Ueber das Wesen der sogenannten Saamenthiere. *N. Notiz. a.d. Geb.*
        d. Natur- und Heilk., Weimar, 1841, **19,** 4-8.
        Demonstration of the cellular origin of spermatozoa.

1221   RETZIUS, ANDERS ADOLF. 1796-1860
        Ueber das Ligamentum pelvoprostaticum oder den Apparat, durch welchen
        die Harnblase, die Prostata und die Harnröhre an den untern Beckenöffnung
        befestigt sind. *Müller's Arch. Anat. Physiol. wiss. Med.,* 1849, 182-96.
        The "cave of Retzius" described.

1222   LEYDIG, FRANZ. 1821-1908
        Zur Anatomie der männlichen Geschlechtsorgane un Analdrüsen der
        Säugethiere. *Z. wiss. Zool.,* 1850, **2,** 1-57.
        Leydig was the first to describe the interstitial cells of the testis ("Leydig
        cells").

1223   ECKHARD, CONRAD. 1822-1915
        Untersuchungen über die Erection des Penis beim Hunde. *Beitr. Anat.*
        Physiol., 1863, **3,** 123-70.
        Important studies of the erector mechanism.

1224   SCHWEIGGER-SEIDEL, FRANZ. 1834-1871
        Ueber die Samenkörperchen und ihre Entwicklung. *Arch. mikr. Anat.,*
        1865, **1,** 309-35.
        Proof that the spermatozöon possesses a nucleus and cytoplasm.

1225   SKENE, ALEXANDER JOHNSTON CHALMERS. 1838-1900
        The anatomy and pathology of two important glands of the female urethra.
        Amer. J. Obstet., 1880, **13,** 265-70.
        "Skene's glands" or "ducts" described.

1226   MACKENRODT, ALWIN KARL. 1859-1925
        Ueber die Ursachen der normalen und pathologischen Lagen des Uterus.
        Arch. Gynäk., 1895, **48,** 393-421.
        "Mackenrodt's ligaments", the uterosacral ligaments.

1227   STIEVE, HERMANN. 1886-1952
        Die Unfruchtbarkeit als Folge unnatürlicher Lebensweise. München, *J. F.*
        Bergmann, 1926.
        Investigation of the effect of starvation and overfeeding on the gonads
        and on sexual capacity.

Kidney: Urinary Secretion

1228   EUSTACHI, BARTOLOMEO [EUSTACHIUS]. *circa* 1510/20-1574
        Opuscula anatomica. Venetiis, *V. Luchinus,* 1564.
        Several of the plates deal with the structure of the kidney.

1229   BELLINI, LORENZO. 1643-1704
Exercitatio anatomica de structura et usu renum. Florentiae, *ex typ. sub signo Stellae,* 1662.

        Classic description of the gross anatomy of the kidney. Bellini discovered the renal excretory ducts ("Bellini's ducts") and advanced a physical theory of the secretion of the urine. A translation of an extract from the 2nd ed. (1663) is in J. F. Fulton's *Selected readings in the history of physiology,* 2nd ed., 1966, pp. 350-52.

1230   MALPIGHI, MARCELLO. 1628-1694
De viscerum structura exercitatio anatomica. Bononiae, *ex typ. J. Montij,* 1666.

        Includes (pp. 71-100) his essay, *De renibus,* in which he described the uriniferous tubules and the "Malpighian bodies". The great detail and clarity of Malpighi's description was unsurpassed until Bowman (No. 1231). The work is reprinted, with translation, in *Ann. med. Hist.,* 1925, **7,** 245-63.

1231   BOWMAN, *Sir* WILLIAM. 1816-1892
On the structure and use of the Malpighian bodies of the kidney with observations on the circulation through that gland. *Phil. Trans.,* 1842, **132,** 57-80.

        "Bowman's capsule". Bowman provided convincing evidence that the glomerular corpuscle is continuous with the renal tubule and gave the first adequate description of the vascular supply of the nephron. He described the afferent and efferent arterioles as they enter and emerge from the capsule which now bears his name. In the same paper he stated his theory of renal secretion. Bowman's work became the basis for all future studies on the physiology of the kidney. Reprinted in *Med. Classics,* 1940, **5,** 258-91.

1232   LUDWIG, CARL FRIEDRICH WILHELM. 1816-1895
Beiträge zur Lehre vom Mechanismus der Harnsecretion. Marburg, *N. G. Elwert,* 1843.

        Ludwig wrote a classic monograph on renal secretion. He theorized that under the hydrostatic pressure of the blood in the capillaries of the glomerulus, protein and cell-free fluid is separated from the blood by a simple physical process of filtration. This theory contradicted Bowman's contention that the glomerulus secretes fluid. See also Ludwig's dissertation, from which the above work is expanded: De viribus physicis secretionem urinae adjuvantibus. Marburg, *Elwert,* 1842.

1233   ISAACS, CHARLES EDWARD. 1811-1860
Researches into the structure and physiology of the kidney. *Trans. N.Y. Acad. Med.,* 1857, **1,** 377-435.

1234   ——. On the function of the Malpighian bodies of the kidney. *Trans. N.Y. Acad. Med.,* 1857, **1,** 437-56.

        Isaacs confirmed and corrected the findings of Bowman; he introduced dye experiments in the study of the kidney, from which he drew the important conclusion that the Malpighian bodies are the most important agency in the secretion of urine.

1234.1   BERNARD, CLAUDE. 1813-1878
Leçons sur les propriétés physiologiques et les altérations pathologiques des liquides de l'organisme. Paris, *J.B. Baillière*, 1859.

     Bernard was the first to describe an effect of the renal nerves on urine flow.

1235   HEIDENHAIN, RUDOLF PETER HEINRICH. 1834-1897
Versuche über den Vorgang der Harnabsonderung. *Pflüg. Arch. ges. Physiol.*, 1874, **9,** 1-27.

     Heidenhain's "secretion" theory of renal function.

1236   TIGERSTEDT, ROBERT ADOLF ARMAND. 1853-1923, & BERGMAN, PER GUSTAF. 1874-1955
Niere und Kreislauf. *Skand. Arch. Physiol.*, 1898, **8,** 223-71.

     Discovery that a pressor substance (renin) is produced by the kidneys and enters the circulation by the renal veins. Abridged English translation in No. 3160.1.

1236.1   MAGNUS, RUDOLF. 1873-1927, & STARLING, ERNEST HENRY. 1866-1927.
The action of pituitary extracts on the kidney. *J. physiol.*, 1901, **27,** ix-x.

     Magnus and Starling reported that pituitary extracts caused expansion of the kidney and a marked and often prolonged diuresis. This was the first indication that the neurohypophysis plays a part in the regulation of urine secretion.

1236.2   STARLING, ERNEST HENRY. 1866-1927
The fluids of the body. London, *Constable*, 1909.

     Starling put forward the idea that renal excretion of salt (and water) was conditioned by the volume of body fluids, particularly the blood volume. He suggested that the sum total of body fluids was arranged so that the blood supply to the brain was maintained at a point just equal to its need.

1237   CUSHNY, ARTHUR ROBERTSON. 1866-1926
The secretion of the urine. London, *Longmans, Green & Co.,* 1917.

     Cushny's theory of urinary secretion was similar to that of Ludwig, with some modifications. Subsequent work of Richards and his co-workers confirmed his theory.

1237.1   MARSHALL, ELI KENNERLY, JR. 1889-1966, and VICKERS, J.L.
The mechanism of the elimination of phenolsulphonephthalein by the kidney – a proof of secretion by the convoluted tubules. *Bull. Johns Hopkins Hosp.*, 1923, **34,** 1-6.

     Proof of tubular secretion in mammals.

1238   RICHARDS, ALFRED NEWTON. 1876-1966, & SCHMIDT, CARL FREDERIC. 1893-1988
A description of the glomerular circulation in the frog's kidney and observations concerning the action of adrenalin and various other substances upon it. *Amer. J. Physiol,* 1924, **71,** 178-208.

     Richards made many experiments concerning the secretion of urine. Among other things he collected and analysed the fluid from a single glomerulus; his work confirmed the theories of Ludwig and Cushny.

1239   WEARN, JOSEPH TRELOAR. 1893-1984, & RICHARDS, ALFRED NEWTON. 1876-1966
         Observations on the composition of glomerular urine with particular
         reference to the problem of reabsorption in the renal tubules. *Amer. J.
         Physiol.,* 1924, **71,** 209-27.
             Experimental proof that the initial step in urine production is the
         formation in Bowman's space of a protein-free ultrafiltrate of plasma and
         that reabsorption of certain substances must occur in the tubules since they
         were present in the filtrate but absent from the final urine. One of the most
         significant of all publications in renal physiology.

1240   STARLING, ERNEST HENRY. 1866-1927, & VERNEY, ERNEST BASIL. 1894-1967
         The secretion of urine as studied on the isolated kidney. *Proc. roy. Soc. B,*
         1924-25, **97,** 321-63.
             Demonstration that the anti-diuretic action of vasopressin is exerted
         directly on the kidney, and that tubules of the kidney reabsorb water.

1241   REHBERG, POUL BRANDT. 1895-1985
         Studies on kidney function. *Biochem. J.,* 1926, **20,** 447-82.
             First attempt to determine the glomerular filtration rate in man.

1242   HAYMAN, JOSEPH MARCHANT. 1896-
         Estimation of afferent arteriole and glomerular capillary pressures in the
         frog kidney. *Amer. J. Physiol.,* 1927, **79,** 389-409.

1243   MARSHALL, ELI KENNERLY, JR. 1889-1966
         The aglomerular kidney of the toadfish (Opsanus tau). *Bull. Johns Hopk.
         Hosp.,* Baltimore, 1929, **45,** 95-101.
             Proof that the tubules of the kidney of a vertebrate could secrete foreign
         substances.

1244   RHOADS, CORNELIUS PACKARD. 1898-1959
         A method for explantation of the kidney. *Amer. J. Physiol.,* 1934, **109,** 324-28.

1244.1   WALKER, ARTHUR M. & OLIVER, JEAN REDMAN. 1889-1976 *et al*
         Methods for the collection of fluid from single glomeruli and tubules of the
         mammalian kidney, *and* The collection and analysis of fluid from single nephrons
         of the mammalian kidney. *Am. J. Physiol.,* 1941, **134,** 562-89; 580-95.
             This was the first (and for many years) the only application of the
         Wearn-Richards procedure (No. 1239) to the mammalian kidney.

1244.2   VERNEY, ERNEST BASIL. 1894-1967
         The antidiuretic hormone and the factors which determine its release.
         Proc. Roy. Soc. B, 1947, **135,** 26-106.
             Verney elucidated the factors that determine the release of antidiuretic
         hormone, and introduced the osmoreceptor concept.

1245   TRUETA, JOSEP. 1897-1977, *et al.*
         Studies of the renal circulation. Oxford, *Blackwell,* 1947.
             With A. E. Barclay, P. M. Daniel, K. J. Franklin, and M. M. L. Prichard. In
         studying the anurias which follow injury, especially crushing injuries and
         burns, Trueta's team demonstrated that both the processes of filtration and
         of re-absorption are subject to nervous control, leading to the development
         of a more rational therapy for these conditions.

1246   SMITH, Homer William. 1895-1962
The kidney: structure and function in health and disease. New York, *Oxford University Press,* 1951.
An encyclopaedic presentation of kidney physiology, including the many contributions of the author.

1246.01   HARGITAY, B. and KUHN, Werner. 1899-1963
Das Multiplikationsprinzip als Grundlage der Harnkonzentrierung in der Niere. *Zeit. f. Elektrochemie,* 1951, **55**, 539-558.
A theoretical treatment of the countercurrent hypothesis accompanied by data from a working model.

1246.1   WIRZ, Heinrich. 1914- , *et al.*
Lokalisation des Konzentrierungsprozesses in der Niere durch direkte Kryoskopie. *Helv. physiol pharmacol. Acta,* 1951, **9**, 196-207.
The initial experimental evidence advanced in support of the countercurrent hypothesis. With B. Hargitay and W. Kuhn.

1246.2   GOTTSCHALK, Carl W. 1922- , & MYLLE, Margaret.
Micropuncture study of the mammalian urinary concentrating mechanism: evidence for the countercurrent hypothesis. *Am. j. physiol.*, 1959, 196, 927-36.
Proof that tubular fluid is first concentrated in the loop of Henle, then diluted in the ascending limb of the loop before its final concentration in the collecting ducts, as predicted by the countercurrent hypothesis.

NERVOUS SYSTEM

1247   ARIENS KAPPERS, Cornelius Ubbo. 1877-1946
Die vergleichende Anatomie des Nervensystems der Wirbeltiere und des Menschen. 2 vols. Haarlem, *Bohn,* 1920-21.
Ariëns Kappers was Professor of Neuroanatomy at Amsterdam. English translation, 1936, reprinted New York, *Hafner Press,* 1967.

1248   FULTON, John Farquhar. 1899-1960
Physiology of the nervous system. London, *Oxford Univ. Press,* 1938.
Includes excellent bibliography.

*Peripheral Nerves
(including Nervous Impulses)*

1249   MECKEL, Johann Friedrich, *the elder.* 1724-1774
Tractatus anatomico-physiologicus de quinto pare nervorum cerebri. Gottingae, *A. Vandenhoeck,* 1748.
Meckel's graduation thesis, a classic description of the sphenopalatine (Meckel's) ganglion and the dural space lodging the Gasserian ganglion ("Meckel's cave").

1250   JOHNSTONE, James. 1730-1802
Essay on the use of the ganglions of the nerves. *Phil. Trans.,* (1764), 1765, **54,** 177-84.
See also his supplementary papers on the subject, in *Phil. Trans.,* (1767), 1768, **57,** 118-31; (1770), 1771, **60,** 30-35. Revised edition in book form, Shrewsbury, 1771.

1251   HIRSCH, ANTON BALTHASAR RAYMUND.
        Pars quinti nervorum encephali disquisitio anatomica. Vienna, [n.p.], 1765.
        The "Gasserian ganglion", already described by Santorini and others,
        was named after Johann Ludwig Gasser (*fl.* 1757-65), Professor of Anatomy
        at Vienna, by his pupil Hirsch. Also published in Ludwig, C. F., *Scriptores,*
        1791, vol. 1, pp. 244-62.

1252   WRISBERG, HEINRICH AUGUST. 1739-1808
        Observationes anatomicae de quinto pare nervorum encephali. Gottingae,
        J. C. Dieterich, 1777.
        Wrisberg, Professor of Anatomy at Göttingen, is remembered for his
        discovery of the nervus intermedius ("nerve of Wrisberg"), described in the
        above treatise.

1253   SCARPA, ANTONIO. 1752-1832
        Tabulae nevrologicae, ad illustrandum historiam anatomicam cardiacorum
        nervorum, noni nervorum cerebri, glossopharyngaei et pharyngaei ex
        octavo cerebri. Ticini, *apud B. Comini,* 1794.
        This elegantly illustrated anatomical atlas, is regarded as Scarpa's
        greatest work. The result of 20 years of research, it includes the first proper
        delineation of the glossopharyngeal, vagus, hypoglossal, and cardiac
        nerves, and the first demonstration of cardiac innervation. Scarpa was a
        skilful draughtsman. He personally trained Faustino Anderloni, the artist
        who made the drawings and engraved the copperplates for his books.

1254   BELL, *Sir* CHARLES. 1774-1842
        Idea of a new anatomy of the brain. London, *Strahan & Preston,* [1811].
        Contains first reference to experimental work on the motor functions of
        the ventral spinal nerve-roots, without, however, establishing the sensory
        functions of the dorsal roots. This very rare privately printed pamphlet is
        reproduced in *Med. Classics,* 1936, **1,** 105-20. Facsimile reprint, Lon-
        don, 1966. Bell's own annotated copy, preserved in the library of The Royal
        Society, is reproduced in Cranefield, *The way in and the way out: François
        Magendie, Charles Bell and the roots of the spinal nerves,* Mt. Kisco, N.Y.,
        Futura Publishing, 1974. *See* No. 1588.9. Cranefield proves that Magendie
        (No. 1256) discovered the "Bell-Magendie law".

1255   ——. On the nerves; giving an account of some experiments on their
        structure and functions, which lead to new arrangement of the system.
        Phil. Trans., 1821, **111,** 398-424.
        "Bell's nerve", the long thoracic, described.

1256   MAGENDIE, FRANÇOIS. 1783-1855
        Expériences sur les fonctions des racines des nerfs rachidiens. *J. Physiol.
        exp. path.,* 1822, **2,** 276-79.
        Magendie definitely discovered that the anterior root is motor and that
        the dorsal root is sensory, although Romberg, Flourens, Sherrington, and
        others credited the discovery to Charles Bell. In this paper Magendie
        announced that "section of the dorsal root abolishes sensation, section of
        ventral roots abolishes motor activity, and section of both roots abolishes
        both sensation and motor activity" (Cranefield, No. 1588.9.). This discov-
        ery has been called "the most momentous *single* discovery in physiology
        after Harvey". This work was confirmed by Müller in 1831 (No. 1259). For

a translation of the paper, see J. F. Fulton's *Selected readings in the history of physiology,* 2nd ed., 1966, pp. 280-85.

1256.1 ———. Expériences sur les fonctions des racines des nerfs qui naissent de la moelle épinière. *J. Physiol. exp. path.,* 1822, **2**, 366-71.

Further experiments, including, most probably, "the first use of strychnine as part of a study of the localization of function in the nervous system as well as being a very early example of the rational use of a known property of a drug as a tool in physiological investigation"(Cranefield, No. 1588.9).

1257 MÜLLER, JOHANNES. 1801-1858
Zur vergleichenden Physiologie des Gesichtssinnes des Menschen und der Thiere. Leipzig, *C. Cnobloch,* 1826.

Includes Müller's law of specific nerve energies. For an English translation, see his *Elements of physiology,* transl. W. Baly, London, 1838, vol. 1, pp. 766-67.

1258 BELL, *Sir* CHARLES. 1774-1842
The nervous system of the human body. [2nd ed.], London, *Longmans,* 1830.

Records Bell's demonstration that the fifth cranial nerve has a sensory-motor function, his discovery of "Bell's nerve" and the motor nerve of the face, lesion of which causes facial paralysis (Bell's palsy). Bell was preceded in some of these discoveries by Mayo (No. 1390). Also includes the first description of myotonia. First edition, 1824.

1259 MÜLLER, JOHANNES. 1801-1858
Bestätigung des Bell'schen Lehrsatzes, das die doppelten Wurzeln der Rückenmarksnerven verschiedene Fuctionen haben, durch neue und Entscheidende Experimente. *[Froriep's] Notiz. a. d. Geb. d. Natur- u. Heilk.,* Weimar, 1831, **30,** 113-117, 129-34.

Experimental proof of the Bell–Magendie law (*see* Nos. 1254 & 1256) of the spinal nerve roots.

1260 REMAK, ROBERT. 1815-1865
Vorläufige Mittheilungen microscopischer Beobachtungen über den innern Bau der Cerbrospinalnerven und über die Entwickelung ihrer Formelemente. *Arch. Anat. Physiol. wiss. Med.,* 1836, 145-61.

Discovery of the non-medullated nerve-fibres ("fibres of Remak"). Fuller account in his *Observationes anatomicae* (No. 1262).

1261 BURDACH, ERNST. 1801-1876
Beitrag zur mikroskopischen Anatomie der Nerven. Königsberg, *gebr. Bornträger,* 1837.

1262 REMAK, ROBERT. 1815-1865
Observationes anatomicae et microscopicae de systematis nervosi structura. Berolini, *sumtibus et formis Reimerianis,* 1838.
    See No. 1260.

1263 PACINI, FILIPPO. 1812-1883
Nuovi organi scoperti nel corpo humano. Pistoja, *tipog. Cino,* 1840.
    "Pacini's corpuscles", end organs of sensory nerves, earlier described by Vater in 1717.

1264   BERNARD, CLAUDE. 1813-1878
Recherches expérimentales sur les fonctions du nerf spinal, étudié spécialement dans ses rapports avec le pneumogastrique. *Arch. gén. Méd.,* 1844, 4 sér., **4,** 397-426; **5,** 51-93.

1265   HELMHOLTZ, HERMANN LUDWIG FERDINAND VON. 1821-1894
Vorläufiger Bericht über die Fortpflanzungsgeschwindigkeit der Nervenreizung. *Arch. Anat. Physiol. wiss. Med.,* 1850, [71]-73.

Helmholtz succeeded in measuring the velocity of the nervous impulse, by applying the knowledge and techniques of ballistics to the problem. Using a pendulum-myograph of his own invention, he measured the duration of an electric current through a galvanometer from the moment the nerve was stimulated to its interruption when the muscle contracted. A more detailed report "Messungen über deri zeitlichen Verlauf der Zukkung animalischer Muskeln und die Fortpflanzungsgeschwindigkeit der Reizung in den Nerven", appeared in the same journal volume , [276]-364, with its second part in the volume for 1852, 199-216.

1266   WALLER, AUGUSTUS VOLNEY. 1816-1870
Experiments on the section of the glossopharyngeal and hypoglossal nerves of the frog, and observations of the alterations produced thereby in the structure of their primitive fibres. *Phil. Trans.,* 1850, **140,** 423-29.

The "law of Wallerian degeneration". The experiments recorded in the above paper were the starting-point of the neuron theory. Waller showed that if glosso-pharyngeal and hypoglossal nerves are severed, the outer segment, containing the axis-cylinders cut off from the cells, undergoes degeneration, the central stump remaining intact for a long period. From this he inferred that nerve-cells nourish nerve-fibres.

1267   ——. Recherches sur la système nerveux. *C. R. Acad. Sci. (Paris).* 1851, **33,** 370-74; 606-11.

1267.1 TÜRCK, LUDWIG. 1810-1868
Ueber den Zustand der Sensibilität nach theilweiser Trennung des Rückenmarkes. *Z. k. k. Ges. Aerzte Wien,* Abt. I, 1851, **7,** 189-201.

Türck showed that degeneration in a nerve track corresponds to the direction in which it conducts nerve impulses – ascending tracks degenerate above the lesion and descending tracks below it.

1268   VIRCHOW, RUDOLF LUDWIG KARL. 1821-1902
Ueber eine im Gehirn und Rückenmark des Menschen aufgefundene Substanz mit der chemischen Reaction der Cellulose. *Virchows Arch. path. Anat.,* 1854, **6,** 135-38.
Discovery of the neuroglia.

1269   KÜHNE, WILLY. 1837-1900
Ueber die peripherischen Endorgane der motorischen Nerven. Leipzig, *W. Engelmann,* 1862.
Kühne described the neuromuscular end organ ("Kühne's spindle") and introduced the term "telolemma" for the outer covering of its sheath.

1270   ——. Die Muskelspindeln. Ein Beitrag zur Lehre von der Entwickelung der Muskeln und Nervenfasern. *Virchows Arch. path. Anat.,* 1863, **28,** 528-38.
The best early description of proprioceptive receptors in muscles.

1271 DEITERS, OTTO FRIEDRICH CARL. 1834-1863
Untersuchungen über Gehirn und Rückenmark des Menschen und der Säugethiere. Braunschweig, *F. Vieweg u. Sohn,* 1865.
 Deiters discovered glia cells. He showed that each nerve-cell possesses an axis-cylinder or nerve-fibre process. His name is perpetuated in "Deiters' cells" and "nucleus".

1271.1 BISCHOFF, ERNST PHILIPP EDUARD.
Mikroskopischische Analyse der Anastomosen der Kopfnerven. München, J. J. Lentner, 1865.
 Bischoff demonstrated conclusively that there are many interconnections between the trigeminal, facial, nervus intermedius, acoustico-vestibular complex, glosso-pharyngeal, vagus, spinal-accessory, hypoglossal and the upper three cervical nerves. English translation by E. Sachs, Jr. and E.W. Valtin, Hanover, N.H., 1977.

1272 DICKINSON, WILLIAM HOWSHIP. 1832-1913
On the changes in the nervous system which follow the amputation of limbs. *J. Anat. Physiol. (Lond.),* 1869, **3,** 88-96.
 Demonstration that the proximal end of a severed nerve eventually atrophies.

1273 BERNSTEIN, JULIUS. 1839-1917
Untersuchungen über den Erregungsvorgang im Nerven- und Muskelsysteme. Heidelberg, *C. Winter,* 1871.

1274 ——. Ueber die Ermüdung und Erholung der Nerven. *Pflüg. Arch. ges. Physiol.,* 1877, **15,** 289-327.
 After successfully tetanizing a nerve-muscle preparation, Bernstein inferred, from this and additional data, that nerve is exhausted in the process. This conflicted with the findings of Bowditch (No. 1281-82) and Vvedenskii (No. 1280).

1276 RANVIER, LOUIS ANTOINE. 1835-1922
Leçons sur l'histologie du système nerveux. 2 vols. Paris, *F. Savy,* 1878.
 Includes his description of the "nodes of Ranvier", interruptions of the medullary nerve sheaths.

1277 GOLGI, CAMILLO. 1844-1926
Sulla struttura delle fibre nervosa midollate periferiche e centrali, *Arch. Sci. med. (Torino),* 1880, **4,** 221-46.
 "Golgi cells" first described.

1278 TIGERSTEDT, ROBERT ADOLF ARMAND. 1853-1923
Studien über mechanische Nervenreizung. *Acta Soc. Scient. fenn.,* 1880, **11,** 569-660.
 Contains important work on the effects of mechanical stimulation of nerve.

1279 WALLER, AUGUSTUS DÉSIRÉ. 1856-1922, & WATTEVILLE, ARMAND DE. 1846-1925
On the influence of the galvanic current on the excitability of the motor nerves of man. *Phil. Trans.,* (1882), 1883, **173,** 961-91.

1280   VVEDENSKII, Nikolai Evgenevich [Wedenskii]. 1852-1922
Wie rasch ermüdet der Nerv? *Zbl. med. Wiss.*, 1884, **22**, 65-68.
Although Bernstein considered that nerve could be exhausted, Vvedenskii was able, in this paper, to show that such is not the case. Further proof was supplied by Bowditch (No. 1281).

1281   BOWDITCH, Henry Pickering. 1840-1911
Note on the nature of nerve-force. *J. Physiol. (Lond.)*, 1885, **6**, 133-35.

1282   ——. Ueber den Nachweis der Unermüdlichkeit des Säugethiernerven. *Arch. Anat. Physiol., Physiol. Abt.*, 1890, 505-08.
Bowditch demonstrated the indefatigability of nerve ("Bowditch's law").

1283   MARCHI, Vittorio. 1851-1908, & ALGERI, Giovanni.
Sulle degenerazioni descendenti consecutive a lesioni sperimentale in diverse zone della corteccia cerebrale. *Riv. sper. Freniat.*, 1885, **11**, 492-94, 1886, **12**, 208-52.
Marchi's stain, osmic acid, for degenerating myelin sheaths.

1284   BURDON-SANDERSON, Sir John Scott. 1828-1905
Photographic determination of the time-relations of the changes which take place in muscle during the period of so-called 'latent stimulation.' *Proc. roy. Soc. (Lond.)*, 1890, **48**, 14-19.
Measurement by means of photography, of the speed of the nervous impulse.

1286   NISSL, Franz. 1860-1919
Ueber die Veränderungen der Ganglienzellen am Fascialiskern des Kaninchens nach Ausreissung der Nerven. *Allg. Z. Psychiat.*, 1892, **48**, 197-98.

1287   RAMÓN Y CAJAL, Santiago. 1852-1934
Nuevo concepto de la histologia de los centros nerviosos. *Rev. Cienc. méd. Barcelona*, 1892, **18**, 457-76.
Ramón y Cajal, son of a struggling Aragonese doctor, lived to become one of the greatest of all histologists. He devised many staining methods for nervous tissue and did work of fundamental importance to neuro-anatomy. He shared the Nobel Prize in Physiology with Golgi in 1906. By this and later work Cajal provided evidence to support the neuron doctrine. French translation including 2 additional papers, Paris, 1894.

1288   SHERRINGTON, Sir Charles Scott. 1857-1952
Notes on the arrangement of some motor fibres in the lumbo-sacral plexus. *J. Physiol. (Lond.)*, 1892, **13**, 621-772.
Association of the lateral horn cells with the sympathetic outflow. An analysis of the distribution of the ventral nerve roots. Sherrington showed the association of the lateral horn cells with the sympathetic outflow.

1288.1   ——. Further experimental note on the correlation of antagonistic muscles. *Proc. roy. Soc. (Lond.)*, 1893, **53**, 407-20.

The first of Sherrington's papers investigating reciprocal innervation of muscles.

1289   LENHOSSEK, MIHALY. 1863-1937
Beiträge zur Histologie des Nervensystems und der Sinnesorgane. Wiesbaden, *J. F. Bergmann*, 1894.

1290   LANGLEY, JOHN NEWPORT. 1852-1925, & ANDERSON, *Sir* HUGH KERR. 1865-1928
On reflex action from sympathetic ganglia. *J. Physiol. (Lond.)*, 1894, **16,** 410-40.

1291   NISSL, FRANZ. 1860-1919
Ueber eine neue Untersuchungsmethode des Centralorgans speciell zur Feststellung der Localisation der Nervenzellen. *Neurol. Zbl.*, 1894, **13,** 507-08.
Nissl's stain.

1292   DOGIEL, ALEXANDER STANISLAVOVICH. 1852-1922
Die sensiblen Nervenendigungen im Herzen und in den Blutgefässen der Säugethiere. *Arch. mikr. Anat.*, 1898, **52,** 44-70.
"Dogiel's end-bulbs" – sensory nerve-endings.

1293   ——. Ueber den Bau der Ganglien in den Geflechten des Darmes und der Gallenblase des Menschen und der Säugethiere. *Arch. Anat. Physiol., Anat. Abt.*, 1899, 130-58.
Classification of the neurones of spinal and other ganglia.

1293.1 RAMÓN Y CAJAL, SANTIAGO. 1852-1934.
Textura del sistema nervioso del hombre y de los vertebrados. 2 vols. in 3. Madrid, *Moya*, 1899-1904.
From publication in fascicules, 1897-1904 (vol. 1 in 3 pts., vol. 2 in 4 pts.) This monumental work sets out the cytological and histological foundations of modern neurology. Ramón y Cajal's research confirmed the neuron doctrine; his classification of neurons provided a histological basis for cerebral localization. His descriptions of the cerebral cortex are still the most authoritative. Illustrated from Cajal's own drawings. Revised and enlarged French translation, 2 vols, Paris, 1909; reprinted Madrid, 1972.

1294   BAYLISS, *Sir* WILLIAM MADDOCK. 1860-1924
On the origin from the spinal cord of the vaso-dilator fibres of the hind-limb, and on the nature of these fibres. *J. Physiol. (Lond.)*, 1901, **26,** 173-209.

1295   HALLIBURTON, WILLIAM DOBINSON. 1860-1931
The Croonian Lectures on the chemical side of nervous activity. *Lancet,* 1901, **1,** 1659-60, 1741-42.

1296   BIELSCHOWSKY, MAX. 1869-1940
Die Silberimprägnation der Axencylinder. *Neurol Zbl.*, 1902, **21,** 579-84.
Bielschowsky's method of silver staining of nerve fibres. Further paper in the same journal, 1903, **22,** 997-1006.

1297   HERRING, PERCY THEODORE. 1872-1967
        The spinal origin of the cervical sympathetic nerve. *J. Physiol. (Lond.),*
        1903, **29,** 282-85.
            Section of the white rami caused retrograde degeneration of the lateral
        column cells.

1298   HEAD, *Sir* HENRY. 1861-1940, *et al.*
        The afferent nervous system from a new aspect. *Brain,* 1905, **28,** 99-115.
            This paper opened up a new field in the study of the sensory functions
        of the skin, and the theories put forward in it dominated neurological
        thought until 1940. With W. H. R. Rivers and J. Sherren.

1299   ——. & SHERREN, JAMES. 1872-1945
        The consequences of injury to the peripheral nerves in man. *Brain,* Lon-
        don, 1905, **28,** 116-38.

1300   MACALLUM, ARCHIBALD BYRON. 1858-1934, & MENTEN, MAUD LENORE. 1879-
        1960
        On the distribution of chlorides in nerve cells and fibres. *Proc. roy. Soc. B,*
        1906, **77,** 165-93.

1300.1 SHERRINGTON, *Sir* CHARLES SCOTT. 1857-1952
        On the proprio-ceptive system, especially in its reflex aspect. *Brain,* 1906,
        29, 467-82.
            Sherrington investigated and explained the proprioceptive system.

1301   DOGIEL, ALEXANDER STANISLAVOVIC. 1852-1922
        Der Bau der Spinalganglien des Menschen und der Säugetiere. Jena, *G.
        Fischer,* 1908.

1302   RIVERS, WILLIAM HALSE RIVERS. 1864-1922, & HEAD, *Sir* HENRY. 1861-1940
        A human experiment in nerve division. *Brain,* 1908, **31,** 323-450.
            Head submitted to the division of his own left radial and external
        cutaneous nerves. His subsequent study of the loss and restoration of
        sensation thus brought about, led to a reclassification of the sensory
        pathways. Head was for many years editor of the journal *Brain.*

1302.1 TASHIRO, SHIRO. 1882-1963
        Carbon dioxide production from nerve fibres when resting and when
        stimulated; a contribution to the chemical basis of irritability. *Amer. J.
        Physiol.,* 1913, **32,** 107-36.
            Tashiro showed that the production of the nervous impulse depends on
        the metabolic activity of the nerve fibre.

1303   LUCAS, KEITH. 1879-1916
        The conduction of the nervous impulse. London, *Longmans, Green & Co.,*
        1917.
            Gotch (No. 1420.1), Adrian, and Keith Lucas made important discoveries
        concerning the "all-or-nothing" responses of individual nerve fibres. Their
        work is summarized in the above monograph.

1304   HEAD, *Sir* HENRY. 1861-1940, *et al.*
        Studies in neurology. 2 vols. London, *H. Frowde, Hodder & Stoughton,*
        1920.

Reprint, with modifications and additions, of seven papers published in the journal *Brain* between 1905 and 1918 by H. Head, W. H. R. Rivers, G. Holmes, J. Sherren, H. T. Thompson, and G. Riddoch.

1305 ERLANGER, JOSEPH. 1874-1965, & GASSER, HERBERT SPENCER. 1888-1963
The compound nature of the action current of nerve as disclosed by the cathode ray oscillograph. *Amer. J. Physiol.,* 1924, **70,** 624-66.
Nobel Prize winners, 1944, for their discoveries regarding the highly differentiated functions of single nerve fibres.

1306 KATO, GENICHI. 1890-1979
The theory of decrementless conduction in narcotised region of nerve. Tokyo, *Nankodo,* 1924.
Kato made valuable investigations on nerve conduction. A second volume, *Further studies,* appeared in 1926.

1307 ADRIAN, EDGAR DOUGLAS, 1st *Baron Adrian.* 1889-1977, & ZOTTERMAN, YNGVE. 1899-
The impulses produced by sensory nerve-endings. Part 2. The response of a single end-organ. *J. Physiol. (Lond.),* 1926, **61,** 151-71.
The observations of Adrian and Zotterman on the response of single sensory end-organs to a natural stimulus led them to formulate their conception of "adaptation" of receptors to stimuli.

1308 ———. The basis of sensation. The action of the sense organs. London, *Christophers,* 1928.
Adrian shared with Sherrington the Nobel Prize in 1932 for their work on the physiology of the nervous system. Reprinted, New York, *Hafner,* 1964.

1309 MÜLLER, LUDWIG ROBERT. 1870-
Lebensnerven und Lebenstriebe. 3te. Aufl. Berlin, *J. Springer,* 1931.

1309.1 YOUNG, JOHN ZACHARY. 1907-
The structure of nerve fibres in Cephalopods and Crustacea. *Proc. roy. Soc. B,* 1936, **121,** 319-37.
Young's discovery of the giant nerve fibres of the squid *Loglio forbesi* made possible the study of the electrical phenomena of the nervous impulse in the interior as well as on the surface of a nerve fibre. It led to the work of Hodgkin and Huxley (No. 1310.1).

1310 KIRKMAN, HADLEY. 1901- , & SEVERINGHAUS, AURA EDWARD. 1894-
A review of the Golgi apparatus. *Anat. Rec.,* 1937-38, **70,** 413-31, 557-73; 1938, **71,** 79-103.

1310.1 HODGKIN, *Sir* ALAN LLOYD. 1914- , & HUXLEY, *Sir* ANDREW FIELDING. 1917-
Action potentials recorded from inside a nerve fibre. *Nature (Lond.),* 1939, **144,** 710-11.
Hodgkin and Huxley were the first to succeed in inserting electrodes into a living giant nerve fibre and to measure directly the action potential within it. They shared the Nobel Prize with Sir John Eccles in 1963 "for their discoveries concerning the ionic mechanisms involved in the excitation and inhibition in the peripheral and central portions of the nerve cell membrane".

1310.2   ECCLES, *Sir* JOHN CAREW. 1903-
The ionic mechanism of postsynaptic inhibition. *Prix Nobel in 1963,* pp. 261-83.
Eccles shared the Nobel Prize with A. L. Hodgkin and A. F. Huxley in 1963 *See* No. 1310.1.

Peripheral Autonomic Nervous System

1311   WILLIS, THOMAS. 1621-1675
Practice of physick. London, *T. Dring, C. Harper, and J. Leigh,* 1684.
In Treatise III, pp. 128-158 is to be found Willis's description of the intercostal and spinal nerves. Willis described the ganglion chain as the "intercostal nerve" and thought it came from the head. The *Practice of physick* contains translations of all his works except his *Affectionum quae dicuntur hystericae,* 1671.

1312   EUSTACHI, BARTOLOMEO [EUSTACHIUS]. *circa* 1510/20-1574
Tabulae anatomicae. Roma, *F. Gonzaga,* 1714.
Plate XVIII is a drawing of the sympathetic nervous system. Eustachius was the first to describe the ganglion chain but made the mistake of tracing the origin of the cervical portion to the brain-stem.

1313   POURFOUR DU PETIT, FRANÇOIS. 1664-1741
Mémoire dans lequel il est démontré que les nerfs intercostaux fournissent des rameaux que portent des esprits dans les yeux. *Hist. Acad. roy. Sci. (Paris), (Mém.),* 1727, 1-19.
By cutting the intercostal nerves in the neck, du Petit found that disturbances occurred in the eyes and face of the same side; this disproved earlier views of the cerebral origin of the intercostal nerves.

1314   WINSLOW, JACQUES BÉNIGNE. 1669-1760
Exposition anatomique de la structure du corps humain. Paris, *G. Desprez,* 1732.
Sect. VI deals with the nerves. Winslow designated the ganglion chain "the grand sympathetic nerve", and the smaller branches "the lesser sympathetic", terms which remain today. English translation by G. Douglas, 2 vols, 1733-34. *See* No. 394.

1315   BICHAT, MARIE FRANÇOIS XAVIER. 1771-1802
Nerfs de la vie organique. In his *Traité d'anatomie descriptive,* Paris, 1802, **3,** 319-68.
Bichat was the creator of descriptive anatomy. He introduced the terms "animal" and "vegetative" system. See Nos. 403-04.

1316   WEBER, ERNST HEINRICH. 1795-1878
Anatomia comparata nervi sympathici. Lipsiae, *C. H. Reclam,* 1817.

1317   LOBSTEIN, JEAN GEORGES CHRÉTIEN FRÉDÉRIC MARTIN. 1777-1835
De nervi sympathetici humani fabrica usu et morbis. Parisiis, *F. G. Levrault,* 1823.
Includes description of "Lobstein's ganglion", an accessory ganglion of the sympathetic nerve above the diaphragm. English translation, 1831.

1318   BIDDER, Friedrich Heinrich. 1810-1894, & VOLKMANN, Alfred Wilhelm. 1800-1877
Die Selbständigkeit des sympathischen Nervensystems durch anatomische Untersuchungen nachgewiesen. Leipzig, *Breitkopf u. Härtel,* 1842.
These writers showed the sympathetic nervous system to consist largely of small, medullated fibres originating from the sympathetic and spinal ganglia.

1319   BECK, Thomas Snow. 1814-1877
On the nerves of the uterus. *Phil. Trans.,* 1846, **136,** 213-35.
Beck showed that in man the thoracic sympathetic chain receives communications from the last cervical, thoracic, and upper 1 or 2 lumbar ganglia.

1320   BERNARD, Claude. 1813-1878
Influence du grand sympathique sur la sensibilité et sur la calorification. *C. R. Soc. Biol. (Paris),* (1851), 1852, **3,** 163-64.
Bernard discovered the existence of vasomotor nerves.

1321   ——. Expérience sur les fonctions de la portion céphalique du grand sympathique. *C. R. Soc. Biol. (Paris),* (1852), 1853, **4,** 155.

1322   BROWN-SÉQUARD, Charles Edouard. 1817-1894
Experimental researches applied to physiology and pathology. *Med. Exam.* (Phila.), 1852, **8,** 481-504.
By applying a galvanic current to the superior part of the divided sympathetic nerve and causing vascular contraction and a fall in temperature, Brown-Séquard inferred that section of the sympathetic paralysed and dilated the blood-vessels (pp. 489-90). *See also* Nos. 1325-26.

1323   BUDGE, Julius Ludwig. 1811-1884
Experimenteller Beweis, dass der Nervus sympathicus aus dem Rückenmark entspringt. *Med. Ztg.,* 1852, **21,** 161.

1324   BERNARD, Claude. 1813-1878
Recherches expérimentales sur le grand sympathique et spécialement sur l'influence que la section de ce nerf exerce sur la chaleur animal. *C. R. Soc. Biol. (Paris), (Mémoires),* (1853), 1854, **5,** 77-107.

1325   BROWN-SÉQUARD, Charles Edouard. 1817-1894
Note sur la découverte de quelques-uns des effets de la galvanisation du nerf grand sympathique au cou. *Gaz. méd. Paris,* 1854, 3 sér., **9,** 22-23.

1326   ——. Sur les résultats de la section et de la galvanisation du nerf grand sympathique au cou. *Gaz. méd. Paris,* 1854, 3 sér., **9,** 30-32.

1327   CAMPBELL, Henry Fraser. 1824-1891
Essays on the secretory and the excito-secretory system of nerves. Philadelphia, *J. B. Lippincott & Co.,* 1857.
Campbell saw in the sympathetic a nervous system related to secretion and nutrition and having intimate connexion with the sensory nerves. He coined the term "excito-secretory" to designate his theory; although this term has fallen into desuetude, the same idea was more recently advanced to explain the action of certain glands of internal secretion.

1328   HORNER, JOHANN FRIEDRICH. 1831-1886
        Ueber eine Form von Ptosis. *Klin. Mbl. Augenheilk,* 1869, **7**, 193-98.
        "Horner's syndrome", due to lesion of the cervical sympathetic. The
        same syndrome was evoked in animals by Pourfour du Petit in 1727 (*see*
        No. 1313). It is a proof that the sympathetic governs the pupillary,
        vasomotor, sudomotor, and pilomotor functions. It was also described by
        Claude Bernard, *Leçons sur la physiologie et la pathologie du système
        nerveux,* 1858, **2**, 473-74, and, less impressively, by E. S. Hare, *Lond. med.
        Gaz.,* 1838-39, **1**, 16-18.

1329   GASKELL, WALTER HOLBROOK. 1847-1914
        On the structure, distribution, and function of the nerves which innervate
        the visceral and vascular system. *J. Physiol. (Lond.),* 1886, **7**, 1-80.
        Gaskell established the origin of the preganglionic neurons (white
        rami).

1329.1 LANGLEY, JOHN NEWPORT. 1852-1925, & DICKINSON, WILLIAM LEE. 1862-1904
        On the local paralysis of peripheral ganglia, and on the connexion of
        different classes of nerve fibres with them. *Proc. roy. Soc.,* 1889, **46**, 423-
        31.
        Langley and Dickinson studied the effect of nicotine on nerve fibres and
        were able by this means to make a thorough investigation of the distribution
        of nerve fibres.

1330   BETHE, ALBRECHT. 1872-1954
        Ueber die Primitivfibrillen in den Ganglienzellen von Menschen und
        andern Wirbelthieren. *Jena Morphol. Arb.,* 1897, **7**, 95-116.

1331   GASKELL, WALTER HOLBROOK, 1847-1914
        The involuntary nervous system. Part 1. London, *Longmans, Green & Co.,*
        1916.
        This book sums up the life work of Gaskell, who laid the histological
        foundation of the modern study of the autonomic nervous system. No
        more published.

1332   LANGLEY, JOHN NEWPORT. 1852-1925
        The autonomic nervous system. Cambridge, *W. Heffer,* 1921.
        Langley divided the autonomic nervous system into (1) the
        orthosympathetic, and (2) the parasympathetic; he defined it as an efferent
        system.

1333   GAGEL, OTTO. 1899-
        Zur Histologie und Topographie der vegetativen Zentren im Rückenmark.
        Z. Anat. EntwGesch., 1928, **85**, 213-50.
        Study of the cells of origin of the white rami.

1334   KUNTZ, ALBERT. 1879-1957
        The autonomic nervous system. 2nd ed. Philadelphia, *Lea & Febiger,* 1934.

1335   WHITE, JAMES CLARKE. 1895- , *et al.*
        The autonomic nervous system. 3rd ed. New York, *Macmillan Co.,* 1952.
        With R. H. Smithwick and F. A. Simeone.

Chemical Mediation of Nervous Impulses

1336   ELLIOTT, THOMAS RENTON. 1877-1961
On the action of adrenalin. *J. Physiol. (Lond.)*, 1904, **31**, Proc. Physiol. Soc., pp. xx-xxi.
The first intimation of the chemical mediation of nerve impulses was given in Elliott's suggestion that when a sympathetic nerve impulse arrives at a smooth-muscle cell it liberates adrenaline, which acts as a chemical stimulator.

1337   HOWELL, WILLIAM HENRY. 1860-1945
Vagus inhibition of the heart in its relation to the inorganic salts of the blood. *Amer. J. Physiol.*, 1905-06, **15**, 280-94.
Howell suggested that nerve impulses act indirectly by increasing the amount of diffusible potassium compounds in the heart tissue.

1338   HUNT, REID. 1870-1948, & TAVEAU, RENÉ DE M.
On the physiological action of certain cholin derivatives and new methods for detecting cholin. *Brit. med. J.*, 1906, **2**, 1788-91.
Discovery of the remarkable hypotensive effect of acetylcholine.

1339   DIXON, WALTER ERNEST. 1871-1931, & HAMILL, PHILIP. 1883-1959
The mode of action of specific substances with special reference to secretin. *J. Physiol. (Lond.)*, 1908-09, **38**, 314-36.
These workers drew attention to the similarity between the effects of nerve stimulation and certain drugs, especially muscarine, on the heart.

1340   DALE, *Sir* HENRY HALLETT. 1875-1968
The action of certain esters and ethers of choline, and their relation to muscarine. *J. Pharmacol.*, 1914, **6**, 147-90.
Demonstration of the inhibitory action of acetylcholine on the heart. Dale shared the Nobel Prize with Loewi (No. 1343) in 1936 for their work on the chemical mediation of nervous impulses.

1341   EWINS, ARTHUR JAMES. 1882-1957
Acetylcholine, a new active principle of ergot. *Biochem. J.*, 1914, **8**, 44-49.
Isolation of acetylcholine in ergot.

1342   HUNT, REID. 1870-1948
Vasodilator reactions. *Amer. J. Physiol.*, 1918, **45**, 197-267.
Showed that tissues are more sensitive to acetylcholine after treatment with eserine (physostigmine).

1343   LOEWI, OTTO. 1873-1961
Ueber humorale Uebertragbarkeit der Herznervenwirkung. *Pflüg. Arch. ges. Physiol.*, 1921, **189**, 239-42; 1922, **193**, 201-13; 1924, **203**, 408-12; **204**, 361-67, 629-40.
Loewi's important experiments firmly established the theory of chemical intermediaries in nervous reactions. He shared the Nobel Prize for physiology with Dale in 1936.

1344   ———. & NAVRATIL, E.
Ueber humorale Uebertragbarkeit der Herznervenwirkung. *Pflüg. Arch. ges. Physiol.*, 1924, **206**, 123-40; 1926, **214**, 678-96.

Established the presence of cholinesterase and that *in vitro* eserine inhibited this esterase.

1345   DALE, *Sir* HENRY HALLETT. 1875-1968, & DUDLEY, HAROLD WARD. 1887-1935
The presence of histamine and acetylcholine in the spleen of the ox and the horse. *J. Physiol. (Lond.),* 1929, **68,** 97-123.
Isolation of acetylcholine from ox and horse spleen.

1346   CANNON, WALTER BRADFORD. 1871-1945, & BACQ, ZÉNON M.
Studies on conditions of activity in endocrine organs. xxvi. A hormone produced by sympathetic action on smooth muscle. *Amer. J. Physiol.,* 1931, **96,** 392-412.
Cannon and Bacq suggested the name "sympathin" for a substance which they considered to be liberated into the blood stream following nerve stimulation and which acted in the same manner as sympathetic impulses. *See also* No. 1350.

1347   ENGELHART, ERICH.
Der humorale Wirkungsmechanismus der Oculomotoriusreizung. *Pflüg. Arch. ges. Physiol.,* 1931, **227,** 220-34.

1348   GIBBS, OWEN STANLEY. 1898- , & SZELÖCZEY, J.
Die humorale Übertragung der Chorda tympani-Reizung. *Arch. exp. Path. Pharmak.,* 1932, **168,** 64-88.
Production of acetylcholine on stimulation of the chorda tympani nerve.

1349   BAIN, WILLIAM ALEXANDER. 1905-
The mode of action of vasodilator and vasoconstrictor nerves. *Quart. J. exp. Physiol.,* 1933, **23,** 381-89.

1350   CANNON, WALTER BRADFORD. 1871-1945, & ROSENBLUETH, ARTURO STEARNS. 1900-1970
Studies on conditions of activity in endocrine organs. xxix. Sympathin E and sympathin I. *Amer. J. Physiol.,* 1933, **104,** 557-74.
Adrenaline and sympathin were suggested to be unidentical substances, and Cannon and Rosenblueth proposed the terms "sympathin E" and "sympathin I".

1351   KIBJAKOW, A. W.
Ueber humorale Uebertragung der Erregung von einem Neuron suf das andere. *Pflüg. Arch. ges. Physiol.,* 1933, **232.** 432-43.
Kibjakow showed that some substance in a muscle perfusate is able to contract muscle during stimulation of nerve.

1352   FELDBERG, WILHELM SIEGMUND. 1900- , & GADDUM, *Sir* JOHN HENRY. 1900-1965
The chemical transmitter at synapses in a sympathetic ganglion. *J. Physiol. (Lond.),* 1934, **81,** 305-19.
These workers produced evidence that a chemical agent (acetylcholine) appears in the transfer of nerve impulses from neuron to neuron in sympathetic ganglia.

1353 BROWN, *Sir* GEORGE LINDOR. 1903-1971, *et al.*
Reactions of the normal mammalian muscle to acetylcholine and to
eserine. *J. Physiol. (Lond.),* 1936, **87,** 394-424.
With H. H. Dale and W. Feldberg.

1354 CANNON, WALTER BRADFORD. 1871-1945, & ROSENBLUETH, ARTURO STEARNS.
1900-1970
Autonomic neuro-effector systems. New York, *Macmillan Co.,* 1937.
The authors hypothesized the existence of two sympathins, one
excitatory and the other inhibitory, now known as epinephrine and
norepinephrine. *See* Nos. 1144 & 1350.

1354.1 EULER, ULF SVANTE VON. 1905-1983
A specific sympathomimetic ergone in adrenergic nerve fibres (sympathin)
and its relations to adrenaline and nor-adrenaline. *Acta physiol. scand.,*
1946, **12,** 73-97.
Noradrenaline shown to be the predominant transmitter of the effects
of sympathetic nerve impulses. Shared Nobel Prize, 1970, with Katz and
Axelrod.

1354.2 KATZ, *Sir* BERNARD. 1911-
The release of neural transmitter substances. Liverpool, *University Press,*
1969.
Katz shared the Nobel Prize in 1970 with U. S. von Euler and J. Axelrod
for his research into the nature of the processes of chemical
neurotransmission.

Spinal Cord

1354.9 BLAES, GERARD [BLASIUS]. 1626-1682
Anatome medullae spinalis, et nervorum. Amstelodami, *Apud Casparum
Commelinum,* 1666.
First separate work on the spinal cord. Blaes "illustrated the separate
origin of the anterior and posterior roots, the dorsal root ganglia and the
differentiation between the gray and white matter of the spinal cord"
(McHenry).

1355 BOHN, JOHANN. 1640-1718
Circulus anatomico-physiologicus. Lipsiae, *J. F. Gleditsch,* 1686.
Bohn experimented on the decapitated frog, declaring the reflex
phenomena to be entirely material and mechanical, the general view of the
time being that "vital spirits" were present in the nerve-fluid. Bohn showed
that the nerves do not contain a "nerve juice". (See p. 460 of the book.)

1356 POURFOUR DU PETIT, FRANÇOIS. 1644-1741
Lettres d'un médecin des hôpitaux du Roy . . . contient un nouveau système
du cerveau, *etc.,* Namur, *C. G. Albert,* 1710.
Theory of contralateral innervation.

1357   UNZER, JOHANN AUGUSTUS. 1727-1799
Erste Gründe einer Physiologie der eigentlichen thierischen Natur thierischer Körper. Leipzig, *bey Weidmanns Erben und Reich,* 1771.

        Unzer was probably the first to employ the work "reflex" in connection with sensory–motor reactions. T. Laycock translated his book into English for the Sydenham Society in 1851.

1358   BURDACH, KARL FRIEDRICH. 1776-1847
Vom Baue und Leben des Gehirns. 3 vols. Leipzig, *in der Dyk'schen Buchhandlung,* 1819-26.

        Includes description of "Burdach's column", the posterior column of the spinal cord. This work is also "an unrivalled source of historical information on macroscopical neuroanatomy" (Meyer).

1359   HALL, MARSHALL. 1790-1857
On the reflex function of the medulla oblongata and medulla spinalis. *Phil. Trans.,* 1833, **123,** 635-65.

        Marshall Hall established the difference between volitional action and unconscious reflexes. This and subsequent work of Hall gave "reflex action" (a term invented by him) a permanent place in physiology.

1360   CLARKE, JACOB AUGUSTUS LOCKHART. 1817-1880
Researches into the structure of the spinal cord. *Phil. Trans.,* 1851, **141,** 607-21.

        Clarke made important researches on the spinal cord. He described the nucleus dorsalis. He introduced the method of mounting sections with Canada balsam.

1361   GOLL, FRIEDRICH. 1829-1903
Beiträge zur feineren Anatomie des menschlichen Rückenmarks. *Denkschr. med.-chir. Ges. Kanton Zürich,* 1860, pp. 130-71.

        Includes description of "Goll's column" or "tract", the posterior column of the spinal cord.

1362   SECHENOV, IVAN MIKHAILOVICH. 1829-1905
Physiologische Studien über die Hemmungsmechanischen für die Reflexthätigkeit des Rückenmarks im Gehirne des Frosches. Berlin, *A. Hirschwald,* 1863.

        Sechenov discovered the cerebral inhibition of spinal reflexes. He was Professor of Physiology at St. Petersburg and Moscow, and the "father of Russian physiology".

1363   LOVÉN, OTTO CHRISTIAN. 1835-1904
Ueber die Erweiterung von Arterien in Folge einer Nervenerregung. *Ber. k. sachs. Ges. Wiss. Lpz.,* 1866, **18,** 85-110.

        The "Lovén reflex", vasodilatation of an organ when its afferent nerve is stimulated.

1364   GOLTZ, FRIEDRICH LEOPOLD. 1834-1902
Beiträge zur Lehre von den Functionen der Nervencentren des Frosches. Berlin, *A. Hirschwald,* 1869.

        Goltz made important observations on the decerebrate frog. He showed it to possess no volitional powers except after stimulation, no memory and no intelligence. His experiments on frogs deprived of their spinal cords showed them to have intelligence but lessened powers of co-ordination and adaptation.

1365 ———. Ueber die Functionen des Lendenmarks des Hundes. *Pflüg. Arch. ges. Physiol.,* 1874, **8,** 460-98.; *See* No. 1364.

1366 LISSAUER, HEINRICH. 1861-1891
Beitrag zur pathologischen Anatomie der Tabes dorsalis und zum Faserverlauf in menschlichen Rückenmark. *Neurol. Zbl.,* 1885, **4,** 245-46.
"Lissauer's tract", the marginal tract in the spinal cord.

1367 MITCHELL, SILAS WEIR. 1829-1914, & LEWIS, MORRIS JAMES. 1852-
Physiological studies of the knee-jerk. *Med. News (Phila.),* 1886, **48,** 169-73, 198-203.
Demonstration that the knee-jerk can be reinforced by sensory stimulation.

1368 NANSEN, FRIDTJOF. 1861-1930
The structure and combination of the histological elements of the central nervous system. *Bergens Mus. Aarsberetning,* 1886, 29-214.
Nansen, better known for his Arctic explorations, was the first to point out that the posterior root fibres divide on entering the spinal cord into ascending and descending branches.

1368.1 HIS, WILHELM, *Snr.* 1831-1904
Zur Geschichte der menschlichen Rückenmarkes und der Nervenwurzeln. *Abh. math.-phys. Cl. k. sächs. Ges Wiss. Leipzig,* (1886), 1887, **13,** 477-514.
He clearly stated the neuron theory in 1886.

1368.2 FOREL, AUGUSTE HENRI. 1848-1931
Einige hirnanatomische Betrachtungen und Ergebnisse. *Arch. Psychiat. Nervenkr.,* 1887, **18,** 162-98.
Independently of His, Forel formulated the neuron theory.

1369 WALDEYER-HARTZ, HEINRICH WILHELM GOTTFRIED. 1836-1921
Ueber einige neuere Forschungen im Gebiete der Anatomie des Centralnervensystems. *Dtsch. med. Wschr.,* 1891, **17,** 1213-18, 1244-46, 1287-89, 1331-32, 1352-56.
A statement of the neuron theory, to which Waldeyer gave the name.

1370 GOLTZ, FRIEDRICH LEOPOLD. 1834-1902
Der Hund ohne Grosshirn. *Pflüg. Arch. ges. Physiol.,* 1892, **51,** 570-614.
Goltz was able to keep dogs alive for eight months after he had performed subtotal decerebration. He found them incapable of purposive movements but able to walk with adequate co-ordination. Frontal decortication caused restlessness; from his experiments Goltz concluded that the site of integration of pseudo-affective mechanisms is subcortical.

1371 ———. & EWALD, ERNST JULIUS RICHARD. 1855-1921
Der Hund mit verkürtzen Rückenmark. *Pflüg. Arch. ges. Physiol.,* 1896, **63,** 362-400.
Goltz and Ewald succeeded in impregnating a bitch after its spinal cord had been severed.

1372   FLATAU, EDUARD. 1869-1932
Atlas des menschlichen Gehirns und des Faserverlaufes. Berlin, *Karger,*
1894.
Flatau's law—"the greater the length of the fibres in the spinal cord the
closer they are situated to the periphery".

1373   BAYLISS, *Sir* WILLIAM MADDOCK. 1860-1924
Further researches on antidromic nerve-impulses. *J. Physiol. (Lond.),* 1902,
28, 276-99.

1374   HEAD, *Sir* HENRY. 1861-1940, & THOMPSON, HAROLD THEODORE. 1878-1935
The grouping of afferent impulses within the spinal cord. *Brain,* 1906, **29,**
537-741.

1375   MONAKOW, CONSTANTIN VON. 1853-1930
Der rote Kern, die Haube und die Regio hypothalamica bei einigen
Säugetieren und beim Menschen. *Arb. hirnanat. Inst. Zürich,* 1909, **3,** 51-
267; 1910, **4,** 103-225.
"Monakow's bundle", the rubrospinal tract.

1376   HEAD, *Sir* HENRY. 1861-1940, & RIDDOCH, GEORGE. 1888-1947
The automatic bladder, excessive sweating and some other reflex condi-
tions, in gross injuries of the spinal cord. *Brain,* 1917, **40,** 188-263.
Classic studies on "spinal man". Republished in book form, 1918.

1377   RIDDOCH, GEORGE. 1888-1947
The reflex functions of the completely divided spinal cord in man,
compared with those associated with less severe lesions. *Brain,* 1917, **40,**
264-402.
Riddoch described in detail the results of complete transection of the
spinal cord in man. With Head (*see* No. 1376) he made one of the most
painstaking investigations of this subject.

1377.1 FOERSTER, OTFRID. 1873-1941
The dermatomes in man. *Brain,* 1933, **56,** 1-39.

Brain, including Medulla: Cerebrospinal Fluid

1377.2 VAROLI, COSTANZO. 1543-1575
De nervis opticis nonnulisque aliis praeter communem opinionem in
humano capite observatis. Patavii, *apud Paulum & Antonium Meiettos,*
1573.
Varoli described a new method of dissection which enabled him for the
first time to observe and describe the pons. As a result of his new method
of dissecting, Varoli was able to make some contributions to the knowledge of the course and termination of the cranial nerves and to trace the
course of the optic nerve approximately to its true termination. His name
is perpetuated in the "pons varolii". Reprinted, Brussels, 1969. *See* No. 1478.

1377.3 BARTHOLIN, CASPAR. 1575-1629
Institutiones anatomicae, novis recentiorum opinionibus & observationibus,
quarum innumerae hactenus editae non sunt, figurisque auctae ab auctoris
filio Thoma Bartholino. Lug. Batavorum, *Apud Franciscum Hackium,* 1641.

In this revision of his father's anatomical treatise, Thomas Bartholin (1616-80) included the first depiction of the fissure of Sylvius, the lateral cerebral fissure, and the only part of the surface of the cerebral hemispheres to be given a name between 1641 and the 19th century. *See* No. 1387. Sylvius (Franciscus de Le Boë, 1614-72) made his neurological observations in 1637 but did not publish until 1663. He collaborated with Bartholin on the above work, publishing in it ten illustrations of the brain after his own drawings.

1378   WILLIS, THOMAS. 1621-1675
Cerebri anatome: cui accessit nervorum descriptio et usus. Londini, *typ. J. Flesher, imp. J. Martyn & J. Allestry,* 1664.
    The most complete and accurate account of the nervous system which had hitherto appeared, and the work that coined the term, "neurology". In its preparation Willis was helped by his students Richard Lower and Thomas Millington, and its illustrations are by the architect, Sir Christopher Wren, making this one of the earliest scientific collaborations in England. Willis's classification of the cerebral nerves held the field until the time of Soemmerring. The book includes (Cap. I and plates 1, 2) the description of the "circle of Willis", and of the eleventh cranial nerve ("nerve of Willis"). Willis recognized the sympathetic system and accepted the brain as the organ of thought. English translation by S. Pordage, 1681. *The anatomy of the brain and nerves. Tercentenary edition,* ed. by W. Feindel, 2 vols, Montreal, 1965, reprints this translation with a complete annotated bibliography of the work. Wepfer (No. 2703) and others preceded Willis in giving a detailed and complete description of the "circle of Willis".

1378.1   STENSEN, NIELS. 1638-1686
Discours sur l'anatomie du cerveau. Paris, *Robert de Ninville,* 1669.
    In this remarkably prescient argument for and critique of anatomical research into brain function Stensen opposed Descartes (No. 574) arguing that it was idle to speculate about cerebral function when so little was known about the anatomical structure of the brain. Stensen proved anatomically that the pineal gland was not the seat of the soul. Latin translation, Leiden, 1671. Reprinted in Winslow (No. 394), and translated in that work. Modern English translation, Copenhagen, 1950.

1379   VIEUSSENS, RAYMOND. 1641-1715
Nevrographia universalis. Lugduni, *J. Certe,* 1684.
    Vieussens, professor at Montpellier, was the first to describe the centrum ovale correctly. The publication of the above work threw new light on the subject of the configuration and structure of the brain, spinal cord, and nerves. With numerous large folding copperplates, it is considered the best illustrated work on the nervous system published in the 17th century. Second issue, identical except dated 1685. Both issues have the words, "editio nova" on the title page.

1379.1   RIDLEY, HUMPHREY. 1653-1708
The anatomy of the brain, London, *Sam. Smith,* 1695.
    The first book on the brain in the English language, including the first account of the circular venous sinus which Ridley names, and the first English account of a pineal tumour.

1380   PACCHIONI, ANTONIO. 1665-1726
Dissertatio epistolaris ad Lucam Schroeckium de glandulis conglobatis durae meningis humanae. Romae, *Francesco Buagni*, 1705.

        Includes a description and illustration of the pacchionian bodies of the arachnoid tissue under the dura, producing by pressure slight depressions ("Pacchionian depressions"). See also Pacchioni's *De durae meningis fabrica et usu disquisito anatomica*, Romae, *D.A. Herculis*, 1701.

1380.1   HENSING, JOHANN THOMAS. 1683-1726
Cerebri examen chemicum. Giessae-Hassorum, *vid. J. R. Vulpii,* 1719.

        First account of the chemical composition of the brain. Hensing discovered the presence of phosphorus. Annotated English translation with biography and historical analysis, by D.B. Tower. New York, *Raven Press,* [1983].

1381   WHYTT, ROBERT. 1714-1766
An essay on the vital and other involuntary motions of animals. Edinburgh, *Hamilton, Balfour & Neill,* 1751.

        Whytt, famous Edinburgh neurophysiologist, was the first to prove that the response of the pupils to light is a reflex action ("Whytt's reflex"). He described this reflex at length and mentioned that its afferent pathways lie in the optic nerve and the efferent pathways in the third pair.

1382   COTUGNO, DOMENICO [COTUNNIUS]. 1736-1822
De ischiade nervosa commentarius. Neapoli, *apud Frat. Simonios,* 1764.

        Valsalva in 1692 briefly mentioned the cerebrospinal fluid, but "Cotugno was the first to describe the fluid surrounding the spinal cord and to suggest tht it was in continuity with the ventricular and cerebral subarachnoid fluids. However, his concept of the cerebral and spinal fluid, which is the beginning of its modern physiology, remained in obscurity until rediscovery by Magendie some 60 years later" (Clarke & O'Malley). For more information regarding this book and a translation of the section dealing with the cerebrospinal fluid, see the article by H. R. Viets in *Bull. Inst. Hist. Med.,* 1935, **3**, 701-38. English translation, London, 1775. *See* Nos. 4515 & 4204.2.

1382.1   MALACARNE, MICHAELE VINCENZO GIACINTO. 1744-1816
Nuova esposizione della vera struttura del cervelletto umano. Torino, *G. Briolo,* 1776.

        The first detailed account of the anatomy of the cerebellum, which introduced the terms, "tonsil", "pyramid", "lingula", and "uvula". Reprinted in his *Encefalotomia nuova universale.* 3 vols., Torino, 1780.

1382.2   SAUCEROTTE, LOUIS SEBASTIAN. 1741-1814
Mémoire sur les contre-coups dans les lésions de la tête [1768]. *Mémoires sur les subjets proposés pour le prix de l'Acad. Roy. de Chir. (Paris),* 1778, 4 (Part 1), 368-438.

        "One of the first achievements of modern brain physiology" (Neuburger). Saucerotte carried out surgical experiments on dogs which convinced him that the anterior part of the cerebrum innervated the lower limbs and the posterior the upper limbs.

1383   SOEMMERRING, SAMUEL THOMAS. 1755-1830
Dissertatio inauguralis anatomica de basi encephali et originibus nervorum cranio egredientium libri quinque. Gottingae, *apud A. Vandenhoeck vid.,* 1778.

The first accurate enumeration of the 12 cranial nerves, superseding that of Willis (No. 1378). Soemmerring is notable for his accuracy in anatomical illustration. This was his thesis. The same publisher issued an edition for commercial circulation the same year, deleting "Dissertatio inauguralis anatomica" from the title.

1384   GENNARI, FRANCISCO. 1750-1797
De peculiari structura cerebri, nonnulisque ejus morbis. Parmai, *ex. reg. typog.*, 1782.
Gennari was the first to demonstrate the laminar structure of the cerebral cortex, discovering (in 1776) the "line of Gennari" ("Gennari's stria").

1385   MONRO, ALEXANDER, *Secundus*. 1733-1817
Observations on the structure and functions of the nervous system. Edinburgh, *W. Creech*, 1783.
Monro discovered the communication between the lateral ventricles of the human brain with each other and with the third ventricle, the "foramen of Monro". Alexander *secundus* was the greatest of the three Monros.

1386   PROCHASKA, GEORG. 1749-1820
Adnotationum academicarum. Fasciculus tertius. III. De functionibus systematis nervosi. 3 pts. Pragae, *W. Gerle*, 1780-84.
Prochaska introduced the idea of a "sensorium commune" in the central nervous system, a consistent and comprehensive theory of reflex action. English translation, London, *Sydenham Society*, 1851.

1386.1   FOURCROY, ANTOINE FRANÇOIS, *Comte de*. 1755-1809
Examen chimique du cerveau de plusieurs animaux. *Ann. Chim. (Paris)*, 1793, **16**, 282-97.
Fourcroy, French physician and chemist, made important researches on the chemistry of the brain. He noted albumen (protein) as a principal constituent.

1387   REIL, JOHANN CHRISTIAN. 1759-1813
Exercitationum anatomicarum fasciculus primus. De structura nervorum [All published]. Halle, *Venalis,* 1796.
Description of the "island of Reil". This was the first part of the surface of the cerebral hemispheres to be given a name since 1641 (No. 1377.3). See also Reil's follow-up paper in *Arch. Physiol. (Halle)*, 1809, **9**, 136-46; Reil was the editor of this journal, the first periodical devoted to physiology.

1388   ROLANDO, LUIGI. 1773-1831
Saggio sopra la vera struttura del cervello dell'uomo e degl'animali e sopra le funzioni del sistema nervoso. Sassari, *Stamp. Privileg.*, 1809.
Includes description of "Rolando's substance", "tubercle", and "funiculus". Rolando described ablation experiments for brain localization similar to Flourens (No.1391). They were largely unknown until Magendie published a French translation of them in his *J. Phys. exper. path.*, 1823, **3**, 95-113, which was reprinted by Flourens in No. 1493. Rolando was correct in allocating motor activity to the cerebral hemispheres; however his views on cerebellar function were replaced by those advanced by Flourens.

1389   GALL, FRANZ JOSEPH. 1758-1828, & SPURZHEIM, JOHANN CASPAR. 1776-1832
        Anatomie et physiologie du système nerveux en général, et du cerveau en
        particulier. 4 vols. and atlas. Paris, *F. Schoell,* 1810-19.
        Introduced the theory of localization of cerebral function, although in
        a somewhat fantastic form. This pioneer attempt to map out the cerebral
        cortex according to function gave rise to the pseudo-science of phrenol-
        ogy. The work also contains some important additions to the knowledge
        of cerebral anatomy. Gall and Spurzheim ended their collaboration after
        the first 146pp. of Vol. 2. The remainder was written by Gall alone. The
        second edition was revised by Gall, and published without the plates, but
        with a collection of replies to his critics as *Sur les fonctions du cerveau et
        sur celles de chacune de ses parties.* 6 vols., Paris, *l'Auteur,* 1822-25. English
        translation of second edition, 6 vols., Boston, 1835.

1389.1 VAUQUELIN, LOUIS NICOLAS. 1763-1829
        Analyse de la matière cérébrale de l'homme et de quelques animaux. *Ann.
        Musée Hist. nat. (Paris),* 1811, **18,** 212-239.
        First complete chemical analysis of the nervous system.

1389.2 LEGALLOIS, JULIEN JEAN CESAR. 1770-1814
        Expériences sur le principe de la vie. Paris, *D'Hautel,* 1812.
        Legallois located the respiratory centre in the medulla oblongata and
        not in the spinal cord, as had been previously believed. "For the first time,
        an area of brain substance within a major subdivision of the brain and
        having a specific function had been defined accurately by experiment"
        (Clarke & Jacyna). *See* No. 928.

1390   MAYO, HERBERT. 1796-1852
        Anatomical and physiological commentaries. Numbers I & II [All published].
        London, *T. & G. Underwood,* 1822-23.
        Mayo discovered and described the functions of the Vth and VIIth
        cranial nerves on pp. 107-120 of Number I, and did much towards the
        clarification of the idea of reflex action. Reprinted, Metuchen, N.J., *Scarecrow
        Press,* 1975.

1391   FLOURENS, MARIE JEAN PIERRE. 1794-1867
        Recherches sur les propriétés et les fonctions du système nerveux dans les
        animaux vertébrés. *Arch. gén. Méd.,* 1823, **2,** 321-70.
        Flourens removed the cerebrum and cerebellum in pigeons, showing
        maintenance of reflexes with loss of cerebration in the former case and
        disturbance of equilibrium in the latter case. Thus he demonstrated that the
        cerebrum is the organ of thought and the cerebellum the organ controlling
        the co-ordination of body movements and of will-power. *See* Nos. 1388 &
        1493.

1392   MAGENDIE, FRANÇOIS. 1783-1855
        Mémoire sur un liquide qui se trouve dans le crâne et le canal vertébral de
        l'homme et des animaux mammifères. *J. Physiol. exp. path.,* 1825, **5,** 27-37;
        1827, **7,** 1-29, 66-82.
        First clear description of the cerebrospinal fluid.

1393   ROLANDO, LUIGI. 1773-1831
        Osservazioni sul cervelletto. *Mem. r. Accad. Sci. Torino,* 1825, **29,** 163-88.

Rolando was the first to investigate the functions of the cerebellum. His name is perpetuated in the "fissure of Rolando", so named by F. Leuret, *Anatomie comparée,* 1839-57, whose attention had been drawn to it previously by Rolando.

1394 ——. Della struttura degli emisferi cerebrali. *Mem. r. Accad. Sci. Torino,* 1829, **35,** 103-47.

1395 BOUILLAUD, JEAN BAPTISTE. 1796-1881
Recherches expérimentales tendant à prouver que le cervelet préside aux actes de la station et de la progression, et non à l'instinct de la propagation. · *Arch. gén. Méd.,* 1827, **15,** 64-91; 225-47.

Bouillaud identified the anterior lobes as the speech centre. Refuting Gall, he showed that the brain controls equilibration, station, and progression. Title of second paper varies. His earlier *Traité clinique et physiologique de l'encéphalite ou inflammation du cerveau,* Paris, 1825, includes some pathological and clinical studies on loss of articulate speech associated with lesions of the anterior lobes, and gives reasons for the localization of this function in the brain. *See* No. 4618.

1396 PURKYNĔ, JAN EVANGELISTA [PURKINJE]. 1787-1869
"Neueste Untersuchungen aus der Nerven-und Hirnanatomie" [title taken from first sentence of otherwise untitled article]. *Ber. Versamml. dtsch. Naturf. u. Aerzte,* Prag, 1837, (1838), **15,** 177-80.

Description of the "flask-shaped ganglionic bodies" known as "Purkinje cells". Reprinted in his *Opera Omnia,* 1939, **3,** 47-9. Also published in *Oken's Isis,* 1838, pp. 582-84.

1396.01 LEURET, FRANÇOIS. 1797-1851, & GRATIOLET, PIERRE. 1815-1865.
Anatomie comparée du système nerveux. 2 vols. and atlas. Paris, *Baillière,* 1839-57.

The first comprehensive systematic investigation of the mammalian brain. Leuret wrote vol. 1 without Gratiolet, who later became his collaborator, publishing vol. 2 and the atlas after Leuret's death.

1396.1 BAILLARGER, JULES GABRIEL FRANÇOIS. 1809-1890
Recherches sur la structure de la couche cortical des circonvolutions du cerveau. *Mém Acad. roy. Méd. (Paris),* 1840, **8,** 149-83.

Baillarger demonstrated that the cortex is made up of layers and that fibres connect the cortex with the internal white matter. English translation in von Bonin. Some papers on the cerebral cortex, Springfield, *C.C. Thomas,* 1960.

1397 MAGENDIE, FRANÇOIS. 1783-1855
Recherches physiologiques et cliniques sur le liquide céphalo-rachidien ou cérébro-spinal. 1 vol. and atlas. Paris, *Méquignon-Marvis,* 1842.
"Foramen of Magendie" described.

1398 FAIVRE, ERNEST. 1827-1879
Des granulations méningiennes. Paris, *Thèse No. 142,* 1853.
See also his paper in *Ann. Sci. nat.,* 1853, **20,** 321-33 (Zool.).

1399   BERNARD, CLAUDE. 1813-1878
        Leçons sur la physiologie et la pathologie du système nerveux. 2 vols. Paris,
        J. Baillière, 1858.

1400   BROCA, PIERRE PAUL. 1824-1880
        Remarques sur le siège de la faculté du langage articulé, suivie d'une
        observation d'aphémie (perte de la parole). *Bull. Soc. anat., Paris,* 1861,
        36, 330-57.
        Broca claimed the third left frontal convolution of the brain as the centre
        of articulate speech – a point now disputed. He was first to trephine for a
        cerebral abscess diagnosed by this theory of localization of function. He
        introduced the term "aphemia" ("motor aphasia", "Broca's aphasia").English
        translation in von Bonin. Some papers on the cerebral cortex, Springfield,
        C.C. Thomas, 1960. See No. 4619.

1401   DALTON, JOHN CALL. 1825-1889
        On the cerebellum, as the centre of co-ordination of the voluntary
        movements. *Amer. J. med. Sci.,* 1861, n.s. **41,** 83-88.

1401.1 AUBURTIN, ERNEST. ?1825-1893
        Considérations sur les localisations cérébrales, et en particulier sur le siège
        de la faculté du language articulé. *Gaz. hebd. Méd. Chir.,* 1863, **10,** 318-21,
        348-51, 397-402, 455-58.
        Auburtin did much to establish the principle of cerebral localization. He
        demonstrated on a patient whose frontal lobe was exposed following a
        gunshot wound that merely touching the uninjured lobe with a spatula
        would abolish speech, which would return immediately when the spatula
        was removed.

1402   LUYS, JULES BERNARD. 1828-1897
        Recherches sur le système nerveux cérébro-spinal; sa structure, ses
        fonctions, et ses maladies. 1 vol. and atlas. Paris, *J. B. Baillière,* 1865.
        The beginning of knowledge of thalamic function. This work contains
        Luys's descriptions of the two structures which bear his name: the
        subthalamic nucleus and the centre median of the thalamus.

1403   MEYNERT, THEODOR HERMANN. 1833-1892
        Der Bau der Gross-Hirnrinde und seine örtlichen Verschiedenheiten,
        nebst einem pathologisch-anatomischen Corollarium. *Vjschr. Psychiat.,*
        1867, **1,** 77-93, 198-217; 1868, **2,** 88-113.
        Meynert described the fountain decussation of the tegmental tract
        ("Meynert's decussation") and several other structures in the brain. Pub-
        lished in book form, 1868.

1404   MITCHELL, SILAS WEIR. 1829-1914
        Researches on the physiology of the cerebellum. *Amer. J. med. Sci.,* 1869,
        n.s. **57,** 320-38.
        Mitchell, leading American neurologist of his time, performed over 350
        experiments upon the cerebellum. He emphasized its co-ordinating
        function, first postulated by Flourens, and he proposed his "augmentor"
        theory of cerebellar function.

1405   FRITSCH, GUSTAV THEODOR. 1838-1891, & HITZIG, EDUARD. 1838-1907
Ueber die elektrische Erregbarkeit des Grosshirns. *Arch. Anat. Physiol. wiss. Med.*, 1870, 300-32.

      These workers showed that electrical stimulation of the frontal cortex in various experimental animals caused movements of the extremities of the opposite side of the body, thus proving the existence of a motor area in the cerebral cortex, predicted earlier in the same year by Hughlings Jackson. Translation in *J. Neurosurg.*, 1963, **20**, 905-16. Reprinted, with translation, in R. H. Wilkins, *Neurosurgical classics,* New York, 1965.

1406   GUDDEN, BERNHARD ALOYS VON. 1824-1886
Experimentaluntersuchungen über das peripherische und centrale Nervensystem. *Arch. Psychiat. Nervenkr.*, 1870, **2**, 693-723.

      Modern study of the functions of the thalamus began with the important investigations of Gudden. He is remembered eponymically by "Gudden's commissure" and "Gudden's atrophy" – specific thalamic nuclei degenerate when certain areas of the cerebral cortex are destroyed. His collected works were published in 1889. He was drowned in a lake at Starnberg by his patient Ludwig II, the mad king of Bavaria.

1406.01   LUYS, JULES BERNARD. 1828-1897
Iconographie photographique des centres nerveux. Paris, *Baillière*, 1873.

      Contains 70 photographs of brain sections taken by Luys himself, with 64 lithographed schemas based on his drawings. Luys undertook this work when the evidence of his lithographs published in 1865 (No. 4012) was disputed. It is the first large-scale photographic atlas of the anatomy of the brain.

1406.1   BARTHOLOW, ROBERTS. 1831-1904
Investigations into the functions of the human brain. *Amer. J. med. Sci.*, 1874, **67,** 305-13.

      Bartholow confirmed in man the findings of Fritsch and Hitzig (No. 1405) that electrical stimulus of the cortex on one side stimulated muscles on the other side of the body.

1407   BETS, VLADIMIR ALEKSANDROVIC [BETZ, W.]. 1834-1894
Anatomischer Nachweis zweier Gehirncentra. *Zbl. med. Wiss.*, 1874, **12,** 578-80, 595-99.

      Discovery of the giant pyramidal cells of the motor cortex.

1408   HITZIG, EDUARD. 1838-1907
Untersuchungen über das Gehirn. Berlin, *A. Hirschwald,* 1874.

      Hitzig accurately defined the limits of the motor area in the cerebral cortex of the dog and the monkey.

1408.1   CATON, RICHARD. 1842-1926
The electric currents of the brain. *Brit. med. J.*, 1875, **2**, 278.

      Caton succeeded in leading off action potentials from the brains of animals, a first step towards the development of the electroencephalograph. See also *Brit. med. J.*, 1877, **1**, Suppl. 62-75.

1408.2   KEY, AXEL. 1832-1901, & RETZIUS, MARCUS GUSTAF. 1842-1919.
Studien in der Anatomie des Nervensystems und des Bindegewebes. Erste Hälft und zweite Hälfte, erste Abtheilung. 2 vols. Stockholm, *Samons & Wallin,* 1875-76.

One of the most strikingly beautiful neuroanatomies ever published, with exquisite reproductions of the colour dye injection experiments. The authors confirmed the existence of the foramina of Magendie and Luschka, and studied the movement of the cerebrospinal fluid. All published.

1409   FERRIER, *Sir* DAVID. 1843-1928
The functions of the brain. London, *Smith, Elder & Co.,* 1876.
Ferrier may be said to have laid the foundations of our knowledge concerning the localization of cerebral function. His book includes his earlier work published in the *West Riding Lunatic Asylum Reports.* Facsimile reprint, 1966.

1410   FLECHSIG, PAUL EMIL. 1847-1929
Die Leitungsbahnen im Gehirn und Rückenmark des Menschen auf Grund entwicklungsgeschichtlicher Untersuchungen. Leipzig, *W. Engelmann,* 1876.
Flechsig mapped out the motor and sensory areas of the cerebral cortex, and named the "pyramidal tract".

1411   FOREL, AUGUSTE HENRI. 1848-1931
Untersuchungen über die Haubenregion und ihre oberen Verknüpfungen im Gehirne des Menschen und einiger Säugethiere, mit Beiträgen zu den Methoden der Gehirnuntersuchung. *Arch. Psychiat. Nervenkr.,* 1877, **7,** 393-495.
Forel elucidated the subthalamic region, "campus Foreli".

1412   LEWIS, WILLIAM BEVAN. 1847-1929
On the comparative structure of the cortex cerebri. *Brain,* 1878, **1,** 79-96.
Lewis described the giant cells of the precentral convolution.

1413   EXNER, SIEGMUND. 1846-1926
Untersuchungen über die Localisation der Funktionen in der Grosshirnrinde des Menschen. Wien, *W. Braumuller,* 1881.
Exner identified the superficial tangential fibres of the molecular layer of the cerebral cortex, known eponymically as "Exner's plexus".

1414   MUNK, HERMANN, 1839-1912
Ueber die Functionen der Grosshirnrinde. Berlin, *A. Hirschwald,* 1881.
Munk made important investigations on the functions of the temporal lobes.

1415   OTT, ISAAC. 1847-1916
The relation of the nervous system to the temperature of the body. *J. nerv. ment. Dis.,* 1884, **11,** 141-52.
Ott wrote important papers on the nervous regulation of body temperature. His papers on the heat-centre in the brain and on the thermo-inhibitory apparatus were published in the same journal, 1887, **14,** 150-62, 428-38; 1888, **15,** 85-104.

1415.1   THUDICHUM, JOHANN LUDWIG WILHELM. 1829-1901
A treatise on the chemical constitution of the brain. London, *Baillière, Tindall & Cox,* 1884.
Thudichum, a German emigré, discovered cephalins and myelins in brain tissue. An enlarged German edition of his book was published at

Tübingen, 1901. See biography by D. L. Drabkin, 1958, which includes an annotated bibliography of Thudichum's writings. Reprint of the original work, with historical introduction by Drabkin, 1962.

1416   GOLGI, CAMILLO. 1844-1926
Sulla fina anatomia degli organi centrali del sistema nervoso. Milano, *U. Hoepli, 1886* .

Golgi's histological studies made a clear conception of the nervous system possible for the first time. He demonstrated the existence of multipolar nerve-cells (Golgi cells) by means of his silver nitrate stain, and described the "Golgi apparatus" and "Golgi type II" nerve cells – cells with short axons ramified within the cortex. In 1906 he shared the Nobel Prize with Ramón y Cajal. First published as a series of papers in *Riv. sper. Freniat.,* 1882-85. Chiefly known from the German translation, *Untersuchungen über den feineren Bau des centralen und peripherischen Nervensystems* (1894).

1416.1   BEEVOR, CHARLES EDWARD. 1854-1907, & HORSLEY, *Sir* VICTOR ALEXANDER HADEN. 1857-1916
A minute analysis (experimental) of the various movements produced by stimulating in the monkey different regions of the cortical centre for the upper limb, as defined by Professor Ferrier. *Phil. Trans. B.,* 1887, **178,** 153-68.

Beevor, physician to the National Hospital, Queen Square, London, collaborated with Horsley in an important series of investigations of the localization of cerebral function.

1417   FRANÇOIS-FRANCK, CHARLES EMILE. 1849-1921
Leçons sur les fonctions motrices du cerveau. Paris, *O. Doin,* 1887.

François-Franck's studies on the excitability of the cerebral cortex and the localization of function followed work in collaboration with Pitres; Charcot wrote the preface. *See also* No. 1423.

1418   WESTPHAL, CARL FRIEDRICH OTTO. 1833-1890
Ueber einen Fall von chronischer progressiver Lähmung der Augenmuskeln (Ophthalmoplegia externa) nebst Beschreibung von Ganglien-zellengruppen im Bereiche des Oculomotoriuskerns. *Arch. Psychiat. Nervenkr.,* 1887, **18,** 846-71.

"Westphal's nucleus" – for accommodation – in the third cranial nerve. Called also "Edinger's nucleus" (see the same journal, 1885, **16,** 858-89).

1419   HORSLEY, *Sir* VICTOR ALEXANDER HADEN. 1857-1916, & SHARPEY-SCHAFER, *Sir* EDWARD ALBERT. 1850-1935
A record of experiments upon the functions of the cerebral cortex. *Phil. Trans. B,* (1888), 1889, **179,** 1-45.

A detailed analysis, by means of faradic stimulation, of the motor responses of the cerebral cortex, internal capsule, and spinal cord of higher primates.

1419.1   VAN GIESON, IRA. 1865-1913
Laboratory notes of technical methods for the nervous system. *N.Y. med. J.,* 1889, **1,** 57-60.

Van Gieson's acid fuchsin and picric acid stain for nerve tissue.

1420   PICK, ARNOLD. 1851-1924
Ueber ein abnormes Faserbündel der menschlichen Medulla oblongata.
Arch. Psychiat. Nervenkr., 1890, **21,** 636-40.
"Pick's bundle" of nerve fibres in the medulla oblongata.

1420.1   GOTCH, FRANCIS. 1853-1913, & HORSLEY, *Sir* VICTOR ALEXANDER HADEN. 1857-
1916
On the mammalian nervous system, its functions, and their localisation
determined by an electrical method. *Phil. Trans. B,* 1891, 182, 267-526.
    Gotch and Horsley showed that electric currents are produced in the
mammalian brain, and they recorded them with the string galvanometer of
the capillary electrometer. Their work led eventually to the development
of the electroencephalograph.

1421   LUCIANI, LUIGI. 1840-1919
Il cervelletto. Nuovi studi di fisiologia normale e patologica. Firenze, *Le
Monnier,* 1891.
    Luciani succeeded in keeping dogs alive after total extirpation of the
cerebellum, and initiated the modern study of cerebellar function.

1422   NISSL, FRANZ. 1860-1919
Ueber den sogenannten Granula der Nervenzellen. *Neurol. Zbl.,* 1894, **13,**
676-85, 781-89, 810-14.
    "Nissl's granules".

1423   CHARCOT, JEAN MARTIN. 1825-1893, & PITRES, JEAN ALBERT. 1848-1928
Les centres moteurs corticaux chez l'homme. Paris, *Rueff & Cie.,* 1895.
    Three papers by Charcot and Pitres in 1877, 1878, and 1883 left no doubt
as to the existence of cortical motor centres in man. These were later
published in book form (above).

1424   DEJERINE, JOSEPH JULES. 1849-1917, & DEJERINE-KLUMPKE, AUGUSTA. 1859-
1927
Anatomie des centres nerveux. 2 vols. Paris, *Rueff & Cie.,* 1895-1901.

1425   DONALDSON, HENRY HERBERT. 1857-1938
The growth of the brain. London, *W. Scott,* 1895.

1426   RETZIUS, MAGNUS GUSTAF. 1842-1919
Das Menschenhirn. Studien in der makroskopischen Morphologie. 2 vols.
Stockholm, *P. A. Norstedt,* 1896.
    Retzius studied a large series of subprimate, simian, and human brains,
and clarified some of the more difficult problems of cerebral morphology.

1427   WERNICKE, CARL. 1848-1905
Atlas des Gehirns. 2 pts. Breslau, *Schletter,* 1897-1900.

1428   LOEB, JACQUES. 1859-1924
Einleitung in die vergleichende Gehirnphysiologie und vergleichende
Psychologie. Leipzig, *J. A. Barth,* 1899. English translation with revisions
by the author, New York, 1900.

1428.1   RAMÓN Y CAJAL, Santiago. 1852-1934
Estructura dela corteza cerebral olfativa del hombre y mamíferos. *Trabajos del Laboratorio de Investigaciones biológicas de la Universidad de Madrid,* 1901, **1**, 1-140.

    Ramón y Cajal's descriptions of the limbic cortex are still the most authoritative. The above work and three shorter papers in the same volume were translated by L.M. Kraft as *Studies on the cerebral cortex,* London, 1955.

1429   VOGT, Oskar. 1870-1959
Zur anatomischen Gliederung des Cortex cerebri. *J. Psychol. Neurol. (Lpz.),* 1903, **2**, 160-80.

1430   CAMPBELL, Alfred Walter. 1868-1937
Histological studies on the localisation of cerebral function. Cambridge, *Univ. Press,* 1905.

    The precentral area of the cerebral cortex is known as "Campbell's area". Campbell and Brodmann were pioneers in the study of the architectonics of the cerebral cortex.

1431   DEJERINE, Joseph Jules. 1849-1917, & ROUSSY, Gustave. 1874-1948
Le syndrome thalamique. *Rev. neurol.,* 1906, **14**, 521-32.

    The "thalamic syndrome", investigations of the effect of localized thalamic injury.

1432   SHERRINGTON, *Sir* Charles Scott. 1857-1952
The integrative action of the nervous system. New York, *Charles Scribner's Sons,* 1906.

    Sherrington insisted that the essential function of the nervous system was the co-ordination of activities of the various parts of the organism. His work on the nervous system, especially his experimental studies of reflex action, had a profound influence upon modern physiology. He shared the Nobel Prize with Adrian in 1932. During his period as Professor of Physiology at Oxford (1913-36) he created what was considered to be the best school of physiology in the world. Biography by Lord Cohen, Liverpool, 1958, and Ragnar Granit, London, 1966.

1433   SMITH, *Sir* Grafton Elliot. 1871-1937
A new topographical survey of the human cerebral cortex, being an account of the distribution of the anatomically distinct cortical areas and their relationship to the cerebral sulci. *J. Anat. Physiol. (Lond.),* 1907, **41**, 237-54.

    Elliot Smith, Professor of Anatomy at Cairo, Manchester, and University College, London, initiated modern studies of cerebral function with his work on the cortical pattern of the human brain.

1434   BRODMANN, Korbinian. 1868-1918.
Beiträge zur histologischen Lokalisation der Grosshirnrinde. VI. Die Cortexgliederung des Menschen. *J. Psychol. Neurol. (Lpz.),* 1908, **10**, 231-46.

    "Brodmann's areas", the occipital and pre-occipital area of the cerebral cortex.

1435   ——. Vergleichende Lokalisationslehre der Grosshirnrinde in ihren Prinzipien dargestellt auf Grund des Zellenbaues. Leipzig, *J. A. Barth,* 1909.

Brodmann was a pioneer in the study of cytoarchitectonics. His book was republished in 1925. It was the most comprehensive account of the subject. Brodmann's work first appeared as a series of papers in *J. Psychol. Neurol. (Lpz.),* 1903-08. His map of the human cortex appeared in the same journal, 1907, **10,** 231-46, 287-334.

1435.1   HORSLEY, *Sir* VICTOR ALEXANDER HADEN. 1857-1916, & CLARKE, ROBERT HENRY. 1850-1926
The structure and functions of the cerebellum examined by a new method. *Brain,* 1908, **31,** 45-124.
Stereotactic apparatus for the accurate location of electrodes in the brain.

1436   KARPLUS, JOHANN PAUL. 1866-1936, & KREIDL, ALOIS. 1864-1928
Gehirn und Sympathicus. *Pflüg. Arch. ges. Physiol.,* 1909, **129,** 138-144; 1910, **135,** 401-16; 1912, **143,** 109-27.
First experimental studies on the hypothalamus.

1437   SACHS, ERNEST. 1879-1958
On the structure and functional relations of the optic thalamus. *Brain,* 1909, **32,** 95-186.

1438   BARBOUR, HENRY GRAY. 1886-1943, & ABEL, JOHN JACOB. 1857-1938
Tetanic convulsions in frogs produced by acid fuchsin, and their relation to the problem of inhibition in the central nervous system. *J. Pharmacol.,* 1910, **2,** 169-99.

1438.1   HEAD, *Sir* HENRY. 1861-1940, & HOLMES, *Sir* GORDON MORGAN. 1876-1965
Sensory disturbances from cerebral lesions. *Brain,* 1911, **34,** 102-254.
First systematic account of the functions of the thalamus and its relationship to the cerebral cortex. Reprinted in No. 1304.

1438.2   MONAKOW, CONSTANTIN VON. 1853-1930
Die Lokalisation im Grosshirn und der Abbau der Funktion durch kortikale Herde. Wiesbaden, *J. F. Bergmann,* 1914.
A monumental work on cerebral localization.

1439   WEED, LEWIS HILL. 1886-1952
Studies on cerebro-spinal fluid. III. The pathways of escape from the subarachnoid spaces with particular reference to the arachnoid villi. *J. med. Res.,* 1914, **31,** 51-117.
Weed mapped out the pathways of the circulation of the cerebrospinal fluid.

1440   ——. The development of the cerebro-spinal spaces in pig and man. *Contr. Embryol. Carneg. Instn.,* 1917, **5,** No. 14.

1441   TILNEY, FREDERICK. 1875-1938, & RILEY, HENRY ALSOP. 1887-1966
The form and functions of the central nervous system. New York, *P. B. Hoeber,* 1921.

1442   DUSSER DE BARENNE, JOHANNES GREGORIUS. 1885-1940
Experimental researches on sensory localization in the cerebral cortex of the monkey (Macacus). *Proc. roy. Soc. B,* 1924, **96,** 272-91.

Dusser de Barenne demonstrated the major functional subdivisions of the sensory cortex.

1443   LIDDELL, EDWARD GEORGE TANDY. 1895-1981, & SHERRINGTON, *Sir* CHARLES SCOTT. 1857-1952
Reflexes in response to stretch (myotatic reflexes). *Proc. roy. Soc. B,* 1924, **96,** 212-42; 1925, **97,** 267-83.
This investigation of the stretch reflex was of value in elucidating muscle tone and posture.

1444   ECONOMO, CONSTANTIN, *Freiherr von San Serff.* 1876-1931, & KOSKINAS, GEORG N.
Die Cytoarchitektonik der Hirnrinde des erwachsenen Menschen. 1 vol. and atlas. Wien & Berlin, *J. Springer,* 1925.
Abridged English translation, 1929.

1445   PAVLOV, IVAN PETROVITCH. 1849-1936
Lectures on conditioned reflexes. 2 vols. New York, *International Publishers,* 1928-41.
Besides his important work on digestion, Pavlov is remembered for his investigations upon conditioned reflexes. He is one of the greatest physiologists of all time. An English translation of another work by Pavlov, entitled *Conditioned reflexes* appeared in 1927. *See* No. 1022.

1446   BERGER, JOHANNES ["HANS"]. 1873-1941
Über das Elektrenkephalogramm des Menschen. *Arch. Psychiat. Nervenkr.,* 1929, **87,** 527-70.
First description of the electroencephalogram. Berger showed that the electrical activity of the human brain could be recorded from the intact scalp.

1446.1 LASHLEY, KARL SPENCER. 1890-1958
Brain mechanisms and intelligence: a quantitative study of injuries to the brain. Chicago, *Univ. of Chicago Press,* 1929.
Lashley related nervous function and behaviour with well-defined areas of the brain, particularly in connexion with cerebral lesions.

1446.2 KELLER, ALLEN DUDLEY. 1901- , & HARE, WILLIAM KENDRICK. 1908-
The hypothalamus and heat regulation. *Proc. Soc. exp. Biol., (N.Y.),* 1932, **29,** 1069-70.
Location of the heat-regulating centre in the hypothalamus.

1447   ADRIAN, EDGAR DOUGLAS, 1*st Baron Adrian.* 1889-1977, & MATTHEWS, *Sir* BRYAN HAROLD CABOT. 1906-
The interpretation of potential waves in the cortex. *J. Physiol. (Lond.),* 1934, **81,** 440-71.
Confirmation of Berger's findings (No. 1446). See also *Brain,* 1934, **57,** 355-85.

1448   CLARK, *Sir* WILFRID EDWARD LE GROS. 1895-1971
The structure and connections of the thalamus. *Brain,* 1932, **55,** 406-70.

1449   ——. The topography and homologies of the hypothalamic nuclei in man. *J. Anat. (Lond.),* 1936, **70,** 203-14.

1450 FOERSTER, OTFRID. 1873-1941
The motor cortex in man in the light of Hughlings Jackson's doctrines. *Brain,* 1936, **59,** 135-59.
In this Hughlings Jackson Lecture, Foerster published his famous cytoarchitectonic map of the human cerebral cortex.

1451 WALKER, ARTHUR EARL. 1907-
The primate thalamus. Chicago, *Univ. Press,* (1938).

1451.1 HESS, WALTER RUDOLF. 1881-1973
Die funktionelle Organisation des vegetativen Nervensystems. Basel, *B. Schwabe,* 1948.
Hess shared the Nobel Prize with Egas Moniz in 1949 for his discovery of the functional organization of the interbrain as a co-ordinator of the activities of the internal organs.

For history, see 1574, 1574.1, 1577, 1586-87, 1588.4, 1588.7-1588.9, 1588.32,1588.14, 1588.15, 1588.19, 1588.21, 1588.24.

ORGANS OF SPECIAL SENSES

1452 SCHNEIDER, CONRAD VIKTOR. 1614-1680
Dissertatio de osse cribriforme, et sensu ac organo odoratus. Wittebergae, *Mevi,* 1655,
"Schneider's membrane", the pituitary membrane of the nasal chamber and sinuses.

1453 SCARPA, ANTONIO. 1752-1832
Anatomicae disquisitiones de auditu et olfactu. Ticini, *typog. P. Galeatius,* 1789.
Scarpa made important researches concerning the auditory and olfactory apparatus of fishes, birds, reptiles, and man. See L. Sellers and B. Anson, [Scarpa's] Anatomical observations on the round window, *Arch. Otolaryng.,* 1962, **75,** 2-45.

1454 SOEMMERRING, SAMUEL THOMAS. 1755-1830
Abbildungen der menschlichen Organe des Geruches. Frankfurt A.M., *Varrentrapp u. Wenner,* 1809.

1455 ———. Abbildungen der menschlichen Organe des Geschmackes und der Stimme. Frankfurt a.M., *Varrentrapp u. Wenner,* 1806.

1456 MÜLLER, JOHANNES. 1801-1858
Ueber die phantastischen Gesichtserscheinungen. Coblenz, *J. Hölscher,* 1826.
Müller's early studies on specific nerve energies are included in the above work. Later he stated, in his *Handbuch der Physiologie,* Coblenz, 1840, **2,** 258, his law of specific nerve energies – each nerve of special sense, however excited, gives rise to its own peculiar sensation.

1456.1 SCHLEMM, FRIEDRICH. 1795-1858
Arteriarum capitis superficialium icon nova. Berolini, *J. W. Boike,* 1830.
Includes description of the "canal of Schlemm", the circular canal at the junction of the cornea and the sclerotic.

1457   WEBER, ERNST HEINRICH. 1795-1878
         De pulsu, resorptione, auditu et tactu. Annotationes anatomicae et
         physiologicae. Lipsiae, *C. F. Koehler,* 1834.
         Includes Weber's law on the relationship between stimulus and sen-
         sation. English translation of *De tactu,* New York *Academic Press,* 1978.

1458   MÜLLER, JOHANNES. 1801-1858
         Ueber die Compensation der physischen Kräfte am menschlichen
         Stimmorgan, mit Bemerkungen über die Stimme der Säugethiere, Vögel
         und Amphibien. Berlin, *A. Hirschwald,* 1839.

1459   WEBER, ERNST HEINRICH. 1795-1878
         Der Tastsinn und das Gemeingefühl. In Wagner's *Handwörterbuch der
         Physiologie,* Braunschweig, 1846, **3,** Abt. 2, 481-588.
         English translation of *Tastsinn, Academic Press,* 1978.

1460   WAGNER, RUDOLF. 1805-1864, & MEISSNER, GEORG. 1829- 1903
         Ueber das Vorhandensein bisher unbekannter eigenghümlicher
         Tastkörperchen (Corpuscula tactus) in den Gefühlswärzchen der
         menschlichen Haut, und über die End-Ausbreitung sensitiver Nerven.
         Nachr. Georg-Augusts Univ. kgl. Ges. Wiss. Göttingen, 1852, 17-32.
         First published account of the tactile nerve endings – "Wagner's
         corpuscles".

1461   BRÜCKE, ERNST WILHELM VON, *Ritter.* 1819-1892
         Grundzüge der Physiologie und Systematik der Sprachlaute für Linguisten
         und Taubstummenlehrer. Wien, *C. Gerold's Sohn,* 1856.

1462   MERKEL, CARL LUDWIG. 1812-1876
         Anatomie und Physiologie des menschlichen Stimm- und Sprach-Organs
         (Anthropophonik). Leipzig, *A. Abel,* 1857.

1463   WUNDT, WILHELM MAX. 1832-1920
         Beiträge zur Theorie der Sinneswahrnehmung. *Z. rat. Med.,* 1858, **4,** 229-
         93; 1859, **7,** 279-318, 321-96; 1861, **12,** 145-262; 1862, **14,** 1-77; 1863, **15,**
         104-79.
         Sensory perception. Wundt was one of the founders of experimental
         psychology.

1464   FECHNER, GUSTAV THEODOR. 1801-1887
         Ueber ein wichtiges psychophysisches Grundgesetz und dessen Beziehung
         zur Schätzung der Sterngrössen. *Abh. k. sächs. Ges. Wiss. (Lpz.), maths.-
         phys. Cl.,* (1858), 1859, **4,** 455-532.
         Fechner–Weber law on stimulus and sensation. *See also* Nos. 1457 &
         4972.

1465   BROWN-SÉQUARD, CHARLES EDOUARD. 1817-1894
         Recherches sur la transmission des impressions de tact, de chatouillement,
         de douleur, de température et de contraction (sens musculaire) dans la
         moëlle épinière. *J. Physiol. (Paris),* 1863, **6,** 124-45, 232-48, 581-646.
         Among Brown-Séquard's best work was his study of the pathways of
         conduction in the spinal cord.

1466   TÜRCK, LUDWIG. 1810-1868
        Ueber die Haut-Sensibilitätsbezirke der einzelnen Rückenmarks-
        nervenpaare. *Denkschr. k. Akad. Wiss. (Wien), math.-nat. Cl.,* 1868, **29,**
        299-326.
        Investigation of the cutaneous distribution of the separate pairs of
        spinal nerves.

1467   DONDERS, FRANS CORNELIS. 1818-1889
        De physiologie der spraakklanken. Utrecht, *C. van der Post, jr.,* 1870.
        Donders's most important work was performed in the field of ophthal-
        mology, but he wrote a classic treatise on the physiology of speech. Also
        published in *Onderzoekingen gedaan in het Physiologisch Laboratorium
        der Utrechtsche Hoogeschool,* 1870, **3,** 354-73.

1468   BLIX, MAGNUS GUSTAV. 1849-1904
        Experimentelle Beiträge zur Lösung der Frage über die specifische Energie
        der Hautnerven *Z. Biol.,* 1884, **20,** 141-56; 1885, **21,** 145-60.
        Besides his investigation of the specific energies of cutaneous nerves,
        Blix is remembered for his work on the thermodynamics of muscular
        contraction; he designed a muscle indicator diagram; he was also the first
        to suggest centrifugal force in the separation of red and white blood cells.

1469   GOLDSCHEIDER, JOHANNES KARL AUGUST EUGEN ALFRED. 1858-1935
        Die spezifische Energie der Temperaturnerven. *Mh. prakt. Derm.,* 1884, **3,**
        198-208, 225-41.

1470   ——. Neue Thatsachen über die Hautsinnesnerven. *Arch. Anat. Physiol.,
        Physiol. Abt.,* 1885, Suppl. Bd., 1-110.
        Goldscheider recorded important investigations on the nerves conveying
        the sensation of temperature and on the nerves of cutaneous sensation.

1471   TARCHANOFF, IVAN ROMANOVICH [TARKHANOFF]. 1848-1909
        Ueber die galvanischen Erscheinungen in der Haut des Menschen bei
        Reizungen der Sinnesorgane und bei verschiedenen Formen der
        psychischen Thätigkeit. *Pflüg. Arch. ges. Physiol.,* 1890, **46,** 46-55.
        Psycho-galvanic reflex described.

1472   EWALD, ERNST JULIUS RICHARD. 1855-1921
        Physiologische Untersuchungen über das Endorgan des Nervus octavus.
        Wiesbaden, *J. F. Bergmann,* 1892.
        Ewald clarified the function of the eighth cranial nerve.

1473   FERRY, ERVIN SIDNEY. 1868-1956
        Persistence of vision. *Amer. J. Sci.,* 1892, 3 ser. **44,** 192-207.
        Ferry modified Weber's law on the relationship between stimulus and
        sensation. Following the work of Porter, *Proc. roy. Soc. (Lond.),* 1898, **63,**
        347; 1902, **70,** 313, the term "Ferry–Porter Law" came into being.

1474   ZWAARDEMAKER, HENDRIK. 1857-1930
        Die Physiologie des Geruchs. Leipzig, *W. Engelmann,* 1895.
        For his studies on olfaction and olfactometry Zwaardemaker developed
        the so-called "camera inodorata" (odourless chamber). His instrument to
        check the patency of the nasal passages is still in use.

1475   FREY, MAX VON. 1852-1932
Untersuchungen über die Sinnesfunctionen der menschlichen Haut. I.
Druckempfindung und Schmerz. *Abh. k. sächs. Ges. Wiss. (Lpz.), math.-
phys. Cl.,* (1896), 1897, **23**, 169-266.
In his investigations on cutaneous sensibility Frey introduced his
method of testing the sensitiveness of pressure points by means of bristles
mounted in a handle.

1476   WINKLER, CORNELIS. 1855-1941
The central course of the nervus octavus and its influence on motility. *Verh.
kon. Akad. Wet. (Amst.),* 1907, **14**, 1-202.
Winkler was Professor of Neurology and Psychiatry at Amsterdam and
Utrecht. He published more than 200 papers, among the most important
being that on the central pathways of the eighth nerve.

1477   HOFFMANN, ERICH. 1868-1959
Ueber eine nach innen gerichtete Schützfunktion der Haut (Esophylaxie)
nebst Bemerkungen über die Entstehung der Paralyse. *Dtsch. med. Wschr.,*
1919, **45**, 1233-36.
Hoffmann stressed the role of the skin as a secretory organ, producing
hormone-like substances; he suggested the term "esophylaxis" for this
function.

Eye: Vision

1478   VAROLI, COSTANZO. 1543-1575
De nervis opticis nonnulisque aliis praeter communem opinionem in
humano capite observatis. Patavii, *apud Paulum & Antonium Meiettos,*
1573.
Varoli described a new method of dissection which enabled him for the
first time to observe and describe the pons. As a result of his new method
of dissecting, Varoli was able to make some contributions to the knowledge of the course and termination of the cranial nerves and to trace the
course of the optic nerve approximately to its true termination. His name
is perpetuated in the "pons varolii". Reprinted, Brussels, 1969. *See* No. 1377.2.

1479   CARCANO LEONE, GIOVANNI BATTISTA. 1536-1606
Anatomici libri II ... In altero de musculis, palpebrarum atque oculorum
motibus deservientibus, accurate disseritur. Ticini, *apud H. Bartholum,*
1574.
First exact description of the lacrimal duct. Carcano gave the true
position of the lacrimal gland and showed the route taken by the tears.

1480   SCHEINER, CHRISTOPH. 1575-1650
Oculus, hoc est: fundamentum opticum. Oeniponti, *apud D. Agricolam,*
1619.
Scheiner, a Jesuit astronomer, was a pioneer in physiological optics. He
demonstrated how images fall on the human retina, noting the change in
curvature of the lens during accommodation, and devised the pin-hole test
("Scheiner's test") to illustrate accommodation and refraction.

1481   MEIBOM, Heinrich. 1638-1700
De vasis palpebrarum novis epistola. Helmstadi, *typ. H. Mulleri,* 1666.
    Meibom described the conjunctival (Meibomian) glands; they were, however, already known to Galen and were figured by Casserius in 1609.

1481.1   MARIOTTE, Edmé. d. 1684
Nouvelle découverte touchant la veüe. Paris, *Frederic Leonard,* 1668.
    Discovery of the blind spot in the retina, the existence of which Mariotte deduced from his experiments investigating the fate of light rays striking the base of the optic nerve. Facsimile reprint in J. Brons, *The blind spot of Mariotte...,* Copenhagen & London, 1939.

1481.2   BRIGGS, William. 1642-1704
Ophthalmo-graphia; sive, oculi eiusque partium descriptio anatomica. Cantabridgiae, *J. Hart,* 1676.
    First English treatise on the anatomy of the eye. Briggs described the papilla of the optic disc and hypothesized that vibrations caused by rays of light striking fibres of the retina were conveyed to the papilla and thence to the optic thalami, on the model of a spider's web.

1481.3   ———. Nova visionis theoria. In: *Philosophical Collections,* 1682, **No. 6,** 167-78.
    Briggs' treatise on the physiology of vision influenced Sir Isaac Newton who reprinted it in book form with his own introduction, London, 1685.

1482   DUDDELL, Benedict.
A treatise of the diseases of the horny coat of the eye, and the various kinds of cataracts. London, *J. Clark,* 1729.
    "Descemet's membrane" was first described by Duddell. Descemet described it in 1758; see No. 1484.1.

1483   ZINN, Johann Gottfried. 1727-1759
De ligamentis ciliaribus. Gottingae, *typ. J. C. L. Schulzii,* 1753.

1484   ———. Descriptio anatomica oculi humani. Gottingae, *apud vid. A. Vandenhoeck,* 1755.
    The first complete study of the anatomy of the eye, including the first description of the "zonule of Zinn" and the "annulus of Zinn".

1484.1   DESCEMET, Jean. 1732-1810
An sola lens crystallina cataracte sedes? [Paris, *Veuve de Quillau,* 1758].
    "Descemet's membrane", the posterior membrane of the cornea; *see* No. 1482.

1484.2   PORTERFIELD, William. 1695-1771
A treatise on the eye. The manner and phenomena of vision. 2 vols. Edinburgh, *G. Hamilton & J. Balfour,* 1759.
    Porterfield was Professor of the Institutes and Practice of Medicine at Edinburgh from 1724-26. His book included many original observations. It was the first important British work on the anatomy and physiology of the eye.

1485   FONTANA, Felice. 1730-1805
Ricerche de motu del iride. Lucca, *Giusta,* 1765.
        An investigation of how and why the iris contracts. See P.K. Knoefel, *Felice Fontana: life and works,* Trento, [1984]. *See also* No.2103.

1486   YOUNG, Thomas. 1773-1829
Observations on vision. *Phil. Trans.,* 1793, **83,** 169-81.
        The versatile Young is regarded as one of the greatest of all scientists. In the above work he showed that the act of accommodation is due to a change of curvature of the crystalline lens, whereby light rays of various lengths can be brought to a focus on the retina.

1487   ——. On the mechanism of the eye. *Phil. Trans.,* 1801, **91,** 23-28
        Includes the first description of astigmatism, with measurements and optical constants.

1488   ——. On the theory of light and colours. *Phil. Trans.,* 1802, **92,** 12-48.
        Young, the "Father of physiological optics", established the wave theory of light, explaining the phenomena of interference and dispersion.

1489   SOEMMERRING, Samuel Thomas. 1755-1830
Abbildungen des menschlichen Auges. *Frankfurt a.M., Varrentrapp u. Wenner,* 1801.
        Soemmerring is best remembered for his fine anatomical illustrations, of which those devoted to the human eye are a good example. In 1791 he made important observations on the macula lutea: De foramine centrali limbo luteo cincto retinae humanae, *Comment. Soc. reg. Sci. Gotting.,* 1795-98 (1799), **13,** 3-13; on p. 4 he states that he made these observations on January 27, 1791. French translation in Demours, No. 5842.1.

1490   TENON, Jacques René. 1724-1816
Observations anatomiques sur quelques parties de l'oeil et des paupières. In his *Mémoires et observations sur l'anatomie, la pathologie, et la chirurgerie.* Paris, *Nyon,* 1806, pp.193-207.
        Although Tenon did not discover the fibrous capsule and the interfascial space of the orbit, they are named after him.

1491   JACOB, Arthur. 1790-1874
An account of a membrane in the eye, now first described. *Phil. Trans.,* 1819, **109,** 300-07.
        "Jacob's membrane", the layer of the retina containing the rods and cones.

1492   PURKYNĚ, Jan Evangelista [Purkinje], 1787-1869
Beiträge zur Kenntniss des Sehens in subjectiver Hinsicht. Prag, *Fr. Vetterl von Wildenkron,* 1819.
        Purkyně's graduation dissertation on the subjective visual phenomena earned for him the appreciation of Goethe and the chair of physiology at Breslau. Reprinted in his *Opera omnia,* vol. 1, pp. 1-56, 1918. There were two issues of the first edition published the same year. The second edition was published in 1823.

1492.1   ——. Commentatio de examine physiologico organi visus et systematis cutanei. Vratislaviae, *typis Universitatis,* 1823.

Purkyně was first to examine the interior of the human eye and the dog eye, using only a candle and a concave spherical lens. He thus invented the ophthalmoscope three decades before Helmholtz (1851; No. 5866). Reprinted in his *Opera* (No. 82), 1918, **1**, 163-94. English trans. in John, *Jan Evangelista Purkyne*, Philadelphia, 1959. See Albert & Miller, Jan Purkinje and the ophthalmoscope, *Amer. J. Ophth.*, 1973, **76**, 494-99.

1493   FLOURENS, MARIE JEAN PIERRE. 1794-1867
Recherches expérimentales sur les propriétés et les fonctions du système nerveux, dans les animaux vertébrés. Paris, *Crevot,* 1824.
    Experimental proof that vision depends on the integrity of the cerebral cortex. *See* No. 1391 for his first paper on the subject. Partial English translation in von Bonin, Some papers on the cerebral cortex, Springfield, *C.C. Thomas,* 1960.

1494   HORNER, WILLIAM EDMONDS. 1793-1853
Description of a small muscle of the internal commissure of the eyelids. *Philad. J. med. phys. Sci.,* 1824, **8**, 70-80.
    Horner described the tensor tarsi (Horner's) muscle, supplying the lacrimal apparatus. It was first described by Du Verney in 1749.

1494.1 PURKYNĚ, JAN EVANGELISTA [PURKINJE]. 1787-1869
Beobachtungen und Versuche zur Physiologie der Sinne. Neue Beiträge zur Kenntniss des Sehens in subjectiver Hinsicht. 2 vols., Berlin, *Reimer,* 1825.
    "Purkyně phenomenon" or "Purkyně shift", a change in the apparent relative luminosity of colours in a dim light (scotopic vision) compared with that in full daylight (photopic vision). Also published in *Rust's Mag. ges. Heilk.,* 1825, **20**, 3-83, 199-276, 391-423. See V. Kruta, *J.E. Purkyně, physiologist. A short account of his contributions. . . with a bibliography of his works.* Prague, *Academia Publishing House,* 1969.

1495   MÜLLER, JOHANNES. 1801-1858
Zur vergleichenden Physiologie des Gesichtssinnes des Menschen und der Thiere. Leipzig, *C. Cnobloch,* 1826.
    Includes (p. 73) his explanation of the colour sensations produced by pressure upon the retina.

1496   FIELDING, GEORGE HUNSLEY. 1801-1871
On a new membrane in the eye. Hull, *I. Wilson,* 1832.
    "Fielding's membrane", the tapetum of the retina.

1497   DALRYMPLE, JOHN. 1804-1852
The anatomy of the human eye. London, *Longmans,* 1834.
    First English work on ocular anatomy.

1498   WHEATSTONE, *Sir* CHARLES. 1802-1875
Contributions to the physiology of vision. *Phil. Trans.,* 1838, **128**, 371-94; 1852, **142**, 1-17.

1499   BREWSTER, *Sir* DAVID. 1781-1868
On the conversion of relief by inverted vision. *Trans. roy. Soc. Edinb.,* 1840-44, **15**, 657-62.

1500   ———. On the knowledge of distance given by binocular vision. *Trans. roy. Soc. Edinb.,* 1840-44, **15**, 663-75.

1501   BRUCH, KARL WILHELM LUDWIG. 1819-1884
Untersuchungen zur Kenntniss des körnigen Pigments der Wirbelthiere in physiologischer und pathologischer Hinsicht. Zürich, *Meyer u. Zeller*, 1844.
Includes a description of "Bruch's membrane" of the choroid.

1502   KUSSMAUL, ADOLF. 1822-1902
Die Farbenerscheinungen im Grunde des menschlichen Auges. Heidelberg, *K. Groos*, 1845.
An important description of colour phenomena in the fundus oculi. This paper won for Kussmaul the Karl Friedrich Medal of the University of Heidelberg.

1503   LISTING, JOHANN BENEDICT. 1808-1882
Beitrag zur physiologischen Optik. Göttingen. *Vandenhoeck & Rupprecht*, 1845.

1504   MACKENZIE, WILLIAM. 1791-1868
On the vision of objects on and in the eye. *Edinb. med. surg. J.*, 1845, **64**, 38-97.
An introduction to the then little-known subject of catoptrics.

1505   BOWMAN, *Sir* WILLIAM. 1816-1892
Lectures on the parts concerned in the operations on the eye, and on the structure of the retina. London, *Longmans*, 1849.
Bowman did more than any other man to advance ophthalmic surgery in England. The above work is the first to include a sound description of the microscopical anatomy of the eye and the ciliary ("Bowman's") muscle. The book consists of several lectures given at the London Ophthalmic Hospital and published in the *Lond. med. Gaz.* in 1847. Part of it is reprinted in *Med. Classics*, 1940, **5**, 292-336.

150μ6   MÜLLER, HEINRICH. 1820-1864
Zur Histologie der Netzhaut. *Z. wiss. Zool.*, 1851, **3**, 234-37.
Discovery of visual purple.

1507   BUDGE, JULIUS LUDWIG. 1811-1884
Ueber den Einfluss des Nervensystems auf die Bewegung der Iris. *Arch. physiol. Heilk.*, 1852, **11**, 773-826.

1508   HELMHOLTZ, HERMANN LUDWIG FERDINAND VON. 1821-1894
Ueber die Theorie der zusammengesetzten Farben. *Arch. Anat. Physiol. wiss. Med.*, 1852, 461-82; *Ann. Phys. Chem.*, 1852, **87**, 45-66

1509   ———. Ueber die Accommodation des Auges. *v. Graefes Arch. Ophthal.*, 1854-55, **1**, 2 Abt., 1-74.
Helmholtz determined the optical constants and explained the mechanism of accommodation, with the help of the ophthalmometer which he had invented in 1852.

1510   BUDGE, JULIUS LUDWIG. 1811-1884
Ueber die Bewegung der Iris. Braunschweig, *F. Vieweg u. Sohn*, 1855.

1511   PANIZZA, BARTOLOMEO. 1785-1867
Osservazioni sul nervo ottico. *G. r. Ist. Lomb. Sci.*, 1855, 237-52.
Panizza localized visual function in the posterior part of the cerebellum.

1511.1   HOLMGREN, ALARIK FRITHIOF. 1831-1897
           Method att objectivera effecten av ljusintryck pa retina. *Upsal Läkaref. Förh.*,
           1865, **1**, 177-91.
           Discovery of the electroretinogram, the beginning of the use of
           electrophysiological methods for studying visual systems.

1512   SCHULTZE, MAXIMILIAN JOHANN SIGISMUND. 1825-1874
           Zur Anatomie und Physiologie der Retina. Bonn, *M. Cohen u. Sohn,* 1866.
           One of the greatest of all histologists, Max Schultze is remembered by
           ophthalmologists for his monograph on the nerve-endings in the retina.

1513   HELMHOLTZ, HERMANN LUDWIG FERDINAND VON. 1821-1894
           Handbuch der physiologischen Optik. 1 vol. and atlas. Leipzig, *L. Voss,* 1867.
           One of the greatest books on physiological optics. It includes Helmholtz's
           revival of the Young theory of colour vision. English translation by J.P.C.
           Southall of 3rd German edition, 3 vols., Menasha, Wis., 1924-25.

1513.1   HERING, KARL EDWALD KONSTANTIN. 1834-1918
           Die Lehre vom binokularen Sehen. Leipzig, *Wilhelm Engelmann,* 1868.
           Hering's law: that the corresponding muscles of the two eyes are always
           equally innervated. The book includes classic experiments and observa-
           tions on eye movement control. Engl. trans. by B. Bridgeman and L. Stark,
           New York, *Plenum,* 1977.

1514   HOLMGREN, ALARIK FRITHIOF. 1831-1897
           Om retinaströmmen. *Upsala LäkFören. Förh.,* 1870-71, **6**, 419-55.
           First demonstration of retinal action currents.

1515   HERING, KARL EWALD KONSTANTIN. 1834-1918
           Zur Lehre vom Lichtsinne. *S. B. k. Akad. Wiss. (Wien), math.-nat. Cl.,* 3
           Abt., 1872, **66,** 5-24; 1873, **68,** 186-201, 229-44; 1874, **69,** 85-104, 179-217;
           1875, **70,** 169-204.
           Hering's theory of colour sense.

1515.1   LEBER, THEODOR. 1840-1917
           Studien über den Flüssigkeitswechsel im Auge. *v. Graefes Arch. Ophthal.,*
           1873, **19,** Abt. II, 87-185.
           Leber discovered how the ciliary body excretes intraocular fluid.

1516   GUDDEN, BERNHARD ALOYS VON. 1824-1886
           Ueber die Kreuzung der Fasern im Chiasma nervorum opticorum. *v. Graefes
           Arch. Ophthal.,* 1874, **20,** 2 Abt., 249-68; 1879, **25,** 1 Abt., 1-56.
           Important studies on the partial decussation of optic paths.

1517   BOLL, FRANZ CHRISTIAN. 1849-1879
           Zur Physiologie des Sehens und der Farbenempfindung. *Mber. k. preuss.
           Akad. Wiss. Berlin,* 1877, 2-7, 72-74.
           Boll noted that visual purple is bleached on exposure to light.

1518   SATTLER, HUBERT. 1844-1928
           Ueber den feineren Bau der Chorioidea des Menschen nebst Beiträgen zur
           pathologischen und vergleichenden Anatomie der Aderhaut. *v. Graefes
           Arch. Ophthal.,* 1876, **22,** Abt. 2, 1-100.
           "Sattler's layer" of the choroid.

1519 KÜHNE, WILLY. 1837-1900
Ueber den Sehpurpur. *Untersuch. physiol. Inst. Univ. Heidelberg,* 1878, **1,** 15-103.

Kühne was Professor of Physiology at Amsterdam and Heidelberg. Among his best work is his investigation of visual purple (rhodopsin) which he was first to extract from the retina. Several other papers by him on the same subject appear in the above volume.

1520 LOCKWOOD, CHARLES BARRETT. 1856-1914
The anatomy of the muscles, ligaments and fasciae of the orbit, including an account of the capsule of Tenon, the check ligaments of the recti, and the suspensory ligaments of the eye. *J. Anat. Physiol., (Lond.),* 1885, **20,** 1-25.

"Lockwood's suspensory ligament" of the globe of the eye.

1521 HENSCHEN, SALOMON EBERHARD. 1847-1930
Kort öfversigt af läran om lokalisationen i hjernbarken. *Upsala LäkFören. Förh.* 1888, **27,** 507-25, 601-12.

Discovery of the cortical visual centre.

1522 LADD-FRANKLIN, CHRISTINE. 1847-1930
Eine neue Theorie der Licht-Empfindung. *Z. Psychol. Physiol. Sinnesorg.,* 1893, **4,** 211-21.

Ladd-Franklin theory of vision.

1523 RAMÓN Y CAJAL, SANTIAGO. 1852-1934
Die Retina der Wirbelthiere...In Verbindung mit dem Verfasser zusammengestellt, übersetzt und mit Einleitung versehen von Dr. Richard Greeff...Wiesbaden, *J. F. Bergmann,* 1894.

Classic account of the vertebrate retina. First published in the Belgian review *La Cellule,* and later translated with extensive additions by Ramón y Cajal. Engl. trans., *The structure of the retina,* Springfield, [1972].

1524 KRIES, JOHANNES ADOLF VON. 1853-1928
Ueber die Funktion der Netzhautstäbchen. *Z. Psychol. Physiol. Sinnesorg.,* 1896, **9,** 81-123.

Important paper on the function of the retinal rods.

1525 EDRIDGE-GREEN, FREDERICK WILLIAM. 1863-1953
Some observations on the visual purple of the retina. *Trans ophthal. Soc. U.K.,* 1902, **22,** 300-02.

Edridge-Green first put forward his theories on the function of the retinal rods and of the visual purple about 1889. See also his *Physiology of vision,* 1920.

1525.1 GOTCH, FRANCIS. 1853-1913
The time relations of the photo-electric changes in the eyeball of the frog. *J. Physiol. (Camb),* 1903, **29,** 388-410.

First correct electroretinograms.

1525.2 GULLSTRAND, ALVAR. 1862-1930
Demonstration eines Instrumentes zur Erzeugung von Strahlengebilden um leuchtende Punkte. *Ber. ophthal. Ges.* (1902), 1903, 290-92.

Gullstrand invented the slit-lamp, making possible the microscopic study of the living eye.

1526   ——. Einführung in die Methoden der Dioptrik des Auges des Menschen. Leipzig, *S. Hirzel,* 1911.
Discovery of the intracapsular mechanism of accommodation. Gullstrand received the Nobel Prize in 1911 for his work on the dioptrics of the eye.

1527   VOGT, ALFRED. 1879-1943
Atlas der Spaltlampenmikroskopie des lebenden Auges. Berlin, *J. Springer,* 1921.
An important work on the biomicroscopy of the eye. Second ed. greatly revised and enlarged, vol. 1-2, *Springer,* 1930-31; vol. 3, Stuttgart, *F. Enke,* 1942; vol. 3 (English translation) Zurich, 1947. Second ed. reprinted, Bonn, *J. P. Wayenborgh,* 1977. English trans. by F.C. Blodi, 3 vols., Bonn, *J.P. Wayenborgh,* 1978-81.

1528   ADRIAN, EDGAR DOUGLAS, 1*st Baron Adrian.* 1889-1977, & MATTHEWS, RACHEL.
The action of light on the eye. *J. Physiol. (Lond.),* 1927, **63,** 378-414; **64,** 279-301; 1928, **65,** 273-308.
Adrian and Matthews made important researches on the electrical discharges from the vertebrate optic nerve.

1529   PARSONS, *Sir* JOHN HERBERT. 1868-1957
An introduction to the theory of perception. Cambridge, *University Press,* 1927.

1530   DUKE-ELDER, *Sir* WILLIAM STEWART. 1898-1978
The nature of the intra-ocular fluids. London, *G. Pulman,* 1927.

1531   ——. Text-book of ophthalmology. Vol. 1. The development, form, and function of the visual apparatus. London, *H. Kimpton,* 1932.

1532   HARTLINE, HALDON KEFFER. 1903-1983
The responses of single optic nerve fibers of the vertebrate eye to illumination of the retina. *Amer. J. Physiol.,* 1938, **121,** 400-15.
Hartline continued and extended the work initiated by Adrian and Matthews on electrical discharges from the optic nerve. See also his later papers in the same journal, 1940, **130,** 690-711. For his work on visual mechanisms he shared the Nobel Prize in 1967 with Granit (No. 1534) and G. Wald (No. 1535). Reprinted with historical introduction by Hartline in F. Ratliff (ed.). *Studies on excitation and inhibition in the retina,* New York, [1974].

1533   RIGGS, LORRIN ANDREWS. 1912-
Continuous and reproducible records of the electrical activity of the human retina. *Proc. Soc. exp. Biol. (N.Y.),* 1941, **48,** 204-7.
Electroretinography.

1533.1   POLYAK, STEPHEN. 1889-1955
The anatomy and the histology of the retina in man, ape, and monkey. Chicago, *University of Chicago Press,* 1941.
A scholarly tour-de-force with a bibliography of over 700 references.

1534   GRANIT, RAGNAR ARTHUR. 1900-
Sensory mechanisms of the retina: with an appendix on electroretinography.
London, *Geoffrey Cumberlege*, 1947.
An account of twenty years' work on the electrical responses of the
retina, a discussion of visual purple and visual violet, and an exposition of
Granit's hypothesis of colour vision. His researches have done much to
elucidate the mechanism of visual processes. In 1967 he shared the Nobel
Prize with Hartline (No. 1532) and G. Wald.

1535   WALD, GEORGE. 1906-
The molecular basis of visual excitation. *Les Prix Nobel en 1967,* Stockholm, 1968, pp. 260-80.
Shared Nobel Prize in 1967 for research on the photosensitive pigments
in the visual receptor apparatus.

Ear: Hearing

1536   MASSA, NICCOLÓ. 1489-1569
Anatomiae liber introductorius. Venetiis, *F. Bindoni ac M. Pasini,* 1536.
Massa described the action of the ossicles. English translation in No.
461.2.

1537   FALLOPPIO, GABRIELE [FALLOPIUS]. 1523-1562
Observationes anatomicae. Venetiis, *apud M. A. Ulmum,* 1561.
Includes first clear description of the membrana tympani. Fallopius
discovered the "aqueduct of Fallopius".

1538   EUSTACHI, BARTOLOMEO [EUSTACHIUS]. *circa* 1510/20-1574
De auditus organis. In his *Opuscula anatomica,* Venetiis, 1564, pp. 148-64.
Eustachius is credited with several anatomical discoveries, among them
the tensor tympani muscle and the Eustachian tube. In the last respect,
however, he was anticipated by Alcmaeon, about 500 B.C. Eustachius was
the first to describe the chorda tympani as a nerve.

1539   COITER, VOLCHER. 1534-1576
De auditus instrumento. In his *Externarum et internarum principalium
humani corporis partium tabulae,* Noribergae, *in off. T. Gerlatzeni,* 1572,
88-105.
The first monograph on the ear. A compendium of contemporary
knowledge of the anatomy and physiology of the ear. Most copies are
dated 1573. *See* Nos. 284 & 464.1. English translation, Amsterdam, 1955.

1540   CASSERI, GIULIO [JULIUS CASSERIUS *Placentinus*]. 1552-1616
De vocis auditusque organis historia anatomica. 2 pts. Ferrariae, *exc. V.
Baldinus, typ. Cameralis,* 1600-01.
A masterpiece of book illustration and the most beautiful book ever
published on the ear and throat in man and in lower animals. Like his
teacher, Fabrizio, who studied the development of the chick for clues to
human embryology, Casseri endeavoured to explain the human larynx
and ear by reference to the lower animals.   In addition to elegant
illustrations and beautiful book design the work describes numerous
important discoveries.

1541 INGRASSIA, GIOVANNI FILIPPO. 1510-1580
In Galeni librum de ossibus. Panormi, *ex typog. J. B. Maringhi,* 1603.
  Ingrassia is by some accredited with the discovery of the stapes; he also observed the sound-conducting capacity of the teeth.

1542 FOLLI, CECILIO [FOLIUS]. 1615-1660
Nova auris internae delineatio. Venetiis, 1645.
  Announces the discovery of the long process of the malleus. Folius "accurately discussed the general configuration of the middle ear, described the round and oval windows, delineated the three ossicles with the so-called fourth ossicle, the semicircular canals and cochlea" (Mettler). Also in A. Haller, *Disputationes ad morborum historiam,* etc. 1749, **4,** 365-68.

1543 STENSEN, NIELS [STENO]. 1638-1686
Observationes anatomicae, quibus varia oris, oculorum, et narium vasa describuntur. Lugduni Batavorum, *J. Chouët,* 1662.
  Ceruminous glands first mentioned.

1544 WILLIS, THOMAS. 1621-1675
De anima brutorum. Oxonii, *R. Davis,* 1672.
  Chap. XIV is devoted to the sense of hearing; in it Willis described the "paracusis of Willis" (p. 73). English translation, 1683.

1545 DU VERNEY, GUICHARD JOSEPH. 1648-1730
Traité de l'organe de l'ouie; contenant la structure, les usages et les maladies de toutes les parties de l'oreille. Paris, *E. Michallet,* 1683.
  First scientific account of the structure, function and diseases of the ear. Du Verney showed that the bony external meatus develops from the tympanic ring and that the mastoid air cells communicate with the tympanic cavity. He it was who first suggested the theory of hearing later developed by, and accredited to, Helmholtz. English translation, 1737. See also *A bibliography of editions of Du Verney's Traité ... published between 1683 and 1750,* compiled by N. Asherson, *J. Laryng. Otol.,* 1979, Suppl. No. 2, and book-form edition, London, *H. K. Lewis,* 1979.

1545.1 SCHELHAMMER, GUNTHER CHRISTOPHER. 1649-1712
De auditu liber unus. Lugduni Batavorum, *P. de Graaf,* 1684.
  An early account of the anatomy, physics and physiology of hearing, preceded by a historical summary of earlier work.

1546 VALSALVA, ANTONIO MARIA. 1666-1723
De aure humana tractatus. Bononiae, *typ. C. Pisarii,* 1704.
  Valsalva, a pupil of Malpighi and teacher of Morgagni, is best remembered for his work upon the ear, in which he described and depicted its most minute muscles and nerves. He divided the ear into "external", "middle", and "internal"; his method of inflating the middle ear (Valsalva's manoeuvre) is still practised. The book includes a description of "Valsalva's dysphagia".

1547 CASSEBOHM, JOHANN FRIEDRICH. 1699?-1743
Tractatus quatuor anatomici de aure humana. Tractatus quintus anatomicus de aure humana. Cui accedit tractatus sextus de aure monstri humani. Halae Magdeburgi, *sumtibus Orphanotrophei,* 1734-35.
  Important tracts on the anatomy and physiology of the ear. See No. 469.1.

1548   PYL, THEODOR.
Dissertatio medica de auditu in genere et de illo que fit per os in specie. Gryphiswald, 1742.

       Pyl was the first (page 20) to record the labyrinthine fluid and to discuss its rôle in the transmission of sound.

1549   COTUGNO, DOMENICO [COTUNNIUS]. 1736-1822
De aquaeductibus auris humanae internae. Neapoli, *ex typ. Simoniana,* 1761.

       Cotugno is sometimes accredited with the discovery of the "liquor Cotunnii", the labyrinthine fluid, first noted by Pyl in 1742. He did, however, make important contributions to the knowledge on the structure and function of the ear, including the discovery of the aural aqueducts. The naso-palatine nerve and the columns in the osseous spiral lamina are named after him.

1550   SCARPA, ANTONIO. 1752-1832
De structura fenestrae rotundae auris, et de tympano secundario anatomicae observationes. Mutinae, *apud Soc. typog.,* 1772.

       Scarpa's first scientific work, a comparative anatomical investigation of the ear, in which he offered a more accurate and complete description of the osseous labyrinth and demonstrated the true function of the round window. *See also* No. 1553.

1551   GEOFFROY, E:TIENNE LOUIS, *le comte.* 1725-1810
Dissertations sur l'organe de l'ouie. 1. De l'homme. 2. Des reptiles. 3. Des poissons. Amsterdam & Paris, *Cavelier,* 1778.

1552   COMPARETTI, ANDREA. 1746-1801
Observationes anatomicae de aure interna comparata. Patavii, *S. Bartholomaeus,* 1789.

1553   SCARPA, ANTONIO. 1752-1832
De penitiori ossium structura commentarius. Lipsiae, *J. F. Hartknoch,* 1799.

1554   SOEMMERRING, SAMUEL THOMAS. 1755-1830
Abbildungen des menschlichen Hoerorganes. Frankfort a.M., *Varrentrapp u. Wenner,* 1806.

1555   JACOBSON, LUDWIG LEVIN. 1783-1843
Supplementa ad otojatriam. Supplementum primum de anastomosi nervorum nova in aure detecta. *Acta. reg. Soc. Med. Havnien.,* 1818, **5,** 293-303.

       Jacobson described the tympanic canal, nerve, and plexus, all of which are named after him. In 1809 he discovered "Jacobson's organ", as reported two years later by G. Cuvier.

1556   WEBER, ERNST HEINRICH. 1795-1878
De aure et auditu hominis et animalium. Lipsiae, *apud G. Fleischerum,* 1820.

1556.1 WHEATSTONE, *Sir* CHARLES. 1802-1875
Experiments on audition. *Quart. J. Sci. Lit. Arts,* 1827, **24,** 67-72.
Occlusion effect on sound perception.

1557 FLOURENS, MARIE JEAN PIERRE. 1794-1867
Expériences sur les canaux semi-circulaires de l'oreille chez les oiseaux.
Ann. sci. nat., 1828, **15,** 113-24.
Flourens showed that lesion of the semicircular canals produces motor
incoordination and loss of equilibrium. Menière based his work (No. 3372)
on Flourens's crucial experiments.

1558 SHRAPNELL, HENRY JONES. *d.* 1834
On the form and structure of the membrana tympani. *Lond. med. Gaz.,*
1832, **10,** 120-24.
Description of the pars flaccida ("Shrapnell's membrane") of the tympanic membrane.

1559 CORTI, ALFONSO, *Marchese.* 1822-1888
Recherches sur l'organe de l'ouïe des mammifères. *Z. wiss. Zool.,* 1851, **3,**
109-69.
Corti made important investigations on the finer anatomy of the
mammalian cochlea. The "organ of Corti" in the cochlea is named after
him.

1560 REISSNER, ERNST. 1824-1878
De auris internae formatione. Dorpati Livonorum, *H. Laakmann,* 1851.
Description of the vestibular membrane ("Reissner's membrane").

1561 SCHULTZE, MAXIMILIAN JOHANN SIGISMUND. 1825-1874
Ueber die Endigungsweise des Hörnerven im Labyrinth. *Arch. Anat. Physiol.
wiss. Med.,* 1858, 343-81.
Schultze's great monographs on the nerve-endings of the sense organs
were of prime importance in the development of the science of histology.
Besides that dealing with the internal ear, he wrote others dealing with the
nose and the retina. *See* Nos. 936, 1512.

1562 HELMHOLTZ, HERMANN LUDWIG FERDINAND VON. 1821-1894
Die Lehre von der Tonempfindungen als physiologische Grundlage für die
Theorie der Musik. Braunschweig, *F. Vieweg u. Sohn,* 1863.
Helmholtz's theory of hearing, upon which all modern theories of
resonance are based. This exhaustive study of acoustics ranks as one of the
greatest books on the subject and shows that Helmholtz was, besides being
a great physicist and physician, an accomplished musician. English
translation of 3rd edition, London, 1875.

1563 ———. Die Mechanik der Gehörknöchelchen und des Trommelfells. *Pflügers
Arch. ges. Physiol.* 1868, **1,** 1-60. .
Helmholtz's study of the mechanism of the tympanum and ossicles of
the middle ear did much to elucidate the phenomenon of audition. It
includes a description of "Helmholtz's ligament" of the malleus. Separate
offprint, Bonn, 1869. English translation, London, 1873.

1564 GOLTZ, FRIEDRICH LEOPOLD. 1834-1902
Ueber die physiologische Bedeutung der Bogengänge des Ohrlabyrinths.
Pflüg. Arch. ges. Physiol., 1870, **3**, 172-92.
  Goltz demonstrated the relation of vertigo and vestibular disturbance,
showing that the former is a result of disease or irritation of the semicircular
canals.

1566 RETZIUS, MAGNUS GUSTAF. 1842-1919
Das Gehörorgan der Wirbelthiere. 2 vols. Stockholm, *Samson & Wallin,*
1881-84.
  The most magnificent of all comparative anatomical studies of the ear,
and the most beautiful studies of the ear after those of Casseri (No.1540).
Retzius described the "Retzius bodies" in the labyrinth.

1567 STEIN, STANISLAV ALEKSANDR FYODOROVICH. 1855-
Die Lehren von den Funktionen der einzelnen Theile des Ohrlabyrinths.
Jena, *G. Fischer,* 1894.
  Stein studied the functions of separate parts of the labyrinth. This is a
translation from the Russian.

1568 EWALD, ERNST JULIUS RICHARD. 1855-1921
Zur Physiologie des Labyrinths. 3. Mittheilung. Das Hören der labyrinthlosen
Tauben. *Pflüg. Arch. ges. Physiol.*, 1894, **59**, 258-75.

1569 ——. Zur Physiologie des Labyrinths. 4. Mittheilung. Die Beziehungen des
Grosshirns zum Tonuslabyrinth. *Pflüg. Arch. ges. Physiol.*, 1895, **60**, 492-
508.

1569.1 BEAUREGARD, EMMANUEL HENRI. 1851-1900, & DUPUY, PIERRE EDMOND.
1855-1904
Note sur la variation éléctrique (courant d'action) déterminée dans le nerf
acoustique par le son. *C. R. Soc. Biol. (Paris),* 1896, **48**, 690-92.
  Beauregard and Dupuy recorded the action potential in the auditory
nerve of the frog.

1569.2 GRAY, ALBERT ALEXANDER. 1869-1936
The labyrinth of animals. 2 vols., London, *Churchill,* 1907-08.
  "An important and elaborate work designed to give the anatomy of the
labyrinth, or inside of the ears of vertebrates, with the exception of fishes"
(Casey Wood). Illustrated with stereoscopic photographs.

1570 WILKINSON, GEORGE. 1867-1956, & GRAY, ALBERT ALEXANDER. 1869-1936
The mechanism of the cochlea. A restatement of the resonance theory of
hearing. London, *Macmillan & Co.,* 1924.

1570.1 BÉKÉSY, GEORG VON. 1899-1972
Über den Knall und die Theorie des Hörens. *Phys. Z.,* 1933, **34**, 577-82.
  In 1961 Békésy was awarded a Nobel Prize for his discoveries concerning
the physical mechanisms of stimulation within the cochlea. English
translation in Békésy, *Experiments in hearing,* 1960.

1571   DALTON, JOHN CALL. 1825-1889
The experimental method in medical science. New York, *G. P. Putnam's Sons,* 1882.
    Dalton, Professor of Physiology at the universities of Buffalo and Vermont, and the College of Physicians and Surgeons, New York, was the first American to devote his time exclusively to that subject. He was present at the first demonstration of ether as an anaesthetic, Oct 16, 1846, and was quick to see its possibilities as a means of illustrating his lectures with experiments on living animals. As a result of the opposition to this method of teaching he published the above book. Reprint, New York, 1980.

1572   ——. Doctrines of the circulation. Philadelphia, *H. C. Lea's Son & Co.,* 1884.

1573   MARCET, WILLIAM. 1829-1900
A contribution to the history of the respiration of man. London, *J. & A. Churchill,* 1897.

1574   NEUBURGER, MAX. 1868-1955
Die historische Entwicklung der experimentellen Gehirn- und Rückenmarksphysiologie vor Flourens. Stuttgart, *F. Enke,* 1897.
    Unsurpassed coverage of the experimental physiology of the brain and spinal cord up to the work of Flourens. The best edition is the extensively annotated English translation by E. S. Clarke, Baltimore, *Johns Hopkins University Press,* 1981.

1574.1 SOURY, JULES. 1842-1915
Le système nerveux centrale structure et fonctions. Histoire critique des théories et des doctrines. 2 vols., Paris, *Carré & Naud,* 1899.
    Massive history of the anatomy and physiology of the nervous system from ancient Greece to the end of the 19th century, limited in its historical analysis. The second volume is a survey of end of 19th century opinions on the structure and function of the nervous system.

1575   FOSTER, *Sir* MICHAEL. 1836-1907
Lectures on the history of physiology. Cambridge, *Univ. Press,* 1901.
    Reprinted 1924 and (*Dover Pubs.*), 1970.

1576   STIRLING, WILLIAM. 1851-1932
Some apostles of physiology. London, *Waterlow & Sons,* 1902.
    Well illustrated, and finely printed, but dated history, by a pupil of Ludwig. *See* No. 629.

1577   FEARING, FRANKLIN. 1892-
Reflex action. A study in the history of physiological psychology. Baltimore, *Williams & Wilkins,* 1930.
    Reprinted, New York, *Hafner,* 1964.

1580   CANNON, WALTER BRADFORD. 1871-1945
The story of the development of our ideas of chemical mediation of nerve impulses. *Amer. J. med. Sci.,* 1934, **188,** 145-59.

1581   LIEBEN, Fritz. 1890-1966
        Geschichte der physiologischen Chemie. Leipzig, *Deuticke,* 1935.
        Reprinted, Hildesheim, 1970.

1583   FRANKLIN, Kenneth James. 1897-1966
        A short history of physiology. 2nd ed. London, *Staples Press,* 1949.

1584   BASTHOLM, Egvind Borge Martin Marius. 1904-
        The history of muscle physiology from the natural philosophers to Albrecht
        von Haller. Copenhagen, *Munksgaard,* 1950.
        Acta Historica Scientiarum Naturalium et Medicinalium, Vol. 7.

1586   POYNTER, Frederick Noel Lawrence. 1908-1979
        The history and philosophy of knowledge of the brain and its functions: an
        Anglo-American symposium. Edited by F. N. L. Poynter. Oxford, *Blackwell,*
        1958.

1586.1 BROOKS. Chandler McCuskey. 1905- , & CRANEFIELD, Paul Frederick.
        1925-
        The historical development of physiological thought. New York, *Hafner,*
        1959.

1587   LIDDELL, Edward George Tandy. 1895-1981
        The discovery of the reflexes. Oxford, *Clarendon Press,* 1960.

1588   BÖTTCHER, Helmuth Maximilian. 1895-
        Hormone: Die Geschichte der Hormonforschung. Köln, *Kiepenheuer &
        Witsch,* 1963.

1588.1 FISHMAN, Alfred Paul. 1918- , & RICHARDS, Dickinson Woodruff. 1895-
        1973
        Circulation of the blood: men and ideas. New York, *Oxford University Press,*
        1964. Reprint, Bethesda, 1982.

1588.2 FULTON, John Farquhar. 1899-1960
        Selected readings in the history of physiology. Compiled by John F. Fulton,
        completed by Leonard G. Wilson. Springfield, *C. C. Thomas,* 2nd ed., 1966.
            These readings extend from Aristotle to contemporary writers; they
        give access to many classical works that might otherwise be unobtainable
        to students of the history of physiology. Foreign material is translated into
        English. First edition 1930.

1588.3 KEILIN, David. 1887-1963
        The history of cell respiration and cytochrome, edited by Joan Keilin,
        Cambridge, *Cambridge University Press,* 1966.
            See No. 968.

1588.4 CLARKE, Edwin Sisterson. 1919- & O'MALLEY, Charles Donald. 1907-1970
        The human brain and spinal cord. A historical study illustrated by writings
        from antiquity to the twentieth century. Berkeley, *University of California
        Press,* 1968.

Massive anthology of primary source material on neuroanatomy and neurophysiology. Excellent commentaries and bibliographies.

1588.5   RAPP, D.
Die Entwicklung der physiologischen Methodik von 1784 bis 1911. Eine qualitative Untersuchung. Münster, *Inst. Gesch. d. Med.,* 1970.

1588.6   HALL, Thomas Steele. 1909-
Ideas of life and matter; studies in the history of general physiology 600 b.c. to a.d. 1900. 2 vols. Chicago, *University of Chicago Press,* 1969.

1588.7   YOUNG, Robert M.
Mind, brain and adaptation in the nineteenth century. Cerebral localization and its biological context from Gall to Ferrier. Oxford, *Clarendon Press,* 1970.

1588.8   MEYER, Alfred.
Historical aspects of cerebral anatomy. London, *Oxford University Press,* 1971.
A highly detailed, very technical, but well-documented study.

1588.9   CLARKE, Edwin Sisterson. 1919- , & DEWHURST, Kenneth Eastham. 1919-1985
An illustrated history of brain function. Oxford, *Sandford Pubs.,* 1972.

1588.10   FLORKIN, Marcel. 1900-1979
A history of biochemistry. 5 vols. Amsterdam, *Elsevier,* 1972-
Forms vols. 30-34 of *Comprehensive biochemistry,* edited by M. Florkin and E. H. Stotz.

1588.11   NEEDHAM, Dorothy Mary Moyle. 1896-1988
Machina carnis: the biochemistry of muscular contraction in its historical development. Cambridge, *University Press,* 1972.
A definitive history of the development of knowledge on muscle biochemistry; valuable bibliography.

1588.12   ROTHSCHUH, Karl Eduard. 1908-1984
History of physiology. Translated and edited, with a new English bibliography, by G. B. Risse. Huntington, N.Y., *Krieger Publishing Co.,* 1973.
A revised and expanded translation of *Geschichte der Physiologie,* Berlin, 1953.

1588.13   HARRIS, C.R.S.
The heart and the vascular system in ancient Greek medicine from Alcmaeon to Galen. Oxford, *Clarendon Press,* 1973.

1588.14   CRANEFIELD, Paul Frederick. 1925-
The way in and the way out. François Magendie, Charles Bell and the roots of the spinal nerves. With a facsimile of Charles Bell's annotated copy of his Idea of a new anatomy of the brain. Mount Kisco, N.Y., *Futura Publishing,* 1974.
An annotated bibliography of the literature documenting the history of this controversy together with reproductions of the texts of the crucial papers. *See* Nos. 1254-1259.

1588.15 WORDEN, FREDERIC GARFIELD. 1918- , *et al.*
The neurosciences: paths to discovery. Cambridge, Mass., *Massachusetts Institute of Technology,* 1975.
Thirty-one contributions to a symposium in honour of F. O. Schmitt. Edited by Worden, J. P. Swazey and G. Adelman.

1588.16 WEST, JOHN B. 1928-
Translations in respiratory physiology. Edited by John B. West. Stroudsberg, PA, *Dowden, Hutchinson & Ross,* [1975].
English translations of 22 classic papers (some quite lengthy) with introductions by various experts.

1588.17 FRANK, ROBERT G., JR.
Harvey and the Oxford physiologists. A study of scientific ideas. Berkeley, *Univ. of California Press,* 1980.

1588.18 FRUTON, JOSEPH STEWART. 1912-
A bio-bibliography for the history of the biochemical sciences since 1800. Philadelphia, *American Philosphical Society,* 1982.
An index to bio-bibliographical articles listed alphabetically by scientist. Supplement published, Philadelphia, 1985.

1588.19 BRAZIER, MARY AGNES BURNISTON. 1904-
A history of neurophysiology in the 17th and 18th centuries. From concept to experiment. A history of neurophysiology in the 19th century. 2 vols., New York, *Raven Press,* [1983-88].

1588.20 LESCH, JOHN E.
Science and medicine in France. The emergence of experimental physiology, 1790-1855. Cambridge, Mass., *Harvard Univ. Press,* 1984.

1588.21 JEANNEROD, MARC.
The brain machine: The development of neurophysiological thought. Cambridge, Mass., *Harvard University Press,* 1985.
Translation of *Le cerveau-machine: physiologie de la volonté,* Paris, 1983.

1588.22 ASTROUP, POUL. 1915-, & SEVERINGHAUS, JOHN W. 1922-
The history of blood gases, acids and bases. Copenhagen, *Munksgaard,* 1986.
The authors are prominent investigators in the field.

1588.23 GOTTSCHALK, CARL W. 1922- , BERLINER, ROBERT W. 1915-, & GIEBISCH, GERHARD H. 1927- (Eds.)
Renal physiology: People and ideas. Bethesda, *American Physiological Society,* [1987].
A collective work on the history of renal physiology with thematic chapters by the editors and other prominent investigators.

1588.24 CLARKE, EDWIN SISTERSON. 1919- , & JACYNA, L.S.
Nineteenth century origins of neuroscientific concepts. Berkeley, *University of California Press,* 1987.
Detailed analysis, emphasizing first half of 19th century, with detailed bibliographies, and bibliographical notes.

STATE MEDICINE: PUBLIC HEALTH: GERIATRICS: HYGIENE

1589   FRONTINUS, Sextus Julius. A.D. 35-104
The two books on the water supply of the city of Rome of Sextus Julius
Frontinus, water commissioner of the city of Rome, A.D. 97. A photographic
reproduction of the sole original Latin manuscript and its reprint in Latin;
also, a translation into English, and explanatory chapters by Clemens
Herschel. Boston, *Dana, Estes & Co.,* 1899.
The *De aquis urbis Romae* of Frontinus gives a history and description
of the water supply of ancient Rome, and the laws governing its use and
maintenance.

1589.1   ZERBI, Gabriele. 1485-1505
[Gerontocomia.] [Rome, *Eucharius Silber,* alias Franck, 1489.]
The first printed book on geriatrics – a guide to the proper hygiene,
physical and mental, as well as particularly to the diet of the aged, Zerbi was
the founder of the science of geriatrics. English translation by L.R. Lind,
Philadelphia, *American Philosophical Society,* 1988. *See also* Nos. 363.4
and 1758.1.

1590   PHAER, Thomas [Phayer; Phayr]. 1510-1560
A new booke entyteled the regiment of lyfe. London, *E. Whytchurch,* 1544.
Translation of a book by Jehan Goeurot published in 1530. Garrison
states that it is a version of the *Regimen Sanitatis.*

1591   BOORDE, Andrew [Borde]. ?1490-1549
The breviary of helthe, for all manner of syckenesses and diseases the
whiche may be in man, or woman doth folowe. London, *W. Middleton,*
1547.
This, probably the earliest "modern" work on hygiene, throws some
light on the condition of that subject in the 16th century.

1592   CORNARO, Luigi. 1467-1566
Trattato de la vita sobria. Padova, *G. Perchacino,* 1558.
Garrison considers this "the best treatise on personal hygiene and the
simple life in existence". Cornaro was called the Apostle of Senescence. A
good English edition was published in 1903.

1594   HARINGTON, *Sir* John. 1560-1612
A new discourse of a stale subject, called the Metamorphosis of Aiax.
Written by Misacmos to his friend Philostilpnos. London, *R. Field,* 1596.
Harington invented a water-closet in which the disposal of excreta was
for the first time controlled by mechanical means. He published several
tracts on the device, the first appearing in 1596. These were elegantly
reprinted by the Chiswick Press in an edition limited to 100 copies (1814).
"Ajax" is a pun on "a jakes", an Elizabethan name for a privy. Critical,
annotated edition by E. S. Donno, New York, *Columbia Univ. Press,* 1962.

1595   FLOYER, *Sir* John. 1649-1734
Medicina gerocomica; or the Galenic art of preserving old men's healths.
London, *F. Isted,* 1724.
First English book devoted to geriatrics.

1596   HALES, Stephen. 1677-1761
A description of ventilators. London, *W. Innys,* 1743.
Hales devised a ventilator, by means of which fresh air could be introduced into gaols, mines, hospitals, the holds of ships, etc. The invention met with immediate approval and contributed much towards health of those for whom it was employed. Hales was the inventor of artificial ventilation.

1597   TISSOT, Simon André. 1728-1797
Avis au peuple sur la santé. Lausanne, *J. Zimmerli pour F. Grasset,* 1761.
A tract on medicine written for the lay public; it ran through several editions and was translated into all European languages. English translation in 1765.

1598   HOWARD, John. 1726-1790
The state of the prisons in England and Wales. Warrington, *W. Eyres,* 1777.
Howard devoted much of his life to the improvement of the conditions then prevailing in prisons. The publication of his book led to legislation abolishing abuses in prisons and providing for their proper cleaning. The Howard League for Penal Reform is one result of his charitable work. Reprint of 4th ed. (1792), Montclair, N.Y., 1973. See L. Baumgartner, John Howard (1726-1790) hospital and prison reformer: a bibliography. *Bull. Hist. Med.,* 1939, **7**, 486-534, 595-626.

1599   FRANK, Johann Peter. 1745-1821
System einer vollständigen medicinischen Polizey. 9 vols. Mannheim, Tübingen, Wien, 1779-1827.
First systematic treatise on public hygiene. In his classic work, Frank, the "Father of Public Hygiene", considered the ruler of a state to stand in the relation of a father to his children, among his duties being the safeguarding of the people's health and the preservation of a healthy race by appropriate laws. The last two volumes were edited by G. C. G. Voigt. Selections from an English translation, with introduction by Erna Lesky, was published by the Johns Hopkins Press, Baltimore, 1976.

1600   TENON, Jacques René. 1724-1816
Mémoires sur les hôpitaux de Paris. Paris, *P. D. Pierres,* 1788.
Reforms quickly followed Tenon's disclosures of the dreadful conditions prevailing in the hospitals of Paris in the 18th century. He was also instrumental in the foundation of a special hospital for children.

1601   HOWARD, John. 1726-1790
An account of the principle lazarettos in Europe. Warrington, *T. Cadell,* 1789.
Following on his work for the improvement of the conditions in prisons, Howard travelled extensively in Europe, carrying out an elaborate investigation into the conditions of hospitals. Reprint of 2nd ed. (1791), Montclair, N.Y., 1973.

1601.1   DAZILLE, Jean B.D. 1732-1812
Observations sur les maladies des nègres...2 vols., Paris, *l'Auteur,* 1792.
A pioneer study of the health conditions and diseases of black slaves in the Americas, perhaps the first of its kind. The first edition (1776) did not include the second volume.

1602   HUFELAND, Christoph Wilhelm. 1762-1836
Die Kunst das menschliche Leben zu verlängern, Jena, *Akad. Buchhandlung,* 1797.
    Hufeland's "Makrobiotik", one of the most popular books of its time on personal hygiene. It was translated into all European languages. Hufeland was court physician at Weimar. English translation, 1797.

1602.1   SINCLAIR, *Sir* John. 1754-1835
The code of health and longevity; or, a concise view of the principles calculated for the preservation of health, and the attainment of long life. 4 vols., Edinburgh, *A. Constable & Co.,* 1807.
    One of the most comprehensive works on gerontology ever written, with a bibliography of 1800 references, supplemented by abstracts, translated excerpts from ancient authors, national data, etc.

1603   ROBERTON, John.
A treatise on medical police. 2 vols. Edinburgh, *J. Moir,* 1809.
    First notable work on the subject in English.

1604   WELLS, William Charles. 1757-1817
An essay on dew. London, *Taylor & Hessay,* 1814.
    For this important work, Wells was awarded the Rumford Medal of the Royal Society. His researches on the subject were of major importance in the development of the science of ventilation, particularly in its relation to relative humidity and the influence of the latter on the comfort of the occupants of factories, ships, theatres, etc. Wells was physician to St. Thomas's Hospital, London, from 1800 until his death.

1604.1   CARLISLE, *Sir* Anthony. 1868-1840
An essay on the disorders of old age, and on the means of prolonging life. London, *Longmans,* 1817.
    Carlisle, a distinguished surgeon and anatomist, advised young people to adopt a sound regimen early in life in order to secure longevity. Addressing himself directly to old people he described diseases common to the elderly and paid particular attention to the problems of performing surgical operations on the aged.

1604.2   ACCUM, Friedrich. 1769-1838
A treatise on the adulterations of food. London, *Longman,* 1820.
    One of the earliest exposures of food adulteration. This sensational but scientific work embroiled the author in such scandal that he finally had to flee England.

1605   FODÉRÉ, François Emmanuel. 1764-1835
Leçons sur les épidémies et l'hygiène publique. 4 vols. Paris, *F. G. Vevrault,* 1822-24.

1605.1   CANSTATT, Carl Friedrich. 1807-1850
Die Krankheiten des höhren Alters und ihre Heilung. 2 vols. Erlangen, *Enke,* 1839.
    Canstatt's book is one of the most important in the history of geriatrics, summarizing all previous work on the subject. Canstatt himself only lived to the age of 43.

1606   PARENT-DUCHÂTELET, ALEXANDRE JEAN BAPTISTE. 1790-1836
Hygiène publique. 2 vols. Paris, *J. B. Baillière*, 1836.

1607   ——. De la prostitution dans la ville de Paris. 2 vols. Paris, *J. B. Baillière*, 1836.

1608   CHADWICK, *Sir* EDWIN. 1800-1890
Report ... from the Poor Law Commissioners on an inquiry into the sanitary conditions of the labouring population of Great Britain. London, *W. Clowes & Sons*, 1842.

Chadwick devoted his life to social reform. He was secretary to the Poor Law Commission when he made the above report to Parliament. In it he included a careful analysis of causes of death in 1838 and 1839 and gave a vivid picture of insanitary conditions in England and Wales. The complete report was issued in 3 vols. in 1842 (though the 2nd and 3rd volumes are infrequently found) plus a supplementary summary volume published in 1843. As a result of this and an earlier (1833) report, the foundations of later systems of government inspection were laid, a Public Health Act was passed (1848) and a General Board of Health was established. Reprinted, Edinburgh, 1965. *See also* No. 1625.

1609   SHATTUCK, LEMUEL. 1793-1859
Report of a general plan for the promotion of public and personal health, devised, prepared, and recommended by the commissioners appointed under a resolve of the legislature of Massachusetts relating to a sanitary survey of the State. Boston, *Dutton & Wentworth*, 1850.

Compiled by a team, but entirely written by Shattuck, this report was the first general blueprint for the promotion of public health presented to an American governmental body. Its first proposal was for the creation of state and local boards of health in an era when such state commissions were non-existent. A Board of Health was not set up until 1869, however. Shattuck has been called "the Chadwick of America". An abridged version of this famous Report appears in G. C. Whipple's *State sanitation*, Cambridge, [Mass.], 1917; a facsimile reproduction was published in 1948.

1610   CHEVALLIER, JEAN BAPTISTE ALPHONSE. 1793-1879
Dictionnaire des altérations et falsifications des substances alimentaires, médicamenteuses et commerciales. 2 vols. Paris, *Béchet jeune*, 1850.

Chevallier, a chemist, was a prolific writer. Above is probably his most important publication.

1610.1   INTERNATIONAL SANITARY CONFERENCE.
Procès-verbaux de la conférence sanitaire internationale ouverte à Paris le 27 juillet 1851. Paris, *Imprimerie Nationale*, 1852.

First international sanitary conference; it prepared an international sanitary code dealing with cholera, plague, and yellow fever.

1611   NIGHTINGALE, FLORENCE. 1820-1910
Notes on hospitals. London, *John W. Parker & Son*, 1859.

Includes four plans of hospitals. A third edition, completely revised, was published by Longmans, Green & Co., London, 1863.

1612   ——. Notes on nursing: what it is, and what it is not. London, *Harrison & Sons*, [1860].

After receiving training in Germany and France, Florence Nightingale had some nursing experience in England. The Crimean war gave her an opportunity to demonstrate the value of trained nurses. Within a few months of her arrival at Scutari, the mortality rate among soldiers there fell from 42% to 2%. Florence Nightingale lived to become the greatest figure in the history of nursing. Facsimile reproduction (? of first edition), Philadelphia, 1946. Biographies by Sir E. T. Cook, 1913, and Cecil Woodham-Smith, 1950. See also *Bio-bibliography of Florence Nightingale,* by W. J. Bishop & S. Goldie, 1962.

1613   PETTENKOFER, MAX JOSEF VON. 1818-1901
Ueber eine Methode die Kohlensäure in der atmosphärischen Luft zu bestimmen. *J. prakt. Chem.,* 1862, **85,** 165-84.
Pettenkofer was the founder of experimental hygiene; he was the first to institute a laboratory for hygienic investigation.

1614   PARKES, EDMUND ALEXANDER. 1819-1876
A manual of practical hygiene. London, *John Churchill & Sons,* 1864.
First important English treatise on hygiene.

1615   BAZALGETTE, *Sir* JOSEPH WILLIAM. 1819-1891
Metropolitan Board of Works Report on experiments with respect to the ventilation of sewers. 3 parts. London, *Brickhill & Bateman,* [1866-69].
Bazalgette planned the sewers of London.

1616   VIRCHOW, RUDOLF LUDWIG KARL. 1821-1902
Ueber die Canalisation von Berlin. *Vjschr. gerichtl. öff. Med.,* 1868, n.F. **9,** 1-43.
Virchow advocated a canal sewer system for Berlin. Such a system was constructed by Hobrecht. *See* No. 1624.

1617   ———. Ueber gewisse, die Gesundheit benachtheiligende Einflüsse der Schulen. *Virchows Arch. path. Anat.,* 1869, **46,** 447-70.
Improvements in school hygiene and the regular inspection of school children were brought about by the efforts of Virchow. English translation, New York, 1871. Virchow's papers on public health were collected, annotated, and translated into English by L.J.Rather as *Collected essays on public health and epidemiology,* 2 vols., [Canton, Mass.,1985].

1618   PETTENKOFER, MAX JOSEF VON. 1818-1901
Das Kanal- oder Siel-System in München. München, *H. Manz,* 1869.
Pettenkofer was responsible for the installation of the modern system of sewage disposal in Munich, and thus succeeded in almost completely ridding that city of typhoid.

1619   LISTER, JOSEPH. 1*st Baron Lister.* 1827-1912
On the effects of the antiseptic system of treatment upon the salubrity of a surgical hospital. *Lancet,* 1870, **1,** 4-6, 40-42.

1620   BELGRAND, MARIE FRANÇOIS EUGÈNE. 1810-1878
La Seine. Etudes hydrologiques. Régime de la pluie, des sources, des eaux courantes. (Les travaux souterrains de Paris.) 4 vols. and atlas. Paris, *Vve. C. Dunod,* 1872-87.
Belgrand designed the Paris sewers.

1621   GALTON, *Sir* Douglas Strutt. 1822-1899
Observations on the construction of healthy dwellings. Oxford, *Clarendon Press,* 1880.
      Galton spent some years in the army; he had a variety of interests, chief among them being railways, education and sanitary science. He designed the Herbert Hospital at Woolwich and he invented a ventilating fire grate.

1622   COHN, Hermann Ludwig. 1838-1906
Die Hygiene des Auges in den Schulen. Wien, Leipzig, *Urban & Schwarzenberg,* 1883.
      Cohn did much to promote school hygiene. He advocated regular examination of the eyes of school children, an idea which was put into practice in 1885. An English translation of the book appeared in 1886.

1623   BOLTON, *Sir* Francis John. 1831-1887
London water supply, including a history and description of the London waterworks. London, *W. Clowes,* 1884.

1624   HORBRECHT, James. 1825-1902
Die Canalisation von Berlin. Berlin, *Ernst u. Korn,* 1884.
      Hobrecht was responsible for the construction of the Berlin sewers.

1625   RICHARDSON, *Sir* Benjamin Ward. 1828-1896
The health of nations. A review of the works of Edwin Chadwick. 2 vols. London, *Longmans, Green & Co.,* 1887.
      Chadwick may be said to have initiated the public health era. Largely through his efforts the Public Health Act 1848 came into existence in England. He was the greatest sanitarian of the 19th century; among other things he was responsible for the introduction of glazed earthenware pipes for drains. See also R. A. Lewis's *Edwin Chadwick and the public health movement, 1832-54,* London, 1952. Facsimile reprint, 1965.

1626   SIMON, *Sir* John. 1816-1904
Public health reports. 2 vols. London, *J. A. Churchill,* 1887.
      Simon was the first medical officer for the City of London. Together with his *English sanitary institutions,* the above work played a great part in paving the way for modern reforms in the sphere of hygiene and public health. Next to Chadwick, Simon was the greatest sanitary reformer of the 19th century. *See also* No. 1650. Biography by R. Lambert, 1963.

1627   BILLINGS, John Shaw. 1838-1913
Description of the Johns Hopkins Hospital. Baltimore, *I. Friedenwald,* 1890.
      Billings was responsible for the designing of the Johns Hopkins Hospital, Baltimore. "It marked a new departure in hospital construction...It was the most perfect and best equipped institution of its time" (Kelly & Burrage).

1628   BURDETT, *Sir* Henry Charles. 1847-1920
Hospitals and asylums of the world. 4 vols. and atlas. London, *J. & A. Churchill,* 1891-93.
      This great work deals with the history, administration, and planning of hospitals, and includes a bibliography.

1629   STEVENSON, *Sir* Thomas. 1838-1908, & MURPHY, Shirley Foster. 1849-1923
A treatise on hygiene and public health. Edited by T. Stevenson and S. F.
Murphy. 3 vols. London, *J. & A. Churchill,* 1892-94.
A co-operative work.

1631   DIBDIN, William Joseph. 1850-1925
The purification of sewage and water. London, *Sanitary Publ. Co.,* 1897.
    Dibdin introduced the bacterial system of sewage purification. Previously he had devised the contact system.

1632   STODDART, Frederick Wallis. 1860-1917
Some points in the construction of the continuous sewage filter. *Proc. incorp.
Ass. munic. County Engrs,* 1901, **28,** 278-90.

1633   GREAT BRITAIN. *Parliament.*
Royal Commission on sewage disposal. Reports 1-8. London, *Eyre &
Spottiswoode,* 1902-12.

1634   CALMETTE, Leon Charles Albert. 1863-1933
Recherches sur l'épuration biologique et chimique des eaux d'égout. 8
vols. Paris, *Masson & Cie.,* 1905-08.

1635   FOREL, Auguste Henri. 1848-1931
Die sexuelle Frage. München, *E. Reinhardt,* 1905.
    Forel's best work; translated into 16 languages; 16th edition in 1931.

1636   WASSERMANN, August von. 1866-1925
Die Bedeutung der Bakterien für die Gesundheitspflege. München, *R.
Oldenbourg,* 1905.

1637   WINSLOW, Charles-Edward Amory. 1877-1957, & PHELPS, Earle Bernard.
1876-
Investigation on the purification of Boston sewage, with a history of the
sewage-disposal problem. Washington, *Govt. Printing Office,* 1906.

1638   HENRI, Victor, *et al.*
Stérilisation de grandes quantités d'eau par les rayons ultraviolets. *C. R.
Acad. Sci. (Paris),* 1910, **150,** 932-34; **151,** 677-80.
    With A. Helbronner and M. de Recklinghausen.

1639   RUBNER, Max. 1854-1932, *et al.*
Handbuch der Hygiene. 6 vols. Leipzig, *S. Hirtzel,* 1911-13.
    With Max Gruber and P. M. Ficker.

1640   FOWLER, Gilbert John. 1868-1953
Sewage disposal by oxidation methods. Trans. XV. Int. Congr. Hyg.
Demog., 1912, Washington, 1913, **4,** 375-83.

1641   ROSENAU, Milton Joseph. 1869-1946
Preventive medicine and hygiene. New York, *D. Appleton & Co.,* 1913.
    6th edition, 1935.

1641.1   NASCHER, IGNATZ LEO. 1863-1944
          Geriatrics: The diseases of old age and their treatment, including physi-
          ological old age, home and institutional care, and medico-legal relations.
          Philadelphia, *P. Blakiston's Sons,* 1914.
               The first modern treatise on the subject. Nascher coined the term
          "geriatrics" in a paper of that name in *N.Y. med. J.,* 1909, **90,** 358-59.

1641.2   STOPES, MARIE CHARLOTTE CARMICHAEL. 1880-1958
          Contraception (birth control). Its theory, history and practice. A manual for
          the medical and legal professions. London, *John Bale,* 1923.
               The first important English handbook on birth control.

1642   IMHOFF, KARL. 1876-
          Fortschritte de Abwasserreinigung. Berlin, 1925.
               In 1909 Imhoff devised the system of sewage purification which bears
          his name.

History of State Medicine, Public Health, Geriatrics, and Hygiene

1646   VIOLLET LE DUC, EUGÈNE EMMANUEL. 1814-1879
          Histoire de l'habitation humaine. Paris, 1875.

1647   UFFELMANN, JULIUS AUGUST CHRISTIAN. 1837-1894
          Die öffentliche Hygiene im alten Rom. Berlin, 1881.

1648   FORT, GEORGE FRANKLIN.
          Medical economy during the Middle Ages; a contribution to the history of
          European morals, from the time of the Roman Empire to the close of the
          14th century. New York, *J. W. Bouton,* 1883.

1650   KOTELMANN, LUDWIG WILHELM JOHANNES. 1839-1908
          Gesundheitspflege im Mittelalter. Hamburg, Leipzig, *L. Voss,* 1890.

1650   SIMON, *Sir* JOHN. 1816-1904
          English sanitary institutions, reviewed in their course of development, and
          in some of their political and social relations. London, *Cassell & Co.,* 1890.
          One of the best accounts of the development of public health in Great
          Britain in the 19th century. It is a mine of information and greatly
          influenced modern developments and legislation on public health.

1651   RUBNER, MAX. 1854-1932
          Zur Vorgeschichte der modernen Hygiene. Berlin, *O. Francke,* 1905.

1652   DELAUNAY, HENRI. 1865-
          L'hygiène publique à travers les âges. Paris, *Vigot frères,* 1906.

1653   MORRIS, *Sir* MALCOLM ALEXANDER. 1849-1924
          The story of English public health. London, *Cassell & Co.,* 1919.

1654   RÁVENEL, MAZYCK PORCHER. 1861-1946
          A half-century of public health. Jubilee historical volume of the American
          Public Health Association. New York, *Amer. Publ. Health Assoc.,* 1921.

1654.1   LA CROIX, PAUL. 1806-1884
History of prostitution among all the peoples of the world, from the most remote antiquity to the present day. Translated from the original French by SAMUEL PUTNAM. 3 vols. Chicago, *Pascal Covici,* 1926.

1655   GARRISON, FIELDING HUDSON. 1870-1935
The history of heating, ventilation, and lighting. *Bull. N.Y. Acad. Med.,* 1927, 2 ser., **3,** 57-67.

1656   NEWSHOLME, *Sir* ARTHUR. 1857-1943
Evolution of preventive medicine. London, *Baillière, Tindall & Cox,* 1927.

1657   McCURRICH, HUGH JAMES. 1890-
The treatment of the sick poor of this country and the preservation of the health of the poor in this country. London, *Humphrey Milford,* 1929.

1657.1   NEWMAN, *Sir* GEORGE. 1870-1948
The rise of preventive medicine. London, *Oxford University Press,* 1932.

1658   WILLIAMS, JOHN HARGREAVES HARLEY. 1901-1974
A century of public health in Britain, 1832-1929. London, *A. & C. Black,* 1932.

1659   FILBY, FREDERICK A.
A history of food adulteration and analysis. London, *Allen & Unwin,* 1934.

1660   NEWSHOLME, *Sir* ARTHUR. 1857-1943
Fifty years in public health: a personal narrative with comments. London, *George Allen & Unwin,* (1935).

1661   ——. The last thirty years in public health. London, *Allen & Unwin,* 1936.

1662   HIMES, NORMAN EDWIN. 1899-1949
Medical history of contraception. Baltimore, *Williams & Wilkins,* 1936.
    Reprinted with updating preface, 1963, 1970.

1664   CANADIAN PUBLIC HEALTH ASSOCIATION.
The development of public health in Canada: a review of the history and organization of public health in the provinces of Canada, with an outline of the present organization of the National Health Section of the Department of Pensions and National Health, Canada. Edited by R. D. DEFRIES. Toronto, *Canad. Pub. Hlth. Assoc.,* 1940.

1664.1   CODMAN, ERNEST AMORY. 1869-1940
Study in hospital efficiency. [Boston, *Privately Printed,* 1916.]
    Pioneer application of efficiency engineering principles to hospital administration, made over a five year period. Codman was responsible for the "end result idea". This revolutionary concept, which seems so obvious today, was that a hospital should follow every patient it treats long enough to determine whether or not the treatment was successful. If the treatment was not successful the cause of failure should be determined in order to prevent similar failures in the future. Codman was exceptionally outspoken in his views. *See* No. 4400.5.

1665   REYNOLDS, REGINALD. 1905-
        Cleanliness and godliness. London, *Allen & Unwin,* 1943.
            A history of sewage disposal, the privy, and related matters.

1666   WINSLOW, CHARLES-EDWARD AMORY. 1877-1957
        The conquest of epidemic diseases. A chapter in the history of ideas.
        Princeton, *University Press,* 1943.
            Reprinted 1980.

1667   ROBINS, FREDERICK WILLIAM.
        The story of water supply. London, *Oxford University Press,* 1946.

1668   LEONARD, FRED EUGENE. 1866-1922
        A guide to the history of physical education. 3rd edition, revised and
        enlarged by GEORGE AFFLECK. Philadelphia, *Lea & Febiger,* 1947.

1669   FERGUSON, THOMAS. 1900-
        The dawn of Scottish social welfare. A survey from medieval times to 1863.
        London, *Nelson,* 1948.

1670   FRAZER, WILLIAM MOWLL. 1888-1958
        A history of English public health, 1834-1939. London, *Baillière, Tindall &
        Cox,* 1950.

1671   WILLIAMS, RALPH CHESTER. 1888-
        The United States Public Health Service, 1798-1950. Washington, *Com-
        missioned Officers Association of the United States Public Health Service,*
        1951.

1671.1 SAND, RENÉ. 1877-1953
        The advance to social medicine. London, *Staples Press,* 1952.
            Originally published in French, 1948.

1671.11 SHOCK, NATHAN WETHERILL. 1906-
        A classified bibliography of gerontology and geriatrics. Stanford, *Univer-
        sity Press,* (1951).
            Supplements, in 1957 and 1963.

1671.2 BROCKINGTON, COLIN FRASER. 1903-
        A short history of public health. London, *Churchill,* 1956.
            2nd edition, 1966.

1671.3 ROSEN, GEORGE. 1910-1977
        A history of public health. New York, *MD Publications,* 1958.

1671.4 DAINTON, COURTNEY.
        The story of England's hospitals. London, *Museum Press,* 1961.

1671.5 HENRIQUES, LOUIS FERNANDO. 1916-
        Prostitution and society. A survey. 3 vols. London, *MacGibbon & Kee,* 1962-
        68.
            Vol. 1: Primitive, classical and oriental. Vol. 2: Prostitution in Europe
        and the New World. Vol 3: Modern sexuality.

1671.6   FINCH, Bernard Ephraim, & GREEN, Hugh.
Contraception through the ages. London, *Peter Owen,* 1963.

1671.61   LÜTH, Paul.
Geschichte der Geriatrie. Dreitausend Jahre Physiologie, Pathologie und Therapie des alten Menschen. Stuttgart, *Ferdinand Enke,* 1965.

1671.62   LEISTIKOW, Dankwart.
Ten centuries of European hospital architecture. Ingelheim am Rhein, *C. H. Boehringer Sohn,* 1967.

1671.7   GOODMAN, Neville Marriot. 1898-1980
International health organizations and their work. 2nd ed. Edinburgh, *Churchill-Livingstone,* 1971.
    A systematic account of international health work from its beginnings to modern times. First published 1952.

1671.8   HOWARD-JONES, Norman. 1909-1985
The scientific background of the International Sanitary Conferences, 1851-1938. Geneva, *World Health Organization,* 1975.
    First published in *WHO Chronicle,* 1974. **28,** 159-71, 229-47, 369-84, 414-26, 455-70, 475-508.

1671.9   FREEMAN, Joseph T.
Aging: Its history and literature. New York, *Human Sciences Press,* [1979].
    Includes bibliographies of classic works, of the history of geriatrics, and of periodicals devoted to the subject.

EPIDEMIOLOGY

See also 1767-1782.1, Climatic & Geographical Factors in Medicine.

1672   HIPPOCRATES, 460-375 B.C.
Epidemics I and III. *In:* [Works] with an English translation by. W. H. S. Jones. London, *W. Heinemann,* 1923, **1,** 139-287.
    Hippocrates introduced the inductive method of studying epidemics.

1673   BAILLOU, Guillaume de [Ballonius]. 1538-1616
Epidemiorum et ephemeridum libri duo. Paris, *J. Quesnel,* 1640.
    De Baillou was a follower of Hippocrates in his advancement of the doctrine of "epidemic constitutions". Crookshank regards him as the first modern epidemiologist.

1674   CLEGHORN, George. 1716-1789
Observations on the epidemical diseases in Minorca. From the year 1744 to 1749. London, *D. Wilson,* 1751.
    Cleghorn left a good account of several diseases and conditions not previously observed, among them epidemic jaundice. He included in his book accounts of many post-mortems.

1675 HUXHAM, JOHN. 1692-1768
Observationes de aëre et morbis epidemicis. 3 vols. Londini, *J. Hinton,* 1752-70.

 Huxham made daily records of the weather and prevailing diseases; his aim was to establish a relationship between atmospheric conditions and disease. The work was first published in 1728; vol. 1 and 2 of the edition given above are second edition, which was rounded off by a third volume published posthumously. English translation of vol. 1 and 2, 1758-67.

1675.1 WEBSTER, NOAH. 1758-1843
A brief history of epidemic and pestilential diseases. 2 vols., Hartford, Conn., *Hudson & Goodwin,* 1799.

 "The best general summary of epidemiological opinion at the beginning of the nineteenth century; and few works surpass it as a compendium of earlier speculations in this field". (Winslow). A great linguist, Webster was the author of the famous dictionary. Osler considered the above work the most important American medical work written by a layman.

1676 VILLALBA, JOAQUIN DE.
Epidemiologia española. 2 vols. Madrid, *M Repullés,* 1802.

 A chronological history of epidemics occurring in Spain to the end of the 17th century.

1677 HAESER, HEINRICH. 1811-1884
Bibliotheca epidemiographica. Jenae, *F. Mauke,* 1843.

 A second edition was published in 1862.

1678 HECKER, JUSTUS FRIEDRICH KARL. 1795-1850
Die grossen Volkskrankheiten des Mittelalters. Historischpathologische Untersuchungen. Gesammelt und in erweiteter Bearbeitung hrsg. von A. HIRSCH. Berlin, *T. C. F. Enslin,* 1865.

 A collection of essays on the Black Death, the dancing mania, and the English sweat, published 1832-34 and later in a collective English edition, *The epidemics of the Middle Ages,* 2 pts., London, 1833-35; reprinted 1844, 1846, 1859. In the first English edition the general title accompanies Part 2 only; the work entitled "The sweating sickness", which completes the series, was not included in this edition.

1679 HAESER, HEINRICH. 1811-1884
Geschichte der epidemischen Krankheiten. Jena, *H. Dufft,* 1882.

 Forms vol. 3 of his *Lehrbuch der Geschichte der Medizin,* 3te. Aufl.

1680 CREIGHTON, CHARLES. 1847-1927
A history of epidemics in Britain, 2 vols. Cambridge, *University Press,* 1891-94.

 The most important work on the subject and a classical contribution to modern epidemiology, of which Creighton may be said to have been the founder. Reprinted with new introductory material, 1965.

1681 STICKER, GEORG. 1860-1960
Abhandlungen aus der Seuchengeschichte und Seuchenlehre. 2 vols. [in 3]. Giessen, *A. Töpelmann,* 1908-12.

1682   PRINZING, FRIEDRICH. 1859-
Epidemics resulting from wars. Edited by HARALD WESTERGAARD. Oxford, *Clarendon Press,* 1916.

1683   GREENWOOD, MAJOR. 1880-1949
Epidemiology, historical and experimental. Baltimore, *Johns Hopkins Press,* 1932.

1683.1   ——. Epidemics and crowd diseases; an introduction to the history of epidemiology. London, *Williams & Norgate,* 1935.

1684   MAJOR, RALPH HERMON. 1884-1970
War and disease. Garden City, N.Y., *Doubleday,* 1941.

1685   WINSLOW, CHARLES-EDWARD AMORY. 1877-1957
Man and epidemics. Princeton, N.J., *University Press,* 1952.

1685.1   ACKERKNECHT, ERWIN HEINZ. 1906-1988
History and geography of the most important diseases. New York, *Hafner,* 1965.
    Originally published in German, 1963.

DEMOGRAPHY: STATISTICS

1686   GRAUNT, JOHN. 1620-1674
Natural and political observations mentioned in a following index, and made upon the Bills of Mortality. London, *T. Roycroft for J. Martin, J. Allestry and T. Dicas,* 1662.
    The first book on vital statistics. Graunt, a draper, studied the Bills of Mortality, which began as weekly lists of deaths and their causes, compiled by parish clerks. They gained much in importance after Graunt's work, and in 1838 merged into the Registrar-General's returns. Graunt was a friend of Sir William Petty. Some authorities attribute authorship of the above work to Petty. In his *A bibliography of Sir William Petty F.R.S. and of Observations on the bills of Mortality by John Graunt, F.R.S,* (1971) Geoffrey Keynes traces the interrelationship of these authors.

1687   HALLEY, EDMUND. 1656-1742
An estimate of the degrees of mortality of mankind, drawn from curious tables of the births and funerals at the city of Breslaw, with an attempt to ascertain the price of annuities upon lives. *Phil Trans.,* 1693, **17,** 596-610.
    Halley, the astronomer, compiled the "Breslau tables" to show "the proportion of men able to bear arms ... to estimate mortality rates, to ascertain the price of annuities upon lives, and was thus the virtual founder of vital statistics" (Garrison). The data on which Halley based his conclusions were supplied to him by Caspar Neumann, a pastor of Breslau.

1688   PETTY, *Sir* WILLIAM. 1623-1687
Several essays in political arithmetic. London, *Robert Clavel and Henry Mortlock,* 1699.
    A pioneer statistician, Petty took the first census of Ireland. He was Professor of Anatomy at Oxford and later Graham Professor of Music. *See* No. 1686.

1689   JURIN, JAMES. 1684-1750
A letter ... containing, a comparison between the mortality of the natural small pox, and that given by inoculation. London, *W. J. Innys*, 1723.

Jurin was an enthusiastic supporter of inoculation against smallpox and proved statistically that the fatality of inoculated smallpox is very much less than the fatality of natural smallpox. This is one of the earliest applications of statistics to a particular socio-medical problem.

1690   MOIVRE, ABRAHAM DE. 1667-1754
Annuities upon lives; or, the valuation of annuities upon any number of lives; as also, of reversions. To which is added, an appendix concerning the expectations of life and probabilities of survivorship. London, *F. Fayram, B. Motte, and W. Pearson*, 1725.

De Moivre, French Huguenot mathematician and demographer, formulated the hypothesis that among a body of persons over a certain age the successive annual decreases by death are nearly equal.

1691   SÜSSMILCH, JOHANN PETER. 1707-1767
Die göttliche Ordnung in denen Veränderungen des menschlichen Geschlechts. Berlin, *D. A. Gohl*, 1742.

Süssmilch, a German army chaplain, produced an important book on vital statistics. Among other things, he showed the necessity of a healthy and industrious population for the survival of a nation. His work was the most important until the time of Malthus.

1691.1   DEPARCIEUX, ANTOINE. 1703-1768
Essai sur les probabilités de la durée de la vie humaine: d'où l'on déduit la manière de déterminer les rentes viagères, tant simples qu'en tonintes. Paris, *Guérin Frères*, 1746.

Deparcieux was the first to construct correct life tables. Appendix in 1760.

1692   SHORT, THOMAS. 1690?-1772
New observations, natural, moral, civil, political, and medical, on city, town, and country Bills of Mortality. London, *T. Longman & A. Millar*, 1750.

Original and suggestive work on vital statistics, showing vividly the changing conditions of life as he saw it (Greenwood).

1692.1   HEBERDEN, WILLIAM. 1710-1801
A collection of the yearly bills of mortality, from 1657 to 1758 inclusive. Together with several other bills of an earlier date...London, *A. Millar*, 1759.

The only collected edition of early bills of mortality, which were generally published as broadsides and are not available separately. Includes reprints of Nos. 1686 and 1688. This work has traditionally been attributed to Thomas Birch, but Hull (1899) gives strong evidence that Heberden was the author.

1693   MALTHUS, THOMAS ROBERT. 1766-1834
An essay on the principle of population, as it affects the future improvement of society. London, *J. Johnson*, 1798.

Malthus laid down the principle that populations increase in geometrical ratio, but that subsistence increases only in arithmetical ratio. He argued that a stage is reached where increase of populations must be limited by sheer want, and he advocated checks on population increase in order to reduce misery and want. His work was an important influence on both Darwin and Wallace in their formulation of the concept of natural selection. It also had a profound influence on the decrease in size of families down to the present time. The book was at first published anonymously, but Malthus attached his name to the greatly expanded second edition of 1803. Malthus continued to revise the work through the sixth edition, 2 vols., 1826. All editions but the fourth contain significant new material.

1694   KING, GREGORY. 1648-1712
        Natural and political observations and conclusions upon the state and condition of England. *In:* CHALMERS, G.: *An estimate of the comparative strength of Great Britain.* 2nd ed., London, *J. Stockdale,* 1802.
        King attempted to estimate the population by statistical methods. The above paper was written in 1696 but not published until 1802, when it appeared as an appendix to Chalmers's books. As a statistician King surpassed Petty.

1695   DUVILLARD, E. E.
        Analyse et tableaux de l'influence de la petite vérole sur la mortalité à chaque âge, et de celle qu'un préservatif tel que la vaccine peut avoir sur la population et la longevité. Paris, *Imprimerie Impériale,* 1806.
        Duvillard showed statistically the effect of smallpox vaccination on the mortality rate.

1696   CASPER, JOHANN LUDWIG. 1796-1864
        Beiträge zur medizinischen Statistik un Staatsarzneikunde. 2 vols. Berlin, *F. Dümmler,* 1825-35.

1696.1 PLACE, FRANCIS. 1771-1854
        Illustrations and proofs of the principle of population including an examination of the proposed remedies of Mr. Malthus, and a reply to the objections of Mr. Godwin and others. London, *Longman,* 1822.
        Place was the first important proponent of birth control in any English-speaking country. The above work openly advocates contraception, though without indicating how it was to be achieved. Reprinted with additional material collected by N.E. Himes, London, 1930.

1697   HAWKINS, FRANCIS BISSET. 1796-1894
        Elements of medical statistics. London, *Longman,* 1829.
        First English book devoted specifically to medical statistics. Hawkins was instrumental in obtaining the insertion of a column for the names of diseases or other causes of death, in connexion with the first Act for the registration of births and deaths.

1698   LOUIS, PIERRE CHARLES ALEXANDRE. 1787-1872
        Recherches sur les effets de la saignée dans quelques maladies inflammatoires, et sur l'action de l'émétique et des vésicatoires dans la pneumonie. Paris, *J. B. Baillière,* 1835.
        Broussais's system of medicine, his "médicine physiologique", was refuted by Louis, who, by his introduction of statistical methods into medicine, exposed its fallacies. Besides his important work on tuberculosis, Louis was instrumental in establishing medicine as an exact science by the introduction of the numerical or statistical method. English translation, Boston, 1836.

1698.1   QUETELET, Lambert Adolphe Jacques. 1796-1874
Sur l'homme et le développement des facultés, ou essai de physique sociale. 2 vols. Paris, *Bachelier*, 1835.

     Quetelet's statistical researches on the development of the physical and intellectual qualities of man, and an exposition of his concept of the "average man", which became the by-word of quantitative studies. English translation, Edinburgh, 1842. *See* No. 171.

1699   FARR, William. 1807-1883
Vital statistics. In McCulloch, J. R., *A statistical account of the British Empire*, 2nd ed., London, 1839, **2**, 521-90.

     Ranks with Graunt's *Observations* as an original contribution to medical statistics. First edition, 1837. Reprinted, Farnborough, *Gregg*, 1974.

1700   GAVARRET, Louis Denis Jules. 1809-1890
Principes généraux de statistique médicale. Paris, *Bechet jeune & Labé*, 1840.

     In his work on medical statistics Gavarret improved and systematized the method of Louis and gave special consideration to therapeutic problems.

1700.1   FARR, William. 1807-1883
English life table. Tables of lifetimes, annuities, and premiums. London, *Longman*, 1864.

     First application of computers to medical statistics. The appendix details the use of the Scheutz version of Charles Babbage's calculating machine in the construction of English Life Table No. 3. However, the machine required constant attention, and the G.R.O. soon reverted to manual calculations employing logarithms until conversion to mechanical calculation methods in 1911. See J.M. Eyler, *Victorian social medicine: the ideas and methods of William Farr*, Baltimore, *Johns Hopkins Press*, [1979].

1701   KÖRÖSI, Josef von. 1844-1906
Plan einer Mortalitäts-Statistik für Grossstädte. Wien, *C. Gerold*, 1873.

     The modern methods of interpreting vital statistics of large cities were devised by von Körösi.

1702   RUMSEY, Henry Wyldbore. 1809-1876
Essays and papers on some fallacies of statistics concerning life and death, health and disease. London, *Smith, Elder & Co.*, 1875.

1703   FARR, William. 1807-1883
Supplement to the thirty-fifth annual report of the Registrar-General of Births and Marriages in England. London, *Eyre & Spottiswoode*, 1875.

     Includes statistical calculations of the effect on life expectation if certain preventable diseases were eliminated.

1704   ———. Vital statistics. A memorial volume of selections from the reports and writings of William Farr. London, *E. Stanford*, 1885.

     Farr applied statistical methods to epidemiology and was the first mathematically to express the rise and fall of epidemic diseases, thus making possible the more accurate prediction of the occurrence of epidemics.

1705   BILLINGS, JOHN SHAW, 1838-1913
On vital and medical statistics. New York, *Trow,* 1889.

1706   PEARSON, KARL. 1857-1936
The chances of death and other studies in evolution. 2 vols. London, *E. Arnold,* 1897.

1707   DAVENPORT, CHARLES BENEDICT. 1866-1944
Statistical methods, with special reference to biological variation. New York, *J. Wiley & Sons,* 1899.
        Davenport introduced statistical methods into American evolutionary studies.

1709   GALTON, *Sir* FRANCIS. 1822-1911
Probability: The foundation of eugenics. Oxford, *H. Frowde,* 1907.

1710   BERTILLON, JACQUES. 1851-1914
La dépopulation de la France. Paris, *F. Alcan,* 1911.

1711   PEARSON, KARL. 1857-1936
On the handicapping of the first-born. London, *Dulau & Co.,* 1914.

1712   PEARL, RAYMOND. 1879-1940, & REED, LOWELL JACOB. 1886-1966
On the rate of growth of the population of the United States since 1790 and its mathematical representation. *Proc. nat. Acad. Sci. (Wash.),* 1920, **6,** 275-88.

1713   CARR-SAUNDERS, *Sir* ALEXANDER MORRIS. 1886-1966
The population problem; a study in human evolution. Oxford, *Clarendon Press,* 1922.

1714   PEARL, RAYMOND. 1879-1940
The natural history of population. Oxford, *University Press,* 1939.

History of Demography: Statistics

1715   WESTERGAARD, HARALD.
Contributions to the history of statistics. London, *P. S. King,* 1932.

1716   GREENWOOD, MAJOR. 1880-1949
Medical statistics from Graunt to Farr. Cambridge, *University Press,* 1948.
        FitzPatrick Lectures, 1941 and 1943.

1716.1   PEARSON, KARL. 1857-1936
The history of statistics in the 17th and 18th centuries against the changing background of intellectual, scientific and religious thought. Lectures by Karl Pearson given at University College London during the academic sessions 1921-1933. Edited by E.S. Pearson. New York, *Macmillan,* [1978].

1716.2   STIGLER, STEPHEN M.
The history of statistics. The measurement of uncertainty before 1900. Cambridge, Mass., *Belknap Press of Harvard University Press,* 1986.
        The first comprehensive history of statistics from about 1700 to 1900.

MEDICAL JURISPRUDENCE

See also 2069-2117, TOXICOLOGY.

1717 CONSTITUTIO CRIMINALIS CAROLINA. 1533
Kaiser Karl's des Fünften Peinlich Gerichtsordnung ... Hrsg. von R. SCHMID.
Jena, *A. Schmid*, 1835.
The Constitutio Criminalis of Charles V is probably the oldest European
document of any importance dealing with medical jurisprudence. It
authorized judges to call expert witnesses in medico-legal cases.

1718 CODRONCHI, GIOVANNI BATTISTA. 1547-1628
Methodus testificandi, inquibusvis casibus medicis oblatis. In his: *De vitiis
vocis, libri duo,* Francofurti, *A. Wechel,* 1597, pp. 148-232.
First important work on forensic medicine.

1719 FIDELI, FORTUNATO. 1550-1630
De relationibus medicorum. Panormi, *apud I. A. de Franciscis,* 1602.

1720 ZACCHIAS, PAOLO. 1584-1659
Quaestiones medico-legales. 9 vols. Romae, Amstelaedami, 1621-61.
Zacchias, a Papal physician, was one of the founders of medical
jurisprudence. His treatise includes information concerning injuries of the
eye, etc., and contains section on the medico-legal aspects of insanity. The
last two volumes were published in Amsterdam.

1721 SEBIISCH, MELCHIOR. 1578-1674?
De notis virginitatis. Lipsiae, 1630.
Details the methods of previous and contemporary writers concerning
the determination of virginity.

1722 WELSCH, GOTTFRIED. 1618-1690
Rationale vulnerum lethalium judicium. Lipsiae, *sumpt. Ritzschianis,* 1660.
Welsch stressed the need for autopsy in medico-legal cases.

1723 GARMANN, CHRISTIAN FRIEDERICH. 1640-1708
De gemellis et partu numerosiore. Lipsiae, *typ. vid. H. Coleri,* 1667.
Medico-legal aspects of multiple births.

1724 SWAMMERDAM, JAN. 1637-1680
Tractatus physico-anatomico-medicus de respiratione usuque pulmonum.
Lugduni Batavorum, *apud Danielem, Abraham. et Adrian. à Gaasbeeck,*
1667.
Swammerdam's earliest published work. In it he recorded his discovery
that the lungs of newborn infants will float on water if respiration has taken
place, an important medico-legal point.

1725 BLÉGNY, NICOLAS DE. 1652-1722
La doctrine des rapports de chirurgie, fondées sur les maximes d'usage et
sur la disposition des nouvelles ordonnances. Lyon, *T. Amaubry,* 1684.

De Blégny explained the obligation of surgeons to report any suspicion of crime, and explained how to prepare expert opinion for presentation before the court.

1726   BOHN, JOHANN. 1640-1718
De renunciatione vulnerum, seu vulnerum lethalium examen. Lipsiae, *J. F. Gleditsch,* 1689.
"The best work on fatal injuries, with frequent references of medico-legal importance" (Nemec).

1727   SCHREYER, JOHANN.
Erörterung und Erläuterung der Frage: Ob es ein gewiss Zeichen wenn, eines todten Kindes Lunge im Wasser untersincket, dass solches in Mutter-Leiber gestorben sey? Zu Rettung seiner Ehre in Druck befördert. Zeitz, *J. H. Ammersbachen,* 1690.
Swammerdam's discovery that the foetal lungs will float on water if respiration has taken place was first put to practical use by Schreyer, who thereby secured the acquittal of a girl accused of infanticide.

1728   VALENTINI, MICHAEL BERNHARD. 1657-1729
Corpus juris medico-legale. Francofurti ad M., *sumpt. J. A. Jungii,* 1722.
This reprints Valentini's *Pandectae medico legales* (1701) and *Novellae medico-legales* (1711) with the addition of *Authentica jatro-forensia.*

1729   ALBERTI, MICHAEL. 1682-1757
Systema jurisprudentiae medicae. 2 vols. Halae, *imp. Orphanotrophei,* 1725.
A work covering the whole field of medical jurisprudence as then understood, and ranking in importance with the work of Valentini. Second edition in 6 vols., *Halae,* 1733-47.

1730   LOUIS, ANTOINE. 1723-1792
Mémoire sur une question anatomique relative à la jurisprudence; dans lequel on établit les principes pour distinguer, à l'inspection d'un corps trouvé pendu, les signes du suicide d'avec ceux de l'assassinat. Paris, *P. G. Cavelier,* 1763.
Louis was a pioneer of French medical jurisprudence. Above is a classic discussion on the differential signs of murder and suicide in cases of hanging.

1731   ——. Mémoire contre la légitimité des naissances prétendues tardives. Paris, *P. G. Cavelier,* 1764.
An attempt to set the minimum and maximum time limits of duration of human pregnancy. Supplement published in 1764.

1732   HUNTER, WILLIAM. 1718-1783
On the uncertainty of the signs of murder, in the case of bastard children. *Med. Obs. & Inqu.,* London, 1784, **6,** 266-90.
This essay on the signs of murder in illegitimate children is, in Garrison's view, the most important early contribution to forensic medicine by a British writer.

1733   FARR, SAMUEL. 1741-1795
Elements of medical jurisprudence. London, *T. Becket,* 1788.
First textbook in English on medical jurisprudence.

1734   FODÉRÉ, FRANÇOIS EMMANUEL. 1764-1835
Les lois éclairées par les sciences physiques, ou traité de médecine légale et hygiène publique. 3 vols. Paris, *chez Croullebois et chez Deterville,* and VII [1799].
This important publication was for many years the authoritative textbook on the subject in France.

1735   BECK, THEODORIC ROMEYN. 1791-1855
Elements of medical jurisprudence. 2 vols. Albany, *Websters & Skinners,* 1823.
First notable American text on forensic medicine.

1736   HEINROTH, JOHANN CHRISTIAN AUGUST. 1773-1843
System der psychisch-gerichtlichen Medizin. Leipzig, *C. H. F. Hartmann,* 1825.
The first important work exclusively on medico-legal aspects of insanity.

1737   GROSS, SAMUEL DAVID. 1805-1884
Observations on manual strangulation, illustrated by cases and experiments. *West J. med. phys. Sci.,* 1836, **9,** 25-38.
After performing an autopsy on a strangulation case, Gross set out to study the physiology involved in manual strangulation. He set up a series of experiments on dogs for this purpose and provides autopsy reports on each as well as guidelines for medical examiners investigating strangulations.

1738   TAYLOR, ALFRED SWAINE. 1806-1880
Elements of medical jurisprudence. London, *Deacon,* 1836.
One of the best-known English texts on the subject; thirteenth edition, *Principles and practice of medical jurisprudence,* appeared in 1984.

1739   RAY, ISAAC. 1807-1881
A treatise on the medical jurisprudence of insanity. Boston, 1838.
The first authoritative and comprehensive treatise in English on the relation between law and psychiatry. Ray became the most influential American writer on forensic psychiatry in the 19th century. He put the above work through five editions, the last of which appeared in 1871. Reprint of 1st edition with introduction and notes by W. Overholser, Cambridge, Mass., *Harvard Univ. Press,* 1962.

1740   GUY, WILLIAM AUGUSTUS. 1810-1885
Principles of forensic medicine. London, *H. Renshaw,* 1844.

1741   CASPER, JOHANN LUDWIG. 1796-1864
Gerichtliche Leichenöffnungen. Berlin, *A. Hirschwald,* 1850.
Casper was a great authority on forensic medicine. He also wrote on medical statistics. Above is an important compilation on judicial autopsies.

1742   HAMILTON, FRANK HASTINGS. 1813-1886
Deformities after fractures. *Trans. Amer. med. Ass.,* 1855, **8,** 347-443.
Hamilton was a medical inspector of the U.S. Army and later became Professor of Surgery at Bellevue Hospital. *See* No. 4420.

1743   CASPER, JOHANN LUDWIG. 1796-1864
        Practisches Handbuch der gerichtlichen Medicin. 2 vols. Berlin, *A. Hirschwald,* 1857-58.
        Casper was the greatest name in forensic medicine in his time. His book was published in English by the New Sydenham Society in 1861-65; it was unsurpassed for many years.

1744   ——. Klinische Novellen zur gerichtlichen Medizin. Berlin, *A. Hirschwald,* 1863.

1745   TARDIEU, AUGUSTE AMBROISE. 1818-1879
        Etude médico-légale et clinique sur l'empoisonnement. Paris, *J. B. Baillière,* 1867.

1746   DRAGENDORFF, GEORG JOHANN NOEL. 1836-1898
        Die gerichtlich-chemische Ermittelung von Giften in Nahrungsmitteln, Luftgemischen, Speiseresten, Körpertheilen, etc. St. Petersburg, *H. Schmitzdorff,* 1868.
        Dragendorff, Professor of Pharmacy at Dorpat, Marburg, and Vienna, contributed an important book on forensic chemistry. He was responsible for the introduction of several methods for the detection of poisons in the human body.

1747   ——. Beiträge zur gerichtlichen Chemie einzelner organischer Gifte. St. Petersburg, *H. Schmitzdorff,* 1872.

1748   KRAFFT-EBING, RICHARD VON. 1840-1902
        Lehrbuch der gerichtlichen Psychopathologie. Stuttgart, *F. Enke,* 1875.

1749   HOFMANN, EDUARD VON, *Ritter.* 1837-1897
        Lehrbuch der gerichtlichen Medicin. Wien, *Urban & Schwarzenberg,* 1877-78.
        An important German work on the subject. Hofmann's book went through many editions and was translated into several European languages.

1750   MANN, JOHN DIXON. 1840-1912
        Forensic medicine and toxicology. London, *C. Griffin & Co.,* 1893.

1751   BROUARDEL, PAUL CAMILLE HIPPOLYTE. 1837-1906
        La mort et la mort subite. Paris, *J. B. Baillière,* 1895.
        Brouardel was Professor of Forensic Medicine, Paris. He was to a great extent responsible for the development of that subject in France; he instituted courses of practical instruction at the Paris morgue, and wrote several monographs on forensic medicine. English translation, London, 1897.

1752   ——. L'infanticide. Paris, *J. B. Baillière,* 1897.

1753   ——. La pendaison, la strangulation, la suffocation, la submersion. Paris, *J. B. Baillière,* 1897.

1754   UHLENHUTH, Paul Theodor. 1870-1957
Eine Methode zur Unterscheidung der verschiedenen Blutarten, im besonderen zum differentialdiagnostischen Nachweise des Menschenblutes. *Dtsch. med. Wschr.*, 1901, **27**, 82-83, 260-61.

Uhlenhuth was the first to use precipitins in medico-legal tests for human blood.

1755   MERCIER, Charles Arthur. 1852-1919
Criminal responsibility. Oxford, *Clarendon Press,* 1905.

1756   OTTENBERG, Reuben. 1882-
Medicolegal application of human blood grouping. *J. Amer. med. Ass.*, 1921, **77,** 682-83; 1922, **78,** 873-77; **79,** 2137-43.

An important series of papers on blood-grouping and the jurisprudence of paternity. Ottenberg performed the first matched-blood transfusion.

1757   McINDOE, *Sir*Archibald Hector. 1900-1960, & FRANCES-CHETTI, Adolphe. 1896-
Reciprocal skin homografts in a medico-legal case of familial identification of exchanged identical twins. *Brit. J. plast. Surg.*, 1950, **2,** 283-89.

Skin grafting used to decide the relationship of identical twins who had been accidentally separated at birth.

History of Medical Jurisprudence

1757.1   NEMEC, Jaroslav.
Highlights in medicolegal relations. Revised & enlarged ed. Washington, D.C., *Govt. Printing Office,* 1976.

1757.2   FORBES, Thomas Rogers. 1911-1988
Surgeons at the Bailey. English forensic medicine to 1878. New Haven, *Yale University Press,* 1985.

MEDICAL ETHICS

1757.90   HIPPOCRATES. 460-375 b.c.
Iusiurandum *In* Nicholaus Perottus, De generibus metrorum.[Verona, *Boninus de Boninis,* c. 1475-83].

First printing of the Hippocratic Oath. This also appeared at about the same time in Franciscus Argilagnes (ed.) (Articella), Venice, *Hermannus Liechtenstein Levilapis,* 1483. First English translation of the oath by John Read appeared in Francisco Arceo, *A most excellent and compendious method of curing woundes in the head, and in other partes of the body,* London, *Thomas East,* 1588.

1758   JONES, William Henry Samuel. 1876-1963
The doctor's oath, an essay in the history of medicine. Cambridge, *Univ. Press,* 1924.

The Hippocratic Oath forms the basis of medical ethics. It was probably an ancient temple oath of the Asclepiadae, and not a genuine Hippocratic document. In the above work the various manuscripts of the Oath are enumerated and critically discussed.

1758.1   ZERBI, Gabriele. 1445-1505
          De cautelis medicorum. [Venice, *Christophorus de Pensis, de Mandello*, not
          before 1495.]
              The first practical treatise on medical ethics. *See also* Nos. 363.2 and
          1589.1.

1759   CASTRO, Rodericus A. 1546-1627
          Medicus-politicus: sive de officiis medico-politicis tractatus. Hamburgi, *ex*
          bibl. Frobeniano, 1614.
              One of the first "modern" works on medical ethics.

1760   HOERNIGK, Ludwig von. 1600-1667
          Politia medica. Franckfurt a.M., *bey C. Schleichen u. Mitverwandten*, 1638.

1761   HARVEY, Gideon. ?1640-1700
          The conclave of physicians, detecting their intrigues, frauds, and plots,
          against their patients. London, *J. Partridge*, 1683.

1762   FRITSCH, Ahasuerus. 1629-1701
          Medicus peccans, sive tractatus de peccatis medicorum. Norimbergae,
          apud W. M. Endterum, 1684.

1763   BARD, Samuel. 1742-1821
          A discourse upon the duties of a physician. New York, *A. & J. Robertson*,
          1769.
              The first American treatise on medical ethics. Samuel Bard was one of
          the founders of King's College, New York. Facsimile reprint, New York,
          1921.

1764   PERCIVAL, Thomas. 1740-1804
          Medical ethics; or, a code of institutes and precepts, adapted to the
          professional conduct of physicians and surgeons. Manchester, *printed by*
          S. Russell for J. Johnson and R. Bickerstaff, London, 1803.
              First published for private circulation, 1794. The British and American
          medical professions have adopted much of "Percival" in their ethical
          codes. An edition of the book published in 1927 was reprinted in 1975.

1765   BELL, John. 1763-1820
          Letters on professional character and manners. Edinburgh, *J. Moir*, 1810.

1766   PAGEL, Julius Leopold. 1851-1912
          Medicinische Deontologie. Berlin, *O. Coblentz*, 1897.

MEDICAL EDUCATION AND THE MEDICAL PROFESSION

1766.500 MORGAN, John. 1735-1789
          A discourse upon the institution of medical schools in
          America....Philadelphia, *William Bradford*, 1765.
              The first American publication on medical education. Morgan founded
          the first medical school in the United States, in connection with what is now
          the University of Pennsylvania.

1766.501   BERNARD, Claude. 1813-1878
Introduction à l'étude de la médicine expérimentale. Paris, *J.-B. Baillière*, 1865.
     Probably the greatest classic on the principles of physiological investigation and of the scientific method as applied to the life sciences. The English translation, New York, 1927, has been frequently reprinted. See P.F. Cranefield, *Claude Bernard's revised edition of his Introduction à l'étude de la médecine expérimentale*, New York, 1976.

1766.502   FLEXNER, Abraham. 1866-1959
Medical education in the United States and Canada. New York, *Carnegie Foundation*, 1910.
     This report caused massive reforms in North American medical education, including the closure or merging with stronger institutions, of 76 medical schools between 1910 and 1920. Part 1 is a history and analysis of medical education with recommendations for improvement. Part 2 describes, state by state, each medical school in existence at the time the report was prepared.

1766.503   ———. Medical education in Europe, New York, *Carnegie Foundation*, 1912.
     Flexner wrote the first systematic and thorough comparisons of the major systems of medical education.

1766.504   ———. Medical education: A comparative study. New York, *Macmillan*, 1925.

History of Medical Education and the Medical Profession

1766.600   RIVINGTON, Walter. 1835-1897
The medical profession. Dublin, *Fannin & Co.*, 1879.
     A history of the organization of the medical profession with particular reference to Britain.

1766.601   PUSCHMANN, Theodor. 1844-1899
Geschichte des medizinischen Unterrichtes von den ältesten Zeiten bis zur Gegenwart. Leipzig, *Veit & Co.*, 1889.
     The only comprehensive multinational study of the development of medical education, and of limited value for coverage of the 19th century. English translation, 1891, reprinted, with introduction by Erwin Ackerknecht, New York, *Hafner*, 1966.

1766.602   BAAS, Johann Hermann. 1838-1909
Die geschichtliche Entwicklung des ärztlichen Standes. Berlin, *F. Wreden*, 1896.

1766.603   BILLROTH, Christian Albert Theodor. 1829-1894
The medical sciences in the German Universities: a study in the history of civilization. Translated by William H. Welch. New York, *Macmillan*, 1924.
     German edition first published in 1876.

1766.604   SHAFER, Henry Burnell. 1906-
The American medical profession, 1783 to 1850. New York, *Columbia Univ. Press*, 1936.

1766.605   NORWOOD, WILLIAM F.
Medical education in the United States before the Civil War, Philadelphia, *University of Pennsylvania Press*, 1944.
Reprint, New York, *Arno Press*, 1971.

1766.606   NEWMAN, CHARLES EDWARD. 1900-1989
The evolution of medical education in the nineteenth century. London, *Oxford Univ. Press*, 1957.
Covers medical education in England.

1766.607   ACKERKNECHT, ERWIN HEINZ. 1906-1988
Medicine at the Paris Hospital 1794-1848. Baltimore, *Johns Hopkins Press*, 1967.

1766.608   O'MALLEY, CHARLES DONALD. 1907-1970
History of medical education: an international symposium. Edited by C.D. O'MALLEY. Berkeley, *Univ. of California Press*, 1970.

1766.609   KAUFMAN, MARTIN.
American medical education: the formative years, 1765-1910. Westport, Conn., *Greenwood Press*, 1976.

1766.610   PETERSON, M. JEANNE.
The medical profession in mid-Victorian London. Berkeley, *Univ. of California Press*, 1978.

CLIMATIC & GEOGRAPHICAL FACTORS IN MEDICINE

1767   HIPPOCRATES.460-375 B.C.
On airs, waters, and places. *In* [Works] with an English translation by W. H. S. JONES. London, *W. Heinemann*, 1923, **1,** 65-137.
"The first book ever written on medical geography, climatology, and anthropology" (Garrison). The Latin translation of this text was first published in Rhazes' *Liber ad Almansorem*, Milan, 1481. *See* No. 39.1. The standard Greek edition is *Hippokrates über die Umwelt*. Herausgegeben und übersetzt von H. Diller, Corpus Medicorum Graecorum, I, 1,2, Berlin, 1970.

1768   ABDOLLATIF [ABU MUHAMMAD ABDU'L-LATIF]. 1162-1231
Historiae Aegypti compendium. Oxonii, *typ. Academicis,* 1800.
Arabic-Latin bilingual text. Abdollatif gave a good description of the fauna and flora of Egypt, its inhabitants and some of its diseases. He was the first writer, according to Hirsch, to dispute the accuracy of Galen. The first printed version of his work appeared in 1789 (Tübingen, Arabic text).

1769   CLERMONT, CHARLES [CLAROMONTIUS].
De aere, locis, et aquis terrae Angliae; deque morbis Anglorum vernaculis. Londini, *T. Roycroft et J. Martyn,* 1672.
An outline of the medical topography of England.

1770   HILLARY, WILLIAM. 1697-1763
Observations on the changes of the air and the concomitant epidemical diseases, in the Island of Barbados. London, *C. Hitch & L. Hawes,* 1759.
Hillary included good accounts of lead colic and infective hepatitis, and probably the first description of sprue.

1771   CASAL Y JULIAN, CASPAR. 1679-1759
        Historia natural, y medica de el Principado de Asturias. Madrid, *M. Martin*,
        1762.
            Includes the first clear description of pellagra. Casal wrote the book in
        1735, but it was not published until 1762; a reprint was published in Oviedo
        in 1900.

1772   RUTTY, JOHN. 1698-1775
        A chronological history of the weather and seasons, and of the prevailing
        diseases in Dublin. London, *Robinson & Roberts,* 1770.
            Rutty's book includes a description of relapsing fever.

1773   CHALMERS, LIONEL. 1715-1777
        An account of the weather and diseases of South-Carolina. 2 vols. London,
        E. & C. Dilly, 1776.
            Originally published in the *Gentleman's Magazine,* 1751-54.

1774   FOTHERGILL, JOHN. 1712-1780
        Observations on the weather and diseases of London. In his *Works.* Lon-
        don, 1783, **1,** 145-240.

1775   CURRIE, WILLIAM. 1754-1828
        An historical account of the climates and diseases of the United States of
        America. Philadelphia. *T. Dobson,* 1792.

1776   FINKE, LEONHARD LUDWIG. 1747-1837
        Versuch einer allgemeinen medicinisch-praktischen Geographie. 3 vols.
        Leipzig. *Weidmann,* 1792-95.

1776.1 ANNESLEY, *Sir* JAMES. 1780-1847
        Researches into...the more prevalent diseases of India, and of warm
        climates generally. 2 vols., London, *Longman,* 1828.
            A landmark in geographical pathology, superbly illustrated. Annesley's
        cases, collected over many years' service throughout India, represented
        the most complete treatment of diseases on the sub-continent to date.

1777   DRAKE, DANIEL. 1785-1852
        A systematic treatise, historical, etiological, and practical, on the principal
        diseases of the interior valley of North America. Cincinnati, *W. B. Smith &
        Co.,* 1850.
            Vol. 2 posthumously published as 2nd series, ed. S. H. Smith & F. G.
        Smith, Philadelphia, Lippincott, Grambo & Co., 1854. This classical contri-
        bution to the social history of N. America includes the most important work
        on the natural history of malaria published up to that time.

1778   HIRSCH, AUGUST. 1817-1894
        Handbuch der historisch-geographischen Pathologie. 2 vols. Erlangen, *F.
        Enke,* 1860-64.
            This is perhaps the greatest work on the subject. The best edition is the
        English translation prepared from the second edition, by Charles Creighton,
        3 vols., London, *New Sydenham Society,* 1883-86.

1779 LOMBARD, HENRI CLERMOND. 1803-1895
Traité de climatologie médicale, 4 vols. and 1 atlas. Paris, *J. B. Baillière,*
1877-80.

1780 McKINLEY, EARL BALDWIN. 1894-1938
A geography of disease. Washington, *George Washington Univ. Press,*
1935.
  Published as supplement to *Amer. J. trop. Med.,* 1935, **15**, No. 5.

1781 PETERSEN, WILLIAM FERDINAND. 1887-1950
The patient and the weather. With the assistance of Margaret E. Milliken.
4 vols. [in 7]. Ann Arbor, *Edwards Bros.,* 1934-38.

1782 KÖPPEN, WLADIMIR PETER. 1846-1940, & GEIGER, RUDOLF.
Handbuch der Klimatologie. Vol. 1-5. Berlin, *Gebr. Bornträger,* 1930-38.

1782.1 BARKHUS, ARNE.
Medical geographies. *Ciba Symp.,* 1945, **6**, 1997-2016.
A historical survey of the classical works.

MATERIA MEDICA: PHARMACY: PHARMACOLOGY

For drugs with specific action, see under the diseases concerned

1783 THEOPHRASTUS *of Eresos. circa* 371 – *circa* 287 B.C.
[De historia et causis plantarum.] [Treviso. *B. Confalonerius,* 1483.]
  Theophrastus, a pupil of Aristotle, succeeded him as head of the Athens
Peripatetic School. He also inherited Aristotle's library. This is the earliest
work of scientific botany, a subject not addressed in any of the writings of
Aristotle. Part of the book is devoted to plant-lore and the gathering of
drugs for medicinal purposes. Theophrastus collated and systematized the
existing botanical knowledge and described about 500 plants. A Greek-
English bilingual edition appeared in the *Loeb Classics* series in 1916, in 2
vols., edited by Sir A. Hort. *See* No. 87.1.

1784 KRATEUAS [CRATEVAS]. *fl.* 100 B.C.
[Singer, C. The herbal in antiquity and its transmission to later ages. *J. Hellen.
Stud.,* 1927, **47**, 1-52.]
  Krateuas, personal physician to Mithridates VI, Eupator of Pontus (120-
63 BC), was one of the first to issue botanical illustrations in the form of
picture-books with very brief annotations. Only fragments of his works
have come down to us, second-hand, through the writings of others,
particularly Dioscorides. The MS of Dioscorides known as the *Codex
Vindobonensis* is a magnificent copy of his *De materia medica (See* No.
1786). It was written in Constantinople about AD 512, for Patricia Juliana
Anicia, daughter of the Emperor Flavius Anicius Olybrius. It contains
nearly 400 coloured paintings of plants, including versions of some
drawings attributed to Krateuas, which were reproduced in Singer's paper.
The *Codex Vindobonensis* is now in the Austrian National Library, Vienna.
Facsimile edition, Graz, *Akademische Druck,* 1965-70.

1785   SCRIBONIUS LARGUS. *fl.* A.D. 40
De compositionibus medicamentorum liber unus. Parisiis, *ap. C. Wechel,*
1528.
First written in A.D. 47. This is an important compilation of drugs and
prescriptions. Among other things, it records the drinking of one's own
blood as a therapeutic rite. Scribonius was the first to describe accurately
the preparation of true opium. G. Helmreich edited a Latin edition of the
book, published in 1887, while a German version by W. Schonack
appeared in 1913. The standard Latin edition is by S. Sconocchia, Leipzig,
1983. *See* No. 1984.1.

1786   DIOSCORIDES, PEDANIUS, *Anazarbeus. fl.* A.D. 54-68
De materia medica. Edidit MAX WELLMANN. 3 vols. Berolini, *Weidmann,* 1906-
14.
Dioscorides' work is the authoritative source on the materia medica of
antiquity. He described over 600 plants and plant principles. His *De materia
medica* was first printed in Greek by Aldus Manutius in 1499; the first Latin
translation was published in Colle, 1478. The above edition by Wellman is
the definitive Greek text. John Goodyer made an English translation
between 1652 and 1655, which remained in manuscript until R. T. Gunther
edited and published it as *The Greek herbal of Dioscorides* (Oxford, 1934,
reprinted New York, *Hafner,* 1959). The above also contains the *Fragmenta*
of Krateuas. *See* No. 1784.

1787   THOMPSON, REGINALD CAMPBELL. 1876-1941
The Assyrian herbal. London, *Luzac & Co.,* 1924.
A study of ancient Assyrian medical drugs.

1788   ABU MANSUR MUWAFFAK BIN ALI HARAWI. *fl.* 970
Liber fundamentorum pharmacologiae ... Primus Latio donavit R. SELIGMANN.
2 pts. Vindobonae, *Antonius Nob. de Schmid,* 1830-1833.
The most important Persian pharmacological work. It was written
about A.D. 970. The above epitome is taken from a MS of 1055; a German
version appeared in 1893 under the direction of R. Kobert.

1789   NICOLAUS *Salernitanus. fl.* 1140
Antidotarium. Venetiis, *N. Jensen,* 1471.
This work, which first appeared in 1140, was the first formulary to be
printed. It consists of 139 prescriptions and includes the original formula
for the "anaesthetic sponge" (spongia somnifera), the earliest sources of
which are MSS of the 8th century, and a table of weights and measures
which formed the basis of the modern grain, scruple, drachm etc. The book
must have been of great contemporary value, as it was one of the first
medical works to be printed.

1790   PLATEARIUS, MATTHAEUS. *fl.* 1130-1150
De simplici medicina seu Circa instans. *In* Nicolaus Praepositus,
Dispensarium, Lugduni, 1537, ff. 70-96.
The original of the first French herbal, this derived from Dioscorides
and first appeared about 1140. A French translation was published by P.
Dorveaux in 1913.

1791   MACER FLORIDUS.
De virtutibus herbarum. Neapoli, *imp. per Arnoldum de Bruxella,* 1477.

The earliest printed herbal. A later edition (Milano, 1482) is a contender for the honour of being the first printed herbal with illustrations. *Macer Floridus,* a poem describing the virtues of 88 simples, was written in the 12th century and is ascribed variously to Aemilius Macer, Hugo of Tours, and to Odo of Meudon. It was the original of the earliest known Scandinavian medical writing, the *Laegebog* of Henrik Harpestreng. Many editions and translations are available.

1792   ALBERTUS MAGNUS [ALBERT VON BOLLSTÄDT]. 1193-1280
De vegetabilibus libri vii. Berolini, *G. Reimeri,* 1867.
    One of Albertus's most important publications and the best work on natural history produced during the Middle Ages. It was written about 1250, and is based on his own accurate botanical observations, containing also some therapeutic material. C. Jessen edited the above edition.

1793   NICOLAUS *Myrepsus. circa* 1280
Medicamentorum opus. Basileae, *per Jo. Oporinum,* 1549.
    The "Antidotarium magnum" of Nicolaus Myrepsus. It was the largest strictly pharmaceutical work that had appeared (it was written about 1270-1280) and contained more than 2,500 formulae. The above is a Latin translation by Leonhart Fuchs.

1794   ORTOLFF VON BAYRLANT. *circa* 1400
Artzneibuch. [Augsburg, *G. Zainer*], 1477.
    First German pharmacopoeia. Ortolff was a physician in Würzburg. The book was an important German text of popular medicine in its day. *See also* Hain (No. 6752), 12111.

1795   HERBARIUS
Herbarius latinus. Mainz, *Peter Schoeffer,* [14]84.
    The first herbal printed in Germany and the prototype for most of the herbals printed during the remainder of the 15th century. With text in Latin and with German synonyms, this is often called the *Latin Herbarius.* It was the first printed book to be issued with a title page bearing a complete imprint. Also known as "Herbarius Moguntinus". *See also* No. 95.

1796   HERBAL.
Herbarius zu deutsch. Mainz, *P. Schoeffer,* [1485].
    The first herbal written and printed in a modern language, and sometimes called the "German Herbarius". It is also referred to as "Gart der Gesundheit", although it was never issued under this title. The anonymous compiler probably received advice on medical matters from a Dr. Johann Wonnecke of Kaub, town physician of Frankfurt. This is the first printed book with some plant illustrations drawn from nature (65 out of 379 woodcuts). The scientific illustrations have been attributed to Erhard Rewich of Utrecht. Reproduced in facsimile, Munich, 1924, and Stuttgart, 1968.

1797   HORTUS SANITATIS.
Ortus sanitatis. Moguntiae, *J. Meydenbach,* 1491.
    The plant illustrations in this work are for the most part copied from the German Herbarius (No. 1796). 150 illustrations of animals and minerals are new or borrowed from models in manuscripts or playing cards, etc. It is one of the most important of the early herbals. Facsimile edition, with W. L.

Schreiber's *Die Kräuterbücher des XV. and XVI. Jahrhunderts,* Munich, 1924. An English translation of *c.* 1521 (S.T.C. 22367) was reprinted London, *Quaritch,* 1954, edited by N. Hudson. *See* No. 96.

1798   LEONICENO, Niccolo. 1428-1524
De Plinii et plurium aliorum in medicina erroribus. [Ferrara, *L. de Valentia et A. de Castronovo,* 1492.]
A correction of the botanical errors of Pliny. Remembering the times in which Leoniceno lived, Garrison considers this work "a feat of the rarest intellectual courage". It was accepted by later botanists and thus made possible scientific description of the materia medica. The second edition, [Ferrara, *per Joannem Maciochium,* 1509,] contains the first printings of Leoniceno's responses to his critics in 1493, 1503, and 1507, which apparently circulated in manuscript until 1509.

1799   BANCKES' HERBAL.
Here begynnyth a new mater, the whiche sheweth and treateth of ye vertues & proprytes of herbes, the whiche is called an Herball. London, *Rycharde Banckes,* 1525.
Earliest English printed herbal. Published anonymously, it is usually referred to as "Banckes' Herbal". The text was derived from a medieval manuscript, and although the work had no claim to originality it was the basis of most English herbals until Turner, No. 1811. Only two copies are known. Reproduced with modern transcription by S. V. Larkey and T. Pyles, New York, 1941.

1800   OVIEDO Y VALDÉS, *Don* Gonçalo Fernández de. 1478-1557
Sumaria de la historia natural de las Indias. Toledo, *R. de Petras,* 1525.
First known description of the medicinal plants of Central America. Oviedo first described *chigoe* ("jiggers"?) in this book. A 3-volume edition was published at Madrid in 1851-53.

1801   GRANT HERBIER
Le grant herbier en francoys, contenant les qualitez, vertus et proprietez des herbes, arbres, gommes & semences, etc. [Paris, *par Guillaume Nyverd pour Jehan Petit, et pour Michel le Noir,* ca. 1520].
The "Grant Herbier" or Arbolayre was probably derived from Platearius (No. 1790), and the "Grete Herball" (No. 1802) is a translation of it.

1802   GRETE HERBAL.
The grete herball whiche geveth parfyt knowlege and understandyng of all maner of herbes and there gracyous vertues. Southwarke, *P. Treveris,* 1526.
First illustrated English herbal. It is mainly a translation of the French "Grant Herbier".

1803   BRUNFELS, Otto. 1488-1534
Herbarum vivae eicones. 3 vols. Argentorati, *apud I. Schottum,* 1530-36.
Brunfels was first in time and importance among the German botanists of the 16th century. For the illustrations in this work he went direct to nature instead of the earlier writers. The result was a new standard in botanical illustration and the first book on the subject which relied wholly on personal observation. The drawings were by Hans Weiditz.

1804   BRASAVOLA, Antonio Musa. 1500-1555
Examen omnium simplicium medicamentorum, quorum in officinis usus est. (Romae, *A. B. de Asula*), 1536.

Brasavola introduced some new drugs into the pharmacopoeia. The book is written in the form of a dialogue.

1805   TURNER, William. 1508-1568
Libellus de re herbaria novus. [Londini, *apud Ioannem Byddellum,* 1538].

An alphabetical catalogue of plants and medicines made from them. Turner, the "Father of English Botany", treated plants as simples, and did not attempt to show their relationships. He was a much travelled man and a friend of Conrad Gesner. He introduced lucerne into England. Reproduced in facsimile, London, 1877, and London, *Ray Society,* 1965. *See* Nos. 1810.2 & 1811.

1806   BOCK, Jerome [Tragus, Hieronymus]. 1498-1554
New Kreütter Buch. Strassburg, *W. Rihel,* 1539.

Bock was the first to describe the local flora of Germany, discovering many new species. His work gave a fresh impetus to plant description, With Brunfels and Fuchs he was one of the three "German fathers of botany". See B. Hoppe, *Das Kräuterbuch des Hieronymus Bock,* Stuttgart, A. Hiersemann, 1969.

1807   GESNER, Conrad. 1516-1565
Historiae plantarum et vires ex Dioscoride, Paulo Aegineta, *etc.* Parisiis, *apud Ioannem Lodoicum Tiletanum,* 1541.

A pocket dictionary of plants. Gesner, the "German Pliny", is remarkable for his encyclopaedic bibliographies. He attempted a *Historia plantarum,* which was unfinished at his death. *See* No. 1809.1.

1808   FUCHS, Leonhart. 1501-1566
De historia stirpium commentarii. Basileae, *in off. Isingriniana,* 1542.

The most famous herbal of the 16th century. Besides its accurate and detailed account of medical plants, it contains over 500 fine woodcuts, some of which are of interest as being the first European figures of certain American plants. A Flemish edition of the book, 1543, contains woodcuts of such excellence that many prefer it to the earlier edition. The name of Fuchs is preserved in the American "fuchsias". A collection of drawings made for *De historia stirpium,* and two further volumes that Fuchs was never able to publish, are now in the Austrian National Library, Vienna. A facsimile of a coloured copy of the German edition, 1543, was published in Zurich, 1981-85.

1809   GESNER, Conrad. 1516-1565
Enumeratio medicamentorum purgantium. Basileae, *per H. Frobenium,* 1543.

An index of purgatives.

1809.1   ———. Opera botanica per duo aecula desiderata, ex bibliotheca C.J. Trew. Nunc primum in lucem edidit et prefatus est C. C. Schmidel. 2 vols., Norimbergae, *J.M. Seligmann,* [1753-] 1754-59.

Stricken with the plague at the age of 49, Gesner was unable to complete his *Historia plantarum (See* No. 1807.) His collection of botanical watercolours changed hands several times until they were acquired by the physician-scholar, Cristoph J. Trew (d. 1769) who arranged to have them published as woodcuts and engravings in 1754-59. A second edition appeared in 1771. The watercolours then disappeared from view until they were "rediscovered" at the University of Erlangen in 1929. More recently 187 of the 700 watercolours were published in colour facsimile with extensive commentary, and transcription of the manuscript notes as: *Conradi Gesneri historia plantarum. Faksimileausgabe*, hg. von H. Zoller, M. Steimann & K. Schmid. 8 vols., Dietikon-Zürich, *Urs Graf*, 1972-80. The same publishers are also issuing the complete series of 700 watercolours in facsimile as *Historia plantarum, Gesamtausgabe*. 2 vols., 1987- .

1810   CORDUS, VALERIUS. 1515-1544
Pharmacorum omnium, quae quidem in usu sunt, conficiendorum ratio, vulgo vocant dispensatorium pharmacopolarum.Norimbergae, *apud J. Petreium,* 1546.
    The first real pharmacopoeia to be published. It was recognized as the official pharmacopoeia of Nuremberg. Facsimile edition, 1934.

1810.1   VESALIUS, ANDREAS. 1514-1564
Epistola, rationem modumque propinandi radicis Chynae decocti...Basileae, [*Ex off. Joannis Oporini*, 1546].
    In this work on the discovery and therapeutic use of the china root in the treatment of syphilis, Vesalius described the first attempt to formulate methods of identification of an exotic drug. He also offered physicians an opportunity to determine whether or not a drug coming into common use might be adulterated. The work contains Vesalius's defence of his anatomical methods and doctrines as described in the *Fabrica* (No. 375), as well as important autobiographical data.

1810.2   TURNER, WILLIAM. 1508-1568
The names of herbes in Greke, Latin, English, Duche & Frenche wyth the commune names that herbaries and apotecaries use. [London, *John Day*, 1548].
    A much-expanded English translation of Turner's *Libellus* (No. 1805). That and the above work mark the beginning of scientific botany in England. They contain the first records of the occurrence of some 238 species of flowering plants, a few of them precisely localized. Reprinted with introduction and bibliography, London, *Ray Society*, 1965.

1811   ———. A new herball. 3 vols. London, *S. Mierdman;* Collen, *A. Birckman,* 1551-68.
    The first original scientific herbal written by an Englishman, and the first scientific herbal published in the English language. The illustrations were taken from the blocks cut for the 8vo edition of Fuchs (1546). Turner was a strongly unorthodox thinker whose stubborn Protestant convictions forced him into exile on the Continent during the Catholic reaction at the end of the reign of Henry VIII, and again during the reign of Mary. He had a varied and turbulent career as naturalist, theologian and physician. Parts 2 and 3 were produced in English in Cologne, 1562 and 1568, while Turner was an exile in Germany. Part 3 was issued only with a reprint of Parts 1 and 2.

1811.1   CRUZ, MARTIN DE LA.
          The Badianus manuscript. (Codex Barberini, Latin, 241) Vatican Library.
          An Aztec Herbal of 1552. Introduction, translation and annotations by
          Emily W. Emmart. Baltimore, *Johns Hopkins Press,* 1940.
          The earliest complete Mexican medical text and the only medical text
          known to be the work of Aztec Indians. Written by an Aztec physician,
          Martin de la Cruz, and translated into Latin by another Indian, Juan Badia,
          around the time of the Spanish Conquest, the work is the earliest extant
          medical treatise written by a native American, and of course, the earliest
          herbal written in the Americas. Fine colour reproductions.

1812   DODOENS, REMPERT [DODONAEUS]. 1517-1585
          Cruÿdeboeck. Tantwerpen, *Jan ver der Loe,* 1554.
          Dodoens was the first Belgian botanist of international repute. Drawing
          on the illustrations of Fuchs, but preparing his own text, Dodoens improved
          on the alphabetical Fuchs organization scheme by grouping plants accord-
          ing to their properties and reciprocal affinities. With this work he provided
          a national herbarium of species indigenous to the Flemish provinces.
          English translation, London, 1578. Facsimile reprint Nieuwendijk, *Forel,*
          [1978].

1813   ANGUILLARA, LUIGI. *circa* 1512-1570
          Semplici dell'eccellente ... liquali in piu pareri à diversi nobili huomini
          scritti appaiono, et nuovamente da G. Marinello mandati in luce. Vinegia,
          V. Valgrisi, 1561.
          Anguillara was one of the best of many commentators of Dioscorides.

1814   CORDUS, VALERIUS. 1551-1544
          Annotationes in Pedacii Dioscoridis Anazarbei de medica materia.
          Argentorati, *excud. I. Rihelius,* 1561.
          This work not only modernizes the species listed by Dioscorides, but in
          addition lists about 500 new species of plants. Published posthumously,
          the work was carefully edited by Conrad Gesner. Cordus was the inventor
          of phytography and the discoverer of ethyl (sulphuric) ether.

1815   GARCIA D'ORTA. 1501-1568
          Coloquios dos simples, e drogas he cousas mediçinais da India. Goa,
          Joannes, 1563.
          The first account of Indian materia medica and the first textbook on
          tropical medicine written by a European. It includes a classic account of
          cholera. It is the third book printed in India and is almost priceless. For an
          account of its author, see L. H. Roddis, *Ann. med. Hist.,* 1929, **1,** 198-207.
          English translation by Sir Clements R. Markham, London, 1913.

1816   OCCO, ADOLPH. 1524-1606
          Enchiridion, sive ut vulgo vocant dispensatorium, compositorum
          medicamentorum, pro Reipub. Augstburgensis pharmacopoeia. [Augsburg,
          1564].
          One of the earliest pharmacopoeias, and one which exerted a great
          influence on later pharmacopoeias. Several new editions followed the first,
          and that of 1613 was adopted as the official pharmacopoeia of Augsburg,
          the famous *Pharmacopoeia Augustana.* Occo, the third of a famous
          medical family, was town physician of Augsburg. The book has been

reprinted in facsimile, with notes, by the State Historical Society of Wisconsin, 1927, and is edited by T. Husemann.

1817   MONARDES, NICOLÁS. 1493-1588
Dos libros. El uno trata de todas las cosas que traen nuestras Indias Occidentales, *etc*. Sevilla, *S. Trugillo,* 1565.
First treatise on Central American drugs, and for many years the most important work on the medicinal plants of the New World. A second part to the book appeared in 1571, and a third, together with the first two, in 1574. English translation by John Frampton: *Joyfull newes out of the newe found world,* 1577 (reprinted 1925).

1818   PARACELSUS [BOMBASTUS VON HOHENHEIM, THEOPHRASTUS PHILIPPUS AUREOLUS]. 1493-1541
De gradibus, de compositionibus, et dosibus receptorum ac naturalium libri septem. Myloecii, *Excudebat Petrus Fabricius,* 1562.
Paracelsus has been called by some "the pioneer of modern chemists" and by others "uncouth, boorish, vain, ignorant and pretentious". His *De gradibus* contains most of his innovations in chemical therapeutics. A definitive edition of the works of Paracelsus was published by K. Sudhoff. *See* No. 57.

1819   ACOSTA, CRISTOBAL. [COSTA, (CHRISTOVAL DA)]. *ca* 1540-1599
Tractado delas drogas, y medicinas de las Indias Orientales, con sus plantas debuxadas al bivo. Burgos, *Martin de Victoria,* 1578.
This is mainly a translation of Garcia d'Orta's *Coloquios* (No. 1815) with the addition of some illustrations. Acosta travelled to India where he met Garcia d'Orta.

1819.1   FARFAN, AGUSTIN. 1531/32-1604
Tractado breve de anathomia y chirurgia. Mexico, *Antonio Ricardo,* 1579.
Includes the first work on the plants and botanic remedies of the New World. Second edition, *Tractado brebe de medicina* (1592). This is an abridgement of manuscripts left in Mexico by Francisco Hernández. *See* Nos. 1820.1 & 1821.1.

1820   GERARD, JOHN. 1545-1612
The herball or generall historie of plantes. London (*E. Bollifant for B. and J. Norton*), 1597.
Gerard is perhaps the best remembered of all the English herbalists. The most important edition of his book is the second, published by T. Johnson in 1633 (reprinted in facsimile, New York, *Dover,* 1975). Johnson greatly enlarged the book, correcting many mistakes and bringing the number of plants included to a total of 2850. Gerard plagiarized much of his work from Dodoens (No. 1812). See B. Henrey, *British botanical and horticultural literature before 1800,* Vol. 1, pp. 35-54, 1975.

1820.1   HERNÁNDEZ, FRANCISCO. 1517-1587
Quatro libros de la naturaleza, y virtudes de las plantas, y animales que estan receuidos en el uso de medicina en la Nueua España...Mexico, *Viuda de Lopez Davalos,* 1615.
Physician to Philip II of Spain, Hernández travelled to Mexico by order of the king, and studied the natural history of the region from 1570-77. His works, which filled more than 20 manuscript volumes, were deposited in

the library of the Escorial, and in Mexico City, but never published in Hernández's lifetime. Many of them have since been lost. A manuscript of this summary in Latin, edited for the king by N.A. de Recchi, found its way to Mexico where it was revised and translated into Spanish-Aztec and published by F. Ximenez. It is the second work on the natural history, plants, and botanic medicines of Mexico to be published in the New World. *See* Nos. 1819.1 & 1821.1.

1821   PHARMACOPOEIA.
Pharmacopoeia Londinensis. London, *E. Griffin for J. Marriott*, 1618.
   The first London pharmacopoeia, issued by the (Royal) College of Physicians. The first edition was published on May 7, but contained many typographical errors; a corrected edition appeared on December 7, 1618. In the first issue the name of the publisher is printed "Marriot". Facsimile reprint of both versions, with introduction by G. Urdang, Madison, 1944.

1821.1   HERNÁNDEZ, FRANCISCO. 1517-1587
Rerum medicarum Novae Hispaniae thesaurus...Romae, *Ex typographeio Jacobi Mascardi*, 1628.
   This summary of Hernández's very extensive manuscript account of the natural history of Mexico (*see* No. 1820.1) was edited by N.A. de Recchi, and published at the expense of Prince Federico Cesi with notes by G. Terrentio, J. Faber, F. Colonna, and Cesi. Publication of the work was discontinued with the death of Cesi in 1628. It is usually seen in the reissue of 1649 or 1651, for which Francesco Stelluti was responsible. The remainder of Hernandez's extant manuscripts were finally published in the *Obras completas*, 4 vols., Mexico City, 1959-66. *See* Nos. 1819.1 & 1820.1.

1822   PARKINSON, JOHN. 1567-1650
Paradisi in sole paradisus terrestris. Or a garden of all sorts of pleasant flowers. London, *H. Lownes and R. Young*, 1629.
   The title is a pun on the author's name (park-in-sun).

1823   ——. Theatrum botanicum: The theater of plants. Or, an universall and compleate herball. London, *T. Cotes*, 1640.
   Parkinson, the last of the old English herbalists, was Apothecary to James I. His massive herbal of 1,755 pages describes nearly 3,800 plants, nearly double the number described in the first edition of Gerard. Parkinson was more original than either Gerard or Johnson. Rohde calls the *Theatrum botanicum* the "largest herbal in the English language".

1824   PHARMACOPOEIA.
Codex medicamentarius seu pharmacopoeia Parisiensis. Lutetiae Parisiorum, *sumpt. Olivarii de Varennes*, 1639.
   First Paris pharmacopoeia.

1825   PISO, WILLEM. 1611-1678
De Indiae utriusque re naturali et medica libri quatuordecim. Amstelaedami, *apud L. et D. Elzevirios*, 1658.
   Piso introduced ipecacuanha into Europe. Reproduced in part, with translation, in *Opuscula Selecta Neerlandicorum de Arte Medica*, 1937, No. 14. This is an extensively revised and enlarged second edition of Piso's *Historia naturalis Brasiliae* (1648). *See* Nos. 2263.1 & 5303.

1826   BADO, SEBASTIANO [BALDI] *fl.* 1640-1676
Anastasis corticis Peruviae, seu chinae defensio. Genuae, *typ. P. I. Calenzani,* 1663.
A defence of the virtues of Peruvian bark. Bado includes evidence to show that "fever bark" was introduced into Spain in 1632.

1826.1   JOSSELYN, JOHN. *fl.* 1675.
New-Englands rarities discovered: in birds, beasts, fishes, serpents, and plants of that country. Together with the physical and chyrurgical remedies wherewith the natives constantly use to cure their distempers, wounds, and sores...London, *G. Widdowes,* 1672.
The first detailed account of the natural history and botany of North America, including the first extensive study of North American Indian medicine.

1827   WELSCH, GOTTFRIED. 1618-1690
De medicis et medicamentis Germanorum. Lipsiae, 1688.

1827.1   POMET, PIERRE. 1658-99
Histoire générale des drogues...Paris, *Loyson...,* 1694.
The most complete materia medica of the time, compiled by the druggist/botanist Pomet. English translation, London, 1712.

1828   RIVINUS, AUGUSTUS QUIRINUS. 1652-1723
Censura medicamentorum officinalium. Lipsiae, *J. Fritsch,* 1701.
A list of officially recognized drugs, with a classification of useless and undesirable ones. Rivinus also noted incompatibles.

1828.1   CULPEPER, NICHOLAS. 1616-54
The English physician. Boston, *Nicholas Boone,* 1708.
This reprint of Culpeper's popular work on herbal remedies was the first medical book (94pp.) printed in North America.

1828.2   ———. Pharmacopoeia Londinensis; or the London dispensatory...Boston, *Nicholas Booone* [sic], 1720.
The first herbal printed in North America, and the first full-length medical book published in North America. From the 1653 London edition.

1829   LINNÉ, CARL VON [LINNAEUS]. 1707-1778
Genera plantarum. Lugduni Batavorum *apud Conradum Wishoff,* 1737.
Linnaeus's botanical classification, the starting-point of modern systematic botany. The book is dedicated to Boerhaave. English translation by Erasmus Darwin, Lichfield, 1787.

1830   GAUB, HIERONYMUS DAVID. 1705-1780
Libellus de methodo concinnandi formulas medicamentorum. Lugduni Batavorum, *C. Wishoff,* 1739.
A treatise on prescriptions. Gaub was professor of chemistry at Leiden.

1831   HEBERDEN, WILLIAM, *Snr.* 1710-1801
Αυτιθηεριακά. An essay on mithridatium and theriaka. [London], 1745.
Heberden's first printed work. His criticism of current superstitions concerning these two concoctions resulted ultimately in their removal from the pharmacopoeia.

1832   BARTRAM, JOHN. 1699-1777
          Descriptions, virtues, and uses of sundry plants of these northern parts of
          America. [Philadelphia], 1751.
              Bartram founded the first botanical garden in America (at Kingsessing).
          Linnaeus refers to him as the "greatest natural botanist in the world".

1833   HALLER, ALBRECHT VON. 1708-1777
          Bibliotheca botanica. 2 vols., Tiguri, *apud Orell, Gessner, Fuessli et socc.,*
          1771-72.
              This was the first of the several bibliographies compiled by Haller, one
          of the greatest figures in the history of medicine. The work contains the
          most exhaustive and thorough information of the writings in the field of
          botany then extant. Choulant considered that the bibliographies on botany
          and anatomy were the best of Haller's works.

1833.1   WITHERING, WILLIAM. 1741-1799
          A botanical arrangement of all the vegetables naturally growing in Great
          Britain. 2 vols. London, *T. Cadell,* 1776.
              The first flora of Great Britain using Linnean binomial nomenclature,
          and the first complete scientific classification and description of British
          plants in the English language. Withering included much information on
          natural places of growth, time of flowering, economic uses as foods and
          drugs, and poisonous properties.

1834   BROWN, WILLIAM. 1752-1792
          Pharmacopoeia simpliciorum et efficaciorum. Philadelphiae, *ex. off. Styner
          & Cist,* 1778.
              The first original pharmacopoeia published in the USA. Reproduced in
          facsimile, with translation, in *The Badger Pharmacist,* 1938. No. 22-25.

1835   PERCIVAL, THOMAS. 1740-1804
          Observations on the medical uses of the oleum jecoris aselli, or cod liver
          oil, in the chronic rheumatism, and other painful disorders. *Lond. med. J.,*
          1782, **3,** 392-401.
              First record of the clinical use of cod liver oil in England.

1836   WITHERING, WILLIAM. 1741-1799
          An account of the foxglove, and some of its medical uses. Birmingham, *G.
          G. J. & J. Robinson,* 1785.
              Withering was one of the greatest medical botanists and his book is a
          pharmacological classic. Before his time digitalis was a widely used folk
          remedy, occasionally mentioned in the literature, but it was due to him that
          correct dosages were established and the action of digitalis in dropsy and
          on the heart became generally recognized. He did not know of the
          distinction between renal and cardiac dropsy. Facsimile reprint, London,
          1949. Facsimile reprint, with marginal notes on relevant points in the text,
          and a history of digitalis since Withering's day, by J.K. Aronson, London,
          Oxford Univ. Press, 1985. *See* No. 2734.31.

1836.1   MARSHALL, HUMPHREY. 1722-1801.
          Arbustrum Americanum: the American grove, or, an alphabetical catalogue
          of forest trees and shrubs...Philadelphia, *Joseph Crukshank,* 1785.
              Like his cousin, John Bartram (No. 1832), Marshall maintained a private
          botanical garden. According to W. Darlington the above work is "the first

truly indigenous botanical essay published in the Western Hemisphere".
It contains some information about medicines.

1837 SCHOEPFF, JOHANN DAVID. 1752-1800
Materia medica Americana, potissimum regni vegetabilis. Erlangae, *J. J. Palmii*, 1787.

Schoepff came to America in 1777 as a surgeon with the Hessian troops employed by the British Forces. He returned to Germany in 1784 and compiled the first full American materia medica, describing about 400 plants, including a few references to American Indian remedies.

1838 CULLEN, WILLIAM. 1710-1790
A treatise of the materia medica. 2 vols. Edinburgh, *C. Elliot,* 1789.
An expansion of Cullen's "Lectures on materia medica", 1773.

1838.1 WOODVILLE, WILLIAM. 1752-1805
Medical botany...3 vols. & Supplement. London, *Phillips for the author,* 1790-94[95].

Issued in numbers from 1790-1795, this is the first edition in book form. Probably the finest of all colour-plate medical botanies in English, containing systematic and general descriptions of all the plants in the materia medica of the Royal Colleges of Physicians of London and Edinburgh. It remained the standard work on the plants of the British pharmacopoeia until the 1880s.

1838.2 STEARNS, SAMUEL. 1747-1819.
The American herbal, or materia medica. Walpole, New Hampshire, *Thomas & Thomas,* 1801.

The first herbal both produced and printed in the United States, as opposed to those which were reprints of European works. Includes information on American Indian remedies.

1838.3 DEROSNE, CHARLES LOUIS. 1780-1846
Sur l'opium. *Ann. Chim.,* 1802, **45,** 257-85.
Isolation of alkaloids from opium.

1839 SERTÜRNER, FRIEDRICH WILHELM ADAM. 1783-1841
Darstellung der reinen Mohnsäure (Opiumsäure); nebst einer chemischen Untersuchung des Opiums, mit vorzüglicher Hinsicht auf einen darin neu entdeckten Stoff. *J. Pharm. (Lpz.),* 1805, **14,** 47-93.
Isolation of morphine.

1840 GOMES, BERNARDINO ANTONIO. 1769-1823
Ensaio sobre o cinchonino, e sobre sua influencia em a virtude da quina, e de outras cascas. *Mem. Acad. reale Sci. Lisboa,* 1810, **3,** 202-217.

Gomes obtained a substance, which he named *cinchonino,* from cinchona bark. That it contained the active principle of cinchona was later proved by Pelletier and Caventou. For an English translation of the paper, see *Edinb. med. surg. J.,* 1811, **7,** 420-31.

1841 BARTON, WILLIAM PAUL CRILLON. 1786-1856
Vegetable materia medica of the United States. 2 vols. Philadelphia, *M. Carey & Son,* 1817-[19].

Barton served as a naval surgeon and, in 1815, became Professor of Botany at Philadelphia. Along with Bigelow (No. 1842) Barton's work shares the distinction of being the first botanical work with coloured plates issued in the United States.

1842   BIGELOW, JACOB. 1786-1879
American medical botany. 3 vols. Boston, *Cummings & Hilliard,* 1817-20.
Bigelow, one of America's greatest botanists, was professor of materia medica at Harvard. This is the first book printed in the United States to include colour plates printed in colour. See R.J. Wolfe, *Jacob Bigelow's American medical botany, 1817-1821*...Boston, *Boston Medical Library,* 1979.

1843   PELLETIER, PIERRE JOSEPH. 1788-1842, & MAGENDIE, FRANÇOIS. 1783-1855
Recherches chimiques et physiologiques sur l'ipécacuanha. *Ann. Chim. Phys., (Paris),* 1817, **4,** 172-85.
Isolation of emetine.

1844   ——. & CAVENTOU, JOSEPH BIENAIME. 1795-1877
Mémoire sur un nouvel alcali végétal (la strychnine) trouvé dans la fève de Saint-Ignace, la noix vomique, *etc. J. Pharm. (Paris),* 1819, **5,** 145-174.
Isolation of strychnine.

1845   PHARMACOPOEIA.
Pharmacopoeia of the United States of America. Boston, *C. Ewer,* 1820.
First official US pharmacopoeia.

1846   MAGENDIE, FRANÇOIS. 1783-1855
Formulaire pour la préparation et l'emploi de plusieurs nouveaux médicamens, tels que la noix vomique, la morphine, *etc.* Paris, *Méquignon-Marvis,* 1822.
Magendie was the pioneer of experimental physiology in France. His *Formulaire* introduced into medical practice several of the newly discovered alkaloids, notably morphine, veratrine, brucine, piperine, emetine, as well as quinine and strychnine. An English translation of this book appeared in 1824.

1847   SCHENK, JOHANN HEINRICH.
Erfahrungen über die grossen Heilkräfte des Leberthrans gegen chronische Rheumatismen und besonders gegen das Hüft- und Lendenweh., *J. pract. Heilk.,* 1822, **55,** 6 St., 31-58; 1826, **62,** 3 St., 3-40.
Schenk's account of his experience with cod liver oil led to its general use on the continent of Europe. Author's name incorrectly given as Scherer in original.

1848   SÉRULLAS, GEORGES SIMON. 1774-1832
Mémoire sur l'iodure de potassium, l'acide hydriodique et sur un composé nouveau de carbone, d'iode et d'hydrogène. *Ann. Chim. Phys.,* 1822, 2 sér., **20,** 163-68.
Iodoform discovered.

1848.1   BALARD, ANTOINE JÉROME. 1802-1876
Sur une substance particulière contenue dans l'eau de la mer. *Ann. Chim. (Paris),* 1826, **32,** 337-81.
Isolation of bromine.

1849 RAFINESQUE, CONSTANTIN SAMUEL. 1783-1840
   Medical flora. 2 vols. Philadelphia, *Atkinson, etc.* 1828-30.
   Rafinesque was a great botanist, conchologist, archaeologist, and
   economist. Born in a suburb of Istanbul, he was also a world citizen and
   a prolific writer with 939 works to his credit. He died in extreme poverty
   in Philadelphia and, but for the intervention of a few friends, his body
   would have been sold for dissection purposes. This work describes for the
   first time a number of American Indian remedies.

1849.1 LUGOL, JEAN GUILLAUME AUGUST. 1786-1851
   Mémoire sur l'emploi de l'iode dans les maladies scrofuleuses. Paris,
   Baillière, 1829.
   Lugol's solution.

1850 GUTHRIE, SAMUEL. 1782-1848
   New mode of preparing a spirituous solution of chloric ether. *Amer. J. Sci.*
   Arts, 1832, **21,** 64-65; **22,** 105-06.
   Guthrie, Liebig and Soubeiran discovered chloroform independently of
   one another. Guthrie discovered the modern method of making chloroform by distilling alcohol with chlorinated lime. Second paper has title: On
   pure chloric ether.

1851 SOUBEIRAN, EUGÈNE. 1793-1858
   Recherches sur quelques combinaisons du chlore. *Ann. Chim. (Paris),*
   1831, 2e sér., **48,** 113, 57.
   Soubeiran, like Liebig and Guthrie, discovered chloroform; it is difficult
   to determine who was first, as each may have allowed an interval of time
   to elapse between discovery and publication.

1852 LIEBIG, JUSTUS VON. 1803-1873
   Ueber die Verbindungen, welche durch die Einwirkung des Chlors auf
   Alkohol, Aether, ölbildenes Gas und Essiggeist entstehen. *Ann. Pharm.*
   (Heidelberg), 1832, **1,** 182-230.
   Discovery, in 1831, of chloroform and chloral. Independently chloroform
   was discovered by Souberian and by Guthrie.

1853 ROBIQUET, PIERRE JEAN. 1780-1840
   Nouvelles observations sur les principaux produits de l'opium. *Ann. Chim.*
   (Paris), 1832, 2e sér. **51,** 225-67.
   Isolation of codeine.

1854 MEIN.
   Ueber die Darstellung des Atropins in weissen Krystallen. *Ann. Chem.*
   Pharm., 1833, **6,** 67-72.
   Mein isolated atropine in pure form in 1831.

1855 RUNGE, FRIEDLIEB FERDINAND. 1795-1867
   Ueber einige Producte der Steinkohlendestillation. *Ann. Phys. Chem. (Lpz.),*
   1834, **31,** 65-77, 513-24; **32,** 308-32.
   Carbolic acid first prepared from coal-tar.

1856 PEREIRA, JONATHAN. 1804-1853
   The elements of materia medica. 2 vols. London, *Longman,* 1839-40.

The first great English work on the subject. Pereira was Professor of Materia Medica at the School of Pharmacy set up by the Pharmaceutical Society of Great Britain.

1857   PIRIA, RAFFAELE. 1815-1865
Recherches sur la salicine et les produits qui en dérivent. *C. R. Acad. Sci., (Paris)*, 1839, **8,** 479-85.
Piria made salicylic acid from salicin.

1858   BENNETT, JOHN HUGHES. 1812-1875
Treatise on the oleum jecoris aselli, or cod liver oil. Edinburgh, *Maclachlan, Stewart & Co.,* 1841.
Bennett visited Paris and Germany, and learned there of the beneficial effects of cod liver oil. His book drew the attention of English medical men to the value of the oil.

1859   BALARD, ANTOINE JEROME. 1802-1876
Mémoire sur l'alcool amylique. *C. R. Acad. Sci. (Paris)*, 1844, **19,** 634-41.
Discovery of amyl nitrite.

1860   HOMOLLE, AUGUSTIN EUGÈNE. 1808-1875
Mémoire sur la digitale pourprée. *J. Pharm. Chim.*, 1845, 3me. sér., **7,** 57-83.
Isolation of an active principle in digitalis, amorphous digitalin, more potent than the plant itself.

1861   MERCK, GEORG FRANZ. 1825-1873
Vorläufige Notiz über eine neue organische Base im Opium. *Ann. Phys. Chem. (Lpz.)*, 1848, **66,** 125-28.
Isolation of papaverine.

1861.1   GERLAND, H.
New formation of salicylic acid. *J. chem. Soc.*, 1852, **5,** 133-35.
Synthesis of salicylic acid.

1862   PORCHER, FRANCIS PEYRE. 1825-1895
The medicinal, poisonous and dietetic properties of the cryptogamic plants of the United States. New York, *Baker, Godwin & Co.,* 1854.

1862.1   BUCHHEIM, RUDOLF. 1820-1879
Lehrbuch der Arzneimittellehre. Leipzig, *L. Voss,* 1856.
Buchheim was the most important of the early teachers of pharmacology.

1863   BERNARD, CLAUDE. 1813-1878
Leçons sur les effets des substances toxiques et médicamenteuses. Paris, *J. B. Baillière,* 1857.
Bernard included a summary of his experiments with curare in the *Leçons* to establish his priority in researching its effects. He demonstrated in these experiments the susceptibility of the nerve-muscle preparation to a chemical (pharmacological) effect.

1864   LEMAIRE, FRANÇOIS JULES. 1814-1886
        Du coaltar saponiné, désinfectant énergique. Paris, *Germer-Baillière,* 1860.
        Lemaire was first to point out the antiseptic properties of carbolic acid.

1865   NIEMANN, ALBERT. 1834-1861
        Ueber eine neue organische Base in den Cocablättern. Göttingen, *E. A. Huth,* 1860.
        Isolation of cocaine, 1859, from the coca leaf, brought from Peru by Scherzer.

1865.1 PORCHER, FRANCIS PEYRE. 1825-1895
        Resources of the Southern fields and forests...Being a medical botany of the Confederate States...Charleston, *Evans & Cogswell,* 1863.
        The first extensive treatise on the botany of the Southern states of the US and the only Confederate manual of materia medica. This is also a manual of "survival information", teaching how live off the land and how to make medicines from indigenous plants, because the Union blockade of Confederate ports prevented the importation of medicines from Europe.

1866   PHARMACOPOEIA.
        British Pharmacopoeia, published pursuant to the Medical Act, 1858. London, *General Medical Council,* 1864.
        First official British pharmacopoeia.

1866.1 FRASER, *Sir* THOMAS RICHARD. 1841-1919
        On the physiological action of the Calabar bean (Physostigma venenosum, *Balf.*). *Trans. roy. Soc. Edinb.* (1866), 1867, **24,** 715-88.
        Isolation of eserine (physostigmine).

1867   BROWN, ALEXANDER CRUM. 1838-1922, & FRASER, *Sir* THOMAS RICHARD. 1841-1919
        On the connection between chemical constitution and physiological action. *Trans. roy. Soc. Edinb.,* 1868-69, **25,** 151-203, 693-739.
        Brown and Fraser were the first to investigate the relationship between the chemical constitution of substances and their action upon the body.

1868   MORÉNO Y MAÏZ, THOMAS.
        Recherches chimiques et physiologiques sur l'Erythroxylum coca du Pérou et la cocaïne. Paris, *L. Leclerc,* 1868.
        This, the first study of the pharmacological action of cocaine, contains the earliest suggestion of its use as a local anaesthetic.

1869   LIEBREICH, OSCAR. 1839-1908
        Das Chloral, ein neues Hypnoticum. *Arch. dtsch. Ges. Psychiat.,* 1869, **16,** 237.
        Demonstration of the value of chloral hydrate as a hypnotic. See also his monograph *Das Chloralhydrat,* Berlin, 1869.

1869.1 SCHMIEDEBERG, JOHANN ERNST OSWALD. 1838-1921
        Untersuchungen über die pharmakologisch wirksamen Bestandtheile der Digitalis purpurea *L. Arch. exp. Path. Pharmak.,* 1875, **3,** 16-43.
        Schmiedeberg isolated digitoxin from digitalis.

1869.2   BUSS, CARL EMIL.
Ueber die Anwendung der Salicylsäure als Antipyreticum. *Dtsch. Arch. klin. Med.*, 1875, **15**, 457-501.
Buss introduced the clinical use of salicylic acid as an antipyretic.

1870   BENTLEY, ROBERT. 1825-1893, & TRIMEN, HENRY. 1843-1896
Medicinal plants, being descriptions with original figures of the principal plants employed in medicine. 4 vols. London, *J. & A. Churchill,* 1880.

1871   ANREP, VASILI KONSTANTINOVICH. 1852-1918
Ueber die physiologische Wirking des Cocaïn. *Pflüg. Arch. ges. Physiol.,* 1880, **21**, 38-77.
Anrep studied the action of cocaine and, like Moréno y Maïz, suggested that it might be used as a local anaesthetic.

1873   LADENBURG, ALBERT. 1842-1911
Die natürlich vorkommenden mydriatisch wirkenden Alkaloïde. *Ann. Chem. Pharm.*, 1881, **206**, 274-307.
Isolation of hysocine (scopolamine).

1874   MARTINDALE, WILLIAM. 1840-1902
The extra pharmacopoeia of unofficial drugs ... With references to their use abstracted from the medical journals by W. Wynn Westcott. London, *H. K. Lewis,* 1883.
29th edition, 1989.

1875   SCHMIEDEBERG, JOHANN ERNST OSWALD. 1838-1921
Grundriss der Arzneimittellehre. Leipzig, *F. C. W. Vogel,* 1883.
Schmiedeberg, leading German pharmacologist, was professor at Dorpat and Strasburg. Among his many valuable investigations may be mentioned his study of the effect of drugs on the circulation.

1877   CERVELLO, VINCENZO. 1854-1919
Recherches cliniques et physiologiques sur la paraldéhyde. *Arch. ital. Biol.,* 1884, **6**, 113-34.
Introduction of paraldehyde into therapeutics as a narcotic.

1878   FILEHNE, WILHELM. 1844-1927
Ueber das Antipyrin, ein neues Antipyreticum. *Z. klin. Med.,* 1884, **7**, 641-42.
Introduction of antipyrine.

1879   UNNA, PAUL GERSON. 1850-1929
Eine neue Form medicamentöser Einverleibung. *Fortschr. Med.,* 1884, **2**, 507-09.
Unna introduced specially coated pills for local absorption in the intestine.

1880   BINZ, CARL. 1832-1913
Vorlesungen über Pharmakologie. Berlin, *A. Hirschwald,* 188[4]-86.
Includes his test for quinine in urine. English translation of second edition, 1895-97. Binz was Professor of Pharmacology at Bonn. His most important work was perhaps the demonstration that quinine in low concentrations kills numerous micro-organisms.

1880.1   FREUD, SIGMUND. 1856-1939
          Ueber coca. *Centralblatt. ges. Ther.*, 1884, **2**, 289-314.
          Freud described his observations (with himself as subject) on the effects
          of cocaine, including its abolition of hunger and fatigue, the "exhilaration and
          lasting euphoria". He also described its supposed non-addictiveness, calling
          it "absolutely harmless in long use". He later bitterly regretted this miscon-
          ception, as he himself nearly became addicted, and misuse of the drug
          contributed to the death of one of his dearest friends. Freud's suggestion that
          cocaine might act by abolishing the effect of agencies that depress bodily
          feeling has since been confirmed, and his recognition of the drug's anaes-
          thetizing qualities may have given Koller the idea to revolutionize eye surgery
          by using cocaine as the first local anaesthetic. *See* No. 5678. English transla-
          tion in *St. Louis med. & surg. J.*, 1884, **47**, 502-05. Revised second edition by
          Freud, Vienna, 1885. Also translated in Freud, *The cocaine papers*, Vienna/
          Zurich, 1963 and Freud, *Cocaine Papers*, R. Byck (ed.), New York, 1974.

1881   BRUNTON, *Sir* THOMAS LAUDER, *Bart*. 1844-1916
          A text-book of pharmacology, therapeutics and materia medica. London,
          Macmillan & Co., 1885.
          Brunton was physician to St. Bartholomew's Hospital and an eminent
          pharmacologist. He is notable for his introduction of amyl nitrite in the
          treatment of angina pectoris and for a vast amount of other work concerning
          the action of drugs on the cardiovascular system.

1882   BAUMANN, EUGEN. 1846-1896
          Ueber Disulfone. *Ber. dtsch. chem. Ges.*, 1886, **19**, 2806-14.
          Preparation of sulphonal.

1883   UNNA, PAUL GERSON. 1850-1929
          Ichthyol und Resorcin als Repräsentanten der Gruppe reduzierender
          Heilmittel. Hamburg, Leipzig, *L. Voss,* 1886.
          Unna introduced ichthyol and resorcinol into medicine. Supplement to
          Mh. prakt. Derm., No. 1.

1883.01   LANGE, CARL GEORG. 1834-1900
          Om Periodiske Depressionstilstande og deres Patogenese. Copenhagen,
          Jacob Lunds Forlag, 1886.
          Lange was the first to use a mixture of drugs containing lithium
          carbonate for the preventive treatment of periodic depression. This work
          contains the "first unequivocal account of prophylactic drug treatment for
          an exclusively psychiatric – as distinct from physical – condition" (Johnson).

1883.1   NAGAI, NAGAJOSI. 1844-1929
          Ephedrin. *Pharm. Ztg.,* 1887, **32,** 700.
          Isolation of ephedrine.

1883.2   CAHN, ARNOLD, & HEPP, PAUL.
          Sur l'action de l'antifébrine (acétanilide) et de quelques corps analogues.
          Progrès méd., 1887, **5,** 43-46.
          Introduction of acetanilide (antifebrin).

1883.3   HINSBERG, OSCAR HEINRICH DANIEL.1857-1939, & KAST, ALFRED. 1856-1903
          Ueber die Wirkung des Acetphenetidins. *Zbl. med. Wiss.,* 1887, **25,** 145-8.
          Introduction of phenacetin.

1884 KAST, ALFRED. 1856-1903
Sulfonal, ein neues Schlafmittel.2 *Berl. klin. Wschr.*, 1888, **25,** 309-14.
Introduction of sulphonal, previously discovered by Baumann.

1885 FRASER, *Sir* THOMAS RICHARD. 1841-1919
Strophanthus hispidus; its natural history, chemistry, and pharmacology.
Trans. roy. Soc. Edinb., 1890, **35,** 955-1027; 1892, **36,** 343-457.
Introduction of Strophanthus hispidus.

1886 CASH, JOHN THEODORE. 1854-1936, & DUNSTAN, *Sir* WYNDHAM ROWLAND. 1861-
1949
The physiological action of the nitrites of the paraffin series, considered in
connection with their chemical constitution. *Phil. Trans. B,* (1893), 1894,
184, 505-639.

1887 PAUL, BENJAMIN HORATIO. 1828-1902, & COWNLEY, ALFRED JOHN.
The chemistry of ipecacuanha. *Pharm. J.,* 1894-95, **54,** 111-15, 373-74, 690-
92.
Emetine first obtained in pure form.

1888 FISCHER, EMIL. 1852-1919, & ACH, LORENZ. 1868-1948
Neue Synthese der Harnsäure und ihrer Methylderivate. *Ber. dtsch. chem.
Ges.,* 1895, **28,** 2473-80.

1889 FILEHNE, WILHELM. 1844-1927
Ueber das Pyramidon, ein Antipyrinderivat. *Berl. klin. Wschr.,* 1896, **33,**
1061-63.
Filehne was responsible for the introduction of amindopyrine
(pyramidon).

1890 KRÖNIG, CLAUS LUDWIG THEODOR BERNHARD. 1863-1918, & PAUL, THEODOR.
1862-1928
Die chemischen Grundlagen der Lehre von der Giftwirkung und
Desinfection. *Z. Hyg. InfektKr.,* 1897, **25,** 1-112.
Krönig and Paul described a new method for the quantitative study of
disinfection and laid the foundation of modern knowledge of disinfectants.

1890.1 HEFFTER, KARL WILHELM ARTHUR. 1859-1925
Ueber Pellote. Beiträge zur chemischen und pharmakologischen Kenntniss
der Cacteen. Zweite Mitteilung. *Arch. exp. Path. Pharmak.,* 1898, **40,** 385-
429.
Isolation of mescaline, the active agent in peyote. One of the first
scientific investigations of a psychedelic drug.

1891 DRESER, HEINRICH. 1860-1925
Pharmakologisches über Aspirin (Acetylsalicylsäure). *Pflüg. Arch. ges.
Physiol.,* 1899, **76,** 306-18.
Acetylsalicylic acid (aspirin) introduced into medicine.

1892 FISCHER EMIL. 1852-1919, & MERING, JOSEPH VON. 1849-1908
Ueber eine neue Klasse von Schlafmitteln. *Therap. Gegenw.,* 1903, **44,** 97-
101.
Synthesis of barbitone.

1893 RIDEAL, SAMUEL. 1863-1929, & WALKER, J. T. AINSLIE. 1868-1930
Standardisation of disinfectants. *J. sanit. Inst.,* 1903, **24,** 424-41.
Rideal–Walker method for testing disinfectants.

1893.1 CLOETTA, MAX. 1868-1940
Ueber Digalen (Digitoxinum solubile). *Münch. med. Wschr.,* 1904, **51,** 1466-68.
Introduction of digalen.

1893.2 LANGLEY, JOHN NEWPORT. 1852-1925
On the reaction of cells and of nerve-endings to certain poisons, chiefly as regards the reaction of striated muscle to nicotine and to curari. *J. Physiol. (Lond.),* 1905, **33,** 374-413.
Langley introduced the concept of a receptor substance present in the biological object with which a drug has to interact in order to exert its biological effect.

1894 MELTZER, SAMUEL JAMES. 1851-1920, & AUER, JOHN. 1875-1948
Physiological and pharmacological studies of magnesium salts. *Amer. J. Physiol.,* 1905, **14,** 366-88; 1906, **15,** 387-405; **16,** 233-51.
A study of the anaesthetic and other effects of magnesium salts.

1895 BARGER, GEORGE. 1878-1939, *et al.*
An active alkaloid from ergot. *Brit. med. J.,* 1906, **2,** 1792.
Isolation of ergotoxine. With F. H. Carr and H. H. Dale.

1895.1 WINDAUS, ADOLF. 1876-1959, & VOGT, KARL. 1880-
Synthese des Imidazolyläthylamins. *Ber. dtsch. chem. Ges.,* 1907, **40,** 3691-95.
Synthesis of histamine.

1896 ABEL, JOHN JACOB. 1857-1938, & ROWNTREE, LEONARD GEORGE. 1883-1959
On the pharmacological action of some phthaleins and their derivatives. *J. Pharmacol.,* 1909, **1,** 231-64.
This work led to the universal clinical use of phenolsulphonephthalein in renal function tests and of phenoltetrachlorphthalein in hepatic function tests.

1897 HUNT, REID. 1870-1948, TAVEAU, RENÉ DE M.
On the relation between the toxicity and chemical constitution of a number of derivatives of choline and analogous compounds. *J. Pharmacol.,* 1909, **1,** 303-39.

1898 BARGER, GEORGE. 1878-1939, & DALE, *Sir* HENRY HALLETT. 1875-1968
Chemical structure and sympathomimetic action of amines. *J. Physiol. (Lond.),* 1910, **41,** 19-59.
Discovery of histamine in an ergot extract.

1899 DALE, *Sir* HENRY HALLETT. 1875-1968, & LAIDLAW, *Sir* PATRICK PLAYFAIR. 1881-1940
The physiological action of ß-iminoazolylethylamine. *J. Physiol. (Lond.),* 1910, **41,** 318-44.
Study of the effect of histamine.

1900 MEYER, HANS HORST. 1853-1939, & GOTTLIEB, RUDOLPH. 1864-1924
Die experimentelle Pharmakologie als Grundlage der Arzneibehandlung.
Berlin, *Urban & Schwarzenberg*, 1910.

1901 ABEL, JOHN JACOB. 1857-1938, & MACHT, DAVID ISRAEL. 1882-1961
Two crystalline pharmacological agents obtained from the tropical toad,
Bufo agua. J. Pharmacol., 1911-12, **3**, 319-77.
  Isolation of bufagin. Preliminary communication in *J. Amer. med. Assoc.*,
1911, **56**, 1531-35.

1901.1 BARGER, GEORGE. 1878-1939, & DALE, *Sir* HENRY HALLETT. 1875-1968
ß-iminazolylethylamine a depressor constituent of intestinal mucosa. *J. Physiol. (Lond.)*, 1911, **41**, 499-503.
  Isolation of histamine from animal tissues.

1901.2 HARTWICH, CARL. 1851-1917
Die menschlichen Genussmittel. Ihre Herkunft, Verbreitung, Geschichte,
Anwendung, Bestandteile und Wirkung. Leipzig, *Tauchnitz*, 1911.
  A monumental encyclopaedia of ethnopharmacology.

1903 BOURQUELOT, EMILE. 1851-1921
La synthèse des glucosides par les ferments. *J. Pharm. Chim.*, 1913, 7 sér.,
8, 337-59.
  Bourquelot did important work on the synthesis of glucosides; several
more papers followed the one given above.

1903.1 HENRY, THOMAS ANDERSON. 1873-1958
The plant alkaloids. London, *J. & A. Churchill*, 1913.

1903.2 DAKIN, HENRY DRYSDALE. 1880-1952
On the use of certain antiseptic substances in the treatment of infected
wounds. *Brit. med. J.*, 1915, **2**, 318-20.
  Eusol and chloramine-T.

1904 STRAUB, WALTER. 1874-1944
Digitaliswirkung am isolierten Vorhof des Frosches. *Arch. exp. Path.
Pharmak.*, 1916, **79**, 19-29.
  An important analysis of the action of digitalis on the isolated heart.

1905 BROWNING, CARL HAMILTON. 1881-1972, *et al.*
Flavine and brilliant green, powerful antiseptics with low toxicity to the
tissues: their use in the treatment of infected wounds. *Brit. med. J.*, 1917,
1, 73-79.
  Introduction of acriflavine. With R. Gulbransen, E. L. Kennaway, and L.
H. D. Thornton.

1906 TSCHIRCH, ALEXANDER. 1856-1939
Handbuch der Pharmakognosie. 3 vols. and Register. Leipzig, *C. H.
Tauchnitz*, 1917-27.
  Includes detailed accounts of the history of each drug.

1907   JACOBS, Walter Abraham. 1883-1967, & HEIDELBERGER, Michael. 1888-
Chemotherapy of trypanosome and spirochete infections. Chemical series. I.
N-phenylglycineamide-*p*-arsonic acid. *J. exp. Med.,* 1919, **30,** 411-15.
Introduction of tryparsamide.

1908   YOUNG, Hugh Hampton. 1870-1945, *et al.*
A new germicide for use in the genito-urinary tract; "mercurochrome-220".
J. Amer. med. Assoc., 1919, **73,** 1483-91.
Introduction of mercurochrome. With E. C. White and E. O. Swartz.

1909   HEFFTER, Karl Wilhelm Arthur. 1859-1925
Handbuch der experimentellen Pharmakologie ... Hrsg. von A. Heffter.
Vol. 1- . Berlin, *J. Springer,* 1920- .

1910   SPIRO, Karl. 1867-1932, & STOLL, Arthur. 1887-1971
Ueber die wirksamen Substanzen des Mutterkorns. *Schweiz. med Wschr.*
1921, **2,** 525-29.
Isolation of ergotamine.

1910.1 FLEMING, *Sir* Alexander. 1881-1955.
On a remarkable bacteriolyte substance found in secretions and tissues.
Proc. roy. Soc. B., 1922, **93,** 306-17.
Lysozyme.

1911   CHURCHMAN, John Woolman. 1877-1937
Intravenous use of dyes. *J. Amer. med. Assoc.,* 1925, **85,** 1849-53.
Churchman demonstrated the selective bactericidal action of gentian
violet against staphylococci. See also *J. exp. Med.,* 1912, **16,** 221-47; *J. Urol.,*
1924, **11,** 1-18.

1912   CUSHNY, Arthur Robertson. 1866-1926
The action and uses in medicine of digitalis and its allies. London,
Longmans, Green & Co., 1925.

1912.1 ——. Biological relations of optically isomeric substances. Baltimore,
Williams & Wilkins, 1926.
Cushny made important contributions concerning the pharmacological
action of optical isomers over a period of nearly twenty years. He summarized
this work and that of others in his Charles E. Dohme Lectures, 1925.

1913   GOTTLIEB, Rudolf. 1864-1924
Vergleichende Messungen über die Gewöhnung des Atemzentrums an
Morphin, Dicodid und Dilaudid. *Münch. med. Wschr.,* 1926, **73,** 595-96.
Introduction of dilaudid.

1914   HANZLIK, Paul John. 1885-1951
Actions and uses of the salicylates and cinchophen in medicine. *Medicine,*
1926, **5,** 197-373.
Republished in book form, Baltimore, 1927.

1915   LOEVENHART, Arthur Salomon. 1878-1929, & STRATMAN-THOMAS,
Warren Kidwell. 1894-
On the chemotherapy of neurosyphilis and trypanosomiasis. *J. Pharmacol.,*
1926, **29,** 69-82.

Study of the effect of twelve different substances in neurosyphilis and trypanosomiasis.

1916   BEST, CHARLES HERBERT. 1899-1978, *et al.*
The nature of the vaso-dilator constituents of certain tissue extracts. *J. Physiol. (Camb.),* 1927, **62,** 397-417.
Proof that histamine occurs in certain organs in amounts sufficient to account for the depressant action of extracts of these organs. With H. H. Dale, H. W. Dudley, and W. V. Thorpe.

1917   GADDUM, *Sir* JOHN HENRY. 1900-1965
The action of adrenalin and ergotamine on the uterus of the rabbit. *J. Physiol. (Lond.),* 1926, **61,** 141-50.
Gaddum produced concentration-effect curves of antagonistic drugs, showing the dose-ratio linearly related to antagonistic concentration. *See also* No. 1925.1

1918   CHEN, KO KUEI. 1898- , & SCHMIDT, CARL FREDERIC. 1893-
Ephedrine and related substances. Baltimore, *Williams & Wilkins Co.,* 1930.
A digest of the literature, together with an excellent bibliography. By their earlier work (*J. Pharmacol.,* 1924, **24,** 339-57) Chen and Schmidt aroused worldwide interest in ephedrine.

1919   FELDBERG, WILHELM SIEGMUND. 1900- , & SCHILF, ERICH.
Histamin: seine Pharmakologie und Bedeutung für die Humoralphysiologie. Berlin, *J. Springer,* 1930.

1920   SMITH, SYDNEY.
Digoxin, a new digitalis glucoside. *J. chem. Soc.,* 1930, 508-10.
Isolation of digoxin from *Digitalis lanata.*

1921   FISCHL, VIKTOR, & SCHLOSSBERGER, HANS. 1887-
Handbuch der Chemotherapie. 2 vols. Leipzig, *Fischer,* 1932-34.

1923   CHOPRA, RAM NATH. 1882- , *et al.*
The pharmacological action of an alkaloid obtained from *Rauwolfia serpentina* Benth. A preliminary note. *Indian J. med. Res.,* 1933, **21,** 261-71.
R. N. Chopra, J. C. Gupta, and B. Mukherjee demonstrated the sedative and hypotensive effect of an alkaloid isolated from *Rauwolfia serpentina* (reserpine).

1924   CLARK, ALFRED JOSEPH. 1885-1941
The mode of action of drugs on cells. London, *E. Arnold & Co.,* 1933.

1924.1   TILLETT, WILLIAM SMITH. 1892-1974, & GARNER, RAYMOND LORAINE. 1906-
The fibrinolytic activity of hemolytic streptococci. *J. exp. Med.,* 1933, **58,** 485-502.
Tillett and Garner discovered a substance elaborated by a strain of haemolytic streptococcus which promoted lysis of fibrin and is now known as streptokinase.

1924.2   VIALLI, MAFFO, & ERSPAMER, VITTORIO. 1909-
Cellule enterocromaffini e cellule basigranulose acidofile nei vertebrati.
(Ricerche istochimiche.) *Z. Zellforsch. mikr. Anat.*, 1933, **19**, 743-73.
   Vialli and Erspamer reported "enteramine", which Erspamer and B.
Asero (*Nature, Lond.*, 1952, **169**, 800-01) found to be identical with 5-
hydroxytryptamine, isolated and named serotonin by M. M. Rapport *et al.*
in 1948 (*J. biol. Chem.*, **176**, 1243-51).

1924.3   EULER, ULF SVANTE HANSSON VON. 1905-1983
Zur Kenntnis der pharmakologischen Wirkungen der Natursekreten und
Extrakten männlicher accessorischer Geschlechtsdrüsen. *Arch. exp. Path.
Pharmak.*, 1934, **175**, 78-84.
   Prostaglandins. Von Euler reported that a lipid fraction of human
seminal fluid had potent activities on smooth muscle, hence the name.
Later, prostaglandins were found to be widely distributed in mammalian
tissues and body fluids.

1925   BOVET, DANIEL. 1907- , & STAUB, ANNE-MARIE.
Action protectrice des éthers phénoliques au cours de l'intoxication
histaminique. *C. R. Soc. Biol. (Paris)*, 1937, **124**, 547-49.
   First description of structure and action of an antihistamine.

1925.1   GADDUM, *Sir* JOHN HENRY. 1900-1965
The quantitative effect of antagonistic drugs, *J. Physiol.(Lond.)*, 1937, **89**,
7P-9P.
   Gaddum was the first to formulate the theory of competitive drug
antagonism. *See also* No. 1917.

1926   BUTTLE, GLADWIN ALBERT HURST. 1899-1983, *et al.*
The action of substances allied to 4:4'-diaminodiphenylsulphone in
streptococcal and other infections in mice. *Biochem. J.*, 1938, **32**, 1101-10.
   G. A. H. Buttle, T. Dewing, G. E. Foster, W. H. Gray, S. Smith, and D.
Stephenson discovered the potency of dapsone.

1927   EISLER, O. & SCHAUMANN, O.
Dolantin, ein neuartiges Spasmolytikum und Analgetikum. (Chemisches
und pharmakologisches.) *Dtsch. med. Wschr.*, 1939, **65**, 967-69.
   Synthesis of pethidine (dolantin).

1928   GUNN, JAMES ANDREW. 1882-1958
The pharmacological actions and therapeutic uses of some compounds
related to adrenaline. *Brit. med. J.*, 1939, **2**, 155-60, 214-19.

1928.1   STOLL, ARTHUR, 1887-1971, & HOFMANN, ALBERT. 1906-
Partialsynthese von Alkaloiden vom Typus des Ergobasins. *Helv. chim.
Acta*, 1943, **26**, 944-65.
   Synthesis of lysergic acid diethylamide (LSD).

1928.2   DODD, MATTHEW CHARLES. 1910- , & STILLMAN, WILLIAM BARLOW. 1904-
The in vitro bacteriostatic action of some simple furan derivatives. *J.
Pharmacol.*, 1944, **82**, 11-18.
   Nitrofuran (nitrofurazone).

1928.3   LÄUGER, P., *et al.*
Über Konstitution und toxische Wirkung von natürlichen und neuen synthetischen insektentötenden Stoffen. *Helv. chim. Acta,* 1944, **27,** 892-928.
With H. Martin and P. Müller. Dichlordiphenyltrichlorethane (DDT) was introduced as an insecticide by Paul Müller (1899-1965). He received the Nobel Prize in 1948 for his discovery of the high efficacy of DDT against several varieties of arthropod.

1928.4   CHRISTENSEN, LAURITZ ROYAL. 1914-
Streptococcal fibrinolysis. A proteolytic reaction due to a serum enzyme activated by streptococcal fibrinolysin. *J. gen. Physiol.,* 1945, **28,** 363-83.
Purification and concentration of Tillett and Garner's (No. 1924.1) substance to produce streptokinase.

1929   PETERS, *Sir* RUDOLPH ALBERT. 1889-1982, *et al.*
British anti-lewisite (*BAL*). *Nature (Lond.),* 1945, **156,** 616-19.
With L. A. Stocken and R. H. S. Thompson. BAL (dimercaprol) was discovered during the 1939-45 war.

1929.1   SNYDER, MARSHALL LOVEJOY. 1907- , *et al.*
Effectiveness of a nitrofuran in the treatment of infected wounds. *Milit. Surg.,* 1945, **97,** 380-84.
First clinical use of "furacin" (nitrofuran). With C. L. Kiehn and J. W. Christopherson.

1929.2   McCARTY, MACLYN. 1911-
The occurrence of nucleases in culture filtrates of group A hemolytic streptococci. *J. exp. Med.,* 1948, **88,** 181-88.
Streptodornase. See also W. S. Tillett *et al., Proc. Soc. exp. Biol. (N.Y.),* 1948, **68,** 184-88.

1929.3   PATON, *Sir* WILLIAM DRUMMOND MACDONALD. 1917- , & ZAIMIS, ELEANOR. 1915-1982
Curare-like action of polymethylene *bis*-quaternary ammonium salts. *Nature (Lond.),* 1948, **161,** 718-19.
Methonium compounds. See also the same journal, 1948, **162,** 810.

1929.4   AHLQUIST, RAYMOND PERRY. 1914-
A study of the adrenotropic receptors. *Am. J. Physiol.,* 1948, **153,** 586-600.
Described the concept of α and ß adrenergic receptors in the sympathetic nervous system, and placed specific receptors into pharmacologic mechanisms.

1930   ROCHA E SILVA, MAURICIO. 1910- , *et al.*
Bradykinin, a hypotensive and smooth muscle stimulating factor releases from plasma globulin by snake venoms and by trypsin. *Amer. J. Physiol.,* 1949, **156,** 261-73.
Discovery of bradykinin. With W. T. Beraldo and G. Rosenfeld.

1930.1   CADE, JOHN FREDERICK JOSEPH. 1912-
Lithium salts in the treatment of psychotic excitement. *Med. J. Austral.,* 1949, **36,** 349-52.
The first clinical trial of lithium.

1931   MÜLLER, J. M., *et al.*
Reserpin, der sedative Wirkstoff aus *Rauwolfia serpentina* Benth.
Experientia (Basel), 1952, **8,** 338.
Isolation of reserpine. With E. Schlittler and H. J. Bein.

1931.1   COURVOISIER, S., *et al.*
Propriétés pharmacodynamiques du chlorhydrate de chloro-
3(diméthylamino-3'propyl)-10 phénothiazine (4.560 R.P.). *Arch. int.
Pharmacodyn.,* 1953, **92,** 305-61.
Chlorpromazine. With J. Fournel, R. Ducrot, M. Kolsky, and P. Koetschet.

1931.2   PINCUS, GREGORY GOODWIN. 1903-1967, & CHANG, MIN CHUEH. 1908-
The effects of progesterone and related compounds on ovulation and early
development in the rabbit. *Acta physiol. latinoamer.,* 1953, **3,** 177-83.
First practical demonstration of an oral contraceptive.

1931.3   RANDALL, LOWELL ORLANDO. 1910- , *et al.*
The psychosedative properties of methaminodiazepoxide. *J. Pharmacol.,*
1960, **129,** 163-71.
Librium. With four co-authors.

1931.4   BERGSTRÖM, SUNE. 1916- , *et al.*
The structure of prostaglandin E, F_1 and F_2. *Acta chem. scand.,* 1962, **16,**
501-2.
With R. Ryhage, B. Samuelsson and J. Sjovall. In this and subsequent
papers Bergström and colleagues elucidated the chemical structure of
prostaglandins. Nobel Prize, 1982.

1931.5   BLACK, JAMES WHYTE. 1924- , *et al.*
A new adrenergic beta-receptor antagonist. *Lancet,* 1964, **1,** 1080-81.
Propranolol. With A. F. Crowther, R. G. Shanks, L. H. Smith and A. C.
Dornhorst.

1931.6   AXELROD, JULIUS. 1912-
Noradrenaline: fate and control of its biosynthesis. *Le Prix Nobel en 1970,*
189-208.
Shared Nobel Prize with Katz and von Euler in 1970 for his studies on
the pharmacology of central transmitter substances. His work is summed
up in his Nobel lecture.

1931.7   HAMBERG, MATS., *et al.*
Thromboxanes: a new group of biologically active compounds derived
from prostaglandin endoperoxides. *Proc. nat. Acad. Sci. (Wash.),* 1975,
72, 2994-98.
With J. Stevenson and B. Samuelsson.

1931.71   BOREL, J.F. *et al.*
Biological effects of cyclosporin A: a new antilymphocytic agent. *Agents &
Actions* (Basel), 1976, **6,** 468-75.
The immunosuppressive cyclosporin A, instrumental in the success of
organ transplants. With C. Feurer, H.U. Gubler & H. Strähelin.

1931.8   GOODMAN, Louis Sanford. 1906- , & GILMAN, Alfred. 1908-
The pharmacological basis of therapeutics. 7th ed. New York, *Macmillan Co.*, 1985.
Includes useful historical information.

Antibiotics

1932   TYNDALL, John. 1820-1893
The optical deportment of the atmosphere in relation to the phenomena of putrefaction and infection. *Phil Trans.*, 1876, **166**, 27-74.
Tyndall observed the selective bacteria-inhibiting effect of *Penicillium* and the resistance of *Ps. pyocyanea* to it. *See* No. 2495.

1932.1   PASTEUR, Louis. 1822-1895, & JOUBERT, Jules François.
Charbon et septicémie. *C. R. Acad. Sci. (Paris)*, 1877, **85**, 101-15l.
Pasteur and Joubert were probably the first to realize the practical implications of antibiosis. They noted the antagonism between *Bacillus anthracis* and other bacteria in cultures.

1932.2   EMMERICH, Rudolf. 1852-1914, & LÖW, Oscar. 1844-
Bakteriolytische Enzyme als Ursache der erworbenen Immunität und die Heilung von Infectionskrankheiten durch dieselben. *Z. Hyg. Infekt.- Kr.*, 1889, **31**, 1-65.
Emmerich and Löw prepared a water-soluble antibiotic substance, pyocyanase, from *Pseudomonas pyocanea.* It inhibited pathogenic cocci and the organisms responsible for diphtheria, plague, cholera, and typhoid.

1932.3   GOSIO, Bartolomeo. 1863-1944
Ricerche batteriologische e chimiche sulle alterazioni del mais; contributo all'etiologia della pellagra. *Riv. Ig. San. pubbl.*, 1896, **7**, 825, 869, 961.
First recorded scientific observations on the action of a penicillin. Gosio produced an antibacterial crystalline substance from *Penicillium glaucum.*

1933   FLEMING, *Sir* Alexander. 1881-1955
On the antibacterial action of cultures of a penicillium, with special reference to their use in the isolation of *B. influenzae. Brit. J. exp. Path.*, 1929, **10**, 226-36.
Discovery of the growth-inhibiting action of *Pennicillium* on certain bacteria. Nobel Prize (with Florey and Chain) 1945. The only book which Fleming ever wrote concerning his discovery was Fleming (ed.), *Penicillin: its practical application.* London, *Butterworth*, 1946. Biography of Fleming by G. Macfarlane, 1984. For historical references to bacterial inhibition by moulds and "antibiosis" see G. Papacostas & J. Graté, *Les associations microbiennes.* Paris, *Doin*, 1928.

1933.1   DUBOIS, Rene Jules. 1901-1982
Bactericidal effect of an extract of a soil bacillus on gram-positive cocci. *Proc Soc. exp. Biol. (N.Y.)*, 1939, **40**, 311-12.
Isolation of gramicidin.

1933.2   OXFORD, ALBERT EDWARD, *et al.*
          Studies in the biochemistry of micro-organisms. LX. Griseofulvin,
          $C_{17}H_{17}O_6Cl$, a metabolic product of *Penicillium griseo-fulvum* Dierckx.
          Biochem. J., 1939, **33**, 240-48.
          Isolation of griseofulvin. With H. Raistrick and P. Simonart.

1933.3   ABRAHAM, *Sir* EDWARD PENLEY. 1913- , & CHAIN, *Sir* ERNST BORIS. 1906-1979
          An enzyme from bacteria able to destroy penicillin. *Nature (Lond.)*, 1940,
          146, 837.
          Penicillinase.

1934   CHAIN, *Sir* ERNST BORIS. 1906-1979, *et al.*
          Penicillin as a chemotherapeutic agent. *Lancet*, 1940, **2**, 226-28.
          Proof of the therapeutic action *in vivo* of penicillin against streptococcal
          and other bacterial infections. Building upon Fleming's work (No.1933),
          the consequences of which had originally been widely unappreciated,
          even by Fleming himself, Chain and his co-workers concentrated penicil-
          lin and showed that it was probably the most effective chemotherapeutic
          drug known, and that it was relatively non-toxic. This led to mass production
          of the drug, which has saved untold millions of lives. With H. W. Florey, A.
          D. Gardner, N. G. Heatley, M. A. Jennings, J. Orr-Ewing and A. G. Sanders.
          Chain and Florey shared the Nobel Prize with Fleming (No. 1933) in 1945.
          Biography of Florey by G. Macfarlane, 1979.

1934.1   ABRAHAM, *Sir* EDWARD PENLEY. 1913- , *et al.*
          Further observations on penicillin. *Lancet*, 1941, **2**, 177-89.
          First report of the chemotherapeutic action of penicillin on humans (10
          cases). With E. Chain, C. M. Fletcher, H. W. Florey, A. D. Gardner, N. G.
          Heatley and M. A. Jennings.

1934.2   ABRAHAM, *Sir* EDWARD PENLEY. 1913- *et al.*
          Penicillamine, a characteristic degradation product of penicillin. *Nature
          (Lond.)*, 1943, **151**, 107 (only).
          With E. Chain, W. Baker and R. Robinson.

1935   SCHATZ, ALBERT. 1920- , *et al.*
          Streptomycin, a substance exhibiting antibiotic activity against Gram-
          positive and Gram-negative bacteria. *Proc. Soc. exp. Biol. (N.Y.)*, 1944, **55**,
          66-69.
          Introduction of streptomycin. With E. Bugie and S. A. Waksman.

1936   JOHNSON, BALBINA A., *et al.*
          Bacitracin: a new antibiotic produced by a member of the *B. subtilis* group.
          Science, 1945, **102**, 376-77.
          With H. Anker and F. L. Meleney.

1937   AINSWORTH, GEOFFREY CLOUGH. 1905- , *et al.*
          "Aerosporin", an antibiotic produced by *Bacillus aerosporus* Greer. *Na-
          ture (Lond.)*, 1947, **160**, 263.
          Discovery of aerosporin (polymyxin). With A. M. Brown and G.
          Brownlee.

1938   EHRLICH, JOHN. 1907- , *et al.*
Chloromycetin, a new antibiotic from a soil actinomycete. *Science*, 1947,
106, 417.
        Production of chloramphenicol from *Streptomyces venezuelae*. With Q.
R. Bartz, R. M. Smith, D. A. Joslyn and P. R. Burkholder.

1939   HERRELL, WALLACE EDGAR. 1909- , *et al.*
Procaine penicillin G (duracillin); a new salt of penicillin which prolongs
the action of penicillin. *Proc. Mayo Clin.*, 1947, **22**, 567-70.
        With D.R. Nichols and F.R. Heilman.

1940   SMADEL, JOSEPH EDWIN. 1907-1963, & JACKSON, ELIZABETH B.
Chloromycetin, an antibiotic with chemotherapeutic activity in experimental
rickettsial and viral infections. *Science*, 1947, **106**, 418-19.
        Introduction of chloramphenicol.

1941   STANSLY, PHILIP GERALD. 1912- , *et al.*
Polymyxin: a new chemotherapeutic agent. *Bull. Johns Hopk. Hosp.*, 1947,
81, 43-54.
        With R. G. Shepherd and H. J. White.

1942   SYMPOSIUM
Aureomycin—a new antibiotic. *Ann. N. Y. Acad. Sci.*, 1948, **51**, 175-342.
        Discovery and clinical application of chlortetracycline (aureomycin).

1943   BROTZU, GIUSEPPE. 1895-1976
Ricerche su di un nuovo antibiotico. *Lav. Ist. Ig. Univ. Cagliari*, 1948, pp.
1-11.
        Brotzu showed that a *Cephalosporium acremonium* filtrate inhibited
the growth of Gram-positive and -negative organisms.

1944   WAKSMAN, SELMAN ABRAHAM. 1888-1973, & LECHEVALIER, HUBERT ARTHUR.
1926-
Neomycin, a new antibiotic active against streptomycin-resistant bacteria,
including tuberculosis organisms. *Science*, 1949, **109**, 305-07.
        Isolation of neomycin.

1945   HANSON, FREDERICK REUBEN. 1921- , & EBLE, THOMAS EUGENE. 1923-
An antiphage agent isolated from *Aspergillus* sp. *J. Bact.*, 1949, **58**, 527-9.
        Isolation of fumagillin, an antibiotic with amoebicidal activity. See also
Science, 1951, **113**, 202-3.

1945.1 FINLAY, ALEXANDER CARPENTER. 1906- , *et al.*
Terramycin, a new antibiotic. *Science*, 1950, **111**, 85.
        Oxtetracycline (terramycin).

1945.2 BURTON, H. S., & ABRAHAM, *Sir* EDWARD PENLEY. 1913-
Isolation of antibiotics from a species of *Cephalosporium*. Cephalosporins
P_1, P_2, P_3, P_4 and P_5. *Biochem. J.*, 1951, **50**, 168-174.

1945.3 FINLAY, ALEXANDER CARPENTER. 1906- , *et al.*
Viomycin, a new antibiotic active against mycobacteria. *Amer. Rev. Tuberc.*,
1951, **63**, 1-3.
        Isolation of viomycin. With 11 co-authors.

1945.4   HAZEN, Elizabeth Lee. 1885-1975, & BROWN, Rachel Fuller. 1898-1980
          Fungicidin, an antibiotic produced by a soil actinomycete. *Proc. Soc. exp.
          Biol. (N.Y.)*, 1951, **76**, 93-97.
          Isolation of nystatin (fungicidin).

1946   McGUIRE, James Myrlin. 1909- , *et al.*
          "Ilotycin", a new antibiotic. *Antibiot. and Chemother.*, 1952, **2**, 281-83.
          Discovery of erythromycin. With R. L. Bunch, R. C. Anderson, H. E.
          Boaz, E. H. Flynn, H. M. Powell, and J. W. Smith.

1947   ABRAHAM, *Sir* Edward Penley. 1913- , *et al.*
          Purification and some properties of cephalosporin N, a new penicillin.
          Biochem. J., 1954, **58**, 94-102.
          With G. G. F. Newton and C. W. Hale.

1947.1   NEWTON, Guy G. F. 1920-1969, & ABRAHAM, *Sir* Edward Penley. 1913-
          Cephalosporin C, a new antibiotic containing sulpher and d-x aminoadipic
          acid. *Nature (Lond.).*, 1955, **175**, 158 (only).

1947.2   GOLD, W., *et al.*
          Amphotericins A and B, antifungal antibiotics produced by a streptomycete.
          Antibiot. Ann., 1955-6, 579-91.
          With six co-authors.

1947.3   HATA, Toju, *et al.*
          Mitomycin, a new antibiotic from streptomyces. *J. Antibiot. (A).*, 1956, **9**,
          141-6.
          Isolation of mitomycin C, effective in Hodgkin's disease and lymphoma.
          With six co-authors.

1947.4   UMEZAWA, Hamao, *et al.*
          Production and isolation of a new antibiotic, kanamycin. *J. Antibiotics Japan,
          Ser. A*, 1957, **10**, 181-88.
          With nine co-authors.

1947.5   WEINSTEIN, Marvin Joseph. 1916- , *et al.*
          Gentamicin, a new antibiotic complex from *Micromonospora. J. medicinal
          Chem.*, 1963, **6**, 463-4.
          With nine co-authors.

Sulphonamides

1948   GELMO, Paul. 1879-1961
          Ueber Sulfamide der *p*-Amidobenzolsulfonsäure. *J. prakt. Chem.*, 1908, **77**,
          369-82.
          Para- aminobenzenesulphonamide (sulphanilamide) first prepared.

1949   DOMAGK, Gerhard. 1895-1964
          Ein Beitrag zur Chemotherapie der bakteriellen Infektionen. *Dtsch. med.
          Wschr.*, 1935, **61**, 250-53.
          Prontosil, the first drug containing sulphanilamide, was introduced into
          medicine by Domagk. He was awarded the Nobel Prize in 1939.

1950   TRÉFOUËL, JACQUES. 1897-1977, *et al.*
Activité du *p*-aminophénylsulfamide sur les infections streptococciques expérimentales de la souris et du lapin. *C. R. Soc. Biol. (Paris)*, 1935, **120**, 756-58.
    J. Tréfouël, Mme Tréfouël, F. Nitti, and D. Bovet assumed that the sulphonamide group was responsible for the results obtained with Domagk's prontosil. Their work led them to introduce sulphanilamide.

1951   WHITBY, *Sir* LIONEL ERNEST HOWARD. 1895-1956
Chemotherapy of pneumococcal and other infections with 2-(*p*-aminobenzenesulphonamido) pyridine. *Lancet*, 1938, **1**, 1210-12.
    Experimental proof of the efficacy of sulphapyridine (M & B 693) in pneumococcal pneumonia.

1952   EVANS, GLADYS MARY, *Mrs. Jenks*, & GAISFORD, WILFRID FLETCHER. 1902-
Treatment of pneumonia with 2-(*p*-aminobenzenesulphonamido) pyridine. *Lancet*, 1938, **2**, 14-19.
    Clinical proof of the value of sulphapyridine.

1953   GSELL, OTTO. 1902-
Chemotherapie akuter Infektionskrankheiten durch Ciba 3714 (Sulfanilamidothiazol). *Schweiz. med. Wschr.*, 1940, **70**, 342-50.
    First important clinical trial of sulphathiazole.

1954   MARSHALL, ELI KENNERLY. 1889-1966, *et al.*
Sulfanilylguanidine: a chemotherapeutic agent for intestinal infections. *Bull. Johns Hopk. Hosp.*, 1940, **67**, 163-88.
    Sulphaguanidine was introduced by E. K. Marshall, A. C. Bratton, H. J. White, and J. T. Litchfield.

1955   ROBLIN, RICHARD OWEN. 1907- , *et al.*
Chemotherapy, II. Some sulfanilamido heterocycles. *J. Amer. chem. Soc.*, 1940, **62**, 2002-05.
    Synthesis of sulphamerazine, by R. O. Roblin, J. H. Williams, P. S. Winnek, and J. P. English.

1955.1   WOODS, DONALD DEVEREUX. 1912-1964
The relation of *p*-amniobenzoic acid to the mechanism of the action of sulphanilamide. *Brit J. exp. Path.*, 1940, **21**, 74-90.
    Isolation of *p*-aminobenzoic acid, a structural analogue of sulphanilamide.

1956   FINLAND, MAXWELL. 1902- , *et al.*
Sulfadiazine. Therapeutic evaluation and toxic effects on four hundred and forty-six patients. *J. Amer. Med. Assoc.*, 1941, **116**, 2641-47.
    Introduction of sulphadiazine. With E. Strauss and O. L. Peterson.

1957   POTH, EDGAR JACOB. 1899- , & KNOTTS, FRANK LOUIS. 1912-
Succinyl sulfathiazole, a new bacteriostatic agent locally active in the gastrointestinal tract. *Proc. Soc. exp. Biol. (N. Y.)*, 1941, **48**, 129-30.
    Introduction of sulphasuxidine.

1958   MACARTNEY, Donald William, *et al.*
Sulphamethazine: clinical trial of a new sulphonamide. *Lancet,* 1942, **1,** 639-41.
Sulphadimidine; with G. S. Smith, R. W. Luxton, W. A. Ramsay, and J. Goldman.

For history of pharmacy and therapeutics, see 2029-2068.21

THERAPEUTICS

1959   GALEN, A.D. 130-200
De methodo medendi. *In his:* Opera, ed. C. G. Kuhn, Lipsiae, 1825, **10,** 1-1021.
The Greek *editio princeps* of Methodus medendi was published at Venice from the press of Z. Callierges in 1500. Books 3-6 of the 14 were published in an English translation by T. Gale, in London, 1566. Galen's shorter textbook of therapy, *Ad Glauconem de medendi methodo,* was translated into French by C. Daremberg in *Oeuvres anatomiques, phsyiologiques et médicales de Galien,* Paris, 1856, **2,** 706-784.

1959.1   CAELIUS AURELIANUS. *fl.* 500 A.D.
Tardarum passionum libri V. Basel, *Heinrich Petri,* 1529.
From a clinical point of view, the two works of Caelius Aurelianus, based on Greek originals by Soranus of Ephesus now lost, represent the high-point of Graeco-Roman medical achievement. The first edition of *Chronic diseases* was edited by J. Sichart. The first edition of *Acute diseases — Liber celerum vel acutarum passionum,* was edited by J. Winter of Andernach and published in Paris at the press of Simon de Colines in 1533. Both editions were based on Latin manuscripts which have since disappeared. The standard modern edition is *On acute diseases. On chronic diseases,* edited and translated by I.E. Drabkin. Chicago, *University of Chicago Press,* [1950]. *See also* Nos. 4805.1 & 4915.1.

1959.2   ARNALD OF VILLANOVA. *circa* 1240-1311
Von Bewahrung und Bereitung der Weine. [Esslingen, *Konrad Fyner,* 1478].
The first printed book on wine discusses the value of wine in diet and as a medication. Translated from the Latin by W. von Hirnkofen. Facsimile with English translation by Henry Sigerist, 1943.

1959.3   SCHOOL OF SALERNO
Regimen sanitatis Salernitanum necnon Arnaldi de Villa Nova. [Louvain, *Johann de Paderborn* (Westphalia), *circa* 1480].
Probably originating about 1160, the *Regimen sanitatis* from the medical school at Salerno (where medicine was first treated as a separate science) had greater popular influence than virtually any other medieval medical tract. The first edition of this collection of very sensible dietary and hygienic precepts was printed with the famed commentary on the Regimen by Arnald of Villanova. It is one of three undated editions, all probably printed around 1480, but to which no order of priority can be established. English translation by Thomas Paynel, [London, 1535]. *See* Nos. 49-51.

1960   PETRUS HISPANUS, *Pope John XXI.* ?1226-1277
Thesaurus pauperum. [Florence, *F. Bonaccorsi, circa* 1485.]

One of the most popular medical books of the Middle Ages; first written about 1260. After its first printing about 1584 it was many times reprinted in the next 100 years. Petrus Hispanus was the only medical man to become Pope.

1961   ISAAC JUDAEUS [ISHAQ IBN SULAIMAN AL ISRA'ILI'] ?880-932
De particularibus diaetis. Padua, *Cerdonis*, 1487.
First separately printed work on diet.

1962   ELSHOLTZ, JOHANN SIGMUND. 1623-1688
Clysmatica nova; oder newe Clystier-Kunst. Berlin, *D. Reichel*, 1665.
Elsholtz's book on the venous infusion of medicaments was one of the first works to deal with blood transfusion. Latin edition in 1667; English translation in 1677. Reprint of Latin 1667 edition, Hildesheim, *G. Olms*, 1966.

1963   MAJOR, JOHANN DANIEL. 1634-1693
Chirurgia infusoria. Kiloni, *J. Reumannus*, 1667.
Major, the first Professor of Medicine at Kiel, was the first to make successful intravenous injections of drugs into the human body, in 1662. Sir Christopher Wren in 1656 had injected wine and ale into the veins of a dog.

1964   STOLL, MAXIMILIAN. 1742-1788
Rationis medendi in nosocomico practico Vindobonensi. 7 pts. Vienae Austriae, 1777-90.

1965   FRANK, JOHANN PETER. 1745-1821
De curandis hominum morbis epitome. 6 vols., Mannhemii, *C.F. Schwan*, 1792-94.

1966   HAHNEMANN, CHRISTIAN FRIEDRICH SAMUEL. 1755-1843
Organon der rationellen Heilkunde. Dresden, *Arnold*, 1810.
Hahnemann, the founder of homoeopathy, embodied his theories in the *Organon*. The minute doses set down by him did much to correct the evils of the polypharmacy of his time, in which overdosage was pervasive. He professed to base medicine on a knowledge of symptoms, regarding investigation of the causes of symptoms as useless; he thus rejected all the lessons of pathology and morbid anatomy. There are several English translations, the first of which appeared in 1833.

1967   TROUSSEAU, ARMAND. 1801-1867, & PIDOUX, HERMANN. 1808-1882
Traité de thérapeutique et de matière médicale. 2 vols. Paris, *Béchet jeune*, 1836-39.
"A valuable work of reference, containing a large amount of information on the various articles or the materia medica, collected from the best authorities, interspersed with much original matter" (Waring).

1968   RYND, FRANCIS. 1801-1861
Neuralgia - introduction of fluid to the nerve. *Dublin med. Press*, 1845, **13**, 167-68.
First hypodermic infusions were made possible by an invention of Rynd. The description of his instrument is given in *Dublin Quart. J. med. Sci.*, 1861, **32**, 13.

1969   WOOD, ALEXANDER. 1817-1884
         New method of treating neuralgia by the direct application of opiates to the
         painful joints. *Edinb. med. surg. J.*, 1855, **82**, 265-81.
              Wood of Edinburgh was the first (1853) to employ hypodermic injec-
         tion as a therapeutic procedure. See also *Brit. med. J.*, 1858, 721-23, for a
         later paper by him. A full account of his work is given by Howard-Jones
         (No. 2063).

1972   WOOD, HORATIO CHARLES. 1841-1920
         A treatise on therapeutics. Philadelphia, *J. B. Lippincott*, 1874.
              Wood was a professor of botany (1866-76), therapeutics (1875-1907)
         and nervous diseases (1875-1901) in the University of Pennsylvania. In his
         book the effects of various drugs in small doses was first discussed; it also
         contains a standard classification of drugs.

1973   BRUNTON, *Sir* THOMAS LAUDER, *Bart*. 1844-1916
         An introduction to modern therapeutics, being the Croonian Lectures on
         the relationship between chemical structure and physiological action.
         London, *Macmillan & Co.*, 1892.
              One of the best known of Lauder Brunton's works.

1975   HUCHARD, HENRI. 1844-1910, & FIESSINGER, CHARLES ALBERT. 1857-1942
         La thérapeutique en vingt médicaments. Paris, *A. Maloine*, 1910.
              Huchard and Fiessinger suggested that actual drug therapy should be
         limited to 20 medicaments.

1976   ABEL, JOHN JACOB. 1857-1938, *et al.*
         Plasma removal with return of corpuscles (plasmaphaeresis), *J. Pharmacol.*,
         1914, **5**, 625-41.
              Report of a method of removal of plasma from the living animal, with
         return of the corpuscles after washing and separation by centrifugalization.
         With L. G. Rowntree and B. B. Turner. See also their earlier papers in the
         same journal, 1914, **5**, 275-316, 611-23.

1977   HALDANE, JOHN SCOTT. 1860-1936
         The therapeutic administration of oxygen. *Brit. med. J.*, 1917, **1**, 181-83.
              Haldane initiated oxygen therapy.

1978   DRINKER, PHILIP. 1894-1972, & McKHANN, CHARLES F.
         The use of a new apparatus for the prolonged administration of artificial
         respiration. I. A fatal case of poliomyelitis. *J. Amer. med. Ass.*, 1929, **92**, 1658-
         60.
              The Drinker respirator ("iron lung").

1979   EVE, FRANK CECIL. 1871-1952
         Actuation of the inert diaphragm by a gravity method. *Lancet*, 1932, **2**, 995-
         97.
              Eve's method of artificial respiration.

1981   LOVELACE, WILLIAM RANDOLPH. 1907-1965
         Oxygen for therapy and aviation: an apparatus for the administration of
         oxygen or oxygen and helium by inhalation. *Proc. Mayo Clin.*, 1938, **13**,
         646-54.

1982 BULBULIAN, ARTHUR H. 1900-
Design and construction of the masks for the oxygen inhalation apparatus.
Proc. Mayo Clin., 1938, **13**, 654-56.
 The B. L. B. (Boothby-Lovelace-Bulbulian) mask. *See also* the previous
entry.

1983 TOCANTINS, LEANDRO MAUES. 1901-
Rapid absorption of substance injected into the bone marrow. *Proc. Soc.
exp. Biol. (N. Y.)*, 1940, **45**, 292-96.
 Tocantins demonstrated the possibility of transfusion of fluids via the
bone marrow. See also later paper with J. F. O'Neill, *Surg. Gynec. Obstet.*,
1941, **73**, 281-87.

PHYSICAL THERAPY: ELECTROTHERAPY: HYDROTHERAPY

1984 ASCLEPIADES *of Bithynia*. 124-56 B.C.
Ὑγιεινά Παραυγελματα Gesundheitsvorschriften ... bearbeitet ... von
Robert Ritter von Welz. Würzburg, *Vogt u. Mocker*, 1842.
 The Greek physician Asclepiades acquired a great reputation in Rome.
His remedies included change of diet, friction, bathing, and exercise. The
above edition includes Greek, Latin, and German texts. English translation,
New Haven, 1955. *See* No. 19.

1984.1 SCRIBONIUS LARGUS. *fl.* A.D. 40
De compositionibus medicamentorum liber unus. Parisiis, *ap. C. Wechel*,
1528.
 First written in A.D. 47. This is an important compilation of drugs and
prescriptions. Among the 271 remedies are the first use of electrotherapy
(for headaches) using the shock of the torpedo fish. *See* No. 1785.

1985 GALEN, A.D. 130-200
De sanitate tuenda ed. K. KOCH. Corpus Medicorum Graecorum V, 4,2.
Lipsiae et Berolini, *B.G. Teubner*, 1914, 1-198.
 English translation by R. M. Green, Springfield, Ill., 1951.

1986 DE BALNEIS.
De balneis omnia quae extant apud Graecos, Latinos, et Arabas. Venetiis,
apud Iuntas, 1553.
 This is a collective work, incorporating the writings of more than 70
authorities, among whom may be mentioned Avicenna, Averroës,
Avenzohar, Guainerio, Gesner, Savonarola, Petrus de Abano, and
Maimonides. It gives an extensive history of balneology and an exact
description of all the then known watering-places (about two hundred).

1986.1 MERCURIALI, GIROLAMO. 1530-1606
Artis gymnasticae apud antiquos celeberrimae, nostris temporibus ignoratae.
Venetiis, *apud Iuntas*, 1569.
 One of the earliest books to discuss the therapeutic value of gymnastics
and sports generally for the cure of disease and disability, and an important
study of gymnastics in the ancient world. The second edition, *De arte
gymnastica libri sex*, Venice, *Juntas*, 1573 is the first illustrated book on
gymnastics. It contains 20 woodcuts by Coriolan. Partial English translation

of 2nd ed.in *The muscles and their story... including the whole text of Mercurialis...*by J.W.F. Blundell, London, 1864. *See* No. 4478.100.

1986.2   BACCI, ANDREA. 1550?-1600
De thermis.... Venice, *Valgrisi*, 1571.
A comprehensive study of mineral waters, dealing with all the spas of the then-known world. Besides exhaustive coverage of the baths of antiquity and of Bacci's own time, the work gives considerable attention to wines, especially in relation to their medical use.

1986.3   FULLER, FRANCIS. 1670-1706
Medicina gymnastica; or, a treatise concerning the power of exercise. London, *Knaplock*, 1705.
The first English book on the power of exercise in treating disease. Fuller also recommended exercise for aid in the recovery from psychological and emotional disorders. In this he preceded Cheyne (No. 4840).

1987   HAHN, JOHANN SIGMUND. 1696-1773
Unterricht von der wunderbare Heilkraft des frischen Wassers bei dessen innerlichem und äusserlichem Gebrauche durch die Erfahrung bestätigt. Breslau, Leipzig, *D. Pietsch*, 1737.
The treatment of fevers by means of the cold pack was revived by S. Hahn and by his son J. S. Hahn; in his treatise, the latter advised the use of water in all diseases. A seventh edition of the book appeared as recently as 1938.

1987.1   KRATZENSTEIN, CHRISTIAN GOTTLIEB. 1723-1795.
Abhandlung von dem Nutzen der Electricität in der Artzneywissenschaft. Halle, *Carl Hermann Hemmerde*, 1744?
A student of Johann Gottlob Krüger (No.1987.2), Kratzenstein was apparently the first to publish a treatise on electrotherapy, although he may have been publishing experiments devised by Krüger. Second edition, Halle, *C.H. Hemmerde*,1745. English translation in E. Snorrason, *C.G. Kratzenstein and his studies on electricity during the eighteenth century*, Odense, 1974.

1987.2   KRÜGER, JOHANN GOTTLOB. 1715-1759
Zuschrifft an seine Zuhörer worinnen er ihnen seine Gedancken von der Electricität mittheilet und ihnen zugleich seine künftige Lectionen bekant macht. Halle, *Hermann Hemmerde*, 1744.
This is the first work to discuss the possible therapeutic uses of electricity. Krüger predicted that the best results would be with paralysed limbs. *See* No. 1987.1. Second edition, with additions, 1745.

1987.3   JALLABERT, JEAN. 1712-1768
Experiences sur l'électricité... Geneva, *Barrillot & Fils*, 1748.
Discovery of stimulation of muscles by electricity, and the first proof that paralysis could be successfully treated by electricity.

1987.4   TISSOT, CLEMENT JOSEPH. 1750-1826
Gymnastique médicinale et chirurgicale, ou essai sur l'utilité du mouvement, ou des différens excercice du corps, et du repos dans la cure des maladies. Paris, *Bastien*, 1780.

The first book on therapeutic exercise as the term is understood today. English translation with facsimiles in reduced format of 18th century translations into German, Italian and Swedish, New Haven, [1964].

1988   CURRIE, JAMES. 1756-1805
Medical reports, on the effects of water, cold and warm, as a remedy in fever and febrile diseases. Liverpool, *Cadell & Davies*, 1797.
Currie was among the first in Britain to use cold water packs in the treatment of fever. He made some original observations on the clinical use of the thermometer. It was Currie who first edited Robert Burns's Collected Works.

1988.1   GRAPENGIESSER, CARL JOHANN CHRISTIAN. 1764-1846
Versuche des Galvanismus zur Heilung einiger Krankheiten. Berlin, *Myliussi*, 1801.
Grapengiesser was the first physician to use Volta's "pile", the first battery, which Volta first described in print in 1800. Grapengiesser "noted that in paralyzed muscle excitability could be so poor that 150 elements were necessary to produce contraction. He placed conductors on moistened skin and found by trial and error that the best results were obtained with the zinc pole placed over the nerve trunk and the other pole over the branches of the nerve. He also noted that contraction occurred on the make and break of the circuit". (Licht).

1989   CARPUE, JOSEPH CONSTANTINE. 1764-1846
An introduction to electricity and galvanism. London, *A Phillips*, 1803.
One of the first works in the English language entirely devoted to medical electricity. Carpue also played a key role in the development of rhinoplasty. *See* No. 5737.

1989.1   ALDINI, GIOVANNI. 1762-1834
An account of the late improvements in galvanism...London, *Cuthell & Martin*, 1803.
Nephew of Galvani (*see* No. 593), Aldini developed and promoted animal electricity. His sensational experiments on the body of a criminal executed at Newgate, conducted with Carpue (No. 1989) were significant for the development of cardiac electrostimulation. He also was among the first to treat melancholy (schizophrenia) with electricity, precursing modern shock therapy.

1990   DÖBEREINER, JOHANN WOLFGANG. 1780-1849
Anleitung zur Darstellung und Anwendung aller Arten der kräftigsten Bäder und Heilwässer welche von Gesunden und Kranken gebraucht werden. Jena, 1816.
Döbereiner was the first to treat the subject of light therapy on a scientific basis.

1991   EDWARDS, WILLIAM FREDERIC. 1776-1842
De l'influence des agents physiques sur la vie. Paris, *Crochard*, 1824.
Includes account of Edwards' important experimental work regarding the effect of light on the body. English translation in 1832. *See* No. 598.1.

1992   PRIESSNITZ, VINCENZ. 1799-1851
        The coldwater cure, its principles, theory, and practice. London, *W. Strange*, [183-?].
        Priessnitz, a layman, became famous for his successful use of cold water as a therapeutic.

1993   LING, PER HENRIK. 1776-1839
        Gymnastikens allmänna grunder. Upsala, *Palmblad & Co.*, 1834; *Leffler & Sebell*, 1840.
        The foundation of modern gymnastics and therapeutic massage. Ling established the Swedish school of physiotherapy with his institute for training gymnastics teachers in Stockholm in 1813. He developed the ancient Greek art of calisthenics into a science based on sound anatomic and physiological principles. "After Ling, scientific body building by rational calisthenics became a recognized procedure not only for the weak child or adult, but, of even greater consequence, as an integral part of the plans for preventative medicine which were taking form in the schools and gymnasia of all civilized nations" (Bick).

1994   CRUSELL, GUSTAF SAMUEL. 1810-1858
        Ueber den Galvanismus als chemisches Heilmittel gegen örtliche Krankheiten. St. Petersburg, *K. Kray*, 1841-43.
        Crusell began to use electrolysis as a cauterizing agent in 1839. *See* No. 5604.

1995   DUCHENNE DE BOULOGNE, GUILLAUME BENJAMIN ARMAND. 1806-1875
        De l'électrisation localisée et de son application à la physiologie, à la pathologie, et à la thérapeutique. Paris, *J. B. Baillière*, 1855; atlas, 1862.
        Duchenne, most famous of the electrotherapists, employed faradic current in treating patients as early as 1830. An English translation of the third edition of his book appeared in 1871. (*See also* No. 614.)

1995.1 REMAK, ROBERT. 1815-1865
        Ueber methodische Electrisirung gelähmter Muskeln, Berlin, *A. Hirschwald*, 1855.
        Discovery of the motor points, the entry points of the nerves into the muscles – essential for stimulating the muscles by electricity.

1996   ZIEMSSEN, HUGO WILHELM VON. 1829-1902
        Die Electricität in der Medicin. Berlin, *A. Hirschwald*, 1857.
        Ziemssen confirmed Remak's discovery of the motor points, established their exact location, and published exact instructions for finding the motor points for stimulating the various muscles of the body.

1996.1 REMAK, ROBERT. 1815-1865
        Galvanotherapie der Nerven- und Muskelkrankheiten. Berlin, *A. Hirschwald*, 1858.
        Having treated some 700 patients with galvanic current, Remak believed that it was superior to faradic current for electrotherapy.

1996.2 BUSQUÉ Y TORRO, SEBASTIAN
        Gimnástica, hygiénica, medica, y ortopédica. Madrid, *M. Galiano*, 1865.
        Busqué developed the modern concept of rehabilitation.

1996.3   ALTHAUS, JULIUS. 1833-1900
On the electrolytic treatment of tumors, and other surgical diseases. London, *J. Churchill*, 1867.
> Althaus introduced Duchenne's methods into England. He was the first to employ electrolysis for medical purposes. Greatly expanded third edition, 1873.

1996.4   BEARD, GEORGE M. 1838-1883, & ROCKWELL, ALPHONSE DAVID. 1840-1933
A practical treatise on the medical and surgical uses of electricity, including localized and general electrization. New York, *William Wood*, 1871.
> Beard and Rockwell were the leading American electrotherapists of the 19th century. This is the most influential American treatise ever published on electrotherapy. It is of especial value today for its comprehensive and carefully documented historical analysis. In a nontherapeutic application of medical electricity Rockwell invented the electric chair.

1997   DOWNES, *Sir* ARTHUR HENRY. 1851-1938, & BLUNT, THOMAS PORTER.
Researches on the effect of light upon bacteria and other organisms. *Proc. roy. Soc. (Lond.)*, 1877, **26**, 488-500.
> Downes and Blunt were the first to demonstrate the bactericidal action of sunlight; they regarded the germicidal property of light as depending on oxidation.

1998   WINTERNITZ, WILHELM. 1835-1917
Die Hydrotherapie. 2 vols. Wien, *Urban & Schwarzenberg*, 1877.

1999   D'ARSONVAL, JACQUES ARSÈNE. 1851-1940
Recherches d'électrothérapie: la voltaisation sinusoïdale. *Arch Physiol. norm. path.*, 1892, 5 sér., **4**, 69-80.
> Introduction of high-frequency currents in electrotherapy.

2000   FINSEN, NIELS RYBERG. 1860-1904
Om anvendelse medicinen af koncentrerede kemiske lysstraaler. Kjobenhavn, *Gyldendal*, 1896.
> Finsen was the founder of modern phototherapy. He demonstrated the value of invisible light, the actinic or chemical ray, the ultra-violet ray, as therapeutic measures. He received the Nobel Prize for Medicine in 1903.

2001   BECQUEREL, ANTOINE HENRI. 1852-1908
Sur les radiations émises par phosphorescence. *C. R. Acad. Sci. (Paris)*, 1896, **122**, 420-21.
> The discovery of radioactivity. Becquerel shared the Nobel Prize for Physics in 1903 with Pierre and Marie Curie.

2002   FREUND, LEOPOLD. 1868-1944
Demonstration eines mit Röntgenstrahlen behandelten Falles von Naevus pigmentosus pilosus. *Wien. klin. Wschr.*, 1897, **10**, 73-74.
> First use of *x* rays for deep irradiation therapy.

2003   CURIE, PIERRE. 1859-1906, & CURIE, MARIE SKLODOWSKA. 1867-1934
Sur une substance nouvelle radio-active, contenue dans la pechblende. *C. R. Acad. Sci. (Paris)*, 1898, **127**, 175-78, 1215-17.
> The Curies, studying the radioactivity of minerals containing uranium and thorium, isolated from pitchblend a substance which they called

radium and which they showed to possess an astonishing degree of radioactivity. Since then radium has proved to be a valuable agent in the treatment of cancer. They shared the Nobel Prize for Physics with Becquerel in 1903 and Marie Curie received the Nobel Prize for Chemistry in 1911.

2003.1 LEDUC, STEPHANE ARMAND NICOLAS. 1853-1939
Introduction électrolytique des ions dans l'organisme vivant. *C. R. Ass. franç. Avance. Sci.* (1900), 1901, **29**, pt. 2, 1111-25.
Introduction of ionic medication.

2003.2 ———. L'électrisation cérébrale. *Rev. int. Electrothér.*, 1903-04, **13**, 143-49.
Leduc reported the effects of a galvanic current on the brain. His work led the way to electric convulsion therapy, introduced by Carletti and Bini (No. 4962).

2005 BERGONIÉ, JEAN. 1857-1925, & TRIBONDEAU, LOUIS MATHIEU FRÉDÉRIC ADRIEN. 1872-1918.
Interprétation de quelques résultats de la radiothérapie et essai de fixation d'une technique rationelle. *C. R. Acad. Sci. (Paris)*, 1906, **143**, 983-85.
Bergonié–Tribondeau law, "the sensitivity of cells to radiation varies directly with the reproductive capacity of the cells and inversely with their degree of differentiation" (Dorland).

2006 WEBER, *Sir* HERMANN DAVID. 1823-1918, & WEBER, FREDERICK PARKES. 1863-1962
Climatology and balneotherapy. London, *Smith, Elder & Co.*, 1907.

2007 NAGELSCHMIDT, KARL FRANZ. 1875-1952
Ueber Diathermie. (Transthermie, Thermopenetration.) *Münch med. Wschr.*, 1909, **56**, 2575-76.
Nagelschmidt employed high frequency currents in treatment after the suggestions of Tesla and the work of Nernst, claiming priority over the latter in the use of this method. Nagelschmidt named this form of treatment "diathermy".

2008 REGAUD, CLAUDE. 1870-1940, & FERROUX, R.
Discordance des effets des rayons X, d'une part dans la peau, d'autre part dans le testicule, par le fractionnement de la dose: diminution de l'efficacité dans la peau, maintien de l'efficacité dans le testicule. *C. R. Soc. Biol. (Paris)*, 1927, **97**, 431-4.
Dose fractionation.

2009 SCHLIEPHAKE, ERWIN. 1894-
Therapeutische Versuche im elektrischen Kurzwellenfeld. *Klin. Wschr.*, 1930, **9**, 2333-36.
Introduction of short-wave diathermy.

2010 PIÉRY, ANTOINE MARIUS. 1873-1957
Traité de climatologie biologique et médicale. Publié sous la direction de M. Piéry. 3 vols. Paris, *Masson*, 1934.

2010.1   POHLMANN, R., *et al.*
Ueber die Ausbreitung und Absorption des Ultraschalls im menschlichen Gewebe und seine therapeutische Wirkung an Ischias und Plexusneuralgie. *Dtsch. med. Wschr.*, 1939, **65**, 251-54.
First therapeutic use of ultrasonics. With R. Richter and E. Parow.

2010.2   KERST, Donald William. 1911-
The acceleration of electrons by magnetic induction. *Physical Rev.*, 1941, **60**, 47-52.
The betatron.

2010.3   GINZTON, Edward Leonard. 1915- , *et al.*
A linear electron accelerator. *Rev. sci. Instrum.*, 1948, **19**, 89-108.
With K. B. Mallory and H. S. Kaplan.

2010.4   NEWBERRY, G. R.
The microwave linear electron accelerator. *Brit. J. Radiol.*, 1949, **22**, 473-86.

2010.5   WAKIM, Khalil Georges. 1970- , *et al.*
Therapeutic possibilities of microwaves. *J. Amer. med. Ass.*, 1949, **139**, 989-93.
Introduction of microwave radiation therapy. With J. F. Herrick, G. M. Martin, and F. H. Krusen.

For history of physical therapy, see 2029, 2043, 2046-47, 2056, 2057.1, 2068.17, 2068.21

BLOOD TRANSFUSION

See also 860-913, Haematology

2011   COLLE, Giovanni. 1558-1631
Methodus facile parandi iucunda tuta et nova medicamenta. Venetiis, 1628.
Page 170 includes the first definite description of a blood transfusion.

2012   LOWER, Richard. 1631-1691
The method observed in transfusing the blood out of one live animal into another. *Phil. Trans.*, 1665-66, **1**, 353-58.
In February 1665 Lower successfully transfused dogs with blood.

2013   DENIS, Jean Baptiste [Denys]. *c.* 1625-1704
Lettre ... touchant deux expériences de la transfusion faites sur des hommes. Paris, *J. Cusson*, 1667.
The first transfusion of blood into a human was performed by Denis on June 15, 1667; he transfused lamb's blood into a youth. For partial translation, see G. L. Keynes's *Blood transfusion*, Bristol, 1949, pp. 14-15. Denis also wrote: "a letter concerning a new way of curing sundry diseases by transfusion of blood", which was published in some copies of *Phil. Trans.*, 1667, **2**, 489-504; for reprint and a paper on the subject, see A. D. Farr, *Med. Hist.*, 1980, **24**, 143-62.

2014   LOWER, RICHARD. 1631-1691, & KING, *Sir* EDMUND.1629-1707
An account of the experiment of transfusion, practised upon a man in London. *Phil Trans.*, 1667, **2**, 557-64.
First transfusion of blood performed on a human in England, Nov. 23, 1667.

2015   BLUNDELL, JAMES. 1790-1877
Experiments on the transfusion of blood by the syringe. *Med.-chir. Trans.*, 1818, **9**, 56-92.
Blundell invented a syringe by means of which he was able to transfuse dogs.

2015.1   ——. Some account of a case of obstinate vomiting, in which an attempt was made to prolong life, by the injection of blood into the veins. *Med.-chir. Trans.*, 1819, **10**, 296-311.
Records the first human to human transfusion. A man received 12 to 14 oz. of blood from several donors by means of Blundell's funnel and syringe. He died 56 hours after the transfusion.

2016   PRÉVOST, JEAN LOUIS. 1790-1850, & DUMAS, JEAN BAPTISTE ANDRÉ. 1800-1884
Examen du sang et de son action dans les divers phénomènes de la vie. *Ann. Chim. (Paris)*, 1821, **18**, 280-97.
First successful use of defibrinated blood for animal transfusions. This was the first attempt to prevent coagulation during transfusion.

2017   BLUNDELL, JAMES. 1790-1877
Observations on transfusion of blood. *Lancet*, 1828-29, **2**, 321-24.
The first human to human transfusion in which the patient did not die. Blundell established the most fundamental points in transfusion, including the incompatibility of interspecies transfusion and the method of indirect transfusion. With his descriptions of about ten cases over a ten-year period, Blundell revived interest in blood transfusion after a century-long hiatus.

2017.1   HICKS, JOHN BRAXTON. 1823-1897
Cases of transfusion, with some remarks on a new method of performing the operation. *Guy's Hosp. Rep.*, 1869, **14**, 1-14.
Sodium phosphate used as anticoagulant in blood transfusion.

2017.2   AVELING, JAMES HOBSON. 1828-1892
Immediate transfusion in England: seven cases, and the author's method of operating. *Obstet. J. Gt. Britain*, 1873, **1**, 289-311.
Portable transfusion apparatus.

2018   LANDOIS, LEONARD. 1837-1902
Auflösung der rothen Blutzellen. *Zbl. med. Wiss.*, 1874, **12**, 419-22.
Landois discovered the haemolysing effect of blood serum of one species when transfused into another.

2018.1   KIMPTON, ARTHUR RONALD. 1881- , & BROWN, JAMES HOWARD. 1884-
A new and simple method of transfusion. *J. Amer. med. Assoc.* 1913, **61**, 117-8.
In order to prevent blood coagulation during transfusion, Kimpton and Brown used apparatus lined with paraffin wax. See also *Boston med. surg. J.*, 1915, **173**, 425-7.

2019   HUSTIN, ALBERT. 1882-1967
        Note sur une nouvelle méthode de transfusion. *Bull. Soc. roy. Sci. méd. Brux.*, 1914, **72**, 104-11.
           Hustin demonstrated the anticoagulant powers of sodium citrate and glucose in blood transfusion.

2020   AGOTE, LUIS. 1868-1954
        Nuevo procedimiento para la transfusion de la sangre. *An. Inst. mod. Clin. méd. (B. Aires)*, 1914, **1**, 24-31.
           Agote was the first to transfuse citrated blood. Text in Spanish and French.

2021   LEWISOHN, RICHARD. 1875-1962
        A new and greatly simplified method of blood transfusion. A preliminary report. *Med. Rec. (N.Y.)*, 1915, **87**, 141-42.
           About the same time as Agote, Lewisohn introduced the citrate method of blood transfusion. See also his later paper in *Surg. Gynec. Obstet.*, 1915, **21**, 37-47.

2021.1 ROBERTSON, OSWALD HOPE. 1886-1966
        Transfusion with preserved red blood cells. *Med. Bull. (Paris)*, 1917-1918, **1**, 436-40.
           Robertson stored blood and used it with good results to treat casualties on the battlefield.

2022   FLOSDORF, EARL WILLIAM. 1904-1958, & MUDD, STUART. 1893-
        Procedure and apparatus for preservation in "lyophile" form of serum and other biological substances. *J. Immunol.*, 1935, **29**, 389-425.

2023   MARRIOTT, HUGH LESLIE. 1900-1983, & KEKWICK, ALAN. 1909-1974
        Continuous drip blood transfusion. *Lancet*, 1935, **1**, 977-81.
           Introduction of the slow-drip method of blood transfusion.

2024   HEDENIUS, PER JOHANNES. 1906-
        A new method of blood transfusion. *Acta med. scand.*, 1936, **89**, 263-267.
           Heparin used in blood transfusion. See also the same journal, **88**, 443-49.

2025   YUDIN, SERGEI SERGEIEVICH. 1891-1954
        Transfusion of cadaver blood. *J. Amer. med. Ass.*, 1936, **106**, 997-99.
           Cadaver blood used in human transfusions. Prof. Shamov of Kharkov carried out the first experimental work on transfusion of cadaver blood in 1927.

2026   FANTUS, BERNARD. 1874-1940
        The therapy of the Cook County Hospital. Blood preservation. *J. Amer. med. Assoc.*, 1937, **109**, 128-31.
           Described the establishment of the first blood bank (at the Cook County Hospital).

2027   GOODALL, JAMES ROBERT. 1878-1947, *et al.*
        An inexhaustible source of blood for transfusion, and its preservation. Preliminary report. *Surg. Gynec. Obstet.*, 1938, **66**, 176-78.

J. R. Goodall, F. O. Anderson, G. T. Altimas, and F. L. MacPhail pointed out the possibility of using placental blood for transfusion purposes.

2027.1   LOUTIT, JOHN FREEMAN. 1910- , & MOLLISON, PATRICK LOUDON. 1914-
Advantages of a disodium-citrate-glucose mixture as a blood preservative. *Brit. med. J.*, 1943, **2**, 744-5.
This work made possible the storage of whole blood for up to three weeks.

2028   GRÖNWALL, ANDERS JOHAN TROED. 1912- , & INGLEMAN, BJÖRN.
Untersuchungen über Dextran und sein Verhalten bei parenteraler Zufuhr. *Acta physiol. scand.*, 1944, **7**, 97-107.
Introduction of dextran as plasma substitute.

2028.1   SMITH, AUDREY URSULA. 1915-1981
Prevention of haemolysis during freezing and thawing red blood-cells. *Lancet*, 1950, **2**, 910-11.
Demonstration that human blood diluted with equal volumes of 30% glycerol in Ringer's lactate solution could be frozen at -79° C and thawed after eight weeks without damage.

History of Blood Transfusion

2028.40   SCHEEL, PAUL. 1773-1811
Die Transfusion des Blutes und Einsprützung der Arzneyen in die Adern. Historisch und in Rücksicht auf die practische Heilkunde bearbeitet. 2 vols. Copenhagen, *F. Brummer*, 1802-03.
The first major work on transfusion since the 17th century and an excellent early history of the subject. Scheel reviewed both transfusion and intravenous injection. A third volume by J. F. Dieffenbach, *Die Transfusion des Blutes und die Infusion der Arzeneien in die Blutgefässe*, was published in Berlin, 1828.

2028.41   SIMILI, ALESSANDRO.
Origine e vicende della trasfusione del sangue. Considerazioni storico-critche. Bologna, *Cooperativa Tipografica Azzoguidi*, 1933.

2028.42   MALUF, NOBEL SUYDAM R. 1913-
History of blood transfusion. *J. Hist. Med.*, 1954, **9**, 59-107.

2028.43   PEUMERY, JEAN JACQUES.
Les origines de la transfusion sanguine. Amsterdam, *B. M. Israël*, 1974.
Reprinted from *Clio Medica*, Vol. 9, 1974.

2028.50   RÉAUMUR, RENÉ ANTOINE FERCHAULT DE. 1683-1757
Avis pour donner du secours à ceux que l'on croit noyez. [Montpellier, *Imprimérie d'Augustin F. Rochard*, 1740.]
In this unsigned 4-page pamphlet Réaumur argued that those who had been drowned for several hours could be resuscitated. His ideas inspired the formation of the Amsterdam Society (No. 2028.51). This anonymous

work was attributed to Réaumur by various contemporary writers on drowning.

2028.51 AMSTERDAM SOCIETY.
Historie en Gedenkschriften van de Maatschappy, tot Redding von Drenkelingen, Opgerecht Binnen Amsterdam 1768. Amsterdam, *Pieter Meijer*, 1768.
The first of many volumes of reports by the first society to save people drowned in the waterways of Amsterdam, established in 1767. Before 1767 anyone taken from the water was presumed dead and no attempts were made at resuscitation. News of the success of this organization spread rapidly through Europe, and similar societies were formed in other countries. French translation, Amsterdam, 1768. English translation by T. Cogan, London, 1773. *See* No. 2028.52.

2028.52 JOHNSON, ALEXANDER. 1715/16-1799.
A short account of a society at Amsterdam instituted in the year 1767 for the recovery of drowned persons...London, *John Nourse*, 1773.
An English summary of No. 2028.51, and the first detailed report on the society's work published in England. Johnson proposed the formation of a similar society in England. The Royal Humane Society was formed by T. Cogan and W. Hawes in 1774.

2028.53 GOODWYN, EDMUND. 1756-1829
The connexion of life with respiration; or, an experimental inquiry into the effects of submersion, strangulation, and several kinds of noxious airs, on living animals. London, *J. Johnson*, 1788.
Goodwyn emphasized the importance of ventilation in resuscitation.

2028.54 KITE, CHARLES. 1768-1811
An essay on the recovery of the apparently dead. London, *C. Dilly*, 1788.
Kite recommended the use of artificial ventilation and was probably the first to recommend electric shock for resuscitation.

2028.55 LEROY D'ETOILLES, JEAN JACQUES JOSEPH. *b.* 1798
Recherches sur l'asphyxie. *J. Physiol.*, 1827, **7**, 45-65.
"Leroy invented a two-bladed instrument to aid in the insertion of a laryngeal tube by the ability to control the direction of its tip. He also invented a limiting mechanism for the bellows, to enable given amounts of air to be inflated, after he noticed at post-mortem where bellows had been used for inflation, that emphysema and tension pneumothorax were not uncommon. This research eventually led to the abandonment of bellows in resuscitation kits. Leroy also advocated chest and abdominal compression" (Huston).

2028.56 HALL, MARSHALL. 1790-1857
On a new mode of effecting artificial respiration. *Lancet*, 1856, **1**, 229.
Marshall Hall's method of artificial respiration.

2028.57 SILVESTER, HENRY ROBERT. 1828-1908
A new method of resuscitating still-born children, and of restoring persons apparently drowned or dead. *Brit. med. J.*, 1858, 576-79.
Silvester's method of artificial respiration.

2028.58   HOWARD, Benjamin. *d.* 1900.
Plain rules for the restoration of persons apparently dead from drowning. New York, *E.B. Treat & Co.*, 1869.
Howard's method of artificial ventilation is taught for resuscitation from drowning.

2028.59   SHARPEY-SCHAFER, *Sir* Edward Albert. 1850-1935
Description of a simple and efficient method of performing artificial respiration on the human subject especially in cases of drowning. To which is appended instruction for the treatment of the apparently drowned. *Med.-chir. Trans.*, 1904, **87**, 609-23.

2028.60   NIELSEN, Holger. 1866-1955
En oplivingsmethode. *Ugeskr. Laeg.*, 1932, **94**, 1201-03.
Holger Nielsen ("arm-lift") method of artificial respiration.

History of Resuscitation

2028.90   HUSTON, Kenneth Garth, *Sr.* 1926-1987
Resuscitation: an historical perspective. Catalogue of an exhibit at the annual meeting of the American Society of Anesthesiologists...Park Ridge, *Wood Library-Museum*, 1976.

History of Pharmacology & Therapeutics

2029   FLOYER, *Sir* John. 1649-1734
The ancient Ψυχρολουσια revived; or, an essay to prove cold bathing both safe and useful. London, *S. Smith & B. Walford*, 1702.
A history of cold bathing.

2030   GUIBOURT, Nicholas Jean Baptiste Gaston. 1790-1867
Histoire abrégée des drogues simples. 2 vols. Paris, *L. Colas*, 1820.

2031   HOEVEN, Cornelis Pruys van der. 1792-1871
De historia medicamentorum. Lugduni Batavorum, *S. & J. Luchtmans*, 1846.

2032   FLÜCKIGER, Friedrich August. 1828-1894, & HANBURY, Daniel. 1825-1875
Pharmacographia. A history of the principal drugs of vegetable origin met with in Great Britain and British India. London, *Macmillan & Co.*, 1874.

2033   PETERSEN, Jacob Julius. 1840-1912
Hauptmomente in der geschichtlichen Entwickelung der medicinischen Therapie. Kopenhagen, *A. F. Höst*, 1877.
Reprinted Hildesheim, 1966.

2034   WARING, Edward John. 1819-1891
Bibliotheca therapeutica, or bibliography of therapeutics, chiefly in reference to articles of the materia medica, with numerous critical, historical, and therapeutical annotations, and an appendix containing the bibliography of British mineral waters. 2 vols. London, *New Sydenham Soc.*, 1878-79.
References to over 10,000 items, 'arranged under 660 separate headings or articles,' some with comments by the compiler.

2035   BELL, JACOB. 1810-1859, & REDWOOD, THEOPHILUS.1806-1892
Historical sketch of the progress of pharmacy in Great Britain. London, *Butler & Tanner,* 1880.

2036   PETERS, HERMANN. 1847-1920
Aus pharmazeutischer Vorzeit in Bild und Wort. 2 vols. Berlin, *J. Springer.* 1889-91.
    English translation, Chicago, 1899.

2037   FEISSINGER, CHARLES ALBERT. 1857-1942
La thérapeutique des vieux maîtres. Paris, *Soc. d'Editions Sci.,* 1897.

2038   BERENDES, JULIUS. 1837-1914
Geschichte der Pharmazie. Leipzig, *E. Gunther,* 1898.

2039   DRAGENDORFF, GEORG JOHANN NOEL. 1836-1898
Die Heilpflanzen der verschiedenen Völker und Zeiten. Stuttgart, *F. Enke,* 1898.

2040   ANDRÉ-PONTIER, L.
Histoire de la pharmacie. Paris, *O. Doin,* 1900.

2040.1   MORTIMER, W. GOLDEN.
Peru: the history of coca, "the divine plant of the Incas". New York, *J.H. Vail,* 1901.
    The most comprehensive work on the coca plant and the history of its use by the Incas and their descendants. Reprinted, San Francisco, *And/Or Press,* 1974.

2041   SCHELENZ, HERMANN. 1846-1922
Geschichte der Pharmazie. Berlin, *J. Springer,* 1904.
    Reprinted Hildesheim, 1964.

2043   MARTIN, FERDINAND HEINRICH ALFRED. 1874-
Deutsches Badewesen in vergangenen Tagen. Jena, *E. Diederichs,* 1906.

2044   HOEFLER, MAX. 1848-1914
Die volkmedizinische Organotherapie und ihr Verhältnis zum Kultopfer. Stuttgart, [1908?].

2045   WOOTTON, A. C. 1843-1910
Chronicles of pharmacy. 2 vols. London, *Macmillan & Co.,* 1910.
    From antiquity to time of writing, with chapters on pharmacy in mythology, in Shakespeare, in the Bible, and in popular medicine. Reprinted Boston, *Milford House,* 1972.

2046   GRASSET, HECTOR.
La médecine naturiste à travers les siècles. Histoire de la physiothérapie. Paris, *J. Rousset,* 1911.

2047   COLWELL, HECTOR ALFRED. 1875-1946
An essay on the history of electrotherapy and diagnosis. London, *W. Heinemann,* 1922.

2048 ROHDE, Eleanor Sinclair. *d.* 1950
The old English herbals. London, *Longmans, Green & Co.*, 1922.
Reprinted London, *Minerva Press*, 1972.

2049 BENEDICENTI, Alberico. 1866-1961
Malati medici e farmacisti. Storia dei rimedi traverso i secoli e delle teorie
che ne spiegano l'azione sull'organismo. 2 vols. Milano, *V. Hoepli*, 1924-
25.
Second edition, 1947-51.

2050 KLEBS, Arnold Carl. 1870-1943
Catalogue of early herbals. Lugano, *L'Art Ancien*, 1925.

2051 URDANG, George. 1882-1960
Der Apotheker als Subjekt und Objekt der Literatur. Berlin, *J. Springer*, 1926.

2052 LA WALL, Charles Herbert. 1871-1937
Four thousand years of pharmacy; an outline history of pharmacy. Philadelphia, *J. B. Lippincott*, 1927.
First history of pharmacy by an American. Reprinted as *The curious lore
of drugs and medicines*, New York, *Garden City Publ. Co.*, 1936.

2053 SINGER, Charles Joseph. 1876-1960
The herbal in antiquity and its transmission to later ages. *J. Hellen. Stud.*,
1927, **47**, 1-52.
In this paper Singer showed the methods by which ancient herbals are
studied and the results achieved by such study.

2054 THOMPSON, Charles John Samuel. 1862-1943
The mystery and art of the apothecary. London, *John Lane*, [1929].

2055 REUTTER DE ROSEMONT, Louis. 1876-
Histoire de la pharmacie à travers les âges. 2 vols. Paris, *Peyronnet*, 1931.

2056 COULTER, John Stanley. 1885-1949
Physical therapy. New York, *P. B. Hoeber*, 1932.
"Clio medica" series.

2056.1 TISCHNER, Rudolf. 1879-
Geschichte der Homöopathie. 1 vol. [in 4]. Leipzig, *B. Schwabe*, 1932-39.

2057 ADLUNG, Alfred. 1875- , & URDANG, George. 1882-1960
Grundriss der Geschichte der deutschen Pharmazie. Berlin, *J. Springer*, 1935.

2057.1 BRAUCHLE, Alfred.
Naturheilkunde in Lebensbildern. Leipzig, *Reclam*, 1937.
Mainly 19th-20th century: includes hydrotherapy, massage, and dietetics.
Second edition, 1951.

2058 GRIER, James.
A history of pharmacy. London, *Pharmaceutical Press*, 1937.

2059   ARBER, Agnes Robertson. 1879-1960
        Herbals: their origin and evolution. A chapter in the history of botany,
        1470-1670. 2nd edition. Cambridge, *University Press*, 1938.
            Includes an invaluable bibliography. Reprinted,with new introduction
        and additional references, 1987.

2060   HAGGIS, Alec William James. 1889-1946
        Fundamental errors in the early history of cinchona. *Bull. Hist. Med.*, 1941,
        10, 417-59, 568-92.

2061   TAYLOR, Norman. 1883-
        Cinchona in Java: the story of quinine. New York, *Greenberg*, [1945].

2062   BUESS, Heinrich. 1911-
        Die Injektion, *Ciba Z.*, 1946, **9**, 3594-3642.
            Deals exhaustively with the history of intravenous and intramuscular
        injection.

2063   HOWARD-JONES, Norman. 1909-1985
        A critical study of the origins and early development of hypodermic
        medication. *J. Hist. Med.*, 1947, **2**, 201-49.

2064   BOUSSEL, Patrice.
        Histoire illustrée de la pharmacie. Paris, *Guy Le Prat*, [1949].

2065   JARAMILLO-ARANGO, Jaime. 1897-1962
        A critical review of the basic facts in the history of cinchona. *J. Linn. Soc.
        (Botany)*, 1949, **53**, 272-309.

2067   URDANG, George. 1882-1960
        The development of pharmacopoeias. *Bull. Wld Hlth Org.*, 1951, **4**, 577-
        603.

2068   MOLDENKE, Harold Norman. 1909- , & MOLDENKE, Alma Lance. 1908-
        Plants of the Bible. Waltham, Mass., *Chronica Botanica Co.*, 1952.
            The most comprehensive treatise available on plants and plant prod-
        ucts mentioned in the Bible.

2068.2 MATTHEWS, Leslie Gerald.
        History of pharmacy in Britain. Edinburgh, *E. & S. Livingstone*, 1962.

2068.3 BÖTTCHER, Helmuth Maximilian. 1895-
        Miracle drugs. A history of antibiotics. London, *Heinemann*, 1963.
            First published in German, 1959.

2068.4 HOLMSTEDT, Bo, & LILJESTRAND, Goran.
        Readings in pharmacology. Selected and edited by B. Holmstedt and G.
        Liljestrand. Oxford, *Pergamon Press*, 1963.
            An anthology of outstanding achievement in the growth of pharma-
        cology.

2068.5 KREMERS, Edward. 1865-1941, & URDANG, George. 1882-1960
        History of pharmacy. 3rd ed. Philadelphia, *Lippincott*, 1963.
            4th ed., 1976, revised by G. Sonnedecker.

2068.6   THOMAS, Kenneth Bryn. 1916-1978
Curare, its history and usage. London, *Pitman*, [1964].

2068.7   TREASE, George Edward. 1902-
Pharmacy in history. London, *Baillière, Tindall and Cox*, 1964.
       Traces the origins of pharmacy in ancient civilizations and its development in England from medieval to modern times.

2068.8   VELLARD, J.
Histoire du curare. Les poisons de chasse en Amérique du Sud. Paris, *Gallimard*, [1965].

2068.9   HEILMANN, Karl Eugen.
Kräuterbücher in Bild und Geschichte. München-Allach, *K. Kölbl*, 1966.

2068.10   LICHT, Sidney.
History of electrotherapy. In: *Therapeutic electricity and ultraviolet radiation*, ed. by S. Licht. New Haven, *E. Licht*, 1967.

2068.11   CRELLIN, John.
Medical ceramics: a catalogue of the English and Dutch collections in the Museum of the Wellcome Institute for the History of Medicine, London, *Wellcome Institute for the History of Medicine*, 1969.

2068.12   BOVÉ, Frank James.
The story of ergot. Basel, *S. Karger*, 1970.
       Exhaustive and well-documented, but no index.

2068.13   CRELLIN, John. & SCOTT, J.R.
Glass and British pharmacy, 1600-1900: a survey and guide to the Wellcome Collection of British Glass. London, *Wellcome Institute for the History of Medicine*, 1972.

2068.14   LEAKE, Chauncey Depew. 1896-1978
An historical account of pharmacology to the 20th century. Springfield, *C. C. Thomas*, 1975.

2068.15   HARE, Ronald. 1899-1986
The birth of penicillin. London, *Allen & Unwin*, 1970.
       "Disposes of many myths deeply embedded in the literature" (Macfarlane, *see* No. 1934) and is the best available account.

2068.16   ACKERKNECHT, Erwin Heinz. 1906-1988
Therapeutics from the Primitives to the 20th century, with an appendix: history of dietetics. New York, *Hafner Press*, 1973.
       Includes a valuable bibliography. First published in German, Stuttgart, 1970.

2068.17   SCHIÖTZ, Eiler H., & CYRIAX, James Henry. 1904-1985
Manipulation past and present, with an extensive bibliography. London, *W. Heinemann*, 1975.

2068.18   HENREY, Blanche.
British botanical and horticultural literature before 1800. 3 vols., London, *Oxford University Press*, 1975.

A complete history and bibliography of the subject, including a revised history of the English herbal literature, and accounts of other books of medical and pharmaceutical interest.

2068.19 DREY, Rudolf E.A.
Apothecary jars. Pharmaceutical pottery and porcelain in Europe and the East 1150-1850, with a glossary of terms used in apothecary jar inscriptions. London, *Faber & Faber*, [1978]
The most comprehensive study in English.

2068.20 JOHNSON, F. Neil.
The history of lithium therapy. London, *Macmillan*, [1984].

2068.21 ROWBOTTOM, Margaret & SUSSKIND, Charles.
Electricity and Medicine: a history of their interaction. San Francisco, *San Francisco Press*, [1984].

TOXICOLOGY

See also 1717-1757, Medical Jurisprudence

2069 NICANDER [Nikander]. 185-135 b.c.
Theriaca et alexipharmaca. Venetiis, *apud Aldum Manutium*, 1499.
Nicander was a Greek poet and physician. His *Theriaca* deal in 958 hexameters, with the symptoms and treatment of poisoning by the bites of poisonous animals; the *Alexipharmaca* consider intoxications through animal, vegetable, and mineral poisoning and their suitable antidotes. He is the first writer to mention the medicinal use of the leech. The above work has a Greek text; a Latin translation appeared at Cologne in 1531. Modern edition and translation by A.S.F. Gow and A.F. Schofield, Cambridge, 1953. Reprinted, 1979.

2070 PETRUS *de Abano*. 1250-1315
Tractatus de venenis. Mantua, [*Thomas of Hermannstadt*], 1472.
The first printed book on toxicology, and one of the most elegantly printed of medical incunabula. For an English translation, see *Ann. med. Hist.*, 1924, **6**, 26-53.

2070.1 JONES, John. 1645-1709
The mysteries of opium revealed. London, *Richard Smith*, 1700.
Includes the earliest English description of drug addiction, and withdrawal. Jones attempted to use wine as a partial substitute until withdrawal was complete.

2071 LETTSOM, John Coakley. 1744-1815
Some remarks on the effects of lignum quassiae amarae. *Mem. med. Soc. Lond.*, 1779-87, **1**, 128-65.
Includes (p. 151) "original account of alcoholism, which is incidentally the first paper on the drug habit" (Garrison).

2071.1 TROTTER, Thomas. 1761-1832
An essay, medical, philosophical, and chemical, on drunkenness, and its effects on the human body. London, *T. N. Longman & O. Rees*, 1804.
First book on alcoholism.

2072   ORFILA, MATHIEU JOSEPH BONAVENTURE. 1787-1853
Traité des poisons. 2 vols. Paris, *Crochard*, 1814-15.
     Orfila, pioneer toxicologist, was the leading medico-legal expert of his time. He was born in Minorca, studied at Valencia, Barcelona, and Paris, and was one of the founders of the Académie de Médecine. He was a popular teacher, and is particularly remembered for his writings on toxicology. English translation, 1815-17.

2073   PARIS, JOHN AYRTON. 1785-1856
Pharmacologia; or the history of medicinal substances, with a view to establish the art of prescribing. 3rd ed. London, *W. Phillips*, 1820.
     First description of arsenic cancer (p. 133).

2074   WATERTON, CHARLES. 1782-1865
Wanderings in South America. London, *J. Mawman*, 1825.
     Includes a detailed description of the paralysing effects of curare. Reprinted, London, *O. U. P.*, 1973, edited by L. H. Matthews.

2075   ADDISON, THOMAS. 1793-1860, & MORGAN, JOHN. 1797-1847
An essay on the operation of poisonous agents upon the living body. London, *Longman, Rees*, 1829.
     First book in English on the action of poisons on the living body.

2076   CHRISTISON, *Sir* ROBERT. 1797-1882
A treatise on poisons. Edinburgh, *A. Black*, 1829.
     Christison, a famous toxicologist, was a Professor of Medical Jurisprudence at Edinburgh. During the trial of Burke and Hare he performed an autopsy on the body of one of the victims and gave evidence as to the cause of death.

2077   MARSH, JAMES. 1794-1846
Account of a method of separating small quantities of arsenic from substances with which it may be mixed. *Edinb. new phil. J.*, 1836, **21**, 229-36.
     Marsh method for the detection of arsenic.

2077.1   SLEEMAN, *Sir* WILLIAM HENRY. 1788-1856
Rambles and recollections of an Indian official. 2 vols. London, *Hatchard & Son*, 1844.
     Lathyrism, a disease occuring in India, and parts of Africa, was known to Hippocrates. Sleeman, an Indian official and major general who presided over the suppression of Thuggi, had no special knowledge of medicine, but gave the first detailed account of lathyrism in vol. 1.

2077.2   MOREAU, JACQUES-JOSEPH. 1804-1884
Du hachische et de l'aliénation mentale: études psychologiques. Paris, *Fortin, Masson*, 1845.
     Classic monograph on cannabis intoxication, and a most important scientific work on the subject. English translation, New York, *Raven Press*, [1973].

2078   KÖLLIKER, RUDOLPH ALBERT VON. 1817-1905
Physiologische Untersuchungen über die Wirkung einiger Gifte. *Virchows Arch. path. Anat.*, 1856, **10**, 3-77, 235-96.
     First investigation of the effects of poisons on muscular contraction.

2079   BERNARD, Claude. 1813-1878
Analyse physiologique des propriétés des systèmes musculaires et nerveux au moyen du curare. *C. R. Acad. Sci. (Paris)*, 1856, **43**, 825-29.
    Bernard showed that curare acted by stopping the transmission of impulses from motor nerves to voluntary muscles.

2080   WORMLEY, Theodor George. 1826-1897
Micro-chemistry of poisons. New York, *Baillière Bros.*, 1867.
    The first American book entirely devoted to toxicology and an important contribution to the identification of poisons.

2081   LEWIN, Louis. 1850-1929
Die Nebenwirkungen der Arzneimittel. Berlin, *A. Hirschwald*, 1881.
    This is the first book of its kind. It deals with the borderline between the pharmacological and the toxicological action of drugs with the untoward or side-effects of all kinds of medicaments. For details regarding this book and its author, see D. I. Macht, *Ann. med. Hist.*, 1931, **3**, 179-94, which includes a bibliography of Lewin's writings. English translation, with the author's revisions, Detroit, 1883.

2082   SULLIVAN, William Charles. 1869-1926
A note on the influence of maternal inebriety on the offspring. *J. ment. Sci.*, 1899, **45**, 489-503.
    Foetal alcohol syndrome – first serious study.

2083   KOBERT, Eduard Rudolf. 1854-1918
Lehrbuch der Intoxikationen. 2te. Aufl. 2 vols. Stuttgart, *F. Enke*, 1902-06.

2084   ABEL, John Jacob. 1857-1938, & FORD, William Webber. 1871-1941
On the poisons of Amanita phalloides. *J. biol. Chem.*, 1906-07, **2**, 273-88.
    Abel and Ford showed that there were two poisons in the fungus *Amanita phalloides,* and that immunity against them could be attained. A further study on the subject by the same authors is in *Arch. exp. Path. Pharmak.*, 1908, Suppl., 8-15.

2085   SCOTT, *Sir* Henry Harold. 1874-1956
On the 'vomiting sickness' of Jamaica. *Ann. trop. Med. Parasit.*, 1916, **10**, 1-78.
    Discovery of the cause of the "vomiting sickness of Jamaica", ackee poisoning.

2086   LEWIN, Louis. 1850-1929
Phantastica. Berlin, *G. Stilke*, 1924.
    The classic of psychoactive drug classification. Lewin established the following categories: Euphorics, Phantastics, Inebriants, Hypnotics, and Excitants. English translation, 1931.

2086.1   BERINGER, Kurt. 1893-1949
Der Meskalinrausch. Seine Geschichte und Erscheinungsweise. Berlin, *Julius Springer,* 1927.
    The most comprehensive treatise on peyote and its active agent, mescaline, which was synthesized in 1919.

2089   LESCHKE, Erich Friedrich Wilhelm. 1877-1933
Die wichtigsten Vergiftungen. Fortschritte in deren Erkennung und Behandlung. München, *J. F. Lehmann*, 1933.

2090   McINTYRE, Archibald Ross. 1902-
Curare, its history, nature, and clinical use. Chicago, *University Press*, 1947.

2091   HALD, Jens, *et al.*
The sensitizing effect of tetraethylthiuramdisulphide (Antabuse) to ethylalcohol. *Acta pharmacol. (Kbh.)*, 1948, **4**, 285-96.
    Introduction of "antabuse" in the treatment of alcoholism. With E. Jacobsen and V. Larsen. See also *Lancet*, 1948, **2**, 1004.

See also 2118-2137.02, Occupational and Aviation Medicine; 2069-2091, Toxicology

2092   CITOIS, François [Citesius]. 1572-1652
De novo et populari apud Pictones dolore colico bilioso diatriba. Augustoriti Pictonum, *apud Antonium Mesnier*, 1616.
    Citois described Poitou colic, "colica Pictonum", in great detail, and it was this description which was responsible for the condition being recognized as a definite syndrome. Partial English translation in No. 2241.

2093   HUXHAM, John. 1692-1768
De morbo colico Damnoniensi. Londini, *S. Austen*, 1739.
    Huxham left a vivid account of the "Devonshire colic". He was at fault, however, in ascribing it to the tartar extracted from apples in the process of making cider.

2094   CADWALADER, Thomas. 1708-1779
An essay on the West-India dry-gripes ... to which is added, an extraordinary case in physick. Philadelphia, *B. Franklin*, 1745.
    Cadwalader, an American pupil of Cheselden, left a classical account of lead colic and lead palsy. This was later shown by Benjamin Franklin, printer of the above work, to be due to the consumption of Jamaica rum which had been distilled through lead pipes. The "extraordinary case" mentioned in the title refers to a case of osteomalacia. Cadwalader's autopsy of the victim's body is one of the earliest recorded in the United States. The above work is probably the first medical book containing significant original research to be published by an American physician in America.

2095   TRONCHIN, Theodore. 1709-1781
De colica pictonum. Genevae, *apud fratres Cramer*, 1757.
    Tronchin, sometime physician to Voltaire, showed that the so-called "Poitou colic" was caused by drinking water which had passed through lead gutters. Tronchin introduced inoculation into Holland, France, and Switzerland; he was Boerhaave's favourite pupil and became a very wealthy practitioner. Partial English translation in No. 2241.

2096   BAKER, *Sir* George. 1722-1809
An essay concerning the cause of the endemial colic of Devonshire. London, *J. Hughs*, 1767.
    Baker demonstrated that the cider of Devonshire contained lead, while that made in other parts of England did not. He further showed that it was common practice in Devon to line cider presses with lead. He proved that

lead poisoning was the cause of Devonshire colic. He was responsible for the abandonment of lead in the making of cider presses, and thus for the disappearance of the colic. See also his paper in *Med. Trans. Coll. Phys. Lond.*, 1768, **1**, 175-256. Facsimile reprint, 1958.

2097 MÉRAT DE VAUMARTOISE, François Victor. 1780-1851
Sur la colique, vulgairement appelée colique des peintres, des plombiers, du plomb, etc. Paris, *P. F. Rigot*, an XI [1803].

2098 TANQUEREL DES PLANCHES, Louis Jean Charles Marie. 1810-1862
Traité des maladies de plomb ou saturnines. 2 vols. Paris, *Ferra*, 1839.
Classical description of the diseases found among lead workers. Reporting on 1200 cases of lead poisoning, Tanquerel's studies were so complete that later studies added little to knowledge of the symptoms and signs of the disease. English translation, Lowell, Mass., 1848.

2099 BURTON, Henry. 1799-1849
On a remarkable effect upon the human gums produced by the absorption of lead. *Med.-chir. Trans.*, 1840, **23**, 63-79.
Burton was the first to note the blue line on the gums in lead poisoning – "Burton's blue line" – an important diagnostic sign. He was physician to St. Thomas's Hospital, London.

2100 DEJERINE-KLUMPKE, Augusta. 1859-1927
Des polynévrites en général et des paralysies et atrophies saturnines en particulier. Paris, *F. Alcan*, 1889.
Madame Dejerine-Klumpke, famous neurologist, contributed an important work on lead palsies.

2101 LEGGE, *Sir* Thomas Morison. 1863-1932, & GOADBY, *Sir* Kenneth Weldon. 1873-1958
Lead poisoning and lead absorption. London, *E. Arnold*. 1912.

VENOMS

2102 REDI, Francesco. 1626-1697
Osservazioni intorno alle vipere. Firenze, *Stella*, 1664.
The first methodical work on snake-poison. Redi demonstrated for the first time that, for the poison to produce its effect, it must be injected under the skin.

2103 FONTANA, Felice. 1730-1805
Ricerche fisiche sopra il veleno della vipera. Lucca, *J. Giusti*, 1767.
The starting point of modern investigations of serpent venoms. This work also includes Fontana's description of the ciliary canal in the eye of an ox. This structure does not appear in the human eye, but certain spaces in the trabecular meshwork are often referred to as the spaces of Fontana. The greatly expanded French translation, 2 vols., 1781, includes Fontana's work on the anatomy of the nerves and nerve regeneration. Vol. 2 discusses American poisons. English translation prepared from French edition, 2 vols., 1787.

2104   MITCHELL, Silas Weir. 1829-1914, & REICHERT, Edward Tyson. 1855-
Researches upon the venom of the rattlesnake. Washington, *Smithsonian Inst.*, 1860.
See No. 2106.

2105   FAYRER, *Sir* Joseph. 1824-1907
The thanatophidia of India. London, *J. & A. Churchill*, 1872.
Describes all the venomous snakes of India. One of the finest books on the subject.

2106   MITCHELL, Silas Weir. 1829-1914, & REICHERT, Edward Tyson. 1855-
Researches upon the venoms of poisonous serpents. Washington, *Smithsonian Inst.*, 1886.
Mitchell (*see also* No. 2104) and Reichert showed snake venom to be protein in nature, and demonstrated the presence of toxic albumins. Mitchell was one of the first to investigate the snake venoms.

2107   CALMETTE, Léon Charles Albert. 1863-1933
Contribution à l'étude du vénin des serpents. *Ann. Inst. Pasteur*, 1894, **8**, 275-91; 1895, **9**, 225-51; 1898, **12**, 343-47.
Calmette carried out extensive investigations on the immunization of animals to venoms. He obtained antivenom sera with therapeutic properties.

2108   FRASER, *Sir* Thomas Richard. 1841-1919
On the rendering of animals immune against the venom of the cobra and other serpents; and on the antidotal properties of the blood serum of the immunised animals. *Brit. med. J.*, 1895, **1**, 1309-12.
Fraser investigated the possibilities of immunization against cobra venom and obtained "antivenene", an antivenom serum.

2109   CALMETTE, Léon Charles Albert. 1863-1933
Le vénin des serpents. Paris, *Soc. d'éd. Scient.*, 1896.

2110   FLEXNER, Simon. 1863-1946, & NOGUCHI, Hideyo. 1876-1928
Snake venom in relation to haemolysis, bacteriolysis, and toxicity. *J. exp. Med.*, 1902, **6**, 277-301.

2111   KYES, Preston. 1875-1949
Ueber die Wirkungsweise des Cobragiftes. *Berl. Klin. Wschr.*, 1902, **39**, 886-90, 918-22.
While in Germany Kyes published an important series of papers on venoms. He showed lecithin to be a complement of cobra-haemolysin. English translation in Ehrlich, *Studies in immunity*, 1910.

2112   ——. & SACHS, Hans. 1877-1945
Zur Kenntniss der Cobragift activirenden Substanzen. *Berl klin. Wschr.*, 1903, **40**, 21-23, 57-60, 82-85.
English translation in Ehrlich, *Studies in immunity*, 1910.

2113   ——. Ueber die Isolirung von Schlangengift-Lecithiden. *Berl. klin. Wschr.*, 1903, **40**, 956-59, 982-84.
English translation in Ehrlich, *Studies in immunity*, 1910.

2114 NOGUCHI, Hideyo. 1876-1928
Snake venoms. Washington, *Carnegie Inst.*, 1909.

2115 BRAZIL, Vital. 1865-1950
A defensa contra o ophidismo. São Paulo, 1911.
  Brazil founded the Instituto Butantan, São Paulo, one of the first institutes to produce antivenin sera on a large scale. French translation, 1911.

History of Toxicology

2116 LEWIN, Louis. 1850-1929
Die Gifte in der Weltgeschichte. Berlin, *J. Springer*, 1920.
  Lewin was a prolific writer, producing more than 200 books and papers. The above is perhaps his best work, and contains a history of poisonings from the most ancient times to the present century, enhanced by innumerable citations from ancient and modern literature.

2117 ———. Die Pfeilgifte, nach eigenen toxikologischen und ethnologischen Untersuchungen. Leipzig, *J. A. Barth*, 1923.

OCCUPATIONAL MEDICINE

See also 2069-2117, Toxicology

2118 ELLENBOG, Ulrich. 1440-1499
Von den gifftigen besen Tempffen und Reuchen. Augsburg, *M. Ramminger*, 1524.
  Written in 1473 but not published until 1524, this pamphlet on the diseases of miners is the first known work on industrial hygiene and toxicology. A reprint of the text appears in *Münch. Beitr. Lit. Naturwiss. Med.*, 1927, **2**, Sonderheft; and an English translation in *Lancet*, 1932, **1**, 270-71.

2118.1 PARACELSUS, [Bombastus von Hohenheim, Theophrastus Philippus Aureolus]. 1493-1541
Von der Bergsucht oder Bergkranckheiten drey Bücher...[Dilingen, *Durch Sebaldum Mayer,*] 1567.
  Paracelsus's book on the diseases of miners was the first monograph on the diseases of an occupational group. The first section covers the diseases, mainly pulmonary affections, of miners, including the etiology, pathogenesis, symptomatology and therapy. The second book describes the diseases of smelter workers and metallurgists, and the third section discusses diseases caused by mercury. English translation by G. Rosen in *Four treatises of Theophrastus von Hohenheim, called Paracelsus*, ed. by H.E. Sigerist, Baltimore, *Johns Hopkins Press*, 1941.

2119 PANSA, Martinus. *b. circa* 1580
Consilium peripneumoniacum. Leipzig, *T. Schürer*, 1614.

Martin Pansa, a pupil of Georg Agricola, wrote the most important work on occupational disease before Ramazzini. He described the symptoms of the lung diseases of miners and smelters.

2120   STOCKHAUSEN, SAMUEL. *fl.* 1619-1656
Libellus de lythargyrii fumo morbifico. Goslar, 1656.
Stockhausen had considerable experience in treating the diseases of miners. His book on industrial diseases did much to clarify contemporary knowledge regarding the relative toxicity of lead, mercury, arsenic, cobalt, and other metals, although he claimed that lead colic was caused only by lead fumes. French translation, Paris, 1776.

2121   RAMAZZINI, BERNARDINO. 1633-1714
De morbis artificum diatriba. Mutinae, *A. Capponi*, 1700.
Ramazzini wrote the first comprehensive and systematic treatise on occupational diseases. It deals with pneumoconiosis and other diseases of miners, with lead poisoning in potters, with silicosis in stonemasons, diseases among metal workers, and even a chapter devoted to the "diseases of learned men". It was translated into English in 1705; a new English translation by Wilmer Cave Wright appeared in 1940. The French edition by the noted chemist, Fourcroy, Paris, 1777 contains significant additions. The second French edition by Philibert Patissier, Paris, *Baillière*, 1838, provides so much new material on the diseases of workers in France as to virtually double the length of Ramazzini's text. *See* No. 4478.101.

2122   POTT, PERCIVALL. 1714-1788
Chirurgical observations relative to the cataract, the polypus of the nose, the cancer of the scrotum, *etc.* London, *for L. Hawes, W. Clarke, and R. Collins*, 1775.
First description of an occupational cancer (chimney-sweeps' cancer of the scrotum).

2123   THACKRAH, CHARLES TURNER. 1795-1833
The effects of the principal arts, trades and professions, and of civic states and habits of living on health and longevity. London, *Longman*, 1831.
The first systematic publication in Great Britain on industrial disease and its prevention. For comprehensiveness, first-hand clinical experience and constructive proposals for improvements, Thackrah's monograph is superior to that of Ramazzini. It attracted attention from both medical men and laymen at the time that it appeared, and played an important part in stimulating the factory and health legislation which mitigated some of the worst features of the Industrial Revolution. The book also includes important information on the harmful effects of child labour. The second edition (1832) was doubled in length. A reprint of the 2nd edition, with a life of the author by A. Meiklejohn, was published in 1957.

2123.1   McCREADY, BENJAMIN WILLIAM. 1813-1892
On the influence of trades, professions, and occupations, in the United States in the production of disease. *Trans. Med. Soc. St. of N.Y.*, 1836-37, **3**, 91-150.
The first American work devoted entirely to occupational diseases. Reprinted with introduction, Baltimore, *Johns Hopkins Press*, 1943.

2123.1   TARDIEU, AUGUSTE AMBROISE. 1818-1879
Mémoire sur les modifications physiques et chimiques que détermine dans certaines parties du corps l'exercice des diverse professions, pour servir à la recherche médico-légale de l'identité. *Ann. Hyg. publ. Méd. lég.*, 1849, **42**, 388-423; 1850, **43**, 131-44.

In this comprehensive work on occupational marks, Tardieu states that Corvisart, Dupuytren, and Trousseau would take pride in identifying the professions of their patients at first sight, using knowledge of occupational marks and other physical signs of occupations.

2124   POL, B., & WATELLE, T. J. J.
Mémoire sur les effets de la compression de l'air. *Ann. Hyg. publ.*, 1854, 2 sér., **1**, 241-79.

An early paper on "caisson sickness".

2125   THIERSCH, CARL. 1822-1895
De maxillarum necrosi phosphorica. Lipsiae, *apud A. Edelmannum*, 1867.

A classical description of phosphoric necrosis of the jaw.

2125.1   ZENKER, FRIEDRICH ALBERT. 1825-1898
Ueber Staubinhalationskrankheiten der Lungen. *Dtsch. Arch. klin. Med.*, 1867, **2**, 116-72.

Zenker described siderosis and suggested the term "pneumonokoniosis" as a suitable general title for diseases due to inhaled dust.

2126   VOLKMANN, RICHARD VON. 1830-1889
Beiträge zur Chirurgie, anschliessend an einen Bericht über die Thätigkeit der chirurgischen Universitäts-Klinik zu Halle im Jahre 1873. Leipzig, *Breitkopf u. Härtel*, 1875.

Contains (pp. 370-81) first description of industrial tar and paraffin cancer.

2127   HIRT, LUDWIG. 1844-1907
Die Krankheiten der Arbeiter. 4 vols. Breslau, Leipzig, *F. Hirt u. Sohn*, 1871-78.

2127.1   BELL, JOSEPH. 1837-1911
Paraffin epithelioma of the scrotum. *Edinb. med. J.*, 1876, **22**, 135-37.

Shale oil shown to be a cause of skin cancer. A teacher of Sir Arthur Conan Doyle, Bell was the model for the character of Sherlock Holmes.

2128.1   REHN, LUDWIG. 1849-1930
Blasengeschwülste bei Fuchsin-Arbeitern. *Arch. klin. Chir.*, 1895, **50**, 588-600.

Rehn noted the frequent appearance of papilloma and carcinoma of the bladder among men employed in the aniline dye industry.

2129   OLIVER, *Sir* THOMAS. 1853-1942
Dangerous trades: the historical, social, and legal aspects of industrial occupations as affecting health, by a number of experts. Edited by T. OLIVER. London, *John Murray*, 1902.

2130   MURRAY, HUBERT MONTAGUE. 1855-1907
In Report of the Departmental Committee on Compensation for Industrial
Diseases. Cd. 3495 and 3496. London, *Wyman and Sons, for His Majesty's
Stationery Office*, 1907.

            The first reported case of asbestosis was observed by Murray at Charing
Cross Hospital, London, in 1899 and reported to the Committee (Report, p.
14: Minutes of Evidence, p. 127) in 1907.

2131   HILL, *Sir* LEONARD ERSKINE. 1866-1952
Caisson sickness, and the physiology of work in compressed air. London,
E. Arnold, 1912.

2132   MOCK, HARRY EDGAR. 1880-1959
Industrial medicine and surgery. Philadelphia, *W. B. Saunders*, 1919.

2133   VERNON, HORACE MIDDLETON. 1870-1951
Industrial fatigue and efficiency. London, *G. Routledge*, 1921.

2134   HAMILTON, ALICE. 1869-1970
Industrial poisons in the United States. New York, *Macmillan Co.*, 1925.

2134.1   SEILER, HENRY EDMUND. 1899-1978.
A case of pneumoconiosis. Result of the inhalation of asbestos dust. *Brit.
med. J.*, 1928, **2**, 982 (only).

            Seiler established an unequivocal relationship between asbestos and
pulmonary fibrosis.

2135   BREZINA, ERNST.
Die gewerblichen Vergiftungen und ihre Bekämpfung. Stuttgart, *F. Enke*,
1932.

2135.1   RONCHESE, FRANCESCO
Occupational marks and other physical signs. A guide to personal identification. New York, *Grune & Stratton*, 1948.

            Calluses, other dermatological and physical signs of professions and
occupations illustrated and described, with an annotated bibliography that
includes some historical references.

History of Industrial Hygiene and Medicine

2136   ROSEN, GEORGE. 1910-1977
The history of miners' diseases. A medical and social interpretation. New
York, *Schuman's*, 1943.

2137   TELEKY, LUDWIG. 1872-1957
History of factory and mine hygiene. New York, *Columbia University Press*,
1948.

2137.01   HUNTER, DONALD. 1898-1978.
The diseases of occupations. London, *English Univ. Press*, 1955.

            A classic textbook on the subject with valuable historical chapters and
references. Hunter put the text through six editions to 1978. The work was
rewritten as *Hunter's Diseases of occupations*, ed. by P.A.B. Raffle, W.R.

Lee, R.I. McCallum, and R. Murray., Boston, *Little, Brown*, [1987]. In this form it includes the most authoritative history of occupational medicine.

2137.02   WHITTACKER, Alfred Heacock & SELLECK, Henry B.
Occupational health in America. Detroit, *Wayne State University Press*, 1962.
Written under the auspices of the Industrial Medical Association, this history emphasizes 20th century achievements.

AVIATION MEDICINE

See also Nos. 914-971.1, respiratory system.

2137.1   LEULIER DUCHÉ, Louis.
Tentamen medicum de aerostatum usu medicinae applicando...Montpellier, *Picot*, 1784.
The first work on aviation medicine, published one year after Montgolfier. Leulier Duché speculated on ways that ballooning might be used in medicine, quoting an anecdote privately communicated to him by Montgolfier describing the "high" experienced by the aeronauts on a particular ascent.

2137.2   JEFFRIES, John. 1744/45-1819
A narrative of the two aerial voyages of Dr. Jeffries with Mons. Blanchard; with meteorological observations and remarks. London, *J. Robson*, 1786.
The first flight by a physician, the first crossing of the English channel by balloon, and the first international flight. Jeffries, an American, made a series of carefully planned scientific observations, emphasizing meteorology.

2137.3   HENDERSON, Yandell. 1873-1944.
Effects of altitude on aviators. *Aviat. & Aeronaut. Engineering*, 1917, **2**, 145-47.
The first discussion of decompression sickness in flying personnel.

2137.4   BROCA, André. & GARSAUX, Paul.
Note préliminaire sur l'étude des effets de la force centrifuge sur l'organisme. *Bull. Acad. Méd. (Paris)*, 1919, **82**, 75-77.
The first anti-blackout device. Proposed the use of the *g* belt to prevent the flow of blood to the abdomen.

2137.5   ANDERSON, H. Graeme.
The medical and surgical aspects of aviation. London, *Henry Frowde*, 1919.
The first textbook on aviation medicine.

2137.6   BAUER, Louis Hopewell. 1888-1964
Aviation medicine. Baltimore, *Williams & Wilkins*, 1926.
Bauer established the first school for flight surgeons in the United States. His book discusses the question of oxygen supply and its essential partial pressure, and discusses the effect of hight degrees of acceleration on the circulatory system. Includes the first significant bibliography on the subject. See J.F. Fulton, Louis H. Bauer and the rise of aviation medicine, *J. Aviation med.*, 1955, **26**, 92-103.

2137.7 BARCROFT, JOSEPH. 1872-1947
Muscular exercise at low barometric pressures. *Arch. Sci. Biol.*(Napoli), 1931, **16**, 609-15.
With C.G. Douglas, L.P. Kendal, & R. Margaria. The first recorded attack of bends pain experienced at low barometric pressures. The authors atttempted to find the maximum altitude at which work could be done effectively with the subject breathing pure oxygen.

2137.8 JONGBLOED, J. & NOYONS, A.K.
Der Einfluss von Beschleunigungen auf den Kreislaufapparat. *Pflüg. Arch. ges. Physiol.*, 1933-34, **233**, 67-97.
Determination of the effect of high acceleration on blood pressure, establishing that the systolic pressure in arteries going to the head falls progressively as acceleratory forces increase.

2137.9 BOOTHBY, WALTER MEREDITH. 1880-1953, & LOVELACE, WILLIAM RANDOLPH. 1907-1965.
Oxygen in aviation. The necessity for the use of oxygen and a practical apparatus for its administration to both pilots and passengers. *J. Aviat. Med.*, 1938, 9, 172-198.
First acute case of decompression sickness recognized.

2137.10 ARMSTRONG, HARRY G.
Principles and practice of aviation medicine. Baltimore, *Williams & Wilkins*, 1939.
Used by all American flight surgeons during World War II.

History of Aviation Medicine

2137.30 HOFF, EBBE CURTIS. 1906-1985, & FULTON, JOHN FARQUHAR. 1899-1960
A bibliography of aviation medicine. Springfield, *C.C. Thomas*, 1942.

2138 FULTON, JOHN FARQUHAR. 1899-1960
Aviation medicine in its preventive aspects: an historical survey. London, *Oxford University Press*, 1948.

2138.1 SERGEYEV, A. A.
Essays on the history of aviation medicine. Translation of Ocherki po istorii aviatsionnoy meditsiny...Moscow, 1962. Washington, *National Aeronautics and Space Administration*, [1965].
Primarily useful for the history of aviation medicine in Russia, with a very extensive bibliography.

2138.2 ROBINSON, DOUGLAS H.
The dangerous sky. A history of aviation medicine. Seattle, *University of Washington Press*, 1973.

2138.3 BENFORD, ROBERT J.
The heritage of aviation medicine. An annotated directory of early artifacts. Washington, D.C., *Aerospace Medical Association*, [1979].
Descriptions and photographs of notable artifacts, including the original clothing worn by John Jeffries (No.2137.2).

MILITARY AND NAVAL HYGIENE AND MEDICINE

See also 5547-5813.15, SURGERY

2139   PARÉ, AMBROISE. 1510-1590
La méthode de traicter les playes faictes par hacquebutes et aultres bastons
à feu; et de celles qui sont faictes par flèches, dardz et semblables. Paris,
Chés viuant Gaulterot, 1545.
Among Paré's most important work is his treatise on gunshot wounds.
He is one of the greatest of the military surgeons, and is particularly
remembered for his abandonment of the practice of cauterization of
gunshot wounds with boiling oil, until his time a universal procedure.

2139.1   MAGGI, BARTOLOMEO. 1477-1552
De vulnerum sclopetorum et bombardarum curatione tractatus. Bononiae,
per B. Bonardum, 1552.
Maggi, Professor of Surgery at Bologna, wrote an important work on
military surgery. He showed that not all gunshot wounds suppurated and
he discarded cauterization, treating such wounds with white of egg and salt
water.

2140   GALE, THOMAS. 1507-1587
An excellent treatise of wounds made with gonneshot. London, *R. Hall,*
(1563).
Gale, a contemporary of Paré, was surgeon in Henry VIII's army at
Montreuil. His book supported the views of Paré regarding the treatment of
gunshot wounds, denying the poisonous effect of bullets; Gale, however,
applied messy and complicated unguents to wounds, doing more harm than
good. Forms part 3 of his *Certaine workes of chirurgerie* (No. 2371).

2141   CLOWES, WILLIAM. 1544-1604
A prooved practise for all young chirurgians, concerning burnings with
gunpowder, and woundes made with gunshot. London, *T. Orwyn for T.
Cadman,* 1588.
An interesting picture of Elizabethan surgery is given by William
Clowes in this book on gunshot wounds. Clowes, the best surgical writer
in Elizabethan times, was surgeon to St. Bartholomew's Hospital. In
amputation he covered the stump with integument – an earlier form of the
flap method. The *Selected Writings of William Clowes* were edited by F. N.
L. Poynter, London, 1949.

2142   FABRY, WILHELM [FABRICIUS *Hildanus*]. 1560-1634
New Feldt Arztny Buch von Kranckheiten und Schäden, so in Kriegen den
Wundartzten gemeinlich fürfallen. Basel, *L. König,* 1615.
Fabry's book includes an early description of a field drug chest for army
use. He was one of the most eminent surgeons of his time, although not
prepared to adopt all the teachings of Paré. He had considerable mechanical
ingenuity and devised many pieces of apparatus. English translation, 1674.

2143   MAGATI, CESARE. 1579-1647
De rara medicatione vulnerum. Venetiis, *apud A. & B. Dei, fratres,* 1616.
Like Paré, Magati believed that gunshot wounds were not in themselves
poisonous. He suggested a bandage moistened with plain water in place
of the various salves then in vogue.

2144 WOODALL, JOHN. 1570-1643
The surgions mate. London, *E. Griffin*, 1617.
  Woodall was the surgeon-general to the East India Company. This is the first textbook for naval surgeons. Woodall was an early advocate of limes and lemons as a preventive measure against scurvy. He was surgeon to St. Bartholomew's Hospital. The second edition (London, 1639) includes the first edition of Woodall's collected works. That edition was made required reading for all naval surgeons in the East India Company. Facsimile reprint, Bath, *Kingsmead Press*, 1978. Biography by J. H. Appleby, *Med. Hist.*, 1981, **25**, 251-68. *See* No. 3711.

2145 MINDERER, RAYMUND. *c.* 1570-1621
Medicina militaris, seu libellus castrensis. Augspurg, *A. Aperger*, 1620.
  Minderer's book gives a good idea of the position of military surgery during the Thirty Years' War. He published a pharmacopoeia in 1621; he also discovered ammonium acetate. An English edition appeared in 1674.

2146 PURMANN, MATTHÄUS GOTTFRIED. 1649-1711
Der rechte und warhafftige Feldscher. Franckfurt & Leipzig, *M. Rohrlach*, 1690.
  Purmann was a skilful army surgeon – one of the most famous of the period. Despite this he believed in the efficacy of the weapon-salve and the sympathetic powder.

2147 COCKBURN, WILLIAM. 1669-1739
An account of the nature, causes, symptoms, and cure of the distempers that are incident in seafaring people. With observations on the diet of the sea-men in his Majesty's navy. London, *Hugh Newman*, 1696.
  Cockburn studied medicine at Leiden; he became famous on account of his secret remedy for dysentery. The book is a record of two years spent as a ship's doctor.

2148 ATKINS, JOHN. 1685-1757
The navy-surgeon, or a practical system of surgery. London, *C. Ward and R. Chandler*, 1734.
  Atkins was an English naval surgeon. His book includes some useful case reports and contains the first English description of African trypanosomiasis.

2149 LE DRAN, HENRI FRANÇOIS. 1685-1770
Traité ou reflexions tirées de la pratique sur les playes d'armes à feu. Paris, *C. Osmont*, 1737.
  English translation, 1743.

2150 PRINGLE, *Sir* JOHN. 1707-1782
Observations on the diseases of the army. London, *A. Millar & D. Wilson*, 1752.
  Pringle, founder of modern military medicine, was Physician-General of the British Army from 1744 to 1752. His books lay down the principles of military sanitation and the ventilation of barracks, gaols, hospital ships, etc. He did much to improve the lot of soldiers, and it was due to remarks in his book that foot-soldiers were given blankets when on service. The preface of the book includes an account of the origin of the Red Cross idea

(the neutrality of military hospitals on the battlefield); for a further note on this, see *Lancet*, 1943, **2**, 234.

2151   LIND, JAMES. 1716-1794
An essay on the most effectual means, of preserving the health of seamen, in the Royal Navy. London, *A. Millar*, 1757.
Lind is regarded as the founder of naval hygiene in England. Besides his work on scurvy (*see* No.3713), he is notable for the above book, which deals not only with the men but also with the appalling conditions in which they lived afloat. He advocated measures to improve ships' ventilation and to prevent the spread of disease aboard ship. He also caused great improvements to be made in the food on board ships of the British Navy. L. H. Roddis published a biography of Lind in 1951.

2152   SWIETEN, GERARD L. B. VAN. 1700-1772
Kurze Beschreibung und Heilungsart der Krankheiten, welche am öftesten in dem Feldlager beobachtet werden. Wien, Prag, Triest, *J. T. Trattnern*, 1758.
An essay on diseases of military camps. English translation, 1762.

2153   BROCKLESBY, RICHARD. 1722-1797
Oeconomical and medical observations ... tending to the improvement of military hospitals, and to the cure of camp diseases, incident to soldiers. London, *T. Becket & P. A. De Hondt*, 1764.
The best book of the century regarding military sanitation.

2154   RAVATON, HUGUES.
Chirurgie d'armée. Paris, *P. F. Didot le jeune*, 1768.
One of the most important works on military surgery during the 18th century. Ravaton, a skilful army surgeon, was the first to employ a tin boot, suspended on four rings, for the "hanging" position of broken bones. He was also first to adopt the double-flap method in amputations.

2155   JONES, JOHN. 1729-1791
Plain, concise, practical remarks, on the treatment of wounds and fractures; to which is added an appendix, on camp and military hospitals; principally designed for the use of young military surgeons in North America. New York, *John Holt*, 1775.
The first surgical work written by an American and printed in North America. Jones's work was the accepted guide to surgical practice during the American Revolutionary War.

2156   PRINGLE, *Sir* JOHN. 1707-1782
A discourse upon some late improvements of the means for preserving the health of mariners. London, *Royal Society*, 1776.
Besides his pioneer work in military medicine, Pringle did much to improve the conditions of sailors afloat. *See also* Nos. 2150 & 3714.

2157   RUSH, BENJAMIN. 1745-1813
Directions for preserving the health of soldiers: recommended to the consideration of the officers of the Army of the United States. Published by order of the Board of War. Lancaster, *John Dunlap*, 1778.
A reprint from the *Philadelphia Packet*, No. 284. The pamphlet was reprinted by the Massachusetts Temperance Alliance in Boston, 1865, for distribution to the Union soldiers.

2158   BLANE, *Sir* GILBERT. 1749-1834

Observations on the diseases incident to seamen. London, *J. Cooper*, 1785.

William Hunter recommended Blane as private physician to Admiral Rodney; Blane sailed with him to the W. Indies and became physician to the British Fleet. He was held in great esteem in the navy and was instrumental in effecting improvements in living conditions among seamen. He strongly supported Lind's views on scurvy. In 1799 he made recommendations which formed the basis of the Quarantine Act of that year. Later he became physician to St. Thomas's Hospital. With Lind he stands predominant in the history of naval medicine.

2158.1   PERCY, PIERRE FRANÇOIS, *le Baron*. 1754-1825

Manuel du chirurgien-d'armée. Paris, Méquignon, 1792.

One of Napoleon's leading surgeons, Percy laid down his principles of the practice of military surgery in the same year he was appointed *médecin consultant* of the Army of the North. He devised his own instrument for bullet extraction, the *tribulcon*. He was responsible, with Larrey, for the invention of special ambulances and squads of litter-bearers, including a "super-ambulance" capable of carrying 8 surgeons, 8 attendants, and dressings for 1200.

2159   TROTTER, THOMAS. 1761-1832

Medicina nautica; an essay on the diseases of seamen. 3 vols. London, *T. Cadell, jun. and W. Davies (T. N. Longman and O. Rees)*, 1797-1803.

Trotter has left an excellent account of the conditions of seamen at the beginning of the 19th century. His book includes an interesting theory of the causation of fevers. He worked hard to improve the conditions of the ship's medical officer and the seaman.

2159.1   ROBERTSON, JAMES. 1742-1814

Remarks on the management of the scalped-head. *Phil. med. surg. J.*, 1805-06, **2, pt.2**, 27-30.

Treatment for the quintessential American war injury suffered by troops and settlers alike on the American frontier.

2160   LARREY, DOMINIQUE JEAN, *le baron*, 1766-1842

Mémoires de chirurgie militaire, et campagnes.(Vol. 5 entitled Relation médicale de campagnes et voyages.) 5 vols. Paris, *J. Smith*, 1812-17; *Baillière*, 1841.

Larrey was the greatest military surgeon in history. Of him Napoleon said: "C'est l'homme le plus vertueux que j'ai connu". He was present at all Napoleon's great battles and one of the few who stood by him on his abdication, and was waiting for him on his return in 1815. Larrey was one of the first to amputate at the hip-joint (No. 4442), the first to describe the therapeutic effect of maggots on wounds, gave the first description of "trench foot", invented the "ambulante volonte", used advanced first-aid posts on the battlefield, and devised several new operations. He was familiar with the stomach tube, with *débridement*, and with the infectious nature of granular conjunctivitis (*see* No. 5837). He was a kindly man, who devoted much of his life to the well-being of the soldiers, among whom not even Napoleon commanded more love and respect. Larrey states on page 1 of vol. 5, published 24 years after vol. 4, that he intended it to complete his campaign memoirs. Vol. 5 includes his account of the Battle of Waterloo and Napoleon's exile. English translation with notes by R.W. Hall of vols.

1-3 in 2 vols., Baltimore, 1814. English translation of vol. 4 by J.C. Mercer, Philadelphia, 1832.

2161   GUTHRIE, GEORGE JAMES. 1785-1856
On gun-shot wounds of the extremities, requiring the different operations of amputation, with their after treatment. London, *Longman*, 1815.
Guthrie was the leading British military surgeon during the first half of the 19th century. He served in the Napoleonic Wars; his book is one of the most important in the history of the subject.

2161.1 MANN, JAMES. 1759-1832
Medical sketches of the campaigns of 1812, 13, 14. To which are added, surgical cases, observations on military hospitals; and flying hospitals attached to a moving army. Dedham, Mass., *H. Mann*, 1816.
The primary record of medicine during the War of 1812.

2162   HENNEN, JOHN. 1779-1828
Observations on some important points in the practice of military surgery. Edinburgh, *A. Constable & Co.*, 1818.
"A valuable surgical record of the Napoleonic period" (Garrison).

2162.1 DOUGLAS, JOHN. 1788-1861
Medical topography of Upper Canada. London, *Burgess & Hill*, 1819.
The only book on the War of 1812 by a British or Canadian surgeon, and the first medical book on the Province of Ontario, Canada. This and the work of Mann (No. 2161.1) are the only books on medicine in the War of 1812. Reprint with introduction by C.G. Roland, 1985.

2163   DUPUYTREN, GUILLAUME, *le baron*. 1777-1835
Traité théorique et pratique des blessures par armes de guerre. 2 vols. Paris, *J. B. Baillière*, 1834.

2163.1 UNITED STATES, War Dept. *Surgeon General's Office.*
Statistical report on the sickness and mortality in the Army of the United States. Vol. 1 (1819-1839), Vol. 2 (1839-1855), Vol. 3 (1855-1860). Washington, D.C, 1840, 1856, 1860.
Volume one by Thomas Lawson (1781/5-1861), volume two by Richard H. Coolidge (1820-66).

2164   STROMEYER, GEORG FRIEDRICH LUDWIG. 1804-1876
Maximen der Kriegsheilkunst. Hannover, *Hahn*, 1855.
A landmark in military surgery, written by the founder of modern military surgery in Germany. Stromeyer, surgeon-general to the army of Hanover, is also notable for his important contributions to orthopaedics. *See* Nos. 4320-21.

2165   GREAT BRITAIN. War Office, *Medical Services.*
Medical and surgical history of the British Army which served in Turkey and the Crimea during the war against Russia, in the years 1854-56. 2 vols. London, *Harrison & Sons*, 1858.
First official medical and surgical history of a war.

2166   DUNANT, JEAN HENRI. 1828-1910
Un souvenir de Solferino. Genève, *J. G. Fick*, 1862.

Dunant's account of the great sufferings endured by the wounded at Solferino resulted in the Geneva Convention of 1864. In 1901 he was awarded the first Nobel Peace Prize. English translations, Washington, 1939 and London, 1947.

2166.1   BILL, JOSEPH HOWLAND, JR. 1835?-1885
Notes on arrow wounds. *Am. J. med. Sci.*, 1862, **154**, 365-87.
The definitive work on American Indian arrow wounds suffered by U.S. troops and settlers in frontier warfare during the Western expansion of the United States. Bill eventually developed an instrument for extraction of arrows, which he described in *Med. Rec.*, 1876, **11**, 245.

2167   MITCHELL, SILAS WEIR. 1829-1914, *et al.*
Gunshot wounds and other injuries of nerves. Philadelphia, *J. B. Lippincott & Co.*, 1864.
Mitchell, G. R. Morehouse, and W. W. Keen were army surgeons during the American Civil War; their book was the first exhaustive study of the traumatic neuroses. Reprinted, San Francisco, *Norman Publishing*, 1989. *See* No. 4544.

2168   ESMARCH, JOHANN FRIEDRICH AUGUST VON. 1823-1908
Der erste Verband auf dem Schlachtfelde. Kiel, *Schwers*, 1869.
Esmarch introduced the first-aid bandage on the battlefield.

2169   MAAS, HERMANN. 1842-1886
Kriegschirurgische Beiträge aus dem Jahre 1866. Breslau, *Maruschke & Berendt*, 1870.
A surgical history of the Seven Weeks War between Germany and Austria.

2170   LISTER, JOSEPH, 1st *Baron Lister.* 1827-1912
A method of antiseptic treatment applicable to wounded soldiers in the present war. *Brit. med. J.*, 1870, **2**, 243-44.
In 1870, for the first time on the battlefield, French and German army surgeons applied antiseptic methods in the management of wounds. Lister published the above short paper describing the simplest method he could devise to use carbolic as an antiseptic.

2171   UNITED STATES. War Dept. *Surgeon General's Office.*
The medical and surgical history of the War of the Rebellion, 1861-65. 6 vols. Washington, *Govt. Printing Office*, 1870-88.
Written by Joseph. J. Woodward (1833-84), Charles Smart (1841-1905), George A. Otis (1830-81), and David. L. Huntington (1834-99) under the direction of Joseph K. Barnes (1817-83), Surgeon General of the Army. This massive, graphically illustrated set has been called the "first comprehensive American medical book". It is one of the most remarkable works ever published on military medicine. An index of operators and reporters appears at the end of the third surgical volume. This index makes it possible to look up any surgeon and find the patients he treated. *See* No. 5185.

2172   VIRCHOW, RUDOLF LUDWIG KARL. 1821-1902
Ueber Lazarette und Barracken. *Berl. klin. Wschr.*, 1871, **8**, 109-11, 121-24, 133-35, 157-59.

On the best way of setting up military hospitals to prevent the spread of infectious diseases. For English translation *see* No. 1617 (note).

2173   KLEBS, THEODOR ALBRECHT EDWIN. 1834-1913
Beiträge zur pathologischen Anatomie der Schusswunden. Leipzig, *F. C. W. Vogel*, 1872.
    Klebs filtered the discharges from gunshot wounds, found the filtrate to be non-infectious, and from that reasoned that traumatic septicaemia is of bacterial origin. He was the first to filter bacteria and to experiment with the filtrate.

2174   LANGENBECK, BERNHARD RUDOLPH CONRAD VON. 1810-1887
Chirurgische Beobachtungen aus dem Kriege. Berlin, *A. Hirschwald*, 1874.

2175   LAVERAN, CHARLES LOUIS ALPHONSE. 1845-1922
Traité des maladies et épidémies des armées. Paris, *G. Masson*, 1875.

2176   REYHER, KARL KARLOVICH. 1856-1890
Ueber primäres Debridement der Schusswunden. *Trans. 7th Int. Med. Congr.*, London, 1881, **2**, 587-97.
    Reyher, a Russian surgeon, reintroduced *débridement* and made a controlled study of its value in contaminated gunshot wounds during the Russo-Turkish War of 1877. *See* No. 2177.

2177   GRAY, HENRY MCILREE WILLIAMSON. 1870-1938
Treatment of gunshot wounds by excision and primary suture. *Brit. med. J.*, 1915, **2**, 317.
    Gray revived *débridement* of wounds, with primary suture. This procedure has been traditionally credited to Larrey and Desault. Larrey (No. 2160) employed excision and primary suture only for treatment of wounds of the mouth which might otherwise result in a salivary fistula. However, Larrey, and his predecessor, Desault, "both treated extremity wounds by *incision*, as needed, to relieve tissue tension and establish free wound drainage, not by wound excision and primary suture" (Fackler).

2178   GREAT BRITAIN. War Office. *Medical Services.*
History of the Great War [First World War]. Medical Services. 12 vols. London, *H. M. Stationery Office*, 1921-29.

2179   UNITED STATES. War Dept. *Surgeon General's Office.*
The medical department of the U.S. Army in the First World War. Prepared under the direction of M. W. Ireland. 15 vols. [in 17]. Washington, *Govt. Printing Office*, 1921-29.

2180   GREAT BRITAIN.
History of the second world war. Medical series. 13 vols. London, *H. M. Stationery Office*, 1952-62.

2180.1   UNITED STATES ARMY MEDICAL SERVICE.
The Medical Department of the United States Army in World War II. 30 vols. in 33. Washington, *Office of the Surgeon General*, 1952-68.
    Since 1968 this series of unnumbered volumes or multi-volume sets devoted to particular subjects has continued under the name of U.S. Army Medical Department.

History of Military & Naval Hygiene & Medicine

2181   BILLROTH, CHRISTIAN ALBERT THEODOR. 1829-1894
        Historische Studien über die Beurtheilung und Behandlung der
        Schusswunden vom fünfzehnten Jahrhundert bis auf die neueste Zeit.
        Berlin, *G. Reimer*, 1859.
            English translation in *Yale J. Biol. Med.*, 1931, **4**, 16-36, 119-48, 225-57;
        reprinted in book form, New Haven, 1933.

2182   KÖHLER, ALBERT. 1850-1936
        Grundriss einer Geschichte der Kriegschirurgie. Berlin, *A. Hirschwald*, 1901.

2183   BRUNNER, CONRAD. 1859-1927
        Die Verwundeten in den Kriegen der alten Eidgenossenschaft. I. *Beitr. klin.
        Chir.*, 1903, **37**, 1-174.
            History of the care of the wounded during the Wars of the Swiss
        Confederation. Brunner shows that the Swiss were the first nation in
        Europe to organize state care of the wounded. Part 2 of the above work was
        published in book form, Tübingen, 1903.

2184   CABANÈS, AUGUSTIN. 1862-1928
        Chirurgiens et blessés à travers l'histoire. Paris, *A. Michel*, [1918].
            In this well-illustrated book Cabanès deals exhaustively with the
        transportation and surgical treatment of the wounded.

2185   GARRISON, FIELDING HUDSON. 1870-1935
        Notes on the history of military medicine. Washington, *Assoc. Mil. Surg.*,
        1922.

2186   ASHBURN, PERCY MOREAU. 1872-1940
        A history of the Medical Department of the United States Army. Boston,
        Houghton Mifflin, 1929.

2187   RODDIS, LOUIS HARRY. 1886-1969
        A short history of nautical medicine. New York, *P. B. Hoeber*, [1941].

2187.1 ADAMS, GEORGE WORTHINGTON.
        Doctors in blue. The medical history of the Union Army in the [United
        States] civil war. New York, *Henry Schuman*, 1952.

2188   KEEVIL, JOHN JOYCE. 1901-1957
        Medicine and the navy, 1200-1900. 4 vols. Edinburgh, *E. & S. Livingstone
        Ltd.*, 1957-63.
            Vol. 3-4 by C. Lloyd and J. L. S. Coulter.

2188.1 CUNNINGHAM, H. H.
        Doctors in gray: the Confederate Medical Service. Baton Rouge, *Louisiana
        State University Press*, 1958.

2188.2 GORDON, MAURICE BEAR. 1916-
        Naval and maritime medicine during the American revolution. Ventnor, N.
        J., *Ventnor Publishers*, 1978.

2188.3   GILLETT, Mary C.
           The [United States] Army Medical Department, 1775-1818. Washington, D.C.,
           Center of Military History, 1981.

2188.4   ———. The United States Army Medical Department, 1818-1865. Wash-
           ington, D.C., *Center of Military History*, 1987.

MEDICINE: GENERAL WORKS

See also 1-86.7, Collected Works; Opera Omnia

2189   GALEN. A.D. 130-200
           Galen on medical experience. First edition of the Arabic version with
           English translation and notes, by R. Walzer. London, *Oxford University Press*,
           1944.

2190   RABANUS MAURUS [Hrabanus], *Archbishop of Mayence*. 776?-856.
           De sermonum proprietate sive Opus de universo. [Strassburg, *Adolf Rusch*,
           1467?]
               This is the earliest known printed book to include a section dealing with
           medicine. It is a general encyclopaedia – the first of all printed encyclopae-
           dias – and devotes Book 18, Chap. V to medicine and diseases. It is known
           to have been printed by Rusch, the "R" printer, before July 20, 1467, from
           the first roman type ever cast. For an interesting paper on the book,
           including a translation of the chapter dealing with medicine, see E. C.
           Jessup, *Ann. med. Hist.*, 1934, n.s., **6**, 35-41.

2191   JOHN *of Gaddesden* [Johannes Anglicus]. ?1280-1361
           Rosa anglica practica medicine a capite ad pedes. (Papie, *J. A. Birreta*, 1492.)
               First printed medical book of an Englishman. John of Gaddesden was
           a prebendary of St. Paul's Cathedral and physician to Edward II. The work,
           to quote Garrison, "consists mainly of Arabist quackeries and countryside
           superstitions"; it was compiled about 1314. For information regarding the
           various printed editions, see the article by Dock in *Janus (Amsterdam)*, 1907,
           51, 425. See also H. P. Cholmeley: *John of Gaddesden and the Rosa
           medicinae*, Oxford, 1912.

2192   FERRARI DA GRADI [Giovanni Matteo]. ?1392-1472
           Practica, sive commentarium textuale in Nonum Almansoris cum
           ampliationibus et additionibus materierum. 2 vols. [Pavia, 1472.]
               For bibliographical and other details regarding this, the first large
           medical book to be printed, see the essay by Arnold C. Klebs in: *Essays on
           the history of medicine presented to Karl Sudhoff, on his seventieth
           birthday*, 1923, London, 1924.

2193   DE FEBRIBUS.
           De febribus opus sane aureum non magis utile, quam rei medicae
           profitentibus necessarium. Venetiis, *apud Gratiosum Perchacinum*, 1576.
               Includes writings on fever by Hippocrates, Galen, Paul of Aegina, Alexander
           of Tralles, Aetius, Oribasius, Nonus, Actuarius, Avicenna, Rhazes, Avenzoar,
           Averroës, Isaac Judaeus, Serapion, Haly Abbas, Celsus, Serenus, Pliny,
           Gariopontus, Constantinus Africanus, Gordon, Peter of Abano, Arnold of
           Villanova, Nicolaus Nicolus, and the medical writings attributed to Philonius.

2194   ALPINI, Prospero [Alpinus]. 1553-1617
De praesagienda vita et morte aegrotantium. Venetiis, *M. Sessa*, 1601.
A classical work on prognosis. English translation, London, 1746.

2195   PLATTER, Felix [Plater]. 1536-1614
Praxeos seu de cognoscendis, praedicendis, praecavendis, curandisque
affectibus homini incommodantibus. 2 vols. Basileae, *typ. C. Waldkirchius*,
1602-03.
The first attempt at a classification of diseases according to symptoms.
Over a period of 50 years Platter dissected more than 300 bodies and made
many observations of value to pathological anatomy.

2196   SENNERT, Daniel. 1572-1637
De febribus libri iv. Accessit ad calcem; ejusdem de dysenteria tractatus.
Lugduni, *J. Lautret*, 1627.
An important monograph on fevers.

2197   LE BÖE, Franciscus de [Sylvius]. 1614-1672
Praxeos medicae idea nova. 4 vols. Lugdani Batavorum, *apud viduam J.*
Le Carpentier (Hagae Comitum, *apud Henricum Scheuleer*), 1671-74.
Sylvius was a supporter of the Iatrochemical School. He established at
Leiden the first university chemical laboratory in Europe.

2198   SYDENHAM, Thomas. 1624-1689
Observationes medicae circa morborum acutorum historiam et curationem.
Londini, *G. Kettilby*, 1676.
Sydenham recorded important observations on dysentery, scarlet fever, scarlatina, measles and other conditions. He stressed the clinical study
of medicine and kept careful case records. English translation in No. 64 and
prior English editions. The above book is really a third edition of his
Methodus curandi febres, 1666; second edition, 1668. The Latin texts of
both editions of *Methodus curandi* were reprinted, with Latham's translation, an introduction and notes by G.G. Meynell, Folkstone, *Winterdown*
Books, 1987.

2199   BOERHAAVE, Herman. 1668-1738
Aphorismi de cognoscendis et curandis morbis. Lugduni Batavorum, *J.*
vander Linden, 1709.
The *Aphorisms* represent one of Boerhaave's best works. English
translation, 1715.

2199.1   MATHER, Cotton. 1663-1728.
The angel of Bethesda [1724] edited, with introduction and notes, by
Gordon W. Jones. Barre, Mass., *American Antiquarian Society & Barre*
Publishers, 1972.
The only large systematic compilation of medical knowledge prepared
in the Thirteen Colonies before the American revolution. The manuscript,
which Mather finished in 1724, remained unpublished in the American
Antiquarian Society until the above edition.

2200   SWIETEN, Gerard L. B. van. 1700-1772
Commentaria in Hermanni Boerhaave aphorismos, de cognoscendis et
curandis morbis. 6 vols. Lugduni Batavorum, *J. & H. Verbeek*, 1742-76.

A pupil of Boerhaave, van Swieten transplanted the latter's method of teaching to Vienna and founded the Vienna School of Medicine. He spent many years on the preparation of his great *Commentaria*. English translation, 18 vols., 1771-76.

2201   HUXHAM, JOHN. 1692-1768
An essay on fevers. London, *S. Austen*, 1750.
Huxham's best work. He was well known in the west of England and wrote important monographs on diphtheria and on Devonshire colic. Huxham seemed to appreciate that a difference existed between typhus and typhoid, at that time usually regarded as one condition. This book included the first use of the word "influenza" by an English physician.

2202   LINNE, CARL VON. [LINNAEUS]. 1707-1778
Genera morborum, sistens morborum classes, genera et species. 5 vols. Amstelodami, *frat. de Tournes*, 1763.
Sauvages adopted the botanical system of Linnaeus for a classification of diseases; his book exerted a wide influence on his contemporaries. He enumerated 2,400 different diseases.

2204   CULLEN, WILLIAM. 1710-1790
Synopsis nosologiae methodicae. Edinburgi, 1769.
This work made Cullen's reputation. In it he divided diseases into fevers, neurosis, cachexias and local disorders. Cullen was the foremost British clinical teacher of his time, one of the first to give clinical lectures in Great Britain. (*See also* No. 76.) Several English translations are available.

2205   CLARK, JOHN. 1744-1805
Observations on fevers. London, *T. Cadell*, 1780.

2207   HEBERDEN, WILLIAM. *Snr*. 1710-1801
Commentarii de morborum historia et curatione. Londini, *T. Payne*, 1802.
Samuel Johnson called Heberden "the last of our learned physicians". The above work included all his important papers which had earned him his great reputation and which are dealt with elsewhere in the present book (*see* Nos. 2887, 2291, 5438, 5831).
The book was published by Heberden's son and at once acquired a European reputation; "it had the distinction of being the last important medical treatise written in Latin" (Rolleston). An English translation which appeared in the same year as the original work was reprinted in 1962.

2208   PINEL, PHILIPPE. 1745-1826
Adynamie. *Dict. Sci. méd.*, Paris, 1812, **1**, 161-63.

2209   BLACKALL, JOHN. 1771-1860
Observations on the nature and cure of dropsies. London, *Longman*, 1813.
Blackall was before Bright in detecting albuminuria in association with dropsy. His book, of which the second edition is more important than the first, includes reports on cases of angina pectoris.

2210   PARRY, CALEB HILLIER. 1755-1822
Collections from the unpublished writings. 2 vols. London, *Underwoods*, 1825.

Includes Parry's interesting description of eight cases of exophthalmic goitre, the first of which was observed in 1786 (*see* No. 3813), and his notes on four cases of angina pectoris. Parry was a copious note-taker, and many of these notes are here published for the first time. His careful records of many years' observation in practice were intended to form a large work, *Elements of pathology and therapeutics*, of which only the first volume appeared, in 1815; this was republished, together with the unfinished vol. 2, in 1825. *See* No. 4522.

2211   SMITH, THOMAS SOUTHWOOD. 1788-1861
A treatise on fever. London, *Longman, etc.*, 1830.
Both a doctor and a minister, Smith called himself, "physician to body and soul". He has been called "the intellectual father of our modern public health system".

2212   BIGELOW, JACOB. 1786-1879
A discourse on self-limited diseases. Boston, *N. Hale*, 1835.
Bigelow was attached to the Massachusetts General Hospital. The above "did more than any other work or essay in our own language to rescue the practice of medicine from the slavery of the drugging system which was part of the inheritance of the profession" (Oliver Wendell Holmes).

2213   STOKES, WILLIAM. 1804-1878
A treatise on the diagnosis and treatment of diseases of the chest. Dublin, *Hodges & Smith*, 1837.
Stokes, most prominent of the Irish school of medicine, established his reputation by his book on diseases of the chest. Important among its contents are his discovery of a stage of pneumonia prior to that described by Laennec as the first, his observations that contraction of the side has sometimes followed the cure of pneumonia and that paralysis of the intercostal muscles and diaphragm may result from pleurisy, and his employment of the stethoscope as an aid to the detection of foreign bodies in the air passages.

2215   BRIGHT, RICHARD. 1789-1858, & ADDISON, THOMAS. 1793-1860
Elements of the practice of medicine. Vol. 1. [pts. 1-3, all published.] London, *Longmans*, 1839.
Originally issued in three parts from 1836 to 1839 when the authors were joint lecturers on medicine at Guy's Hospital.

2217   MAGENDIE, FRANÇOIS. 1783-1855
Leçons sur les phénomènes physiques de la vie. 4 vols. Paris, *J. B. Baillière*, 1836-38.
Magendie, pioneer experimental physiologist, regarded pathology as only a modification of physiology, "medicine the physiology of the sick man". By him clinical medicine was reconstructed on physiological lines.

2218   GRAVES, ROBERT JAMES. 1796-1853
A system of clinical medicine. Dublin, *Fannin & Co.*, 1843.
Graves was one of the founders of the Irish school of medicine and one of the most important figures in Irish medicine at the middle of the 19th century. Second edition of the book (as *Clinical lectures on the practice of medicine*) in 1848.

2219   WATSON, *Sir* THOMAS, *Bart.* 1792-1882
        Lectures on the principles and practice of physic. 2 vols. London, *J. W. Parker*, 1843.
        First published in the *Medical Times & Gazette*, 1840-42, Watson's famous lectures appeared in book form and formed the most important treatise of medicine for a quarter-century. Watson wrote in a fine style, and his book was reorganized as a sound guide to clinical medicine. Watson suggested (vol. 2, p. 349) rubber gloves for antisepsis; he also instructed his students to wash their hands in a solution of chloride of lime before assisting at deliveries.

2220   MURCHISON, CHARLES. 1830-1879
        A treatise on the continued fevers of Great Britain. London, *Parker, Son, & Bourn*, 1862.
        Murchison was one of the greatest clinical teachers London has ever known; of his many writings his book on the continued fever is probably the most important.

2221   TROUSSEAU, ARMAND. 1801-1867
        Clinique médicale de l'Hôtel Dieu de Paris. 2 vols. Paris, *J. B. Baillière*, 1861.
        Trousseau, great clinician of the Hôtel-Dieu, made important advances in the treatment of diphtheria, typhoid, scarlet fever and other conditions. In his book he emphasized the value of bedside observation. He supported the doctrine of the specific nature of disease and realized the significance of Pasteur's work on fermentation. English translation, 1868-72.

2222   CHARCOT, JEAN MARTIN. 1825-1893
        Leçons sur les maladies des vieillards et les maladies chroniques. Paris, *A. Delahaye*, 1867.
        Charcot inaugurated a course of study of geriatrics, at the Salpêtrière, in 1866; his lectures are embodied in the above work. English translation, 1881.

2223   ADDISON, THOMAS. 1793-1860
        A collection of the published writings. London, *New Sydenham Soc.*, 1868.
        Addison was a contemporary of Bright at Guy's Hospital and a fine lecturer.

2224   TRAUBE, LUDWIG. 1818-1876
        Zur Fieberlehre. In his *Gesammelte Beiträge*, Berlin, 1871, **2**, pt. 1, 624-56, 679-83; 1878, **3**, 503-05, 582-87.

2225   SENATOR, HERMANN. 1834-1911
        Untersuchungen über den fieberhaften Process und seine Behandlung. Berlin, *A. Hirschwald*, 1873.
        Senator was a director of the Charité Hospital in Berlin and later at the university polyclinic. His study of fever represents his best work.

2226   LIEBERMEISTER, CARL VON. 1833-1901
        Handbuch der Pathologie und Therapie des Fiebers. Leipzig, *F. C. W. Vogel*, 1875.

2227   LATHAM, PETER MERE. 1789-1875
        The collected works. 2 vols. London, *New Sydenham Soc.*, 1876-78.
        Latham, successively physician to Middlesex and St. Bartholomew's
        hospitals, was an authority on cardiac disease and among the earliest in
        England to advocate auscultation. He held progressive views on medical
        education and championed clinical study in the wards. His clinical lectures
        are among the very best.

2229   STRÜMPELL, ERNST ADOLF GUSTAV GOTTFRIED. 1853-1925
        Lehrbuch der speciellen Pathologie und Therapie der inneren Krankheiten.
        2 vols. Leipzig, *F. C. W. Vogel*, 1883-84.
        More than 30 editions of this book appeared, many translated into other
        languages. English translation in 1887. *See* No. 4349.

2230   FAGGE, CHARLES HILTON. 1838-1883
        The principles and practice of medicine. 2 vols. London, *J. & A. Churchill*,
        1886.
        Fagge was physician to Guy's hospital and editor of *Guy's Hospital
        Reports*. His important textbook was published posthumously.

2231   OSLER, *Sir* WILLIAM, *Bart*. 1849-1919
        The principles and practice of medicine. New York, *D. Appleton*, 1892.
        Osler's textbook was the best English work on medicine of its time. He
        became Regius Professor of Medicine at Oxford in 1904. Besides being one
        of the greatest of all clinicians, he was possessed of a fine literary style and
        an extensive knowledge of medical bibliography. Garrison has written of
        him: "When he came to die, Osler was, in a very real sense, the greatest
        physician of our time ... Good looks, distinction, blithe, benignant man-
        ners, a sunbright personality, radiant with kind feeling and good will
        toward his fellow men, an Apollonian poise, swiftness and surety of
        thought and speech, every gift of the gods was his; and to these were added
        careful training, unsurpassed clinical ability, the widest knowledge of his
        subject, the deepest interest in everything human, and a serene hold upon
        his fellows that was as a seal set upon them". For Osler's own account of
        the preparation of his textbook, see the *Bibliotheca Osleriana* (No. 6772),
        item 3544. See also R.L. Golden & C.G. Roland, *Sir William Osler: an an-
        notated bibliography with illustrations*, San Francisco, *Norman Publish-
        ing*, 1988; and Harvey Cushing's *Life of Sir William Osler*, 2 vols. Oxford,
        Oxford University Press, 1925.

2232   GULL, *Sir* WILLIAM WITHEY. 1816-1890
        A collection of the published writings. 2 vols. London, *New Sydenham Soc.*,
        1894-96.
        Gull, one of the best clinicians of his time, spent most of his working life
        at Guy's Hospital. He described the spinal lesion of tabes and left an
        important account of aneurysm. His best works are his description of
        myxoedema and his original description of arteriolosclerotic atrophy of
        the kidney.

2233   STILLER, BERTHOLD. 1837-1922
        Die asthenische Konstitutionskrankheit. Stuttgart, *F. Enke*, 1907.
        "Stiller's disease" – habitus asthenicus.

2234   EPPINGER, HANS. 1879-1946, & HESS, LEO. 1879-1963
Vagotonie: klinische Studie. Berlin, *A. Hirschwald,* 1910.
English translation, 1915.

2235   HURRY, JAMIESON BOYD. 1857-1930
Vicious circles in disease. London, *J. Churchill,* 1911.

2236   BAEHR, GEORGE, *et al.*
A diffuse disease of the peripheral circulation (usually associated with lupus erythematosus and endocarditis). *Trans. Ass. Amer. Phycns.,* 1935, **50**, 139-55.
See No. 2237. With P. Klemperer and A. Schifrin.

2237   KLEMPERER, PAUL. 1887-1964, *et al.*
Diffuse collagen disease; acute disseminated lupus erythematosus and diffuse scleroderma. *J. Amer. med. Assoc.,* 1942, **119**, 331-32.
P. Klemperer, A. D. Pollack, and G. Baehr combined a number of diseases, hitherto regarded as unrelated, into an entity which they termed diffuse collagen disease.

2237.01   THOREK, MAX. 1880-1960
The face in health and disease. Philadelphia, *F.A. Davis,* 1946.

2237.1   HARGRAVES, MALCOLM MCCALLUM. 1903- , *et al.*
Presentation of two bone marrow elements: The "Tart" cell and the "L. E". cell. *Proc. Mayo Clin.,* 1948, **23**, 25-28.
The Hargraves "L. E". cell, a diagnostic aid in acute disseminated lupus erythematosus. With H. Richmond and R. J. Morton. First reported by Morton in *A study of the bone marrow in cases of disseminated lupus erythematosus,* his Univeristy of Minnesota thesis, 1947, prepared under the guidance of Hargraves.

2238   SELYE, HANS. 1907-1982
The physiology and pathology of exposure to stress. Montreal, *Acta Inc.,* 1950.
In his study of the aetiology of the collagen disease Selye developed the idea that animals react to stress or injury by a certain sequence of physiological reactions – the "general adaption syndrome".

History of Internal Medicine

See also 6375-6668, HISTORY OF MEDICINE, and under individual subjects.

2239   FABER, KNUD HELGE. 1862-1956
Nosography, the evolution of clinical medicine in modern times. 2nd ed., New York, *P. B. Hoeber,* 1930.
A well-illustrated and reliable account. Reprinted 1976.

2240   ROLLESTON, *Sir* HUMPHRY DAVY, *Bart.* 1862-1944
Internal medicine. New York, *P. B. Hoeber,* 1930.
A short history of the subject; one of the *Clio Medica* series. Reprinted, 1976.

2241   MAJOR, Ralph Hermon. 1884-1970
        Classic descriptions of disease. Springfield, *C. C. Thomas*, 1932.
        A collection of classic descriptions of disease by 179 different writers,
        from ancient times to the present. Foreign papers are translated into
        English. A second edition of this most interesting and useful book appeared
        in 1939, the principal additions being on the subjects of malaria and yellow
        fever, and a third edition was published in 1945.

2243   BETT, Walter Reginald. 1903-1968
        The history of internal medicine. Selected diseases. Chicago, *University of
        Chicago Press*, 1960.
        Attempts to list and annotate every reference of fundamental importance
        in the development of 21 selected diseases.

2243.2 KEELE, Kenneth David. 1909-1987
        The evolution of clinical methods in medicine. London, *Pitman*, [1963].
        FitzPatrick Lectures 1960-61. This book traces the changing clinical
        methods throughout the centuries to show how they arose and how they
        have grown into their present forms.

CONDITIONS DUE TO PHYSICAL FACTORS

2244   ACOSTA, José de, 1539-1600
        Historia natural y moral de las Indias. Sevilla, *Juan de Léon*, 1590.
        Lib. 3, chap. 9 contains his description of mountain sickness, "Acosta's
        disease", which he experienced during his crossing of the Peruvian Andes.
        This was the first description of what is more often called altitude sickness
        today.   English translation, London, 1604. Facsimile reprint, Valencia,
        Albatros, 1977. English translation, London, 1604.

2245   FABRY, Wilhelm [Fabricius *Hildanus*]. 1560-1634
        De combustionibus. Basileae, *sumpt. Ludovici Regis*, 1607.
        First book devoted entirely to burns. Fabry was the first to classify burns.
        English translation, London, 1643.

2246   HORST, Georg. ?-1688
        De siriasi. Basileae, *typ. J. J. Deckeri*, 1665.
        A treatise on sunstroke.

2247   DUPUYTREN, Guillaume, *le baron*. 1777-1835
        Leçons orales de clinique chirurgicale. Tom. 1, Paris, *Germer-Baillière*, 1832.
        Dupuytren's classification of burns (p. 424). English translation by A.S.
        Doane, Boston, 1833.

2248   LONGMORE, *Sir* Thomas. 1816-1895
        Remarks upon a tabular return (No. 1), or synopsis of sixteen cases of heat-
        apoplexy. *Indian Ann. med. Sci.*, 1859, **6**, 396-406.
        Longmore was an army surgeon in India; he gave an excellent account
        of heat-stroke.

2248.1   POLLOCK, GOERGE DAVID. 1817-1897
          Cases of skin-grafting and skin-transplantation. *Trans. clin. Soc. Lond.*, 1871,
          4, 37-47.
          Pollock used Reverdin's skin-grafting technique in the treatment of
          burn contractures.

2249   BARCLAY, ALEXANDER. 1822-1874
          Contributions to the natural history of insolatio. *Madras quart. J. med. Sci.*,
          1860, **1**, 347-95.
          Barclay, an army surgeon, wrote an important paper on heat-stroke.

2250   WOOD, HORATIO CHARLES. 1841-1920
          Thermic fever, or sunstroke. Philadelphia, *J. B. Lippincott*, 1872.
          A study of the pathology of sunstroke. Wood held the chairs of botany,
          therapeutics, and neurology at the University of Pennsylvania.

2250.1   COPELAND, WILLIAM PRESTON.
          The treatment of burns. *Med. Rec. (N.Y.)*, 1887, **31**, 518 (only).
          Introduction of the open or exposure method for the treatment of
          burns.

2250.2   WILMS, MAX. 1867-1918
          Studien zur Pathologie der Verbrennung. Die Ursache des Todes nach
          ausgedehnter Hautverbrennung. *Mitt. Grenzgeb. Med. Chir.*, 1901, **8**, 393-
          442.
          Wilms was first to carry out full excision of burnt tissue, and sometimes
          grafted excised areas.

2251   BARTHE DE SANDFORT, EDMOND.
          La kérithérapie (nouvelle balnéation thermocireuse). *J. Méd. intern.*, 1913,
          17, 211-14.
          Treatment of burns with ambrine (paraffin-resin solution); keritherapy.

2252   UNDERHILL, FRANK PELL. 1877-1932, *et al.*
          Blood concentration changes in extensive superficial burns, and their
          significance for systemic treatment. *Arch. intern. Med.*, 1923, **32**, 31-49.
          F. P. Underhill, G. L. Carrington, R. Kapsinow, and G. T. Pack made
          important studies on the blood concentration following burns.

2253   DAVIDSON, EDWARD CLARK. 1894-1933
          Tannic acid in the treatment of burns. *Surg. Gynec. Obstet.*, 1925, **41**, 202-
          21.
          Introduction of tannic acid in the treatment of burns.

2254   RIEHL, GUSTAV. 1855-1943
          Zur Therapie schwerer Verbrennungen. *Wien. klin. Wschr.*, 1925, **38**, 833-
          34.
          Riehl was an early advocate of blood transfusion in the treatment of
          shock after burns.

2255   GOLDBLATT, DAVID. 1894-
          Contribution to the study of burns, their classification and treatment. *Ann.
          Surg.*, 1927, **85**, 490-501.
          Goldblatt's classification of burns.

2256   PACK, George Thomas. 1898- , & DAVIS, Andrew Hobson. 1899-
         Burns. Types, pathology and management. Philadelphia, *Lippincott, Co.*,
         1930.

2257   JELLINEK, Stefan. 1871-
         Elektrische Verletzungen. Klinik und Histopathologie. Leipzig, *J. A. Barth*,
         1932.

2258   ALDRICH, Robert Henry. 1902-
         The role of infection in burns; the theory and treatment with special
         reference to gentian violet. *New Engl. J. Med.*, 1933, **208**, 299-309.
         Introduction of gentian violet in the treatment of burns.

2259   BETTMAN, Adalbert Goodman. 1883-
         The tannic acid–silver nitrate treatment of burns: a method of minimizing
         shock and toxemia and shortening convalescence. *Northw. Med.*, 1935, **34**,
         46-51.
         Bettman introduced the tannic acid–silver nitrate method of treating
         burns.

2260   BUNYAN, John. 1907-1983
         Envelope method of treating burns. *Proc. roy. Soc. Med.*, 1940, **34**, 65-70.
         Bunyan bag.

2261   HARKINS, Henry Nelson. 1905-1967
         The treatment of burns. Springfield, Baltimore, *C. C. Thomas*, 1942.
         Contains some history of the subject and includes a valuable bibliography
         of 1,320 entries.

TROPICAL MEDICINE

See also under the names of individual tropical diseases

2262   WHETSTONE, George. [WATESTONE] 1544?-1587?
         The cures of the diseased, in remote regions. Preventing mortalitie,
         incident in forraine attempts, of the English nation. London, *F. K[ingston]
         for H. L[ownes]*, 1598.
         Written under the anonymity of initials and attributed to Whetsone,
         Elizabethan poet, soldier, and traveller, this book is the earliest work in
         English devoted to tropical medicine. It discusses sunstroke, tabardilla
         (possibly typhus or yellow fever), prickly heat, dysentery, erysipelas and
         scurvy. Facsimile reproduction, with introduction and notes by Charles
         Singer, Oxford, 1915.

2262.1   ABREU, Alexo de. 1568-1630
         Tratado de las siete enfermedades, de la inflammacion universal del
         higado, zirbo, pyloron, y riñones, y de la obstrucion, de la satiriasi, de la
         terciana y febre maligna, y passion hipocondriaca. Lleva otros tres tratados,
         del mal de Loanda, del guzano, y de las fuentes y sedales. Lisboa, *P.
         Craesbeeck*, 1623.

The first important work on tropical disease. Only six copies of this book are known. It includes full accounts of malaria, typhoid, and scurvy, and the first accurate descriptions of yellow fever, amoebic hepatitis, dracontiasis, trichuriasis, and tungiasis. For a study of the book see F. Guerra, *Clio Medica*, 1968, **1**, 59-60.

2263 BONDT, Jacob de [Bontius]. 1592-1631
De medicina Indorum. Lugduni Batavorum, *F. Hackium*, 1642.

Bontius was probably the first to regard tropical medicine as an independent branch of medical science. He spent the last four years of his life in the Dutch East Indies, and his book incorporates the experience he gained there. It is the first Dutch work on tropical medicine and includes the first modern description of beri-beri and cholera. English translation, 1769. *See* No. 3736.

2263.1 PISO, Willem. 1611-1678
Historia naturalis Brasiliae. Lugduni Batavorum, *apud F. Hackius*; Amstelodami, *apud L. Elzevirium*, 1648.

A pioneer work on tropical medicine and the largest work from the standpoint of format published by the Elzeviers. The folio includes *De medicina brasiliensi* by Piso and *Historia rerum naturalium brasiliae* by Georg Marggraf (1610-44). The second edition entitled *De Indiae utriusque re naturali et medica libri xiv* (Amsterdam, 1658) included additional material by Piso and by de Bondt (*see* No. 2263). *See also* Nos. 1825 & 5303.

2264 LIND, James. 1716-1794
An essay on diseases incidental in Europeans in hot climates. London, *T. Becket & P. A. DeHondt*, 1768.

Lind came near to discovering the connection between malaria and mosquitoes. He is best remembered for his work on scurvy (No. 3713), but the above book is one of the more important early works on tropical medicine.

2265 PRUNER-BEY, Franz. 1808-1882
Die Krankheiten des Orient's. Erlangen, *Palm u. enke*, 1847.

2266 MANSON, *Sir* Patrick. 1844-1922
Tropical diseases. London, *Cassell & Co.*, 1898.

Manson has been called the "father of modern tropical medicine". He had vast experience of disease in the Tropics and himself made many valuable contributions to the knowledge of this subject. He described tinea nigra and tinea imbricata, found filaria in elephantiasis and discovered *Filaria hominis*. In 1898 he founded the London School of Tropical Medicine. The 16th edition of his book, edited by P. H. Manson-Bahr, appeared in 1966.

2267 CASTELLANI, Aldo. 1877-1971, & CHALMERS, Albert John. 1870-1920
Manual of tropical medicine. London, *Baillière, Tindall & Cox*, 1910.

Castellani made several discoveries of great importance in tropical medicine. The above work is a standard text on tropical medicine in English. Third edition, 1919.

History of Tropical Medicine

2268   SCOTT, *Sir* HENRY HAROLD. 1874-1956
A history of tropical medicine. 1 vol. [in 2]. London, *Arnold*, 1939.
     This is an exhaustive history of the subject, and one of the best histories of special subjects yet produced. The book is furnished with a most useful bibliography.

2268.1   KEAN, BENJAMIN HARRISON. 1912- , *et al.*
Tropical medicine and parasitology: classic investigations. 1 vol. [in 2]. Ithaca, London, *Cornell Univ. Press*, 1978.
     About 200 key papers, reproduced in whole or in part, in English translation where necessary. Includes useful biographical notes. With K. E. Mott and A. J. Russell.

PATHOLOGY

2269   GALEN, A.D. 130-200
De affectorum locorum notitia libri vi. Parisiis, *Officina Henrici Stephani*, [1513].
     First separate dated Latin translation of *De locis affectis*, made by Guillaume Copp of Basel. In this work devoted to pathology, Galen made many valuable deductions on inflammation and on tumours. He was familiar with cholera, hydrophobia, and malaria, the relations of urinary calculi to the kidney, ureter, and bladder. He recognized bronchitis, empyema, consumption, and pyuria. English translation by R.E. Siegel, Basel, 1976.

2270   BENIVIENI, ANTONIO. 1443-1502
De abditis nonnulus ac mirandis morborum et sanationum causis. Florentiae, *P. Giuntae*, 1507.
     To our knowledge Benivieni was the first physician to request permission of his patient's relatives to perform necropsies in obscure cases. His posthumously published, unorganized collection of cases entitled *The hidden causes of disease* stands out as the first book to give extensive consideration to the practice of post–mortem examinations, by which he hoped to explain the hidden or internal causes of disease. The work includes the results of 20 post–mortems. The bodies were incised, not dissected, and the results are correspondingly sketchy. Nevertheless Benivieni has been called "the father of pathological anatomy". A facsimile reproduction and English translation, 1954.

2271   FERNEL, JEAN FRANÇOIS. 1497-1558
Medicina. 3 pts. [in 1]. Lutetiae Parisiorum, *apud A. Wechelum*, 1554.
     The first systematic treatise on pathology, which also introduced the names for the sciences of pathology and physiology. In the second part, entitled "Pathologia", Fernel provided the first systematic essay on the subject, methodically discussing the diseases of each organ. Fernel was the first to describe appendicitis, endocarditis, etc. He believed aneurysms to be produced by syphilis, and differentiated true from false aneurysms. He was physician to Henri II of France. The first section of the above work is the second edition of Fernel's classic treatise on physiology (No. 572).

2272   SCHENCK, Johann, *von Grafenberg*. 1530-1598
Observationum medicarum, rararum, novarum, *etc*. 2 vols. Francofurti, *sumpt. J. Rhodii*, 1600.
   Schenck was the greatest compiler of his day. His *Observationes* form the easiest source-book for the pathological observations of Sylvius, Vesalius, and Columbus, and represent a lifetime of medical reading and experience. They were first published at Basle, 1584-97.

2273   SEVERINO, Marco Aurelio. 1580-1656
De recondita abscessuum natura. Neapoli, 1632.
   The first textbook of surgical pathology. It treats of all kinds of swelling under the term "abscess" and describes neoplasms of the genital organs and sarcomata of bones. Tumours of the breast are classified into four groups, the section devoted to them being one of the most important in the book. This was also the first book to include illustrations of lesions with the text.

2274   BONET, Theophile. 1620-1689
Sepulchretum, sive anatomia practica ex cadaveribus morbo denatis. 2 vols., Genevae, *L. Chouët*, 1679.
   This is the first collection of systematized pathological anatomy. It contains clinical and pathological descriptions of nearly 3,000 cases selected from the literature from the time of Hippocrates, but mainly from the 16th and 17th centuries. It is the most useful reference book for early descriptions of pathological conditions.

2275   HOFFMANN, Friedrich. 1660-1742
De metastasi sive sede morbo mutata. Halae, 1731.
   In Allbutt's opinion Hoffmann was the first to perceive that pathology is an aspect of physiology.

2276   MORGAGNI, Giovanni Battista. 1682-1771
De sedibus, et causis morborum per anatomen indagatis libri quinque. 2 vols. Venetiis, *typog. Remondiniana*, 1761.
   By this great work, one of the most important in the history of medicine, Morgagni was the true founder of modern pathological anatomy. The work was completed in Morgagni's 79th year and consists of a series of 70 letters reporting about 700 cases and necropsies. As best he could, he correlated the clinical record with the post–mortem finding. Morgagni gave the first descriptions of several pathological conditions. He was Professor of Anatomy at Padua. Selections from the above work are reproduced in *Med. Classics*, 1940, **4**, 640-839. English translation by B. Alexander, 3 vols., London, 1769, (facsimile reprint, New York, *Hafner,* 1960; Mount Kisco, N.Y., *Futura*, 1980).

2277   HUNTER, John. 1728-1793
On the digestion of the stomach after death. *Phil Trans.*, 1772, **62**, 447-54.

2278   SANDIFORT, Eduard. 1742-1814
Observationes anatomicae-pathologicae. 4 vols. Lugduni Batavorum, *P. v. d. Eyk & D. Vygh*, 1777-81.
   Sandifort's beautifully illustrated work on pathological anatomy included records of ulcerative aortic endocarditis, renal calculi, herniae, bony

ankyloses, and congenital abnormalities. His work is comparable with that of Morgagni. *See* No. 2734.2.

2279 WALTER, JOHANN GOTTLEIB. 1734-1818
Von den Krankheiten des Bauchfells und dem Schlagfluss. Berlin, *G. J. Decker*, 1785.
  Text in Latin and German. Includes an accurate description of peritonitis.

2280 BAILLIE, MATTHEW. 1761-1823
An account of a remarkable transportation of the viscera. *Phil. Trans.*, 1788, **78**, 350-63.
  Baillie recorded a case of congenital dextrocardia with complete situs inversus viscerum. Reprinted in Willius & Keys, *Cardiac classics*, 1941, pp. 257-62.

2281 ———. The morbid anatomy of some of the most important parts of the human body. London, *J. Johnson & G. Nicol*, 1793.
  Baillie was a nephew and pupil of W. Hunter. The above is the first systematic textbook of morbid anatomy, treating the subject for the first time as an independent science. *See also* Nos. 2736, 3167.1, 3218, & 3427. Baillie was the last and most eminent owner of the famous gold-headed cane (No. 6709).

2282 ———. A series of engravings, accompanied with explanations, which are intended to illustrate the morbid anatomy of some of the most important parts of the human body. London, *W. Bulmer & Co.*, 1799-1803.
  The first systematic atlas of pathology. This work was intended to illustrate No. 2281, but, with its extensive descriptive text for each plate, it may be appreciated separately. The black & white engravings were prepared by John Hunter's artist and amanuensis, William Clift (1775-1849), and depict numerous specimens from Hunter's collection. A colour facsimile edition of Clift's personal copy reproducing his original watercolours, including some loaned by the Royal College of Physicians, was published in Melbourne, *Univ. of Melbourne Press*, 1985.

2283 HUNTER, JOHN. 1728-1793
A treatise on the blood, inflammation, and gun-shot wounds. London, *G. Nicol*, 1794.
  It was while serving with the army at Belle Isle during the Seven Years' War that Hunter collected the material for his epoch-making book on inflammation and gunshot wounds. His studies on inflammation in particular are fundamental for pathology.

2284 MECKEL, JOHANN FRIEDRICH, *the younger*. 1781-1833
Tabulae anatomico-pathologicae. 4 pts. Lipsiae, *I. F. Gleditsch*, 1817-26.
  Meckel's work on embryology brought a better understanding of congenital malformations, which had previously been attributed by many to supernatural influence. This work illustrates a number of anomalies and other diseases. It is a supplement to his *Handbuch der pathologischen Anatomie*. *See* No. 534.56.

2284.1 HOOPER, ROBERT. 1773-1835
The morbid anatomy of the human brain. London, *For the author*, 1826.

Based on over 4000 autopsies performed over 30 years, and illustrated with fine hand-coloured plates.

2285   BRIGHT, RICHARD. 1789-1858
Reports of medical cases, selected with a view of illustrating the symptoms and cure of diseases by a reference to morbid anatomy. 2 vols. [in 3]. London, *Longmans*, 1827-31.
Although the name of Bright is perpetuated by his classic description of chronic non-suppurative nephritis, known eponymically as "Bright's disease", the *Reports* contain numerous other outstanding contributions to general pathology, neuropathology, as well as nephrology. Bright differentiated renal from cardiac dropsy (oedema) and was first to correlate this and the previously observed albuminuria with the nephritic changes observed at autopsy. Vol. 2, published in 2 parts, is one of the earliest and most important atlases of neuropathology. Superbly illustrated throughout with hand-coloured plates. Facsimile reprint of vol. 1, London, *Gower Publishers & Royal Society of Medicine*, 1985. *See* No. 4206.

2285.1 BILLARD, CHARLES MICHEL. 1800-1832
Traité des maladies des enfans nouveau-nés et à la mamelle. 1 vol. and atlas. Paris, *J. B. Baillière*, 1828.
The first significant work on the pathological anatomy of infants. Billard performed several hundred autopsies on infants and children and correlated the data obtained with clinical observations he had made. The work includes the "first classification of infantile diseases of any importance" (Abt/Garrison). English translation of the third edition, 1839. *See* No. 6332.

2285.2 ABERCROMBIE, JOHN. 1781-1844
Pathological and practical researches on diseases of the brain and spinal cord. Edinburgh, *Waugh and Innes*, 1828.
First textbook of neuropathology. Originally published in a series of articles in *Edin. med. surg. J.*, 1818-19, and first collected into book form in the German translation, with appendix, by C. Nasse, Bonn, *E. Weber*, 1821.

2286   CRUVEILHIER, JEAN. 1791-1874
Anatomie pathologique du corps humain. 2 vols. Paris, *J. B. Baillière*, 1829-42.
The fine hand-coloured lithographs of gross pathology make this one of the greatest works of its kind. Cruveilhier, first Professor of Pathological Anatomy in Paris, gave the first description of multiple sclerosis (in vol. 2 above), and an early description of "Cruveilhier's palsy" (*see* No. 4734). Hypertrophic pyloric stenosis and ulceration of the stomach due to hyperacidity were also for the first time described in the above work; to each the name "Cruveilhier's disease" has been attached. From publication in fascicules, 1829-42.

2287   HORNER, WILLIAM EDMONDS. 1793-1853
A treatise on pathological anatomy. Philadelphia, *Carey*, 1829.
First American work on the subject. Horner was Professor of Anatomy at Pennsylvania, and made several anatomical discoveries.

2288   LOBSTEIN, JEAN GEORGE CHRÉTIEN FRÉDÉRIC MARTIN. 1777-1835
Traité d'anatomie pathologique. 2 vols. and atlas. Paris, *F. G. Levrault*, 1829-33.

Includes a historical review of the subject from the time of the Ancient Egyptians to Corvisart, and showed the advances in pathology during the preceding 50 years. Lobstein was the first to use the word "arteriosclerosis". He was professor at Strasburg.

2289   HOPE, James. 1801-1841
Principles and illustrations of morbid anatomy. London, *Whittaker & Co.*, 1834.
Hope left a fine pathological atlas with brilliantly hand-coloured lithographs from his own drawings. While the book does not equal the atlases of Cruveilhier and Carswell, it is important as being a great stimulus to the study of pathology in England.

2290   HODGKIN, Thomas. 1798-1866
Lectures on the morbid anatomy of the serous and mucous membranes. 2 vols. London, *Sherwood,* 1836; *Simpkin, Marshall & Co.*, 1840.
Important work which stimulated the study of tissue pathology in England. Hodgkin was the first in England to give a regular lecture course in morbid anatomy, which he began at Guy's in 1827. Vol. 2, pt. 2 was never published.

2291   CARSWELL, *Sir* Robert. 1793-1857
Illustrations of the elementary forms of disease. London, *Longman, etc.* 1838.
Carswell was Professor of Morbid Anatomy at University College, London, and one of the leading English pathologists of his day. A fine artist, he personally painted 2,000 water-colours of pathological specimens. His great pathological atlas contains splendid hand-coloured lithographs which he selected from his collection of water-colours and personally drew on stone.

2292   GROSS, Samuel David. 1805-1884
Elements of pathological anatomy. 2 vols. Boston, *Marsh*, 1839.
In his day Gross was the most famous surgeon in the U.S.A. He was for a time Professor of General Anatomy, Physiology, and Pathological Anatomy at Cincinnati Medical College and while there published his *Elements*, the first exhaustive, systematic study of pathological anatomy in English. Gross was the first to precede each description of the morbid anatomy of an organ with an account of its healthy colour, weight, size and consistence founded on original research. The second edition of 1845 was considerably revised and enlarged, while the third edition of 1857 was abridged. Horner's book (No. 2287) was the only important work on pathology to precede it in America.

2293   ROKITANSKY, Carl, *Freiherr von.* 1804-1878
Handbuch der pathologischen Anatomie. 3 vols. Wien, *Braumüller u. Seidel*, 1842-46.
Rokitansky ranks with Morgagni as among the greatest of all writers on gross pathology. He is said to have performed over 30,000 autopsies himself. His *Handbuch* was for many years pre-eminent among its contemporaries. Although Rokitansky embraced more than one false doctrine, he was quick to admit and correct his mistakes. Virchow's criticism of the first edition of the *Handbuch* led Rokitansky to re-write it. He foresaw the eventual importance of chemical pathology, at that time non-existent. Vol.

1 of the first edition was published last; vol. 3 was published first. English translation, 4 vols., London, 1849-54.

2294   ADDISON, WILLIAM. 1802-1881
Experimental and practical researches on the structure and function of blood corpuscles; on inflammation; and on the origin and nature of tubercles in the lungs. *Trans. prov. med. surg. Ass.*, 1843, **11**, 233-306.
   Addison gave an important account of the process of inflammation. See L.J. Rather, *Addison and the white corpuscles: An aspect of nineteenth-century biology.* London, *Wellcome Institute*, 1972. *See also* No. 3059.

2294.1   GOODSIR, JOHN. 1814-1867, & GOODSIR, HENRY D.S.
Anatomical and pathological observations. Edinburgh, *Myles Macphail*; London, *Simpkin, Marshall*, 1845.
   John Goodsir's paper on "Centres of nutrition" anticipates to a certain extent the cell doctrine afterwards developed by Virchow (*see* No. 2299). Virchow dedicated the first edition of his *Cellularpathologie* to Goodsir. Goodsir's paper on the bone-forming properties of certain corpuscles found within osseous tissue represent the foundation of the study of osteogenesis, as distinct from descriptive osteology.

2295   WALLER, AUGUSTUS VOLNEY. 1816-1870
Microscopic examination of some of the principal tissues of the animal frame, as observed in the tongue of the living frog, toad, etc. *Phil. Mag.*, 1846, **29**, 271-87, 397-405.
   Waller observed the penetration and migration of leucocytes through the endothelial vessel walls.

2296   VIRCHOW, RUDOLF LUDWIG KARL. 1821-1902
Die pathologischen Pigmente. *Virchows Arch. path. Anat.*, 1847, **1**, 379-404, 407-86.
   On the origin and chemical composition of extracellular and intracellular pigments, and on the supposed formation of new cells by the membranous envelopment of pigmented blood corpuscles or pigment granules.

2297.1   LEBERT, HERMANN. 1813-1878
Traité d'anatomie pathologique générale et spéciale. 4 vols., Paris, *Baillière*, 1857-61.
   Lebert set out to cover both general and special pathology. The superb hand-coloured copperplate engravings of macro- and micropathology in this work are among the finest ever published.

2298   LISTER, JOSEPH, 1*st Baron Lister.* 1827-1912
On the early stages of inflammation. *Phil Trans.*, 1858, **148**, 645-702.
   This paper reports the results of one of Lister's most valuable researches; his conclusions still hold today.

2299   VIRCHOW, RUDOLPH LUDWIG KARL. 1821-1902
Die Cellularpathologie in ihrer Begründung auf physiologische und pathologische Gewebelehre. Berlin, *A. Hirschwald*, 1858.
   Virchow was the greatest figure in the history of pathology. His best work, *Die Cellularpathologie*, is one of the most important books in the history of medicine and the foundation stone of cellular pathology. Reprinted Hildesheim, 1966. The English translation, London, 1860, was

reprinted several times in the 19th century, and in recent years. Virchow, Professor of Pathology at Würzburg and Berlin, founded the *Archiv für pathologische Anatomie und Physiologie ("Virchow's Archiv")*. Biography by E. H. Ackerknecht, 1953. See L. J. Rather, *A commentary on the medical writings of Rudolf Virchow*, San Francisco, *Norman Publishing*, 1990.

2300   CORNIL, ANDRÉ VICTOR. 1837-1908, & RANVIER, LOUIS ANTOINE. 1835-1922
Manuel d'histologie pathologique. 3 pts. Paris, *Germer-Baillière*, 1869-76.
English translations, Philadelphia, 1880, and London, 1882-86.

2301   BERNARD, CLAUDE. 1813-1878
Leçons de pathologie expérimentale. Paris, *J. B. Baillière*, 1872.
An elaboration of his lectures on the subject at the Collège de France.

2302   COHNHEIM, JULIUS FRIEDRICH. 1839-1884
Neue Untersuchungen über die Entzündung. Berlin, *A. Hirschwald*, 1873.
Cohnheim was the master experimental pathologist of the 19th century. He was a pupil of Virchow and Kölliker; in contradiction of the former, he showed the essential feature of inflammation to be the passage of leucocytes through the capillary walls and their accumulation at the site of the injury – "ohne Gefässe keine Entzündung". His first article on the subject will be found in *Virchows Arch. path. Anat.*, 1867, **40**, 1-79.

2303   ———. Vorlesungen über allgemeine Pathologie. 2 vols. Berlin, *A. Hirschwald*, 1877-80.
Apart from Virchow's *Cellularpathologie*, this was the most influential textbook of pathology during the 19th century. It includes (vol. 1, p. 38) a report on the experimental production of heart murmours. English translation, New Sydenham Society, 3 vols., 1889-90.

2304   VIRCHOW, RUDOLF LUDWIG KARL. 1821-1902
Die Sections-Technik im Leichenhause des Charité-Krankenhauses. Berlin, *A. Hirschwald*, 1876.
On the technique of dissection. English translation, London, 1876.

2305   ZIEGLER, ERNST. 1849-1905
Lehrbuch de allgemeinen und speciellen pathologischen Anatomie und Pathogenese. Jena, *G. Fischer*, 1881-82.
An outstanding textbook which today remains of value to pathologists. Ziegler was Professor of Pathology at Freiburg, and founded the *Beiträge zur pathologischen Anatomie ("Ziegler's Beiträge")*.

2306   WILD, CARL.
Beitrag zur Kenntnis der amyloiden und der hyalinen Degeneration des Bindegewebes. *Beitr. path. Anat. Physiol.*, 1886, **1**, 175-200.
First reported case of primary amyloidosis.

2307   METCHNIKOFF, ELIE [MECHNIKOV, ILYA ILYICH]. 1845-1916
Lektsii o sravnitelnoi patologii vospaleniy. St. Petersburg, *K. L. Rikker*, 1892.
Metchnikoff's classic lectures on the pathology of inflammation. The book was translated into French in the same year, and in 1893 an English version appeared. An English edition was also published New York, *Dover*, 1968.

2308   WELCH, WILLIAM HENRY. 1850-1934
Adaptation in pathological processes. *Trans. Congr. Amer. Phys. Surg.*, 1897, **4**, 284-310; also in *Amer. J. med. Sci.*, 1897, **113**, 631-55.
Reproduced in *Bibliotheca Medica Americana*, Baltimore, 1937, Vol. 3.

2309   ADAMI, JOHN GEORGE. 1862-1926
The principles of pathology. 2 vols. Philadelphia, *Lea & Febiger*, [1908-09].
Vol. 2 written with A. G. Nicholls.

2310   MARCHAND, FELIX JACOB. 1846-1928
Ueber die Entzündung. *Med. Klin.*, 1911, **7**, 1921-27.
A notable paper on inflammation. Marchand succeeded Ziegler as editor of the latter's *Beiträge*.

2311   HENKE, FRIEDRICH. 1868-1943, & LUBARSCH, OTTO. 1860-1933
Handbuch der speziellen pathologischen Anatomie und Histologie. 12 vols. Berlin, *J. Springer*, 1924-52.

2312   MENKIN, VALY. 1901-
Isolation and properties of the factor responsible for increased capillary permeability. *Proc. Soc. exp. Biol. (N.Y.)*, 1937, **36**, 164-66.
Leukotaxine isolated.

PALEOPATHOLOGY

2312.1   ESPER, JOHANN FRIEDRICH. 1732-1781
Ausfürliche Nachricht von neuentdeckten Zoolithen, unbekannter vierfüsiger Thiere...Nuremberg, *Georg Knorrs*, 1774.
The first published description of disease in ancient bones, a possible bone tumour affecting a fossil cave bear. *See* No. 203.7.

2312.2   RUFFER, *Sir* MARC ARMAND. 1859-1917
Studies in the palaeopathology of Egypt. Edited by R. L. MOODIE. Chicago, *Univ. Press*, 1921.
A collection of papers published previously in various journals. Ruffer spent many years in Egypt in the study of palaeopathology.

2312.3   MOODIE, ROY LEE. 1880-1934
Paleopathology; an introduction to the study of ancient evidences of disease. Urbana, *Univ. of Illinois Press*, 1923.
Surveys the ancient evidence of disease in plants, invertebrates and vertebrates, including man. Reprint, 1975.

2312.4   WILLIAMS, HERBERT U. 1866-1938
Human paleopathology, with some original observations on symmetrical osteoporosis of the skull. Arch. Pathol., 1929, **7**, 839-902.

2312.5   JARCHO, SAUL. 1906-
Human palaeopathology. Edited by Saul Jacho. New Haven, *Yale University Press*, 1966.
Includes material on the history of paleopathology in the United States.

2312.6   BROTHWELL, Don Reginald, & SANDISON, Andrew Tawse. -1982
          Diseases in antiquity: a survey of the diseases, injuries and surgery of early
          populations. Springfield, *C. C. Thomas*, [1967].

2312.7   STEINBOCK, Robert Ted. 1952-
          Paleopathological diagnosis and interpretation: bone diseases in ancient
          human populations. Springfield, *C.C. Thomas*, 1976.
              The first text providing diagnostic criteria for evaluating ancient skeletal
          remains.

2312.8   COCKBURN, Aidan. 1912-1981, & COCKBURN, Eve.
          Mummies, disease, and ancient cultures. Cambridge, *Cambridge Univer-
          sity Press*, 1980.

History of Pathology

2313   CHIARI, Hans. 1851-1916
          Geschichte der pathologischen Anatomie des Menschen. *In*: Puschmann,
          T.: *Handbuch der Geschichte der Medizin*, 1903, **2**, 473-559.

2316   GOLDSCHMID, Edgar. 1881-1957
          Entwicklung und Bibliographie der pathologisch-anatomischen Abbildung.
          Leipzig, *K. W. Hiersemann*, 1925.
              Traces the development of pathological anatomical illustration and
          includes a chronological bibliography of all important publications con-
          taining illustrations of pathological conditions, and an index of artists,
          printers, and publishers. Fine colour plates.

2317   LONG, Esmond Ray. 1890-1979
          A history of pathology. Baltimore, *Williams & Wilkins*, 1928.
              The first systematic history of the subject in the English language.
          Revised edition, New York, *Dover Publications*, 1965.

2318   ———. Selected readings in pathology. Springfield, *C. C. Thomas*, 1929.
              This work makes it possible to read many of the classical writings on the
          subject which previously, through language difficulties, were beyond the
          reach of many. The book forms a valuable companion to Long's history of
          the subject. 2nd ed., 1961.

2319   KRUMBHAAR, Edward Bell. 1882-1966
          Pathology. New York, *P. B. Hoeber*, 1937.
              Krumbhaar edited the *Clio Medica* series of volumes on the history of
          medicine, and contributed a history of pathology to it.

2319.1   FOSTER, William Derek. 1925-1981
          A short history of clinical pathology. Edinburgh, *E. & S. Livingstone Ltd.*, 1961.

2319.2   MAULITZ, Russell Charles. 1944-
          Morbid appearances: the anatomy of pathology in the early nineteenth
          century. Cambridge, *Cambridge University Press*, 1987.

TUBERCULOSIS

See also 3216-3243, PULMONARY TUBERCULOSIS, and under the names of infected organs.

2320   SMITH, *Sir* GRAFTON ELLIOT. 1871-1937, & RUFFER, *Sir* MARC ARMAND. 1859-1917
        Pott'sche Krankheit an einer ägyptischen Mumie. Giessen, *A. Töpelmann,* 1910.
        The fact that tuberculosis was present among the ancient Egyptians was proved when Elliot Smith and Ruffer described a genuine case of Pott's disease in a mummy of 1000 B.C.

2321   LE BOE, FRANCISCUS DE [SYLVIUS]. 1614-1672
        Opera medica. Amstelodami, *apud D. Elsevirium et A. Wolfgang,* 1679.
        Tuberculosis was known to the ancients only in its advanced form, and little progress was made in the knowledge of the condition until the time of Sylvius. He asserted that tubercles are often to be found in the lung and that they softened and suppurated to form cavities.

2322   BAYLE, GASPARD LAURENT. 1774-1816
        Recherches sur la phthisie pulmonaire. Paris, *Gabon,* 1810.
        The beginning of the modern clinical conception of tuberculosis. Bayle gave the best description to date of the varieties of tuberculosis. He was first to use the term "miliary" to describe small tubercles and first to speak of tuberculous diathesis. He left an original description of the coarse character of the tubercle and its identity with the pulmonary, granular, and other varieties of tuberculosis. He recognized six types of pulmonary lesion. English translation, Liverpool, 1815.

2323   KLENCKE, PHILIPP FRIEDRICH HERMANN. 1813-1881
        Ueber die Ansteckung und Verbreitung der Scrophelkrankheit bei Menschen durch den Genuss der Kuhmilch. Leipzig, *C. E. Kollmann,* 1846.
        Klencke showed the possibility of the transmission of tuberculosis to man by cow's milk. In 1843 he succeeded in inoculating rabbits with tuberculosis.

2324   VILLEMIN, JEAN ANTOINE. 1827-1892
        Etudes sur la tuberculose; preuves rationelles et expérimentales de sa spécifité et de son inoculabilité. Paris, *J. B. Baillière,* 1868.
        Villemin inoculated guinea-pigs and rabbits with sputum, caseous material, and miliary tubercles, with resulting development of tuberculosis. His brilliant experimental work proved tuberculosis to be a specific infection transmissible by an inoculable agent.

2325   BUHL, LUDWIG VON. 1816-1880
        Lungenentzündung, Tuberkulose und Schwindsucht. München, *R. Oldenbourg,* 1872.
        Buhl stated that disseminated miliary tuberculosis is always associated with the presence of a caseous focus in some part of the body, which is the centre from which infection starts (Buhl–Dittrich law). English translation, 1874.

2326   GRANCHER, JACQUES JOSEPH. 1843-1907
De l'unité de la phthisie. Paris, *Thèse No.* 50, 1873.
      Confirmation of Villemin. Grancher in 1903 instituted the "Grancher system" – the boarding out of children from tuberculous households in France.

2327   KLEBS, THEODOR ALBRECHT EDWIN. 1834-1913
Die künstliche Erzeugung der Tuberkulose. *Arch. exp. Path. Pharmak.*, 1873, **1**, 163-80.
      Klebs was the first to produce experimental bovine tuberculosis (by feeding cattle with infected milk). His work confirmed the earlier researches of Villemin.

2328   THAON, LOUIS ALBERT. 1846-1886
Recherches sur l'anatomie pathologique de la tuberculose. Paris, *Thèse No.* 45, 1873.

2329   COHNHEIM, JULIUS FRIEDRICH. 1839-1884
Die Tuberkulose vom Standpunkte der Infectionslehre. Leipzig, *A. Edelmann*, 1880.
      Cohnheim, a pioneer pathologist, was Virchow's most distinguished pupil. Among his many valuable experiments, the greatest was perhaps his successful inoculation of tuberculosis in the anterior chamber of the rabbit's eye, 1877, an account of which is included in the above work. This proved that tuberculous material derived from different sources owed its infectiveness to the same contagious factor. The book first appeared in quarto, 29 pp., 1879, with a Latin imprint: Lipsiae, *typis A. Edelmanni.* This scarce version was followed by the more common octavo (44 pp.) recorded above. An English translation is included in D. U. Cullimore's *Consumption as a contagious disease*, London, [1880].

2330   CONCATO, LUIGI MARIA. 1825-1882
Sulla poliorromennite scrofolosa, o tisi delle sierose. *G. int. Sci. med.*, 1881, n.s. **3**, 1037-53.
      Concato's excellent description of tuberculous inflammation of the serous membranes resulted in the eponym "Concato's disease".

2331   KOCH, ROBERT. 1843-1910
Die Aetiologie der Tuberkulose. *Berl, klin. Wschr.*, 1882, **19**, 221-30.
      Discovery of the tubercle bacillus announced March 24, 1882. This paper also contains a statement of "Koch's postulates". *See also* Nos. 2536 and 5167. Koch published a fuller account in *Mitt. k. Gesundh-Amte*, 1884, **2**, 1-88, in which he reported how he had succeeded in producing experimental tuberculosis in animals after cultivating the bacillus. Reprinted with translation in *Med. Classics*, 1938, **2**, 821-80. Koch received the Nobel Prize in 1905.

2331.1   ZIEHL, FRANZ. 1859-1926
Zur Färbung des Tuberkelbacillus. *Dtsch. med. Wschr.*, 1882, **8**, 451.
      Ziehl–Neelsen stain.

2331.2   NEELSEN, FRIEDRICH CARL ADOLF. 1854-1894
Ein casuistischer Beitrag zur Lehre von der Tuberkulose. *Zbl. med. Wiss.*, 1883, **21**, 497-501.

Includes (p. 500) details of his stain for the tubercle bacillus (*see* No. 2331.1).

2332   KOCH, ROBERT. 1843-1910
Weitere Mittheilungen über ein Heilmittel gegen Tuberkulose. *Dtsch. med. Wschr.*, 1890, **16**, 1029-32; 1891, **17**, 101-102, 1189-92.
Introduction of tuberculin in the treatment of tuberculosis. The second paper describes "Koch's phenomenon", and tuberculin skin test. Koch showed that tuberculin injected intradermally would elicit a severe local inflammatory reaction in tuberculous patients. This was the first diagnostic skin test.

2333   ———. Ueber neue Tuberkulinpräparate. *Dtsch. med. Wschr.*, 1897, **23**, 209-13.
Koch's new tuberculin (Tuberculin R).

2334   ARLOING, SATURNIN. 1846-1911
Sur l'obtention de cultures et d'émulsions homogènes du bacille de la tuberculose humaine en milieu liquide et "sur une variété mobile de ce bacille". *C. R. Acad. Sci. (Paris)*, 1898, **126**, 1319-21.
Sero-agglutination for the diagnosis of tubercle bacillus.

2335   SMITH, THEOBOLD. 1859-1934
A comparative study of bovine tubercle bacilli and of human bacilli from sputum. *J. exp. Med.*, 1898, **3**, 451-511.
First clear differentiation between the bovine and human types of tubercle bacillus.

2336   CALOT, JEAN FRANÇOIS. 1861-1944
Les maladies qu'on soigne à Berck. Paris, *Masson*, 1900.
An account of the work of the Rothschild Hospital at Berck-sur-Mer, where Calot specialized in the treatment of surgical tuberculosis in children.

2337   CALMETTE, LEON CHARLES ALBERT. 1863-1933
Sur un nouveau procédé de diagnostic de la tuberculose chez l'homme par l'ophtalmo-réaction à la tuberculine. *C. R. Acad. Sci. (Paris)*, 1907, **144**, 1324-26.
Calmette's conjunctival reaction test for tuberculosis.

2338   PIRQUET VON CESENATICO, CLEMENS PETER. 1874-1929
Der diagnostische Wert der kutanen Tuberkulinreaktion bei der Tuberkulose des Kindesalters auf Grund von 100 Sektionen. *Wien. klin. Wschr.*, 1907, **20**, 1123-28.
Introduction of Pirquet's test – a cutaneous reaction employed in the diagnosis of tuberculosis.

2339   MORO, ERNST. 1874-1951
Ueber eine diagnostische verwertbare Reaktion der Haut auf Einreibung mit Tuberkulinsalbe. *Münch. med. Wschr.*, 1908, **55**, 216-18; 2025-28.
Moro's percutaneous tuberculin reaction, employed as a diagnostic measure.

2340   WOLFF-EISNER, ALFRED. 1877-1948
Die kutane und konjunktivale Tuberkulinreaktion, ihre Bedeutung für
Diagnostik und Prognose der Tuberkulose. *Z. Tuberk.,* 1908, **12**, 21-25.
Wolff-Eisner's conjunctival tuberculin reaction.

2341   MANTOUX, CHARLES. 1877-1947
Intradermo-réaction de la tuberculine. *C. R. Acad. Sci. (Paris)*, 1908, **147**,
355-57.
Mantoux's intradermal tuberculin skin test.

2342   ROLLIER, AUGUSTE. 1874-1954
Die Heliotherapie der Tuberkulose. Berlin, *J. Springer*, 1913.
In 1903 Rollier introduced ultra-violet light and Alpine sunlight in the
treatment of surgical tuberculosis. Heliotherapy for chronic affections was
advocated as early as the 5th century A.D. by Caelius Aurelianus.

2343   CALMETTE, LÉON CHARLES ALBERT. 1863-1933, *et al.*
Essai d'immunisation contre l'infection tuberculeuse. *Bull. Acad. Med.
(Paris),* 1924, 3 sér., **91**, 787-96.
With C. Guérin and B. Weill-Hallé, B.C.G. (Bacille Calmette–Guérin)
vaccine was first produced in 1906 and subcultured for 13 years. It was
used as a prophylactic against tuberculosis in children in 1921. *See also* No.
2346.

2334   MOLLGAARD, HOLGER. 1885-?
Ueber die experimentellen Grundlagen für die Sanocrysin-Behandlung
der Tuberkulose. *Tuberk.-Bibl.*, 1925, Heft 20, 1-72.
Mollgaard was responsible for the introduction of sanocrysin.

2345   SAUERBRUCH, ERNST FERDINAND. 1875-1951, *et al.*
Ueber Versuche, schwere Formen der Tuberkulose durch diätetische
Behandlung zu beeinflussen. *Münch. med. Wschr.*, 1926, **73**, 47-51.
Gerson introduced a salt-restricted diet in the treatment of tuberculosis;
this was subsequently modified by Sauerbruch and Herrmannsdorfer,
becoming known as the "Gerson–Sauerbruch–Hermannsdorfer diet". With
A. Hermannsdorfer and M. Gerson.

2346   CALMETTE, LÉON CHARLES ALBERT. 1863-1933, *et al.*
Sur la vaccination préventive des enfants nouveau-nés contre la tuberculose
par le B.C.G. *Ann. Inst. Pasteur*, 1927, **41**, 201-32.
With C. Guérin, L. Négre, and A. Boquet.

2347   WELLS, HENRY GIDEON. 1875-1943, & LONG, ESMOND RAY. 1890-1979.
The chemistry of tuberculosis. Second edition. Baltimore, *Williams &
Wilkins*, 1932.

2348   VOLLMER, HERMANN. 1896-1959, & GOLDBERGER, ESTHER WHITE. 1905-
A new tuberculin patch test. *Amer. J. Dis. Child.*, 1937, **54**, 1019-24.

2349   FELDMAN, WILLIAM HUGH. 1892- , *et al.*
The effect of promin (sodium salt of P. P'-diamino-diphenyl-sulfone-N, N'-
dextrose sulfonate) on experimental tuberculosis: a preliminary report.
Proc. Mayo Clin., 1940, **15**, 695-99.

Experimental evidence of the value of promin (sodium glucosulphone) in tuberculosis. With H. C. Hinshaw and H.E. Moses. See also *Amer. Rev. Tuberc.*, 1942, **45**, 303-33.

2349.1   RICH, ARNOLD RICE. 1893-1968
The pathogenesis of tuberculosis. Springfield, *C.C. Thomas*, 1944.
Classic work on the pathogenesis of tuberculosis and its immunology and hypersensitivity.

2350   HINSHAW, HORTON CORWIN. 1902- , & FELDMAN, WILLIAM HUGH. 1892-1974
Streptomycin in treatment of clinical tuberculosis: a preliminary report. *Proc. Mayo Clin.*, 1945, **20**, 313-18.

2351   DOMAGK, GERHARD. 1895-1964, *et al.*
Ueber eine neue, gegen Tuberkelbazillen in vitro wirksame Verbindungsklasse. *Naturwissenschaften*, 1946, **33**, 315.
Introduction of thiosemicarbazone in treatment of tuberculosis. With R. Behnisch, F. Mietzsch, and H. Schmidt.

2352   FRAPPIER, ARMAND. 1904- , & GUY, ROLAND. 1913-
A new and practical B.C.G. skin test (the B.C.G. scarification test) for the detection of the total tuberculous allergy. *Canad. J. publ. Hlth.*, 1950, **41**, 72-83.

2352.1   HEAF, FREDERICK ROLAND GEORGE. 1894-1973
The multiple-puncture tuberculin test. *Lancet*, 1951, **2**, 151-53.
The Heaf multiple-puncture tuberculin test.

2353   ROBITZEK, EDWARD HEINRICH. 1912-1984, *et al.*
Chemotherapy of human tuberculosis with hydrazine derivatives of isonicotinic acid. (Preliminary report of representative cases.) *Quart. Bull. Sea View Hosp.*, 1952, **13**, 27-51.
Introduction of isoniazid. With I. J. Selikoff and G. G. Ornstein. See also *Amer. Rev. Tuberc.*, 1952, **65**, 257-442.

2353.1   GRIFFITHS, MARGARET ISABEL, & GAISFORD, WILFRED FLETCHER. 1902-
Freeze-dried B.C.G. Vaccination of newborn infants with a British vaccine. *Brit. med. J.*, 1956, **2**, 565-8.
Freeze-dried B.C.G. vaccine.

2353.2   RIST, NOEL. *et al.*
Experiments on the antituberculous activity of alpha-ethyl-thioisonicotinamide. *Amer. Rev. Tuberc.*, 1959, **79**, 1-5.
Ethionamide. With F. Grumbach and D. Liberman.

2353.3   THOMAS, J. P., *et al.*
A new synthetic compound with antituberculous activity in mice; ethambutol (dextro-2, 2'-(ethylenediimino)-di-l-butanol). *Amer. Rev. resp. Dis.*, 1961, **83**, 891-3.
With C. O. Baughn, R. G. Wilkinson and R. G. Shepherd.

History of Tuberculosis

2354   FLICK, LAWRENCE FRANCIS. 1856-1938
Development of our knowledge of tuberculosis. Philadelphia, 1925.

2355   PIÉRY, ANTOINE MARIUS. 1873-1957, & ROSHEM, JULIEN.
Historie de la tuberculose. Paris, *G. Doin*, 1931.

2356   MEACHEN, GEORGE NORMAN. 1876-
A short history of tuberculosis. London, *Bale*, 1936.

2357   WEBB, GERALD BERTRAM. 1871-1948
Tuberculosis. New York, *P. B. Hoeber*, 1936.
     Clio Medica series.

2358   KAYNE, GEORGE GREGORY. 1901-1945
The control of tuberculosis in England, past and present. London, *Oxford University Press*, 1937.

2359   HART, PHILIP MONTAGU D'ARCY. 1900-
Chemotherapy of tuberculosis. Researches during the past 100 years. *Brit. med J.*, 1946, **2**, 805-10, 849-55.

2360   BURKE, RICHARD MICHAEL. 1903-
Historical chronology of tuberculosis. 2nd ed. Springfield, *C. C. Thomas*, 1955.

SYPHILIS

See also 4772-4806, NEUROSYPHILIS; 5195-5227.1, SEXUALLY TRANSMITTED DISEASES

2362   GRÜNPECK, JOSEPH. 1473-1532
Tractatus de pestilentia scorra. [?Leipzig, *Boettiger*, 1496].
     Grünpeck was first to record mixed primary lesions, multiple primary lesions, and to note the second incubation period of syphilis. A translation of the above is in *Arch. Derm. Syph. (Chicago)*, 1930, **22**, 430.

2363   LEONICENO, NICCOLO. 1428-1524
Libellus de epidemia, quam vulgo morbum Gallicum vocant. Venetiis, *in domo Aldi Manutii*, 1497.
     One of the earliest treatises on the subject, and one of very few medical books printed by Aldus Manutius. Leoniceno includes a good description of syphilitic hemiplegia. He believed that syphilis was known to classical writers. English translation in Major, *Classic descriptions of disease*, 3rd ed., 1945, p. 15.

2363.1   LOPEZ DE VILLALOBOS, FRANCISCO. 1473-1549
El sumario de la medicina, con un tratado sobre las pestiferas buuas. Salamanca, *Antonio de Barreda*, 1498.
     H. Goodman considers this among the best of all works on the subject in the 15th and 16th centuries. Reprinted Salamanca, 1973. For English translation see *Bull. Inst. Hist. Med.*, 1939, **7**, 1129-39. An English translation was also published in London, 1870.

2364   FRACASTORO, GIROLAMO [FRACASTORIUS]. 1478-1553
Syphilis sive morbus gallicus. Veronae, *[S. Nicolini da Sabbio]*, 1530.

The most famous of all medical poems. It epitomized contemporary knowledge of syphilis, gave to it its present name, and recognized a venereal cause. Fracastorius refers to mercury as a remedy. First complete English translation by Nahum Tate (Later Poet Laureate) was published in 1686; translation by W. van Wyck (1934). L. Baumgartner and J. F. Fulton published a handlist of editions of the poem in 1933 and a bibliography of the poem in 1935.

2365   MASSA, NICCOLO. 1489-1569
Liber de morbo gallico. Venetiis, *in aedibus F. Bindoni ac M. Pasini*, 1507 [1527].

Includes a description of the neurological manifestations of syphilis. P. Krivatsy, *J. Hist. Med.*, 1974, **29**, 230-33, has provided evidence that this edition was printed in 1527. Massa was Professor of Anatomy in Venice.

2366   MATTIOLI, PIETRO ANDREA. 1500-1577
Morbi gallici novum ac utilissimum opusculum quo vera et omnimoda ejus cura percipi potest. [Bononiae, *imp. haered. Hieronymi de Benedictis*, 1533].

Mattioli considered mercury a specific in the treatment of syphilis. He was probably the first to work extensively on syphilis of the newborn. He is better known for his commentary on Dioscorides.

2367   DIAZ DE ISLA, RODRIGO RUIZ. 1462-1542
Tractado cótra el mal serpintino. (Sevilla, *D. de Robertis*, 1539).

Diaz de Isla, a Barcelonese surgeon, wrote of a disease "previously unknown, unseen and undescribed", which appeared in Barcelona in 1493 and which was obviously syphilis. This is probably the earliest reference to the West Indian origin of syphilis (the writer believed that the disease originated in Haiti) and the book is the chief source of the opinions of those who believe in the American origin of syphilis. Text reproduced with German translation in *Janus*, 1901, **6**, 653-55; 1902, **7**, 31-40. Extensively discussed in No. 2430.

2368   HÉRY, THIERRY DE. ?1500-1599
La méthode curatoire de la maladie venerienne. Paris, *M. David*, 1552.

De Héry made a fortune from treating syphilitic patients. He recommended mercurial inunctions and guaiac internally.

2369   PARACELSUS, THEOPRASTUS PHILIPPUS AURELOUS BOMBASTUS VON HOHENHEIM. 1493-1541
Von der frantzösischen kranckheit drey Bücher. Franckfurt am Mayn, *H. Gülfferichen*, 1553.

Paracelsus suggested the hereditary transmission of syphilis and advocated mercury internally, as an antisyphilitic. He called the disease "French gonorrhoea" and thus started the confusion which lasted until the 19th century.

2370   FALLOPPIO, GABRIELE [FALLOPIUS]. 1523-1562
De morbo gallico. Patavii, *apud C. Gryphium*, 1563.

Fallopius was one of the first prominent opponents of the use of mercury in syphilis. He distinguished syphilitic and non-syphilitic condylomata.

2371   GALE, THOMAS. 1507-1587
        Certaine works of chirurgerie. London, *R. Hall*, (1563).
        Includes the first mention of syphilis in the English literature. Facsimile
        reprint, New York, *Da Capo Press*, 1971.

2372   LUIGINI, LUIGI [LUISINUS, ALOYSIUS]. *b.* 1526.
        De morbo gallico omnia quae extant. 3 vols. Venetiis, *apud J. Zilettum*, 1566-
        67.
        A collection of important writings on syphilis to 1500. Boerhaave
        published a revision of this work in 1728, covering the period 1495-1566.

2373   CLOWES, WILLIAM. 1540-1604
        A short and profitable treatise touching the cure of the morbus gallicus by
        unctions. London, *J. Daye*, 1579.
        William Clowes, the greatest of the Elizabethan surgeons, published the
        first original English treatise on syphilis. It was his first work; it demonstrates
        the prevalence of the disease at that time (Clowes says that of every 20
        persons admitted to St. Bartholomew's Hospital, 15 were found to be
        suffering from syphilis). Facsimile reprint, New York, *Da Capo Press*, 1972.

2374   FERNEL, JEAN FRANÇOIS. 1497-1558
        De luis venereae curatione perfectissima liber. Antverpiae, *ex off. C. Plantini*,
        1579.
        French translation, Paris, 1879.

2375   ABERCROMBY, DAVID. 1621-1695
        Tuta, ac efficax luis venereae. Londini, *S. Smith*, 1684.
        Abercromby advanced the idea that syphilis was caused by a parasite.

2376   GRUNER, CHRISTIAN GOTTFRIED. 1744-1815
        Morborum antiquitates. Vratislaviae, *J. F. Korn*, 1774.
        Pp. 85-100: "Lists 191 semeiological varieties of syphilis described in the
        period" (Garrison).

2377   HUNTER, JOHN. 1728-1793
        A treatise on the venereal disease. London, 1786.
        In Hunter's day the venereal diseases were thought to be due to a single
        poison. To test this theory Hunter experimented with matter taken from a
        gonorrhoeal patient who, unknown to Hunter, also had syphilis. Hunter
        maintained that gonorrhoea and syphilis were caused by a single patho-
        gen. Backed by the weight of his authority, this experiment retarded the
        development of knowledge regarding the two diseases. Contrary to
        legend, however, there is no proof that Hunter actually inoculated himself
        with venereal disease. The hard ("Hunterian") chancre eponymizes Hunter.
        This work also makes a major contribution to urological surgery.

2378   BELL, BENJAMIN. 1749-1806
        A treatise on gonorrhoea virulenta, and lues venerea. 2 vols. Edinburgh, *J.
        Watson & G. Mudie*, 1793.
        Bell was the first to differentiate between gonorrhoea and syphilis.

2378.1   BERTIN, RENÉ JOSEPH HYACINTHE. 1757-1828
Traité de la maladie vénérienne chez les enfans nouveau-nés, les femmes
enceintes et les nourrices. Paris, *Chez Gabon*, 1810.
First systematic work on congenital syphilis.

2379   WALLACE, WILLIAM. 1791-1837
Treatment of the venereal disease by the hydriodate of potash, or iodide
of potassium. *Lancet*, 1835-36, **2**, 5-11.
Wallace introduced potassium iodide in the treatment of syphilis,
reporting good results in 139 patients.

2380   COLLES, ABRAHAM. 1773-1843
Practical observations on the venereal disease, and on the use of mercury.
London, *Sherwood, Gilbert & Piper*, 1837.
In this work (p. 304) is stated "Colles's law". Colles introduced small
doses of mercury in the treatment of syphilis. He was Professor of Surgery
at Dublin.

2381   RICORD, PHILLIPPE. 1800-1889
Traité pratique des maladies vénériennes. Paris, *De Just Rouvier & E. Le
Bouvier,* 1838.
Includes the description of "Ricord's chancre", the initial lesion in
syphilis. Ricord re-demonstrated the specific character of syphilis and
divided it into the three stages, primary, secondary, and tertiary. *See also*
No. 5202.

2383   DIDAY, CHARLES JOSEPH PAUL EDOUARD. 1812-1894
Traité de la syphilis des nouveau-nés et des enfants à la mamelle. Paris, *V.
Masson*, 1854.
An important work on congenital syphilis. English translation, 1859.

2384   BETTINGER, JULIUS. 1802-1887
Aerztliches Intelligenz-Blatt, 1856, **3**, 425-28.
First demonstration of the experimental inoculability of syphilis. The
information is given in a discussion on the subject by the Society of
Physicians of the Palatinate; it appeared anonymously, without title, and
identity of the writer was not disclosed until fifty years later. See the
footnote on page 585 of Garrison's *Introduction* for further details; a biographical note appears in *Derm. Z.*, 1913, **20**, 220-23.

2385   VIRCHOW, RUDOLPH LUDWIG KARL. 1821-1902
Ueber die Natur der constitutionell-syphilitischen Affectionen. *Virchows
Arch. path. Anat.*, 1858, **15**, 217-336.
Virchow's great work on the pathology of syphilis confirmed the fact
that it was a disease which involved all organs and tissues of the body and
showed that the causal organism was transferred through the blood to the
various organs and tissues. Issued as offprint, Berlin, 1859.

2386   HUTCHINSON, *Sir* JONATHAN. 1828-1913
Report on the effects of infantile syphilis in marring the development of the
teeth. *Trans path. Soc. Lond.*, 1858, **9**, 449-55.
Hutchinson of St. Bartholomew's Hospital, is memorable for his original
description of the notched incisors ("Hutchinson's teeth") in congenital

syphilis. His name is also associated with "Hutchinson's triad" (interstitial keratitis, notched incisors and labyrinthine disease) in congenital syphilis.

2387 KUSSMAUL, ADOLF. 1822-1902
Untersuchungen über den constitutionellen Mercurialismus und sein Verhältniss zur constitutionellen Syphilis. Würzburg, *Stahel*, 1861.

2388 PELLIZZARI, PIETRO. 1823-1892
Della transmissione delle sifilide mediante l'inoculazione del sangre. [Florence, 1862].
Proof of the possibility of transmission of syphilis by blood transfusion.

2389 WILKS, *Sir* SAMUEL, *Bart.* 1824-1911
On the syphilitic affections of internal organs. *Guy's Hosp. Rep.*, 1863, **24**, 1-63.
Wilks's outstanding work was on visceral syphilis, a subject which he was one of the first to study.

2390 PROFETA, GUISEPPE. 1840-1911
Sulla sifilide per allattamento. *Sperimentale,* 1865, 4 ser., **15**, 328-38, 339-418.
Profeta's law – a non-syphilitic child born of syphilitic parents is immune.

2390.1 LANCEREAUX, ETIENNE. 1829-1910
Traité historique et pratique de la syphilis. Paris, *J. B. Baillière*, 1866.
A complete review of contemporary knowledge. English translation, 2 vols., 1868-69.

2391 MOON, HENRY. 1845-1892
On irregular and defective tooth development. *Trans. odont. Soc. G. B.*, 1876-77, n.s. **5**, 223-43.
"Moon's molars", the first molars in congenital syphilitics.

2392 KLEBS, THEODOR ALBRECHT EDWIN. 1834-1913
Das Contagium der Syphilis. Eine experimentelle Studie. *Arch. exp. Path Pharmea.*, 1878-79, **10**, 161-221.
Klebs inoculated syphilis into apes and probably saw the spirochaete before Schaudinn and Hoffmann.

2393 FOURNIER, JEAN ALFRED. 1832-1915
La syphilis héréditaire tardive. Paris, *G. Masson*, 1886.
Fournier, one of the greatest syphilologists, did more than any other person to develop the knowledge regarding congenital syphilis. Through his writings, the importance of syphilis as a cause of degenerative diseases was recognized.

2394 BALZER, FELIX. 1849-1929
Expériences sur la toxicité du bismuth. *C. R. Soc. Biol. (Paris)*, 1889, 9 sér., **1**, 537-44.
Balzer was the first to suggest bismuth in the treatment of syphillis.

2395 FOURNIER, JEAN ALFRED. 1832-1915
Les chancres extra-génitaux. Paris, *Rueff & Cie.*, 1897.

2396 JARISCH, ADOLF. 1850-1902
Therapeutische Versuche bei Syphilis. *Wien. med. Wschr.*, 1895, **45**, 720-21.
Jarisch–Herxheimer reaction; *see also* No. 2397.

2397 HERXHEIMER, KARL. 1861-1944
Ueber eine bei Syphilitischen vorkommende Quecksilberreaktion. *Dtsch. med. Wschr.*, 1902, **28**, 895-97.
See No. 2396.

2398 METCHNIKOFF, ELIE. 1845-1916, & ROUX, PIERRE PAUL EMILE. 1853-1933
Études expérimentales sur la syphilis. *Ann. Inst. Pasteur*, 1903, **17**, 809-21; 1904, **18**, 1-6.
Metchnikoff and Roux successfully transmitted syphilis from man to the higher apes. Although not the first to do this, they recorded much new information concerning the disease.

2399 SCHAUDINN, FRITZ RICHARD. 1871-1906, & HOFFMANN ERICH. 1868-1959
Vorläufiger Bericht über das Vorkommen von Spirochaeten in syphilitischen Krankheitsprodukten und bei Papillomen. *Arb. k. GesundhAmte.*, 1905, **22**, 527-34.
On March 3, 1905, Schaudinn discovered the causal organism of syphilis *Spirochaeta pallida*, in serum obtained from a genital lesion by Hoffmann. Schaudinn later renamed the spirochaete *Treponema pallidum*.

2399.1 BERTARELLI, ERNESTO. 1873-?
Ueber die Transmission der Syphilis auf das Kaninchen. Vorläufiger Bericht. *Zbl. Bakt.*, 1906, I Abt. Orig., **41**, 320-26.
Transmission of syphilis to rabbits.

2400 LANDSTEINER, KARL. 1868-1943, & MUCHA, VIKTOR. 1877-?
Zur Technik der Spirochaetenuntersuchung. *Wien. klin. Wschr.*, 1906, **19**, 1349-50.
Dark field method of diagnosis for presence of *T. pallidum*.

2401 LEVADITI, CONSTANTIN. 1874-1953
A propos de l'impregnation au nitrate d'argent des spirochètes sur coupes. *C. R. Soc. Biol. (Paris)*, 1906, **60**, 67-68.
Levaditi's method of staining *T. pallidum*.

2402 WASSERMANN, AUGUST VON. 1866-1925, *et al.*
Eine serodiagnostische Reaktion bei Syphilis. *Dtsch. med. Wschr.*, Berlin, 1906, **32**, 745-46.
The "Wassermann reaction", a specific diagnostic blood test for syphilis, and a modification of the complement-fixation reaction of Bordet and Gengou. With A. Neisser and C. Bruck.

2403 EHRLICH, PAUL. 1854-1915, & HATA, SAHACHIRO. 1873-1938
Die experimentelle Chemotherapie der Spirillosen (Syphilis, Rückfallfieber, Hühnerspirillose, Frambösie). Berlin, *J. Springer*, 1910.
After many experiments on the action of synthetic drugs upon spirochaetal diseases, Ehrlich and Hata in 1909 discovered salvarson ("606"), specific in the treatment of syphilis and yaws.

2404 NOGUCHI, HIDEYO. 1876-1928
A method for the pure cultivation of pathogenic Treponema pallidum (Spirochaeta pallida). *J. exp. Med.*, 1911, **14**, 99-108.
Pure culture of *T. pallidum* first obtained.

2405 EHRLICH, PAUL. 1854-1915
Ueber Laboratoriumsversuche und klinische Erprobung von Heilstoffen. *Chem. Ztg.*, 1912, **36**, 637-38.
Introduction of neoarsphenamine (neosalvarsan).

2406 LANGE, KARL FRIEDRICH AUGUST. 1883-?
Die Ausflockung kolloidalen Goldes durch Zerebrospinalflüssigkeit bei luetischen Affektion des Zentralnervensystems. *Z. Chemother.*, 1913, **1**, 44-78.
Lange's colloidal gold test for the diagnosis of cerebrospinal syphilis. See also *Berl. klin. Wschr.*, 1912, **49**, 897-901.

2407 MEINICKE, ERNST. 1878-1945
Ueber ein neue Methode der serologischen Luesdiagnose. *Berl. klin. Wschr.*, 1917, **54**, 613-14.
Meinicke diagnostic reaction.

2408 SACHS, HANS. 1877-1945, & GEORGI, WALTER. 1889-1920
Zur Kritik des serologischen Luesnachweises mittels Ausflockung. *Münch. med. Wschr.*, 1919, **66**, 440-42.
Sachs–Georgi diagnostic reaction.

2409 WEICHARDT, JULIUS WOLFGANG. 1875-1945, & SCHRADER, ERICH.
Über die Serodiagnostik der Syphilis mittels Ausflockung durch cholesterinierte Extrakte. *Med. Klin.*, 1919, **15**, 139-40.
Weichardt's reagent.

2410 WARTHIN, ALDRED SCOTT. 1866-1931, & STARRY, ALLEN CHRONISTER. 1890-
A more rapid and improved method of demonstrating spirochetes in tissues (Warthin and Starry's cover-glass method). *Amer. J. Syph.*, 1920, **4**, 97-103.
Warthin and Starry's method.

2411 SAZERAC, ROBERT 1875- , & LEVADITI, CONSTANTIN. 1874-1953
Traitement de la syphilis par le bismuth. *C. R. Acad. Sci. (Paris)*, 1921, **173**, 338-40.
Introduction of sodium-potassium bismuth tartrate in the treatment of syphilis.

2412 KAHN, REUBEN LEON. 1887-
A simple quantative precipitation reaction for syphilis. *Arch. Derm. Syph. (Chicago)*, 1922, **5**, 570-78.
Kahn test.

2413 KOLMER, JOHN ALBERT. 1886-1962
Studies in the standardization of the Wassermann reaction. XXX. A new complement-fixation test for syphilis based upon the results of studies in the standardization of technic. *Amer. J. Syph.*, 1922, **6**, 82-110.
Kolmer test.

2414   STOKES, JOHN HINCHMAN. 1885- , & CHAMBERS, STANLEY OWEN. 1897-
Bismuth arsphenamine sulphate. *J. Amer. med. Assoc.*, 1927, **89**, 1500-1505.
Clinical introduction of bismarsen, synthesized by G. W. Raiziss in 1924.

2414.1   EAGLE, HARRY. 1905-
Studies in the serology of syphilis. VII. A new flocculation test for the serum
diagnosis of syphilis. *J. Lab. clin. Med.*, 1932, **17**, 787-91.
Eagle flocculation test.

2415   TATUM, ARTHUR LAWRIE. 1884-1955, & COOPER, GARRETT ARTHUR. 1904-
An experimental study of mapharsen (meta-amino para-hydroxy phenyl
arsine oxide) as an antisyphilitic agent. *J. Pharmacol.*, 1934, **50**, 198-215.
Introduction of mapharsen.

2416   FOERSTER, OTTO HOTTINGER. 1876-1965, *et al.*
Mapharsen in the treatment of syphilis. A preliminary report. *Arch. Derm.
Syph. (Chicago)*, 1935, **32**, 868-92.
Clinical use of mapharsen. With R. L. McIntosh, L. M. Wieder, H. R.
Foerster, and G. A. Cooper.

2417   PANGBORN, MARY CANDACE. 1907-
A new serologically active phospholipid from beef heart. *Proc. Soc,. exp.
Biol. (N.Y.)*, 1941, **48**, 484-86.
Cardiolipin antigen for serological diagnosis of syphilis. For isolation
and purification see *J. biol. Chem.*, 1942, **143**, 247-56.

2418   MAHONEY, JOHN FRIEND. 1889-1957, *et al.*
Penicillin treatment of early syphilis. A preliminary report. *Vener. Dis.
Inform.*, 1943, **24**, 355-57; also in *Amer. J. publ. Hlth.*, 1943, **33**, 1387-91.
Introduction of penicillin in treatment of syphilis. With R. C. Arnold and
A. Harris.

2418.1   HARRIS, AD, *et al.*
A microflocculation test for syphilis using cardiolipin antigen: preliminary
report. *J. vener. Dis. Inform.*, 1946, **27**, 169-74.
V. D. Research Laboratory test (Harris test). With A. A. Rosenberg and
L. M. Riedel.

2419   NELSON, ROBERT ARMSTRONG. 1921- , & MAYER, MANFRED MARTIN. 1916-
Immobilization of *Treponema pallidum in vitro* by antibody produced in
syphilitic infection. *J. exp. Med.*, 1949, **89**, 369-93.
Nelson's treponemal immobilization test.

2419.1   CANNEFAX, GEORGE RADFORD. 1911- , & GARSON, WARFIELD. 1918-
Reiter protein complement fixation test for syphilis. *Publ. Hlth. Rep. (Wash.).*,
1957, **72**, 335-40.
See also H. Reiter, *Brit. J. vener. Dis.*, 1960, **36**, 18-20.

2419.2   DEACON, WILBUR EUGENE. 1907- , *et al.*
A fluorescent test for treponemal antibodies. *Proc. Soc. exp. Biol. (N.Y.)*, 1857,
96, 477-80.
Fluorescent treponemal antibody test. With V. H. Falcone and A. Harris.

2419.3   HUNTER, ELIZABETH F. *et al.*
An improved FTA test for syphilis; the absorption procedure (FTA-ABS).
Publ. Hlth. Rep. (Wash.), 1964, **79**, 410-412.
Absorbed fluorescent treponemal antibody (FTA-ABS) test. With W. E.
Deacon and P. E. Meyer.

2419.4   RATHLEV, TARA.
Haemagglutination test utilizing pathogenic *Treponema pallidum* for the
sero-diagnosis of syphilis. *Brit. J. vener. Dis.*, 1967, **43**, 181-5.
Treponemal haemagglutination (TPHA) test.

History of Syphilis

See also 5226-5227.1, HISTORY OF SEXUALLY TRANSMITTED DISEASES

2420   FUCHS, CONRAD HEINRICH. 1803-1855
Die ältesten Schriftseller über die Lustseuche in Deutschland, von 1495 bis
1510. Göttingen, *Dietrich*, 1843.
Gives texts of German tracts on syphilis published between 1495 and
1510.

2421   ROSENBAUM, JULIUS. 1807-1874
Geschichte der Lustseuche in Alterthume. Halle, *Lippert u. Schmidt*, 1845.
Second impression; first published in 1839. French translation, 1847;
English version, 1901. 7th edition (1904) reprinted Munich, *S. Karger*, 1971.

2422   BURET, FRÉDÉRIC.
Syphilis today and among the ancients. 2 vols. Philadelphia, *F. A. Davis*, 1891-
95.

2423   BLOCH, IWAN. 1872-1922
Der Ursprung der Syphilis. 2 pts. Jena, *G. Fischer*, 1901-11.
Bloch is the chief modern supporter of the theory of the Columbian
origin of syphilis.

2424   SUDHOFF, KARL FRIEDRICH JAKOB. 1853-1938
Aus der Frühgeschichte der Syphilis. Leipzig, *Barth*, 1912.
Sudhoff, one of the greatest medical historians, believed in the pre-
Columbian existence of syphilis.

2425   ——. Mal Franzoso in Italien in der ersten Hälfte des 15. Jahrhunderts.
Giessen, *A. Töpelmann*, 1912.
Forms Heft 5 of K. Sudhoff & G. Sticker: *Zur historischen Biologie der
Krankheitserreger.*

2426   DOHI, KEIZO. 1866-1931
Beiträge zur Geschichte der Syphilis; insbesondere über ihren Ursprung
und ihre Pathologie in Ostasien. Tokio, *Nankodo*, 1923.
Gives, in an appendix, a list of writers on syphilis from 1495 to 1829.

2427   SUDHOFF, KARL FRIEDRICH JAKOB. 1853-1938
The earliest printed literature on syphilis. Being ten tractates from the years
1495-98 ... Adapted by CHARLES SINGER. Florence, *R. Lier & Co.*, 1925.

2428   JEANSELME, ANTOINE EDOUARD. 1858-1935
        Histoire de la syphilis. Paris, *G. Doin*, 1931.
        Forms tome I of *Traité de la syphilis*, ed. by E. Jeanselme and E. Shulmann.

2429   PUSEY, WILLIAM ALLEN. 1865-1940
        The history and epidemiology of syphilis. Springfield, Ill., *C. C. Thomas*,
        1933.

2429.1 FLECK, LUDWIK.
        Entstehung und Entwicklung einer wissenschaftlichen Tatsache. Einführung
        in die Lehre vom Denkstil und Denkkollektiv. Basel, *Benno Schwabe*, 1935.
            A very thorough history of the discovery of the Wasserman reaction,
        and its acceptance by the scientific community. English translation: *Gen-
        esis and development of a scientific fact*, Chicago, *Univ. of Chicago Press*,
        1979.

2430   HOLCOMBE, RICHMOND CRANSTON. 1874-
        Who gave the world syphilis? The Haitian myth. New York, *Froeben Press*,
        1937.

2431   WHITWELL, JAMES RICHARD. 1863-1945
        Syphilis in earlier days. London, *H. K. Lewis*, 1940.

2432   GOODMAN, HERMAN. 1894-
        Notable contributors to the knowledge of syphilis. New York, *Froeben Press*,
        1944.

2432.1 DENNIE, CHARLES CLAYTON. 1883-?
        A history of syphilis. Springfield, *C. C. Thomas*, 1962.

LEPROSY

2433   ARETAEUS *the Cappadocian*. A.D. 81-138?
        On elephas, or elephantiasis. In his *Extant Works*, edited by FRANCIS ADAMS,
        London, 1856, 366-73, 494-98.
            Classical description of "elephantiasis Aretaei", nodous leprosy.

2434   DANIELSSEN, DANIEL CORNELIUS. 1815-1894, & BOECK, CARL WILHELM.
        1808-1875
        Om spedalskhed. Udgivet efter Foranstaltning af den Kongelige Norske
        Regjerings Department for det Indre. 1 vol. and atlas. Christiania (Bergen),
        trykt hos C. Gröndahl, 1847.
            First modern description of leprosy ("Danielssen–Boeck disease").
        Danielssen, physician to the leprosy hospital at Bergen, was the founder of
        scientific leprology. The extremely rare *Atlas* was published in Bergen; it
        consists of 24 plates and two pages of text. French translation, Paris, *J. B. Baillière*,
        1848; the atlas was also reproduced in French, Rio de Janeiro, in 1946.

2435   MOUAT, FREDERIC JOHN. 1816-1897
        Notes on native remedies. No. 1. The chaulmoogra. *Indian Ann. med. Sci.*,
        1854, **1**, 646-52.
            Chaulmoogra oil was first introduced into Western medicine by Mouat,
        having been used for many centuries previously by the Chinese.

2436   HANSEN, GERHARD HENRIK ARMAUER. 1841-1912
Indberetning til det Norske mediciniske Selskab i Christiania om en med understottelse af selskabet foretaghen reise for at anstille undersogelser angaende spedalskhedens arsager, tidels udforte sammen med forstander Hartwig. *Norsk. Mag. f Laegevidensk.*, 1874, 3 R., **4**, 9 Heft, 1-88; Case reports, i-liii.

Hansen discovered the leprosy bacillus on 28 February 1873. He had been stimulated by the previous work of Danielssen and Boeck, and his own demonstration of the leprosy bacillus is one of the earliest observations of pathogenic bacteria. For an English translation of the paper see *Brit. for. med. -chir. Rev.*, 1875, **55**, 459-89.

2436.1   NEISSER, ALBERT LUDWIG SIEGMUND. 1855-1916
Über die Ätiologie des Aussatzes. *Jber. akad. nat. Vereins Breslau*, 1879, **57**, 65-72.

Neisser obtained leprosy tissue from Hansen and, using aniline dyes for staining *Myco. leprae*, was able to demonstrate it more convincingly than Hansen.

2436.2   STEFANSKY, W. K.
Eine Lepraähnliche Erkrankung der Haut und der Lymphdrüsen bei Wanderratten. *Zbl. Bakt.*, 1903, I Abt. Orig., **33**, 481-7.
Murine leprosy described.

2437   POWER, FREDERICK BELDING. 1853-1927, & GORNALL, FRANK HOWORTH.
The constituents of chaulmoogra seeds. *J., chem. Soc.*, 1904, **85**, 838-51.

2438   ROST, ERNEST REINHOLD. 1872-?
The cultivation of the Bacillus leprae. *Indian med. Gaz.*, 1904, **39**, 167-69.
Rost cultivated the leprosy bacillus, and he prepared leprolin.

2439   UNNA, PAUL GERSON. 1850-1929
Histotechnik der leprösen Haut. Hamburg, Leipzig, 1910.
Unna was among the first to maintain that the lymphatics were involved in leprosy and that it was curable.

2440   MITSUDA, KENSUKE. 1876-
[On the value of a skin reaction to a suspension of leprous nodules.] *Hifuka Hinyoka Zasshi, [Jap. J. Derm. Urol.]*, 1919, **19**, 697-708.
Mitsuda (lepromin) reaction. English translation by the author in *Int. J. Leprosy*, 1953, **21**, 347-58.

2440.1   WADE, HERBERT WINDSOR. 1886-1968, & LARA, C. B.
A plea for the early recognition of leprosy, with notes on diagnosis and methods. *J. Philippine med. Ass.*, 1924, **4**, 132-40.
The scraped-incision slit-skin method for bacterial examination in leprosy.

2440.2   BUTTLE, GLADWIN ALBERT HURST. 1899-1983, *et al.*
The action of substances allied to 4:4'-diaminodiphenylsulphone in streptococcal and other infections in mice. *Biochem. J.*, 1938, **32**, 1101-10.
Dapsone (DDS). *See also* No. 1926.

2441   FAGET, Guy Henry. 1891-1947, *et al.*
The promin treatment of leprosy. A progress report. *Publ. Hlth Rep. (Wash.)*, 1943, **58**, 1729-41.
Promin (sodium glucosulphone) introduced in the treatment of leprosy. With R. C. Pogge, F. A. Johansen, J. F. Dinan, B. M. Prejean, and C. G. Eccles.

2442   MUIR, Ernest. 1880-1974
Preliminary report on diasone in the treatment of leprosy. *Int. J. Leprosy*, 1944, **12**, 1-6.
Muir found diasone (a sulphone) valuable in the treatment of leprosy.

2442.1   HARKNESS, Arthur Herbert, & BROWNLEE, G.
Leprosy treated with sulphetrone in 1943. *Proc. roy. Soc. Med.*, 1948, **41**, 309-10.
Clinical use of solapsone (sulphetrone).

2442.2   DAVEY, Thomas Frank 1907-1983, & CURRIE , Gordon.
Clinical trials of diphenyl thiourea compound SU 1906 (Ciba 1509E) in the treatment of leprosy. Progress during the first year. *Leprosy Rev.*, 1956, **27**, 94-111.
Introduction of diphenylthiourea (thiambutosine) therapy.

2442.3   ——., & HOGERZEIL, L. M.
Diethyl dithiolisophthalate in the treatment of leprosy (ETIP or "Etisul"); a progress report. *Leprosy Rev.*, 1959, **30**, 61-72.
Ditophal (Etisul) in leprosy.

2442.4   SHEPARD, Charles Carter. 1914-1985
Acid-fast bacilli in nasal excretions in leprosy, and results of inoculation of mice. *Amer. J. Hyg.*, 1960, **71**, 147-57.
Transmission of leprosy to animals. See also *J. exp. Med.*, 1960, **112**, 445.

2442.5   REES, Richard John William. 1917- , *et al.*
Experimental and clinical studies on rifampicin in treatment of leprosy. *Brit. med. J.*, 1970, **1**, 89-92.
With J. M. H. Pearson and M. F. R. Waters.

History of Leprosy

2443   ZAMBACO, Demetrius Alexandre, *Pasha*. 1830-1913
La lèpre à travers les siècles et les contrées. Paris, *Masson & Cie.*, 1914.

2444   MERCIER, Charles Arthur. 1852-1919
Leper houses and mediaeval hospitals. London, *H. K. Lewis*, 1915.

2446   WEYMOUTH, Anthony [*Pseudonym*].
Through the leper-squint. A study of leprosy from pre-Christian times to the present day. London, *Selwyn & Blount*, (1938).

2447   KEFFER, Luiza.
Indice bibliográfico de lepra, 1560-1943. 3 vols. São Paulo, 1944-48.
Supplements 1-5, 1952-62.

2447.1   FEENY, PATRICK.
          The fight against leprosy. London, *Elek*, 1964.

PARASITOLOGY

See also under individual diseases.

2448   TYSON, EDWARD. 1650-1708
          Lumbricus teres, or some anatomical observations on the round worm
          bred in human bodies. *Phil. Trans.*, 1683, **13**, 133-61.
          Tyson gave one of the first descriptions of the anatomy of *Ascaris
          lumbricoides.*

2448.1   REDI, FRANCESCO. 1626-1697
          Osservazioni ... intorno agli animali viventi che si trovano negli animali
          viventi. Firenze, *per P. Matini*, 1684.
          Redi was among the first of the parasitologists. He demonstrated the
          reproductive organs of *Ascaris lumbricoides* and also ascaris eggs. The
          results of his experiments appear in the above work, which also records his
          study and description of 108 different species.

2448.2   ANDRY, NICOLAS. 1658-1742
          De la géneration des vers dans le corps de l'homme. Paris, *d'Houry*, 1700.
          The first medical parasitology text – an exhaustive study of the parasites
          of man, the diseases associated with them and their treatment. Andry's
          views were often ahead of his time. Unlike most of his contemporaries, he
          did not believe in the spontaneous generation of parasites but clearly
          stated that their seeds entered the body from outside sources and that some
          foods were particularly liable to contain them. English translation, London,
          1701.

2449   RUDOLPHI, KARL ASMUND. 1771-1832
          Entozoorum, sive verminum intestinalium, historia naturalis. 2 vols.
          Amstelodami, 1808-10.
          A system of helminthology. Rudolphi gave the name "echinococcus" to
          the common vesicular hydatid, describing three species.

2450   KÜCHENMEISTER, GOTTLOB FRIEDRICH HEINRICH. 1821-1890
          Ueber Cestoden im allgemeinen und die des Menschen insbesondere.
          Zittau, *W. Pahl*, 1853.

2451   DAVAINE, CASIMIR JOSEPH. 1812-1882
          Traité des entozoaires et des maladies vermineuses. Paris, *J. B. Baillière*, 1860.

2452   COBBOLD, THOMAS SPENCER. 1828-1886
          Entozoa. 2 pts. London, *Groombridge & Sons*, 1864-69.
          Cobbold was the most distinguished helminthologist of his time. He
          named *Filaria bancrofti, Bilharzia haematobia*, and several other para-
          sites. He was a friend of Manson, several of whose papers he communi-
          cated to the Linnean Society and the Quekett Microscopical Club.

2453   LEUCKART, Karl Georg Friedrich Rudolf. 1823-1898
Die menschlichen Parasiten und die von ihnen herrührenden Krankheiten.
2 vols. Leipzig, *F. C. Winter*, 1863-76.
> English translation, Edinburgh, 1886.

2454   BRAUN, Maximilian Gustav Christian Carl. 1850-1930
Die thierischen Parasiten des Menschen. Würzburg, *A. Stuber*, 1883.

2455   MANSON, *Sir* Patrick. 1844-1922
The Filaria sanguinis hominis and certain new form of parasitic disease in
India, China and warm countries. London, *H. K. Lewis*, 1883.
> A collection of several papers written by Manson.

2456   BLANCHARD, Raphael Anatole Emile. 1857-1919
Traité de zoologie médicale. 2 vols. Paris, *J. B. Baillière*, 1886-90.

2457   KOCH, Robert. 1843-1910
Reise-Bericht über Rinderpest, Bubonenpest in Indien und Afrika, Tsetse-
oder Surrakrankheit, Texasfieber, tropische Malaria, Schwarzwasserfieber.
Berlin, *J. Springer*, 1898.

2458   CLARKE, James Jackson. 1860-1940
Protozoa and disease. 4 vols. London, *Baillière, Tindall & Cox*, 1903-15.

2459   LEIDY, Joseph. 1823-1891
Researches in helminthology and parasitology. With a bibliography of his
contributions to science. Washington, *Smithsonian Inst.*, 1904.
> In vol. 46 of *Smithsonian Miscellaneous Collections.* Leidy was the
> greatest descriptive naturalist in America.

2460   RANSOM, Brayton Howard. 1879-1925, & FOSTER, Winthrop Davenport.
1880-1918
Life history of *Ascaris lumbricoides* and related forms. *J. Agric. Res.*, 1917,
11, 395-98.

2461   STILES, Charles Wardell. 1867-1941, & HASSALL, Albert. 1862-1942
Key-catalogue of the protozoa reported for man. Washington, *Govt.
Printing Office*, 1925.

2462   WENYON, Charles Morley. 1878-1948
Protozoology. 2 vols. London, *Baillière, Tindall & Cox*, 1926.
> Wenyon was one of the world's foremost authorities on medical
> protozoology.

2463   LEIPER, Robert Thomson. 1881-1969
Landmarks in medical helminthology. *J. Helminth*, 1929, **7**, 101-18.

2463.1   FOSTER, William Derek. 1925-1981
A history of parasitology. Edinburgh, *E. S. Livingstone Ltd.*, 1965.

MICROBIOLOGY

2464   WILLIS, THOMAS. 1621-1675
Diatribae duae medico-philosophicae quarum prior agit de fermentatione sive de motu intestino particularum in quovis corpore. Londini, *T. Roycroft*, 1659.

Contains the earliest suggestion that fermentation is an intestinal or internal motion of particles; the analogy between putrefaction and fermentation is also noted.

2464.1   LEEUWENHOEK, ANTHONY VAN. 1632-1723
An abstract of a letter...Sep. 17, 1683. containing some microscopical observations, about animals in the scurf of the teeth. *Phil. Trans.*, 1684, **14**, 568-74.

Records discovery of bacteria in the mouth, with the first illustrations of the basic types – cocci, bacteria and spiral forms. Although Leeuwenhoek had observed bacteria earlier, this paper has usually been considered to be the first memoir on bacteria.

2465   GLEICHEN, WILHELM FRIEDRICH VON [*Called* RUSSWORM]. 1717-1783
Abhandlung über die Saamen- und Infusionsthierchen, und über die Erzeugung: nebst mikroskopischen Beobachtungen des Saamens der Thiere, und verschiedener Infusionen. Nürnberg, *A. W. Winterschmidt*, 1778.

Gleichen was probably the first to attempt to stain bacteria; he used carmine and indigo.

2466   MÜLLER, OTTO FRIEDRICH. 1730-1784
Animalcula infusoria fluviatilia et marina, quae detexit, systematice descripsit et ad vivum delineari. Hauniae, *N. Mölleri*, 1786.

Müller was the first to attempt a systematic classification of bacteria. He published several papers on the subject, the best being the above posthumous work.

2467   FABBRONI, ADAMO.
Dell'arte de fare il vino. Firenze, 1787.

Fabbroni is considered the first to promote modern ideas on the nature of fermentation. He showed that air was not considered necessary for fermentation to take place; he was first to regard the ferment as an albumenoid substance. Pasteur considered Fabbroni's work the beginning of modern ideas on the subject. Fabbroni's theory of the fermentation of wine was influential throughout the 19th century. Several of the terms used by him are in use today.

2467.1   APPERT, NICHOLAS. 1742-1841
L'Art de conserver, pendant plusieurs années, toutes les substances animales et végétales...Paris, *Patris*, 1810.

The first workable process for canning foods. In 1795 Appert began developing the process under Napoleon's auspices as a way to maintain food on military expeditions. For strategic reasons he was not allowed to publish the secret method until 1810. Appert's method was strictly empirical. Pasteur eventually discovered a scientific explanation for the process and refined its operation. *See* Nos. 2479 & 2480.

2468   KERNER, CHRISTIAN ANDREAS JUSTINUS. 1786-1862
        Neue Beobachtungen über die in Würtemberg so häufig vorfallenden
        tödtlichen Vergiftung durch den Genuss geräuchter Würste. Tübingen, *C.
        F. Osiander*, 1820.
        Botulism first described.

2469   EHRENBERG, CHRISTIAN GOTTFRIED. 1795-1876
        Die Infusionsthierschen als vollkommene Organismen. 1 vol. and atlas.
        Leipzig, *L. Voss*, 1838.
        Includes (p. 80) first description of *B. subtilis*.

2470   DUJARDIN, FÉLIX. 1801-1860
        Histoire naturelle des zoophytes. Paris, *Lib. encyclopéd. de Roret*, 1841.
        Further modification of and improvements in the classification of
        bacteria.

2471   GOODSIR, JOHN. 1814-1867
        History of a case in which a fluid periodically ejected from the stomach
        contained vegetable organisms of an undescribed form. *Edinb. med. surg.
        J.*, 1842, **57**, 430-43.
        First description of *Sarcina ventriculi*, discovered by Goodsir.

2472   PASTEUR, LOUIS. 1822-1895
        Mémoire sur la fermentation appelée lactique. *C. R. Acad. Sci. (Paris)*, 1857,
        45, 913-16.
        First demonstration of the connection between a specific fermentation
        and the activity of a specific living micro-organism. This paper is often
        considered the beginning of bacteriology as a modern science. The above
        work is a very much abridged "Extrait par l'auteur" of the complete text of
        Pasteur's full paper which underwent roughly simultaneous publication in
        Mémoires de la Société des Sciences, de l'Agriculture et des Arts de Lille, 2e
        sér.,1858, **5**, 13-26, and in *Ann. de Chim. et de Phys.*, 3e sér.,1858, **52**, 408-
        18.

2473   ——. Nouveaux faits pour servir à l'histoire de la levure lactique. *C. R. Acad.
        Sci. (Paris)*, 1859, **48**, 337-38.
        This and the preceding entry mark Pasteur's commencement of the
        study of fermentation. This paper described Pasteur's method of cultivat-
        ing micro-organisms in a medium free of organic nitrogen to produce
        fermentations. The method was absolutely fundamental to his work, but
        not developed for his initial paper on lactic fermentation. He found that the
        conversion of sugar to lactic acid in fermentation is due to small corpuscles,
        isolated or grouped.

2474   ——. Expériences relatives aux générations dites spontanées. *C. R. Acad.
        Sci. (Paris)*, 1860, **50**, 303-07, 849-54; **51**, 348-52, 675-78.

2475   ——. Mémoire sur les corpuscles organisés qui existent dans l'atmosphère.
        Examen de la doctrine des générations spontanées. *Ann. Sci. nat. (Zool.)*,
        1861, **16**, 5-98.
        In these easily reproducible experiments, prefaced by an important
        historical introduction, Pasteur demonstrated beyond dispute that fermen-
        tation is caused by the action of minute living organisms, and that if these
        are excluded or killed fermentation does not occur. The heating process

which Pasteur recommended for sterilization was the earliest form of "pasteurization". The above paper marks the downfall of the theory of spontaneous generation. Pasteur's researches on fermentation led him to the discovery of the bacteria and yeasts and hence to the germ theory of disease; from this all modern bacteriology and immunology have developed.

2475.1 ——. Animalcules infusoires vivant sans gaz oxygène libre et déterminant des fermentations. *C. R. Acad. Sci. (Paris)*, 1861, **52**, 344-47

The discovery of strict anaerobiosis, important for general biology since it shows that oxygen gas is not a requisite for life.

2476 ——. Nouvel exemple de fermentation determinée par des animalcules infusoires pouvant vivre sans gaz oxygène libre, et en dehors de tout contact avec l'air de l'atmosphere. *C. R. Acad. Sci. (Paris)*, 1863, **56**, 416-21.

Pasteur confirmed the fact, established by Schwann (No. 674) that putrefaction was a biological process.

2477 ——. Examen du rôle attribué au gaz oxygène atmosphérique dans la destruction des matières et végétales après la mort. *C. R. Acad. Sci. (Paris)*, 1863, **56**, 734-40.

2478 ——. Recherches sur la putréfaction. *C. R. Acad. Sci. (Paris)*, 1863, **56**, 1189-94.

Pasteur was the first to differentiate between aerobic and anaerobic organisms. (*See also* Nos. 2476-77.)

2479 ——. Études sur le vin. Paris, *Imp. impériale*, 1866.

Although Pasteur's method of preserving wine by partial heat sterilization ("pasteurization") turned out to be a revival of Appert's invention (No.2467.1), Pasteur did rescue the method from oblivion and established on the basis of rigorous scientific experiments what had been only a poorly tested and entirely empirical technique.

2480 ——. Études sur le vinaigre. Paris, *Gauthier-Villars*, 1868.

Pasteur proved that a micro-organism was essential to acetification and developed a patented method which greatly increased the efficiency of production.

2481 ——. Études sur la maladie des vers à soie. 2 vols. Paris, *Gauthier-Villars*, 1870.

This work saved the French silk industry, which had been crippled by the disease *pébrine*. After five years of research on the problem, Pasteur found the germs of this disease not only in the silkworms but also in their moths and ova. He demonstrated a successful method of overcoming the plague by a systematic microscopic examination of ova with elimination of all those found to be diseased.

2482 WEIGERT, CARL. 1845-1904
Ueber Bakterien in der Pockenhaut. *Zbl. med. Wiss.*, 1871, **9**, 609-11.

Weigert, famous as pathologist and histologist, was the first to stain bacteria. He introduced many of the best staining methods in use today.

Weigert discovered bacteria in haemorrhagic smallpox. In the same paper is described how carmine will colour cocci.

2483   COHN, FERDINAND JULIUS. 1828-1898
Untersuchungen über Bacterien. *Beitr. Biol. Pflanzen*, 1872, **1**, Heft 2, 127-224; 1875, Heft 3, 141-207; 1876, **2**, Heft 2, 249-76.
Cohn's morphological classification of bacteria. He founded the *Beiträge*.

2484   LISTER, JOSEPH, 1*st Baron Lister*. 1827-1912
A further contribution to the natural history of bacteria and the germ theory of fermentative changes. *Quart. J. micr. Sci.*, 1873, n.s. **13**, 380-408.
Isolation of *Bacterium lactis,* the specific micro-organism responsible for the lactic acid fermentation of milk.

2485   PASTEUR, LOUIS. 1822-1895
Études sur la bière ... avec une théorie nouvelle de la fermentation. Paris, *Gauthier-Villars,* 1876.
Pasteur resumed his studies on fermentation in 1876, and in this book takes into account the developments in this field since his previous publications on the subject. He described a new and perfected method of preparing pure yeast and acknowledged that a limited quantity of oxygen was important for brewing. Facsimile reproduction in 1920; English translation, 1879.

2486   WEIGERT, CARL. 1845-1904
Ueber eine Mykose bei einem neugeborenen Kinde (Bakterienfärbung mit Anilinfarben). *Jber. schles. Ges. vaterl. Cultur*, (1875), 1876, **53**, 229.
In this paper Weigert showed that methyl violet will reveal cocci in tissues.

2487   EHRLICH, PAUL. 1854-1915
Beitrag zur Kenntnis der Anilinfärbungen und ihrer Verwendung in der mikroskopischen Technik. *Arch. mikr. Anat.*, 1877, **13**, 263-77.
Ehrlich's first paper on the staining of specific granulation in white blood corpuscles by means of aniline dyes. His work immensely affected subsequent technical methods of staining.

2488   KOCH, ROBERT. 1843-1910
Verfahrungen zur Untersuchung, zum Conserviren und Photographiren der Bacterien. *Beitr. Biol. Pflanzen*, 1877, **2**, 399-434.
Koch greatly improved staining methods; he laid the foundations of the technical procedures employed today. In the above paper he described his method of making films of bacteria on cover-slips and fixing them gently by heat; he also gave details of his method of photographing bacteria. In some of his plates the cilia are clearly perceptible.

2489   LISTER, JOSEPH, 1*st Baron Lister*. 1827-1912
On the lactic fermentation and its bearings on pathology. *Trans. path. Soc. Lond.*, 1877-78, **29**, 425-67.
Lister was the first to obtain a pure culture of a bacterium *(Bact. lactis).*

2490   PASTEUR, LOUIS. 1822-1895, & JOUBERT, JULES FRANÇOIS.
Charbon et septicémie. *C. R. Acad. Sci. (Paris)*, 1877, **85**, 101-15.
Discovery of *Vibrion septique (Cl. septicum),* the first pathogenic anaerobe to be found.

2491 TYNDALL, JOHN. 1820-1893
Fermentation and its bearings on the phenomena of disease. Glasgow, *W. Collins*, 1877.
See No. 2495.

2492 MAGNIN, ANTOINE.
Les bactéries. Paris, *F. Savy*, 1878.
English translation by G. M. Sternberg, 1880.

2492.1 PASTEUR, LOUIS. 1822-1895
De l'extension de la théorie des germes à l'étiologie de quelques maladies communes. *C.R. Acad. Sci. (Paris)*, 1880, **90**, 1033-44.
In this study of furunculosis ("boils") and osteomyelitis Pasteur left the first recognizable descriptions of staphylococcus and streptococcus. The term *streptococcus* had been coined by Billroth in 1874; however, Pasteur did not use it here. Ogston (*see* No.2494) named staphylococcus in 1881.

2493 EHRLICH, PAUL. 1854-1915
Ueber das Methylenblau und seine klinisch-bakterioskopische Verwerthung. *Z. klin. Med.*, 1881, **2**, 710-13.
Introduction of methylene blue in bacteriological staining.

2494 OGSTON, *Sir* ALEXANDER. 1844-1929
Report upon micro-organisms in surgical diseases. *Brit. med. J.*, 1881, **1**, 369-75.
Ogston showed micrococci to be constantly present in acute and chronic abscesses. He discovered *Staph. aureus*. Ogston named *staphyloccocus* in his paper: Micrococcus poisoning, *J. Anat. Physiol.*, 1882, **16**, 526-6; & 1883, **17**, 24-58.

2495 TYNDALL, JOHN. 1820-1893
Essays on the floating-matter of the air in relation to putrefaction and infection. London, *Longmans, Green & Co.*, 1881.
Tyndall interested himself in atmospheric germs and dust. His experiments on sterilization by heat led him to the discovery in 1877 of fractional sterilization (Tyndallization). His work on the subject is included in the above book, in which he also described the bactericidal effects of moulds. The researches of Tyndall, even more than those of Pasteur, dealt the final blow to the doctrine of spontaneous generation; they were fundamental for the progress of bacteriology. *See* No. 1932.

2495.1 KOCH, ROBERT. 1843-1910
Zur Untersuchungen von pathogenen Organismen. *Mittheil. Kais. Gesundheitsamte*, 1881, **1**, 1-48.
Koch's description of his methods of growing bacterial cultures in gelatine solutions, making films of bacteria on cover slips and fixing them by gentle heat, and staining slides differentially by aniline. These methods are the bases on which bacteriology largely rests.

2496 FEHLEISEN, FRIEDRICH. 1854-1924
Ueber Erysipel. *Dtsch. Z. Chir.*, 1882, **16**, 391-97.
Discovery of *Strep. pyogenes*. English translation, 1886.

2497   GESSARD, CARLE. 1850-1925
        Sur les colorations bleue et verte des linges à pansements. *C. R. Acad. Sci.
        (Paris)*, 1882, **94**, 536-38.
        Isolation of *Pseudomonas aeruginosa (Ps. pyocyanea)*.

2498   MALASSEZ, LOUIS CHARLES. 1842-1909, & VIGNAL, W.
        Sur une forme de tuberculose sans bacilles. *C. R. Soc. Biol.*, 1883, 7 sér., **5**,
        338-41.
        Isolation of *Pasteurella pseudotuberculosis*.

2498.1 CHAMBERLAND, CHARLES. 1851-1908
        Sur un filtre donnant de l'eau physiologiquement pure. *C. R. Acad. Sci.
        (Paris)*, 1884, **99**, 247-48.
        Chamberland filter.

2499   GRAM, HANS CHRISTIAN JOACHIM. 1853-1938
        Ueber die isolirte Färbung der Schizomyceten in Schnitt- und Trocken-
        präparaten. *Fortschr. Med.*, 1884, **2**, 185-89.
        Gram's method of staining bacteria – one of the most widely used today.

2500   BARY, HEINRICH ANTON DE. 1831-1888
        Vorlesungen über Bacterien. Leipzig, *W. Engelmann*, 1885.

2501   CORNIL, ANDRÉ VICTOR. 1837-1908, & BABÈS, VICTOR. 1854-1926
        Les bactéries et leur rôle dans l'anatomie et l'histologie pathologiques des
        maladies infectieuses. 1 vol. and atlas. Paris, *F. Alcan*, 1885.

2502   HAUSER, GUSTAV. 1856-1935
        Ueber Fäulnissbacterien. Leipzig, *F. C. W. Vogel*, 1885.
        Isolation of *Proteus vulgaris*.

2503   HUEPPE, FERDINAND ADOLF THEOPHIL. 1852-1938
        Die Methoden der Bakterienforschung. Wiesbaden, *Kriedel*, 1885.
        Hueppe, a colleague of Koch, wrote an admirable manual on bac-
        teriological methods, a subject to which he gave several original contribu-
        tions. English translation, New York, 1901.

2503.1 MAYER, ADOLF EDUARD MAYDOLF. 1843-?
        Ueber die Mosaikkrankheit des Tabaks. *Landw. VersSta.*, 1886, **32**, 450-67.
        Mayer was first to describe and name the mosaic disease of tobacco and
        to demonstrate its infectious nature. Translation in *Phytopathological
        Classics*, No. 7, pp. 9-24, Ithaca, 1942. *See* No. 2506.2.

2504   CROOKSHANK, EDGAR MARCH. 1858-1928
        An introduction to practical bacteriology based upon the methods of Koch.
        London, *H. K. Lewis*, 1886.
        Crookshank studied under Koch, and later became Professor of Bac-
        teriology at King's College, London.

2505   SALMON, DANIEL ELMER. 1850-1914, & SMITH, THEOBALD. 1859-1934
        The bacterium of swine-plague. *Amer. monthly micr. J.*, 1886, **7**, 204-05.
        Discovery of *Salmonella cholerae-suis*. The Salmonelleae tribe was
        named after Salmon, even though the discovery was made by Smith. See
        Bibel, *Milestones in immunology* (1988) 31-32..

2505.1 PETRI, RICHARD JULIUS. 1852-1921
Eine kleine Modification des Koch'schen Plattenverfahrens. *Zbl. Bakt.*, 1887, **1**, 279-80.
Petri dish. A similar dish was described by Cornil and Babès (*see* No. 2501) and by Nicati and Rietsch, *Arch. Physiol. norm. path.*, 1885, **6**, 72. Petri was an assistant of Koch.

2506 GAERTNER, AUGUST ANTON HIERONYMUS. 1848-1934
Ueber die Fleischvergiftung in Frankenhausen. a.K. und den Erreger derselben. *Korrespbl. ärztl Ver. Thüringen*, 1888, **17**, 573-600.
Discovery of *Salmonella enteritidis*, a cause of food poisoning.

2506.1 NORDTMEYER, H.
Ueber Wasserfiltration durch Filter aus gebrannter Infusorienerde. *Z. Hyg. InfektKr.*, 1891, **10**, 145-54.
Berkefeld kieselguhr filter.

2506.2 IVANOVSKI, DMITRI IOSIFOVICH. 1864-1920
Ueber die Mosaikkrankheit der Tabakspflanze. *Bull. Acad. imp. Sci. St. Petersburg*, 1892, **3**, 67-70.
The Russian botanist Ivanovski demonstrated that the agent responsible for tobacco mosaic disease could pass through the finest filter then available. This was the starting point of research into the aetiology of virus diseases. An English version is in *Phytopathological Classics* (American Phytopathological Society), No. 7, pp. 25-30, Ithaca , N.Y., 1942. *See* No. 2503.1.

2507 LOEFFLER, FRIEDRICH AUGUST JOHANN. 1852-1915
Ueber Epidemieen unter den im hygienischen Institute zu Greifswald gehaltenen Mäusen und über die Bekämpfung der Feldmausplage. *Zbl. Bakt.*, 1892, **11**, 129-41.
Isolation of *Salm. typhi-murium*.

2508 WELCH, WILLIAM HENRY. 1850-1934, & NUTTALL, GEORGE HENRY FALKINER. 1862-1937
A gas-producing bacillus (Bacillus aërogenes capsulatus nov. spec.) capable of rapid development in the blood-vessels after death. *Johns Hopk. Hosp. Bull.*, 1892, **3**, 81-91.
Discovery of the gas gangrene bacillus (Welch bacillus) *Cl. perfringens*. Reprinted in *Med. Classics*, 1941, **5**, 852-85.

2509 STERNBERG, GEORGE MILLER. 1838-1915
A manual of bacteriology. New York, *W. Wood & Co.*, 1892.
Sternberg, U. S. Surgeon General 1893-1902, was a pioneer bacteriologist. Independently of Pasteur he discovered the pneumococcus and was first in America to photograph the tubercle bacillus. He sent Walter Reed off to make his great discoveries regarding yellow fever.

2510 ERMENGEM, EMILE PIERRE MARIE VAN. 1851-1932
Contribution à l'étude des intoxications alimentaires. Recherches sur des accidents à caractères botuliniques provoqués par du jambon. *Arch. Pharmacodyn.*, 1897, **3**, 213-350, 499-601.
Cl. botulinum was discovered by van Ermengem in cases of food poisoning.

2511   LOEFFLER, FRIEDRICH AUGUST JOHANN. 1852-1915, & FROSCH, PAUL. 1860-1928
        Bericht der Kommission zur Erforschung der Maul- und Klauenseuche bei dem Institut für Infektionskrankheiten. *Zbl. Bakt.*, 1898, I. Abt., **23**, 371-91.
        Loeffler and Frosch proved that foot-and-mouth disease is caused by a filter-passing virus; this is the first recognition of such a virus as the cause of animal disease.

2512   BEIJERINCK, MARTINUS WILLEM. 1851-1931
        Ueber ein Contagium vivum fluidum als Ursache der Fleckenkrankheit der Tabaksblätter. *Verb. k. Acad. Wet. Amst.*, 1898, **65** (2), 3-21.
        Beijerinck confirmed the findings of Ivanovski. He showed that the tobacco mosaic virus would diffuse through agar. Translation in *Phytopathological Classics*, 1942, No. 7.

2513   DURHAM, HERBERT EDWARD. 1866-1945
        On an epidemic of gastro-enteritis associated with the presence of a variety of the Bacillus enteritidis (Gaertner), and with positive sero-diagnostic evidence (in vivo and in vitro). *Brit. med. J.*, 1898, **2**, 600-01.
        Discovery of *Salm. aertrycke* in patients suffering from food poisoning.

2514   NOBELE, JULES DE. 1865-?
        Du séro-diagnostic dans les affections gastro-intestinales d'origine alimentaire. *Ann. Soc. Méd. Gand*, 1898, **77**, 281-306.
        Discovery of *Salmonella aertrycke*, independently of Durham.

2515   MORO, ERNST. 1874-1951
        Ueber die nach Gram färbbaren Bacillen des Säuglingsstuhles. *Wien. klin. Wschr.*, 1900, **13**, 114-15.
        Isolation of *Lactobacillus acidophilus*.

2516   WELCH, WILLIAM HENRY. 1850-1934
        Morbid conditions caused by Bacillus aërogenes capsulatus. *Johns Hopk. Hosp. Bull.*, 1900, **11**, 185-204.
        Welch grouped together the diseases caused by *Cl. perfringens*, earlier discovered by him in association with Nuttall (*see* No. 2508).

2517   KOLLE, WILHELM. 1868-1935, & WASSERMANN, AUGUST VON. 1866-1925
        Handbuch der pathogenen Mikroorganismen. 6 vols. Jena, *G. Fischer*, 1903-09.
        Third edition, 10 vols. [in 19], 1929-31.

2518   SMITH, ERWIN FRINK. 1854-1927
        Bacteria in relation to plant diseases. 3 vols. Washington, *Carnegie Inst.*, 1905-14.
        One of the most careful investigations of the bacterial diseases in plants was made by Smith, who conclusively demonstrated the existence of such diseases and proposed a scheme of classification for the bacteria concerned.

2518.1 MORGAN, HARRY DE RIEMER. 1863-1931
        Upon the bacteriology of the summer diarrhoea of infants. *Brit. med. J.*, 1906, **1**, 908-12.
        Morgan's bacillus, *Proteus morgani*.

2518.2 BECHHOLD, HEINRICH. 1866-1937
Kolloidstudien mit der Filtrationsmethode. *Z. phys. Chem.*, 1907, **60**, 257-318.
Bechhold devised ultrafiltration methods for studies in microbiology.

2519 NOGUCHI, HIDEYO. 1876-1928
Pure cultivation of Spirochaeta refringens. *J. exp. Med.*, 1912, **15**, 446-69.
Noguchi obtained pure cultures of spirochaetae. See also his later papers in the same journal, 1912, **16**, 199-210, 620-28.

2520 WEINBERG, MICHEL. 1868-1940, & SEGUIN, P.
Notes bactériologiques sur les infections gazeuses. *C. R. Soc. Biol. (Paris)*, 1915, **78**, 274-79.
Isolation of *Cl. oedematiens.*

2521 ——. Contribution à l'étiologie de la gangrène gazeuse. *C. R. Acad. Sci. (Paris)*, 1916, **163**, 449-51.
Isolation of *Cl. histolyticum.*

2521.1 LIPSCHÜTZ, BENJAMIN. 1878-1931
Untersuchungen über die Ätiologie der Krankheiten der Herpesgruppe (Herpes zoster, Herpes genitalis, Herpes febrilis). *Arch. Derm. Syph. (Wien)*, 1921, **136**, 428-82.
Lipschütz's important account of herpes virus diseases included identification of the characteristic inclusion bodies ("Zosterkörperchen").

2522 BERGEY, DAVID HENDRICKS. 1860-1937
Manual of determinative bacteriology. Baltimore, *Williams & Wilkins Co.*, 1923.
The Society of American Bacteriologists appointed in 1920 a Committee on Characterization and Classification of Bacterial Types. Their reports were incorporated in the above *Manual* issued under the names of Bergey and his associates. 8th ed., 1974.

2522.1 MURRAY, EVERITT GEORGE DUNNE. 1890-1964, *et al.*
A disease of rabbits characterised by a large mononuclear leucocytosis, caused by a hitherto undescribed bacillus *Bacterium monocytogenes* (n. sp.). *J. Path. Bact.*, 1926, **29**, 407-39.
Isolation of *Listeria monocytogenes.* With R. A. Webb and M. B. R. Swann.

2523 THOMSON, DAVID. 1884-1969, & THOMSON, ROBERT. 1888-
The pathogenic streptococci. An historical survey of their role in human and animal disease. *Ann. Pickett-Thomson Res. Lab.*, 1928-29, **4**, pt. 1-2. London, 1928-29.
Documents over 1,600 studies.

2524 ELFORD, WILLIAM JOSEPH. 1900-1952
A new series of graded collodion membranes suitable for general bacteriological use, especially in filterable virus studies. *J. Path. Bact.*, 1931, **34**, 505-21.
In his important studies on the filtration of virus preparations, Elford showed that different viruses possessed different and characteristic sizes.

2524.1   WOODRUFF, ALICE MILES, & GOODPASTURE, ERNEST WILLIAM. 1886-1960
The susceptibility of the chorio-allantoic membrane of chick embryos to
infection with the fowl-pox virus. *Amer. J. Path.*, 1931, **7**, 209-22.

By their demonstration of the infection of the chorio-allantoic membrane
with the virus of fowl pox, Woodruff and Goodpasture initiated widespread adoption of this host for the study of viruses.

2524.2   LANCEFIELD, REBECCA CRAIGHILL. 1895-1981
A serological differentiation of human and other groups of hemolytic
streptococci. *J. exp. Med.*, 1933, **57**, 571-95.

Lancefield determined the principal pathogenic strains of haemolytic
streptococci and subdivided them into types. All important strains
pathogenic to humans fall into Lancefield's Group A.

2524.3   GRIFFITH, FREDERICK. ?1879-1941
The serological classification of *Streptococcus pyogenes. J. Hyg. (Camb.)*,
1934, **34**, 542-84.

Griffith's classification of streptococci.

2524.4   KLIENEBERGER, EMMY. 1892-1985
The natural occurrence of pleuropneumonia-like organisms in apparent
symbiosis with *Streptobacillus moniliformis* and other bacteria. *J. Path.
Bact.*, 1935, **40**, 93-105.

Klieneberger isolated typical strains of pleuropneumonia-like organisms from *Strep. moniliformis.*

2524.5   STANLEY, WENDELL MEREDITH. 1904-1971
Isolation of a crystalline protein possessing the properties of tobacco-
mosaic virus. *Science*, 1935, **81**, 644-45.

Isolation of a virus in the form of a crystalline material, subsequently
shown to be a nucleoprotein.

2524.6   SCHLESINGER, MAX. 1906-1937
The Feulgen reaction of the bacteriophage substance. *Nature (Lond.)*, 1936,
138, 508-09.

Schlesinger showed the fundamental constituents of bacteriophages to
consist mainly of approximately equal amounts of protein and DNA.

2525   McCOY, ELIZABETH FLORENCE. 1903- , & McCLUNG, LELAND SWINT. 1910-
The anaerobic bacteria and their activities in nature and disease. A subject
bibliography. 2 vols. Berkeley, *Univ. of California Press*, 1939. Supplements were published: 1938-1975, 8 vols., 1941-82.

2526   MacCALLUM. *Sir* PETER. 1885-1975, *et al.*
A new mycobacterial infection in man. *J. Path. Bact.*, 1948, **60**, 93-122.

Myco. ulcerans first described. With J. C. Tolhurst, G. Buckle, and H. A.
Sissons.

2526.1   LURIA, SALVADOR EDWARD. 1912- , & DULBECCO, RENATO. 1914-
Genetic recombinations leading to production of active bacteriophage
from ultraviolet inactivated bacteriophage particles. *Genetics*, 1949, **34**, 93-
125.

Luria shared the Nobel Prize in 1969 with M. Delbrück (No. 2578.5) and A. D. Hershey (No. 256) for work on genetics and replication of bacteria.

2526.2   ROWE, WALLACE PRESCOTT. 1926- , *et al.*
Isolation of a cytopathogenic agent from human adenoids undergoing spontaneous degeneration in tissue culture. *Proc. Soc. exp. Biol. (N.Y.)*, 1953, **84**, 570-73.
Discovery of adenoviruses. With R. J. Huebner, L. K. Gilmore, R. H. Parrott, and T. G. Ward.

2527   FRAENKEL-CONRAT, HEINZ LUDWIG. 1910- , & WILLIAMS, ROBLEY COOK. 1908-
Reconstitution of active tobacco mosaic virus from its inactive protein and nucleic acid components. *Proc. nat. Acad. Sci. (Wash.)*, 1955, **41**, 690-98.
First reconstitution of a virus.

2527.1   SCHAFFER, FREDERICK LELAND. 1921- , & SCHWERDT, CARLTON EVERETT. 1917-
Crystallization of purified MEF-1 poliomyelitis virus particles. *Proc. nat. Acad. Sci. (Wash.)*, 1955, **41**, 1020-23.
First crystallization of an animal virus.

2527.2   SMITH, MARGARET G.
Propagation in tissue culture of a cytopathogenic virus from human salivary gland virus (SGV) disease. *Proc. Soc. exp. Biol. Med.*, 1956, **92**, 424-30.
Isolation of cytomegalovirus.

2527.3   SWEET, BENJAMIN HERSH. 1924- , & HILLEMAN, MAURICE RALPH. 1919-
The vacuolating virus SV$_{40}$. *Proc. Soc. exp. Biol. (N.Y.)*, 1960, **105**, 420-27.
Simian virus type 40.

See 2579-2581.9, for history of microbiology

INFECTION: IMMUNOLOGY: SEROLOGY

2527.99   RHAZES [ABU BAKR MUHAMMAD IBN ZAKARIYA AL-RAZI]. *Circa* 824-925 or 935
De variolis et morbillis commentarius. Londini, *G. Bowyer*, 1766.
In his *Treatise on the smallpox and measles*, Rhazes stated that survival from smallpox infection prevented an individual from ever acquiring the disease again. His explanation for why the disease does not strike the same individual twice is the first theory of acquired immunity. *See* No. 5404.

2528   FRACASTORO, GIROLAMO [FRACASTORIUS]. 1478-1553
De sympathia et antipathia rerum liber unus. De contagione et contagiosis morbis et curatione. Venetiis, *apud heredes L. Iuntae*, 1546.
This book represents a landmark in the development of our knowledge of infectious disease. Fracastoro was the first to state the germ theory of infection. He recognized typhus and suggested the contagiousness of tuberculosis. Haeser even describes him as the "founder of scientific epidemiology". An English translation by W. C. Wright appeared in 1930. *See* No. 5371.

2528.1   KIRCHER, Athanasius. 1602-1680
          Scrutinium physico-medicum contagiosae luis, quae pestis dicitur. Romae,
          typ. Mascardi, 1658.
                Kircher was probably the first to employ the microscope in investigat-
          ing the cause of disease. He mentioned that the blood of plague patients
          was filled with a "countless brood of worms not perceptible to the naked
          eye, but to be seen in all putrefying matter through the microscope"
          (Garrison). He could not have seen the plague bacillus with his low-power
          microscope, but he probably saw the larger micro-organisms. He was the
          first to state explicitly the theory of contagion by animalculae as the cause
          of infectious diseases.

2529   NEEDHAM, Marchamont [Nedham]. 1620-1678
          Medela medicinae. London, *R. Lownds*, 1665.
                Needham, a physician better known for his work in journalism, was one
          of the earliest – if not the first – Englishman to write on the germ theory. In
          his book he included an account of Kircher's experiments with the
          microscope.

2529.1   BONOMO, Giovanni Cosimo. 1663-1696 & CESTONI, Giacinto. 1637-1718
          Osservazioni intorno a' pellicelli del corpo umano. Firenze, *Piero Matini*,
          1687.
                First clinical and experimental proof of infection by a microparasite.
          Bonomo observed *Sarcoptes scabiei*, the scabies mite. This gave re-
          searchers grounds to think in terms of objective, exogenous pathogenic
          agents as the cause of disease. *See* No. 4012.

2529.2   COGROSSI, Carlo Francesco. 1682-1769
          Nuovo idea del male contagioso de' buoi. Milano, *Marc'Antonio Pandolfo
          Malatesta*, 1714.
                In this study of an epizootic Cogrossi formulated much of the modern
          theory of infection. He speculated that infection might occur at the
          microscopic level, and argued that infected individuals should be isolated
          and cured, that those believed to have been exposed to the disease should
          be isolated, and that the personal belongings of both groups should be
          disinfected to exterminate the causitive agent and its eggs. He also
          speculated on the entrance routes of the infection and its transmission
          through secretions and excretions of the infected animal. Facsimile reprint
          with English translation by D.M. Schullian and foreword by L. Belloni,
          Roma, *Società Italiana di Microbiologia*, 1953.

2529.3   JENNER, Edward. 1749-1823
          An inquiry into the causes and effects of the variolae vaccinae. London, *S.
          Low*, 1798.
                Jenner established the fact that a "vaccination" or inoculation with
          vaccinia (cowpox) lymph matter protects against smallpox. What is probably
          the first mention of anaphylaxis appears on p. 13. *See* No. 5423.

2530   GASPARD, Marie Humbert Bernard. 1788-1871
          Mémoire physiologique sur les maladies purulentes et putrides, sur la
          vaccine, *etc. J. Physiol. exp. path.*, 1822, **2**, 1-45; 1824, **4**, 1-69.
                Gaspard was one of the first to make experimental studies on pyaemia
          following the injection of putrid fluids. He experimented on dogs, sheep,

foxes, and pigs, injecting putrid infusions pus, vaccine, lymph, blood, bile, urine, saliva, carbolic acid, hydrogen, or sulphuretted hydrogen.

2531   MARX, KARL FRIEDRICH HEINRICH. 1796-1877
Origines contagii. Caroliruhae et Badae, *D. R. Marx*, 1824.
A supplementary "Additamenta" was published in 1826.

2532   BASSI, AGOSTINO. 1773-1856
Del mal del segno calcinaccio o moscardino malattia che affligge i bachi da seta e sul modo di liberarne le bigattaje anche le piu infestate. 2 vols. Lodi, *Orcesi*, 1835-36.
By his demonstration of the parasitic nature of the muscardine disease of silkworms, Bassi is regarded as the founder of the doctrine of pathogenic micro-organisms. He is rather neglected by medical historians. Facsimile reprint, Pavia, 1956. His *Opere* were published in 1925.

2533   HENLE, FRIEDRICH GUSTAV JACOB. 1809-1885
Von den Miasmen und Contagien. In his *Pathologische Untersuchungen*, Berlin, 1840, pp. 1-82.
Bassi's work on the muscardine disease of silkworms (*see* No. 2532), with its prophecy of the discovery of microbes as the causal agents of other diseases, inspired Henle to write his famous essay on miasms and contagions. He laid down postulates on the aetiological relation of microbes to disease which became fundamentals of bacteriology and which did much to check the reckless speculation which had arisen regarding micro-organisms. Koch later developed these postulates (*see* Nos. 2331, 2536, and 5167). English translation in *Bull. Hist. Med.*, 1936, **6**, 911-83.

2534   PANUM, PETER LUDVIG. 1820-1885
Bidrag til Laeren om den saakaldte putride eller septiske Infection. *Bibl. Laeger*, 1856, 4 R., **8**, 253-85.
Panum was the first to investigate the chemical products of putrefaction. His work had great significance for the doctrine of putrid intoxication. An abstract of the above paper is in *Jb. in- u. ausländ. ges. Med.*, 1859, **101**, 213-17.

2535   KLEBS, THEODOR ALBRECHT EDWIN. 1834-1913
Die Ursache der infectiösen Wundkrankheiten. *Cor.-Bl. d. schweiz. Aerzte*, 1871, **1**, 241-46.
Klebs, Professor of Pathology at Berne, Würzburg, Prague, Zurich, and Chicago, preceded Koch in investigations of the pathology of traumatic infection. He found bacteria in gunshot wounds, granulation tissue, etc., and developed his theory of a single organism, *Microsporon septicum*, as the cause of all pathological changes.

2536   KOCH, ROBERT. 1843-1910
Untersuchungen über die Aetiologie der Wundinfectionskrankheiten. Leipzig, *F. C. W. Vogel*, 1878.
Koch's epochal work on the aetiology of traumatic infectious disease established his reputation. He inoculated animals with material from various sources and produced six types of infection, each due to micro-organisms. He carried these infections through several generations of animals. His great work determined the role of bacteria in the aetiology of wound infections and demonstrated for the first time the specificity of

infection. It also contains the first explicit statement of the criteria implicit in Henle (*See* No. 2533) on contagion which later became known as Koch's postulates. *See also* Nos. 2331 and 5167. English translation, *New Sydenham Society*, 1880.

2537   PASTEUR, Louis. 1822-1895
Sur les maladies virulentes, et en particulier sur la maladie appelée vulgairement choléra des poules. *C. R. Acad. Sci. (Paris)*, 1880, **90**, 239-48.

This paper marked the beginning of Pasteur's work on the attenuation of the infective organism. Noting that fowls inoculated with an attenuated form of the chicken cholera bacterium acquired immunity, he developed the idea of a protective inoculation by attenuated living cultures, and subsequently adopted this principle with anthrax, rabies, and swine erysipelas. His work laid the foundations of the science of immunology. Since 1979, the availability to scholars of Pasteur's original laboratory notebooks has provided evidence that Emile Roux played a crucial and previously unacknowledged role in the development of the vaccine. See also his later paper in the same journal, 1880, **91**, 673-80. Abridged English translation of both papers and discussion of Roux's role in Bibel, *Milestones in immunology* (1988). Roux did receive credit from Pasteur for his work on anthrax. *See* No. 5169.

2538   METCHNIKOFF, Elie. 1845-1916
Über eine Sprosspilzkrankheit der Daphnien. Beitrag zur Lehre über den Kampf der Phagocyten gegen Krankheitserreger. *Virchows Arch. path. Anat.*, 1884, **96**, 177-95.

Metchnikoff originated the theory of phagocytosis. He described phagocytes in leucocytes and showed their function as scavengers. Abridged English translation in Bibel, *Milestones in immunology* (1988).

2539   SALMON, Daniel Elmer. 1850-1914, & SMITH, Theobald. 1859-1934
On a new method of producing immunity from contagious diseases. *Proc. biol. Soc. Wash.*, 1884-86, **3**, 29-33.

Smith found that dead virus can induce immunity against the living virulent virus. Although Smith made the discovery on his own, his supervisor, D.E. Salmon, usurped credit. See Bibel, *Milestones in immunology* (1988) 31-32.

2540   EHRLICH, Paul. 1854-1915
Das Sauerstoff-Bedürfniss des Organismus. Eine farbenanalytische Studie. Berlin, *A. Hirschwald*, 1885.

Includes the first statement of Ehrlich's "side-chain" theory.

2541   PASTEUR, Louis. 1822-1895
Méthode pour prévenir la rage après morsure. *C. R. Acad. Sci. (Paris)*, 1885, **101**, 765-74; 1886, **102**, 459-69, 835-38; **103**, 777-85.

Pasteur's papers describing his rabies vaccine, and the results he attained with it gave further proof of the value of attenuated virus as a protective inoculum against infective diseases in man and animals. This is considered Pasteur's greatest triumph. A grateful public subscribed two and a half million francs and made possible the erection of the Institut Pasteur, Paris. English translation in R. Suzor, *Hydrophobia: An account of M. Pasteur's system....* London, 1887. *See* No. 5483.1.

2542   NUTTALL, George Henry Falkiner. 1862-1937
        Experimente über die bacterienfeindlichen Einflüsse des thierischen
        Körpers. *Z. Hyg. InfektKr.* 1888, **4**, 353-94.
        Working with the defibrinated blood of certain animals, Nuttall was the
        first to describe the bactericidal action of blood. Abridged English trans-
        lation in Bibel, *Milestones in immunology* (1988).

2543   BUCHNER, Hans. 1850-1902
        Ueber die bakterientödtende Wirkung des zellenfreien Blutserums. *Zbl.
        Bakt.*, 1889, **5**, 817-23; **6**, 1-11.
        Following Nuttall's work, Buchner demonstrated that the bactericidal
        power of defibrinated blood was possessed by the cell-free serum, and was
        lost on heating the serum to 55˚C for one hour.

2544   BEHRING, Emil Adolf von. 1854-1917, & KITASATO, Shibasaburo. 1852-
        1931
        Ueber das Zustandekommen der Diphtherie-Immunität und der Tetanus-
        Immunität bei Thieren. *Dtsch. med. Wschr.*, 1890, **16**, 1113-14.
        Discovery of diphtheria and tetanus antitoxins, humoral antitoxic
        antibodies, the basis of serotherapy. Behring was the first recipient (1901)
        of the Nobel Prize for Medicine. English translation in Bibel, *Milestones in
        immunology* (1988).

2544.1 KOCH, Robert. 1843-1910
        Weitere Mittheilungen über ein Heilmittel gegen Tuberkulose. *Dtsch. med.
        Wschr.*, 1890, **16**, 1029-32; 1891, **17**, 101-102, 1189-92.
        The second paper describes "Koch's phenomenon", and tuberculin
        skin test. Koch showed that tuberculin injected intradermally would elicit
        a severe local inflammatory reaction in tuberculous patients. This was the
        first diagnostic skin test. Abbreviated English translation of second paper
        in Bibel, *Milestones of immunology* (1988).

2545   ——. Gesammelte Abhandlungen zur ätiologischen Therapie von
        ansteckenden Krankheiten. Leipzig, *G. Thieme*, 1893.

2545.1 STERNBERG, George Miller. 1838-1915
        Practical results of bacteriological researches. *Trans. Ass. Amer. Phycns.*,
        1892, **7**, 68-86.
        Sternberg demonstrated that the serum of an animal recovered from
        vaccinia possesses the property of neutralizing the activity of the causative
        virus. His test was readily adaptable for use in various host-systems.

2546   PFEIFFER, Richard Friedrich Johannes. 1858-1945, & ISAYEV, Vasiliy Isayevich.
        1854-1911
        Ueber die specifische Bedeutung der Choleraimmunität (Bakteriolyse). *Z.
        Hyg. InfektKr.*, 1894, **17**, 355-400; 1895, **18**, 1-16.
        Pfeiffer and Isayev recorded the occurrence of bacteriolysis in cholera
        vibrios under certain conditions: immune bacteriolysis, "Pfeiffer's phenom-
        enon". Abridged English translation of second part in Bibel, *Milestones in
        immunology* (1988).

2547   BORDET, Jules Jean Baptiste Vincent. 1870-1961
        Contribution à l'étude du sérum chez les animaux vaccinés. *Ann. Soc. roy.
        Sci. méd. nat. Brux.*, 1895, **4**, 455-530.

Bordet's classic paper on the properties of the sera of immunized animals. He showed two different substances (now known as sensitizing antibody and complement) to be involved in the phenomenon of bacteriolysis. He was awarded the Nobel Prize in 1919. English translation in J. Bordet *et al., Studies in immunity*, New York, 1909, pp. 8-80.

2548 METCHNIKOFF, ELIE. 1845-1916
Sur la destruction extracellulaire des bactéries dans l'organisme. *Ann. Inst. Pasteur*, 1895, **9**, 433-61.
See No. 2538.

2549 GRUBER, MAX. 1853-1927, & DURHAM, HERBERT EDWARD. 1866-1945
Eine neue Methode zur raschen Erkennung des Choleravibrio und des Typhusbacillus. *Münch. med. Wschr.*, 1896, **43**, 285-86.
 The discovery of bacterial agglutination. Gruber and Durham discovered the agglutinating action of the serum of typhoid patients upon the typhoid bacillus. First briefly reported by Durham: On a special action of serum of highly immunized animals, and its use for diagnostic and other purposes. *Proc. Roy. Soc. Lond.*, 1986, **59**, 224-26.

2550 WIDAL, GEORGES FERNAND ISIDOR. 1862-1929, & SICARD, ARTHUR.
Recherches de la réaction agglutinante dans le sang et le sérum desséchés des typhiques et dans la sérosité des vésicatoires. *Bull. Mém. Soc. méd. Hôp. Paris*, 1896, 3 sér., **13**, 681-82.
 Developing the work of Gruber and Durham, Widal noted that a patient's serum could be tested with bacteria of known type and his disease identified by this means. The "Gruber–Widal test" was the outcome of this work.

2550.1 KRAUS, RUDOLF. 1868-1932
Über specifische Reactionen im keimfreien Filtraten aus Cholera, Typhus und Pestbouillonculturen, erzeugt durch homologes Serum. *Wien. klin. Woch.*, 1897, **10**, 736-38.
 The precipitin reaction, employed for the qualitative identification of antigens and antibodies. English translation in Bibel, *Milestones in immunology,*(1988) pp. 265-68.

2551 BORDET, JULES JEAN BAPTISTE VINCENT. 1870-1961
Sur l'agglutination et la dissolution des globules rouges par le sérum d'animaux injectés de sang défibriné. *Ann. Inst. Pasteur*, 1898, **12**, 688-95; 1899, **13**, 225-50.
 Bordet's important work on immune haemolysis turned the attention of many investigators towards the subject. English translation in J. Bordet *et al., Studies in immunity*, New York, 1909, p. 134.

2552 ——. Les sérums hémolytiques, leurs antitoxines et les théories des sérums cytolytiques. *Ann. Inst. Pasteur*, 1900, **14**, 257-96; 1901, **15**, 303-18.
 English translation in J. Bordet *et al., Studies in immunity*, New York, 1909, p. 186.

2553 ——., & GENGOU, OCTAVE. 1875-1957
Sur l'existence de substances sensibilisatrices dans la plupart des sérums antimicrobiens. *Ann. Inst. Pasteur*, 1901, **15**, 289-302.

The Bordet–Gengou complement-fixation reaction is the basis of many tests for infection, notably the Wassermann test for syphilis, and reactions for gonococcus infection, glanders, hydatid disease. English translation in Bibel, *Milestones in immunology* (1988), pp. 268-71.

2554 NUTTALL, GEORGE HENRY FALKINER. 1862-1937
On the rôle of insects, arachnids and myriapods, as carriers in the spread of bacterial and parasitic diseases of man and animals. A critical and historical study. *Johns Hopk. Hosp. Rep.*, 1900, **8**, 1-154.

2555 METCHNIKOFF, ELIE. 1845-1916
L'immunité dans les maladies infectieuses. Paris, *Masson*, 1901.
  A classic study of the mechanisms concerned in specific antibacterial immunity, and one of Metchnikoff's best works. He was awarded the Nobel Prize in 1908. English translation, London, 1905.

2556 WASSERMANN, AUGUST VON. 1866-1925
Hämolysine, Cytotoxine and Präcipitine. *Samml. klin. Vortr.*, 1902, n.F. 331 (Chir. Nr. 94), 339-84.

2557 UHLENHUTH, PAUL THEODOR. 1870-1957
Zur Lehre von der Unterscheidung verschiedener Eiweissarten mit Hilfe spezifischer Sera. In: *Festschrift zur sechzigsten Geburtstage von Robert Koch.* Jena, *G. Fischer*, 1903, pp. 49-74.
  Demonstration of organ-specific antigens, in this case in the proteins of the lens of the eye.

2558 WRIGHT, *Sir* ALMROTH EDWARD. 1861-1947, & DOUGLAS, STEWART RANKEN. 1871-1936
An experimental investigation of the rôle of the blood fluids in connection with phagocytosis. *Proc. roy. Soc. (Lond.)*, 1903-04, **72**, 357-370; 1904, **73**, 128-42.
  Wright and Douglas showed the existence of thermolabile substances (opsonins) in normal and immune serum.

2558.1 DONATH, JULIUS. 1870-1950, & LANDSTEINER, CARL. 1868-1943.
Über paroxysmale Hämoglobinurie. *Mün. Med. Woch.*, 1904, **51**, 1590-93.
  The first description of an auto-antibody, and of an auto-immune disease, paroxysmal cold hemoglobinuria. See A.M. Silverstein, *A history of immunology*, New York, *Academic Press*, 1989, Ch. 8, The Donanth-Landsteiner autoantibody...English translation in Bibel, *Milestones in immunology, (1988)*.

2559 EHRLICH, PAUL. 1854-1915
Gesammelte Arbeiten über Immunitätsforschung. Berlin, *A. Hirschwald*, 1904.
  Reprints Ehrlich's writings on immunology to date, as well as three papers by Kyes (Nos. 2111-3). English translation, with two more chapters by Ehrlich and Sachs, and one by Ehrlich, New York, 1906.

2560 NEUFIELD, FRED. 1861-1945, & RIMPAU, WILLI. 1877-
Ueber die Antikörper des Streptokokken- und Pneumokokken-Immunserums. *Dtschr. med. Wschr.*, 1904, **30**, 1458-60.
  Bacteriotropins named and described.

2561   NUTTALL, George Henry Falkiner. 1862-1937
         Blood immunity and blood relationship, a demonstration of certain blood
         relationships amongst animals by means of the precipitin test for blood.
         Cambridge, *Univ. Press*, 1904.

2562   KOLLE, Wilhelm. 1868-1935, & HETSCH, Heinrich. 1873-
         Die experimentelle Bakteriologie und die Infektionskrankheiten. Berlin,
         Wien, *Urban & Schwarzenberg*, 1906.
             English translation, 2 vols., London, *Allen & Unwin*, 1934.

2563   METCHNIKOFF, Elie. 1845-1916
         Quelques remarques sur le lait aigri. Paris, *A. Maloine*, 1906.
             Metchnikoff's theory regarding the effect of lactic acid on bacteria.

2564   RICKETTS, Howard Taylor. 1871-1910
         Infection, immunity and serum therapy. Chicago, *A. M. A. Press*, 1906.

2564.1   ARRHENIUS, Svante August. 1859-1927
         Immunochemistry. The application of the principles of physical chemistry
         to the study of the biological antibodies. New York, *Macmillan*, 1907.
             Arrhenius defined immunochemistry, and laid out its frontiers.

2565   EHRLICH, Paul. 1854-1915
         Beiträge zur experimentellen Pathologie und Chemotherapie. Leipzig,
         Akad. Verlag., 1909.

2566   WOLFF-EISNER, Alfred. 1877-1948
         Handbuch der experimentellen Serumtherapie. München, *J. F. Lehmann*,
         1910.

2567   MUCH, Hans. 1880-1932
         Die Immunitätswissenschaft. Würzburg, *C. Kabitzsch*, 1911.

2567.1   SCHÖNE, Georg.
         Die heteroplastiche und homöoplastiche Transplantation. Berlin, *Springer-
         Verlag*, 1912.
             Schöne coined the term "transplantation immunity". He set out general
         rules governing the acceptance or rejection of tumour grafts which are
         essentially the same as the modern "laws of transplantation". This is a
         comprehensive work on skin and organ transplants.

2568   ZINSSER, Hans. 1878-1940
         Infection and resistance. New York, *Macmillan Co.*, 1914.

2569   HEKTOEN, Ludvig. 1863-1951
         The influence of the x-ray on the production of antibodies. *J. infect. Dis.*,
         1915, **17**, 415-22.
             Proof that x rays suppress the antibody response.

2570   LITTLE, Clarence Cook. 1888-1971, & TYZZER, Ernest Edward. 1875-1966
         Further experimental studies on the inheritance of susceptibility to a
         transplantable tumour, carcinoma (J. W. A.) of the Japanese waltzing
         mouse. *J. med. Res.*, 1916, **33**, 393-427.
             Marks the beginning of the study of histocompatibility antigens.

2571   TWORT, FREDERICK WILLIAM. 1877-1950
An investigation on the nature of ultra-microscopic viruses. *Lancet*, 1915, **2**, 1241-43.

The transmissible lysis of bacteria by viruses (Twort–d'Herelle phenomenon) was first pointed out by Twort. The lytic agent has been named *bacteriophage*. It was the first isolation of a filterable virus. *See also* No. 2572.

2571.1   SANARELLI, GIUSEPPE. 1864-1940
Pathogénie du choléra. Reproduction expérimentale de la maladie. *C. R. Acad. Sci. (Paris)*, 1916, **163**, 538-40.

Sanarelli claimed priority in observing the Shwartzman phenomenon (*See* No. 2576). See *Ann. Inst. Pasteur*, 1939, **63**, 105.

2572   D'HERELLE, FÉLIX HUBERT. 1873-1949
Sur une microbe invisible antagoniste des bacilles dysentérique. *C. R. Acad. Sci. (Paris)*, 1917, **165**, 373-75.

The bacteriophage discovered by d'Herelle was considered by him to be a filterable substance capable of bacteriolysis, similar to, if not identical with Twort's precellular ultramicroscopic virus (see No. 2571). D'Herelle later wrote a book *Le bactériophage*, Paris, 1921 (English translation, Baltimore, 1922), using the name he coined for the substance.

2572.1   BORDET, JULES JEAN BAPTISTE VINCENT. 1870-1961, & CIUCA, M.
Exsudats leucocytaires et autolyse microbienne transmissible. *C. R. Soc. Biol. (Paris)*, 1920, **83**, 1293-96.

Lysogeny.

2573   ROSENOW, EDWARD CARL. 1875-1966
Results of experimental studies on focal infection and elective localization. *Med. Clin. N. Amer.*, 1921, **5**, 573-92.

Rosenow showed that focal infection could by caused by bacteria in teeth, etc.

2573.1   LITTLE, CLARENCE COOK. 1888-1971
The genetics of tissue transplantation in mammals. *J. Cancer Res.*, 1924, **8**, 75-95.

Little established that the homograft reaction was due to genetic differences between donor and recipient.

2573.2   HEIDELBERGER, MICHAEL. 1888- , & AVERY, OSWALD THEODORE. 1877-1955
The soluble specific substance of pneumococcus. *J. exp. Med.*, 1923, **38**, 73-79; 1924, **40**, 301-16.

Heidelberger, Avery, and their colleagues made a chemical study of the antigenic constituents of the pneumococcus, separating the polysaccharide antigens.

2574   BESREDKA, ALEXANDRE. 1870-1940
Immunisation locale; pansements spécifiques. Paris, *Masson & Cie.*, 1925.

Besredka's vaccine, sensitized vaccine. English translation, Baltimore, 1927.

2575 WELLS, HARRY GIDEON. 1875-1943
The chemical aspects of immunity. New York, *Chem. Catalog Co.*, 1925.

2576 SHWARTZMAN, GREGORY. 1896-1965
Studies on Bacillus typhosus toxic substances. I. Phenomenon of local skin reactivity to B. typhosus culture filtrate. *J. exp. Med.*, 1928, **48**, 247-68.
"Shwartzman phenomenon."

2576.01 HEIDELBERGER, MICHAEL. 1888- , & KENDALL, FORREST E. 1898-1975
A quantitative study of the precipitin reaction between Type III pneumococcus polysaccharide and purified homologous antibody. *J. exp. Med.*, 1929, **50**, 809-23.
Heidelberger and Kendall adapted the precipitin reaction to permit the quantitative measurement of antibody and antigen. This established the principle of quantitative immunochemistry.

2576.02 SULZBERGER, MARION B. 1895-1983
Hypersensitiveness to arsphenamine in guinea pigs. I. Experiments in prevention and desensitization. *Arch. Dermatol. Syph.*, 1929, **20**, 669-697.
First demonstration of specific, acquired, lasting refractoriness to sensitization. This is the same or a closely related phenomenon to that demonstrated later by Burnet and Medawar under the name *immune tolerance. See* No. 2603.1.

2576.1 BREINL, FRIEDRICH. 1888- , & HAUROWITZ, FELIX.
Chemische Untersuchung des Präzipitates aus Hämoglobin und Anti-Hämoglobin-Serum und Bemerkungen über die Natur der Antikörper. *Hoppe-Seyl. Z. physiol. Chem.*, 1930, **192**, 45-57.
Template or instruction theory of antibody formation.

2576.2 LANDSTEINER, KARL. 1868-1943
Die Spezifizität der serologischen Reaktionen. Berlin, *Springer,* 1933.
Summary of many years of research on antigen–antibody interactions. Landsteiner considered his study of hapten-antibody reactions to be his most significant work. Revised English translation, 1936 (revised 1945).

2576.3 HOSKINS, MEREDITH.
A protective action of neurotropic against viscerotropic yellow fever virus in *Macacus rhesus. Amer. J. trop. Med.*, 1935, **15**, 675-80.
One of the first examples of an animal virus interference phenomenon was demonstrated by Hoskins.

2576.4 IRWIN, M. ROBERT. 1897-1987, & COLE, LEON J. 1877-1948
Immunogenetic studies of species and of species hybrids in doves, and the separation of species-specific substances in the backcross. *J. exp. Biol.*, 1936, **73**, 85-108.
Irwin coined the term, "immunogenetics" to describe the union of immunology with genetics. He attempted to determine the genetic control of antigenicity through genetic cross matings.

2576.5 GORER, PETER ALFRED. 1907-1961
The genetic and antigenic basis of tumour transplantation. *J. Path. Bact.*, 1937, **44**, 691-97; 1938, **47**, 231-52.

Gorer made the initial discoveries which formed the basis of transplantation genetics. He studied mouse blood groups and described an antigen in erythrocytes (antigen II). His studies established the laws of transplantation immunity. See also his later paper in *Proc. roy. Soc. B*, 1948, **135**, 499-505.

2576.6   MARRACK, JOHN RICHARDSON. 1886-1976
The chemistry of antigens and antibodies. *Spec. Rep. Ser. No.194*. med. Res. Coun. (Lond.), 1934.
"The advent of the lattice theory of antibody-antigen coupling" (Bibel, *Milestones in immunology* [1988]pp. 91-94).

2576.7   WOLLMAN, EUGENE. 1883-1943, & WOLLMAN, ELISABETH. 1888-1943
Recherches sur le phénomène de Twort-d'Hérelle (bactériophage ou autolyse hérédo-contagieuse). *Ann. Inst. Pasteur*, 1938, **60**, 13-57.
The Wollmans made important contributions to the knowledge on bacteriophage and lysogeny.

2576.8   TISELIUS, ARNE WILHELM KAURIN. 1902-1971, & KABAT, ELVIN ABRAHAM. 1914-
An electrophoretic study of immune sera and purified antibody preparations. *J. exp. Med.*, 1939, 69, 119-31.
Antibodies shown to be gamma globulins.

2577   HIRST, GEORGE KEBLE. 1909-
The agglutination of red cells by allantoic fluid of chick embryos infected with influenza virus. *Science*, 1941, **94**, 22-23.
Discovery of virus haemagglutination.

2578   McCLELLAND, LAURELLA. 1912- , & HARE, RONALD. 1899-1986
The absorption of influenza virus by red cells and a new in vitro method of measuring antibodies for influenza virus. *Canad. publ. Hlth. J.*, 1941, **32**, 530-38.
Independently of Hirst, McClelland and Hare discovered virus haemagglutination.

2578.1   FREUND, JULES THOMAS. 1891-1960, & McDERMOTT, KATHERINE.
Sensitization to horse serum by means of adjuvants. *Proc. Soc. exp. Biol. (N.Y.)*, 1942, **49**, 548-53.
Freund's adjuvant. Freund's procedure allowed adjuvants to be used for any antigen.

2578.2   FELTON, LLOYD DERR. 1885-1953, & OTTINGER, BARBARA
Pneumococcus polysaccharide as a paralyzing agent on the mechanism of immunity in white mice. *J. Bact.*, 1942, **43**, 94-5.

2578.3   LANDSTEINER, KARL. 1868-1943, & CHASE, MERRILL WALLACE. 1905-
Experiments on transfer of cutaneous sensitivity to simple compounds. *Proc. Soc. exp. Biol. (N. Y.)*, 1942, **49**, 688-90.
Cellular transfer of delayed hypersensitivity, establishing the criticial role of mononuclear cells in cellular immunity.

2578.4 GIBSON, THOMAS. 1915- , & MEDAWAR, *Sir* PETER BRIAN. 1915-1987
The fate of skin homografts in man. *J. Anat. (Lond),* 1943, **77**, 299-310.
Gibson and Medawar placed the laws of transplantation on a firm scientific basis. A later paper by Medawar (*J. Anat. [Lond.],* 1944, **78**, 176-99) demonstrated that the mechanism of rejection of transplanted tissues is immunological in character.

2578.5 DELBRÜCK, MAX. 1906-1981 , & BAILEY, W. T.
Induced mutations in bacterial viruses. *Cold Spring Harbor Symp. quant. Biol.,* 1946, **11**, 33-37.
Genetic recombination in bacteriophages. Delbrück shared the Nobel Prize with A. D. Hershey and S. E. Luria in 1969 for his work on replication mechanisms and genetic structure of viruses.

2578.6 OUCHTERLONY, ÖRJAN THOMAS GUNNERSSON. 1914-
In vitro method for testing the toxin-producing capacity of diphtheria bacteria. *Acta Path. Microbiol. Scand.,* 1948, **25**, 186-91.
Agar gel immunodiffusion.

2578.7 BURNET, *Sir* FRANK MACFARLANE. 1899-1985, & FENNER, FRANK JOHN. 1914-
The production of antibodies. 2nd ed. Melbourne, *Macmillan,* 1949.
Burnet and Fenner introduced the "self-marker" concept – natural tolerance to one's own body constituents depended on their presence at a critical stage of embryonic development. For his work on immunological tolerance Burnet shared the Nobel Prize with Medawar in 1960.

2578.8 COONS, ALBERT HEWETT. 1912-1978 , & KAPLAN, MELVIN H. 1920-
Localization of antigen in tissue cells. II. Improvements in a method for the detection of antigen by means of fluorescent antibody. *J. exp. Med.,* 1950, **91**, 1-13.
Fluorescent antibody technique.

2578.9 BRUTON, OGDEN CARR. 1908-
Agammaglobulinemia. *Pediatrics,* 1952, **9**, 722-27.
First report.

2578.10 DAUSSET, JEAN. 1917- , & NENNA, ANDRÉ.
Presence d'une leuco-agglutinine dans le sérum d'un cas d'agranulocytose chronique. *C. R. Soc. Biol. (Paris),* 1952, **146**, 1539-41.
Discovery of leuco-agglutinins.

2578.11 BILLINGHAM, RUPERT EVERETT. 1921- , *et al.*
'Actively acquired tolerance' of foreign cells. *Nature (Lond.),* 1953, **172**, 603-06.
Proof of Burnet and Fenner's theory of immunity. With L. Brent and P. B. Medawar. For their discovery of acquired immunological tolerance Medawar and Burnet (No. 2578.7) shared the Nobel Prize in 1960.

2578.12 ——. Quantitative studies on tissue transplantation immunity. I. The survival times of skin homografts exchanged between members of different inbred strains of mice. II. The origin, strength and duration of actively and adoptively acquired immunity. *Proc. roy. Soc. B,* 1954, **143**, 43-80.

Experimental production of immunological tolerance. Paper II distinguished adoptive from passive immunization. With L. Brent, P. B. Medawar, and (Paper I) E. M. Sparrow.

2578.13   GRABAR , PIERRE. 1898-1986 , & WILLIAMS, CURTIS A.
Méthode permettant l'étude conjugée des propriétés éléctrophorétiques et immunochimiques d'un mélange de protéines. Application au sérum sanguin. *Biochem. biophys. Acta*, 1953, **10**, 193-94.
Immunoelectrophoresis.

2578.14   MAYER, MANFRED MARTIN. 1916-1984, & LEVINE, LAWRENCE. 1924-
Kinetic studies on immune hemolysis. III-IV. *J. Immunol.*, 1954, **72**, 511-30.
Complement fixation.

2578.15   MITCHISON, NICHOLAS AVRION. 1928-
Passive transfer of transplantation immunity. *Proc. roy. Soc. B.*, 1954, **142**, 72-87.
Preliminary notice in *Nature (Lond.)*, 1953, **171**, 267-68.

2578.16   PORTER, RODNEY ROBERT. 1917-1985
The fractionation of rabbit -globulin by partition chromatography. *Biochem. J.*, 1955, **59**, 405-10.
Preliminary note in *Biochem. J.*, 1954, **58**, xxxix-xl. Porter received the Nobel Prize in 1972. *See* No. 2578.25.

2578.17   GIERER, ALFRED, & SCHRAMM, GERHARD.
Infectivity of ribonucleic acid from tobacco mosaic virus. *Nature (Lond.)*, 1956, **177**, 702-03.
Proof that nucleic acid produces infectivity. See also *Z. Naturf.*, 1956, **11b**, 138-42.

2578.18   GLICK, BRUCE. 1927- , *et al.*
The bursa of Fabricius and antibody production in the domestic fowl. *Poultry Sci.*, 1956, **35**, 224-25.
The relationship of the bursa of Fabricius to antibody formation was discovered by Glick, T. S. Chang, and R. G. Jaap. Its removal in early life led to inability to produce antibodies.

2578.19   ROITT, IVAN MAURICE 1927- , *et al.*
Autoantibodies in Hashimoto's disease (lymphadenoid goitre). *Lancet*, 1956, **2**, 820-21.
Demonstration of autoantibodies. With D. Doniach, P. N. Campbell, and R. V. Hudson.

2578.20   WITEBSKY, ERNEST. 1901-1969, & ROSE, NOEL RICHARD. 1927-
Studies on organ specificity. IV. Production of rabbit thyroid antibodies in the rabbit. *J. Immunol.*, 1956, **76**, 408-16.
Autoimmune thyroiditis.

2578.21   GOWANS, *Sir* JAMES LEARMONTH. 1924-
The effects of the continuous re-infusion of lymph and lymphocytes on the output of lymphocytes from the thoracic duct of unanaesthetized rats. *Brit. J. exp. Path.*, 1957, **38**, 67-78.

Gowans's work, particularly between 1957 and 1962, was mainly responsible for the fusion of studies on the lymphocytes with the mainstream of immunology. The above paper dealt with the recirculation of lymphocytes. See also *J. Physiol. (Lond.)*, 1959, **146**, 54-69.

2578.22   ISAACS, ALICK. 1921-1967, & LINDENMANN, JEAN. 1924-
Virus interference. I. The interferon. *Proc. roy. Soc. B*, 1957, **147**, 258-67.
    Discovery of interferon, a protein produced from the interaction of virus and cells and having the property of interfering with the multiplication of viruses.

2578.23   PAYNE, ROSE MARISE. 1909-
Leukocyte agglutinins in human sera. Correlations between blood transfusions and their development. *Arch. intern. Med.*, 1957, **99**, 587-606.
    Leucocyte typing.

2578.24   MEDAWAR, *Sir* PETER BRIAN. 1915-1987
The homograft reaction. *Proc. roy. Soc. B*, 1958, **149**, 145-66.
    Medawar showed grafting to be unsuccessful when donor and recipient animals came from the same litter, unless the two are genetically identical – another instance of the delayed hypersensitivity reaction.

2578.25   PORTER, RODNEY ROBERT. 1917-1985
Separation and isolation of fractions of rabbit gamma-globulin containing the antibody and antigenic combining sites. *Nature (Lond.)*, 1958, **182**, 670-71.
    Porter shared the Nobel Prize with G. M. Edelman (No. 2578.39) in 1972 for his work on the separation of antibody molecules.

2578.26   DAUSSET, JEAN. 1917-
Iso-leuco-anticorps. *Acta haemat. (Basel)*, 1958, **20**, 156-66.
    Discovery of the first histocompatibility antigen. Dausset shared the Nobel Prize with B. Benacerraf and G. D. Snell in 1980.

2578.27   ROOD, J. J. VAN, *et al.*
Leucocyte antibodies in sera from pregnant women. *Nature (Lond.)*, 1958, **181**, 1735-36.
    Leucocyte typing and matching of histocompatibility determinants. *See also* Payne (No. 2578.23). With J. G. Eernisse and A. van Leeuwen.

2578.28   YALOW, ROSALYN SUSSMAN. 1921- , & BERSON, SOLOMON A. 1918-1972
Immunosassay of endogenous plasma insulin in man. *J. clin. Invest.*, 1960, **39**, 1157-75.
    First radioimmunoassay of a hormone, a test capable of estimating nonogram or even picogram quantities. For this technique Yalow shared the 1977 Nobel Prize with R. Guillemin and A. Schally.

2578.29   BENACERRAF, BARUJ. 1920- , & McDEVITT, HUGH O'NEILL.
Histocompatibility-linked immune response genes. *Science*, 1972, **175**, 273-79.
    The capacity to mount certain immune responses is genetically determined. Benacerraf shared the 1980 Nobel Prize with J. Dausset and G. D. Snell.

2578.30 SNELL, GEORGE DAVIS. 1903-
Histocompatibility genes of the mouse. *J. nat. Cancer Inst.*, 1958, **20**, 787-824; **21**, 843-75.

Snell has made the greatest contribution to the fundamentals of transplanting genetics. At his suggestion genes governing transplantation were called histocompatibility genes and Gorer's Antigen II became Histocompatibility-2 (H-2). He shared the Nobel Prize with B. Benacerraf and J. Dausset in 1980.

2578.31 BURNET, *Sir* FRANK MACFARLANE. 1899-1985
The clonal selection theory of acquired immunity. Nashville, *Vanderbilt University Press*, & Cambridge, *Cambridge University Press*, 1959.

Theory first published in *Aust. J. Sci.*, 1957, **20**, 67-.

2578.32 MILLER, JACQUES FRANCIS ALBERT PIERRE. 1931-
Immunological function of the thymus. *Lancet*, 1961, **2**, 748-49.

Miller demonstrated the immunological function of the thymus.

2578.33 GOWANS, *Sir* JAMES LEARMONTH. 1924- , *et al.*
Initiation of immune responses by small lymphocytes. *Nature (Lond.)*, 1962, **196**, 651-55.

The lymphocyte shown to be the immunologically competent cell. With D. D. McGregor and D. M. Cowen.

2578.34 JERNE, NEILS KAJ. 1911- , & NORDIN, ALBERT A. 1934-
Plaque formation in agar by single antibody-producing cells. *Science*, 1963, **140**, 405.

Hemolytic plaque assay for enumerating antibody-forming cells.

2578.35 KUNKEL, HENRY GEORGE. 1916-1983 *et al*
Individual antigenic specificity of isolated antibodies. *Science*, 1963, **140**, 1218-19.

Idiotypes. With M. Mannik and R.C. Williams. Kunkel and his team discovered idiotypy independently of Jacques Oudin and Philip Gell.

2578.36 DAVID, JOHN R. 1930-
Delayed hypersensitivity in vitro: its mediation by cell-free substances formed by lymphoid cell-antigen interaction. *Proc. Nat. Acad. Sci. (USA)*, 1966, **56**, 72-77.

Lymphokines (MIF). Simultaneously discovered by Barry R. Bloom (1937-) & B. Bennett. See *Science*, 1966, **153**, 80-82.

2578.37 CLAMAN, HENRY N. 1930- & CHAPERON, EDWARD A. 1920-
Thymus-marrow cell combinations, Synergism in antibody production. *Proc. Soc. Exp. Biol. & Med.*, 1966, **122**, 1167-71.

T cell subsets. With R.F. Triplett.

2578.38 SNELL, GEORGE DAVIS. 1903-
The H-2 locus of the mouse: observations and speculations concerning its comparative genetics and its polymorphism. *Folia biol. (Praha)*, 1968, **14**, 335-58.

Antigen II, discovered by Gorer (No. 2576.5), was studied by Snell and became known as the product of the H-2 locus, the fundamental locus in the history of mammalian transplant biology.

2578.39   EDELMAN, GERALD MAURICE. 1929- , *et al.*
The covalent structure of an entire ÁG immunoglobulin molecule. *Proc. nat. Acad. Sci. (Wash.)*, 1969, **63**, 78-85.
Complete sequence of an immunoglobulin molecule. With five co-authors. Edelman shared the Nobel Prize with R. R. Porter in 1972. See also G.M.Edelman & Miroslav Dave Poulik (1923-), Studies on structure units of the γ-globulins. *J. exp. Med.*, 1961, **113**, 861-884.

2578.40   WU, TAI TE. 1935- , & KABAT, ELVIN A. 1914-
An analysis of the sequences of the variable regions of Bence Jones proteins and myeloma light chains and their implications for antibody complementarity. *J. exp. Med.*, 1970, **132**, 211-50.
Hypervariable regions of "Ig".

2578.41   GERSON, RICHARD K. 1932-1983 & KONDO, K.
Cell interactions in the induction of tolerance: The role of thymic lymphocytes. *Immunology*, 1970, **18**, 723-37.
Suppressor T cells.

2578.42   JERNE, NEILS KAJ. 1911-
Towards a network theory of the immune system. *Ann. Immunol. (Paris)*, 1974, **125C**, 373-389.
Idiotype networks. Jerne shared the 1984 Nobel Prize with Milstein and Köhler for his theoretical contributions to our concept of the immune system.

2578.43   KÖHLER, GEORGES F. 1946- & MILSTEIN, CESAR. 1927-
Continuous cultures of fused cells secreting antibody of predefined specificity. *Nature*, 1975, **256**, 495-97.
Hybridomas. Köhler and Milstein shared the 1984 Nobel Prize with Jerne for the technique of monoclonal antibody formation.

History of Microbiology: Immunology: Allergy

2579   LOEFFLER, FRIEDRICH AUGUST JOHANN. 1852-1915
Vorlesungen über die geschichtliche Entwickelung der Lehre von den Bacterien. Teil 1.[All published]. Leipzig, *F. C. W. Vogel*, 1887.
Loeffler, Professor of Hygiene at Greifswald, made many discoveries in bacteriology. His history of the subject was unfortunately left unfinished.

2580   BULLOCH, WILLIAM. 1868-1941
The history of bacteriology. London, *Oxford Univ. Press*, 1938.
This pioneering and classic history includes brief biographical notes of the more important workers (arranged in a separate section), and an extensive bibliography. Reprinted, *Dover Pub.*, 1979.

2581   FORD, WILLIAM WEBBER. 1871-1941
Bacteriology. New York, *Hoeber*, 1939.
A much briefer history than Bulloch's but with a thorough and accurate bibliography.

2581.1   GRAINGER, THOMAS HUTCHINSON. 1913-
A guide to the history of bacteriology. New York, *Ronald Press*, 1958.
A selective annotated bibliography.

2581.2   DOETSCH, RAYMOND NICHOLAS. 1920-
          Microbiology. Historical contributions from 1776-1908. New Brunswick,
          Rutgers University Press, [1960].

2581.3   BROCK, THOMAS DALE. 1926-
          Milestones in microbiology. Englewood Cliffs, N. J., *Prentice-Hall*, 1961.
          Readings from primary sources, with commentary.

2581.4   HAHON, NICHOLAS. 1924-
          Selected papers on virology. Englewood Cliffs, N.J., *Prentice-Hall*, 1964.
          A source of not-readily available early material.

2581.5   LECHEVALIER, HUBERT ARTHUR. 1926- , & SOLOTOROVSKY, MORRIS.
          Three centuries of microbiology. New York, *McGraw Hill*, 1965.

2581.6   PARISH, HENRY JAMES.
          A history of immunization. Edinburgh and London, *E. & S. Livingstone*, 1965.

2581.7   HAHON, NICHOLAS. 1924-
          Selected papers on the pathogenic rickettsiae. Cambridge, Mass., *Harvard
          University Press*, 1968.

2581.8   FOSTER, WILLIAM DEREK. 1925-1981
          A history of medical bacteriology and immunology. London, *W. Heinemann
          Medical Books*, 1970.

2581.9   WATERSON, ANTHONY PETER. 1923-1983, & WILKINSON, LISE.
          An introduction to the history of virology. Cambridge, *University Press*, 1978.

2581.10   SCHADEWALDT, HANS. 1923-
          Geschichte der Allergie. 4 vols., Diessenhofen, *Dustri-Verlag Fiestle*, 1979-
          83.

2581.11   WHITCOMB, DOROTHY.
          Immunology to 1980. An illustrated bibliography of titles in the Middleton
          Health Sciences Library, including the Julius M. Cruse collection. Madison,
          University of Wisconsin, Center for Health Sciences Libraries, 1985.
              Citations, with paginations, of 3480 items. Author and subject indices.

2581.12   BIBEL, DEBRA JAN.
          Milestones in immunology: A historical exploration. Madison, Wisconsin,
          Science-Tech Publishers, [1988].
              Readings from primary sources from 1884 to 1975 with expert intro-
          ductions, commentaries, and bibliographies.

2581.13   FENNER, FRANK. 1914- , & GIBBS, ADRIAN J.
          Portraits of viruses: A history of virology. Basel, *Karger*, 1988.
              Well-documented essays on specific families of viruses by expert
          researchers, reprinted from *Intervirology*, 1979, **11**- 1986, **26**.

2581.14   SILVERSTEIN, ARTHUR M.
          A history of immunology. San Diego, Calif., *Academic Press*, [1989].
              Carefully documented, well-written, analytical history from the ancient
          world to c. 1975 by an expert researcher in the field. Includes biographical

dictionary of notable contributors, list of "seminal discoveries" from 1714 to 1975 with bibliographical references, list of important books in immunology, 1892-1968, and glossary of technical terms.

ALLERGY AND ANAPHYLAXIS

2581.99   BOTALLO, Leonardo. *circa* 1519-1587/88
De catarrho commentarius. Parisiis, *apud B. Turrisanum*, 1564.
   Summer catarrh (hay fever) first described. Partial English translation in No. 2241.

2582   BOSTOCK, John. 1773-1846
Case of periodical affection of the eyes and chest. *Med. -chir. Trans.*, 1819, **10**, 161-65.
   Bostock's classical description of the "catarrhus aestivus," hay fever, is also referred to as "Bostock's catarrh". It begins the modern era in the clinical recognition of hay fever. The case he described was in fact himself. He was physician to Guy's Hospital, London.

2583   ———. Of the catarrhus aestivus, or summer catarrh. *Med. -chir. Trans.*, 1828, **14**, 437-46.
   On the history and aetiology of hay fever.

2584   ELLIOTSON, John. 1791-1868
Hay fever. *Lond. med. Gaz.*, 1831, **8**, 411-16; 1832-33, **12**, 164-71.
   Elliotson was the first to ascertain that pollen was the cause of hay fever.

2585   MAGENDIE, François. 1783-1855
Lectures on the blood. Philadelphia, *Harrington, Barrington & Haswell*, 1839.
   Pp. 244-49: Magendie showed that secondary or subsequent injections of egg/albumin caused death in rabbits who had tolerated an initial injection. This was the first experiment in anaphylaxis, though Jenner in 1798 had observed the phenomenon in various inoculations. These lectures were delivered at the Collège de France in 1837-38. This English translation is the first edition in book form.

2586   SALTER, Henry Hyde. 1823-1871
On asthma: its pathology and treatment. London, *J. Churchill*, 1860.
   The best work on asthma to appear during the 19th century. Salter, who had suffered from asthma from childhood, may be considered the first modern student of the condition. He called special attention to asthma from animal emanations (cats, rabbits, horses, dogs, cattle, etc.). *See* No. 3169.1.

2587   LIVEING, Edward. 1832-1919
On megrim, sick-headache, and some allied disorders. London, *J. & A. Churchill*, 1873.
   See No. 4549.

2588   BLACKLEY, Charles Harrison. 1820-1900
Experimental researches on the causes and nature of catarrhus aestivus. London, *Baillière, Tindall & Cox*, 1873.

Blackley showed that pollen can produce hay fever in both the asthmatic and catarrhal forms; he also showed that skin reactions were evoked in sensitive persons. Facsimile reproduction, 1959.

2589 ———. Hay fever. London, *Baillière, Tindall & Cox*, 1880.

2590 PORTIER, Paul. 1866-1962, & RICHET, Charles Robert. 1850-1935
De l'action anaphylactique de certains venins. *C. R. Soc. Biol. (Paris)*, 1902, **54**, 170-72.
First full description of the phenomenon of "anaphylaxis," the name itself being coined by Richet. Abbreviated English translation in Bibel, *Milestones of immunology* (1988).

2591 ARTHUS, Nicolas Maurice. 1862-1945
Injections répétées de sérum de cheval chez le lapin. *C. R. Soc. Biol. (Paris)*, 1903, **55**, 817-20.
The "Arthus phenomenon" – a symptom of anaphylaxis. Arthus showed that "antibody-mediated inflammation could be elicited in the skin of sensitized animals upon local introduction of an appropriate antigen" (Silverstein). Abbreviated English translation in Bibel, *Milestones of immunology* (1988).

2591.1 HAMBURGER, Franz. 1874-1954, & MORO, Ernst. 1874-1951
Ueber die biologisch nachweisbaren Veränderungen des menschlichen Blutes nach den Seruminjektion. *Wien. klin. Wschr.*, 1903, **16**, 445-47.
Serum sickness first described.

2592 DUNBAR, William Philipps. 1863-1922
Ursache und Behandlung des Heufiebers. Leipzig, *J. J. Weber*, 1905.
Dunbar studied the relationship of pollen to hay fever, separated the active substances responsible for producing the condition, and introduced a specific therapy.

2593 PIRQUET VON CESENATICO, Clemens Peter. 1874-1929, & SCHICK, Bela. 1877-1967
Die Serumkrankheit. Wien, *F. Deuticke*, 1905.
An excellent description of serum sickness and its significance. English translation, Baltimore, *Williams & Wilkins*, 1951.

2594 OTTO, Richard. 1872-1952
Das Theobald Smithsche Phänomen der Serum-Ueberfindlichkeit. In *Gedenkschr. f.d. verstorb. Generalstabsarzt ... von Leuthold*, Berlin, 1906, **1**, 153-72.
The "Theobald Smith phenomenon" was not reported by Smith but communicated by him to Ehrlich. Later Otto published details of the results obtained in his study of the phenomenon.

2594.1 ———. Zur Frage der Serum-Ueberempfindlichkeit. *Münch. med. Wschr.*, 1907, **54**, 1665-70.
Otto discovered that a state of tolerance developed in animals that survived anaphylactic shock. He induced passive transfer of hypersensitivity.

2595 ROSENAU, Milton Joseph. 1869-1946, & ANDERSON, John F. 1873-1958
A study of the cause of sudden death following the injection of horse serum. Washington, *Govt. Printing Office*, 1906.

Forms Bulletin No. 29 of the Hygienic Laboratory, U. S. Marine Hospital Service. Rosenau and Anderson drew attention to the fact that animals receiving an injection of a foreign protein became sensitive to a second dose of the same protein. This reaction is similar to the anaphylaxis of Richet and the "Theobald Smith phenomenon."

2596   BESREDKA, ALEXANDRE. 1870-1940, & STEINHARDT, EDNA.
De l'anaphylaxie et de l'anti-anaphylaxie vis-à-vis du sérum de cheval. *Ann. Inst. Pasteur*, 1907, **21**, 117-27, 384-91.
"Anti-anaphylaxis" was the term given by Besredka and Steinhardt to the specific desensitization of sensitized animals.

2597   NICOLLE, MAURICE. 1862-1932
Contribution à l'étude du "phénomène d'Arthus." *Ann. Inst. Pastuer*, 1907, **21**, 128-37.
"Passive" anaphylaxis first demonstrated.

2598   PIRQUET VON CESENATICO, CLEMENS PETER. 1874-1929
Klinische Studien über Vakzination und vakzinale Allergie. Leipzig, Wien, *F. Deuticke*, 1907.
Pirquet suggested the word "Allergie"; see also his paper with this title in *Münich. med. Wschr.*, 1906, **53**, 1457-58.

2599   RICHET, CHARLES ROBERT. 1850-1935
De l'anaphylaxie en général et de l'anaphylaxie par la mytilocongestine en particulier. *Ann. Inst. Pasteur*, 1907, **21**, 497-524; 1908, **22**, 465-95.
Nobel Prize winner, 1913, in recognition of his work on anaphylaxis.

2600   AUER, JOHN. 1875-1948, & LEWIS, PAUL A. 1879-1929
The physiology of the immediate reaction of anaphylaxis in the guinea-pig. *J. exp. Med.*, 1910, **12**, 151-75.
First adequate account of the physiological reactions leading to fatal anaphylactic shock.

2600.1   MELTZER, SAMUEL JAMES. 1851-1920
Bronchial asthma as a phenomenon of anaphylaxis. *J. Amer. med. Assoc.*, 1910, **55**, 1021-24.
The work of Auer and Lewis (*see* No. 2600) led Meltzer to the conclusion that bronchial asthma was due to anaphylaxis, although he did not appreciate that not all cases of asthma were so caused.

2600.2   SCHULTZ, WILLIAM HENRY. 1873-1947
Physiological studies in anaphylaxis. I. The reaction of smooth muscle of the guinea-pig sensitized with horse serum. *J. Pharmacol.*, 1910, **1**, 549-67.
Schultz–Dale test for anaphylaxis. *See also* No. 2600.5

2600.3   NOON, LEONARD. 1878-1913
Prophylactic inoculation against hay fever. *Lancet*, 1911, **1**, 1572-73.
Noon and Freeman introduced the treatment of hay fever by means of injections of pollen extract.

2600.4   FREEMAN, JOHN. 1877-1962
         Further observations on the treatment of hay fever by hypodermic in-
         oculations of pollen vaccine. *Lancet,* 1911, **2**, 814-17.
             See No. 2600.3.

2600.5   DALE, *Sir* HENRY HALLETT. 1875-1968
         The anaphylactic reaction of plain muscle in the guinea-pig. *J. Pharmacol.,*
         1913, **4**, 167-223.
             See No. 2600.2. Dale concluded that histamine induced hypersensitivity
         reactions.

2600.6   COOKE, ROBERT ANDERSON. 1880-1960, & VANDER VEER, ALBERT. 1879-
         Human sensitization. *J. Immunol.,* 1916, **1**, 201-305.
             The concept of atopy had its origin in the report by Cooke and Vander
         Veer in 1916.

2601   BESREDKA, ALEXANDRE. 1870-1940
         Anaphylaxie et antianaphylaxie. Paris, *Masson & Cie.,* 1917.
             English translation, 1919.

2601.1   PRAUSNITZ, OTTO CARL WILLY. 1876-1963, & KÜSTNER, HEINZ. 1897-
         Studien über die Ueberempfindlichkeit. *Zbl. Bakt., I Abt. Orig.,* 1921, **86**,
         160-69.
             Prausnitz–Küstner reaction. These workers demonstrated antibodies in
         the blood of persons suffering from atopic allergic diseases. They produced
         local passive sensitization by intracutaneous injection of serum from a
         hypersensitive subject. Prausnitz spent his later years in England, where he
         adopted the surname Prausnitz Giles. Translated by Prausnitz in *Clinical
         aspects of immunology* (P.G.H. Gell & R.R.A. Coombs, eds.) Oxford, 1962,
         pp. 808-16.

2602   LEWIS, *Sir* THOMAS. 1881-1945, & GRANT, RONALD THOMSON. 1892-1989
         Vascular reactions of the skin to injury. II. The liberation of a histamine-like
         substance in injured skin; the underlying cause of factitious urticaria and
         of wheals produced by burning; and observations upon the nervous
         control of certain skin reactions. *Heart,* 1924, **11**, 209-65.
             Lewis postulated that a histamine-like substance ("H-substance") was
         responsible for the anaphylaxis symptom-complex. *See also The blood-
         vessels of the human skin and their responses,* 1927 (No. 797).

2603   STORM VAN LEEUWEN, WILLEM. 1882-1933
         Allergic diseases; diagnosis and treatment of bronchial asthma, hay fever,
         and other allergic diseases. Philadelphia, *J. B. Lippincott,* 1925.
             In his important studies of asthma, Storm van Leeuwen demonstrated
         that in the great majority of patients allergens are the cause of the condition
         and also that patients are sensitive to mould spores. He experimented with
         an allergen-proof chamber and showed the benefit of high altitude to
         asthmatics.

2603.1   SULZBERGER, MARION B. 1895-1903
         Arsphenamine hypersensitiveness in guinea pigs. II. Experiments dem-
         onstrating the role of the skin, both as originator and as site of the
         hypersensitiveness. *Arch. Dermatol. Syph.,* 1930, **22**, 839-849.

Sulzberger showed that allergens gaining access to the epidermis are processed there in some manner (Langerhans cells?) that determines their allergenicity. *See* No. 2576.02

2604   FRANKLIN, Philip. 1880-1951
Treatment of hay fever by intranasal zinc ionization. *Brit. med. J.*, 1931, **1**, 1115-16.
Introduction of the method.

2605   DRAGSTEDT, Carl Albert. 1895- , & GEBAUER-FUELNEGG, Erich.
Studies in anaphylaxis. *Amer. J. Physiol.*, 1932, **102**, 512-26.
Detection of the release of histamines into the circulation during anaphylactic reaction. Thereafter histamine was identified as Lewis's "H-substance."

2605.1   SULZBERGER, Marion B. 1895-1983
Experiments in silk hypersensitivity and the inhalation of allergen in atopic dermatitis (neurodermatitis disseminatus). *J. Allergy*, 1934, **5**, 554-569.
Proof that inhaled allergens can reach the skin in a quantity and quality capable of eliciting urticarial reactions. With W.T. Vaughn. Coca and Sulzberger coined the term, "atopic dermatitis."

2605.2   ———. Penetration of allergens into the human skin. *N.Y. State J. Med.*, 1944, **44**, 2452-2459.
Proof that allergens that produce urticarial reactions can penetrate the skin from external contact and thus produce the reaction that the authors named "contact urticaria." With F. Herrmann and R. Baer.

See No. 2581.10 for HISTORY OF ALLERGY

ONCOLOGY IN GENERAL

2606   GALEN. A.D. 130-200
De tumoribus praeter naturam. In his Opera omnia, ed. cur. C. G. Kühn, Lipsiae, *C. Cnobloch*, 1824, **7**, 705-32.
Galen's classification of tumours persisted for more than 1,000 years. He considered neoplasms to be due to an excess of black bile, which solidified in certain sites. He advocated purges to dissolve the black bile, and if these were unsuccessful, the knife. He was not familiar with internal tumours. Critical edition and English translation by J. Reedy, Diss,(not published,) University of Michigan, 1968.

2607   LE DRAN, Henri François. 1685-1770
Mémoire avec un précis de plusieurs observations sur le cancer. *Mém. Acad. roy. Chir. (Paris)*, 1757, **3**, 1-54.
Le Dran's important discussion on cancer for the first time discarded the humoral conception of the disease. He regarded cancer as a local disease in its early stage and knew that it spread via the lymphatics to regional nodes, and from there into the general circulation. He described with great clarity the path of metastasis in breast carcinoma, including involvement of the lungs.

2607.1   HILL, JOHN. 1714-1775
          Cautions against the immoderate use of snuff; and the effects it must
          produce when this way taken into the body, *etc.* London, *R. Baldwin & J.
          Jackson,* 1761.
          First clinical report (pp. 30-31) of an association between tobacco and
          cancer, in this case "polypusses" of the nose caused by taking snuff. Hill
          was a distinguished botanist and apothecary although regarded by some
          as a quack. See D.E. Redmond, Jr., Tobacco and cancer: the first clinical
          report. *New Eng.J. Med.,* (1970), **282**, 18-23.

2608   PEYRILHE, BERNARD. 1735-1804
          Dissertatio academica de cancro. Parisiis, *De Hansy Jeune,* 1774.
          Peyrilhe was the first to attempt an experimental study to determine the
          nature of cancer. He injected fluid from human mammary cancer into a
          dog; however, the dog howled and aggravated his housekeeper, who
          drowned it. Peyrilhe recognized for the first time the essential unity of the
          many different forms of cancer. French edition, 1776.

2609   POTT, PERCIVALL. 1714-1788
          Chirurgical observations relative to the cataract, the polypus of the nose,
          the cancer of the scrotum, *etc.* London, *Hawes, Clarke & Collins,* 1775.
          First description of an occupational cancer (chimney-sweeps' cancer of
          the scrotum).

2609.1   SOEMMERRING, SAMUEL THOMAS. 1755-1830
          De morbis vasorum absorbentium corporis humani. Trajecti ad Moenum,
          Varrentrapp & Wenner, 1795.
          Soemmerring noted an association between pipe smoking and cancer
          of the lip (p. 109).

2610   RÉCAMIER, JOSEPH CLAUDE ANTHELM. 1774-1852
          Recherches sur le traitement du cancer par la compression méthodique. 2
          vols. Paris, *Gabon,* 1829.
          Récamier was the first to recognize the process of metastasis. He also
          described for the first time invasion of veins by cancer.

2611   HOME, *Sir* EVERARD. 1756-1832
          A short tract on the formation of tumours. London, *Longman,* 1830.
          Contains the first illustrations of microscopic sections of cancer. Home
          drew no worthwhile conclusion from his microscopic studies.

2611.1   WARREN, JOHN COLLINS. 1778-1856
          Surgical observations on tumours, with cases and operations. Boston,
          Crocker & Brewster, 1837.
          First North American book on tumours. Contains 16 hand-coloured
          plates by David Claypoole Johnston (1799-1865).

2612   MÜLLER, JOHANNES. 1801-1858
          Ueber den feinern Bau und die Formen der krankhaften Geschwülste. Lief.
          1. Berlin, *G. Reimer,* 1838.
          This classic work showed that Müller realized the necessity of the cell
          theory for the comprehension of the nature of cancer. He recognized cells,
          their nuclei and nucleoli, and could distinguish various types of tumours
          microscopically. Only Lieferung 1 of the book was published; C. West

translated it into English in 1840. Improved translation with important commentary in L.J. Rather, P. Rather, & J.B. Frerichs, *Johannes Müller and the nineteenth-century origins of tumor cell theory*, Canton, Mass, *Science History Publications*, [1986].

2612.1   WALSHE, WALTER HAYLE. 1812-1892
On the nature and treatment of cancer. London, *Taylor & Walton*, 1846.
Earliest account of the recognition of fragments of malignant tissue.

2613   VIRCHOW, RUDOLF LUDWIG KARL. 1821-1902
Zur Entwickelungsgeschichte des Krebses. *Virchows Arch. path. Anat.*, 1847, **1**, 94-201.
While still a young man Virchow founded the above journal. He wrote a fine paper on cancer and suggested that the exciting cause is local irritation.

2614   LEIDY, JOSEPH. 1823-1891
Transplantation of malignant tumors. *Proc. Acad. nat. Sci. Philad.*, 1851, **5**, 212.
First experimental transplantation of tumours.

2615   HANNOVER, ADOLPH. 1814-1894
Das Epithelioma. Leipzig, *L. Voss*, 1852.
Hannover coined the word "epithelioma." He did not recognize its malignant character but maintained that metastases were produced by cancer cells arriving by way of the blood stream.

2616   BRIGHT, RICHARD. 1789-1858
Clinical memoirs on abdominal tumours and intumescence. London, *New Sydenham Soc.*, 1860.

2617   VIRCHOW, RUDOLF LUDWIG KARL. 1821-1902
Die krankhaften Geschwülste. Vol. 1-3, Heft 1. Berlin, *A. Hirschwald*, 1863-67.
Although tumours were perhaps his greatest interest, Virchow never completed this work which was intended to have 30 lectures. Instead he stopped with the 25th lecture, on carcinoma, probably because of the vigorous attack which Remak and others were making on his conception of the histogenesis of epithelioma. Virchow's 25th lecture records one of his mistakes – his theory of the connective-tissue origin of carcinoma. So great was Virchow's influence that this error was not generally recognized until the work of Waldeyer (*see* No. 2620).

2618   THIERSCH, CARL. 1822-1895
Der Epithelialkrebs namentlich der Haut. 1 vol. and atlas. Leipzig, *W. Engelmann*, 1865.
Thiersch, Professor of Surgery at Erlangen and inventor of the method of skin grafting which bears his name, also made an important contribution to the knowledge of the histogenesis of cancer. He disproved Virchow's theory of the connective-tissue origin of cancer, and advanced evidence of its epithelial cell origin.

2619 MOORE, CHARLES HEWITT. 1821-1870
On the influence of inadequate operations on the theory of cancer. *Med.-chir. Trans.*, 1867, **50**, 245-80.

Modern surgical treatment of cancer is based upon principles laid down by Moore. For cancer of the breast he showed that recurrence was not due to the development of an entirely new tumour because of constitutional susceptibility, as was then generally theorized, but to incomplete removal of the original tumour. He insisted that the entire breast be carefully removed in every case of breast cancer.

2620 WALDEYER-HARTZ, HEINRICH WILHELM GOTTFRIED. 1836-1921
Die Entwicklung der Carcinome. *Virchows Arch. path, Anat.*, 1867, **41**, 470-523; 1872, **55**, 67-159.

Waldeyer confirmed the work of Thiersch (No. 2618) on the epithelial origin of cancer, disproving Virchow's theory (No. 2617). So great was the authority of the latter that it was not until the appearance of the second of the above papers that Virchow's error was finally recognized.

2620.1 NOVINSKY, MSTISLAV ALEXANDROVICH. 1841-1914
O privivanii rakovikh novoobrazovanii. [On the inoculation of cancerous neoplasms.] *Med. Vestn.*, 1876, **16**, 289-90.

Novinsky successfully transplanted two tumours in dogs. German translation in *Zbl. med. Wiss.*, 1876, **14**, 790-91. A fuller report appeared in his thesis *K voprosu o privivanii zlokachestvennich novoobrazovanii (eksperimentalnoi issledovanii). [On the question of inoculation of malignant neoplasms (experimental investigations)].* St. Petersburg, 1877.

2620.2 WEHR, V.
Demonstration der durch Impfung von Hund auf Hund erzeugten Carcinomknötchen. *Verh. dtsch. Ges. Chir.*, 1888, **17**, 52-53.

A tumour transplant from dog to dog was reported by Wehr.

2621 HANAU, ARTHUR NATHAN. 1858-1900
Erfolgreiche experimentelle Uebertragung von Carcinom. *Fortschr. Med.*, 1889, **7**, 321-39.

Hanau successfully transplanted cancer in mammals.

2622 RUSSELL, WILLIAM. 1852-1940
An address on a characteristic organism of cancer. *Brit. med. J.*, 1890, **2**, 1356-60.

"Russell's bodies."

2622.1 MORAU, HENRI. 1860-
Inoculation en série d'une tumeur épithéliale de la souris blanche. *C. R. Soc. Biol.*, 1891, **43**, 289-90.

In 1889 Morau transferred epitheliomata in mice and by 1893 had carried his experiments through 17 generations, the first systematic survey of tumour-host relationships from a purely biological viewpoint.

2623 KUNDRAT, HANS. 1845-1893
Ueber Lympho-Sarkomatosis. *Wien. klin. Wschr.*, 1893, **6**, 211-13, 234-39.

"Kundrat's lymphosarcoma."

2624   SJÖGREN, TAGE ANTON ULTIMUS. 1859-1939
        Fall af epiteliom behandladt med Roentgenstraler. *Förh. Svenska Läkare-Sallskapets Sammankomster,* Stockholm, 1899, p. 208.
        In June 1899 Sjögren was the first successfully to use Roentgen rays in the treatment of cancer.

2624.1 LOEB, LEO. 1869-1959
        On transplantation of tumours. *J. med. Res.,* 1901, **6**, 28-38.
        Loeb successfully transplanted cystic sarcoma of the thyroid in rats. He established the fact that growth of the transplant occurred through proliferation of its peripheral cells.

2625   BORST, MAXIMILIAN. 1869-1946
        Die Lehre von den Geschwülsten. 2 vols. Wiesbaden, *J. F. Bergmann,* 1902.
        "With this book the microscopical epoch in the evolution of the knowledge of cancer may be said to have been brought to a close" (Haagensen).

2625.1 FRIEBEN, ERNST AUGUST FRANZ ALBERT. 1875-
        Cancroid des rechten Handrückens. *Dtsch. med. Wschr.,* 1902, **28**, Vereins-Beilage, 335.
        Frieben reported the carcinogenic effect of x rays in man.

2626   HANSEMANN, DAVID PAUL VON. 1858-1920
        Die mikroskopische Diagnose der bösartigen Geschwülste. 2te. Aufl. Berlin, *A. Hirschwald,* 1902.
        Hansemann originated the theory of anaplasia.

2627   GOLDBERG, S. W., & LONDON, EFIM SEMENOVIC. 1869-1939
        Zur Frage der Beziehungen zwischen Becquerelstrahlen und Hautaffectionen. *Derm. Z.,* 1903, **10**, 457-62.
        Records the first successful employment of radium in the treatment of cancer.

2627.1 PERTHES, GEORG CLEMENS. 1869-1927
        Ueber den Einfluss der Röntgenstrahlen auf epitheliale Gewebe, insbesondere auf das Carcinom. *Arch. klin. Chir.,* 1903, **71**, 955-1000.
        Perthes was among the first to study the inhibitory effect of x rays on carcinoma; he was a pioneer in radiotherapy.

2628   JENSEN, CARL OLUF. 1864-1934
        Experimentelle Untersuchungen über Krebs bei Mäusen. *Zbl. Bakt.,* 1903, Abt. I, Orig., **34**, 28-34, 122-43.
        Jensen carried rat sarcoma through as many as 40 generations of rodents without change in microscopic structure. His classic study discredited the theory of the infectivity of cancer, and established its inoculability. See also *Z. Krebsforsch.,* 1909, **7**, 45-54.

2629   SCHMIDT, MARTIN BENNO. 1863-1949
        Die Verbreitungswege der Karzinome und die Beziehung generalisierter Sarkome zu den leukämischen Neubildungen. Jena, *G. Fischer,* 1903.
        Schmidt supported the theory of the haematogenous origin of carcinoma metastases.

2630   SJÖGREN, TAGE ANTON ULTIMUS. 1859-1939
Om Röntgenbehandling af sarkom. *Hygiea*, 1904, 2 F., **4**, 1142-49.

2631   ———. Om Röntgenbehandling af maligna svulster. *Nord. T. Terapi*, 1904-05, **3**, 8-23.
See No. 2624.

2632   RIBBERT, MORITZ WILHELM HUGO. 1855-1920
Die Entstehung des Carcinoms. Bonn, *F. Cohen*, 1905.
Ribbert was the modern protagonist of the theory of the embryonal origin of cancer.

2633   TYZZER, ERNEST EDWARD. 1875-1965
A study of heredity in relation to the development of tumours in mice. *J. med. Res.*, 1907-08, **17**, 199-211.
First experimental study of the heredity of mouse cancer.

2634   SCHLOFFER, HERMANN. 1868-1937
Chronisch entzündliche Bauchdeckengeschwülste nach Bruchoperationen. *Zbl. Chir.*, 1908, **35**, Beilage, 113-15.
"Schloffer's tumour" – an inflammatory tumour of the abdomen following herniotomy.

2635   LAZARUS-BARLOW, WALTER SYDNEY. 1865-1950
The Croonian Lectures on radioactivity and carcinoma. *Brit. med. J.*, 1909, **1**, 1465-70, 1536-44.

2636   CARREL, ALEXIS. 1873-1944, & BURROWS, MONTROSE THOMAS. 1884-1947
Cultures de sarcome en dehors de l'organisme. *C. R. Soc. Biol. (Paris)*, 1910, **69**, 332-34.
Using the Rous chicken sarcoma, Carrel and Burrows were the first to grow tumour tissue *in vitro*.

2637   ROUS, FRANCIS PEYTON. 1879-1970
A transmissible avian neoplasm (sarcoma of the common fowl). *J. exp. Med.*, 1910, **12**, 696-705; 1911, **13**, 397-411.
Original description of the chicken sarcoma (Rous sarcoma). More than 50 years later (1966) Rous shared the Nobel Prize with Charles Huggins for work on cancer. Rous demonstrated that sarcomatous tumours in hens could be transmitted to normal hens by the injection of cell-free filtrates of the original tumour.

2637.1   CLUNET, JEAN. 1878-1917
Le cancer expérimental. *J. méd. franç.*, 1911, **5**, 299-305.
Experimental production of malignant tumours by means of *x* rays.

2638   FREUND, ERNST. 1863-1946, & KAMINER, GISA. 1883-1941
Zur Diagnose des Karzinoms. *Wien. klin. Wschr.*, 1911, **24**, 1759-64.
A serum reaction, employed by Freund and Kaminer in 1910 for the diagnosis of cancer.

2639   BAYON, HENRY PETER GEORGE. 1876-1952
Epithelial proliferation induced by the injection of gasworks tar. *Lancet*, 1912, **2**, 1579.
Experimental production of cancer by the injection of tar.

2640   FIBIGER, JOHANNES. 1867-1928
Untersuchungen über eine Nematode (Spiroptera sp. n.) und deren
Fähigkeit papillomatöse und carcinomatöse Geschwulstbildungen im
Magen der Ratte hervorzurufen. *z. Krebsforsch.*, 1913, **13**, 217-80; 1914, **14**,
295-326.
    Fibiger demonstrated in rodents the effect of nematodes in the devel-
opment of carcinoma. He was awarded the Nobel Prize in 1926. His results
have subsequently not been confirmed and are no longer accepted.

2641   HOFFMAN, FREDERICK LUDWIG. 1865-1946
The mortality from cancer throughout the world. Newark, N.J., *Prudential
Press*, 1915.

2642   LATHROP, A. E. C., & LOEB, LEO. 1869-1959
Further investigations on the origin of tumours in mice. III. On the part
played by internal secretion in the spontaneous development of tumours.
J. Cancer Res., 1916, **1**, 1-19.
    Demonstration of the influence of an internal secretion on the devel-
opment of spontaneous cancer. Castration of female mice of a strain in
which mammary cancer was frequent reduced its incidence and delayed
its growth.

2643   YAMAGIWA, KATSUSABURO. 1863-1930, & ICHIKAWA, KOICHI. 1888-1948
Ueber die künstliche Erzeugung von Karzinom. *Verh. jap. path. Ges.*, 1916,
6, 169-78; 1917, **7**, 191-96.
    First experimental production of tar cancer in rabbits by painting with
tar products.

2644   EWING, JAMES. 1866-1943
Neoplastic diseases. Philadelphia, *W. B. Saunders*, 1919.
    Fourth edition, 1940.

2645   BRODERS, ALBERT COMPTON. 1885-1964
Squamous-cell epithelioma of the lip. A study of five hundred and thirty-
seven cases. *J. Amer. med. Assoc.*, 1920, **74**, 656-64.
    Broders's classification of tumours, an index of malignancy.

2645.1 BULLOCK, FREDERICK DABNEY. 1878- , *et al.*
A preliminary report on the experimental production of sarcoma of the
liver of rats. *Proc. Soc. exp. Biol. (N.Y.)*, 1920, **18**, 29-30.
    Proof that cancer can be caused by a parasite, *Cysticercus fasciolaris*,
the larval stage of *Taenia crassicolis*. With M. R. Curtis and G. L. Rohdenberg.
See also *Proc. N.Y. path. Soc.*, 1920, **20**, 149-75.

2646   KENNAWAY, *Sir* ERNEST LAURENCE. 1881-1958
The formation of a cancer-producing substance from isoprene (2-methyl-
butadiene). *J. Path. Bact.*, 1924, **27**, 233-38.
    Kennaway produced carcinogenic tars by submitting acetylene or
isoprene to high temperatures in an atmosphere of hydrogen, thus proving
that some carcinogens are pure hydrocarbons.

2647   GYE, WILLIAM EWART. 1884-1952
The aetiology of malignant new growths. *Lancet*, 1925, **2**, 109-17.
Gye advanced the theory that an ultramicroscopic virus combined with an intrinsic chemical factor were concerned in the production of the Rous sarcoma.

2648   BARNARD, JOSEPH EDWIN. 1870-1949
The microscopical examination of filterable viruses associated with malignant new growths. *Lancet*, 1925, **2**, 117-23.
Barnard supported, with photomicrographs, Gye's theory concerning the origin of cancer.

2649   DAWSON, JAMES WALKER. 1870-1927
The melanomata. *Edinb. med. J.*, 1925, **32**, 501-732.
A classic account.

2650   BENDIEN, S. G. T. *d.* 1942
Haemagglutinegehalte van het bloedserum bij carcinoompatiënten. *Ned. T. Geneesk.*, 1926, **70**, i, 2856-58.
Bendien test for the diagnosis of cancer. He published books in German and English on this subject in 1931. Modification by E. C. Lowe, *Brit. med. J.*, 1932, **2**, 1060.

2651   WARBURG, OTTO HEINRICH. 1883-1970
Ueber den Stoffwechsel der Tumoren. Berlin, *J. Springer*, 1926.
In his important studies of the metabolism of tumours, Warburg was first to observe that malignant tissue utilizes glucose by glycolysis, whether or not oxygen is available (aerobic glycolysis). English translation, 1930.

2652   SLYE, MAUD. 1879-1954
Cancer and heredity. *Ann. intern. Med.*, 1928, **1**, 951-76.
By selective breeding over a period of 15 years, Slye produced generations of mice absolutely resistant to, or particularly susceptible to, cancer. She demonstrated that resistance is a Mendelian dominant and susceptibility a recessive, either of which can be bred into or out of susceptible or resistant generations, according to the laws of genetics. Her earlier papers are in *J. med. Res.*, 1914, **25**, 281; 1915, **27**, 159; *J. Cancer Res.*, 1916, **1**, 479, 503; 1921, **6**, 139; 1922, **7**, 107.

2652.1   WIDERÖE, R.
Über ein neues Prinzip zur Herstellung höher Spannungen. *Arch. Elektrotech.*, 1928, **21**, 387-406.
RF-powered linear accelerator.

2653   PIRQUET VON CESENATICO, CLEMENS PETER. 1874-1929
Allergie des Lebensalters, die bösartigen Geschwülste. Leipzig, *G. Thieme*, 1930.
Important study of the age and sex incidence of cancer.

2654   COOK, *Sir* JAMES WILFRED. 1900-1975, *et al.*
The production of cancer by pure hydrocarbons. *Proc. roy. Soc. B*, 1932, **111**, 455-96.
Discovery of the carcinogenic properties of dibenzanthracene compounds. With I. Hieger, E. L. Kennaway, and W. V. Mayneord.

2655   PANCOAST, HENRY KHUNRATH. 1875-1939
        Superior pulmonary sulcus tumor. Tumor characterized by pain. Horner's
        syndrome, destruction of bone and atrophy of hand muscles. *J. Amer. med.
        Assoc.*, 1932, **99**, 1391-96.
        "Pancoast's tumour."

2656   SHOPE, RICHARD EDWIN. 1901-1966
        A transmissible tumor-like condition in rabbits. *J. exp. Med.*, 1932, **56**, 793-
        802.
        Shope papilloma, a benign infectious tumour due to a virus.

2657   LACASSAGNE, ANTOINE MARCELLIN. 1884-1971
        Apparition de cancers de la mamelle chez la souris mâle, soumise à des
        injections de folliculine. *C. R. Acad. Sci. (Paris)*, 1932, **195**, 630-32.

2658   BITTNER, JOHN JOSEPH. 1904-1961
        Some possible effects of nursing on the mammary gland tumor incidence
        in mice. *Science*, 1936, **84**, 162.
        Bittner's "milk factor," the murine mammary tumour involved in the
        transmission of cancer in mice. See also *Amer. J. clin. Path.*, 1937, **7**, 430-
        35.

2659   BONSER, GEORGIANA MAY. 1898-1979, *et al.*
        The carcinogenic action of oestrone: induction of mammary carcinoma in
        female mice of a strain refractory to the spontaneous development of
        mammary tumours. *J. Path. Bact.*, 1937, **45**, 709-14.
        With L. H. Stickland and K. I. Connal.

2659.1 KERST, DONALD WILLIAM. 1911-
        Acceleration of electrons by magnetic induction. *Phys. Rev.*, 1940, **58**, 841.
        Betatron.

2659.2 LEUCHTENBERGER, CECILE. 1906- , *et al.*
        "Folic acid" a tumour growth inhibitor. *Proc. Soc. exp. Biol. (N.Y.)*, 1944,
        55, 204-05.
        Inhibition of tumour growth by a folic acid concentrate. With R.
        Lewisohn, D. Laszlo, and R. Leuchtenberger. These workers later (*Proc. Soc.
        exp. Biol. N.Y.*, 1944, **56**, 144-45) obtained similar results with xanthopterin.

2659.3 HADDOW, *Sir* ALEXANDER. 1907-1976, *et al.*
        Influence of synthetic oestrogens upon advanced malignant disease. *Brit.
        med. J.*, 1944, **2**, 393-98.
        Administration of synthetic oestrogens in advanced mammary cancer
        caused regression of tumours. With J. M. Watkinson, E. Paterson, and P. C.
        Koller.

2659.4 McMILLAN, EDWIN MATTISON. 1907-
        The synchrotron: a proposed high energy particle accelerator. *Phys. Rev.*,
        1945, **68**, 143-144.

2659.5 ALVAREZ, LUIS WALTER. 1911-1988
        The design of a proton linear accelerator. *Phys. Rev.*, 1946, **70**, 799-800.
        Linear ion accelerator. Alvarez received the Nobel Prize for Physics in
        1968.

2659.6   GOODMAN, LOUIS SANFORD. 1906- , *et al.*
Nitrogen mustard therapy. Use of methyl-bis (beta-chloroethyl)amine
hydrochloride and tris (beta-chloroethyl)amine hydrochloride for Hodgkin's
disease, lymphosarcoma, leukemia, and certain allied and miscellaneous
disorders. *J. Amer. med. Assoc.*, 1946, **105**, 475-76.
    With M. M. Wintrobe, W. Dameshek, M. J. Goodman, and M. T.
McLennan.

2660   BEARD, HOWARD HORACE. 1894- , *et al.*
Effect of intraperitoneal injection of malignant urine extracts in normal and
hypophysectomized rats. *Science*, 1947, **105**, 475-76.
    Test for diagnosis of cancer. With B. Halperin and S. H. Libert.

2660.1   FARBER, SIDNEY. 1903-1973, *et al.*
Temporary remissions in acute leukemia in children produced by folic acid
antagonist 4-amethopteroylglutamic acid (aminopterin). *New Engl. J. Med.*,
1948, **238**, 787-93.
    With L. K. Diamond, R. D. Mercer, R. F. Sylvester, and V. A. Wolff.

2660.2   CASSEN, BENEDICT. 1902- , *et al.*
A sensitive directional gamma-ray detector. *Nucleonics*, 1950, **6**, 78-81.
    Scintillation counters for tumour location. With L. Curtis and C. W. Reed.

2660.3   BERGMANN, WERNER, & FEENEY, ROBERT J.
Contributions to the study of marine products. XXXII. The nucleosides of
sponges. I. *J. org. Chem.*, 1951, **16**, 981-7.
    Cytosine arabinoside, a pyramidine antagonist, used in acute
myeloblastic anaemia.

2660.4   EVERETT, JAMES LIONEL, *et al.*
Aryl-2-halogenoalkylamines. Part XII. Some carboxylic derivatives of *NN*-
Di 2-chloroethylaniline. *J. chem. Soc.*, 1953, 2386-92.
    Chlorambucil (a nitrogen mustard) used in the chemotherapy of can-
cer. With J. R. Roberts and W. J. C. Ross.

2660.5   FARBER, SIDNEY. 1903-1973, *et al.*
Clinical studies on the carcinolytic action of triethylenephosphoramide.
Cancer, 1953, **6**, 135-41.
    TEPA. With five co-authors.

2660.6   GRAY, LOUIS HAROLD. 1905-1965, *et al.*
The concentration of oxygen dissolved in tissues at the time of irradiation
as a factor in radiotherapy. *Brit. J. Radiol.*, 1953, **26**, 638-48.
    The sensitivity of tumour cells to x rays shown to be much enhanced
when irradiated in a well-oxygenated medium. With A. D. Conger, M.
Ebert, S. Hornsey, and O. C. A. Scott.

2660.7   BERGEL, FRANZ. 1900- , & STOCK, J. A.
Cytoactive amino-acid and peptide derivatives. I. Substituted
phenylalanines. *J. chem. Soc.*, 1954, 2409-17.
    Melphalan (a nitrogen mustard) later used in the chemotherapy of
cancer.

2660.8   FARBER, SIDNEY. 1903-1973
           Carcinolytic action of antibiotics: puromycin and actinomycin. D. *Amer. J. Path.*, 1955, **31**, 582 (only).

2660.9   HEIDELBERGER, CHARLES. 1920- , *et al.*
           Fluorinated pyrimidines, a new class of tumour-inhibitory compounds. *Nature (Lond.),* 1957, **179**, 663-6.
           Synthesis of 5-fluorouracil. With eight co-authors.

2660.10   STEWART, SARAH ELIZABETH. 1906- , *et al.*
           The induction of neoplasms with a substance released from mouse tumors by tissue culture. *Virology,* 1957, **3**, 380-400.
           Isolation of polymavirus (papovavirus). With B. E. Eddy, A. M. Gochenour, N. G. Borgese, and G. E. Grubbs.

2660.11   ARNOLD, HERBERT. *et al.*
           Neuartige Krebs-Chemotherapeutica aus der Gruppe der zyklischen N-Lost-Phosphamidester. *Naturwissenschaften,* 1958, **45**, 64-66.
           Cyclophosphamide. With F. Bourseaux and N. Brock.

2660.12   BURKITT, DENIS PARSONS. 1911- .
           A sarcoma involving the jaws in African children. *Brit J. Surg.,* 1958-59, **46**, 218-23.
           "Burkitt's tumour" (African lymphoma), first described in detail by Sir Albert Cook, a medical missionary, but not published by him.

2660.13   VOGT, MARGUERITE, & DULBECCO, RENATO. 1914-
           Virus-cell interaction with a tumour-producing virus. *Proc. nat. Acad. Sci. (Wash.),* **46**, 365-70.
           Polyomavirus (papovavirus) shown to be capable of transforming cells in culture.

2660.14   BROOME, JOHN DENIS.
           Evidence that the L-asparaginase of guinea pig serum is responsible for its antilymphoma effects. *J. exp. Med.,* 1963, **118**, 99-148.

2660.15   FOWLER, J. F. *et al.*
           Pre-therapeutic experiments with the fast neutron beam from the Medical Research Council cyclotron. A symposium. *Brit. J. Radiol.,* 1963, **36**, 77-121.

2660.16   JOHNSON, IRVING STANLEY. 1925- , *et al.*
           The Vinca alkaloids: a new class of oncolytic agents. *Cancer Res.,* 1963, **23**, 1390-1427.
           Includes vinblastine and vincristine. With J. G. Armstrong, M. Gorman and J. P. Burnett jr.

2660.17   EPSTEIN, MICHAEL ANTHONY. 1921- , & BARRY M.
           Cultivation in vitro of human lymphoblasts from Burkitt's malignant lymphoma. *Lancet,* 1964, **1**, 252-3.
           Discovery of a human herpes virus causing infectious mononucleosis and implicated in Burkitt's lymphoma and other forms of cancer.

2660.18   ——., *et al.*
Virus particles in cultured lymphoblasts from Burkitt's lymphoma. *Lancet,* 1964, **1**, 702-3.
Presence of herpes-like virus particles in Burkitt's tumour cells reported. With B. G. Achong and Y. M. Barr.

2660.19   PULVERTAFT, ROBERT JAMES VALENTINE. 1897-
Cytology of Burkitt's tumour (African lymphoma). *Lancet,* 1964, **1**, 238-40.

2660.20   TEMIN, HOWARD MARTIN. 1934-
Nature of the provirus of Rous sarcoma. *National Cancer Institute Monograph 17.* Bethesda, Md., *National Cancer Institute,* 1964, pp. 557-70.
Temin proposed a DNA intermediate in Rous sarcoma virus infection – after infection a DNA provirus is synthesized which contains all the genetic information of the RNA viral genome. Temin shared the Nobel Prize with D. Baltimore and R. Dulbecco in 1975.

2660.21   CLEMMESEN, JOHANNES. 1908-
Statistical studies in the aetiology of malignant neoplasms. 5 vols. Kobenhavn, *Ejnar Munksgaard,* 1965-77.
Acta path. microbiol. scand., Suppl. 174 (Pts. 1-2), 209, 247, 261.

2660.22   BALTIMORE, DAVID. 1938-
RNA-dependant DNA polymerase in virions of RNA tumour viruses. *Nature (Lond.),* 1970, **226**, 1209-11.
Baltimore shared the Nobel Prize with R. Dulbecco and H. M. Temin in 1975 for discoveries concerning the interaction between tumour viruses and the genetic material of the cell.

2660.23   TEMIN, HOWARD MARTIN. 1934- , & MIZUTANI, SATOSHI.
RNA-dependent DNA polymerase in virions of Rous sarcoma virus. *Nature (Lond.),* 1970, **226**, 1211-13.
See No. 2660.22

2660.24   DE VITA, VINCENT T. 1935- , *et al.*
Combination chemotherapy in the treatment of advanced Hodgkin's disease. *Ann. intern. Med.,* 1970, **73**, 881-95.
Combination chemotherapy with nitrogen mustard (mustine hydrochloride), vincristine sulphate, procarbazine hydrochloride and prednisone, introduced in 1964 for the treatment of advanced Hodgkin's disease. With A. A. Serpick and P. P. Carbone.

2660.25   SHOPE, THOMAS, *et al.*
Malignant lymphoma in cottontop marmosets after inoculation with Epstein–Barr virus. *Proc. nat. Acad. Sci. (Wash.),* 1973, **70**, 2487-91.
Epstein–Barr virus as a cause of Burkitt's lymphoma. With D. DeChairo and G. Miller.

2660.26   BIGGS, PETER MARTIN. 1926- , *et al.*
Field trials providing immunity against the Marek's disease (of chickens) herpes virus demonstrated the aetiological relationship of this virus with cancer. With six co-authors.

2660.27   DULBECCO, RENATO. 1914-
           From the molecular biology of oncogenic DNA viruses to cancer. *Les Prix
           Nobel en 1975*, Stockholm, pp. 172-80.
               Dulbecco shared the Nobel Prize in 1975 with D. Baltimore and H. M.
           Temin for his discoveries concerning the interaction between tumour
           viruses and the genetic material of the cell.

2660.28   VARMUS, HAROLD E. 1942- , & BISHOP, J. MICHAEL. 1936- *et al.*
           DNA related to the transforming gene(s) of avian sarcoma viruses is
           present in normal avian DNA. *Nature*, 1976, **260**, 170-73.
               Discovery of the first "oncogene." Varmus and Bishop shared the Nobel
           Prize for medicine in 1989. The paper was co-authored by D. Stehelin and
           P. Vogt, neither of whom shared in the prize.

History of Oncology

2661   BEHLA, ROBERT. 1850-1921
           Die Carcinomlitteratur. Eine Zusammenstellung der in- und ausländischen
           Krebsschriften bis 1900. Berlin, *R. Schoetz*, 1901.

2661.1   WOLFF, JACOB. 1861-1938
           Die Lehre von der Krebskrankheit von den ältesten Zeiten bis zur Gegenwart.
           4 vols. Jena, *Fischer*, 1907-28.
               Exhaustive and accurate review of all the available information on
           cancer.

2662   HAAGENSEN, CUSHMAN DAVIS. 1900-
           An exhibit of important books, papers, and memorabilia illustrating the
           evolution of the knowledge of cancer. *Amer. J. Cancer*, 1933, **18**, 42-126.

2662.1   DONNER FOUNDATION.
           Index to the literature of experimental cancer research 1900-1935. Lancaster,
           Pa., *Wickersham Printing Co.*, 1948.
               Divided into author and subject sections.

2662.2   VAILLANCOURT, PAULINE M.
           Bibliographic control of the literature of oncology 1800-1960. Metuchen,
           N.J., *Scarecrow Press*, 1969.
               Includes a short, well-documented history.

2662.3   SHIMKIN, MICHAEL BORIS. 1912-
           Contrary to nature. Being an illustrated commentary on some persons and
           events of historical importance in the development of knowledge con-
           cerning cancer. Washington, *Dept. Health, Education & Welfare*, 1977.

2662.4   RATHER, LELLAND JOSEPH. 1913-1989
           The genesis of cancer. A study in the history of ideas.
           Baltimore, *Johns Hopkins Press*, 1978.

2662.5   RAVEN, RONALD WILLIAM.
           The theory and practice on oncology. Historical evolution and present
           principles. Carnforth, Lancs., *Parthenon Publishing*, [1990].

PHYSICAL DIAGNOSIS : MEDICAL INSTRUMENTATION

See also under the names of individual organs and regions

2663   GALEN. A.D. 130-200
        De usu repirationis. An in arteriis natura sanguis contineatur. De usu
        pulsuum. De causis respirationis. An edition with English translation and
        commentary by D.J. FURLEY and J.S. WILKIE. Princeton, *Princeton University
        Press*, 1984.
            These texts illustrate Galen's views on respiration and the arteries.
        Galen established a system of medicine on the minutiae of pulse variations,
        which persisted into the 18th century.

2664   ———. De differentiis morborum libri ii...Parisiis, *Officina Henrici Stephani*,
        [1514].
            First Renaissance Latin translation of this work, made by Niccolo
        Leoniceno of Vicenza.

2665   ———. De morborum symptomatis. London, *R. Pynson*, 1522.
            This volume of Galen's selected works includes Thomas Linacre's Latin
        translation of *De symptomatum differentiis.*

2666   JOANNES ACTUARIUS. *fl.* 1350
        De urinis libri vii. Basileae, *apud. A. Cratandrum*, [1529].
            The most complete medieval treatise on uroscopy. Actuarius was first
        to use a graduated glass for its examination. Joannes Actuarius was the last
        of the great Byzantine physicians. This is the first complete Latin transla-
        tion. An abridged edition appeared in 1519. Partial English translation in
        No. 2241.

2667   SILVATICO, GIAMBATTISTA. 1550-1621
        De iis qui morborum simulant deprehendendis liber. Mediolani, *ex off
        quondam P. Pontii*, 1595.
            The first treatise on feigned diseases.

2668   SANTORIO, SANTORIO [SANCTORIUS]. 1561-1636
        Commentaria in primam fen primi libri canonis Avicennae. Venetiis, *Jacobus
        Sarcina*, 1625.
            The chief value of this work is in its cautious revelation of the principles
        of construction of various instruments that Santorio had invented, including
        a hygrometer, a pendulum for measuring pulse rate, a syringe for extracting
        bladder stones, and a bathing bed. The instruments are depicted in
        woodcut diagrams, the earliest illustrations of Santorio's instruments. For
        the first description of Santorio's pulse-clock *see* No. 572.1.

2670   FLOYER, *Sir* JOHN. 1649-1734
        The physician's pulse-watch. 2 vols. London, *S. Smith & B. Walford*, 1707-
        10.
            Before watches had hands to record the seconds, Floyer invented a
        pulse-watch which divided the minute. He was the first to count the pulse
        with the aid of a watch and to make regular observations on the pulse-rate.
        The second volume contains the first English translation of Cleyer's book
        on Chinese pulse-lore, *Specimen medicinae Sinicae. (see* No. 6492).

2671   MARTINE, George. 1702-1741
Essays medical and philosophical. London, *A. Millar*, 1740.
First important work on clinical thermometry, and the only scientific treatment of the subject before Wunderlich.

2672   AUENBRUGGER, Leopold, *Edler von Auenbrugg*. 1722-1809
Inventum novum ex percussione thoracis humani ut signo abstrusos interni pectoris morbos detegendi. Vindobonae, *J. T. Trattner*, 1761.
The greatness of Auenbrugger's discovery of the value of immediate percussion of the chest as a diagnostic measure was not at first recognized. His little book met with a cold reception, while a French translation by Rozière de la Chassagne in 1770 attracted little notice. But Auenbrugger lived to see the appearance in 1808 of J. N. Corvisart's classic translation of the book, after which the value of percussion was universally recognized. English translation by J. Forbes, 1824 (reprinted in Willius and Keys, *Cardiac classics*, 1941., pp. 193-213); also with introduction by H. E. Sigerist, in *Bull. Hist. Med.*, 1936, **4**, 373-403. For bibliography of the *Inventum novum* see P. J. Bishop, *Tubercle*, 1961, **42**, 78. Facsimile reprint by Max Neuburger (Vienna, 1922) includes the original edition, and translations into English, French and German.

2672.1   BOZZINI, Philipp. 1773-1809
Lichtleiter, eine Erfindung zur Anschauung innerer Theile und Krankheiten nebst der Abbildung. *J. pract. Heilk.*, 1806, **24**, 1 St., 107-24.
Bozzini introduced a speculum in which the idea of illumination and reflection by mirrors was utilized. English translation in *Urology*, 1974, **3**, 119-23. Bozzini published his work in book form, *Der Lichtleiter*, Weimar, 1807, which is translated in *Quart. Bull. Northw. Univ. med. Sch.*, 1949, **23**, 332-54.

2672.2   DOUBLE, François Joseph. 1776?-1842
Séméiologie générale, ou traité des signes et de leur valeur dans les maladies. Vol. 2. Paris, *Croullebois*, 1817.
Double introduced and applied auscultation (pp. 31 and 186).

2673   LAENNEC, René Theophile Hyacinthe. 1781-1826
De l'auscultation médiate, ou traité du diagnostic des maladies des poumons et du coeur. 2 vols. Paris, *J. A. Brosson & J. S. Claudé*, 1819.
Auscultation in the instrumental sense dates from Laennec's invention of the stethoscope (at first merely a roll of stiff paper) with a view to amplifying the sound of the heart's action. The publication of this book revolutionized the study of disease of the thoracic organs. The work illustrates his wooden stethoscope, which could be purchased from the publishers, and which was advertised for sale on the original printed wrappers of the first edition. The second edition, 1826, is even more important, since it gives not only the various physical signs elicited in the chest, but adds the pathological anatomy, diagnosis, and treatment of each disease encountered. Laennec, perhaps the greatest clinician of his time, died of tuberculosis. English translation by J. Forbes, 1821. Reprinted, 1962.

2674   STOKES, William. 1804-1878
An introduction to the use of the stethoscope. Edinburgh, *Maclachlan & Stewart*, 1825.

Stokes, famous member of the Irish school of medicine, published the first systematic treatise on the use of the stethoscope – and this before his qualification at Edinburgh. His name is perpetuated in medical literature in connection with "Cheyne–Stokes respiration" and the "Stokes–Adams syndrome."

2675   PIORRY, PIERRE ADOLPHE. 1794-1879
De la percussion médiate. Paris, *J. S. Chaudé*, 1828.
Piorry, pioneer of mediate percussion, introduced the percussor and the pleximeter in 1826. He also developed refinements to Laennec's stethoscope.

2676   SKODA, JOSEF. 1805-1881
Abhandlung über Perkussion und Auskultation. Wien, 1839.
Skoda classified the various sounds obtained on percussion according to their musical pitch and tone. "Skoda's resonance" is an important diagnostic sign in pneumonia and pericardial effusion. Following Skoda's work, percussion at last gained general acceptance as a diagnostic procedure. English translation, 1853.

2676.1   LEARED, ARTHUR. 1822-1879
On the self-adjusting double stethoscope. *Lancet*, 1856, **2**, 138, 202.
Leared demonstrated a binaural stethoscope at the Great Exhibition, London, 1851. Camman introduced the pattern whose main design continues in use today; this was illustrated in the *N.Y. med. Times*, Jan. 1855, and reproduced in *Lancet*, 1856, **1**, 398.

2676.2   NEUMANN, ERNST. 1834-1918
Ueber das verschiedene Verhalten gelähmter Muskeln gegen den constanten und inducirten Strom und die Erklärung desselben. *Dtsch. Klinik*, 1864, **16**, 65-69.
One of the first publications on electrodiagnosis.

2677   WUNDERLICH, CARL REINHOLD AUGUST. 1815-1877
Das Verhalten der Eigenwärme in Krankheiten. Leipzig, *O. Wigand*, 1868.
This classic work on temperature in disease laid the foundation of modern knowledge regarding clinical thermometry. Garrison has said of Wunderlich that he "found fever a disease and left it a symptom." The book was translated into English and published by the New Sydenham Society in 1871.

2678   WILKS, *Sir* SAMUEL, *Bart*. 1824-1911
On markings of furrows on the nails as the result of illness. *Lancet*, 1869, **1**, 5-6.

2679   ALLBUTT, *Sir* THOMAS CLIFFORD. 1836-1925
Medical thermometry. *Brit for med.- chir. Rev.*, 1870, **45**, 429-41.
Allbutt introduced the modern clinical thermometer.

2680   BROADBENT, *Sir* WILLIAM HENRY, *Bart*. 1835-1907
The pulse. London, *Cassell & Co.*, 1890.

2680.01   TRUAX, CHARLES. 1852-1918
The mechanics of surgery. Chicago, *Charles Truax & Co.*, 1899.

An encyclopaedic work which describes, illustrates and analyses the entire range of instrumentation employed in medical and surgical practice. No one since Truax has undertaken this ambitious project. Reprinted with introduction by James M. Edmonson, San Francisco, *Norman Publishing*, 1988.

2680.1   HOWRY, Douglas Hamilton. 1920- , & BLISS W. Roderic.
Ultrasonic visualization of soft-tissue structures of the body. *J. Lab. clin. Med.*, 1952, **40**, 579-92.
First tomogram of soft tissue.

2681   WILD, John Julian. 1911- , & REID, J. M.
Progress in the techniques of soft tissue examination by 15 MC pulsed ultrasound. In *Ultrasound in biology and medicine*, ed. E. Kelly. Washington, D. C., *American Institute of Biological Sciences*, 1957, pp. 30-48.

2682   DONALD, Ian. 1910-1987 , *et al.*
Investigation of abdominal masses by pulsed ultrasound. *Lancet*, 1958, **1**, 1188-94.
Donald , J. MacVicar and T. G. Brown used an ultrasound scanner to investigate the pregnant abdomen (*see also* No. 6235.1).

History of Physical Diagnosis: Medical Instrumentation

2682.50   MITCHELL, Silas Weir. 1829-1914
The early history of instrumental precision in medicine. New Haven, *Tuttle, Moorehouse & Taylor*, 1892.

2682.51   MOELLER-CHRISTENSEN, Peter Vilhelm. 1903-88.
The history of the forceps. Trans. by W.E. Calvert. Oxford, *Oxford University Press*, 1938.
Not limited to the obstetric forceps.

2682.52   REISER, Stanley Joel.
Medicine and the rise of technology. Cambridge, *Cambridge University Press*, 1978.

2682.53   BENNION, Elisabeth.
Antique medical instruments. London, *Sotheby Parke Bernet*, 1979.
Covers medical and surgical instruments from the Renaissance to 1870.

2682.54   DAVIS, Audrey B. & APPEL, Toby.
Bloodletting instruments in the National Museum of History and Technology. Washington, D.C., *Smithsonian Institution Press*, 1979.

2682.55   DAVIS, Audrey B.
Medicine and its technology: an introduction to the history of medical instrumentation. Westwood, Conn., *Greenwood Press*, [1981].

2682.56   WEBSTER, John G.
Encyclopedia of medical devices and instrumentation. John G. Webster, editor-in-chief. 4 vols., New York, *John Wiley & Sons*, [1988].

Some of the articles in this work include historical references, useful for the recent history of this rapidly evolving field.

2683   RÖNTGEN, WILHELM CONRAD. 1845-1923
Ueber eine neue Art von Strahlen.(Vorläufige Mittheilung.) *Sitzber. phys. -med. Ges. Würzburg*, 1895, 132-41. Eine neue Art von Strahlen. II. Mittheilung. Ibid, 1896, 11-16, 16-19.
The discovery of *x* rays, which Kölliker later renamed "Roentgen rays"; the foundation stone of the science of roentgenology. For his work, Röntgen was awarded the first Nobel Prize for Physics in 1901. English translation in *Nature*, (February,) 1896, **53**, 274 and 377. See also Röntgen's third paper on the subject: Weitere Beobachtungen über die Eigenschaften der X-Strahlen. *Sitzber. K. Preuss. Akad. Wiss., Ber., Kl. Phys.-Math.*, 1897, 576-592. Facsimile reprint of all three papers, English translation, and bibliography in H. Klickstein, *Wilhelm Conrad Röntgen on a new kind of rays. A bibliographical study*, 2 vols., 1966.

2684   JONES, *Sir* ROBERT. 1858-1933, & LODGE, *Sir* OLIVER JOSEPH. 1851-1940
The discovery of a bullet lost in the wrist by means of the Roentgen rays. *Lancet*, 1896, **1**, 476-77.
This was probably the first published report of the clinical use of *x* rays (February 22).

2684.1   KEEN, WILLIAM WILLIAMS. 1837-1932
The clinical application of the roentgen rays in surgical diagnosis. *Am. J. med. Sci.*, 1896, **111**, 256-61.
First clinical application in America, published in March, 1896.

2684.2   BECQUEREL, ANTOINE HENRI. 1852-1908
Sur les radiations émises par phosphorescence. *C. R. Acad. Sci. (Paris)*, 1896, **122**, 420-21.
The discovery of radioactivity – research stimulated by Roentgen's discovery of *x* rays. Becquerel shared the Nobel Prize for Physics in 1903 with Pierre and Marie Curie.

2684.3   MORTON, WILLIAM JAMES. 1846-1920
The x-ray and its application to dentistry. *Dental Cosmos*, 1896, **38**, 478-86.
First dental radiograph.

2685   PUPIN, MICHAEL IDVORSKY. 1858-1935
A few remarks on experiments with Roentgen rays. *Electricity*, New York, 1896, **10**, 68-69.
Introduction of the intensifying screen.

2686   THOMSON, ELIHU. 1853-1937
Stereoscopic Roentgen pictures. *Electrical World*, New York, 1896, **27**, 280.
Invention of the Roentgen stereoscope.

2686.1   WILLIAMS, FRANCIS HENRY. 1852-1936
          A method for more fully determining the outline of the heart by means of
          the fluorescope together with other uses of this instrument in medicine.
          Boston med. surg. J., 1896, **135**, 335-337.
          Estimation of heart size by fluoroscope, first application of *x* rays to
          cardiology.

2687   MACINTYRE, JOHN. 1857-1928
          X-ray records for the cinematograph. *Arch. Skiagraphy*, 1897, **1**, 37.
          Macintyre was the first to demonstrate *x*-ray cinematography.

2687.1   CANNON, WALTER BRADFORD. 1871-1945
          The movements of the stomach studied by means of the Roentgen rays.
          Amer. J. Physiol., 1898, **1**, 359-82.
          Cannon introduced the bismuth meal. He showed that bismuth, opaque
          to *x* rays, could be of great use in conjunction with roentgenology in the
          investigation of the digestive tract. *See* No. 1029.

2687.2   BORDEN, WILLIAM. 1858-1934.
          The use of the Röntgen ray by the Medical Department of the United States
          Army in the war with Spain (1898). Washington, *Government Printing Office*,
          1900.
          The Spanish-American War was the first war in which *x* rays were used
          for diagnostic purposes. This is the first report on the application of X rays
          to military medicine.

2687.3   WILLIAMS, FRANCIS HENRY. 1852-1936
          The Roentgen rays in medicine and surgery. New York, *Macmillan*, 1901.

2688   HOLZKNECHT, GUIDO. 1872-1931
          Eine neue, einfache Dosirungsmethode in der Radiotherapie (das
          Chromoradiometer). *Wien. klin. Rdsch.*, 1902, **16**, 685-87.
          Holzknecht did important work on Roentgen-ray dosimetry.

2689   ALBERS-SCHÖNBERG, HEINRICH ERNST. 1865-1921
          Die Röntgen-Technik. Hamburg, *L. Gräfe & Sillem*, 1903.
          Albers-Schönberg invented the compression diaphragm, the function
          of which is to intensify the object by cutting out secondary rays.

2690   GROEDEL, FRANZ-MAXIMILIAN. 1881-1951
          Die Technik der Roentgenkinematographie. *Dtsch. med. Wschr.*, 1909, **35**,
          434-35.
          First of an important series of papers by Groedel on Roentgen-
          cinematography.

2691   BUCKY, GUSTAV. 1880-1963
          A grafting-diaphragm to cut off secondary rays from the object. *Arch.
          Roentgen Ray*, 1913-14, **18**, 6-9.
          Bucky devised a diaphragm for roentgenography which, by preventing
          the secondary rays from reaching the plate, secured better contrast and
          definition.

2692   COOLIDGE, WILLIAM DAVID. 1873-1975
A powerful Roentgen ray tube with a pure electron discharge. *Amer J. Roentgenol.*, 1913-14, n.s. **1**, 115-24.
Coolidge invented the high vacuum tube, capable of kilovoltage energies.

2692.1   POTTER, HOLLIS ELMER. 1880-?
Diaphragming Roentgen rays. Studies and experiments. *Amer. J. Roentgenol.*, 1916, **3**, 142-5.
Moving grid.

2692.2   CAMERON, DON FRANKLIN. 1889-
Aqueous solutions of potassium and sodium iodids as opaque mediums in roentgenography. *J. Amer. med. Assoc.*, 1918, **70**, 754-5.

2693   SICARD, JEAN ATHANASE. 1872-1929, & FORESTIER, JACQUES. 1890-
Méthode radiographique d'exploration de la cavité épidurale par le lipiodol. *Rev. neurol.*, 1921, **28**, 1264-66.
Lipiodol first used in radiology.

2694   HOLZKNECHT, GUIDO. 1872-1931
Einstellung der Röntgenologie. Wien, *J. Springer*, 1927.

2695   OKA, MITSUTOMO.
Eine neue Methode zur röntgenologischen Darstellung der Milz. *Fortschr. Röntgenstr.*, 1929, **40**, 497-501.
Thorium dioxide ("thorotrast") first used in radiological diagnosis.

2696   STUMPF, PLEIKART. 1888-
Archiv und Atlas der normalen und pathologischen Anatomie in typischen Röntgenbildern. Das röntgenographische Bewegungsbild und seine Anwendung (Flachenkymographie und Kymoskopie). *Fortschr. Röntgenstr.*, 1931, Ergänzungsband 41.
Introduction of roentgenkymography.

2697   GIANTURCO, CESARE. 1905- , & ALVAREZ, WALTER CLEMENT. 1884-
Roentgen ray motion pictures of the stomach. *Proc. Mayo Clin.*, 1932, **7**, 669-71.
Camera used for direct Roentgen-cinematography.

2698   BARTELINK, D. L.
Röntgenschnitte. *Forschr. Röntgenstr.*, 1933, **47**, 399-407.
Tomography first described.

2699   GROSSMANN, G.
Tomographie. *Fortschr. Röntgenstr.*, 1935, **51**, 61-80, 191-208.
Grossmann improved the tomograph.

2700   WATSON, T.
Differential radiography. *Radiography*, 1939, **5**, 81-88.
Transverse tomography.

2700.01   TREADWELL, ANNE DE G. *et al.*
Metabolic studies on neoplasm of bone with the aid of radioactive strontium. *Am. J. med. Sci.*, 1942, **204**, 521-530.
Radioisotopic bone scanning. With B. Low-Beer, H. Friedell, and J. Lawrence.

2700.1   KINMONTH, JOHN BERNARD. 1916-1982
Lymphangiography in man. A method of outlining lymphatic trunks at operation, *Clin. Sci.*, 1952, **11**, 13-20.
Introduction of lymphangiography.

2700.2   ASTLEY, ROY.
Cineradiography with an image amplifier: a practical technique. *Brit. J. Radiol.*, 1955, **28**, 221-2.
Electron optical image intensifier, 1953.

2700.3   OLDENDORF, WILLIAM HENRY. 1925-
Isolated flying spot detection of radiodensity discontinuities displaying the internal structural pattern of a complex object. *IRE Trans. bio-med. Electron.*, 1961, **8**, 68-72.
Oldendorf described his experimental system for reconstructing the appearance of soft tissues by measuring radiodensity discontinuities (differences in tissue attenuation) but it was not fully recognized that very high efficiencies could be achieved until the work of Hounsfield (*see* No. 2700.4).

2700.4   HOUNSFIELD, *Sir* GODFRY NEWBOLD. 1919-
Computerized transverse axial scanning (tomography). *Brit J. Radiol.*, 1973, **46**, 1016-22.
Computer-assisted tomography (CAT), or computed tomography (CT). Hounsfield received a Nobel Prize in medicine in 1979 for his work. He was the first engineer to receive a Nobel prize in that category.

2700.5   LAUTERBUR, PAUL CHRISTIAN. 1929-
Image formation by induced local interactions: Examples employing nuclear magnetic resonance. *Nature*, 1973, **242**, 190-191.
Lauterbur proposed a workable method for using nuclear magnetic resonance to produce images of tissues.

History of Radiology

2701   GOCHT, HERMANN. 1869-1938
Die Röntgen-Literatur. 2 vols. Stuttgart, *F. Enke*, 1911-12.

2702   GLASSER, OTTO. 1895-1964
Wilhelm Conrad Röntgen and the early history of the Roentgen rays. London, *John Bale, Sons & Danielsson*, 1933.
The standard biography of Roentgen with a detailed history of the discovery of Roentgen rays and the early period of roentgenology. Bibliography of 1044 items published during the first year after Roentgen's discovery.

2702.2   BRUWER, André Johannes. 1918-
Classic descriptions in diagnostic roentgenology. 2 vols. Springfield, *C. C. Thomas*, 1964.
A compilation of pioneer contributions to the technology and methodology of diagnostic roentgenology.

2702.3   GRIGG, Emanuel Radu Newman. 1916-
The trail of the invisible light. From X-Strahlen to Radio(bio)logy. Springfield, *C.C. Thomas*, [1965].
A great deal of valuable information presented in a not always serious manner.

2702.4   BRECHER, Ruth, & BRECHER, Edward.
The rays: a history of radiology in the United States and Canada. Baltimore, *Williams & Wilkins*, 1969.

2702.5   BURROWS, E. H.
Pioneers and early years: A history of British radiology. Alderney, Channel Islands, *Colophon Limited*, [1986].
Well-illustrated and carefully documented, incorporating detailed biographies of pioneers. Covers the history before 1930.

DISEASES OF THE CARDIOVASCULAR SYSTEM

2703   WEPFER, Johann Jacob. 1620-1695
Observationes anatomicae, ex cadaveribus eorum, quos sustulit apoplexia. Schaffhusii, *J. C. Suteri*, 1658.
Wepfer showed apoplexy to be a result of haemorrhage into the brain. He described four cases, with clinical and postmortem findings. Partial English translation in Ruskin, *Classics in arterial hypertension* (1956).

2704   RAYNAUD, Maurice. 1834-1881
De l'asphyxie locale et de la gangrène symétrique des extrémités. Paris, *Rignoux*, 1862.
First description of "Raynaud's disease." For a translation by T. Barlow, see *Selected Monographs*, London, 1888, pp. 1-199, *New Sydenham Society*, which also contains a translation of Raynaud's second paper on the subject.

2705   NOTHNAGEL, Carl Wilhelm Hermann. 1841-1905
Zur Lehre von den vasomotorischen Neurosen. *Dtsch. Arch. klin. Med.*, 1867, **2**, 173-91.
Nothnagel described the vasomotor type of acroparaesthesia, sometimes called after him.

2706   MITCHELL, Silas Weir. 1829-1914
Clinical lecture on certain painful affections of the feet. *Philad. med. Times*, 1872, **3**, 81, 113.
First complete description of erythromelalgia, "Weir Mitchell's disease." See also his paper in *Amer. J. med. Sci.*, 1878, **76**, 17-36.

2707   LEGG, John Wickham. 1843-1921
A case of haemophilia complicated with multiple naevi. *Lancet*, 1876, **2**, 856.
First description of multiple hereditary telangiectasis ("Rendu–Osler–Weber disease").

2708 OERTEL, MAX JOSEPH. 1835-1934
Therapie der Kreislauf-Störungen. Leipzig, *F. C. W. Vogel*, 1884.
 English translation in von Ziemssen's *Handbook of general therapeutics*, Vol. 7, London, 1887.

2709 SCHULTZE, FRIEDRICH, 1848-1934
Ueber Akroparästhesie. *Dtsch. Z. Nervenheilk.*, 1893, **3**, 300-18.
 "Schultze's acroparaesthesia." Schultze described the simple form of acroparaesthesia.

2710 RENDU, HENRI JULES LOUIS. 1844-1902
Epistaxis répété chez un sujet porteur de petits angiomes cutanés et muqueux. *Gaz. Hop. (Paris)*, 1896, **69**, 1322-23.
 Rendu's account of multiple hereditary telangiectasis ("Rendu–Osler–Weber disease").

2711 OSLER, *Sir* WILLIAM *Bart*. 1849-1919
On a family form of recurring epistaxis, associated with multiple telangiectases of the skin and mucous membranes. *Johns Hopk. Hosp. Bull.*, 1901, **12**, 333-37.
 "Rendu–Osler–Weber disease." Multiple hereditary telangiectasis was first described by Legg (No. 2707) in 1876 and later by Rendu (No. 2710) and Weber (No. 2714). Reprinted in *Med. Classics*, 1939, **4**, 243-53.

2712 PAULI, WOLFGANG. 1869-1955
Ueber Ionenwirkung und ihre therapeutische Verwendung. *Münch. med. Wschr.*, 1903, **50**, 153-57.
 Hypotensive action of thiocyanates first noted.

2713 PAL, JAKOB. 1863-1936
Gefässkrisen. Leipzig, *S. Hirzel*, 1905.

2714 WEBER, FREDERICK PARKES. 1863-1962
Multiple hereditary developmental angiomata (telangiectases) of the skin and mucous membranes associated with recurring haemorrhages. *Lancet*, 1907, **2**, 160-62.
 "Rendu–Osler–Weber disease."

2715 MOSCHCOWITZ, ELI. 1879-1964
Hypertension of the pulmonary circulation. *Amer. J. med. Sci.*, 1927, **174**, 388-406.

2716 KEITH, NORMAN MACDONNELL. 1885-1976, *et al*.
Some different types of essential hypertension; their course and prognosis. *Amer J. med. Sci.*, 1929, **197**, 332-43.
 The Keith-Wagener-Barker classification of hypertension. With H. P. Wagener and N. W. Barker.

2717 HINES, EDGAR ALPHONSO. 1906- , & BROWN, GEORGE ELGIE. 1885-1935
A standard stimulus for measuring vasomotor reactions: its application in the study of hypertension. *Proc. Mayo Clin.*, 1932, **7**, 332-35.
 Cold-pressor test.

2718   TARR, LEONARD. 1901- , *et al.*
The circulation time in various clinical conditions determined by the use of sodium dehydrocholate. *Amer. Heart J.*, 1933, **8**, 766-86.
Use of decholin sodium for estimation of circulation time. With B. S. Oppenheimer and R. V. Sagar.

2719   GOLDBLATT, HARRY. 1891-1977 , *et al.*
Studies on experimental hypertension. 1. The production of persistent elevation of systolic blood pressure by means of renal ischemia. *J. exp. Med.*, 1934, **59**, 347-79.
The first of Goldblatt's important papers on experimental hypertension, which established an aetiologic role for renal ischemia in the production of hypertension and established a laboratory basis for its study. Written with J. Lynch, R. F. Hanzal, and W. W. Summerville.

2720   BARKER, MARION HERBERT. 1899-1947
The blood cyanates in the treatment of hypertension. *J. Amer. med. Assoc.*, 1936, **106**, 762-67.
Barker made thiocyanate treatment a practical proposition in hypertension.

2721   HOUSSAY, BERNARDO ALBERTO. 1887-1971, & FASCIOLO, JUAN CARLOS. 1911- Secreción hipertensora del rinón isquemiado. *Rev. Soc. argent. Biol.*, 1937, **13**, 284-94.
Houssay and Fasciolo transplanted an ischaemic kidney into an animal from which both kidneys had been removed. Hypertension resulted after establishment of circulation, supporting the view that hypertension is due to a chemical substance with pressor action produced in the ischaemic kidney. They later showed that the ischaemic kidneys of hypertensive dogs contained an excess of renin. See also *Biol. Acad. nac. Med. B. Aires*, 1937, **34**, 342; *J. Physiol. (Lond.)*, 1938, **94**, 281.

2722   HOMANS, JOHN. 1877-1955
Circulatory diseases of the extremities. New York, *Macmillan Co.*, 1939.

2723   WAGENER, HENRY PATRICK. 1890-1961, & KEITH, NORMAN MACDONNELL. 1885-1976
Diffuse arteriolar disease with hypertension and the associated retinal lesions. *Medicine*, 1939, **18**, 317-430.
Wagener and Keith classified essential hypertension into four groups.

2724   WILSON, CLIFFORD. 1906- , & BYROM, FRANK BURNET.
Renal changes in malignant hypertension; experimental evidence. *Lancet*, 1939, **1**, 136-39.
Production of hypertension in rats by constriction of one renal artery, and important studies of the renal changes produced, which included degeneration of the renal arterioles.

2724.1   BRAUN-MENENDEZ, EDUARDO. 1903- , *et al.*
The substance causing renal hypertension. *J. Physiol. (Lond.)*, 1940, **98**, 283-98.
Angiotensin. With J. C. Fasciolo, L. F. Leloir, and J. M. Muñoz. Independently isolated by Page and Helmer (*see* No. 2724.2) and later named angiotensin.

2724.2   PAGE, IRVING HEINLY. 1901- , & HELMER, O. M.
A crystalline pressor substance (angiotonin) resulting from the reaction
between renin and renin-activator. *J. exp. Med.*, 1940, **71**, 29-42.
Isolation of angiotonin (angiotensin).

2725   KEMPNER, WALTER. 1903-
Treatment of kidney disease and hypertensive vascular disease with rice
diet. *N. Carol. med. J.*, 1944, **5**, 125-33.
Kempner rice diet for the treatment of hypertension.

2725.1   ABEATICI, S., & CAMPI, L.
La visualizzazione radiologica della porta per via splenica. *Minerva med.
(Torino)*, 1951, **42**, i, 593-94.
Introduction of portal venography for investigation of portal hyper-
tension.

HEART AND AORTA

2726   SASSONIA, ERCOLE. [SAXONIA]. 1551-1607
De pulsibus. Francofurti, *Palthenius*, 1604.
Early description of heart block. (Cap. C, p. 152).

2726.1   STENSEN, NIELS. [STENO, NICOLAUS]. 1638-1686.
Embryo monstro affinis Parisiis dissectus. *Acta med. philos. Hafniensia*,
1671-72, **1**, 202-03.
First known description of the "tetralogy of Fallot" (*see* No. 2792). Reprinted in his *Opera philosophica*, ed. W. Maar, Vol. 2, Copenhagen, *V. Tryde*,
1910, pp. 49-53. For translation see *Proc. Mayo Clin.*, 1948, **23**, 317.

2726.2   MAYOW, JOHN. 1643-1679
Tractatus ... de motu musculari et spiritibus animalibus. Oxonii, *e theatro
Sheldoniano*, 1674.
In the second edition of the "Tractatus quinque" Mayow recorded a case
of mitral stenosis, probably the first description. Reprinted in his "Medico-
physical works," Edinburgh, 1907, pp. 295-97.

2727   RIVIÈRE, LAZARE. [RIVERIUS]. 1589-1655
Opera medica universa. Francofurti, *J. P. Zubrodt*, 1674.
Riverius was the first to note aortic stenosis (p. 638 of the above).

2728   GERBEC, MARKO. [GERZEBIUS]. 1658-1718
Pulsus mira inconstantia. *Misc. cur. Ephem. nat. cur.*, 1691, Norimbergae,
1692, **10**, 115-18.
First reported case of temporary cardiac arrest with syncopal attacks,
the syndrome to which the names of Stokes (No. 2756) and Adams (No.
2745) were later attached.

2729   VIEUSSENS, RAYMOND. 1641-1715
Novum vasorum corporis humani systema. Amstelodami, *P. Marret*, 1705.

Vieussens was among the first to describe the morbid changes in mitral stenosis, the throbbing pulse in aortic insufficiency, and the first correctly to describe the structure of the left ventricle, the course of the coronary vessels and the valve in the large coronary vein. He was the first to diagnose thoracic aneurysm during the life of the patient. Vieussens included a classic description of the symptoms of aortic regurgitation in his book. Partial English translation in No. 2241.

2730   COWPER, WILLIAM. 1666-1709
Of ossifications or petrifications in the coats of arteries, particularly in the valves of the great artery. *Phil. Trans.*, 1706, **24**, 1970-77.

    First description of aortic insufficiency. Reproduced in Willius & Keys: *Cardiac classics*, 1941, pp. 109-14.

2731   LANCISI, GIOVANNI MARIA. 1654-1720
De subitaneis mortibus libri duo. Romae, *J. F. Buagni*, 1707.

    In the above work Lancisi noted cardiac hypertrophy and dilatation as causes of sudden death. He was the first to describe valvular vegetation, and his book gives a classification of the cardiac diseases then recognized. Lancisi's work laid the foundation for a true understanding of cardiac pathology. There are three different states of the title page of this work, with no definite order of priority established. See P. Kligfield, Survey of variant title page vignettes in Lancisi's De subitaneis mortibus, *J. Hist. Med. & all. Sci.*, 1983, **38**, 336-39. English translation by P.D. White & A.V. Boursy, New York, *St. John's University Press*, [1971.]

2732   HALLER, ALBRECHT VON. 1708-1777
De aortae venaeque cavae gravioribus quibusdam morbis. Gottingae, *A. Vandenhoeck*, [1749].

2733   SENAC, JEAN BAPTISTE. 1693-1770
Traité de la structure du coeur, de son action, et de ses maladies. 2 vols. Paris, *Chez Briasson*, 1749.

    Senac's valuable treatise on the heart added much to the knowledge of the anatomy and diseases of that organ; he mentioned the leucocytes, which he considered to belong to the chyle, and he described pericarditis. Senac was the first to use quinine for palpitation.

2734   MORGAGNI, GIOVANNI BATTISTA. 1682-1771
De sedibus, et causis morborum per anatomen indagatis. 2 vols. Venetiis, *typ. Remondiniana*, 1761.

    Classic descriptions of mitral stenosis (Letter III) and heart block, Stokes–Adams syndrome (vol. 1, p. 70) are reprinted in English translation in Willius & Keys, *Cardiac classics*, 1941, pp. 177-82.

2734.1   NICHOLLS, FRANK. 1699-1778
Observations concerning the body of his late Majesty, October 26, 1760. *Phil. Trans.* (1761), 1762, **52**, 265-75.

    Nicholls was the first to describe dissecting aneurysm of the aorta, the patient being King George II, to whom he was physician from 1753-60. Nicholls was also the first to give a correct description of the mode of production of aneurysm.

2734.2   SANDIFORT, Eduard. 1742-1814
Observationes anatomicae-pathologicae. Vol. 1 Lugduni Batavorum, *P. v. d. Eyk & D. Vygh*, 1771.
   A good account of the "tetralogy of Fallot" (No. 2792) is given on pp. 1-38. For English translation see *Amer. Heart J.*, 1956, **51**, 9-25. *See* No. 2278.

2734.3   HUNTER, William. 1718-1783
Three cases of mal-conformation of the heart. *Med. Obs. Inqu.*, 1784, **6**, 291-309.
   Three cases of congenital heart disease recorded. Two plates are opposite pp. 417-18 of the journal.

2734.31   WITHERING, William. 1741-1799
An account of the foxglove, and some of its medical uses. Birmingham, *G. G. J. & J. Robinson,* 1785.
   Before Withering's book, digitalis was a widely used folk remedy, occasionally mentioned in the literature. Withering established the correct dosages, and its action in dropsy and on the heart became generally recognized. Withering did not know of the distinction between renal and cardiac dropsy. Facsimile reprint, London, 1949. Facsimile reprint, with marginal notes on relevant points in the text and a history of digitalis since Withering's day by J.K. Aronson, London, *Oxford Univ. Press*, 1985.

2734.4   UNDERWOOD, Michael. 1737-1820
A treatise on the diseases of children. A new edition. 2 vols. London, *J. Matthews*, 1789.
   The second edition of Underwood's book included the first discussion, in a treatise on children's diseases, of congenital heart disease (vol. 2, pp. 122-27).

2735   SPENS, Thomas. 1764-1842
History of a case in which there took place a remarkable slowness of the pulse. *Med. Commentaries* (1792), Edinburgh, 1793, **7**, 458-65.
   Morgagni described a case of "epilepsy with slow pulse" (*see* No. 2734), but Adams has been given the credit for reporting the first clear case of heart block (No. 2745). There is no doubt that Spens reported such a case in 1792.

2736   BAILLIE, Matthew. 1761-1823
The morbid anatomy of some of the most important parts of the human body. 2nd ed. London, *J. Johnson & G. Nicol,* 1797.
   P. 46: Baillie suggested a relationship between rheumatic fever and valvular heart disease. *See also* Nos. 2281, 3167.1, 3218, & 3427.

2737   CORVISART DES MAREST, Jean Nicolas, *Baron.* 1755-1821
Essai sur les maladies et les lésions organiques du coeur et des gros vaisseaux. Paris, *Migneret,* 1806.
   Corvisart really created cardiac symptomatology and made possible the differentiation between cardiac and pulmonary disorders. He was first to explain heart failure mechanically and to describe the dyspnoea of effort. His translation of Auenbrugger's book on percussion resulted in the universal adoption of that procedure. Corvisart was Napoleon's favourite physician. English translation, 1812, reproduced 1962.

2738   BURNS, ALLAN. 1781-1813
        Observations on some of the most frequent and important diseases of the
        heart. Edinburgh, *Bryce & Co.*, 1809.
            Burns described endocarditis and reported three cases of mitral stenosis.
        He recognized the thrill present in the latter condition and seems to have
        understood the mechanism of a cardiac murmur. He also described
        unilateral paralysis of the diaphragm resulting from pressure on the
        phrenic nerve by a thoracic aneurysm. Biography by J. B. Herrick, 1935.

2739   DUNDAS, DAVID.
        An account of a peculiar disease of the heart. *Med.-chir., Trans.*, 1809, **1**,
        37-46.
            Account of nine cases of rheumatic endocarditis.

2740   WELLS, WILLIAM CHARLES. 1757-1817
        On rheumatism of the heart. *Trans. Soc. Improve. med. chir. Knowl.*, 1812,
        3, 373-424.
            David Pitcairn is accredited with the first reference to rheumatism as a
        cause of cardiac disease, in a lecture given in 1788. Jenner read a paper on
        the same subject in 1789, but the first clinical report on the subject to be
        published was that by Wells. Reprinted in Willius & Keys, *Cardiac classics*,
        1941, pp. 294-312.

2740.1 FARRE, JOHN RICHARD. 1775-1862
        Pathological researches. Essay I. On malformations of the human heart. [All
        published.] London, *Longmans*, 1814.
            The first monograph on congenital defects of the heart.

2741   HODGSON, JOSEPH. 1788-1869
        A treatise on the diseases of arteries and veins. 1 vol. and atlas. London, *T.
        Underwood*, 1815.
            Includes the best illustrations of aneurysms and of aortic valvular
        endocarditis so far published, and the first description on non-sacculated
        dilatation of the aortic arch ("Hodgson's disease").

2742   PARRY, CALEB HILLIER. 1755-1822
        An experimental inquiry into the nature, cause and varieties of the arterial
        pulse. London, *Underwood*, 1816.

2743   CHEYNE, JOHN. 1777-1836
        A case of apoplexy in which the fleshy part of the heart was converted into
        fat. *Dublin Hosp. Rep.*, 1818, **2**, 216-23.
            First accurate description of the condition which later became known
        as "Cheyne–Stokes respiration." Reprinted in F. A. Willius & T. E. Keys:
        Cardiac classics, 1941, pp. 317-20.

2744   ROSTAN, LÉON. 1790-1866
        Mémoire sur cette question de l'asthme des vieillards: est-il une affection
        nerveuse? *Nouv. J. Méd. Chir. Pharm.*, 1817, **3**, 3-30.
            Rostan gave an early description of cardiac ("Rostan's") asthma.

2745   ADAMS, ROBERT. 1791-1875
        Cases of diseases of the heart, accompanied by pathological observations.
        Dublin Hosp. Rep., 1827, **4**, 353-453.

On p. 396 commences a classic account of heart block with syncopal attacks, the first complete description of this condition. Following the paper by Stokes (No. 2756) the eponym "Stokes–Adams syndrome" was employed to describe this state. Adams recognized a thrill in mitral regurgitation (p. 423). Adams also understood tricuspid incompetence (p. 436). The paper is reproduced in full in *Med. Classics*, 1939, **3**, 633-96.

2746   HODGKIN, THOMAS. 1798-1866
On the retroversion of the valves of the aorta. *Lond. med. Gaz.*, 1828-29, **3**, 433-43.
Aortic insufficiency is usually associated with the name of Corrigan, but Hodgkin's account antedates Corrigan by three years. This is one of Hodgkin's best publications.

2747   HOPE, JAMES. 1801-1841
A treatise on the diseases of the heart and great vessels. London, *W. Kidd*, 1832.
Hope did much to advance the knowledge of heart murmurs, valvular disease, and aneurysm; he described the second sound of the left side of the sternum in mitral stenosis as "altered" – losing its short, flat clear sound and becoming a prolonged bellows murmur. From his description this became known as "Hope's early diastolic murmur." His classic descriptions of cardiac asthma, valvular disease (pp. 307-45 above), and cardiac neurosis are reprinted in Willius & Keys, *Cardiac classics*, 1941, pp. 405-15. Probably published in 1831 (see review in *Lond. med. phys. J.*, 1831, p. 513-22 (Dec.)) although "all known copies seem to have cancel title page dated 1832" *(Wellcome Catalogue)*.

2748   CORRIGAN, *Sir* DOMINIC JOHN. 1802-1880
On permanent patency of the mouth of the aorta, or inadequacy of the aortic valves. *Edinb. med. surg. J.*, 1832, **37**, 225-45.
In his wonderfully clear account of aortic insufficiency, Corrigan described the "water-hammer pulse" now commonly known as "Corrigan's pulse." He recognized that the hypertrophy of the heart present in this condition is compensatory and not a disease. Corrigan was the last of the famous band forming the "Irish School of Medicine" in the 19th century. Reprinted in *Med. Classics*, 1937, **1**, 703-27.

2748.1 DIEFFENBACH, JOHANN FRIEDRICH. 1792-1847
Physiologisch-chirurgische Beobachtungen bei Cholera-Kranken. *Cholera-Archiv*, 1832, **1**, Heft 1, 86-105.
First recorded example of cardiac catheterization, performed during an unsuccessful attempt to obtain blood from a patient suffering from cholera (p. 100). Reprinted Güstrow, *Fr. Opitz*, 1834.

2748.2 HÉRISSON, JULES.
Le sphygmomètre; instrument qui traduit à l'oeil toute l'action des artères. Paris, *Crochard*, 1834.
Hérisson invented an instrument for recording blood pressure.

2749   BOUILLAUD, JEAN BAPTISTE. 1796-1881
Traité cliniques des maladies du coeur. 2 vols. Paris, *J. B. Baillière*, 1835.
Vol. 2, page 238: "Bouillaud's disease" – rheumatic endocarditis. Although not first to note the cardiac manifestations of acute rheumatism,

Bouillaud was the first to demonstrate the frequency and importance of heart disease co-incident with acute articular rheumatism. The above work includes the first description of a case of mitral disease with articular rheumatism. Translation of the section on the pathology of endocarditis in Willius & Keys, *Cardiac classics*, pp. 446-55. In 1836 Bouillaud published his *Nouvelles recherches* which contain his "law of coincidence" between rheumatism and cardiac disease. This was translated into English, Philadelphia, 1837.

2750 SOBERNHEIM, Joseph Friedrich. 1803-1846
Akute idiopathische Herzentzündung. In his: *Praktische Diagnostik*, Berlin, 1837, pp. 118-20.
 Sobernheim first used the term "myocarditis."

2750.1 MERCIER, Louis Auguste. 1811-1882
Rétrécissement avec oblitération presque complète de la portion thoracique de l'aorte. *Bull. Soc. anat. Paris*, 1839, **14**, 158-60.
 Diagnosis of coarctation of aorta during life. Translation in *Amer. J. Cardiol.*, 1965, **16**, 253-55.

2751 PIGEAUX, Antoine Louis Jules. 1807-?
Traité pratique des maladies du coeur. Paris, *J. Rouvier*, 1839.

2752 CHEVERS, Norman. 1818-1886
Observations on the diseases of the orifice and valves of the aorta. *Guy's Hosp. Rep.*, 1842, **7**, 387-442.
 First clear account of chronic constrictive pericarditis.

2753 BARLOW, George Hilaro. 1806-1866, & REES, George Owen. 1813-1889
Account of observations ... on patients whose urine was albuminous. *Guy's Hosp. Rep.*, 1843, n.s. **1**, 189-316.
 An early description of a case of subacute bacterial endocarditis is reported on pp. 227-32 (Case 8).

2754 FAUVEL, Sulpice Antoine. 1813-1884
Mémoire sur les signes stethoscopiques du rétrécissement de l'orifice auriculo-ventriculaire gauches du coeur. *Arch. gén. Méd.*, 1843, 4 sér., **1**, 1-16.
 First description of the presystolic murmur in mitral stenosis. Partial English translation in No. 2241.

2755 BRICHETEAU, Isidore. 1789-1861
Observation d'hydropneumopéricarde accompagnée d'un bruit de fluctuation perceptible à l'oreille. *Arch. gén. Méd.*, 1844, 4 sér., **4**, 334-39.
 First adequate description of pneumopericardium.

2755.1 LATHAM, Peter Mere. 1789-1875
Lectures on subjects connected with clinical medicine, comprising disease of the heart. Second edition, 2 vols. London, *Longman*, 1846.
 Includes (vol. 2, pp. 373-79) a classic description of coronary thrombosis, although not using the term. The patient was Thomas Arnold, the educationist, and the report was signed by Joseph Hodgson and by S. Bucknill, Arnold's physician.

2756   STOKES, WILLIAM. 1804-1878
Observations on some cases of permanently slow pulse. *Dublin quart. J. med. Sci.*, 1846, **2**, 73-85.
Stokes's celebrated account of heart block with syncopal attacks – the Stokes–Adams syndrome (*see also* No. 2745). Stokes was most interested in the diagnostic value of this condition. The paper is reprinted in *Med. Classics*, 1939, **3**, 727-38. For history of this syndrome see N. Flaxman, *Bull. Inst. Hist. Med.*, 1937, **5**, 115-30.

2757   WALSHE, WALTER HAYLE. 1812-1892
A practical treatise on the diseases of the lungs and heart, including the principles of physical diagnosis. London, *Taylor, Walton & Maberly*, 1851.
Walshe, physician to University College Hospital, London, was one of the first to recognize the presystolic character of the direct mitral murmur in mitral stenosis.

2758   KIRKES, WILLIAM SENHOUSE. 1823-1864
On some of the principal effects resulting from the detachment of fibrinous deposits from the interior of the heart, and their mixture with the circulating blood. *Med.-chir. Trans.*, 1852, **35**, 281-324.
A classic description of embolism resulting from intracardiac coagula. Reprinted in Willius & Keys: *Cardiac classics*, 1941, pp. 474-82.

2759   VIERORDT, KARL. 1818-1884
Die bildliche Darstellung des menschlichen Arterienpulses. *Arch. physiol. Heilk*, 1854, **13**, 284-87.
Vierordt invented a sphygmograph, which acted on the principle that the indirect estimation of the blood-pressure could by accompanied by measuring the counter-pressure necessary to obliterate the arterial pulsation. This was the first instrument with which a tracing of the human pulse could be made. The paper is the first record of a study with an instrument of precision of the pulse in health and disease. It was expanded into book form: *Die Lehre von Arterienpuls*, Braunschweig, Vieweg, 1855.

2760   STOKES, WILLIAM. 1804-1878
The diseases of the heart and aorta. Dublin, *Hodges & Smith*, 1854.
On pp. 320-27 is to be found Stokes's account of fatty degeneration of the heart, in which he so well described the periodic form of respiration now known as "Cheyne–Stokes breathing." Stokes also gave the first description of paroxysmal tachycardia (p. 161).

2761   PEACOCK, THOMAS BEVILL. 1812-1882
On malformations, etc., of the human heart. London, *J. Churchill*, 1858.
Includes an account of the "tetralogy of Fallot" (*see* No. 2792). Peacock's book was "the first comprehensive study covering the whole field" (Maude Abbott). Reprinted, Boston, Mass., 1973.

2761.1 MALMSTEN, PEHR HENRIK. 1811-1883, & DÜBEN, GUSTAV WILHELM JOHANN. 1822-1892
Fall af ruptura cordis. *Hygiea (Stockh.)*, 1859, **21**, 629-30.
An important account of myocardial infarction, with a histological finding of myocardial necrosis. Abbreviated translation, in German, in *Acta med. scand.*, 1930, **73**, 448-50.

2762   DUROZIEZ, Paul Louis. 1826-1897
Du double souffle intermittent crural, comme signe de l'insuffisance
aortique. *Arch. gén. Méd.*, 1861, 5 sér., **17**, 417-43, 588-605.
    The double intermittent murmur over the femoral arteries, diagnostic of
aortic insufficiency, has become known as "Duroziez's sign." Partial
English translation in No. 2241.

2763   GAIRDNER, *Sir* William Tennant. 1824-1907
Short account of cardiac murmurs. *Edinb. med. J.*, 1861, **7**, 438-53.
    The murmur which Fauvel (No. 2754) had called "presystolic" was
described by Gairdner, who called it "auricular-systolic." This paper is
important as being largely responsible for the recognition in Britain of the
presystolic murmur, previously discounted by most authorities.

2764   FLINT, Austin. 1812-1886
On cardiac murmurs. *Amer. J. med. Sci.*, 1862, n.s. **44**, 29-54.
    First description of the "Austin Flint murmur," present at the apex beat
in aortic regurgitation. Reprinted in *Med. Classics*, 1940, **4**, 864-900.

2764.1   EBSTEIN, Wilhelm. 1836-1912
Ueber einen sehr seltenen Fall von Insufficienz der Valvula tricuspidalis,
bedingt durch eine angeborene hochgradige Missbildung derselben. *Arch.
Anat. Physiol. wiss. Med.*, 1866, 238-54.
    "Ebstein's anomaly," a congenital abnormality of the tricuspid valve.
Translation in *Amer. J. Cardiol.*, 1968, **22**, 867-72.

2765   FRIEDREICH, Nikolaus. 1825-1882
Krankheiten des Herzens. 2te. Aufl. Erlangen, *F. Enke*, 1867.
    First appeared in Virchow's *Handbuch der speciellen Pathologie und
Therapie*, Erlangen, 1854, **5**, 1 Abt., 385-530.

2766   POTAIN, Pierre Carl Édouard. 1825-1901
Des mouvements et des bruits qui se passent dans les veines jugulaires.
Bull. Soc. méd. Hôp. Paris (Mémoires), 1867, 2 sér., **4**, 3-27.
    Classic account of the movements and murmurs in the jugular veins,
important in the diagnosis of heart diseases. Potain's writings were models
of clarity and style. A translation of this paper is to be found in Willius &
Keys, *Cardiac classics*, 1941, pp. 533-56.

2767   WINGE, Emanuel Fredrik Hagbarth. 1827-1894
[Mycosis endocardii.] *Norsk Mag. Laegevid. (Förh. Norske med. Selskab)*,
1869, **23**, 78-82.
    Winge first suggested that endocarditis was due to microbial infection.
A translation of part of his paper is in Major, *Classic descriptions of disease*,
3rd ed., 1945, p. 472.

2768   MYERS, Arthur Bowen Richards. 1838-1921
On the etiology and prevalence of diseases of the heart among soldiers.
London, *J. Churchill*, 1870.
    First description of "Da Costa's syndrome" – the "effort syndrome" of Sir
Thomas Lewis.

2769   WILKS, *Sir* SAMUEL, *Bart.* 1824-1911
Capillary embolism or arterial pyaemia. *Guy's Hosp. Rep.*, 1870, 3 sér., **15**, 29-35.
One of the first accounts of bacterial endocarditis was given by Wilks, who, in his classic paper on the subject, called the condition "arterial pyaemia." Reprinted in Willius & Keys, *Cardiac classics*, 1941, pp. 579-84.

2770   DA COSTA, JACOB MENDES. 1833-1900
On irritable heart; a clinical study of a form of functional cardiac disorder and its consequences. *Amer. J. med. Sci.*, 1871, n.s. **61**, 17-52.
"Da Costa's syndrome." This was first described by Myers (No. 2768) and is now known as "effort syndrome," "soldier's heart," "disordered action of the heart."

2771   FAGGE, CHARLES HILTON. 1838-1883
On the murmurs attendant on mitral contraction. *Guy's Hosp. Rep.*, 1871, 3 ser., **16**, 247-342.
Important and exhaustive account of the knowledge of presystolic murmurs. Fagge's paper also includes many clinical observations relating to the rhythm of heart murmurs and the state of the sounds of the heart in 67 cases at Guy's Hospital.

2772   BÄUMLER, CHRISTIAN. 1836-1933
Cases of partial and general idiopathic pericarditis. *Trans. clin. Soc. Lond.*, 1872, **5**, 8-22.
Pericarditis epistenocardiaca described.

2773   BAMBERGER, HEINRICH. 1822-1888
Ueber zwei seltene Herzaffektionen, mit Bezugnahme auf die Theorie des ersten Herztons. *Wien. med. Wschr.*, 1872, **22**, 1-4, 25-28.
"Bamberger's disease" (Pick's disease, No. 2803).

2774   HEIBERG, HJALMAR. 1837-1897
Ein Fall von Endocarditis ulcerosa puerperalis mit Pilzbildungen im Herzen (Mycosis endocardii). *Virchows Arch. path. Anat.*, 1872, **56**, 407-14.
Heiberg suggested the microbic nature of endocarditis. He described what appeared to him to be the mycelia of *Leptothrix* in the vegetations of a case of ulcerative endocarditis.

2775   TRAUBE, LUDWIG. 1818-1876
Ein Fall von Pulsus bigeminus nebst Bemerkungen über die Leberschwellungen bei Klappenfehlern und über acute Leberatrophie. *Berl. klin. Wschr.*, 1872, **9**, 185-88, 221-24.
First clear description of pulsus bigeminus. Translated in Willius & Keys, *Cardiac classics*, 1941, pp. 590-99.

2776   KUSSMAUL, ADOLF. 1822-1902
Ueber schwielige Mediastino-Pericarditis und den paradoxen Puls. *Berl. klin. Wschr.*, 1873, **10**, 433-35, 445-49, 461-64.
Kussmaul introduced the concept of the "paradoxical pulse."

2777 POTAIN, Pierre Carl Édouard. 1825-1901
Du rhythme cardiaque appelé bruit de galop, de son mécanisme et de sa valeur séméiologique. *Bull. Soc. méd. Hôp. Paris,* (1875), 1876, **12**, (Mém.), 137-66.
Analysis of "gallop rhythm." Partial English translation in No. 2241 and No. 3160.1.

2778 ROKITANSKY, Carl, *Freiherr von.* 1804-1878
Die Defecte der Scheidewände der Herzens. Wien, *W. Braumüller,* 1875.
Rokitansky's memoir on defects of the septum of the heart was his last work, and probably his greatest. It represented 14 years' study of the subject.

2779 BALFOUR, George William. 1823-1903
Clinical lectures on diseases of the heart and aorta. London, *J. & A. Churchill,* 1876.
Includes "Balfour's test" to ascertain whether the heart is still active, in cases of apparent death.

2780 DUROZIEZ, Paul Louis. 1826-1897
Du rétrécissement mitral pur. *Arch. gén. Méd.,* 1877, 6 sér., **30**, 32-54, 184-97.
First description of congenital mitral stenosis, "Duroziez's disease."

2781 HAMMER, Adam. 1818-1878
Ein Fall von thrombotischen Verschlusse einer der Kranzarterien des Herzens. *Wien. med. Wschr.,* 1878, **28**, 97-102.
First description of coronary thrombosis with diagnosis before death. English translation of original report, *Amer. J. Cardiol.,* 1978, **42**, 849-52.

2782 ROGER, Henri. 1809-1891
Recherches cliniques sur la communication congénitales des deux coeurs par inocclusion du septum interventriculare. *Bull Acad. Méd. (Paris),* 1879, 2 sér., **8**, 1074-94,, 1189-91.
Roger drew attention to an important anomaly of the septum, interventricular patency ("maladie de Roger"), demonstrating the presence of a murmur in this condition. This is sometimes called "Roger's murmur", although it had been noted by earlier writers. Translated in Willius & Keys, *Cardiac classics,* 1941, pp. 624-38.

2783 WEIGERT, Carl. 1845-1904
Ueber die pathologische Gerinnungs-Vorgänge. *Virchows Arch. path. Anat.,* 1880, **79**, 87-123.
First description (p. 106) of myocardial infarction.

2784 BASCH, Samuel Siegfried von. 1837-1905
Ueber die Messung des Blutdrucks am Menschen. *Z. klin. Med.,* 1881, **2**, 79-96.
Basch's important modifications of the methods of blood-pressure recording mark the beginning of clinical sphygmomanometry. English translation in Ruskin (No. 3160.1).

2785   CONCATO, Luigi Maria. 1825-1882
Sulla poliorromennite scrofolosa, o tisi delle sierose. *G. int. Sci. med.*, 1881, n.s. **3**, 1037-53.
   "Concato's disease" – inflammation of the serous membranes. Involvement of the pericardium was later described by Pick (No. 2803).

2786   LEYDEN, Ernst von. 1832-1910
Ueber Fettherz. *Z. klin Med.*, 1882, **5**, 1-25.
   Fatty infiltration of the heart first described.

2788   PETER, Charles Félix Michel. 1824-1893
Traité clinique des maladies du coeur et de la crosse de l'aorte. Paris, *J. B. Baillière*, 1883.

2789   PAUL, Constantin Charles Théodore. 1833-1896
Diagnostic et traitement des maladies du coeur. Paris, *Asselin & Cie.*, 1883.
   English translation, 1884.

2790   OSLER, *Sir* William, *Bart.* 1849-1919
The Gulstonian Lectures, on malignant endocarditis. *Brit, med. J.*, 1885, **1**, 467-70, 522-26, 577-79.
   First comprehensive description of subacute bacterial endocarditis.

2791   MacWILLIAM, John Alexander. 1857-1937
Fibrillar contraction of the heart. *J. Physiol. (Lond.)*, 1887, **8**, 296-310.
   MacWilliam discovered that fibrillar contraction of the heart is due to "a rapid succession of incoordinated peristaltic contractions." He clearly described auricular and ventricular fibrillation, and showed that ventricular fibrillation could be caused by the injection of certain poisons into the blood stream. His paper is included, with an account of his life, in Willius & Keys, *Cardiac classics*, 1941, pp. 666-678.

2792   FALLOT, Etienne Louis Arthur. 1850-1911
Contribution à l'anatomie pathologique de la maladie bleu (cyanose cardiaque). *Marseille méd*, 1888, **25**, 77-93, 138-58, 207-23, 270-86, 341-54, 403-20.
   The "tetralogy of Fallot." He gave an important, but not the first, account of this condition (*see* Nos. 2726.1 & 2761). Abstract translation in Willius & Keys, *Cardiac classics*, 1941, pp. 689-90.

2793   ROY, Charles Smart. 1854-1897, & ADAMI, John George. 1862-1926
Remarks on failure of the heart from overstrain. *Brit. med. J.*, 1888, **2**, 1321-26.
   Important experimental work on cardiac overstrain was carried out by Roy and Adami who considered that mechanical overstrain caused chronic thickening of the cardiac valves.

2794   STEELL, Graham. 1851-1942
The murmur of high-pressure in the pulmonary artery. *Med. Chron. (Manch.)*, 1888-89, **9**, 182-88.
   First description of the pulmonary diastolic murmur – the "Graham Steell murmur." Reproduced in Willius & Keys, *Cardiac Classics*, 1941, pp. 680-85.

2795   BOUVERET, Léon. 1851-1929
De la tachycardie essentielle paroxystique. *Rev. Médecine*, 1889, **9**, 753-93, 837-55.
Bouveret introduced the term "Paroxysmal tachycardia". Partial English translation in No. 2241.

2796   HUCHARD, Henri. 1844-1910
Maladies du coeur et des vaisseaux. Paris, *O. Doin*, 1889.
In his important monograph on disorders of the cardiovascular system, Huchard was apparently the first to use the designation "Stokes–Adams disease".

2797   MacWILLIAM, John Alexander. 1857-1937
Cardiac failure and sudden death from ventricular fibrillation. Brit. med. J., 1889, **1**, 6-8.
First description of a case of death from ventricular fibrillation.

2798   POTAIN, Pierre Carl Édouard. 1825-1901
Du sphygmomanomètre et de la mésure de la pression artérielle chez l'homme à l'état normale et pathologique. *Arch. Physiol. norm. path.*, 1889, 5 sér., **1**, 556-69.
Potain devised a simple portable air sphygmomanometer for blood-pressure estimation.

2799   ROSENBACH, Ottomar. 1851-1907
Die Krankheiten des Herzens und ihre Behandlung. Wien, Leipzig, *Urban & Schwarzenberg*, 1893-97.

2800   BROADBENT, Walter. 1868-1951
An unpublished physical sign. *Lancet*, 1895, **2**, 200-01.
"Broadbent's sign" – recession of the intercostal spaces as a sign of adherent pericardium.

2801   MOSSO, Angelo. 1846-1910
Sphygmomanomètre pour mésurer la pression du sang chez l'homme. *Arch. ital. Biol.*, 1895, **23**, 177-97.
A sphygmomanometer for registering the blood-pressure in the finger was invented by Mosso.

2802   EWART, William. 1848-1929
Practical aids in the diagnosis of pericardial effusion, in connection with the question as to surgical treatment. *Brit. med. J.*, 1896, **1**, 717-21.
Pulmonary collapse at the left base in pericardial effusion – "Ewart's sign".

2803   PICK, Friedel. 1867-1926
Ueber chronische unter dem Bilde der Leberzirrhose verlaufende Perikarditis (perikarditische Pseudoleberzirrhose) nebst Bemerkungen über die Zuckergussleber. *Z. klin. Med.*, 1896, **29**, 385-410.
"Pick's disease" – pericardial pseudocirrhosis of the liver.

2804   RIVA-ROCCI, Scipione. 1863-1937
Un nuovo sfigmomanometro. *Gaz. med. Torino*, 1896, **47**, 981-96, 1001-17.

Riva-Rocci's sphygmomanometer marked the end of the search for a simple clinical method of estimating the blood-pressure. Abridged English translation in Ruskin (No. 3160.1).

2804.1   WILLIAMS, FRANCIS HENRY. 1852-1936
A method for more fully determining the outline of the heart by means of the fluoroscope together with other uses of this instrument in medicine. *Boston med. surg. J.,* 1896, **135**, 335-337.
Estimation of heart size by fluoroscope, first application of *x* rays to cardiology.

2805   BROADBENT, *Sir*WILLIAM HENRY, *Bart.* 1835-1907, & BROADBENT, *Sir*JOHN FRANCIS HARPIN, *Bart.* 1865-1946
Heart disease. London, *Baillière, Tindall & Cox,* 1897.
Chapter 17 includes J. Broadbent's classic description of adherent pericardium. See Willius & Keys, *Cardiac classics,* 1941, pp. 712-15, for reproduction of part of this chapter.

2806   EISENMENGER, VICTOR.
Die angeborenen Defecte der Kammerscheidewand des Herzens. *Z. klin. Med.,* 1897, **32**, Suppl.- Heft, 1-28.
"Riding aorta", patent interventricular septum and right ventricular enlargement – the "Eisenmenger syndrome".

2807   HILL, *Sir* LEONARD ERSKINE. 1866-1952, & BARNARD, HAROLD LESLIE. 1868-1908
A simple and accurate form of sphygmomanometer or arterial pressure gauge contrived for clinical use. *Brit. med. J.,* 1897, **2**, 904.
Hill and Barnard made an important modification to the Riva-Rocci sphygmomanometer when they substituted a pressure gauge in place of the mercury manometer used for pressure readings.

2808   GIBSON, GEORGE ALEXANDER. 1854-1913
Diseases of the heart and the aorta. Edinburgh, *Y. J. Pentland,* 1898.

2809   RUMMO, GAETANO. 1853-1917
Sulla cardioptosi; primo abbozzo anatomo-clinico. *Arch. Med int. (Palermo),* 1898, **1**, 161-83.
Rummo drew attention to a downward displacement of the heart – "Rummo's disease".

2809.1   WENCKEBACH, KAREL FREDERIK. 1864-1940
Zur Analyse des unregelmässigen Pulses. *Z. klin. Med.,* 1899, **36**, 181-99.
"Wenckebach phenomenon", a form of arrhythmia.

2809.2   FIEDLER, CARL LUDWIG ALFRED. 1835-1921
Ueber akute interstitielle Myokarditis. Dresden, *W. Baensch,* 1899.
"Fiedler's myocarditis".

2810   GAERTNER, GUSTAV. 1855-1937
Ueber einen neuen Blutdruckmesser (Tonometer). *Wien. med. Wschr.,* 1899, **49**, 1412-18.
Gaertner, an Austrian physician, invented an instrument for measuring blood-pressure by means of a compressing ring applied to the finger.

2811   HUCHARD, HENRI. 1844-1910
Traité cliniques des maladies du coeur et de l'aorte. 3 vols. Paris, O. Doin,
1899-1903.

2812   MACKENZIE, Sir JAMES. 1853-1925
The study of the pulse. Edinburgh, Y. J. Pentland, 1902.
    In his classic monograph Mackenzie included (p. 10) a description and
illustration of his polygraph, with which he made simultaneous tracings of
the pulse, apex beat, etc.

2813   MORITZ, FRIEDRICH. 1861-1938
Ueber orthodiagraphische Untersuchungen am Herzen. Münch. med.
Wschr., 1902, 49, 1-8.
    Orthodiagraphy of the heart.

2814   BONNET, L. M.
Sur la lésion dite sténose congénitale de l'aorte dans la région de l'isthme.
Rev. Médecine, 1903, 23, 108-26.
    Distinction of infantile and adult types of coarctation of the aorta.

2815   CHIARI, HANS. 1851-1916
Ueber die syphilitischen Aortenerkrankungen. Verh. dtsch. path. Ges.,
(1903), 1904, 6, 137-63.

2816   ASCHOFF, KARL ALBERT LUDWIG. 1866-1942
Zur Myocarditisfrage. Verh. dtsch. path. Ges., 1904, 8, 46-53.
    In his work on rheumatic myocarditis, Aschoff described the charac-
teristic lesion (Aschoff body or nodule) and presented a histopathological
picture of myocarditis that was to exert a great influence on the classification
of the disease. Translated in Willius & Keys, Cardiac classics, 1941, pp.
733-39.

2817   KÖHLER, ALBAN. 1874-1947
Technik der Herstellung fast orthodiagraphischer Herzphotogramme
vermittelst Röntgeninstrumentarien mit kleiner Elektrizitätsquelle. Wien,
klin. Rdsch., 1905, 19, 279-82.
    Introduction of teleradiography of the heart.

2818   KOROTKOV, NIKOLAI SERGEIEVICH. 1874-1920
[On methods of studying blood pressure.] Izvest. imp. voyenno-med. Akad.
St. Petersburg, 1905, 11, 365.
    Korotkov introduced the modern method of applying the stethoscope
to the brachial artery during blood-pressure examination with Riva-Rocci's
sphygmomanometer, for the purpose of investigating the sounds made by
the blood after release of the air-pressure cuff. For an English translation
of the paper see Bull. N. Y. Acad. Med., 1941, 17, 877-79.

2819   MACKENZIE, Sir JAMES. 1853-1925
New methods of studying affections of the heart. Brit. med J., 1905, 1, 519-
21, 587-89, 702-05, 759-62, 812-15.
    Mackenzie established the remarkable action of digitalis in auricular
fibrillation.

2820   MARTIN, *Sir* CHARLES JAMES. 1866-1955
Remarks on the determination of arterial blood-pressure in clinical practice. *Brit. med. J.*, 1905, **1**, 865-70.

2821   RITCHIE, WILLIAM THOMAS. 1873-1945
Complete heart-block, with dissociation of the action of the auricles and ventricles. *Proc. roy. Soc. Edinb.*, 1905-06, **25**, 1085-91.
Auricular flutter in man first recognized.

2822   CUSHNY, ARTHUR ROBERTSON, 1866-1926, & EDMUNDS, CHARLES WALLIS. 1873-1941
Paroxysmal irregularity of the heart and auricular fibrillation. In: *Studies in pathology written ... to celebrate the quatercentenary of Aberdeen University.* Edited by W. BULLOCH, Aberdeen, 1906, pp. 95-110.
First recognition of auricular fibrillation in man. Cushny and Edmunds had a case under their care in 1901. Hering described the condition in man in *Prag. med. Wschr.*, 1903, **28**, 377.

2823   KRILOFF, DMITRI DMITRIYEVICH. 1879-
[Estimation of blood-pressure by Korotkov's auditory method.] *Izvest. Imp. voyenno-med. Akad. St Petersburg*, 1906, **13**, 113-221, 319.
Kriloff made extensive observations on the sounds which Korotkov had shown to be emitted by the blood after removal of the Riva-Rocci air-pressure cuff during the blood-pressure measurement.

2824   REUTER, KARL.
Ueber Spirochaeta pallida in der Aortenwand bei Hellerscher Aortitis. *Münch med. Wschr.*, 1906, **53**, 778.
Treponema pallidum first discovered in the diseased aorta.

2825   FELLNER, BRUNO, *jnr.*
Neuerung zur Messung des systolischen und diastolischen Druckes. *Verh. Kongr. inn. Med.*, 1907, **24**, 404-07.
Fellner suggested the use of the stethoscope in the measurement of systolic and diastolic pressure.

2826   MACKENZIE, *Sir* JAMES. 1853-1925
Diseases of the heart. London, *H. Frowde*, 1908.
Chapter 30 of the third edition (1914) includes Mackenzie's classic description of the clinical picture of "nodal rhythm" (auricular fibrillation). Reprinted in Willius & Keys, *Cardiac classics*, 1941, pp. 769-93.

2827   OSLER, *Sir* WILLIAM, *Bart.*, 1849-1919
Chronic infectious endocarditis. *Quart. J. Med.*, 1908-09, **2**, 219-30.
The tender subcutaneous nodes in subacute bacterial endocarditis ("Osler's nodes") were first observed by Osler in 1888, and reported in 1909. This paper is the first definite clinical description of subacute bacterial endocarditis.

2828   BRACHT, ERICH. 1882- , & WÄCHTER.
Beitrag zur Aetiologie und pathologischen Anatomie der Myokarditis rheumatica. *Dtsch. Arch. klin. Med.*, 1909, **96**, 493-514.
"Bracht–Wächter bodies" in the myocardium in bacterial endocarditis.

2829   HORDER, Thomas Jeeves, 1st *Baron Horder*. 1871-1955
Infective endocarditis, with an analysis of 150 cases. *Quart. J. Med.*, 1909, **2**, 289-324.
    Classic description of subacute bacterial endocarditis.

2830   LEWIS, *Sir* Thomas. 1881-1945
Auricular fibrillation; a common clinical condition. *Brit. med. J.*, 1909, **2**, 1528.
    First description of auricular fibrillation as a cause of clinical perpetual arrhythmia. See also the paper in *Heart*, London, 1909-10, **1**, 306-72.

2831   ROTHBERGER, Carl Julius. 1871- ,& WINTERBERG, Heinrich. 1867-1929
Vorhofflimmern und Arhythmia perpetua. *Wien. klin. Wschr.*, 1909, **22**, 839-44.
    Independently of Lewis (No. 2830) these workers claimed auricular fibrillation to be the cause of perpetual arrhythmia.

2832   EPPINGER, Hans. 1879-1946, & STOERK, Oscar. 1870-1926
Zur Klinik des Elektrokardiogramms. *Z. klin. Med.*, 1910, **71**, 157-164.
    First clinical and pathological description of bundle-branch block.

2833   JOLLY, William Adam. 1878-1939, & RITCHIE, William Thomas. 1873-1945
Auricular flutter and fibrillation. *Heart*, 1910, **2**, 177-221.
    Auricular flutter first described.

2834   LIBMAN, Emanuel. 1872-1946, & CELLER, Herbert Louis. 1878-1928
The etiology of subacute infective endocarditis. *Amer. J. med. Sci.*, 1910, **140**, 516-27.
    Libman and Celler found *Strep. endocarditidis* to be the most common cause of subacute bacterial endocarditis.

2835   OBRAZTSOV, Vasili Parmenovich. 1849-1920, & STRAZHESKO, Nikolai Dmitrievich. 1876-1952
Zur kenntniss der Thrombose der Koronararterien des Herzens. *Z. klin. Med.*, 1910, **71**, 116-32.
    First complete description of coronary thrombosis, diagnosed before death and confirmed at necropsy. Reprinted in *Klin. Med. (Mosk.)*, 1949, **27**, No. 11, 15-25.

2836   SCHOTTMÜLLER, Hugo. 1867-1936
Endocarditis lenta. Zugleich ein Beitrag zur Artunterscheidung der pathogenen Streptokokken. *Münch. med. Wschr.*, 1910, **57**, 617-20, 697-99.
    First to isolate *Strep viridans* in cases of bacterial endocarditis, Schottmüller named the condition Endocarditis lenta.

2837   VAQUEZ, Louis Henri. 1860-1936
Les arythmies. Paris, *J. B. Baillière*, 1911.

2838   BAEHR, George. 1887-
Glomerular lesions of subacute bacterial endocarditis. *J. exp. Med.*, 1912, **15**, 330-47.
    Baehr drew attention to the renal lesions in subacute bacterial endocarditis.

2839 HERRICK, JAMES BRYAN. 1861-1954
Clinical features of sudden obstruction of the coronary arteries. *J. Amer. med. Ass.*, 1912, **59**, 2015-20.
Outstanding description of coronary thrombosis. Herrick showed that sudden coronary occlusion is not necessarily fatal. Reprint in Willius & Keys, *Cardiac classics*, 1941, pp. 817-29.

2840 LEWIS, *Sir* THOMAS. 1881-1945
Electro-cardiography and its importance in the clinical examination of heart affections. *Brit. med. J.*, 1912, **1**, 1421-23, 1479-82; **2**, 65-67.

2841 LIBMAN, EMANUEL. 1872-1946
A study of the endocardial lesions of subacute bacterial endocarditis. *Amer. J. med. Sci.*, 1912, **144**, 313-27.

2842 HUISMANS, L.
Der Ersatz des Orthiodiagraphen durch der Teleröntgen. *Verh. dtsch. Kongr. inn. Med.*, 1913, **30**, 266-69.
Instantaneous radiography of the heart.

2843 RITCHIE, WILLIAM THOMAS. 1873-1945
Auricular flutter. Edinburgh, London, *W. Green & Son*, 1914.

2844 WENCKEBACH, KAREL FREDERIK. 1864-1940
Die unregelmässige Herztätigkeit und ihre klinische Bedeutung. Leipzig, Berlin, *W. Engelmann*, 1914.
Wenckebach was the first to demonstrate (pp. 173-75) the value of quinine ("Wenckebach's pills") in the treatment of paroxysmal fibrillation. The same work contains a number of excellent descriptions of various forms of cardiac arrythmia. The second edition, written in co-operation with Heinrich Winterberg, was expanded to 2 vols, Leipzig, *Engelmann*, 1927.

2845 CRANE, AUGUSTUS WARREN. 1868-1937
Roentgenology of the heart. *Amer. J. Roentgenol.*, 1916, **3**, 513-24.
Introduction of kymography in clinical cardioloy.

2846 LUTEMBACHER, RENÉ. 1884-
De la sténose mitrale avec communication interauriculaire. *Arch. Mal. Coeur*, 1916, **9**, 237-60.
"Lutembacher syndrome".

2847 LEWIS, *Sir* THOMAS. 1881-1945
Report upon soldiers returned as cases of "disordered action of the heart" (D.A.H.) or "valvular disease of the heart" (V.D.H.). London, *H. M. Stationery Off.*, 1917.
Medical Research Committee Special Rept. No. 8. Sir Thomas Lewis described as "effort syndrome" the condition of disordered action of the heart known as "Da Costa's syndrome".

2848 FREY, WALTER. 1884-
Ueber Vorhofflimmern beim Menschen und seine Beseitigung durch Chinidin. *Berl. klin. Wschr.*, 1918, **55**, 450-52.

Following Wenckebach's discovery of the efficacy of quinine in the restoration of normal rhythm in auricular fibrillation. Frey showed that quinidine was the most effective of the cinchona alkaloids in this respect.

2849   ZONDEK, HERMANN. 1887-1979
Das Myxödemherz. *Münch. med. Wschr.*, 1919, **66**, 274-75.
First attempt to restore the heart's action by intracardiac injection.

2851   LEWIS, *Sir* THOMAS. 1881-1945
The mechanism and graphic registration of the heart beat. London, *Shaw & Sons*, 1920.
See No. 854. Third edition, 1925.

2852   PARDEE, HAROLD ENSIGN BENNETT. 1886-1972
An electrocardiographic sign of coronary artery obstruction. *Arch. intern. Med.*, 1920, **26**, 244-57.
First description of the typical changes in the electrocardiogram in coronary thrombosis.

2853   SAXL, PAUL. 1880-1932
Verhandlungen ärtzlicher Gesellschaften und Kongressberichte. *Wien. klin. Wschr.*, 1920, **33**, 179-80.
Saxl injected a mercurial compound (Novasurol), a powerful diuretic, for the treatment of cardiac failure.

2853.1   MANN, HUBERT. 1891-1975
A method of analyzing the electrocardiogram. *Arch. intern. Med.*, 1920, **25**, 283-94.
Mann developed the monocardiogram while a fourth-year medical student. This was the first vector loop and the beginning of modern vectorcardiography.

2854   COOMBS, CAREY FRANKLIN. 1879-1932
Rheumatic heart disease. Bristol, *John Wright*, 1924.

2855   LIBMAN, EMANUEL. 1872-1946, & SACKS, BENJAMIN. 1896-
A hitherto undescribed form of valvular and mural endocarditis. *Arch. intern. Med.*, 1924, **33**, 701-37.
"Libman–Sacks disease".

2856   ABBOTT, MAUDE ELIZABETH SEYMOUR. 1869-1940
Congenital cardiac disease. In: Osler & McCrea: *Modern medicine*, 3rd ed., Philadelphia, 1927, **4**, 612-812.

2856.1   ROESLER, HUGO. 1899-
Beiträge zur Lehre von den angeborenen Herzfehlern. *Wien. Arch. inn. Med.*, 1928, **15**, 487-538.
Roesler described the most important roentgenologic sign of aortic coarctation.

2857   ERDHEIM, JAKOB. 1874-1937
Medionecrosis aortae idiopathica (cystica). *Virchows Arch. path. Anat.*, 1929, **273**, 454-79; 1930, **276**, 187-229.
Classic description of aortic medionecrosis.

2858 FORSSMANN, WERNER THEODOR OTTO. 1904-1979
Die Sondierung des rechten Herzens. *Klin. Wschr.*, 1929, **8**, 2085-87, 2287.
 The first cardiac catheterization on a living person. Forssmann catheterized his own heart. In 1956 he shared the Nobel Prize with Cournand (No. 2871) and Richards (No. 2883.2) for his work on cardiac catheterization. Historical note by N. Howard-Jones, *Bull. Hist. Med.*, 1973, **47**, 524-6. English translation in Callahan, Keys & Key, *Classics of Cardiology*, Vol. 3, 250-55.

2859 SANTOS, REYNALDO DOS. 1880- , *et al.*
L'artériographie des membres de l'aorte et de ses branches abdominales. *Méd. contemp. (Lisboa)*, 1929, **47**, 93-96.
 Aortography. With A. C. Lamas and J. Pereira Caldas. Also published in *Bull. Soc. méd. chir. Paris*, 1929, **55**, 587-601.

2860 WOLFF, LOUIS. 1898- , PARKINSON, *Sir* JOHN. 1885-1976, & WHITE, PAUL DUDLEY. 1886-1973
Bundle-branch block with short P-R interval in healthy young people prone to paroxysmal tachycardia. *Amer. Heart J.*, 1930, **5**, 685-704.
 Wolff–Parkinson–White syndrome, the best-known of the "pre-excitation syndromes".

2861 GROLLMAN, ARTHUR. 1901-
The cardiac output of man in health and disease. Springfield, *C. C. Thomas*, 1932.

2862 LEWIS, *Sir* THOMAS. 1881-1945
A lecture on vaso-vagal syncope and the carotid sinus mechanism. *Brit. med. J.*, 1932, **1**, 873-76.
 Vaso-vagal syncope.

2863 WOLFERTH, CHARLES CHRISTIAN. 1887-1965, & WOOD, FRANCIS CLARK. 1901-
The electrocardiographic diagnosis of coronary occlusion by the use of chest leads. *Amer. J. med. Sci.*, 1932, **183**, 30-35.
 Introduction of chest leads.

2864 WILSON, FRANK NORMAN. 1890-1952, *et al.*
Electrocardiograms that represent the potential variations of a single electrode. *Amer. Heart J.*, 1934, **9**, 447-58.
 Unipolar leads. With F. D. Johnston, A. G. MacLeod, and P. S. Barker.

2865 ABBOTT, MAUDE ELIZABETH SEYMOUR. 1869-1940
Atlas of congenital cardiac disease. New York, *Amer. Heart Assoc.*, 1936.
 Reprinted 1954.

2865.1 SCHELLONG, FRITZ.
Elektrographische Diagnostik der Herzmuskelerkrankungen. *Verh. Dtsch. Ges. inn. Med.*, 1936, **48**, 288-310.
 Introduction of the vectorcardiogram.

2866 ROESLER, HUGO. 1899-
Clinical roentgenology of the cardiovascular system. Springfield, *C. C. Thomas*, 1937.

2867   LEVY, ROBERT LOUIS. 1888-1974, *et al.*
        Effects of induced oxygen want in patients with cardiac pain. *Amer. Heart J.*, 1938, **15**, 187-200.
            Diagnosis of cardiac pain. With A. L. Barach and H. G. Bruenn.

2868   PRAECORDIAL LEADS.
        Praecordial leads in electrocardiography. A joint memorandum of a committee of the Cardiac Society of Gt. Britain and Ireland and the Committee of the American Heart Association. *Brit. med. J.*, 1838, **1**, 187 (only).
            Also in *Amer. Heart J.*, 1938, **15**, 107-08, 235-39.

2869   ROBB, GEORGE PORTER. 1898- , & STEINBERG, ISRAEL. 1902-
        A practical method of visualization of the chambers of the heart, the pulmonary circulation, and the great vessels in man. *J. clin. Invest.*, 1938, **17**, 507.
            Introduction of angiocardiography, which for the first time revealed the internal structure of the living heart. A fuller account by the same authors is in *Amer. J. Roentgenol.*, 1939, **41**, 1-17.

2870   STARR, ISAAC. 1895- , *et al.*
        Studies on the estimation of cardiac output in man, and abnormalities in cardiac function, from the heart's recoil and the blood's impacts; the ballistocardiogram. *Amer. J. Physiol*, 1939, **127**, 1-28.
            Introduction of the ballistocardiogram. With A. J. Rawson, H. A. Schroeder, and N. R. Joseph.

2871   COURNAND, ANDRÉ FRÉDÉRIC. 1895-1988, & RANGES, HILMERT ALBERT. 1906-1969
        Catheterization of the right auricle in man. *Proc. Soc. exp. Biol. (N.Y.)*, 1941, **46**, 462-66.
            First investigations with the cardiac catheter as a clinical method of investigation. For his work in this field, Cournand in 1956 shared the Nobel Prize with Forssmann (No. 2858) and Richards (No. 2883.2).

2873   SCHROEDER, HENRY ALFRED. 1906-1975
        Studies on congestive heart failure. I. The importance of restriction of salt as compared to water. *Amer. Heart J.*, 1941, **22**, 141-53.
            Low-sodium diet in heart failure.

2875   GOLDBERGER, EMANUEL. 1913-
        A simple indifferent electrocardiographic electrode of zero potential and a technique of obtaining augmented, unipolar, extremity leads. *Amer. Heart J.*, 1942, **23**, 483-92.
            Augmented unipolar leads.

2876   HENNY, GEORGE CHRISTIAN. 1899- , *et al.*
        Electrokymograph for recording heart motion, improved type. *Amer. J. Roentgenol.*, 1947, **57**, 409-16.
            With B. R. Boone and W. E. Chamberlain.

2877   McMICHAEL, *Sir* JOHN. 1904-
        Circulatory failure studied by means of venous catheterization. *Advanc. intern. Med.*, 1947, **2**, 64-101.

2878   TAUSSIG, HELEN BROOKE. 1898-1986
Congenital malformations of the heart. New York, *Commonwealth Fund*, 1947.

2878.1   BECK, CLAUDE SCHAEFFER. 1894-1971, *et al.*
Ventricular fibrillation of long duration abolished by electric shock. *J. Amer. med. Assoc.*, 1947, *135*, 985-86.
     The first successful defibrillation of a surgical patient, with the chest opened, and the paddles applied directly to the heart. With W.H. Pritchard & H.S. Feil.

2879   BRODÉN, BROR LEONHARD JOHAN. 1910- , *et al.*
Thoracic aortography. Preliminary report. *Acta radiol. (Stockh.)*, 1948, **29**, 181-88.
     With H. E. Hanson and J. Karnell.

2880   CHRISTIE, RONALD VICTOR. 1902-
Penicillin in subacute bacterial endocarditis. Report to the Medical Research Council on 269 patients treated in 14 centres appointed by the Penicillin Clinical Trials Committee. *Brit. med. J.*, 1948, **1**, 1-4.

2881   PRINZMETAL, MYRON. 1908- , *et al.*
Mechanism of the auricular arrythmias. *Circulation*, 1950, **1**, 241-45.
     With E. Corday, I. C. Brill, A. L. Seller, R. W. Oblath, W. A. Flieg, and H. E. Kruger.

2882   WOOD, PAUL HAMILTON. 1907-1962
Congenital heart disease. *Brit. med. J.*, 1950, **2**, 639-45, 693-98.
     A new classification proposed.

2883   ZOLL, PAUL MAURICE. 1911-
Resuscitation of the heart in ventricular standstill by external electric stimulation. *New Engl. J. Med.*, 1952, **247**, 768-71.
     External cardiac pacemaker.

2883.01   EDLER, INGE. 1911- , & HERTZ, CARL HELLMUTH. 1920-
The use of ultrasonic reflectoscope for the continuous recording the movements of heart walls. *K. Fysiogr. Sellsk. Lund. Foersh.*, 1954, **24**, 1-19.
     Echocardiography, from which the field of medical ultrasonics has developed.

2883.1   LaDUE, JOHN SAMUEL. 1911-1980, & WROBLEWSKI, FELIX. 1921-
The significance of the serum glutamic oxalacetic transaminase activity following acute myocardial infarction. *Circulation*, 1955, **11**, 871-77.
     Diagnostic test for myocardial infarction.

2883.2   RICHARDS, DICKINSON WOODRUFF. 1895-1973
The contributions of right heart catheterization to physiology and medicine, with some observations on the physiopathology of pulmonary heart disease. *Amer. Heart J.*, 1957, **54**, 161-71.

2883.21   SATOMURA, S.
Ultrasonic Doppler method for the inspection of cardiac functions. *J. Acoust. Soc. Amer.*, 1957, **29**, 1181-85.

Demonstration of the Doppler shift in the frequency of ultrasound backscattered by moving cardiac structures.

2883.3   HUNTER, SAMUEL WYNNE. 1921- , *et al.*
A bipolar myocardial electrode for complete heart block. *J.-Lancet*, 1959, **79**, 506-8.
With N. A. Roth, D. Bernardez, and J. L. Noble.

2883.4   KOUWENHOVEN, WILLIAM BENNETT. 1886-1975, *et al.*
Closed-chest cardiac massage. *J. Amer. med. Assoc.*, 1960, **173**, 1064-67.
Adequate cardiac massage without thoracotomy. With J.R. Jude and G.G. Knickerbocker.

2883.5   LOWN, BERNARD. 1921- , AMARASINGHAM, R., & NEUMAN, J.
New method for terminating cardiac arrythmias; use of synchronized capacitor discharge. *J. Amer. med. Assoc.*, 1962, **182**, 548-555.
Use of transthoracic direct current countershock of very short duration to avoid the vulnerable period in the cardiac cycle.

2883.6   DAY, HUGHES W.
Preliminary studies of an acute coronary care area. *J.Lancet*, 1963, 83, 53-55.
The coronary care unit.

2883.7   HOFFMAN, BRIAN F. & CRANEFIELD, PAUL FREDERICK. 1925-
The physiological basis of cardiac arrhythmias. *Amer.J.Med.*, 1964, **37**, 670-84.

2883.8   SCHERLAG, BENJAMIN J. 1932- *et al.*
Catheter technique for recording His bundle activity in man. *Circulation*, 1969, **39**, 13-18.
With 5 co-authors.

2883.9   SWAN, HAROLD JAMES CHARLES. 1922- *et al.*
Catheterization of the heart in man with use of a flow-directed balloon-tipped catheter. *New Eng. J. Med.*, 1970, **283**, 447-51.
Flow-guided balloon-tipped catheter of flexible construction, which enabled "placement without associated ventricular arrhythmias, prompt and reliable passage to the pulmonary artery and passage without fluoroscopy". With 5 co-authors.

Angina Pectoris

See also 3021-3047.25, CARDIOVASCULAR SURGERY

2884   HYDE, EDWARD, 1st *Earl of Clarendon*. 1609-1674
Life of Edward, 1st Earl of Clarendon, by himself. Oxford, 1759, **1**, 9.
From the description given by the Earl of Clarendon in his autobiography, his father, Henry Hyde, almost certainly suffered from, and died of, angina pectoris. If this is really so, it is the first recorded case. The description is reproduced in *Ann. med. Hist.*, 1922, **4**, 210.

2885   MORGAGNI, GIOVANNI BATTISTA. 1682-1771
De sedibus, et causis morborum. Venetiis, *typ. Remondiniana*, 1761, **1**, 282.
     An authentic case of angina pectoris is recorded by Morgagni; he observed it in 1707.

2886   ROUGNON DE MAGNY, NICOLAS FRANÇOIS. 1727-1799
Lettre de M. Rougnon à M. Lorry, touchant les causes de la mort de feu Monsieur Charles, ancien capitaine de cavalerie, arrivé à Besançon le 23 février 1768. Besançon, *J. F. Charmet*, 1768.
     Osler, Allbutt, and several other authorities believe this to be the description of an authentic case of angina, thus preceding Heberden's classic account. Other eminent authorities consider the patient to have suffered from pulmonary emphysema. This little book of 55 pages is extremely rare; the whereabouts of only 2 copies is known.

2887   HEBERDEN, WILLIAM, *Snr*. 1710-1801
Some account of a disorder of the breast. *Med. Trans. Coll. Phys. Lond.*, 1772, **2**, 59-67.
     This classic description of angina pectoris is the substance of a paper read on July 21, 1768. Although descriptions of angina are to be found in the works of earlier writers, these mention only dyspnoea in their cases. The merit of Herberden's account (in which, incidently, he used the name "angina pectoris") lies in the fact that he was the first to include a description of the paroxysmal oppression in the thorax. His account is so perfect that it might well have been written today.

2888   PARRY, CALEB HILLIER. 1755-1822
An inquiry into the symptoms and causes of the syncope anginosa commonly called angina pectoris. Bath, *R. Cruttwell*; London, *Cadell & Davis*, 1799.
     This was a paper read before the Gloucester Medical Society in 1788, but not published until 1799. Largely confirming the earlier work of Heberden on the condition, Parry stated his conclusion that disease of the coronary arteries is the responsible factor in angina pectoris (which he called "syncope anginosa"). He was the first to observe the slowing of the heart rate folowing pressure on the carotid artery.

2889   BURNS, ALLAN. 1781-1813
Observations on some of the most frequent and important diseases of the heart. Edinburgh, *Bryce & Co.*, 1809.
     Burns was among the first to suggest (see p. 136) that angina pectoris is an expression of coronary obstruction.

2890   BRUNTON, *Sir* THOMAS LAUDER. 1844-1916
On the use of nitrite of amyl in angina pectoris. *Lancet*, 1867, **2**, 97-98.
     Lauder Brunton was responsible for the introduction of amyl nitrite for the alleviation of angina. Reprinted in F. A. Willius & T. E. Keys: *Cardiac classics*, 1941, pp. 561-64.

2891   NOTHNAGEL, CARL WILHELM HERMANN. 1841-1905
Angina pectoris vasomotoria. *Dtsch. Arch. klin. Med.*, 1867, **3**, 309-322.
     Nothnagel, himself a victim of angina, described the vasomotor form of the disease.

2892 MURRELL, WILLIAM. 1853-1912
Nitro-glycerine as a remedy for angina pectoris. *Lancet*, 1879, **1**, 80-81, 113-15, 151-52, 225-27.
Murrell introduced trinitrin (nitroglycerin, glyceryl trinitrate) in the treatment of angina.

2893 ASKANAZY, S.
Klinisches über Diuretin. *Dtsch. Arch. klin. Med.*, 1895, **56**, 209-30.
In 1895 Askanazy proposed diuretin as a remedy for anginal pain.

2894 ALLBUTT, *Sir* THOMAS CLIFFORD. 1836-1925
Diseases of the arteries, including angina pectoris. 2 vols. London, *Macmillan & Co.*, 1915.
Includes his suggestion of the aortic genesis of angina pectoris, and (vol. 2, p. 368) his mechanical theory of cardiac pain in coronary occlusion.

2894.1 BOUSFIELD, GUY WILLIAM JOHN. 1893-1974
Angina pectoris: changes in electrocardiogram during paroxysm. *Lancet*, 1918, **2**, 457-58.
First electrocardiogram recorded (1917) from a patient with angina pectoris.

2895 JONNESCO, THOMAS. 1860-1926
Angine de poitrine guérie par la résection du sympathique cervicothoracique. *Bull. Acad. Méd. (Paris)*, 1920, 3 sér., **84**, 93-102.
Cervical sympathectomy for the treatment of angina pectoris was first carried out by Jonnesco in 1916.

2896 LAEWEN, ARTHUR. 1876-1958
Paravertebrale Novokaininjektionen zur Differentialdiagnose intra-abdomineller Erkrankungen. *Zbl. Chir.*, 1922, **49**, 1510-12.
First paravertebral injection for the treatment of angina pectoris.

2897 MACKENZIE, *Sir* JAMES. 1853-1925
Angina pectoris. London, *H. Frowde*, 1923.
A classic description of angina by "the beloved physician", one of the greatest of all cardiologists. Mackenzie considered the disease to be due to cardiac failure.

2899 BLUMGART, HERMANN LUDWIG. 1895- , *et al.*
Congestive heart failure and angina pectoris: the therapeutic effect of thyroidectomy on patients without clinical or pathologic evidence of thyroid toxicity. *Arch. intern. Med.*, 1933, **51**, 866-77.
Angina pectoris treated by thyroidectomy. With S. A. Levine and D. D. Berlin.

2900 RAAB, WILHELM. 1895-1969
Thiouracil treatment of angina pectoris; rationale and results. *J. Amer. med. Assoc.*, 1945, **128**, 249-56.

2901 LOBSTEIN, JEAN GEORGES CHRÉTIEN FRÉDÉRIC MARTIN. 1777-1835
Traité d'anatomie pathologique. Paris, *F. G. Levrault*, 1833.

Vol. 2, pp. 553-600 deals with diseases of the arteries. Lobstein wrote an important section on ossification of arteries, and was first to use the word "arteriosclérose" (on p. 550).

2902   BRODIE, *Sir* BENJAMIN COLLINS, *Bart.* 1783-1862
Lectures illustrative of various subjects in pathology and surgery. London, *Longman*, 1846.
Page 361 contains the first description of intermittent claudication in man. This was first reported (in the horse) by "Boullay" [? J. Bouley] in *Arch. gén. Méd.*, 1831, **27**, 425. *See also* No. 2995.

2903   VIRCHOW, RUDOLF LUDWIG KARL. 1821-1902
Ueber die acute Entzündung der Arterien. *Virchows Arch. path. Anat.*, 1847, **1**, 272-378.

2904   ROKITANSKY, CARL, *Freiherr von*. 1804-1878
Ueber einige der wichtigsen Krankheiten der Arterien. *Denkschr. k. Akad. Wiss. Wien*, 1852, **4**, 1-72.
One of Rokitansky's best works.

2905   CHARCOT, JEAN MARTIN. 1825-1893
Sur la claudication intermittente. *C. R. Soc. Biol. (Paris)*, (1858), *Mémoires*, 1859, 2 sér., **5**, 225-38.
Charcot was among the first to report intermittent claudication in man.

2906   KUSSMAUL, ADOLF. 1822-1902, & MAIER, RUDOLF. 1824-1888
Ueber eine bisher noch nicht beschriebene eigenthümliche Arterienerkrankung (Periarteritis nodosa), die mit Morbus Brightii und rapid fortschreitender allgemeiner Muskellähmung einhergeht. *Dtsch. Arch. klin. Med.*, 1866, **1**, 484-518.
First description of periarteritis nodosa.

2906.1   MAHOMED, FREDERICK HORATIO AKBAR. 1849-1884
The etiology of Bright's disease and the prealbuminuric stage. *Med. chir. Trans.*, 1874, **57**, 197-228.
Mahomed proved that cases of "arteriocapillary fibrosis" were hypertensive, and showed that they may occur without renal involvement.

2907   WINIWARTER, FELIX VON. 1852-1931
Ueber eine eigenthümliche Form von Endarteriitis und Endophlebitis mit Gangrän des Fusses. *Arch. klin. Chir.*, 1879, **23**, 202-26.
Early description of thrombo-angiitis obliterans (Buerger's disease, No. 2912).

2907.1   LEYDEN, ERNST VON. 1832-1910
Ueber die Sclerose der coronar-Arterien und die davon abhängigen Krankheitszustände. *Z. klin. Med.*, 1884, **7**, 459-86, 539-80.
A comprehensive account.

2908   HUCHARD, HENRI. 1844-1910
L'artério-sclérose subaiguë dans ses rapports avec les spasmes vasculaires et son traitement par la trinitrine (nitroglycérine). *Gaz. Hôp. (Paris)*, 1887, **60**, 1034-35.

"Huchard's disease" – continued hypertension causing arteriosclerosis. Huchard did much to develop the knowledge concerning arteriosclerosis and summarized his work in a classic monograph published in 1909.

2908.1   JASSINOWSKY, ALEXANDER. 1864-
Ein Beitrag zur Lehre von der Gefässnaht. *Arch. klin. Chir.*, 1891, **42**, 816-41.
    Jassinowsky experimented with arterial sutures on animals. His thesis (Dorpat, 1889) was an experimental-surgical study of the subject.

2908.2   DÖRFLER, JULIUS.
Ueber Arteriennaht. *Beitr. klin. Chir.*, 1899, **25**, 781-825.
    All-layer intima-to-intima arterial anastomosis.

2909   CARREL, ALEXIS. 1873-1944
La technique opératoire des anastomoses vasculaires et la transplantation des viscères. *Lyon méd.*, 1902, **98**, 859-64.
    Carrel perfected the operation of arterial suture, end-to-end anastomosis of severed vessels with triple-threaded sutures. *See also* No. 3026.

2910   JOSUE, OTTO. 1869-1923
Athérôme aortique expérimental par injections répétées d'adrénaline dans les veines. *C. R. Soc. Biol. (Paris)*, 1903, **55**, 1374-76.
    Experimental production of arteriosclerosis.

2911   MÖNCKEBERG, JOHANN GEORG. 1877-1925
Ueber die reine Mediaverkalkung der Extremitätenartien und ihr Verhalten zur Arteriosklerose. *Virchows Arch. path. Anat.*, 1903, **171**, 141-67.
    "Mönckeberg's sclerosis". He described a form of medial sclerosis of the blood-vessels of the extremities. See also his later papers in *Klin. Wschr.*, 1942, **52**, 1473-78, 1521-26.

2912   BUERGER, LEO. 1879-1943
Thrombo-angiitis obliterans; a study of the vascular lesions leading to presenile spontaneous gangrene. *Amer. J. med. Sci.*, 1908, **136**, 567-580.
    Buerger's important paper on thrombo-angiitis obliterans gives the first comprehensive report of the clinical and pathological aspects of the disease. Buerger gave the condition its present name; it is also known as "Buerger's disease".

2913   IGNATOVSKI, ALEXANDER. 1875-
[Influence of animal food on the organism of rabbits]. *Izvest. imp. vo.-med. Akad. St. Petersburg*, 1908, **16**, 154-76.
    Experimental arteriosclerosis produced by a diet of milk and egg yolk. French translation in *Arch. Méd. exp. Anat. path.*, 1908, **20**, 1-20.

2914   ARRILAGA, FRANCISCO C.
Cardiacos negros. Buenos Aires, *Thesis No. 2536*, 1912.
    A classical description of "Ayerza's disease" (cor pulmonale), to which Arrilaga gave the name. Corvisart mentioned the condition in 1806. *See* No. 2917.

2915   ANITSCHKOV, NIKOLAI. 1885-1964 ,& CHALATOV, S. S. 1884-
Ueber experimentelle Cholesterinsteatose und ihre Bedeutung für die
Entstehung einiger pathologischer Prozesse. *Zbl. allg. Path. path. Anat..*,
1913, **24**, 1-9.
Experimental production of arteriosclerosis with cholesterol-rich diet.
Translated in *Arteriosclerosis*, 1983, **3**, 178-182.

2915.1   JEGER, ERNEST
Die Chirurgie der Blutgefässe und des Herzens. Berlin, *A. Hirschwald*, 1913.
Jeger was the first to advocate the bypass principle for management of
peripheral aneurysms.

2916   BERBERICH, JOSEF. 1897- , & HIRSCH, S.
Die Röntgenographische Darstellung der Arterien und Venen am lebenden
Menschen. *Klin. Wschr.*, 1923, **2**, 2226-28.
Arteriography. First angiogram of a living patient.

2916.1   BROOKS, BARNEY. 1884-
Intra-arterial injection of sodium iodid: preliminary report. *J. Amer. med.
Assoc.*, 1924, **82**, 1016-19.
Clinical angiography.

2916.2   ——, & JOSTES, F. A.
A clinical study of diseases of the circulation of the extremities; a description
of a new method of examination. *Arch. Surg. (Chicago)*, 1924, **9**, 485-503.
Femoral arteriography.

2917   AYERZA, LUIS.
Consideraciones sobre la denominación de "Enfermedad de Ayerza".
Semana méd., 1925, **32**, pt. 2, 386-88.
In 1901 Abel Ayerza lectured on the syndrome of chronic cyanosis,
dyspnoea, erythraemia, and sclerosis of the pulmonary artery, "Ayerza's
disease" (cor pulmonale). He did not publish this work, but an important
discussion on the nomenclature was given by Luis Ayerza in the above
paper and in a previous paper in the same journal, 1925, **32**, pt.1, 43. *See*
No. 2914.

2918   KLOTZ, OSKAR. 1878-1936
Concerning the pathology of some arterial diseases. *Ann. clin. Med.*, 1925-
26, **4**, 814-28.
Klotz, eminent Canadian pathologist, is particularly remembered for his
contributions to the subject of arteriosclerosis.

2919   SCHMIDT, MAX. 1898-
Intracranial aneurysms. *Brain*, 1930, **53**, 489-540.
Temporal arteritis is first described in Case 24 (p. 532). Schmidt's paper
also appeared in *Bibl. Laeger*, 1930, **122**, 269 (Case 24, p. 320). Temporal
arteritis was also described as a new condition by B. T. Horton, T. B.
Magath, and G. E. Brown, *Proc. Mayo Clin.*, 1932, **7**, 700-01.

2919.1   PEARSE, HERMAN ELWYN. 1899- , & WARREN, STAFFORD L.
The roentgenographic visualization of the arteries of the extremities in
peripheral vascular disease. *Ann. Surg.*, 1931, **94**, 1094-1102.

2920   SANTOS, REYNALDO DOS. 1880- , & CALDAS, J.
Les dérivés du thorium dans l'artériographie des membres. *Medicina contemp. (Lisboa)*, 1931, **49**, 234-36.
Thorotrast first used in arteriography.

2921   WEISS, SOMA. 1898-1942, & BAKER, JAMES PORTER. 1913-
The carotid sinus in health and disease: its rôle in the causation of fainting and convulsions. *Medicine,* 1933, **12**, 297-354.
The carotid sinus syndrome.

2922   WAGENER, HENRY PATRICK. 1890-1961, & KEITH, NORMAN MACDONNELL. 1885-1976
Diffuse arteriolar disease with hypertension and the associated retinal lesions. *Medicine,* 1939, **18**, 317-430.
The Keith–Wagener classification of fundal lesions.

2923   LAUBRY, CHARLES. 1872-1960, *et al.*
Grosse pulmonaire. Petite aorte. Affection congénitale. *Bull. Soc. méd. Hôp. Paris*, 1940, **56**, 847-50.
Idiopathic dilatation of the pulmonary artery reported. With D. Routier and R. Heim de Balsac.

2924   RICH, ARNOLD RICE. 1893-1968
The rôle of hypersensitivity in periarteritis nodosa; as indicated by seven cases developing during serum sickness and sulfonamide therapy. *Bull. Johns Hopk. Hosp.*, 1942, **71**, 123-35.
Rich considered hypersensitivity to be an important factor in the aetiology of periarteritis nodosa.

2924.1   KUNLIN, JEAN.
Le traitement de l'artérite oblitérante par la greffe veineuse. *Arch. Mal. Coeur*, 1949, **42**, 371-2.
Kunlin, an associate of R. Leriche, first reported the use of a bypass venous graft for femoropopliteal occlusive arterial disease.

2924.2   SELDINGER, SVEN IVAR.
Catheter replacement of the needle in percutaneous angiography. A new technique. *Acta radiol. (Stockh).*, 1953, **39**, 368-76.
Percutaneous arterial catheterization.

2924.3   SONES, FRANK MASON, Jr. & SHIREY, EARL K. 1924-
Cine-coronary arteriography. *Mod. Conc. Cardiovasc. Dis.*, 1962, **31**, 735-38.
Coronary arteriography.

2924.4   DOTTER, C.T. & JUDKINS, MELVIN P.
Transluminal treatment of arteriosclerotic obstruction; description of a new technic and a preliminary report of its application. *Circulation*, 1964, **30**, 654-70.
Percutaneous transluminal coronary angioplasty.

2924.5   JUDKINS, MELVIN P.
Selective coronary arteriography. Part I: A percutaneous transfemoral technic. *Radiology*, 1967, **89**, 815-24.

Ligations of Arteries

2925   HOME, *Sir* EVERARD. 1756-1832
        An account of Mr. Hunter's method of performing the operation for the
        popliteal aneurism. *Lond. med. J.*, 1786, **7**, 391-406.
        First description of John Hunter's method of treating popliteal aneurysm.
        This consisted in a single ligature of the artery at a distance high in the
        healthy tissues. Recorded by his brother-in law. See also *Trans. Soc. Im-
        prove. med. Knowl.*, 1793, **1**, 138. Reprinted in *Med. Classics*, 1940, **4**, 449-
        57.

2925.1 KAST, THOMAS. ?1755-1820
        An account of an aneurism in the thigh, perfectly cured by the operation.
        Med. Communications Mass. Med. Soc., 1790, **1**, 96-98.
        The first femoral ligation reported in America, and the first paper on a
        surgical topic to be published in an American medical periodical.

2926   BELL, JOHN. 1763-1820
        The principles of surgery. Edinburgh, 1801, **1**, 421-26.
        First ligation of the gluteal artery.

2927   DESAULT, PIERRE JOSEPH. 1744-1795
        Remarques et observations sur l'opération de l'anévrisme. In his *Œuvres
        chirurgicales*, Paris, 1801, **2**, 553-80.
        Desault developed the technique of tying blood-vessels for the treatment
        of aneurysm. *See* No. 5580.

2928   ABERNETHY, JOHN. 1764-1831
        Surgical observations on the constitution origin and treatment of local
        diseases. London, *Longmans*, 1809, pp. 234-92.
        First ligation of the external iliac artery for aneurysm. Abernethy
        performed the operation in 1796. *See* No. 5584.

2929   COOPER, *Sir* ASTLEY PASTON, *Bart.* 1768-1841
        A case of aneurism of the carotid artery. *Med.-chir. Trans.*, 1809, **1**, 1-12,
        222-33.
        Cooper ligated the common carotid artery on Nov. 1, 1805; the patient
        died, but a second case (June 22, 1808) proved successful. (*See also* No.
        2955).

2930   DORSEY, JOHN SYNG. 1783-1818
        Inguinal aneurism cured by tying the external iliac artery in the pelvis.
        Eclectic Repert., 1811, **2**, 111-15.
        First successful ligation of the external iliac artery in America (Aug. 19,
        1811).

2931   TRAVERS, BENJAMIN. 1783-1858
        A case of aneurism by anastomosis in the orbit, cured by the ligature of the
        common carotid artery. *Med.-chir. Trans.*, 1811, **2**, 1-16.

2932   GOODLAD, WILLIAM.
        Case of inguinal aneurism cured by tying the external iliac artery. *Edinb.
        med. surg. J.*, 1812, **8**, 32-39.
        Goodlad successfully ligated the external iliac on July 29, 1811.

2934   POST, PHILIP WRIGHT. 1766-1828
A case of carotid aneurism successfully treated. *Amer. med. phil. Reg.*, 1814, **4**, 366-77.

        Post, Professor of Surgery and Anatomy at Columbia College, New York, was the first in America to ligate the common carotid artery for aneurysmal disease.

2935   STEVENS, WILLIAM. 1786-1868
A case of aneurism of the gluteal artery, cured by tying the internal iliac. *Med.-chir. Trans.*, 1814, **5**, 422-34.

        First successful ligation of the internal iliac, Dec. 27, 1812. The patient died in 1822 and an account of the autopsy is given by Richard Owen in *Med.-chir. Trans.*, 1830, **16**, 219-35.

2936   COLLES, ABRAHAM. 1773-1843
On the operation of tying the subclavian artery. *Edinb. med. surg. J.*, 1815, **11**, 1-25.

        Colles tied the subclavian artery in 1811 and again in 1813. Garrison reminds us that Colles is accredited with the first successful ligation of the innominate artery in Europe, but is unable to verify this. The paper is reprinted in *Med. Classics*, 1940, **4**, 1043-72.

2937   GUTHRIE, GEORGE JAMES. 1785-1856
Case of a wound of the peroneal artery successfully treated by a ligature. *Med.-chir. Trans.*, 1816, **7**, 330-37.

        On July 2, 1815, Guthrie successfully ligated the peroneal artery of a German soldier wounded at the Battle of Waterloo.

2938   SODEN, JOHN SMITH. 1780-1863
Case of inguinal aneurism cured by tying the external iliac artery. *Med.-chir. Trans.*, 1816, **7**, 536-40.

2939   POST, PHILIP WRIGHT. 1766-1828
Case of brachial aneurism, cured by tying the subclavian artery above the clavicle. *Tr. phys.-med. soc. N. Y.*, 1817, **1**, 387-94.

        Post was the first successfully to ligate the subclavian artery outside the scaleni (Sept. 8, 1817).

2940   SCARPA, ANTONIO. 1752-1832
Memoria sulla legature delle principali arterie degli arti. Pavia, *P. Bizzoni*, 1817.

2941   COOPER, *Sir* ASTLEY PASTON, *Bart*. 1768-1841, & TRAVERS, BENJAMIN. 1783-1858
Surgical essays. London, *Cox & Son*, 1818, **1**, 101-30.

        In 1817 Cooper ligated the abdominal aorta. The patient died next day, but examination showed that his aorta was so diseased that he could never have recovered, while the ligation was so well performed that with a lesser degree of aortic disease the man would probably have survived.

2942   MOTT, VALENTINE. 1785-1865
Reflections on securing in a ligature the arteria innominata, to which is added a case in which the artery was tied by a surgical operation. *Med. surg. Register*, 1818, **1**, 9-54.

First ligation of the innominate artery, May 11, 1818. The artery was tied off half an inch below its bifurcation, and the patient suffered no respiratory or circulatory embarrassment. The ligature separated from the artery on the 14th day, but on the 20th day the patient was able to walk downstairs. A fatal haemorrhage occurred from the wound, however, and the patient died on the 26th day.

2943   DUPUYTREN, GUILLAUME, *le baron*. 1777-1835
Account of the tying of the subclavian artery. *Edinb. med. surg. J.*, 1819, **15**, 476.
    Dupuytren successfully ligated the subclavian artery on March 7, 1819.

2944   GIBSON, WILLIAM. 1788-1868
Case of a wound of the common iliac artery. *Amer. med. Recorder*, 1820, **3**, 185-93.
    Gibson was the first to ligate the common iliac, July 27, 1812.

2945   COGSWELL, MASON FITCH. 1761-1830
Account of an operation for the extirpation of a tumour in which a ligature was applied to the carotid artery. *New Engl. J. Med. Surg.*, 1824, **13**, 357-60.
    Cogswell ligated the primitive carotid on Nov. 4, 1803.

2946   MACGILL, WILLIAM D. 1802-1833
Account of a case in which both carotids were successfully tied. *N. Y. med. phys. J.*, 1825, **4**, 576.
    In 1823 Macgill successfully ligated in continuity both primitive carotid arteries in the same subject within a month. He was the first American to do so.

2947   DUPUYTREN, GUILLAUME, *le baron*. 1777-1835
Observation sur un cas de ligature de l'artère iliaque externe. *Repert. gén. Anat. Physiol. path.*, 1826, **2**, 230-50.
    Successful ligation of the external iliac, Oct. 16, 1815.

2948   KEY, CHARLES ASTON. 1793-1849
Case of axillary aneurism successfully treated by tying the subclavian artery. *Med. -chir. Trans.*, 1827, **13**, 1-11.
    In 1823 Key successfully ligated the subclavian artery for aneurysm at the axilla.

2949   WARDROP, JAMES. 1782-1869
Case of carotid aneurism successfully treated by tying the artery above the aneurismal tumor. *Med.-chir. Trans.*, 1827, **13**, 217-26.
    Wardrop successfully treated aneurysm of the carotid artery by distal ligation, a procedure suggested by Pierre Brasdor (*see* No. 2951). Wardrop expanded this paper into a book: *On aneurism, and its cure by a new operation*, London, *Longman*, 1828.

2950   MOTT, VALENTINE. 1785-1865
Successful ligature of the common iliac artery. *Am. J. med. Sci.*, 1827, 1, 156-61.
    First successful ligation of the common iliac.

2951 ———. Aneurism of the arteria innominata involving the subclavian and the root of the carotid; successfully treated by tying the carotid artery. *Amer. J. med. Sci.*, 1929, **5**, 297-300.

First application in the United States of the Pierre Brasdor (1721-97) operative technique by distal ligation. Second report, 1830, **6**, 532-34.

2953 ———. Case of aneurism of the right subclavian artery, in which that vessel was tied within the scaleni muscles. *Amer. J. med. Sci.*, 1833, **12**, 354-59.

In his day Mott was the ablest exponent of vascular surgery in the U.S.A. This was the first attempt in America to ligate the subclavian within the scaleni muscles. The procedure had been tried at least twice previously in Europe.

2954 COOPER, *Sir* ASTLEY PASTON, *Bart.* 1768-1841
Case of a femoral aneurism, for which the external iliac artery was tied, with an account of the preparation of the limb, dissected at the extirpation of eighteen years. *Guy's Hosp. Rep.*, 1836, **1**, 43-52.

The artery was tied in 1808, and the patient died in 1826.

2955 ———. Account of the first successful operation, performed on the carotid artery, for aneurism, in the year 1808; with the post-mortem examination in 1821. *Guy's Hosp. Rep.*, 1836, **1**, 53-58.

See No. 2929.

2956 ———. Some experiments and observations on tying the carotid and vertebral arteries, and the pneumo-gastric, phrenic, and sympathetic nerves. *Guy's Hosp. Rep.*, 1836, **1**, 457-75, 654.

2957 KEY, CHARLES ASTON. 1793-1849
Femoral aneurism successfully treated by a ligature of the external iliac artery. *Guy's Hosp. Rep.*, 1836, **1**, 59-78.

Successful ligation of external iliac artery for femoral aneurysm, 1822.

2958 MOTT, VALENTINE. 1785-1865
A case of aneurism of either the ischiatic or gluteal artery, in which the right internal iliac artery was successfully tied. *Amer. J. med. Sci.*, 1837, **20**, 13-15.

Second successful reported ligation of the internal iliac artery in the United States.

2959 TWITCHELL, AMOS. 1781-1850
Gun-shot wound of the face and neck; ligature of the carotid artery. *New Engl. quart. J. Med. Surg.*, 1842-43, **1**, 188-93.

First successful ligature of the carotid artery (for secondary haemorrhage) Oct. 18, 1807, eight months before Sir Astley Cooper (No. 2929). Published 35 years after the event, this paper may set some kind of record for late reporting.

2960 BUCK, GURDON. 1807-1877
Case of aneurism of the femoral artery for which ligatures were successively applied to the femoral, profunda, external and common iliac. *N.Y.J. Med.*, 1858, 3 ser., **5**, 305-11.

2961 SYME, JAMES. 1799-1870
Case of iliac aneurism. *Med. -chir. Trans.*, 1862, **45**, 381-87.
Syme treated a case of iliac aneurysm by opening the sac and ligating the
common iliac and the internal and external iliac arteries.

2962 PARKER, WILLARD. 1800-1884
Ligature of the left subclavian inside the scalenus muscle, together with
common carotid and vertebral arteries for subclavian aneurism haemorrhage from the distal end of the subclavian; death on 42nd day. *Amer. Med.
Times*, 1864, **8**, 114-16.

2963 SMYTH, ANDREW WOODS. 1832-1916
Successful operation for subclavian aneurism. *Amer. J. med. Sci.*, 1866, **52**,
280-82.
 First successful ligation of the innominate artery, 1864. A report on the
condition of the patient in 1869 is given in *New Orleans J. Med.*, 1869, **22**,
464-69.

2964 LISTER, JOSEPH, 1st *Baron Lister.* 1827-1912
Observations on ligature of arteries on the antiseptic system. *Lancet*, 1869,
1, 451-55.
 Lister evolved a carbolized catgut ligature, better than any previously
produced. He was able to cut short the ends of his ligature, closing the
wound tightly and eliminating the necessity for bringing the ends of
ligatures out through the wound.

2965 BALLANCE, *Sir* CHARLES ALFRED. 1865-1936, & EDMUNDS, WALTER. 1850-1930
A treatise on the ligation of the great arteries in continuity. London,
Macmillan & Co., 1891.
 Includes Ballance's scale of measurement of calibre of arteries.

2966 HALSTED, WILLIAM STEWART. 1852-1922
Ligation of the first portion of the left subclavian artery and excision of a
subclavio-axillary aneurism. *Johns Hopk. Hosp. Bull.*, 1892, **3**, 93-94.
 First successful ligation of the left subclavian artery. This was the first
"successful ligation of the first part of either subclavian artery and the first
one of complete extirpation of such an aneurysm" (MacCallum).

2967 MURPHY, JOHN BENJAMIN. 1857-1916
Resection of arteries and veins injured in continuity – end to end suture –
experimental and clinical research. *Med. Rec. (N.Y.)* 1897, **51**, 73-88.
 Successful suture of femoral artery, 1896. This was one of the earliest
end-to-end anastomoses of arteries ever performed.

2968 KEHR, HANS.
Der erste Fall von erfolgreicher Unterbindung der Art. hepatica propria
gegen Aneurysma. *Münch. med. Wschr.*, 1861-67.
 Successful ligation of the hepatic artery.

2969 HALSTED, WILLIAM STEWART. 1852-1922
Partial progressive and complete occlusion of the aorta and other large arteries
in the dog by means of the metal band. *J. exp. Med.*, 1909, **11**, 373-91.
 Halsted introduced a metal band in place of a ligature for the occlusion
of arteries.

2970   VAUGHAN, GOERGE TULLY. 1859-1948
        Ligation (partial occlusion) of the abdominal aorta for aneurism. *Ann. Surg.*,
        1921, **74**, 308-12.
        First successful ligation of the abdominal aorta.

Aneurysms

See also 2726-2900, HEART AND AORTA; 2925-2970, LIGATIONS OF ARTERIES

2971   SAPORTA, ANTOINE. ?-1573
        De tumoribus praeter naturam libri V. Lugduni, *P. Ravaud*, 1624.
        Saporta, in 1554, gave the earliest description of an aortic aneurysm.
        The manuscript of his book was discovered many years after his death, and
        was published by a Lyons doctor, named Gras.

2972   VESALIUS, ANDREAS. 1514-1564
        In Welsch, G. H., Sylloge curationum et observationum medicinalum centurias
        iv complectens. Augustae Vindelicorum, *G. Goebelii*, 1667, pt. 4, p. 46.
        In 1555 Vesalius was the first to diagnose aneurysm of the thoracic and
        abdominal aorta in a living person. This was confirmed at autopsy two
        years later.

2973   LANCISI, GIOVANNI MARIA. 1654-1720
        De motu cordis et aneurysmatibus. Romae, *J. M. Salvioni*, 1728.
        Lancisi noted the frequency of cardiac aneurysm and showed the
        importance of syphilis, asthma, palpitation, violent emotions, and excess
        as causes of aneurysms. He was the first to describe cardiac syphilis. Lancisi
        shares with Vieussens the honour of laying the foundation of the pathology
        of heart disease. Revision of 1745 edition of *De aneurysmatibus*, with
        translation and notes, by W. C. Wright, 1952.

2974   HUNTER, WILLIAM. 1718-1783
        The history of an aneurysm of the aorta, with some remarks on aneurysms
        in general. *Med. Obs. Inqu.*, 1757, **1**, 323-57.
        First recorded case of arteriovenous aneurysm.

2975   SCARPA, ANTONIO. 1752-1832
        Sull' aneurisma. Pavia, *tipog. Bolzani*, 1804.
        Scarpa distinguished true from false aneurysms. He introduced the
        concept of arteriosclerosis. English translations, Edinburgh, 1808 and
        1819.

2976   DUPUYTREN, GUILLAUME, *le baron*. 1777-1835
        [Anévrisme à l'artère poplitée par la compression.] *Bull. Fac. Méd. Paris*,
        1818, **6**, 242.
        Dupuytren was the first successfully to treat aneurysm by compression.

2977   VELPEAU, ALFRED ARMAND LOUIS MARIE. 1795-1867
        Mémoire sur la piqûre ou l'acupuncture des artères dans le traitement des
        anévrismes. *Gaz. méd. Paris*, 1831, **2**, 1-4.
        First attempt at operative treatment of aneurysm.

2977.1 PEACOCK, Thomas Bevill. 1812-1882
[Cases]. *Edinb. med. surg. J.*, 1843, **60**, 276-302.
An important account of dissecting aneurysm. Peacock collected all previously published cases and added a few of his own to a total of 19.

2978 BELLINGHAM, O'Bryen. 1805-1857
Observations on aneurism, and its treatment by compression. London, *J. Churchill*, 1847.
Bellingham introduced the "Dublin method" of treating aneurysm by slow compression.

2979 DONDERS, Frans Cornelis. 1818-1889, & JANSEN, Jan Hissink. 1816-1885
Untersuchungen über die Natur der krankhaften Veränderungen der Arterienwände, die als Ursachen der spontanen Aneurysmen zu betrachten sind. *Arch. physiol. Heilk.*, 1848, **7**, 359-402, 530-60.

2980 MOORE, Charles Hewitt. 1821-1870, & MURCHISON, Charles. 1830-1879
On a new method of procuring the consolidation of fibrin in certain incurable aneurisms. *Med.-chir. Trans.*, 1864, **47**, 129-49.
Moore and Murchison introduced the method of treating aneurysm by passing wire into the aneurysmal sac.

2981 RASMUSSEN, Fritz Valdemar. 1833-1877
Om Haemoptyse navnlig den lethale, i anatomisk og klinisk Henseende. *Hospitalstidende*, 1868, **11**, 33-36, 37-40, 41-43, 45-46, 49-52; 1869, **12**, 41-42, 45-48.
Tuberculous aneurysm of the lung ("Rasmussen's aneurysm"). English translation in *Edinb. med. J.*, 1868, **14**, 385-401, 486-503; 1869, **15**, 97-104, 228-36.

2982 QUINCKE, Heinrich Irenaeus. 1842-1922
Ein Fall von Aneurysma der Leberarterie. *Berl. klin. Wschr.*, 1871, **8**, 349-52, 386.
Quincke observed aneurysm of the hepatic artery in 1870.

2983 WELCH, Francis Henry. 1839-1910
On aortic aneurism in the army and the conditions associated with it. *Med.-chir. Trans.*, 1876, **59**, 59-77.
Welch, an Army surgeon, supported the theory of a causal connexion between syphilis and aneurysm.

2984 EPPINGER, Hans. 1846-1916
Pathogenese (Histogenese und Aetiologie) der Aneurysmen einschliesslich des Aneurysma equi verminosum. *Arch. klin. Chir.*, 1887, **35**, Suppl.-Heft, 1-563.

2985 MATAS, Rudolph. 1860-1957
Traumatic aneurism of the left brachial artery. Failure of direct and indirect pressure; ligation of the artery immediately above tumor; return of pulsation on the tenth day; ligation immediately below tumor; failure to arrest pulsation; incision and partial excision of sac; recovery. *Med. News (Phila.)*, 1888, **53**, 462-66.
First aneurysmorrhaphy, April 6, 1888. See also *Trans. Amer. surg. Ass.*, 1902, **20**, 396-434.

2985.1　DÖHLE, KARL GOTTFRIED PAUL. 1855-1928
Ueber Aortenerkrankung bei Syphilitischen und deren Beziehung zur
Aneurysmenbildung. *Dtsch. Arch. klin. Med.*, 1895, **55**, 190-210.
Döhle clearly defined a specific syphilitic lesion of the aorta as a
prerequisite of aortic aneurysm.

2986　CHURTON, THOMAS. 1839-1926
Multiple aneurysms of the pulmonary artery. *Brit. med. J.*, 1897, **1**, 1223.
Churton was the first to recognize this condition at necropsy.

2987　HELLER, ARNOLD. 1840-1913
Die Aortensyphilis als Ursache von Aneurysmen. *Münch. med. Wschr.*, 1899,
46, 1669-71.
Heller established the fact that syphilis is a cause of aortic aneurysm.

2988　BABCOCK, WILLIAM WAYNE. 1872-1963
A new treatment of thoracic aneurysm. *Ann. clin. Med.*, 1926, **4**, 933-42.
Babcock's operation for thoracic aneurysm. See also *Amer. J. Surg.*, 1932,
16, 401-07.

2989　———. Operative decompression of aortic aneurysm by carotid-jugular
anastomosis. *Surg. Clin. N. Amer.*, 1929, **9**, 1031-41.
Babcock's operation for aortic aneurysm.

2990　SAUERBRUCH, ERNST FERDINAND. 1875-1951
Erfolgreiche operative Beseitigung eines Aneurysma der rechten
Herzkammer. *Arch. klin. Chir.*, 1931, **167**, 586-88.
First successful surgical intervention in cardiac aneurysm.

2991　SMITH, HARRY LEROY. 1887- , & HORTON, BAYARD TAYLOR. 1895-1980
Arteriovenous fistula of the lung associated with polycythemia vera: report
of a case in which the diagnosis was made clinically. *Amer. Heart J.*, 1939,
18, 589-92.

2992　HEPBURN, JOHN. 1888- , & DAUPHINEE, JAMES ARNOLD. 1903-
Successful removal of hemangioma of the lung followed by the disap-
pearance of polycythemia. *Amer. J. med. Sci.*, 1942, **204**, 681-85.
First successful excision of arteriovenous aneurysm of the lung.

2992.1　ALEXANDER, JOHN, & BYRON, FRANCIS X.
Aortectomy for thoracic aneurysm. *J. Amer. med. Assoc.*, 1944, **126**, 1139-
45.
Resection of saccular aneurysm of thoracic aorta.

2993　POPPE, JOHN KARL. 1911-
Cellophane treatment of syphilitic aneurysms with report of results in six
cases. *Amer. Heart J.*, 1948, **36**, 252-56.

2993.1　DUBOST, CHARLES. 1914- , *et al.*
A propos du traitement des anévrysmes de l'aorte. Ablation de l'anévrysme.
Rétablissement de la continuité par greffe d'aorte humaine conservée.
Mém. Acad. Chir. (Paris), 1951, **77**, 381-83.
First successful resection of abdominal aortic aneurysm and insertion of
a homologous graft. With M. Allary and N. Oeconomos.

2993.2   COOLEY, DENTON ARTHUR. 1920- , *et al.*
Total excision of the aortic arch for aneurysm. *Surg. Gynec. Obstet.*, 1955,
101, 667-72.
Total excision and replacement by polyvinyl sponge (Ivalon) prosthesis.
With D. E. Mahaffey and M. E. DeBakey.

VEINS

2994   BRODIE, *Sir* BENJAMIN COLLINS, *Bart.* 1783-1862
Observations on the treatment of varicose veins of the legs. *Med.-chir. Trans.*,
1816, **7**, 195-210.
Brodie first operated for varicose veins in 1814.

2995   ——. Lectures illustrative of various subjects in pathology and surgery.
London, *Longman*, 1846.
P. 186: Brodie's test for insuffiency of the valves in varicose veins, later
associated with the name of Trendelenburg. *See also* No. 2902.

2996   PAGET, *Sir* JAMES, *Bart.* 1814-1899
On gouty and some other forms of phlebitis. *St. Barth. Hosp. Rep.*, 1866,
2, 82-92.
Paget–Schroetter syndrome, venous obstruction in the upper extremity.

2997   TRENDELENBURG, FRIEDRICH. 1844-1924
Ueber die Unterbindung der Vena saphena magna bei
Unterschenkelvaricen. *Beitr. klin. Chir.*, 1890, **7**, 195-210.
"Trendelenburg's operation" – ligation of the great saphenous vein for
the treatment of varicose veins in the leg. Reprinted, with translation, in
Med. Classics, 1940, **4**, 989-1023. The paper also describes his test for
insuffiency of the valves, a procedure previously described by Brodie (No.
2995).

2998   MOORE, W.
The operative treatment of varicose veins, with especial reference to a
modification of Trendelenburg's operation. *Intercolon. med. J. Aust.*, 1896,
1 , 393-407.
Moore's operation of high resection of the saphenous vein for treatment
of varicosities.

2999   SCHIASSI, BENEDETTO.
La cure des varices du membre inférieur par l'injection intraveineuse d'une
solution d'iode. *Sem. méd. (Paris)*, 1908, **28**, 601-02.
Schiassi combined operative and sclerosant methods in the treatment
of varicose veins. Translation in *Med. Press*, 1909, **87**, 377.

3000   LINSER, PAUL. 1871-1963
Ueber die konservative Behandlung der Varicen. *Med. Klin.*, 1916, **12**, 897-
98.
Injection treatment of varicose veins was introduced by Linser.

3001   GENEVRIER, J.
        Du traitement des varices par les injection coagulantes, concentrées de sels
        de quinine. *Soc. méd. mil. franç. Bull.*, 1921, **15**, 169-71.
        Injection of quinine urethane for the treatment of varicose veins.

3002   SICARD, Jean Athanase. 1872-1929, *et al.*
        Traitement des varices par les injections phlébo-sclérosantes du salicylate
        de soude. *Gaz. Hôp. Paris*, 1922, **95**, 1573-75.
        Introduction of sodium salicylate injections for the treatment of varicose
        veins. With J. Paraf and J. Lermoyez.

3003   LINSER, Karl.
        Die Behandlung der Krampfadern mit intravarikösen Kochsalzinjektionen.
        Derm. Wschr., 1925, **81**, 1345-51.
        Sodium chloride first used in the injection treatment of varicose veins.

3004   NOBL, Gabor. 1864-1938
        Die Calorose als Verödungsmittel varikös entarteter Venen. *Wien. klin.
        Wschr.*, 1926, **39**, 1217-19.
        Nobl used dextrose in the injection treatment of varicose veins.

3004.1 BIRLEY, James Leatham. 1884-1934
        Traumatic aneurysm of the intracranial portion of the internal carotid
        artery. With a note by Wilfred Trotter. *Brain,* 1928, **51**, 184-208.
        In 1924 Wilfred Trotter (1872-1939) performed the first planned operation
        for intracranial aneurysm diagnosed pre-operatively.

3005   COOPER, William Morris. 1894-
        The treatment of varicose veins. *Ann. Surg.*, 1934, **99**, 799-805.
        Cooper combined ligation with subsequent injection of 5 per cent
        sodium morrhuate in the treatment of varicose veins.

3005.1 JACOBSON, Julius H., II. & SUAREZ, Ernesto L.
        Microsurgery in anastomosis of small vessels. *Surg. Forum*, 1960, **11**, 243-
        45.
        First demonstration of the value of the operating microscope in micro-
        surgery.

THROMBOSIS: EMBOLISM

3006   VIRCHOW, Rudolf Ludwig Karl. 1821-1902
        Thrombose und Embolie. Gefässentzündung und septische Infektion. In
        his *Gesammelte Abhandlungen zur wissenschaftlichen Medicin,* Frank-
        furt a.M., *Meidinger, Sohn u. Co.,* 1856, pp. 219-732.
        Reprints of papers published between 1846 and 1853. Virchow gave the
        first clear description of thrombosis and embolism (see especially *Beitr. exp.
        Path.*, 1846, **2**, 227-380). Reprinted in Sudhoff's *Klassiker der Medizin*, Bd.
        7-8, Leipzig, 1910. *See* No. 3064.

3007   ZENKER, FRIEDRICH ALBERT. 1825-1898
Beiträge zur normalen und pathologischen Anatomie der Lungen. Dresden, G. Schönfeld's Buchhandlung, 1862.
First description of pulmonary fat embolism in man.

3008   PANUM, PETER LUDVIG. 1820-1885
Experimentelle Beiträge zur Lehre von der Embolie. Virchows Arch. path. Anat., 1862, **25**, 308-38, 433-530.
Experimental study of the effects of ligation of coronary vessels.

3009   FELTZ, VICTOR TIMOTHÉE. 1835-1893
Traité clinique et expérimental des embolies capillaires. Paris, J. B. Baillière, 1870.

3010   COHNHEIM, JULIUS FRIEDRICH. 1839-1884
Untersuchungen über die embolischen Processe. Berlin, A. Hirschwald, 1872.
Cohnheim developed the doctrine of infarction as a result of occlusion of terminal arteries. He explained the haemorrhagic nature of certain infarcts on the basis of a reflux flow and diapedesis through the altered capillaries of the infarcted area.

3011   WELCH, WILLIAM HENRY. 1850-1934
Thrombosis and embolism. In Allbutt, C., System of medicine, London, 1899, **4**, 284-310; and in 2nd ed., 1909, **6**, 691-821.

3012   TRENDELENBURG, FRIEDRICH. 1844-1924
Ueber die operative Behandlung der Embolie der Lungenarterie. Arch. klin. Chir., 1908, **86**, 686-700.
Pulmonary embolectomy first attempted, "Trendelenburg's operation" – first successfully performed by Kirschner (see No. 3016).

3013   MOSNY, ERNEST. 1861-1918, & DUMONT, J.
Embolie fémorale au cours d'un rétrécissement mitral pur. Arteriotomie. Guérison. Bull. Acad. Méd. (Paris), 1911, 3 sér., **66**, 358-61.
First successful embolectomy; operation carried out by G. Labey, November 16, 1911.

3014   KEY, EINAR SAMUEL HENRIK. 1872-1954
Ein Fall operierter Embolie der Arteria femoralis. Wien. klin. Wschr., 1913, **26**, 936-39.
Key performed his first successful embolectomy on December 4, 1912, and reported it to a meeting of the Svenska Läkaresällskapet on January 28, 1913. See also his review in Ergebn. Chir. Orthop., 1929, **22**, 1-94.

3014.1   BAUER, FRITZ.
Fall von Embolus aortae abdominalis, Operation, Heilung. Zbl. Chir., 1913, **40**, 1945-46.
First successful aortic embolectomy.

3015   WARTHIN, ALDRED SCOTT. 1866-1931
Traumatic lipaemia and fatty embolism. Int. Clin., 1913, 23 ser., **4**, 171-227.
Classic clinical description of pulmonary fat embolism.

3016   KIRSCHNER, MARTIN. 1879-1942
Ein durch die Trendelenburgsche Operation geheilter Fall von Embolie der Art. pulmonalis. *Arch. klin. Chir.,* 1924, **133**, 312-59.
First successful surgical treatment of pulmonary embolism, a procedure suggested by Trendelenburg in 1908 (*see* No. 3012).

3017   JEFFERSON, *Sir* GEOFFREY. 1886-1961
Report of a successful case of embolectomy. *Brit. med. J.,* 1925, **2**, 985-87.
First successful embolectomy in Britain.

3018   DUCUING, JEAN. 1889-
Phlébites, thromboses et embolies post-opératoires. Paris, *Masson,* 1929.

3019   MURRAY, DONALD WALTER GORDON. 1894-1976, *et al.*
Heparin and the thrombosis of veins following injury. *Surgery,* 1937, **2**, 163-87.
Clinical use of heparin as anticoagulant. With L.B. Jaques, T. S. Perrett, and C. H. Best.

3019.1   SANTOS, JEAN CID DOS. -1970
Sur la désobstruction des thromboses artérielles anciennes. *Mém. Acad. Chir. (Paris),* 1947, **73**, 409-16.
Thromboendarterectomy.

3020   WRIGHT, IRVING SHERWOOD. 1901- , *et al.*
Report of the Committee for the Evaluation of Anticoagulants in the Treatment of Coronary Thrombosis with Myocardial Infarction. *Amer. Heart J.,* 1948, **36**, 801-15.
With C. D. Marple and D. F. Beck.

3020.1   OUDOT, JACQUES.
La greffe vasculaire dans les thromboses du carrefour aortique. *Presse méd.,* 1951, **59**, 234-6.
Arterial homograft on aorta.

3020.2   FOGARTY, THOMAS J., *et al.*
A method for extraction of arterial emboli and thrombi. *Surg. Gynec. Obstet.,* 1963, **116**, 241-44.
Introduction of the balloon catheter in arterial embolectomy. With J. J. Cranley, R. J. Krause, E. S. Strasser and C. D. Hafner.

CARDIOVASCULAR SURGERY

See also 2925-2970, LIGATIONS OF ARTERIES; 2971-2993.2, ANEURYSMS; 3006-3020.2, THROMBOSIS AND EMBOLISM.

3021   ROMERO, FRANCISCO.
Sur l'hydrothorax et l'hydropéricarde. *Bull. Fac. Méd. Paris,* 1814-1815, **4**, 373-76.
First successful pericardiocentesis. The above reference is not to his first writing on the subject, which cannot be traced. See also *Dict. Sci. med.,* 1819, **40**, 370.

3022   HILSMANN, FRIEDERICH ALEXANDER. 1849-
Ueber die Paracentese des Perikardiums. *Schriften Univ. Kiel,* (1875), 1876,
Diss. Nr. 2, pp. 20.
Account of first pericardiocentesis for suppurative pericarditis.

3022.1   FRANÇOIS-FRANCK, CHARLES-EMILE. 1849-1921
Production artificielle d'insuffisances tricuspidienne mitrale et aortique,
isolées ou combinées chez le chien. *C. R. Soc. Biol. (Paris),* 1882, 7 sér., **4**,
108-10.
Experimental valvulotomy. Translation in *Amer. J. Cardiol.,* 1973, **32**,
993.

3022.2   DALTON, HENRY C. 1847-
Stab wound of pericardium; resection of rib; suture of pericardium;
recovery. *Trans. med. Assoc. (Missouri),* 1894, 218-23.
"This was the first report in America and probably world-wide in which
there was a successful evacuation of a traumatic hemopericardium and a
suture placed in the pericardium. Dalton's patient was operated on in
September, 1891... The patient survived his ordeal and was discharged
from the hospital in three and a half months" (Rutkow).

3023   REHN, LUDWIG. 1849-1930
Fall von penetrirender Stichverletzung des rechten Ventrikel's. Herznaht.
Zbl. Chir., 1896, **23**, 1048-49.
Rehn was the first successfully to suture a wound of the human heart.

3023.1   ——. Ueber penetrirende Herzwunden und Herznaht. *Arch. klin. Chir.,*
1897, **55**, 315-29.
Before 1896 wounds of the heart had always been regarded as fatal.
Rehn's work marks the begining of cardiac surgery. English translation in
Callahan, Keys & Key, *Classics of Cardiology,* vol. 3, 34-44.

3024   JABOULAY, MATHIEU. 1860-1913
Chirurgie du grand sympathique et du corps thyroïde. Paris, *O. Doin,* 1900.
Jaboulay was the first to perform the operation of sympathectomy for
the relief of vascular disease.

3025   BRAUER, LUDOLPH. 1865-1951
Ueber chronich adhäsive Mediastino-Perikarditis und deren Behandlung.
Münch. med. Wschr., 1902, **49**, 1072, 1732.
Brauer was first to suggest the operation of cardiolysis, a procedure
carried out by Petersen.

3025.1   CARREL, ALEXIS. 1873-1944, & GUTHRIE, CHARLES CLAUDE, 1880-1963
The transplantation of veins and organs. *Amer. Med.,* 1905, **10**, 1101-2.
Reports experimental heart transplantation in a dog. See also the earlier
paper on pp. 284-5.

3025.2   GOYANES CAPDEVILA, JOSÉ. 1876-1964
Nuevas trabajos de cirugía vascular; substitución plástica de las arteriás por
las venas, ó arterioplastia venosa, aplicada, como nuevo metodo, al
tratamiento de los aneurismas. *Siglo méd.,* 1906, **53**, 546-8, 561-4.
Goyanes used vein grafts to restore arterial flow.

3025.3   MUNRO, JOHN CUMMINGS. 1858-1910
          Ligation of the ductus arteriosus. *Ann. Surg.*, 1907, **46**, 335-38.
          Munro was first to suggest the feasibility of ligation of a patent ductus
          arteriosus.

3026   CARREL, ALEXIS. 1873-1944
          The surgery of blood vessels, etc. *Johns Hopk. Hosp. Bull.*, 1907, **18**, 18-28.
          Carrel's remarkable technique of end-to-end anastomosis of blood
          vessels; *see also* No. 2909.

3027   ———. Results of the transplantation of blood vessels, organs and limbs. *J.
          Amer. med. Assoc.*, 1908, **51**, 1662-67.
          Carrel showed that arteries kept for days or weeks outside the body can
          be transplanted successfully.

3028   ———. Latent life of arteries. *J. exp. Med.*, 1910, **12**, 460-86.
          Carrel's experiments showed that it was possible to preserve portions
          of blood vessels in cold storage for long periods before using them in
          transplantation. For an appreciation of Carrel, see Garrison's *History,* p. 733.

3028.01   ———. Experimental surgery of the aorta and heart. *Ann. Surg.*, 1910, **52**, 83-
          95.
          Carrel attempted the direct placement of a bypass vessel in a dog.

3028.1   DOYEN, EUGENE LOUIS. 1859-1916
          Chirurgie des malformations congénitales ou acquises du coeur. *Congr.
          franç. Chir., Proc.-verb.*, 1913, **26**, 1062-65; *Presse méd.*, 1913, **21**, 860.
          First attempt at surgical relief of valvular disease of the heart (congenital
          pulmonary stenosis). Experimental valvotomy.

3029   TUFFIER, THÉODORE. 1857-1929
          Etude expérimentelle sur la chirurgie des valvules du coeur. *Bull. Acad.
          Méd. (Paris),* 1914, 3 sér., **71**, 293-95.
          Tuffier carried out the first successful experimental operation for the
          relief of chronic valvular disease. He also operated successfully in a case
          of aortic stenosis.

3030   HALLOPEAU, PAUL. 1876-1924
          Un cas de cardiolyse. *Bull. Mém. Soc. Chir. Paris.*, 1921, **47**, 1120-21.
          First pericardiectomy, for constrictive pericarditis.

3030.1   CUTLER, ELLIOTT CARR. 1888-1947, LEVINE, SAMUEL ALBERT. 1891-1966
          Cardiotomy and valvulotomy for mitral stenosis. Experimental observations
          and clinical notes concerning an operated case with recovery. *Boston med.
          surg. J.*, 1923, **188**, 1023-27.
          Successful section of mitral valve for relief of mitral stenosis.

3031   VOLHARD, FRANZ. 1872-1950, & SCHMIEDEN, VIKTOR. 1874-1945
          Ueber Erkennung und Behandlung der Umklammerung des Herzens
          durch schwielige Perikarditis. *Klin. Wschr.*, 1923, **2**, 5-9.
          First complete pericardiectomy for constrictive pericarditis.

3032 SOUTTAR, *Sir* Henry Sessions. 1875-1964
The surgical treatment of mitral stenosis. *Brit. med. J.,* 1925, **2**, 603-06.
Mitral valvotomy; report of a successful case.

3033 BLUMGART, Herman Ludwig. 1895-1977, *et al.*
Congestive heart failure and angina pectoris: the therapeutic effect of
thyroidectomy on patients without clinical or pathogenic evidence of
thyroid toxicity. *Arch. intern. Med.,* 1933, **51**, 866-77.
Thyroidectomy for the treatment of congestive heart failure and angina
pectoris. With S. A. Levine and D. D. Berlin.

3034 BECK, Claude Schaeffer. 1894-1971
The development of a new blood supply to the heart by operation. *Ann.
Surg.,* 1935, **102**, 801-13.
By implantation of the pectoral muscle into the pericardium, Beck
provided a collateral circulation to the heart for the relief of myocardial
ischaemia. This paper recorded the first operation on a man. It was
preceded by Beck's paper, written with V.L. Tichy an A.R. Moritz, recording
operations on dogs: Production of a collateral circulation to the heart, *Proc.
Soc. exp. Biol. Med.,* 1935, **32**, 759-61.

3035 ———., & TICHY, Vladimir Leslie. 1899-1967
The production of a collateral circulation to the heart. I. An experimental
study. *Amer. Heart J.,* 1935, **10**, 849-73.
First cardio-omentopexy.

3036 PEET, Max Minor. 1885-1949
The surgical treatment of hypertension. *Proc. Calif. Acad. Med.,* 1935-36,
5, 58-90.
Peet operation for hypertension. Preliminary communication in *Univ.
Hosp. Bull. (Ann Arbor),* 1935, **1**, 17-18.

3037 O'SHAUGHNESSY, Laurence. 1900-1940
An experimental method of providing a collateral circulation to the heart.
Brit. J. Surg., 1936, **23**, 665-70.
By attaching a pedicled omental graft to the surface of the heart (cardio-
omentopexy), thus providing a collateral circulation to that organ,
O'Shaughnessy made an important advance in the treatment of angina and
cardiac ischaemia generally.

3038 LERICHE, René. 1879-1955, *et al.*
Arterectomy. *Surg. Gynec. Obstet.,* 1937, **64**, 149-55.
Arterectomy in arterial thrombosis. With R. Fontaine and S. M. Dupertuis.

3038.1 GIBBON, John Heysham. 1903-1973
An oxygenator with a large surface–volume ratio. *J. Lab. clin. Med.,* 1939,
24, 1192-98.
First heart–lung machine used successfully on an animal.

3039 GROSS, Robert Edward. 1905-1988, & HUBBARD, John Perry. 1903-
Surgical ligation of a patent ductus arteriosus: report of first successful case.
J. Amer. Med. Surg., 1939, **112**, 729-31.
One of the earliest successful surgical repairs for congenital heart
disease. See also later paper in *Ann. Surg.,* 1939, **110**, 321-56.

3040   LERICHE, RENÉ. 1879-1955
De la résection du carrefour aortico-iliaque avec double sympathectomie
lombaire pour thrombose artéritique de l'aorte; le syndrome de l'oblitération
termino-aortique par artérite. *Presse méd.*, 1940, **48**, 601-04.
Obliteration of the abdominal aorta.

3041   SMITHWICK, REGINALD HAMMERICK. 1899-
A technique for splanchnic resection for hypertension; preliminary report.
Surgery, 1940, **7**, 1-8.
Smithwick operation for hypertension.

3042   KING, EDGAR SAMUEL JOHN.
Surgery of the heart. London, *E. Arnold & Co.,* (1941).
Includes valuable information regarding the history of the subject.

3043   BLALOCK, ALFRED. 1899-1964, & TAUSSIG, HELEN BROOKE. 1898-1986
The surgical treatment of malformations of the heart in which there is
pulmonary stenosis or pulmonary atresia. *J. Amer. med. Assoc.,* 1945, **128**,
189-202.
The "Blalock-Taussig operation" for the relief of congenital defects of
the pulmonary artery.

3044   CRAFOORD, CLARENCE. 1899-1984, & NYLIN, KARL GUSTAV VILHELM. 1892-1961
Congenital coarctation of the aorta and its surgical treatment. *J. thorac. Surg.,*
1945, **14**, 347-61.
Crafoord and Gross (No. 3044.1) pioneered this basic operation in
cardiac and paediatric surgery.

3044.1   GROSS, ROBERT EDWARD. 1905-1988
Surgical correction for coarctation of the aorta. *Surgery,* 1945, **18**, 673-8.
Resection of coarctation and direct anastomosis of remaining ends. See
also his report of 60 cases in *J. Amer. med. Assoc.,* 1949, **139**, 285-92.

3045   POTTS, WILLIS JOHN. 1895-1968, *et al.*
Anastomosis of the aorta to a pulmonary artery. Certain types in congenital
heart disease. *J. Amer. med. Ass.,* 1946, **132**, 627-31.
With S. Smith and S. Gibson.

3046   BROCK, RUSSELL CLAUDE, *Baron Brock of Wimbledon.* 1903-1980
Pulmonary valvulotomy for the relief of congenital pulmonary stenosis.
Report of three cases. *Brit. med. J.,* 1948, **1**, 1121-26.

3046.1   HARKEN, DWIGHT EMARY. 1910- , *et al.*
The surgical treatment of mitral stenosis. 1. Valvuloplasty. *New Engl. J. Med.,*
1948, **239**, 801-09.
Valvuloplasty for mitral stenosis. With L. B. Ellis, P. F. Ware, and L. R.
Norman.

3046.2   SELLORS, *Sir* THOMAS HOLMES. 1902-1987
Surgery of pulmonary stenosis. A case in which the pulmonary valve was
successfully divided. *Lancet,* 1948, **1**, 988-9.
Operation Dec. 4, 1947.

3047   BLAND, EDWARD FRANKLIN. 1901- , & SWEET, RICHARD HARWOOD. 1901-
A venous shunt for marked mitral stenosis. *Amer. Practit.*, 1948, **2**, 756-61.
    First pulmonary-azygos shunt operation for relief of mitral stenosis.
Two further patients were operated upon later the same year; all three are
reported in *J. Amer. med. Ass.*, 1949, **140**, 1259. A similar procedure was
successfully employed independently by F. d'Allaines and his colleagues
in 1949 (*Mém. Acad. Chir., Paris*, 1949, **75**, 318-19).

3047.1 BIGELOW, W.G. *et al.*
Hypothermia: its possible role in cardiac surgery: an investigation of
factors governing survival in dogs at low body temperatures. *Ann. surg.*,
1950, **132**, 849-66.
    Surface-induced whole body hypothermia and temporary cardiac flow
occlusion. With W.K. Lindsay and W.F. Greenwood.

3047.2 HUFNAGEL, CHARLES ANTHONY. 1916-1989
Aortic plastic valvular prosthesis. *Bull. Georgetown Univ. Med. Center*, 1951,
4, 128-30.
    Hufnagel designed and inserted the first workable prosthetic heart
valve in man.

3047.3 VOORHEES, ARTHUR B. 1921- , *et al.* .
The use of tubes constructed from Vinyon "N" cloth in bridging arterial
defects. *Ann. Surg.*, 1952, **135**, 332-6.
    Introduction of plastic material to repair arterial defects. Voorhees later
abandoned this material in favour of Dacron. With A. Jaretzki and A. W.
Blakemore.

3047.4 DeBAKEY, MICHAEL ELLIS. 1908- ,& COOLEY, DENTON ARTHUR. 1920-
    Successful resection of aneurysm of thoracic aorta and replacement by
graft. *J. amer. med. Assoc.*, 1953. **152**, 673-76.

3047.5 GIBBON, JOHN HEYSHAM. 1903-1973
Application of a mechanical heart and lung apparatus to cardiac surgery.
Minn. Med., 1954, **37**, 171-80, 185.
    First pump oxygenator used on humans. Performed on May 6, 1953, this
was the first successful intracardiac operation in a patient with the use of
total heart-lung bypass.

3047.6 WARDEN, HERBERT EDGAR. 1920- ,*et al.*
Controlled cross circulation for open intracardiac surgery; physiologic
studies and results of creation and closure of ventricular septal defects. *J.
thorac. Surg.*, 1954, **28**, 331-43.
    First repair of various cardiac anomalies. With C.W. Lillehei, M. Cohen,
and R.C. Read.

3047.7 LILLEHEI, CLARENCE WALTON. 1918-
Controlled cross circulation for direct-vision intracardiac surgery; correction of ventricular septal defects, atrioventricularis communis, and tetralogy of Fallot. *Postgrad. Med.*, 1955, **17**, 388-96.

Controlled cross circulation (human heart–lung "machine") for intracardiac surgery.

3047.8   MURRAY, DONALD WALTER GORDON. 1894-1976
Homologous aortic-valve-segment transplants as surgical treatment for aortic and mitral insufficiency. *Angiology*, 1956, **7**, 466-71.
    First successful aortic valve homograft. For report of six-year follow-up, see A. J. Kerwin, *et al., New Engl. J. Med.*, 1962, **266**, 852.

3047.9   DEWALL, RICHARD A. 1926-, *et al*
A simple, expendable, artificial oxygenator for open heart surgery. *Surg. Clin. North America*, 1956, **36**, 1025-34.
    DeWall bubble oxygenator. With six co-authors.

3047.10   FURMAN, SEYMOUR. 1931- , & ROBINSON, GEORGE. 1922-
The use of intracardiac pacemaker in the correction of total heart block. *Surg. Forum.*, 1959, **9**, 245-48.
    First use of pacemaker for Stokes–Adams syndrome, using dogs as subjects. External power source. See also Furman and Scawadel, John B. An intracardiac pacemaker for Stokes–Adams seizures. *New Engl. J. Med.*, 1959, **261**, 943-48.

3047.11   WEIRICH, WILLIAM L., *et al.*
The treatment of complete heart block by the combined use of a myocardial electrode and artificial pacemaker. *Surg. Forum*, 1958, **8**, 360-63.
    With V.L. Gott, and C.W. Lillehei. Attachment of a wire to the ventricular epicardium and bringing it out percutaneously to an external pacemaker.

3047.12   SZILAGYI, D. EMERICK. 1910- , *et al.*
Clinical use of an elastic Dacron prosthesis. *Arch. Surg.*, 1958, **77**, 538-51.
    Arterial prosthesis. With L. C. France, R. F. Smith, and J. G. Whitcomb.

3047.13   COOLEY, DENTON ARTHUR. 1920- *et al.*
Ventricular aneurysm following myocardial infarction: Results of surgical treatment. *Ann. Surg.*, 1959, **150**, 595-612.
    Cardiopulmonary bypass and open excision of the aneurysm. With W.S. Henly, K.H. Amad, & D.W. Chapman.

3047.14   LOWER, RICHARD ROWLAND. 1929- , & SHUMWAY, NORMAN E. 1923-
Studies on orthotopic homotransplantation of the canine heart. *Surg. Forum.*, 1960, **11**, 18-19.
    Important experimental technique (Shumway); reported eight heart homotransplants.

3047.15   CHARDACK, WILLIAM M., *et al.*
A transitorized, self-contained, implantable pacemaker for the long-term correction of complete heart block. *Surgery*, 1960, **48**, 643-54.
    The first fully-implantable pacemaker. With Andrew A. Gage and Wilson Greatbatch.

3047.16   STARR, ALBERT. 1926- , & EDWARDS, M. LOWELL.
Mitral replacement: the shielded ball valve prothesis. *J. thorac. cardiovasc. Surg.*, 1961, **42**, 673-82.

First replacement of the mitral valve in a human. See also *Ann. Surg.*, 1961, **154**, 726-40.

3047.17   ROSS, DONALD NIXON. 1922-
Homograft replacement of the aortic valve. *Lancet*, 1962, **2**, 487 (only).
Homograft valve placed below coronary orifice. See also *J. thorac. cardiovasc. Surg.*, 1964, **47**, 713-19.

3047.18   BARRATT-BOYES, *Sir* BRIAN GERALD. 1924-
Homograft aortic valve replacement in aortic incompetence and stenosis. *Thorax*, 1964, **19**, 131-50.
Subcoronary homograft valve; report on 44 patients, of whom 41 survived.

3047.19   HARDY, JAMES DANIEL. 1918- , *et al.*
Heart transplantation in man: developmental studies and report of a case. *J. Amer. med. Assoc.*, 1964, **188**, 1132-40.
Heart transplant from a chimpanzee into a man; unsuccessful. The paper has seven other authors.

3047.20   BARNARD, CHRISTIAAN NEETHLING. 1922-
A human cardiac transplant: an interim report of a successful operation performed at Groote Schuur Hospital, Cape Town. *S. Afr. med. J.*, 1967, **41**, 1271-4.
First human heart transplant. The operation was on Dec. 3, 1967, and the patient died on Dec. 21.

3047.21   FAVALORO, RENÉ G.
Saphenous vein autograft replacement of severe segmental coronary artery occlusion: operative techique. *Ann. Thorac. Surg.*, 1968, **5**, 334-39.
First report on bypass of a human coronary artery. *See* No. 3047.25.

3047.22   RASTELLI, G. C.
A new approach to "anatomic" repair of transposition of the great arteries. *Mayo Clinic Proc.*, 1969, **41**, 1-12.
"Intraventricular rerouting of left ventricular output through the ventricular septal defect to the aorta and establishing of a new right ventricular outflow through the ventriculotomy and an extracardiac conduit to the pulmonary artery". (Callahan, McGoon, & Key, *Classics of Cardiology*).

3047.23   SEALY, WILL C. *et al.*
Surgical treatment of Wolff–Parkinson–White syndrome. *Ann. thorac. surg.*, 1969, **8**, 1-11.
Surgical management of the tachycardia of Wolff–Parkinson–White syndrome.

3047.24   FONTAN, F. & BAUDET, E.
Surgical repair of triscuspid atresia. *Thorax*, 1971, **26**, 240-48.
"Anastomosis between the divided superior vena cava and the right pulmonary artery, anastomosis of the right atrium to the pulmonary artery, and insertion of a homograft valve in the ostium of the inferior vena cava" (Callahan, McGoon & Key, *Classics of Cardiology*).

3047.25   GARRETT, H. EDWARD   *et al.*
Aortocoronary bypass with saphenous vein graft: seven year follow-up. *J. Amer. med. assoc.*, 1973, **223**, 792-94.
The authors may have done the first successful coronary artery bypass graft in 1964. They recognized its significance only later. With E.W. Dennis and M.E. DeBakey. *See* No. 3047.21

See Nos. 3158, 3161.2, & 3215.9 *for history of cardiac surgery,*

DISORDERS OF THE BLOOD

3048   ABUL QASIM [ALBUCASIS]. 936-1013
Liber theoricae nec non practicae Alsaharavii. [Augustae Vindelicorum, *imp. S. Grimm & M. Vuirsung,* 1519.]
This is the first printing of the medical and therapeutic section of Abul Qasim's medical encyclopaedia or *al-Tasrif.* It contains what is probably the earliest description of haemophilia (fol. 145).

3049   RODRIGUES, JOAO DE CASTELLO BRANCO. [AMATUS LUSITANUS] 1511-1568
Curationum medicinalium centuriae quatuor. Basileae, [*H. Frobenius*], 1556.
Contains (Cent. iii, curat. 70, p. 286) first recorded case of purpura as a separate entity, not associated with fever. English translation of this section in Major, *Classic descriptions of disease,* 3rd. ed., 1945, p. 514.

3050   PANAROLI, DOMENICO. ?-1657
Iatrologismorum seu medicinalium observationum pentecostae quinque utilibus praeceptis. Romae, *F. Moneta,* 1652.
Panaroli described haemolytic jaundice of the newborn.

3051   BEHRENS, RUDOLPH AUGUST. ?-1747
Epistolica dissertatio altera pro spicilegio observationum de morbo maculoso haemorrhagico et noxiis nonnulis mytulis perscripta. Brunsvigae, 1735.
Behrens gave the name "morbus maculosus haemorrhagicus" to the disease purpura haemorrhagica. His paper is reprinted in Werlhof's *Opera medica,* Hannover, 1775, **2**, 615-36.

3052   WERLHOF, PAUL GOTTLIEB. 1699-1767
Disquisitio medica et philologica de variolis et anthracibus. Hannoverae, *sumt. haered. Nicolai Foersteri,* 1735.
Werlhof gave a classic description of purpura haemorrhagica ("Werlhof's disease").

3053   HEBERDEN, WILLIAM, *Snr.* 1710-1801
Commentarii de morborum historia et curatione. Londini, *T. Payne,* 1802.
Chap. 78 reports two cases of anaphylactoid (abdominal) purpura. English translation 1802, reprinted 1962. Henoch (No. 3065) and Schönlein (No. 3058) established this condition as a distinct entity.

3054   OTTO, JOHN CONRAD. 1774-1844
An account of an haemorrhagic disposition existing in certain families. *Med. Reposit.,* 1803, **6**, 1-4.

Otto recognized and adequately described haemophilia, noting that females are not affected but may transmit the disease. His paper is one of the first great contributions to medicine in North America. Reproduced in Major, *Classic descriptions of disease*, 3rd ed., 1945, p. 522.

3055   BURNS, ALLAN. 1781-1813
Observations on the surgical anatomy of the head and neck. Edinburgh, *Bryce*, 1811.
First recorded case of chloroma is to be found on p. 396 of this book.

3056   NASSE, CHRISTIAN FRIEDRICH. 1778-1851
Von einer erblichen Neigung zu tödtlichen Blutungen. *Arch. med. Erfahr.*, 1820, **1**, 385-434.
In his description of haemophilia Nasse stressed the immunity of females, despite their ability to transmit the disease. This fact has become known as "Nasse's law".

3057   BOUILLAUD, JEAN BAPTISTE. 1796-1881
Observations sur l'état des veines dans les infiltrations des membres. *J. Physiol. exp. path*, 1823, **3**, 89-93.
Description of venous obstruction and dropsy.

3058   SCHÖNLEIN, JOHANN LUCAS. 1793-1864
Peliosis rheumatica. In his *Allgemeine und specielle Pathologie und Therapie*, 1837, **2**, 48-49.
"Schönlein's disease" (purpura) first described. English translation in No. 2241.

3058.1   LANE, SAMUEL ARMSTRONG. 1802-1892
Successful transfusion of blood. *Lancet*, 1840-41, **1**, 185-88.
Blood transfusion used in treatment of haemophilia.

3059   ADDISON, WILLIAM. 1802-1881
Experimental and practical researches on inflammation and on the origin and nature of tubercles of the lungs. London, *J. Churchill*, 1843.
Addison made important observations on the blood corpuscles. He is by some considered "the world's first haematologist". He gave the first description of leucocytosis, so named by Virchow in 1858, and he anticipated Cohnheim's conception of inflammation. He was first to observe diapedesis. *See Lancet*, 1907, **1**, 182-83. *See also* No. 2294.

3060   ANDRAL, GABRIEL. 1797-1876
Essai d'hématologie pathologique. Paris, *Fortin, Masson & Cie.*, 1843.
The first monograph on haematology. Andral established analysis of the blood on the basis of exact knowledge of the blood components. He analysed the blood fibrin and albumin. He recognized several forms of anaemia, including that due to lead poisoning. English translation, 1844.

3060.1   DONNÉ, ALEXANDRE. 1801-1878
Cours de microscopie. Paris, *J. B. Baillière*, 1844.
Includes (pp. 10-12) a brief description of leukaemia.

3061   BENNETT, JOHN HUGHES. 1812-1875
Case of hypertrophy of the spleen and liver, in which death took place from suppuration of the blood. *Edinb. med. surg. J.*, 1845, **64**, 413-23.

First definite description of leukaemia; a case under the care of Sir R. Christison but reported by Bennett. On p. 400 of the same journal is a report of a case by D. Craigie, referring to a patient seen in 1841 but not recognized as leukaemia until Craigie heard of Bennett's case in the same hospital. Bennett published a monograph on leucocythaemia in 1852, in which he included the first illustrations of the microscopic appearance of the blood in leukaemia.

3062   VIRCHOW, Rudolf Ludwig Karl. 1821-1902
Weisses Blut. *N. Notiz. Geb. Natur- u. Heilk*, 1845, **36**, 151-56.
Only six weeks after Bennett, Virchow independently published a report on the necropsy of a case of leukaemia. He gave the condition its present name. For translation, see Major, *Classic descriptions of disease*, 3rd. ed., 1945, p. 510.

3062.1   FULLER, Henry William. 1820-1873
Particulars of a case in which enormous enlargement of the spleen and liver, together with dilatation of all the blood vessels of the body, were found coincident with a peculiarly altered condition of the blood. *Lancet*, 1846, **2**, 43-44.
Leukaemia diagnosed during life as the result of a blood examination.

3063   GRANDIDIER, Johann Ludwig. 1810-?
Die Haemophilie oder die Bluterkrankheit. Leipzig, *O. Wigand*, 1855.
First full clinical description of haemophilia.

3064   VIRCHOW, Rudolf Ludwig Karl. 1821-1902
Ueber farblose Blutkörperchen und Leukämie. In his *Gesammelte Abhandlungen zur wissenschaftlichen Medicin*, Frankfort a.M., *Meidinger*, 1856, pp. 147-218.
Includes his paper on "weisses Blut" (*see* No. 3062) and three later papers on leukaemia. *See* No. 3006.

3064.1   FRIEDREICH, Nikolaus. 1825-1882
Ein neuer Fall von Leukämie. *Virchows Arch. path. Anat.*, 1857, **12**, 37-58.
Acute leukaemia first described.

3064.2   BABINGTON, Benjamin Guy. 1794-1866
Hereditary epistaxis. *Lancet*, 1865, **2**, 362-63.

3065   HENOCH, Eduard Heinrich. 1820-1910.
Über den Zusammenhang von Purpura und Intestinalstörungen. *Berl. klin. Wschr.*, 1868, **5**, 517-19.
"Henoch's purpura". Henoch described a form of purpura with abdominal symptoms first mentioned by Heberden (No. 3053). See also the same journal, 1874, **11**, 622, 641-43. This paper is translated into English in No. 2241.

3066   NEUMANN, Ernst. 1834-1918
Ein Fall von Leukämie mit Erkrankung des Knochenmarkes. *Arch. Heilk. (Lpz.)*, 1870, **11**, 1-14.
Neumann was the first to note changes in the bone marrow in leukaemia, and he proposed the term "myelogenous leukaemia".

3067   ORTH, JOHANNES. 1847-1923
Ueber das Vorkommen von Bilirubinkrystallen bei neugebornen Kindern.
Virchows Arch. path. Anat., 1875, **63**, 447-62.
    Kernicterus first described.

3067.1   TREVES, *Sir* FREDERICK, *Bart.* 1853-1923
A case of haemophilia: pedigree through five generations. *Lancet*, 1886, **2**,
533-34.
    True haemophilia in a female. The family was the subject of several later
investigations, the last being reported in *Lancet*, 1973, **2**, 734.

3068   HENOCH, EDUARD HEINRICH. 1820-1910
Ueber Purpura fulminans. *Berl. klin. Wschr.*, 1887, **24**, 8-10.
    First description.

3069   KÖNIG, FRANZ. 1832-1910
Die Gelenkerkrankungen bei Blutern mit Berücksichtigung der Diagnose.
Samml. klin. Vortr., 1890, Chir., N.F., Nr. 11, 233-42.
    König gave a detailed description of joint involvement in haemophilia.

3069.1   EHRLICH, PAUL. 1854-1915
Farbenanalytische Untersuchungen zur Histologie und Klink. Berlin, *A.
Hirschwald*, 1891.
    By means of his methods of staining blood cells Ehrlich differentiated
two types of leukaemia, lymphatic and myelogenous.

3070   VAQUEZ, LOUIS HENRI. 1860-1936
Sur une forme spéciale de cyanose s'accompagnant d'hyperglobulie
excessive et persistante. *C. R. Soc. Biol. (Paris)*, 1892, **44**, 384-88.
    Vaquez first described polycythaemia vera (erythraemia). Osler's paper
on the subject (No. 3073) made it generally known in the English-speaking
world, and the condition has since been named "Vaquez–Osler disease".
For translation, see Major, *Classic descriptions of disease*, 3rd ed., 1945, p.
497.

3071   JENNER, LOUIS LEOPOLD. 1866-1904
A new preparation for rapidly fixing and staining blood. *Lancet*, 1899, **1**,
370-71.
    Jenner's methylene blue-eosin stain for blood.

3072   BROWN, PHILIP KING. 1869-1940, & OPHÜLS, WILLIAM. 1871-1933
A fatal case of acute primary infectious pharyngitis. *Trans. Med. Soc. Calif.*,
1901, 93-101.
    First recorded case of extreme leucopenia.

3073   OSLER, *Sir* WILLIAM, *Bart.* 1849-1919
Chronic cyanosis, with polycythaemia and enlarged spleen: a new clinical
entity. *Amer. J. med. Sci.*, 1903, **126**, 187-201.
    When describing polycythaemia with cyanosis, Osler thought it a new
entity, but later acknowledged the priority of Vaquez's description (No.
3070). Reprinted in *Med. Classics*, 1939, **4**, 254-75.

3074   WOLFF-EISNER, ALFRED. 1877-1948
        Ueber eine Methode zur Untersuchung des lebenden Knochenmarks von
        Thieren und über das Bewegungsvermögen der Myelocyten. *Dtsch. med.
        Wschr.*, 1903, **29**, 165-67.
        Wolff-Eisner trephined the tibia and femur of experimental animals and
        suggested biopsy of bone marrow as a clinical procedure.

3075   ARNETH, JOSEPH. 1873-1955
        Die neutrophilen weissen Blutkörperchen bei Infektions-Krankheiten.
        Jena, *G. Fischer*, 1904.
            "Arneth count". Arneth distinguished five groups of polymorphonuclear
        leucocytes and advocated the estimation of these groups as a valuable aid
        in the determination of bone-marrow reaction to infective and other agents
        (plate 8, p. 37).

3076   GEISBÖCK [GAISBOCK], FELIX.
        Die Bedeutung der Blutdruckmessung für die Praxis. *Dtsch. Arch. klin.
        Med.*, 1905, **83**, 363-409.
            Includes (p. 396) description of "Geisböck's disease" – polycythemia
        hypertonica.

3077   STERNBERG, CARL. 1872-1935
        Pathologie der Primärerkrankungen des lymphatischen und
        hämatopoetischen Apparates. Wiesbaden, *J. F. Bergmann*, 1905.
            Includes (p. 151) Sternberg's description of lymphogranulomatosis,
        which has been given the eponym "Sternberg's disease".

3078   NÄGELI, OTTO. 1871-1938
        Blutkrankheiten und Blutdiagnostik. Leipzig, *Veit & Co.*, 1907-08.

3079   TÜRK, WILHELM. 1871-1916
        Septische Erkrankungen bei Verkümmerung des Granulozytensystems.
        Wien. klin. Wschr., 1907, **20**, 157-62.
            First reported case of complete agranulocytosis.

3079.1 ELLERMANN, VILHELM. 1871-1924, & BANG, O.
        Experimentelle Leukämie bei Hühnern. Zbl. Bakt., 1908, Abt. I. Orig., **46**,
        595-609.
            Cell-free transmission of fowl leukaemia. Ellermann and Bang produced
        leukaemia by means of a filterable agent.

3080   GHEDINI, GIOVANNI. 1877-?
        Per la patogenesi e per la diagnosi delle malattie del sangue e degli organi
        emopoietici. Puntura esplorativa del midollo osseo. *Clin. med. ital.*, 1908,
        47, 724-36.
            Introduction of bone marrow biopsy by puncturing the shaft of the
        tibia.

3080.1 PFANNENSTIEL, HERMANN JOHANN. 1862-1909
        Ueber den habituellen Ikterus de Neugeborenen. *Münch. med. Wschr.*,
        1908, **55**, 2169-74, 2233-37.
            First detailed description of familial icterus gravis neonatorum.

3081   BULLOCH, WILLIAM. 1868-1941, & FILDES, *Sir* PAUL. 1882-1971
        Haemophilia, London, *Dulau & Co.*, 1911.
        Bulloch and Fildes, in their detailed account of haemophilia, claimed to
        have established the fact of immunity in females, and denied the authenticity
        of published cases of female haemophilia. They confirmed the law of
        Nasse. This work, one of the most important on the subject, was issued as
        Memoir XII of the Eugenics Laboratory, University of London, and forms
        parts V-VI of the *Treasury of Human Inheritance* series.

3082   PAPPENHEIM, ARTUR. 1870-1916
        Grundriss der hämatologischen Diagnostik. Leipzig, *W. Klinkhardt*, 1911.
        One of the leaders in modern haematology, Pappenheim improved the
        methods of staining blood cells.

3082.1 RESCHAD, HASSAN & SCHILLING-TORGAU, V.
        Ueber eine neue Leukämie durch echte Uebergangsformen
        (Splenozytenleukämie) und ihre Bedeutung für die Selbständigkeit dieser
        Zellen. *Münch. med. Wschr.*, 1913, **60**, 1981-84.
        Monocytic leukaemia reported.

3083   FRANK, ALFRED ERICH. 1884-1957
        Die essentielle Thrombopenie (konstitutionelle Purpura-Pseudo-
        Hämophilie). *Berl. klin. Wschr.*, 1915, **52**, 454-58, 490-94.
        Frank's essential thrombopenia.

3084   EPPINGER, HANS. 1880-1946, & KLOSS, KARL.
        Zur Therapie der Polyzythämie. *Therap. Mh.*, 1918, **32**, 322-26.
        Phenylhydrazine hydrochloride first used in the treatment of
        polycythaemia.

3085   WESTERGREN, ALF VILHELM. 1891-
        Studies of the suspension stability of the blood in pulmonary tuberculosis.
        Acta med. scand., 1921, **54**, 247-82.
        Westergren's method of measuring the erythrocyte sedimentation rate.

3086   SCHULTZ, WERNER. 1878-1944
        Gangräneszierende Prozesse und Defekt des Granulocytensystems. *Dtsch.
        med. Wschr.*, 1922, **48**, 1495-96.
        "Schultz's syndrome" – first description of agranulocytic angina. Schultz
        reported four cases of necrotic ulcerative infection of the throat with
        complete or almost complete disappearance of polymorphonuclears. To
        describe the blood change he introduced the term "agranulocytosis".

3087   SEYFARTH, CARLY PAUL. 1890-
        Die Sternumtrepanation, ein einfache Methode zur diagnostischen
        Entnahme von Knochenmark bei Lebenden. *Dtsch. med. Wschr.*, 1923, **49**,
        180-81.
        Bone marrow biopsy by sternal puncture.

3087.1 HART, ALFRED PURVIS. 1887-1954
        Familial icterus gravis of the new-born and its treatment. *Canad. med. Ass.
        J.*, 1925, **15**, 1008-112.
        Successful exchange transfusion.

3087.2　WILLEBRAND, ERIK ADOLF VON. 1870-1949
Hereditär pseudohemofili. *Fin. Läk.-Sallsk. Handl.*, 1926, **68**, 87-112.
　　Von Willebrand's disease, pseudo-haemophilia type B, an hereditary bleeding disorder affecting both sexes.

3088　ARINKIN, MIKHAIL. 1876-1948
[Methodology of examining bone marrow in live patients, with haemopoietic disease.] *Vestn. Khir.*, 1927, No. 30, 57-60.
　　Needle puncture of bone marrow biopsy.(In Russian.) German account in *Folia haemat. (Lpz.)*, 1929, **38**, 233-40. English translation from the German in Bick, *Classics of orthopaedics*, 339-44.

3089　PELGAR, KAREL. 1885-1931
Demonstratie van een paar zeldzaam voorkomende typen van bloedlichaampjes en bespreking der patiënten. *Ned. T. Geneesk.*, 1928, **72**, 1178.
　　See No. 3092.

3090　WEISS, SOMA. 1898-1942, *et al.*
The velocity of blood flow in health and disease as measured by the effect of histamine on the minute vessels. *Amer. Heart J.*, 1929, **4**, 664-91.
　　Measurement of circulation time. With G. P. Robb and H. L. Blumgart.

3091　WINTERNITZ, M., *et al.*
Eine klinisch brauchbare Bestimmungsmethode der Blutumlaufszeit mittels Decholininjektion. *Med. Klin.*, 1931, **27**, 986-88.
　　The decholin method for estimation of circulation time. With J. Deutsch and Z. Brull.

3092　HUËT, G. J. 1879-
Over een familiaire anomalie der leucocyten. *Ned. T. Geneesk.*, 1931, **75**, 5956-59.
　　Pelger–Huët anomaly of the nuclei of the leucocytes; *see also* No. 3089. German translation in *Klin. Wschr.*, 1932, **11**, 1264-66.

3093　MACFARLANE, ROBERT GWYN. 1907-1987, & BARNETT, BURGESS.
The haemostatic possibilities of snake-venom. *Lancet*, 1934, **2**, 985-87.
　　Snake venom used in the treatment of haemophilia.

3094　SALAH, M.
Sternal puncture; preliminary note. *J. Egypt. med Ass.*, 1934, **17**, 846-50.
　　Needle for sternal puncture.

3095　QUICK, ARMAND JAMES. 1894-1977
The prothrombin in hemophilia and in obstructive jaundice. *J. biol. Chem.*, 1935, **109**, lxxiii-lxxix.
　　Quick's method for determination of prothrombin clotting time. See also *Amer. J. med. Sci.*, 1935, **190**, 501-11.

3096　WINTROBE, MAXWELL MYER. 1901- , & LANDSBERG, J. WALTER. 1907-
A standardized technique for the blood sedimentation test. *Amer. J. med. Sci.*, 1935, **189**, 102-15.
　　Wintrobe's method for the determination of the erythrocyte sedimentation rate.

3096.1 PATEK, ARTHUR JACKSON. 1904- , & TAYLOR, FRANCIS HENRY LASKEY. 1900-1959
Hemophilia. II. Some properties of a substance obtained from normal human plasma effective in accelerating the coagulation of hemophilic blood. *J. clin. Invest.*, 1937, **16**, 113-24.
Antihaemophilic globulin (factor VIII).

3097 BUTT, HUGH ROLAND. 1910- , & SNELL, ALBERT MARKLEY. 1896-1960
The use of vitamin K and bile in treatment of the haemorrhagic diathesis in cases of jaundice. *Proc. Mayo Clin.*, 1938, **13**, 74-80.
Vitamin K used in the treatment of haemorrhagic disease.

3098 LAWRENCE, JOHN HUNDALE. 1904- , *et al.*
Studies on leukemia with the aid of radioactive phosphorus. *New int. Clin.*, 1939, n.s. **2**, vol. 3, 33-58.
Therapeutic use of radioactive isotopes. With K. G. Scott and L. W. Tuttle.

3099. ———. Nuclear physics and therapy: preliminary report on a new method for the treatment of leukemia and polycythemia. *Radiology*, 1940, **35**, 51-60.
Radio-phosphorus in treatment of leukaemia.

3100 LEVINE, PHILIP. 1900-1987, *et al.*
The rôle of iso-immunization in the pathogenesis of erythroblastosis fetalis. *Amer. J. Obstet. Gynec.*, 1941, **42**, 925-37.
Erythroblastosis foetalis due to rhesus incompatibility between mother and child. With L. Burnham, E. M. Katzin, and P. Vogel.

3102 STAHMANN, MARK ARNOLD. 1914- , *et al.*
Studies on the hemorrhagic sweet clover disease. V. Identification and synthesis of the hemorrhagic agent. *J. biol. Chem.*, 1941, 138, 513-27.
Isolation of dicoumarol (3:3-methylene-bis-4-hydroxycoumarin). With C. F. Huebner and K. P. Link.

3103 COMLY, HUNTER HALL. 1919-
Cyanosis in infants caused by nitrates in well water. *J. Amer. med. Assoc.*, 1945, **129**, 112-16.
Methaemoglobinaemia. Comly first suggested the above hypothesis, since proved valid.

3104 COOMBS, ROBIN ROYSTON AMOS. 1921- , *et al.*
Detection of weak and "incomplete" Rh agglutinins: a new test. *Lancet*, 1945,. **2**, 15-16.
Coombs's test. With A. E. Mourant and R. R. Race. A fuller description appears in *Brit. J. exp. Path.*, 1945, **26**, 255-66.

3105 WIENER, ALEXANDER SOLOMON. 1907-1976
Conglutination test for Rh sensitization. *J. Lab. clin. Med.*, 1945, **30**, 662-67.
Conglutination test.

3016 PATERSON, EDITH. *et al.*
Leukaemia treated with urethane compared with deep *x*-ray therapy. *Lancet*, 1946, **1**, 677.
Urethane in treatment of leukaemia. With A. Haddow, I. Ap Thomas, and J. M. Watkinson.

3107   SOULIER, JEAN PIERRE. 1913- , & GUEGUEN, JEAN.
Action hypoprothrombinémiante (anti-K) de la phényl-indanedione étudiée expérimentalement chez le lapin. Son application chez l'homme. *C. R. Soc. Biol. (Paris)*, 1947, **141**, 1007-11.
Introduction of phenylindanedione.

3107.1   DIAMOND, LOUIS KLEIN. 1902-
Replacement transfusion as a treatment for erythroblastosis fetalis. *Pediatrics*, 1948, **2**, 520-24.
Exchange transfusion.

3107.2   GIBSON, QUENTIN HOWIESON. 1918-
The reduction of methaemoglobin in red blood cells and studies on the cause of idiopathic methaemoglobinaemia. *Biochem. J.*, 1948, **42**, 13-23.
Cause of hereditary methaemoglobinaemia elucidated.

3108   REINIS, Z., & KUBIK, MIRKO.
Klinische Erfahrungen mit einem neuen Präparat der Cumarinreihe. *Schweiz. med. Wschr.*, 1948, **78**, 785-90.
Introduction of ethyl biscoumacetate ("tromexan").

3108.1   BIGGS, ROSEMARY PEYTON, *et al.*
Christmas disease, a condition previously mistaken for haemophilia. *Brit. med. J.*, 1952, **2**, 1378-82.
Christmas disease, haemophilia B, due to lack of Factor IX. Named after the patient whose case was the first recorded example. With six co-authors.

3108.2   ELION, GERTRUDE B., *et al.*
Studies on condensed pyrimidine system. IX. The synthesis of some 6-substituted purines. *J. Amer. chem. Soc.*, 1952, **74**, 411-14.
Synthesis of 6-mercaptopurine. With E. Burgi and G. H. Hitchings.

3108.3   BURCHENAL, JOSEPH HOLLAND. 1912- , *et al.*
Clinical evaluation of a new antimetabolite, 6-mercaptopurine, in treatment of leukemia and allied diseases. *Blood*, 1953, **8**, 965-99.
Clinical introduction of 6-mercaptopurine in treatment of acute leukaemia and chronic myelocytic leukaemia. With nine co-authors.

3108.4   HADDOW, *Sir* ALEXANDER. 1907-1976, & TIMMIS, GEOFFREY MILLWARD.
Myleran in chronic myeloid leukaemia: chemical constitution and biological action. *Lancet*, 1953, **1**, 207-08.
Introduction of myleran (busulphan). For results, see pp. 208-13.

3108.5   SHAY, HARRY. 1898- , *et al.*
Treatment of leukemia with triethylenethiophosphoramide (Thio-TEPA); preliminary results in experimental and clinical leukemia. *Arch. int. Med.*, 1953, **92**, 628-45.
With C. Zarafonetis, N. Smith, I. Woldow and D. C. H. Sun.

3108.6   GALTON, DAVID ABRAHAM GOITEN, *et al.*
Clinical trials of *p*-(DI-2-chloroethylamino)-phenylbutyric acid (CB 1348) in malignant lymphoma. *Brit. med. J.*, 1955, **2**, 1172-76.
Clinical use of chlorambucil for chronic lymphatic leukaemia. With L. G. Israels, J. D. N. Nabarro, and M. Till.

3108.7   LILEY, ALBERT WILLIAM.
Intrauterine transfusion of foetus in haemolytic disease. *Brit. med. J.*, 1963, **2**, 1107-09.

3108.8   FREDA, VINCENT J. 1927- , *et al.*
Successful prevention of experimental Rh sensitization in man with an anti-Rh gamma$_2$-globulin antibody preparation. *Transfusion*, 1964, **4**, 26-32.
    With J. G. Gorman and W. Pollack.

3108.9   ELLISON, ROSE RUTH. 1923- , *et al.*
Arabinosyl cytosine: A useful agent in the treatment of acute leukemia in adults. *Blood*, 1968, **32**, 507-23.
    Cytosine arabinoside. With J. P. Holland, M. Weil, *et al.*

Anaemia and Chlorosis

3109   LANGE, JOHANN. 1485-1565
Medicinalium epistolarum miscellanea. Basileae, *J. Oporinus*, 1554.
    Epistle xxi, pp. 74-77, contains the first definite description of chlorosis. "De morbo virgineo". English translation in No. 2241.

3110   HOFFMANN, FRIEDRICH. 1660-1742
De genuina chlorosis indole, origine et curatione. Halis, 1731.
    Classic description of chlorosis. Lange accurately diagnosed this condition, but it was left to Hoffmann to separate it as a definite entity.

3111   LETTSOM, JOHN COAKLEY. 1744-1815
Hints respecting the chlorosis of boarding schools. London, *C. Dilly*, 1795.

3112   COMBE, JAMES SCARTH. 1796-1883
History of a case of anaemia. *Trans. med.-chir. Soc. Edinb.*, 1824, **1**, 194-204.
    First description of pernicious anaemia. Paper read May 1, 1822.

3113   BLAUD, PIERRE. 1774-1858
Sur les maladies chlorotiques et sur un mode de traitement spécifique dans ces affections. *Rev. méd. franç. étrang.*, 1832, **45**, 337-67.
    For the treatment of chlorosis Blaud prescribed a pill (Blaud's pill) composed of sulphate of iron and carbonate of potassium. Preliminary report in *Bull. gén. Thérap.*, 1832, **2**, 154-55.

3114   FOEDISCH, FERDINAND.
Die krankhafte Mischung des Blutes, vorzüglich bei Chlorose, Hysterie und Pneumonie, durch chemische Versuche ausgemittelt, und der Uebergang in den Darmcanal eingebrachten Eisens. *Allg. med. Ztg.*, 1832, No. 97, col. 1537.
    Foedisch showed chlorotic blood to be deficient in iron. See also *Gaz. méd. Paris*, 1837, 2 sér. **5**, 7.

3115   NASSE, HERMANN. 1807-1892
Das Blut in mehrfacher Beziehung physiologisch und pathologisch untersucht. Bonn, *T. Habicht*, 1836.

Nasse gave the first clear description of anaemia in pregnancy; he also noticed erythrocyte sedimentation in certain pathological conditions.

3116   CHANNING, Walter. 1786-1876
Notes on anhaemia, principally in its connections with the puerperal state, and with functional disease of the uterus: with cases. *New Engl. quart. J. Med. Surg.*, 1842, **1**, 157-88.
First description of pernicious anaemia of pregnancy.

3117   BENNETT, H. N.
Puerperal anaemia; or a peculiar anaemic condition, occurring in gestating and lactating females. *N.Y. J. Med.*, 1847, **9**, 45-48, 197-98.
Bennett described the anaemia of pregnancy and defined it as resulting from the process of reproduction.

3118   ADDISON, Thomas. 1793-1860
Anaemia; disease of the supra-renal capsules. *Lond. med. Gaz.*, 1849, **43**, 517-18.
Addison included a classic description of pernicious (Addisonian) anaemia in his papers on the condition later known as "Addison's disease". Although preceded by Combe, his account was more important in bringing the disease to the notice of the medical profession. *See also* No. 3864.

3119   GRIESINGER, Wilhelm. 1817-1868
Ein Fall von Anaemia splenica bei einem Kinde. *Berl. klin. Wschr.*, 1866, **3**, 212-14.
First reported case of infantile splenic anaemia.

3120   DUNCAN, Johann.
Beiträge zur Pathologie und Therapie der Chlorose. *S.B. k. Akad. Wiss.*, math.-nat. Cl. (Wien), II Abt., 1867, **55**, 516-22.
Duncan showed that the essential feature in chlorosis is a quantitative change in the haemoglobin content and not a great reduction in the number of red blood cells.

3121   VALSUANI, Emilio.
Cachessia puerperale raccolta nella clinica ginecologica dell'ospitale Maggiore di Milano. Milano, *G. Bernardoni*, 1870.
"Valsuani's disease" – progressive anaemia in pregnant and lactating women, probably first described by H. N. Bennett (No. 3117).

3122   GUSSEROW, Adolf Ludwig Sigismund. 1836-1906
Ueber hochgradigste Anämie Schwangerer. *Arch. Gynäk.*, 1871, **2**, 218-35.
An important account of pernicious anaemia of pregnancy.

3124   BIERMER, Anton. 1827-1892
Eine eigenthumliche Form von progressiver perniciöser Anämie. *KorespBl. schweiz. Ärz.*, 1872, **2**, 15-18.
In his account of progressive pernicious anaemia, Biermer was first to describe the retinal haemorrhages. He was at one time accredited with the first description of pernicious anaemia; later it was shown that Addison had described the condition in his classic work on the suprarenals (No. 3118) and that Combe (No. 3112) had reported a case of pernicious anaemia as far back as 1822. On the European Continent the condition is referred to

as "Biermer's disease". Preliminary communication in *Versammlung deutscher Naturforscher und Aertze*, 1868, Tageblatt No. 8, IX Sect., p. 173.

3125   PEPPER, WILLIAM. 1843-1898
Progressive pernicious anaemia, or anaematosis. *Amer. J. med. Sci.*, 1875, **70**, 313-47.
Pepper described bone-marrow changes of pernicious anaemia, though his actual description more closely resembles leukaemia.

3125.1   COHNHEIM, JULIUS FRIEDRICH. 1839-1884
Erkrankung des Knochenmarkes bei perniciöser Anämie. *Virchows Arch. path. Anat.*, 1876, **68**, 291-93.
Cohnheim gave a more convincing account than Pepper of the bone-marrow changes in pernicious anaemia.

3125.2   GARDNER, WILLIAM, & OSLER, Sir WILLIAM, Bart. 1849-1919
A case of progressive pernicious anaemia (idiopathic of Addison). *Canada med. surg. J.*, 1877, **5**, 383-404.
First complete account of pernicious anaemia.

3125.3   EICHHORST, HERMANN LUDWIG. 1849-1921
Die progressive perniziöse Anämie. Leipzig, *Veit und Comp.*, 1878.
Comprehensive account.

3125.4   EHRLICH, PAUL. 1854-1915
Über Regeneration und Degeneration der rothen Blutscheiben bei Anämien. *Berl. klin. Wschr.*, 1880, **17**, 405.

3125.5   ——. Über einige Beobachtungen am anämischen Blut. *Berl. klin. Wschr.*, 1881, **18**, 43.
In the above contributions to the knowledge of anaemia, Ehrlich dealt in the first paper with the blood cells in anaemia, and in the second gave the first description of the reticulocyte.

3126   BANTI, GUIDO. 1852-1925
Dell'anemia splenica. Firenze, *succ. Le Monnier*, 1882.
"Banti's disease". Banti described the pathological changes in the spleen in splenic anaemia. A later paper in *Sperimentale*, 1894, **48**, sez. biol., 407-32, gives an account of hepatic cirrhosis as the sequel of the earlier stage of splenic anaemia; this sequel has been named "Banti's syndrome". A translation of this latter paper is in *Med. Classics*, 1937, **1**, 901-27.

3127   GAUCHER, PHILIPPE CHARLES ERNEST. 1854-1918
De l'epithélioma primitif de la rate; hypertrophie idiopathique de la rate sans leucémie. Paris, *Thèse*, 1882.
"Gaucher's disease" – familial splenic anaemia.

3128   LEICHTENSTERN, OTTO. 1845-1900
Ueber progressive perniciöse Anämie bei Tabeskranken. *Dtsch. med. Wschr.*, 1884, **10**, 849.
First description of subacute combined degeneration of the spinal cord, which Leichtenstern termed progressive pernicious anaemia in tabetics.

3129   EHRLICH, PAUL. 1854-1915
        Ueber einen Fall von Anämie mit Bemerkungen über regenerative
        Veränderungen des Knochenmarks. *Charité-Ann.*, 1888, **13**, 300-09.
        Ehrlich was first to distinguish the aplastic type of anaemia.

3130   HAYEM, GEORGES. 1841-1933
        Du sang et de ses altérations anatomiques. Paris, *G. Masson*, 1889.
        Includes (pp. 614-751) an important account of chlorosis; Hayem, by
        his accurate observation, placed knowledge of the disease on a firm basis.

3131   JAKSCH, RUDOLF VON, *Ritter von Wartenhorst.* 1855-1947
        Ueber Leukaemia und Leukocytose im Kindesalter. *Wien. klin. Wschr.*, 1889,
        2, 435-37, 456-58.
        From this classic description of infantile pseudoleukaemic anaemia, the
        condition became known as "von Jaksch's disease".

3131.1 RINDFLEISCH, GEORG EDUARD. 1836-1908
        Ueber die Fehler der Blutkörperchenbildung bei der perniciösen Anämie.
        Virchows Arch. path. Anat., 1890, **121**, 176-81.
        Rindfleisch made the first clear statement of the bone marrow changes
        in pernicious anaemia.

3132   BUNGE, GUSTAV VON. 1844-1920
        Ueber die Eisentherapie. *Verh. Congr. inn. Med.*, 1895, **13**, 133-47.
        Bunge was father to the concept of iron-deficiency anaemia.

3132.1 DRESBACH, M.
        Elliptical human red cell corpuscles. *Science*, 1904, **19**, 469-70.
        Hereditary elliptocytosis.

3133   HERRICK, JAMES BRYAN. 1861-1954
        Peculiar elongated and sickle-shaped red blood corpuscles in a case of
        severe anemia. *Arch. intern. Med.*, 1910, **6**, 517-21; *Trans. Ass. Amer. Phys.*,
        1910, **25**, 553-61.
        Identification of the sickle-cell type of anaemia.

3134   FABER, KNUD HELGE. 1862-1956
        Anämische Zustände bei der chronischen Achylia gastrica. *Berl. klin. Wschr.*,
        1913, **50**, 958-62.
        Simple achlorhydric (idiopathic microcytic) anaemia described. Faber
        advanced the view that achylia gastrica was a cause both of pernicious
        anaemia and of simple chlorotic anaemia.

3135   SCHMIDT, HARRY BURKE. 1882-
        A clinical study of puerperal anaemia. *Surg. Gynec. Obstet.*, 1918, **27**, 596-
        600.
        Four cases of pernicious anaemia of pregnancy treated by blood
        transfusion.

3136   OSLER, *Sir* WILLIAM, *Bart.* 1849-1919
        Observations on the severe anaemias of pregnancy and the post-partum
        state. *Brit. med. J.*, 1919, **1**, 1-3.
        A classic paper, with classification.

3136.1   MASON, Verne Rheem. 1889-
Sickle-cell anemia. *J. Amer. med. Assoc.*, 1922, **79**, 1318-20.
Mason gave sickle-cell anaemia its present name.

3136.2   GUTHRIE, Clyde Graeme. 1880- , & HUCK, John Gardiner. 1891-
On the existence of more than four isoagglutinin groups in human blood.
Bull. Johns Hopk. Hosp., 1923, **34**, 37-48, 80-88.
First genetic study of sickling.

3137   EDELMANN, Adolf. 1885-1939
Ueber Anaemia infectiosa chronica und ihre Aetiologie. *Wien. klin. Wschr.*,
1925, **38**, 268-69.
"Edelmann's disease" – a type of chronic infectious anaemia.

3138   LEDERER, Max. 1885-1952
A form of acute hemolytic anemia probably of infectious origin. *Amer. J.
med. Sci.*, 1925, **170**, 500-10.
"Lederer's anaemia" first described.

3139   ROBSCHEIT-ROBBINS, Frieda Saur. 1893- , & WHIPPLE, George Hoyt.
1878-1976
Blood regeneration in severe anaemia. II. Favourable influence of liver,
heart and skeletal muscle in diet. *Amer. J. Physiol.*, 1925, **72**, 408-18.
These workers showed the beneficial effect of raw beef liver upon
blood regeneration in anaemia. Their work paved the way for the liver diet
treatment of Minot and Murphy.

3140   MINOT, George Richards. 1885-1950, & MURPHY, William Parry. 1892-
Treatment of pernicious anemia by a special diet. *J. Amer. med. Assoc.*, 1926,
87, 470-76.
Introduction of raw liver diet in the treatment of pernicious anaemia.
This treatment ranks as one of the greatest modern advances in therapy.
See also the later paper in the same journal, 1927, **89**, 759-66. Reprinted in
Blood, 1948, **3**, 8-21. Minot and Murphy shared the Nobel Prize with
Whipple (*see* No. 3139) in 1934.

3141   COOLEY, Thomas Benton. 1871-1945, *et al.*
Anemia in children, with splenomegaly and peculiar changes in the bones.
Amer. J. Dis. Child, 1927, **34**, 347-63.
"Cooley's erythroblastic anaemia", thalassaemia. With E. R. Witwer and
O. P. Lee. An earlier brief account by Cooley and Lee appeared in *Trans.
Amer. Pediat. Soc.*, 1925, **37**, 29.

3142   FANCONI, Guido. 1892-1979
Familiäre infantile perniziösaartige Anämie (perniziöses Blutbild und
Konstitution). *Jb. Kinderheilk.*, 1927, **117**, 257-80.
"Fanconi's syndrome", congenital hypoplasia of bone marrow with
multiple congenital defects occurring as a familial disease.

3142.1   PEABODY, Francis Weld. 1881-1927
The pathology of the bone marrow in pernicious anaemia. *Amer. J. Path.*,
1927, **3**, 179-202.
Peabody studied the bone marrow in pernicious anaemia. He suggested
that failure of blood formation rather than haemolysis was the main defect

in the disease, and that the benefit from liver feeding was due to a factor in liver that promoted development and differentiation of mature erythrocytes.

3143 CASTLE, WILLIAM BOSWORTH. 1897-
Observations on the etiologic relationship of achylia gastrica to pernicious anemia. I. The effect of the administration to patients with pernicious anemia of the contents of the normal human stomach recovered after the ingestion of beef muscle. *Amer. J. med. Sci.*, 1929, **178**, 748-64.

Castle showed pernicious anaemia to be due to absence from the gastric juice of a substance (Castle's intrinsic factor, haemopoietin) that reacts with an extrinsic factor present in many foodstuffs to form the anti-pernicious anaemia factor. His experimental work resulted in the introduction of stomach preparations for the treatment of pernicious anaemia. Preliminary communication in *J. clin. Invest.*, 1928, **6**, 2.

3144 STURGIS, CYRUS CRESSEY. 1891-1966, & ISAACS, RAPHAEL. 1891-
Desiccated stomach in the treatment of pernicious anemia. *J. Amer. med. Assoc.*, 1929, **93**, 747-49.

Sturgis and Isaacs showed that stomach tissue contains a factor active in the treatment of pernicious anaemia.

3144.1 GÄNSSLEN, MAX. 1859-1969
Ein hochwirksamer, injizierbarer Leberextrakt. *Klin. Wschr.*, 1930, **9**, 2099-2102.

Gänsslen introduced an injectable liver extract in the treatment of pernicious anaemia.

3145 WINTROBE, MAXWELL MYER. 1901-
Classification of the anemias on the basis of differences in the size and hemoglobin content of the red corpuscles. *Proc. Soc. exp. Biol. (N.Y.)*, 1930, **27**, 1071-73.

Wintrobe's classification of the anemias.

3145.1 CASTLE, WILLIAM BOSWORTH. 1897- , & TAYLOR, FRANCIS HENRY LASKEY. 1900-1959
Intravenous use of extract of liver. *J. Amer. med. Assoc.*, 1931, **96**, 1198-1201.

3146 WILLS, LUCY. 1888-1964
Treatment of "pernicious anaemia of pregnancy" and "tropical anaemia", with special reference to yeast extract as a curative agent. *Brit. med. J.*, 1931, **1**, 1059-64.

First observations of haemopoietic effect of folic acid.

3147 DAVIDSON, *Sir* LEYBOURNE STANLEY PATRICK. 1894-1981
The classification and treatment of anaemia, with special reference to the nutritional factor. *Trans. med.-chir. Soc. Edinb.*, 1932, n.s. **46**, 105-56.

Davidson's classification of the anaemias.

3148 WILKINSON, JOHN FREDERICK. 1897- , & ISRAËLS, MARTIN CYRIL GORDON.
Achresthic anaemia. *Brit. med. J.*, 1935, **1**, 139-43, 194-97.

Achrestic anaemia described.

3148.1   WHIPPLE, GEORGE HOYT. 1878-1976, & BRADFORD, WILLIAM LESLIE. 1898-1983
Mediterranean disease – thalassemia (erythroblastic anemia of Cooley); associated pigment abnormalities simulating hemochromatosis. *J. Pediat.*, 1936, **9**, 279-311.
          Whipple and Bradford contributed a classic paper on the pathology of thalassaemia, a name introduced by them.

3148.2   CAMINOPETROS, J.
Recherches sur l'anémie érythroblastique infantile des peuples de la Méditerranée orientale. Étude anthropologique, étiologique et pathogénique. La transmission héréditaire de la maladie. *Ann. Méd.*, 1938, **43**, 104-25.
          First evidence that thalassaemia is genetically determined. Earlier report in *Kliniki*, Athens, 1936, **12**, No. 5.

3149   WILLS, LUCY. 1888-1964, & EVANS, BARBARA DOROTHY FORDYCE.
Tropical macrocytic anaemia: its relation to pernicious anaemia. *Lancet*, 1938, **2**, 416-21.

3150   SPIES, TOM DOUGLAS. 1902-1960, *et al.*
Observations of the anti-anemic properties of synthetic folic acid. *Sth. med. J. (Nashville)*, 1945, **38**, 707-09.
          Haemopoietic properties of folic acid reported. With C. F. Vilter, M. B. Koch, and M. H. Caldwell.

3151   ANGIER, ROBERT CRANE. 1917- , *et al.*
The structure and synthesis of liver. *L. casei* factor. *Science*, 1946, **103**, 667-69.
          Isolation, determination of structure, and final synthesis of folic acid.

3152   GOETSCH, ANNE CARLTON TOMPKINS. 1917- , *et al.*
Observations on the effect of massive doses of iron given intravenously to patients with hypochromic anemia. *Blood*, 1946, **1**, 129-42.

3153   NISSIM, JOSEPH ABRAHAM.
Intravenous administration of iron. *Lancet*, 1947, **2**, 49-51.

3154   WEST, RANDOLPH. 1890-
Activity of vitamin B_{12} in Addisonian pernicious anemia. *Science*, 1948, **107**, 398.
          First demonstration of the effectiveness of vitamin B12 in pernicious anaemia.

3154.1   PAULING, LINUS CARL. 1901- , *et al.*
Sickle cell anemia, a molecular disease. *Science*, 1949, **110**, 543-48.
          First recognition of a structural haemoglobin variant. With H. A. Itano, S. J. Singer, and I. C. Wells.

3154.2   NEEL, JAMES VAN GUNDIA. 1915-
The inheritance of sickle cell anemia. *Science*, 1949, **110**, 64-66.
          Genetic evidence that sickle-cell disease is inherited in a simple Mendelian manner.

3155   UNGLEY, CHARLES CADY.
Vitamin B_{12} in pernicious anaemia: parenteral administration. *Brit. med. J.*, 1949, **2**, 1370-77.

3155.1   INGRAM, VERNON MARTIN. 1924-
Gene mutations in human haemoglobin: the chemical difference between normal and sickle cell haemoglobin. *Nature (Lond.)*, 1957, **180**, 326-28.
     Sickle-cell haemoglobin differs from normal haemoglobin by a single amino acid (valine for glutamic acid).

3155.2   ——., & STRETTON, ANTONY OLIVER WARD. 1936-
Genetic basis of the thalassaemia diseases. *Nature (Lond.)*, 1959, **184**, 1903-09.

3155.3   LOCK, STEPHEN PENFORD. 1929- , *et al.*
Stomatocytosis: a hereditary red cell anomaly associated with haemolytic anaemia. *Brit. J. Haemat.*, 1961, **7**, 303-14.
     With R. Sephton Smith and R. M. Hardisty.

3155.4   LEHMANN, HERMANN. 1910-1985, & HUNTSMAN, RICHARD GEORGE.
Man's haemoglobins: including the haemoglobinopathies and their investigation. Amsterdam, *North Holland Pub. Co.*, 1966.
     Explains the current distribution of sickling throughout the world.

History of the Study of Cardiovascular Diseases and Haematology

3156   ROLLESTON, *Sir* HUMPHRY DAVY, *Bart.* 1862-1944
Cardio-vascular diseases since Harvey's discovery. Cambridge, *Univ. Press.*, 1928.
     Harveian Oration, 1928.

3157   ——. The history of angina pectoris. *Glasg. med. J.*, 1937, **127**, 205-25.

3158   WILLIUS, FREDERICK ARTHUR. 1888-1972, & KEYS, THOMAS EDWARD. 1908-
Cardiac classics. A collection of classic works on the heart and circulation with comprehensive biographic accounts of the authors. St. Louis, *C. V. Mosby Co.*, 1941.
     Covers the literature up to 1912. Reprinted in 2 vols. as *Classics of cardiology*, New York, *Dover*, 1961. Reprinted again, with volume 3 by John A. Callahan, Thomas E. Keys & Jack E. Key, Malabar, Florida, *Krieger*, 1983. Volume 4 by John A. Callahan, Dwight C. McGoon, and Jack D. Key, Malabar, *Krieger*, 1989. Vol. 3 covers literature from 1912 to 1955 in a style similar to the first 2 vols. Vol. 4 in 2 pts. covers material published up to 1975, with an abbreviated commentary. Part 1 of Vol. 4 covers cardiac surgery; part 2 covers cardiology.

3159   HERRICK, JAMES BRYAN. 1861-1954
A short history of cardiology. Springfield, *C. C. Thomas*, 1942.

3160   WILLIUS, FREDERICK ARTHUR. 1888-1972, & DRY, THOMAS JAN. 1903-
A history of the heart and circulation. Philadelphia, *W. B. Saunders*, 1948.

3160.1 RUSKIN, ARTHUR.
Classics in arterial hypertension. Springfield, *C.C. Thomas*, 1956.

3161 EAST, CHARLES FREDERICK TERENCE. 1894-1967
The story of heart disease. London, *Wm. Dawson*, [1957].

3161.01 MEADE, RICHARD HARDAWAY. 1897-
A history of thoracic surgery. Springfield, *C. C. Thomas*, 1961.
Includes cardiovascular surgery.

3161.1 BURCH, GEORGE EDWARD. 1910-1986, & DePASQUALE, NICHOLAS P. 1927-
The history of electrocardiography. Chicago, *Year Book Medical Publishers*, 1964.
Reprinted with new introduction by Joel D. Howell, San Francisco, *Norman Publishing*, 1990.

3161.2 JOHNSON, STEPHEN L. 1933-
The history of cardiac surgery. Baltimore, *Johns Hopkins Press*, 1970.

3161.3 LEIBOWITZ, JOSHUA O. 1895-
The history of coronary heart disease. London, *Wellcome Institute*, 1970.
A scholarly work with extensive bibliographies.

3161.4 BOROVICZENY, KARL GEORG VON, *et al.*
Einführung in die Geschichte der Haematologie. Stuttgart, *G. Thieme*, 1974.
Thirteen contributions edited by Boroviczény, H. Schipperges, and E. Seidler. Includes chronological table of events in the history of medicine and a bibliography.

3161.41 COMROE, JULIUS H., JR. & DRIPPS, ROBERT D.
The top ten clinical advances in cardiovascular-pulmonary medicine and surgery 1945-1975. Final report. 2 vols. Washington, D.C., *Govt. Printing Office*, 1977.

3161.42 BEDFORD, DAVIS EVAN. 1898-1978
The Evan Bedford library of cardiology. Catalogue of books, pamphlets and journals. London, *Royal College of Physicians*, 1977.
Descriptions of 1112 items with annotations by Bedford, who donated his collection to the Royal College of Physicians.

3161.5 WINTROBE, MAXWELL MYER. 1901-
Blood, pure and eloquent. A story of discovery, of people, and of ideas. New York, *McGraw-Hill*, 1980.
A collective work by 19 authors, edited by M. M. Wintrobe. This is a detailed history of haematology, well documented and well indexed.

3161.6 JARCHO, SAUL. 1906-
The concept of heart failure from Avicenna to Alberti. Cambridge, Mass., *Harvard University Press*, 1980.
Translations of extensive selections from 19 famous and/or obscure works, with commentary and summary.

3161.7 WINTROBE, MAXWELL MYER. 1901-
Hematology, the blossoming of a science: a story of inspiration and effort. Philadelphia, *Lea & Febiger*, 1985.

DISEASES OF THE RESPIRATORY SYSTEM

3162   ARETAEUS, *the Cappadocian. circa* A.D. 81-138
On angina, or quinsey. In his *Extant works,* ed. F. ADAMS, London, 1856, 249-52, 404-07.

3163   ——. On pleurisy. In his *Extant works,* ed. F. ADAMS, London, 1856, 255-58, 410-16.

3164   VESALIUS, ANDREAS. 1514-1564
Pro magni, et illustr. Terraenovae Ducis fistula, ex levi axilla in thoracis concavum pervia, *etc. In* P. Ingrassia, Quaestio de purgatione per medicamentum, Venetiis, *sumpt. A. Patessii,* 1568.
Vesalius's *consilium* to Ingrassia, dated Madrid, 1562, in which he clearly described the operation for empyema (pp. 92-98). Although treatment of empyema by surgery was referred to in classical times, it became unfashionable, and Vesalius seems to have been the first to revive the actual use of surgery for this illness. English translation in O'Malley, *Andreas Vesalius of Brussels*, Berkeley, *Univ. of California Press*, 1965, pp.398-402.

3165   WILLIS, THOMAS. 1621-1675
Of the convulsive cough and asthma. In his: *Practice of physick*, London, *T. Dring, etc.,* 1684, Treatise VIII, pp. 92-96.
The modern treatment of asthma really begins with Willis, who considered it to be of nervous origin.

3166   FLOYER, *Sir* JOHN. 1649-1734
A treatise of the asthma. London. *R. Wilkins,* 1698.
Floyer provided the first clear descriptions of cases of bronchial asthma. Floyer himself suffered from asthma for over 30 years. He recognized the influence of heredity in asthma. The above includes (p. 239) an important early account of emphysema, from a post mortem on a broken-winded horse.

3166.1   WATSON, *Sir*, WILLIAM. 1715-1787
An account of what appeared on opening the body of an asthmatic person. *Phil. Trans.*, 1746, **54**, 239-45.
Probably the earliest comprehensive clinical and pathological account of emphysema.

3167   MILLAR, JOHN. 1733-1805
Observations on the asthma and on the hooping cough. London, *T. Cadell,* 1769.
Includes Millar's original description of laryngismus stridulus ("Millar's asthma").

3167.1   BAILLIE, MATTHEW. 1760-1823
The morbid anatomy of some of the most important parts of the human body. 2nd ed. London, *J. Johnson & G. Nicol,* 1797, vol. 2, p. 72.
First clinical description of chronic obstructive pulmonary emphysema. The lung on which Baillie performed an autopsy before describing this condition is said to have been that of Samuel Johnson. *See also* Nos. 2281, 2736, 3218, & 3427.

3168   BADHAM, CHARLES. 1780-1845
Observations on the inflammatory affections of the mucous membrane of
the bronchiae. London, *J. Callow*, 1808.
    Badham distinguished acute and chronic bronchitis from pneumonia
and pleurisy, with which it had previously been confused. He gave the
disease its present name.

3168.1   BOWDITCH, HENRY INGERSOLL. 1808-1892
On pleuritic effusions, and the necessity of paracentesis for their removal.
Amer. J. med. Sci., 1852, **23**, 320-50.
    Bowditch pioneered the operation for removal of pleural effusions with
trocar and a suction pump devised by Morrill Wyman (1812-1903). See
Bowditch's earlier paper on the subject in the same journal volume, pp.
103-05.

3169   VIRCHOW, RUDOLF LUDWIG KARL. 1821-1902
Beiträge zur Lehre von den beim Menschen vorkommenden pflanzlichen
Parasiten. *Virchows Arch. path. Anat.*, 1856, **9**, 557-93.
    First description of pulmonary aspergillosis.

3169.1   SALTER, HENRY HYDE. 1823-1871
On asthma: its pathology and treatment. London, *J. Churchill*, 1860.
    The best work on asthma to appear during the 19th century. Salter
called special attention to asthma arising from animal emanations (cats,
rabbits, horses, dogs, cattle, etc.) *See* No. 2586.

3170   HEWETT, FREDERICK CHARLES CRESSWELL.
Thoracentesis: the plan of continuous aspiration. *Brit. med. J.*, 1876, **1**, 317.
    Hewett introduced a method of continuous aspiration of the thorax for
emphysema.

3172   PARROT, JOSEPH. 1829-1883
L'organisme microscopique trouvé par M. Pasteur dans la maladie nouvelle
provoquée par la salive d'un enfant mort de la rage. *Bull. Acad. Méd. Paris*,
1881, 2 sér., **10**, 379.
    Probably the earliest record of pneumococcus.

3173   STERNBERG, GEORGE MILLER. 1838-1915
A fatal form of septicaemia in the rabbit, produced by the subcutaneous
injection of human saliva. *Johns Hopk. Univ. Stud. biol. Lab.*, 1882, **2**, No.
2, 183-200.
    In the same year as Pasteur, and independently, Sternberg discovered
a pneumococcus demonstrating its carriage in the healthy human mouth.

3174   FRIEDLÄNDER, CARL. 1847-1887
Ueber die Schizomyceten bei der acuten fibrösen Pneumonie. *Virchows
Arch. path. Anat.*, 1882, **87**, 319-24.
    Isolation of *Klebsiella pneumoniae* ("Friedländer bacillus"), which
Friedländer regarded as the causal organism in all cases of lobar pneumonia.

3174.1   KRÖNLEIN RUDOLPH ULRICH. 1847-1910
Ueber Lungenchirurgie. *Berl. klin. Wschr.*, 1884, **21**, 129-32.
    Resection of portion of a lobe that was invaded by sarcoma of the rib.

3175   FRAENKEL, ALBERT. 1848-1916
        Die Mikrococcen der Pneumonie. *Z. Klin. Med.*, 1886, **10**, 426-49; **11**, 437-58.
        Fraenkel showed definitely that the organism found by Pasteur (No. 3172) and Sternberg (No. 3173) was a cause of pneumonia.

3176   WEICHSELBAUM, ANTON. 1845-1920
        Ueber die Aetiologie der acuten Lungen- und Rippenfellentzündungen. *Med. Jb.*, 1886, n.F. **1**, 483-554.
        Weichselbaum definitely established that Friedländer's bacillus was responsible for pneumonia in a small percentage of cases.

3177   KÜSTER, ERNST GEORG FERDINAND VON. 1839-1930
        Ueber die Grundsätze der Behandlung von Eiterungen in starrwandigen Höhlen, mit besonderer Berücksichtigung des Empyems der Pleura. *Dtsch. med. Wschr.*, 1889, **15**, 185-87.
        First thoracotomy for empyema.

3177.1 SCHEDE, MAX. 1844-1902
        Die Behandlung der Empyeme. *Verh. Dtsch. Congr. inn. Med.*, 1890, **9**, 41-100.
        Schede introduced the method of extensive rib resection for the treatment of empyema.

3178   KLEMPERER, GEORG. 1865-1946, & KLEMPERER, FELIX. 1866-1932
        Versuche über Immunisirung und Heilung bei der Pneumokokkeninfection. *Berl. klin. Wschr.*, 1891, **28**, 833-35, 869-75.
        Old antipneumococcal serum.

3179   FOWLER, GEORGE RYERSON. 1848-1906
        A case of thoracoplasty for the removal of a large cicatricial fibrous growth from the interior of the chest, the result of an old empyema. *Med. Rec. (N.Y.)*, 1893, **44**, 838-39.
        First thoracoplasty.

3180   DELORME, EDMOND. 1847-1929
        Nouveau traitement des empyèmes chroniques. *Gaz. Hôp. (Paris)*, 1894, **67**, 94-96.
        The procedure of decortication of the lung for treatment of chronic empyema was introduced by Delorme. For his later work on the subject, see *Congr. franç. Chir.*, 1896, **10**, 379.

3181   THOREL, CHRISTEN. 1868-1935
        Die Specksteinlunge. Ein Beitrag zur pathologischen Anatomie der Staublungen. *Beitr. path. Anat.*, 1896, **20**, 81-101.
        Talcosis of lung reported.

3182   NOCARD, EDMOND ISIDORE ETIENNE. 1850-1903, & ROUX, PIERRE PAUL EMILE. 1853-1933
        Le microbe de la péripneumonie. *Ann. Inst. Pasteur*, 1898, **12**, 240-62.
        Discovery of the causal organism of bovine pleuropneumonia, then considered a filterable virus but now known to be a mycoplasma.

3183   GROCCO, PIETRO. 1856-1916
Triangolo paravertebrale opposto nella pleurite essudativa. *Lav. Congr. Med. int.* (1902), Roma, 1903, **12**, 190.
"Grocco's triangle". Grocco described paravertebral dullness on the opposite side in pleural effusion.

3184   EMERSON, CHARLES PHILLIPS. 1872-1938
Pneumothorax; a historical, clinical, and experimental study. *Johns Hopk. Hosp. Rep.*, 1903, **11**, 1-450.

3185   SAUERBRUCH, ERNST FERDINAND. 1875-1951
Ueber die physiologischen and physikalischen Grundlagen bei intrathorakalen Eingriffen in meiner pneumatischen Operationskammer. *Verh. dtsch. Ges. Chir.*, 1904, **32**, pt. 2, 105-15.
Sauerbruch's negative pressure chamber for the prevention of pneumothorax.

3186   NOWOTNY, FRANZ. 1872-1925
Bronchoskopie und bronchoskopische Behandlung von Bronchialasthma. *Mschr. Ohrenheilk.*, 1907, **41**, 679-711.
Introduction of therapeutic bronchoscopy, for treatment of asthma.

3187   KÖRTE, WERNER. 1853-1937
Ueber Lungenresektion wegen bronchiektatischer Cavernen. *Verh. Berl. med. Ges.*, (1908), 1909, **39**, 5-9.
Körte was the first successfully to remove bronchiectatic lobes.

3188   PASTEUR, WILLIAM. 1856-1943
The Bradshaw Lecture on massive collapse of the lung. *Lancet*, 1908, **2**, 1351-55.
Pasteur discovered and described massive collapse of the lung.

3189   JACOBAEUS, HANS CHRISTIAN. 1879-1937
Ueber die Möglichkeit die Zystoscopie bei Untersuchungen seröser Höhlungen anzuwenden. *Münch. med. Wschr.*, 1910, **57**, 2090-92.
Jacobaeus adapted the cystoscope for the study of the interior of the body; this led to the introduction of the thoracoscope.

3190   NEUFELD, FRED. 1861-1945, & HAENDEL, LUDWIG. 1869-1939
Weitere Untersuchungen über Pneumokokken-Heilsera. III. Mitteilung. Über Vorkommen und Bedeutung atypischer Varietäten des Pneumokokkus. *Arb. k. GesundhAmte*, 1910, **34**, 293-304.
New antipneumococcus serum.

3191   TUFFIER, THEODORE. 1857-1929
Gangrène pulmonaire ouverte dans les bronches et traitée par décollement pleuro-pariétal, et greffe d'une masse lipomateuse entre la plèvre décollée et les espaces intercostaux. *Bull. Soc. Chir. Paris*, 1910, **36**, 529-38.
Tuffier's method of extrapleural pneumolysis.

3192   ADLER, ISAAC. 1849-1918
Primary malignant growths of the lungs and bronchi. New York, *Longmans*, 1912.

3192.1   DOCHEZ, ALPHONSE RAYMOND. 1882-1964, & GILLESPIE, LOUIS JOHN. 1886-?
A biological classification of pneumococci by means of immunity reactions.
J. Amer. med. Assoc., 1913, **61**, 727-32.
Dochez and Gillespie differentiated four types of pneumococci.

3192.2   KRUSE, WALTHER. 1864-1943
Die Erreger von Husten und Schnopfen. *Münch. med. Wschr.*, 1914, **61**, 1547.
Kruse reported that colds could be produced in volunteers by intranasal
instillation of bacteria-free filtrates of secretions from persons suffering
from colds.

3193   CASTELLANI, ALDO. 1877-1971
Note sur la "broncho-spirochétose" et les "bronchites mycosiques", affections simulant quelquefois la tuberculose pulmonaire. *Presse méd.*, 1917,
25, 377-80.
"Castellani's bronchitis" (bronchospirochaetosis).

3194   JACKSON, CHEVALIER. 1865-1958
Endothelioma of the right bronchus removed by peroral bronchoscopy.
Amer. J. med. Sci., 1917, **153**, 371-75.
First reported case.

3194.1   WATERS, CHARLES ALEXANDER. 1885-?, *et al.*
Roentgenography of the lung; roentgenographic studies in living animals
after intratracheal injection of iodoform emulsion. *Arch. int. Med.*, 1917,
19, 538-49.
Experimental introduction of iodoform (lipiodol) into the bronchial
tree in dogs, obtaining satisfactory bronchograms. With S. Bayne-Jones
and L. G. Rowntree.

3195   SAUERBRUCH, ERNST FERDINAND. 1875-1951
Die Chirurgie der Brustorgane. Zugleich zweite Auflage der Technik der
Thoraxchirurgie. 2 vols. Berlin, *J. Springer*, 1920-25.
Abridged English translation, Baltimore, 1937.

3196   COUTARD, HENRI. 1876-1950
Un cas d'épithélioma spino-cellulaire de la région latérale du pharynx,
avec adénopathie angulo-maxillaire, guéri depuis six mois par la
röntgenthérapie. *Bull. Ass. franç, Etude Cancer*, 1921, **10**, 160-68.
Carcinoma of pharynx cured by the Coutard method of Röntgen
therapy.

3197   LYNAH, HENRY LOWNDES. 1879-1922, & STEWART, WILLIAM HOLMES. 1868-
Roentgenographic studies of bronchiectasis and lung abscess after direct
injection of bismuth mixture through the bronchoscope. *Amer. J.
Roentgenol.*, 1921, **8**, 49-61.
Important studies on bronchiectasis were carried out by Lynah and
Stewart.

3197.1   MACHT, DAVID ISRAEL. 1882-1961, & TING, GIU-CHING.
A study of antispasmodic drugs on the bronchus. *J. Pharmacol.*, 1921, **18**,
373-98.
Laboratory demonstration of the antispasmodic action of theophylline
on bronchial smooth muscle.

3197.2   HIRSCH, SAMSON.
Klinische und experimentelle Beitrag zur krampflösenden Wirkung der Purinderivate. *Klin. Wschr.,* 1922, **1**, 615-18.
Hirsch established the value of theophylline in the management of asthma.

3198   HEIDELBERGER, MICHAEL. 1888- , & AVERY, OSWALD THEODORE. 1877-1955
The soluble specific substance of pneumococcus. *J. exp. Med.,* 1923, **38**, 73-79; 1924, **40**, 301-16.
Heidelberger, Avery, and their colleagues made a chemical study of the antigenic constituents of the pneumococcus, separating the polysaccharide antigens.

3199   SICARD, JEAN ATHANASE. 1872-1929, & FORESTIER, JACQUES. 1890-
L'exploration radiologique des cavités broncho-pulmonaires par les injections intra-trachéales d'huile iodée. *J. méd. franç.,* 1924, **13**, 3-9.
Bronchography was advanced by the work of Sicard and Forestier on the intratracheal introduction of lipiodol.

3200   LAUGHLEN, GEORGE FRANKLIN. 1888-
Studies on pneumonia following naso-pharyngeal injections of oil. *Amer. J. Path.,* 1925, **1**, 407-14.
Lipoid pneumonia first described.

3201   BARNARD, WILLIAM GEORGE. 1892-1956
The nature of the "oat-celled sarcoma" of the mediastinum. *J. Path. Bact.,* 1926, **29**, 241-44.
An important study of the histology of "oat-celled sarcoma" which Barnard showed to be primary carcinoma of the lung.

3202   BRUNN, HAROLD. 1874-1950
Surgical principles underlying one-stage lobectomy. *Arch. Surg.,* 1929, **18**, 490-515.
Brunn's one-stage lobectomy.

3202.1   CAMPS, PERCY WILLIAM LEOPOLD. 1877-1956
A note on the inhalation treatment of asthma. *Guy's Hosp. Rep.,* 1929, **79**, 496-98.
First use of adrenaline by the respiratory route for the treatment of bronchial asthma.

3202.2   COLE, RUFUS IVORY. 1872-1966
Serum treatment in type I lobar pneumonia. *J. Amer. med. Assoc.,* 1929, **93**, 741-47.
Introduction of monovalent antiserum.

3203   NISSEN, RUDOLPH. 1896-
Exstirpation eines ganzen Lungenflügels. *Zbl. Chir.,* 1931, **58**, 3003-06.
Removal of entire bronchiectatic lung; successful.

3203.1   CAMPBELL, JOHN MUNRO.
Acute symptoms following work with hay. *Brit. med. J.,* 1932, **2**, 1143-44.
"Farmer's lung".

3203.2   SHENSTONE, NORMAN STRAHAN. 1881-   , & JANES, ROBERT MEREDITH. 1894-
Experiences in pulmonary lobectomy. *Canad. med. Ass. J.*, 1932, **27**, 138-45.
Introduction of the hilar tourniquet in pulmonary surgery.

3204   THOMSON, DAVID. 1884-1969, & THOMSON, ROBERT. 1888-
The common cold, with special reference to the part played by streptococci,
pneumococci, and other organisms. London, *Baillière, Tindall & Cox*, 1932.
Annals of the Pickett-Thomson Research Lab., Vol. 8.

3205   GRAHAM, EVARTS AMBROSE. 1883-1957, & SINGER, JACOB JESSE. 1882-1954
Successful removal of entire lung for carcinoma of the bronchus. *J. Amer.
med. Assoc.*, 1933, **101**, 1371-74.
First reported case: April 5, 1933.

3206   KARTAGENER, MANES. 1897-
Zur Pathogenese der Bronchiektasien. I. Bronchiektasien bei Situs viscerum
inversus. *Beitr. Klin. Tuberk.*, 1933, **83**, 489-501.
Bronchiectasis and sinus maldevelopment associated with transposition of viscera – "Kartagener's syndrome".

3207   LILIENTHAL, HOWARD. 1861-1946
Pneumonectomy for sarcoma of the lung in a tuberculous patient. *J. thorac.
Surg.*, 1933, **2**, 600-15.
Total pneumonectomy.

3208   MAYTUM, CHARLES KORAN. 1895-
Tetany caused by functional dyspnea with hyperventilation: report of a
case. *Proc. Mayo Clin.*, 1933, **8**, 282-84.
Hyperventilation syndrome.

3209   BARACH, ALVAN LEROY. 1895-1977
Use of helium as a new therapeutic gas. *Proc. Soc. exp. Biol. (N.Y.)*, 1934,
32, 462-64.
Introduction of helium in the treatment of respiratory affections. See
also *Ann. intern. Med.*, 1935, **9**, 739-65.

3209.1   ABREU, MANOEL DE. 1892-1962
Röntgen-photographia. Processo e apparelho de röntgen-photographia.
Tuberculose pulmonar. Cadastro social. Radiographia e radioscopia.
Röntgen-photographia collectiva. *Rev. Assoc. paul. Med.*, 1936, **9**, 313-24.
Introduction of mass chest radiography.

3210   EVANS, GLADYS MARY, & GAISFORD, WILFRID FLETCHER. 1902-
Treatment of pneumonia with 2-(*p*-aminobenzenesulphonamido) pyridine.
Lancet, 1938, **2**, 14-19.
M & B 693 (sulphapyridine) treatment of pneumonia. This followed the
experimental work of L. E. H. Whitby (*see* No. 1951).

3211   REIMANN, HOBART ANSTETH. 1897-
An acute infection of the respiratory tract with atypical pneumonia: a
disease entity probably caused by a filterable virus. *J. Amer. med. Assoc.*,
1938, **111**, 2377-84.
Atypical pneumonia.

3211.1   CHURCHILL, Edward Delos. 1895-1972, & BELSEY, Ronald Herbert Robert.
Segmental pneumonectomy in bronchiectasis. The lingula segment of the
left upper lobe. *Ann. Surg.*, 1939, **109**, 481-99.

3212   HEFFRON, Roderick. 1901-
Pneumonia. With special reference to pneumococcus lobar pneumonia.
London, *Oxford Univ. Press*, 1939.

3213   MÜLLER, Franz Hermann.
Tabakmissbrauch und Lungencarcinom. *Z. Krebsforsch.*, 1939, **49**, 57-85.
    Müller recorded a statistically significant correlation between cigarette
smoking and lung cancer.

3213.1   EATON, Monroe Davis. 1904- , *et al.*
Studies on the etiology of primary atypical pneumonia. A filterable agent
transmissible to cotton rats, hamsters, and chick embryos. *J. exp. Med.*, 1944,
79, 649-68.
    The Eaton agent, isolated from primary atypical pneumonia. With G.
Meiklejohn and W. van Herick.

3214   COMMISSION ON ACUTE RESPIRATORY DISEASES.
Transmission of primary atypical pneumonia to human volunteers. *J. Amer.
med. Assoc.*, 1945, **127**, 146-49.

3215   DIENES, Louis, & EDSALL, Geoffrey.
Observations on L-organism of Kleineberger. *Proc. Soc. exp. Biol. (N.Y.)*,
1937, **36**, 740-44.
    Isolation of a mycoplasma from man.

3215.1   WYNDER, Ernest Ludwig. 1922- , & GRAHAM, Evarts Ambrose. 1883-1957
Tobacco smoking as a possible etiologic factor in bronchogenic carcinoma.
J. Amer. med. Assoc., 1950, **143**, 329-36.
    A case-control study proving an association between heavy prolonged
cigarette smoking and bronchogenic carcinoma. See also the following
paper on pp. 336-38. Reprinted in *J. Amer. med. Assoc.* 1985, **253**, 2986-97.

3215.2   DOLL, *Sir* William Richard Shaboe. 1912- , & HILL, *Sir* Austin Bradford. 1897-
Smoking and carcinoma of the lung. Preliminary report. *Brit. med. J.*, 1950,
2, 739-48.
    A study of 1,465 cases of lung cancer and 1,465 matched controls, which
confirmed and extended the studies of Wynder and Graham, and others.
See also later papers by the same authors in *Brit. med. J.*, 1952, **2**, 1271-86;
1956, **2**, 1071-81; 1964, **1**, 1399-1410.

3215.3   KUROYA, Masahiko, *et al.*
Newborn virus pneumonitis (type Sendai). II. The isolation of a new virus
possessing hemagglutinin activity. *Yokohama med. Bull.*, 1953, **4**, 217-33.
    M. Kuroya, N. Ishida, and T. Shiratori isolated the first recognized
Sendai (para-influenza) virus.

3215.4   CHANOCK, Robert Merritt. 1904- , *et al.*
Recovery from infants with respiratory illness of a virus related to chimpanzee
coryza agent (CCA). *Amer. J. Hyg.*, 1957, **66**, 281-90.
    Respiratory syncytial virus. With B. Roizman and R. Myers.

3215.5 ———. Growth on artificial medium of an agent associated with atypical pneumonia and its identification as a PPLO. *Proc. nat. Acad. Sci. (Wash.)*, 1962, **48**, 41-49.

A mycoplasma shown to be the cause of some cases of primary atypical pneumonia. With L. Hayflick and M. F. Barile.

3215.6 PEPYS, JACK. *et al*
Farmer's lung. Thermophilic actinomycetes as a source of "farmer's lung hay" antigen. *Lancet*, 1963, **2**, 607-11.

Pepys and five co-authors showed that thermophilic actinomycetes, especially *Micropolyspora faeni*, were the cause of farmer's lung due to mouldy hay.

3215.7 FRASER, DAVID WILLIAM, *et al.*
Legionnaires' disease. Description of an epidemic of pneumonia. *New Engl. J. Med.*, 1977, **297**, 1189-97.

First major scientific account. With 11 co-authors.

3215.8 McDADE, JOSEPH E., *et al.*
Legionnaires' disease. Isolation of a bacterium and demonstration of its role in other respiratory disease. *New Engl. J. Med.*, 1977, **297**, 1197-1203.

With five co-authors. See also p. 1218.

3215.9 MEADE, RICHARD HARDAWAY. 1897-
A history of thoracic surgery. Springfield, *C. C. Thomas*, 1961.

Includes cardiovascular surgery.

PULMONARY TUBERCULOSIS

See also 2320-2360, TUBERCULOSIS

3216 MORTON, RICHARD. 1637-1698
Phthisiologia, seu exercitationes de phthisi. Londini, *imp. S. Smith*, 1689.

The first application of the principles of pathology to the study of pulmonary tuberculosis. Morton showed that the formation of tubercles is a necessary part of the development of this lung disease, and pointed out that the tubercles often heal spontaneously. He noted the enlargement of the tracheal and bronchial glands in cases of pulmonary tuberculosis. The book was translated into English in 1694. Chap. I included the first account of anorexia nervosa.

3217 MARTEN, BENJAMIN. *fl.* 18th cent.
A new theory of consumptions: more especially of a phthisis, or consumption of the lungs. London, *R. Knaplock*, 1720.

Marten considered a parasitic micro-organism to be the cause of tuberculosis, thus forecasting the existence of the tubercle bacillus 162 years before its actual discovery.

3218 BAILLIE, MATTHEW. 1761-1823
The morbid anatomy of some of the most important parts of the human body. London, *J. Johnson & G. Nicol*, 1793.

Baillie's clear and comprehensive description of the pulmonary lesions of tuberculosis could hardly be bettered today. He differentiated the nodular and infiltrating types. *See also* Nos. 2281, 2736, 3167.1, & 3427.

3219   LAENNEC, RENÉ THÉOPHILE HYACINTHE. 1781-1826
De l'auscultation médiate. 2 vols. Paris, *J. A. Brosson & J. S. Chaudé,* 1819.
    Laennec is remembered for his invention of the stethoscope and for his book on auscultation. This work is the foundation stone of modern knowledge of diseases of the chest. Himself tuberculous, Laennec was considered the greatest teacher of his time on tuberculosis. Indeed, it was in elaboration of his investigation of the disease that he invented the stethoscope. He established the fact that all phthisis is tuberculous, described pneumothorax and distinguished pneumonia from the various kinds of bronchitis and from pleuritis. *See also* No. 2673.

3220   CARSON, JAMES. 1772-1843
Essays, physiological and practical. Liverpool, *F. B. Wright* 1822.
    Carson proposed the induction of open pneumothorax for the treatment of pulmonary tuberculosis (p. 64). Later he attempted it on a patient (see his *An inquiry into the cause of respiration,* etc. 2nd ed., London, 1833, p. 50). The procedure was carried out by Forlanini (*see* No. 3225).

3221   LOUIS, PIERRE CHARLES ALEXANDRE. 1787-1872
Recherches anatomico-pathologiques sur la phthisie. Paris, *Gabon & Cie.,* 1825.
    Louis' researches were based on 358 dissections and 1,960 clinical cases, and included a numerical study of extra-pulmonary lesions. English translation, Boston, 1836. A translation of the 2nd edition was published by the Sydenham Society in 1844.

3222   MORTON, SAMUEL GEORGE. 1799-1851
Illustrations of pulmonary consumption. Philadelphia. *Key & Biddle,* 1834.
    Morton published an important collection of illustrations delineating pulmonary tuberculosis which epitomized the knowledge of his time. It was also the first book on the subject to be published in the U.S.A.

3223   BODINGTON, GEORGE. 1799-1882
Essay on the treatment of and cure of pulmonary consumption. London. *Longmans & Co.,* 1840.
    Bodington was one of the first to advocate the sanatorium treatment of pulmonary tuberculosis, with "cold dry air for healing and closing cavities and ulcers of the lungs". His idea was much criticized and he was discouraged from pursuing it. The first sanatorium to be run on lines similar to those suggested by Bodington was that established by H. Brehmer at Görbersdorf in 1859. The book was reprinted in 1906.

3224   PARROT, JOSEPH. 1829-1883
Recherches sur les relations qui existent entre les lésions des poumons et celles des ganglions trachéo-bronchiques. *C. R. Soc. Biol. (Paris),* 1876, sér. 6, **3**, 308-09.
    The primary lesion in pulmonary tuberculosis in children ("Ghon's primary focus") was first described by Parrot.

3225   FORLANINI, Carlo. 1847-1918
A contribuzione della terapia chirurgica della tisi; ablazione de polmone? pneumotorace artificiale? *Gazz. Osp. Clin.*, 1882, **3**, 537, 585, 601, 609, 617, 625, 641, 657, 665, 689, 705.

      Forlanini first discussed the induction of artificial pneumothorax in the above papers; he applied it in 1888. For his report on its application, see *Gazz. med. Torino*, 1894, **45**, 381, 401. English translation in *Tubercle*, 1934-35, **16**, 61-87.

3226   CAYLEY, William. 1836-1916
A case of haemoptysis treated by the induction of pneumothorax so as to collapse the lung. *Trans. clin. Soc. Lond.*, 1885, **18**, 278-84.

      Artificial pneumothorax by pleural incision in intractable haemoptysis. See also *Lancet*, 1885, **1**, 894-95.

3227   LOWSON, David. 1850-1907
A case of pneumonectomy. *Brit. med. J.*, 1893, **1**, 1152-54.

      Partial lobectomy in pulmonary tuberculosis.

3228   TUFFIER, Théodore. 1857-1929
Chirurgie du poumon en particulier dans les cavernes tuberculeuses et la gangrène pulmonaire. Paris, *Masson*, 1897.

      Describes (p. 31) first cure of tuberculosis by removal of lung apex.

3229   MACEWEN, *Sir* William. 1848-1924
On some points in the surgery of the lung. *Brit. med. J.*, 1906, **2**, 1-7.

      Removal of left lung for tuberculosis, April 24, 1895. The patient was alive in 1940; see Bowman, A. K.: *Life and teaching of Sir William Macewen*, London, 1942, p. 344.

3230   BRAUER, Ludolph. 1865-1951
Die Behandlung der einseitigen Lungenphthisis mit künstlichem Pneumothorax (nach Murphy). *Münch. med. Wschr.*, 1906, **53**, 338-39.

      Brauer's method of producing artificial pneumothorax by the injection of nitrogen.

3231   ——. Indications du traitement chirurgical de la tuberculose pulmonaire. *Congr. Ass. franç. Chir.*, 1908, **21**, 569-74.

      First radical thoracoplasty.

3232   WILMS, Max. 1867-1918
Eine neue Methode zur Verengung des Thorax bei Lungentuberkulose. *Münch. med. Wschr.*, 1911, **58**, 777-78.

      Wilms's operation.

3233   GHON, Anton. 1866-1936
Der primäre Lungenherd bei der Tuberkulose der Kinder. Berlin & Wien, *Urban & Schwarzenberg*, 1912.

      Ghon described the anatomical distribution and development of the lesions in pulmonary tuberculosis among children – "Ghon's primary focus". His book was translated into English in 1916. *See also* No. 3224.

3234   SAUERBRUCH, ERNST FERDINAND. 1875-1951
Die Beeinflüssung von Lungenerkrankungen durch künstliche Lähmung des Zwerchfells (Phrenikotomie). *Münch. med. Wschr.*, 1913, **60**, 625-26.
Phrenicotomy in the treatment of pulmonary tuberculosis.

3235   JACOBAEUS, HANS CHRISTIAN. 1879-1937
Endopleurale Operationen unter der Leitung des Thorakoskops. *Beitr. Klin. Tuberk.*, 1916, **35**, 1-35.
Jacobaeus introduced adhesion-section with the cautery, to secure collapse in artificial pneumothorax.

3236   VAJDA, LUDWIG.
Ob das Pneumoperitoneum in der Kollapstherapie der beiderseitigen Lungentuberkulose angewandt werden kann? *Z. Tuberk.*, 1933, **67**, 371-75.
Introduction of artificial pneumoperitoneum for the treatment of bilateral pulmonary tuberculosis.

3237   BANYAI, ANDREW LADISLAUS. 1893-
Therapeutic pneumoperitoneum. A review of 100 cases. *Amer. Rev. Tuberc.*, 1934, **29**, 603-27.
Banyai combined artificial pneumoperitoneum with phrenic nerve paralysis.

3238   FREEDLANDER, SAMUEL OSCAR. 1893-
Lobectomy in pulmonary tuberculosis. Report of a case. *J. thorac. Surg.*, 1935, **5**, 132-42.
The modern era in lung resection for tuberculosis begins with the work of Freedlander. He performed the first planned lobectomy for pulmonary tuberculosis.

3239   SEMB, CARL BOYE. 1895-
Thoracoplasty with extrafascial apicolysis. *Acta chir. scand.*, 1935, Suppl. 37, pt. 2., 1-85.
"Semb's operation".

3240   KAYNE, GEORGE GREGORY. 1901-1945, PAGEL, WALTER TRAUGOTT ULRICH. 1898-1983, & O'SHAUGHNESSY, LAURENCE. 1900-1940
Pulmonary tuberculosis. Pathology, diagnosis, management and prevention. London, *Oxford Univ. Press.*, 1939.
Third edition, 1953, by W. Pagel, F. A. H. Simmonds, and N. Macdonald.

3241   LEHMANN, JÖRGEN. 1898-
Para-aminosalicylic acid in the treatment of tuberculosis. *Lancet*, 1946, **1**, 15-16.
p-Aminosalicylic acid used in pulmonary tuberculosis. See also his earlier paper in *Svenska LäkT.*, 1946, **43**, 2029-40.

History of Pulmonary Tuberculosis

See also 2354-2360, *History of Tuberculosis*

3242   PAGEL, WALTER TRAUGOTT ULRICH. 1898-1983
Die Krankheitslehre der Phthise in den Phasen ihrer geschichtlichen Entwicklung. *Beitr. Klin. Tuberk.*, 1927, **66**, 66-98.

3243   BROWN, LAWRASON. 1871-1937
        The story of clinical pulmonary tuberculosis. Baltimore, *Williams & Wilkins*,
        1941.

LARYNGOLOGY: RHINOLOGY

See also 5046-5072, DIPHTHERIA

3244   CODRONCHI, GIOVANNI BATTISTA. 1547-1628
        De vitiis vocis, libri duo. Francofurti, *apud heredes A. Wecheli*, 1597.
        First treatise devoted solely to diseases of the larynx. (*See also* No. 1718.)

3244.1 HABICOT, NICHOLAS. 1550-1624
        Question chirurgicale par laquelle il est demonstré que le chirurgien doit
        assurément practiquer l'opération de la bronchotomie, vulgairement dicte
        Laryngotomie ou perforation de la fluste tuyau du polmon. Paris, *J. Corrozet*, 1620.
            Four successful cases. Scott Stevenson and Guthrie (*see* No. 3342) state
        that Brasavola performed laryngotomy (in 1546) and that Sanctorius also
        did so.

3245   SCHNEIDER, CONRAD VICTOR. 1614-1680
        Liber primus [-liber quintus et ultimus] de catarrhis. 6 vols. Wittebergae, D.
        T. Mevii & E. Schumacheri, 1660-64.
            Schneider put an end to the idea that nasal mucus originated in the
        pituitary. He demonstrated anatomically and clinically that the mucous
        membrane lining the nose ("Schneider's membrane") is the source of nasal
        discharge, and discussed the tonsils, and ocular and lachrymal mucosa in
        the same way. As a result of his work the ancient doctrine of catarrhal
        diseases was overthrown, and the olfactory processes were definitely
        classified as cranial nerves.

3246   LOWER, RICHARD. 1631-1691
        Dissertatio de origine catarrhi in qua ostenditur illum non provenire a
        cerebro. In his: *Tractatus de corde*. Londini, *typ. J. Redmayne*, 1670, pp.
        221-39.
            With Schneider, Lower overthrew the idea that nasal mucus originated
        in the brain. This discovery localized nasal catarrh in the air passages and
        put an end to the use of many recipes for "purging the brain". The
        Dissertatio was reprinted separately in 1672 and this was reprinted with
        translation, biographical notes, and a bibliographical study by R. Hunter
        and I. Macalpine, 1963.

3248   VIRGILI, PEDRO. 1699-1776
        Sur une bronchotomie faite avec succès. *Mém. Acad. roy. Chir.*, 1743, **1**,
        pt. 3, 141-45.
            Virgili is said to have performed successful tracheotomy at Cadiz, for
        quinsy.

3249   JOURDAIN, ANSELME LOUIS BERNARD BERCHILLET. 1734-1816
        Recherches sur les différens moyens de traiter les maladies des sinus
        maxillaires, et sur les avantages qu'il y a, dans certains cas, d'injecter des
        sinus par le nez. *J. Méd. Chir. Pharm.*, 1767, **27**, 52-71, 157-74.

Jourdain reported a method of washing out the antrum of Highmore through the natural opening.

3250   PLAIGNAUD.
Observation sur un fongus du sinus maxillaire. *J. Chir. (Paris)*, 1791, **1**, 111-16.
First successful operation on a tumour of the maxillary sinus, 1789.

3251   DESCHAMPS, JACQUES LOUIS, *fils*. 1740-1824
Dissertation sur les maladies des fosses nasales et de leurs sinus. Paris, *chez Mme veuve Richard*, an XII, 1804.
First important work on diseases of the nose and nasal sinuses.

3252   CHEYNE, JOHN. 1777-1836
The pathology of the membranes of the larynx and bronchia. Edinburgh, *Mundell, Doig & Stevenson*, 1809.
Cheyne's important book deals mainly with the lesions of croup.

3253   CLOQUET, JULES HIPPOLYTE. 1787-1840
Osphrésiologie, ou traité des odeurs, du sens et des organes de l'olfaction. 2me. éd. Paris, *Méquignon-Marvis*, 1821.
An exhaustive work which discusses olfaction, diseases of the nose, membranous occlusion of the nostrils, deviations of the septum, rhinoplasty, coryza, vasomotor rhinitis, rhinorrhoea, etc. The first edition was entitled *Dissertation sur les odeurs...* (Paris, *Feugueray*, 1815).

3254   PORTER, WILLIAM HENRY. 1790-1861
Observations on the surgical pathology of the larynx and trachea. Dublin, *Hodges & M'Arthur*, 1826.
Porter was Professor of Surgery at the Royal College of Surgeons in Ireland. The above includes a description of "Porter's sign", tracheal tugging in aortic aneurysm.

3255   PHYSICK, PHILIP SYNG. 1768-1837
Description of a forceps, employed to facilitate the extirpation of the tonsil. *Amer. J. med. Sci.*, 1828, **2**, 116-17.
Invention of the modern tonsillotome.

3256   ALBERS, JOHANN FRIEDRICH HERMANN. 1805-1867
Die Pathologie und Therapie der Kehlkopfkrankheiten. Leipzig, *C. Cnobloch*, 1829.

3257   LUDWIG, WILHELM FRIEDRICH VON. 1790-1865
Ueber eine Form von Halsentzündung. *Med. Correspbl. württ. ärztl. Vereins*, 1836, **6**, 21-25.
"Ludwig's angina" first described. English translation and biographical note. *Bull. Hist. Med.*, 1939, **7**, 1115-26.

3257.1 RYLAND, FREDERICK. ?-1857
A treatise on the diseases and injuries of the larynx and trachea. London, *Longman*, 1837.
"A clear exposition of diseases of the larynx as known before the invention of the laryngoscope". (Scott Stevenson and Guthrie, *see* No. 3342).

3258   TROUSSEAU, ARMAND. 1801-1867, & BELLOC, HIPPOLYTE.
Traité pratique de la phthisie laryngée, de la laryngite chronique, et des maladies de la voix. Paris, *J. B. Baillière*, 1837.
A laryngological classic. English translation, 1839.

3259   MOTT, VALENTINE. 1785-1865
A nasal operation for the removal of a large tumour filling up the entire nostril and extending to the pharynx. *Amer. J. med. Sci.*, 1843, n.s. **5**, 87-91.
Removal of a fibrous growth from the nostril by division of the nasal and maxillary bones, July 8, 1841. Preliminary note in the same journal, 1842, **3**, 257.

3260   EHRMANN, CHARLES HENRI. 1792-1878
Sur une opération de laryngotomie pratiquée dans un cas de polype du larynx. *C. R. Acad. Sci. (Paris)*, 1844, **18**, 593, 709.
First removal of a laryngeal polyp.

3261   GREEN, HORACE. 1802-1866
A treatise on diseases of the air-passages. New York, *Wiley & Putnam*, 1846.
Green was the "father of laryngology" in America, and this is the first American treatise in otorhinolaryngology. He was the first successfully to introduce medicaments into the larynx, trachea, and bronchi for local treatment, using a probang, a curved instrument of whalebone 25 cm. long tipped with a tiny sponge. His claims in this connexion were the subject of bitter controversy in the U.S.A. It is possible that he somewhat exaggerated the efficacy of the methods he used and advocated.

3262   ——. On the surgical treatment of polypi of the larynx and oedema of the glottis. New York, *G. P. Putnam*, 1852.
Green was one of the few to remove a laryngeal tumour before the invention of the laryngoscope.

3263   BUCK, GURDON. 1807-1877
On the surgical treatment of morbid growths within the larynx, illustrated by an original case and statistical observations, elucidating their nature and forms. *Trans. Amer. med. Ass.*, 1853, **6**, 509-35.
Thyrotomy for removal of cancer of the larynx. The operation took place in May 1851, and the patient died in 1852.

3264   GROSS, SAMUEL DAVID. 1805-1884
A practical treatise on foreign bodies in the air-passages. Philadelphia, *Blanchard & Lea*, 1854.
First systematic study of the subject. In this celebrated work Gross laid down principles concerning symptoms which are still fundamental, despite the advent of roentgenology.

3265   COCK, EDWARD. 1805-1892
Case of pharyngotomy. *Lancet*, 1856, **1**, 125-26.
First pharyngotomy in England. Fuller report in *Guy's Hosp. Rep.*, 1858, 3 ser., **4**, 217.

3267   CATLIN, GEORGE. 1796-1872
The breath of life; or mal-respiration, and its effects upon the enjoyments and life of man. New York, *John Wiley*, 1861.

Catlin, the famous American artist, was the first in America to call attention to the bad effects of mouth-breathing. He based his book on observations of American Indian practices, and illustrated his book with humorous sketches.

3268   BRUNS, VIKTOR VON. 1812-1883
Die erste Ausrottung eines Polypen in der Kehlkopfshöhle durch Zerschneiden ohne blutige Eröffnung der Luftwege. Tübingen, *Laupp & Siebeck*, 1862.

First enucleation of a laryngeal polyp by the bloodless method.

3269   LEWIN, GEORG RICHARD. 1820-1896
Beiträge zur Laryngoscopie. *Allg. med. Cent.-Ztg*, 1862, **31**, 9, 33.

Lewin was probably the first to extirpate a laryngeal growth with the aid of the laryngoscope. Bruns claimed this distinction, but may not have heard of Lewin.

3270   GERHARDT, CARL ADOLPH CHRISTIAN JACOB. 1833-1902
Studien und Beobachtungen über Stimmbandlähmung. *Virchows Arch. path. Anat.*, 1863, **27**, 68-98, 296-321.

An important study of paralysis of the vocal cords was made by Gerhardt. He diagnosed the growth in the larynx of Friedrich III, Emperor of Germany, whose eventual death from this condition was to have such disastrous effects on German history.

3271   BRUNS, VIKTOR VON. 1812-1883
Die Laryngoskopie und die laryngoskopische Chirurgie. 1 vol. and atlas. Tübingen, *H. Laupp*, 1865.

Bruns claimed to have been the first to remove a tumour from the larynx with the aid of the laryngoscope.

3272   SANDS, HENRY BERTON. 1830-1888
Case of cancer of the larynx, successfully removed by laryngotomy. *N.Y. med. J.*, 1865, **1**, 110-26.

Laryngectomy for papillomata.

3273   TÜRCK, LUDWIG. 1810-1868
Klinik der Krankheiten des Kehlkopfes und der Luftröhre. 1 vol. and atlas. Wien, *W. Braumüller*, 1866.

On p. 295 is a classic description of laryngitis sicca – "Türck's trachoma".

3274   SOLIS-COHEN, JACOB DA SILVA. 1838-1927
Removal of a fibrous polyp from the inferior anterior surface of the right vocal cord with the aid of the laryngoscope. *Amer. J. med. Sci.*, 1867, n.s. **53**, 404-07; **54**, 565-66.

First successful operation for cancer of the larynx.

3275   VOLTOLINI, FRIEDRICH EDUARD RUDOLPH. 1819-1889
Die Anwendung der Galvanokaustik im Innern des Kehlkopfes und Schlundkopfes. Wien, *W. Braumüller*, 1867.

Voltolini was the first to use the galvanocautery in laryngeal surgery.

3276   MEYER, HANS WILHELM. 1825-1895
        Om adenoide Vegetationer i Naesesvaelgrummet. *Hospitalstidende*, 1868,
        11, 177-81.
            First clinical description of adenoid growths. For an English translation
        of the paper *see Med. -chir.* Trans., 1870, **53**, 191-215

3277   HEBRA, HANS VON. 1847-1902
        Ueber ein eigenthümliches Neugebilde an der Nase – Rhinosclerom. *Wien.
        med. Wschr.*, 1870, **20**, 1-5.

3278   MACKENZIE, *Sir* MORELL. 1837-1892
        Essay on growths in the larynx. London, *J. & A. Churchill*, 1871.
            An analysis of 100 of Mackenzie's own cases.

3279   GERHARDT, CARL ADOLPH CHRISTIAN JACOB. 1833-1902
        Ueber Diagnose und Behandlung der Stimmbandlähmung. *Samml. klin.
        Vortr.*, 1872, Nr. 36 (Inn. Med., Nr. 13), 271-82.
            See No. 3270. Continuing his study of laryngeal paralysis. Gerhardt
        proposed the term "cadaveric position" to indicate the position of the vocal
        cord in total paralysis of the larynx.

3280   SOLIS-COHEN, JACOB DA SILVA. 1838-1927
        Diseases of the throat: a guide to the diagnosis and treatment of affections
        of the pharynx, oesophagus, trachea, larynx, and nares. New York, *W. Wood
        & Co.*, 1872.
            First American textbook on oto-rhino-laryngology.

3281   FRAENKEL, BERNHARD. 1836-1911
        Fall von gutartiger Mycosis des Pharynx. *Berl. klin. Wschr.*, 1873, **10**, 94.
            Mycosis pharyngitis first reported.

3282   GUSSENBAUER, CARL. 1842-1903
        Ueber die erste durch Th. Billroth am Menschen ausgeführte Kehlkopf-
        Exstirpation und die Anwendung eines künstlichen Kehlkopfes. *Verh. dtsch.
        Ges. Chir.*, 1874, **3**, Heft 2, 76-89.
            The first complete excision of the larynx for cancer, performed by
        Billroth on 31 December 1873 and reported by Gussenbauer. The patient
        left the hospital in good state on 3 March 1874. Also published in *Arch. klin.
        Chir.*, 1874, **17**, 343-56.

3283   WENDT, HERMANN. 1838-1875
        Rareficirender, trockner Katarrh der Nasenrachenhöhle und des Rachens
        (Atrophie). *In* H. von Ziemssen's *Handbuch der speciellen Pathologie*,
        Leipzig, 1874, **7**, I, 313-16,.
            First description of "Tornwaldt's bursitis", an inflammatory condition of
        the pharyngeal tonsil, so named from the latter's description of it in 1885
        (*see* No. 3295).

3284   RIEGEL, FRANZ. 1843-1904
        Ueber respiratorische Paralysen. *Samml. klin Vortr.*, 1875, Nr. 95 (Inn.
        Med., Nr. 33), 761-96.
            Riegel distinguished between respiratory and phonatory paralysis of
        the larynx.

3285   FRAENKEL, BERNHARD. 1836-1911
Rhinitis chronica. Ozaena. Stockschnupfen. Stinknase. In Ziemssen's *Handbuch der speciellen Pathologie und Therapie*, Leipzig, 1876, **4**, I, 125-34.
     Fraenkel established ozaena as a clinical entity.

3285.1   BROWNE, ISAAC LENNOX. 1841-1902
The throat and its diseases, including associated affections of the nose and ear. London, *Baillière, Tindall & Cox*, 1878.

3286   JARVIS, WILLIAM CHAPMAN. 1855-1895
Surgical treatment of hypertrophic nasal catarrh. *Trans. Amer. laryng. Ass.*, (1880), 1881, **2**, 130-41.
     Jarvis nasal snare described.

3287   MACKENZIE, *Sir* MORELL. 1837-1892
A manual of diseases of the throat and nose. 2 vols. London, *J. & A. Churchill*, 1880-84.
     Mackenzie's great reputation earned him the title of Father of British Laryngology. In 1863 he founded the Golden Square Throat Hospital, London, the first hospital in the world devoted solely to diseases of the throat; he was also the founder of the *Journal of Laryngology*. He was called to attend Crown Prince Frederick, afterwards Emperor Ferderick III of Germany, who suffered from, and succumbed to, a cancer of the larynx. Mackenzie was much maligned by a section of the German medical profession for refusing to agree to operation until biopsy had been performed. Three specimens proved negative and operation was delayed until too late. Mackenzie's health was affected by his arduous duties on behalf of the Emperor and he died in 1892. The *Manual* was the standard work on the subject and had an important influence on the development of laryngology.

3288   SEMON, *Sir* FELIX. 1849-1921
Clinical remarks on the proclivity of the abductor fibres of the recurrent laryngeal nerve to become affected sooner than the adductor fibres, or even exclusively, in cases of undoubted central or peripheral injury or disease of the roots or trunks of the pneumogastric, spinal accessory, or recurrent nerves. *Arch. Laryng. (N.Y.)*, 1881, **2**, 197-222.
     "Semon's law". Of German birth, Semon became one of the greatest laryngologists in Britain. He developed the modern operation of laryngo-fissure for early cancer of the larynx.

3289   INGALS, EPHRAIM FLETCHER. 1848-1918
Deflection of the septum narium. *Trans. Amer. laryng. Ass.*, 1882, **4**, 61-69.
     Ingals devised the operation of partial excision of the septum for the correction of septum deflection.

3290   FRENCH, THOMAS RUSHMORE. 1849-1929
On photographing the larynx. *Trans. Amer. laryng. Ass.*, 1882, **4**, 32-35.
     French was the first to obtain good photographs of the larynx.

3291 ———. On a perfected method of photographing the larynx. *N. Y. med. J.*, 1884, **40**, 653-56.

By means of a special camera of his own invention French improved the method of photographing the larynx.

3292 JELINEK, EDMUND. 1852-1928
Das Cocain als Anästheticum und Analgeticum für den Pharynx und Larynx. *Wien. med. Wschr.*, 1884, **34**, col. 1334-37, 1364-67.

Cocaine first employed in laryngology.

3293 OGSTON, SIR ALEXANDER. 1844-1929
Trephining the frontal sinuses for catarrhal diseases. *Med. Chron.*, 1884, **1**, 235-38.

3294 LOEWENBERG, BENJAMIN BENNO. 1836-1905
Die Natur und die Behandlung der Ozaena. *Dtsch. med. Wschr.*, 1885, **11**, 5-8, 22-24.

Loewenberg described a bacillus found in the secretions of ozaena (*see* No. 3307). He made the first attempt at the treatment of this condition.

3295 TORNWALDT, GUSTAV LUDWIG [THORNWALDT]. 1843-1910
Über die Bedeutung der Bursa pharyngea für die Erkennung und Behandlung gewisser Nasenrachenraum-Krankheiten. Wiesbaden, *J. F. Bergmann*, 1885.

"Tornwaldt's [Thornwaldt's] bursitis", first described by Wendt (*see* No. 3283).

3296 FRAENKEL, BERNHARD. 1836-1911
Erste Heilung eines Larynx-Cancroids vermittelst Ausrottung per vias naturales. *Arch. klin. Chir.*, 1887, **34**, 281-86.

First successful intralaryngeal extirpation of a malignant growth.

3297 MIKULICZ-RADECKI, JOHANN VON. 1850-1905
Zur operativen Behandlung des Empyems der Highmorshöhle. *Arch. klin. Chir.*, 1887, **34**, 626-34.

Mikulicz's operation for the treatment of disease of the accessory nasal sinuses.

3298 BOSWORTH, FRANCKE HUNTINGTON. 1843-1925
A treatise on diseases of the nose and throat. 2 vols. New York, *W. Wood & Co.*, 1889-92.

Bosworth, a pioneer of American rhinology, advanced an important theory of the causation of ozaena.

3299 BRYAN, JOSEPH HAMMOND. 1856-1935
Diagnosis and treatment of abscess of the antrum. *J. Amer. med. Assoc.*, 1889, **13**, 478-83.

Classic paper on sinusitis.

3300   KRIEG, ROBERT. 1848-
Beiträge zur Resection der Cartilago quadrangularis narium zur Heilung
der Skoliosis septi. *Berl. klin. Wschr.*, 1889, **26**, 699-701, 717-20.
The operation of partial excision of the cartilage for the treatment of
deflections of the nasal septum was perfected by Krieg.

3301   LUC, HENRY. 1855-1925
Des abscès du sinus maxillaire. Paris, *Steinheil*, 1889.
See No. 3305.

3302   VOLTOLINI, FRIEDRICH EDUARD RUDOLPH. 1819-1889
Die ersten Operationen in der Kehlklopfshöhle vom Munde aus, bei der
Durchleuchtung des Kehlkopfes von aussen. *Dtsch. med. Wschr.*, 1889, **15**,
340-43.
The first laryngeal operation through the mouth with external illumi-
nation.

3303   AVELLIS, GEORG. 1864-1916
Klinische Beiträge zur halbseitigen Kehlkopflähmungen. *Berl. Klinik*, 1891,
Heft 40, 1-26.
"Avellis's syndrome", recurrent paralysis of the soft palate.

3304   BOSWORTH, FRANCKE HUNTINGTON. 1843-1925
Various forms of disease of the ethmoid cells. *N.Y. med. J.*, 1891, **54**, 505-
07.

3305   CALDWELL, GEORGE WALTER. 1834-1918
Diseases of the accessory sinuses of the nose, and an improved method of
treatment of suppuration of the maxillary antrum. *N.Y. med. J.*, 1893, **58**,
526-28.
Caldwell–Luc operation (*see also* No. 3301). Scanes Spicer independently devised a similar operation (*Brit. med. J.*, 1894, **2**, 1359-60).

3306   GRÜNWALD, LUDWIG. 1863-
Die Lehre von den Naseneiterungen. München, Leipzig, *J. F. Lehmann*, 1893.
Grünwald was the first to attempt the surgical treatment of nasal
suppuration and disease involving the ethmoid and sphenoid bones.
English translation, 1900.

3307   LOEWENBERG, BENJAMIN BENNO. 1836-1905
Le microbe de l'ozène. *Ann. Inst. Pasteur*, 1894, **8**, 292-317.
Loewenberg found a bacillus of the Friedländer group in ozaena.

3308   WINGRAVE, VITRUVIUS HAROLD WYATT. 1858-1938
The pathological and clinical features of atrophic rhinitis. *J. Laryng.*, 1894,
8, 96-110.
Classic paper on atrophic rhinitis (ozaena).

3308.1   PLAUT, HUGO KARL. 1858-1928
Studien zur bacteriellen Diagnostik der Diphtherie und der Anginen.
Dtsch. med. Wschr., 1894, **20**, 920-23.
"Plaut's angina". He noted the association of fusiform bacilli in ulcerat-
ing lesions of the tonsils. Vincent (*see* No. 3309) gave the first comprehen-
sive description of this condition.

3309   VINCENT, JEAN HYACINTHE. 1862-1950
Sur l'étiologie et sur les lésions anatomo-pathologiques de la pourriture d'hôpital. *Ann. Inst. Pasteur*, 1896, **10**, 488-510.

Vincent described a fusiform bacillus and a spirillum which, in association, were responsible for hospital gangrene. Later, in *Arch. int. Laryng.*, 1898, **11**, 44-48, he showed these two organisms to be present in "Vincent's angina".

3309.1   McBRIDE, PETER. 1854-1946
Photographs of a case of rapid destruction of the nose and face. *J. Laryng.*, 1897, **12**, 64-66.

Malignant granuloma of the nose first described.

3310   GLUCK, THEMISTOKLES. 1853-1942
Kehlkopfchirurgie und Laryngoplastik. *Therap. Gegenw.*, 1899, **40**, 169-79, 202-11.

Gluck improved the technique of laryngectomy.

3311   HAJEK, MARKUS. 1861-1941
Pathologie und Therapie der entzündlichen Erkrankungen der Nebenhöhlen der Nase. Leipzig, *F. Deuticke*, 1899.

Hajek, Professor of Laryngology in Vienna, particularly distinguished himself by his classic work on the acccessory nasal sinuses. A fifth American edition of the book appeared in 1926.

3312   PEREZ, FERNANDO. 1863-1935
Recherches sur la bactériologie de l'ozène. *Ann. Inst. Pasteur*, 1899, **13**, 937-50.

Perez isolated an organism from the nose of patients suffering from ozaena. He named it *Cocco-bacillus foetidus ozaenae* and considered it to be causally related to the disease.

3313   FREER, OTTO TIGER. 1857-1932
The correlation of deflections of the nasal septum with a minimum of traumatism. *J. Amer. med. Assoc.*, 1902, **38**, 636-42; 1903, **41**, 1391-98.

Improvement of Ingals's operation (*see* No. 3289).

3314   KILLIAN, GUSTAV. 1860-1921
Die Killian'sche Radicaloperation chronischer Stirnhöhleneiterungen. *Arch. Laryng. Rhin. (Berl.)*, 1903, **13**, 28-88.

Killian devised an operation for the treatment of pathological conditions in the nasal sinuses. It consists of excision of the anterior wall of the frontal sinus, removal of the diseased tissue, and formation of a permanent communication with the nose.

3315   ———. Die submucöse Fensterresektion der Nasenscheidewand. *Arch. Laryng. Rhin. (Berl.)*, 1904, **16**, 362-87.

3316   KUTTNER, ARTHUR. 1862-
Die entzündlichen Nebenhöhlenerkrankungen der Nase im Röntgenbild. Berlin, Wien, *Urban & Schwarzenberg*, 1908.

The first important work on the radiology of the accessory nasal sinuses.

3317   WAUGH, GEORGE ERNEST. 1875-1940
        A simple operation for the complete removal of tonsils, with notes on 900
        cases. *Lancet*, 1909, **1**, 1314-15.
             Waugh introduced blunt dissection tonsillectomy.

3318   WHILLIS, SAMUEL SHORT. 1870-1953, & PYBUS, FREDERICK CHARLES. 1882-1975
        The enucleation of tonsils with the guillotine. *Lancet*, 1910, **2**, 875-78.
             Reverse guillotine tonsillectomy.

3319.1 TROTTER, WILFRED BATTEN LEWIS. 1872-1939
        On certain clinically obscure malignant tumours of the naso-pharyngeal
        wall. *Brit. med. J.*, 1911, **2**, 1057-59.
             "Trotter's syndrome"; deafness, palatal paralysis, and facial neuralgia,
        usually due to a nasopharyngeal carcinoma.

3320   PLUMMER, HENRY STANLEY. 1874-1937
        Diffuse dilatation of the esophagus without anatomic stenosis (cardio
        spasm): a report of ninety-one cases. *J. Amer. med. Assoc.*, 1912, **58**, 2013-
        15.
             See No. 3321.

3321   VINSON, PORTER PAISLEY. 1890-1959
        A case of cardiospasm with dilatation and angulation of the esophagus.
        Med. Clin. N. Amer., 1919, **3**, 623-27.
             See also his later paper in *Minnesota Med.*, 1922, **5**, 107-08. The syn-
        drome of dysphagia, glossitis, and hypochromic anaemia has become
        known as the Plummer–Vinson syndrome (*see* No. 3320). A. Brown Kelly
        and D. R. Paterson drew attention to it in *J. Laryng.*, 1919, **34**, 285, 289.

3322   HOWARTH, WALTER GOLDIE. 1879-1962
        Operations on the frontal sinus. *J. Laryng. Otol.*, 1921, **36**, 417-21.
             Conservative treatment of sinusitis.

3323   ULLMANN, EGON VICTOR. 1894-
        On the aetiology of the laryngeal papilloma. *Acta oto-laryng. (Stockh.)*, 1923,
        5, 317-34.
             In this classic paper Ullmann reported the transmission of the virus to
        animals.

3324   LYNCH, ROBERT CLYDE. 1880-
        Technic of a pan-sinus operation. *South. med. J.*, 1924, **17**, 289-92.
             Independently of Howarth (No. 3322), Lynch devised an operation for
        the conservative treatment of sinusitis.

3325   PROETZ, ARTHUR WALTER. 1888-1966
        Displacement irrigation of nasal sinuses; a new procedure in diagnosis and
        conservative treatment. *Arch. Otolaryng. (Chicago)*, 1926, **4**, 1-13.
             Displacement method of treatment of nasal sinusitis; published in book
        form, St. Louis, 1931.

3326   THOMSON, *Sir* ST CLAIR. 1859-1943, & COLLEDGE, LIONEL. 1883-1948
        Cancer of the larynx. London, *Kegan Paul*, 1930.

Thomson's technique in the laryngofissure procedure for intrinsic cancer of the larynx was published in his *Diseases of the nose and throat*, London, 1911, pp. 732-37.

Laryngoscopy: Bronchoscopy

3327   BABINGTON, Benjamin Guy. 1794-1866
[Description of the glottiscope.] *Lond. med. Gaz.*, 1829, **3**, 555.
Babington was responsible for the introduction of laryngoscopy. He demonstrated a crude "glottiscope" to the Hunterian Society on March 18, 1829, but his effort attracted little attention.

3328   LISTON, Robert. 1794-1847
Practical surgery. London, *J. Churchill*, 1837.
On p. 350 Liston suggested the use of a mirror which could be used for viewing oedematous tumours of the larynx.

3329   GARCIA, Manuel Patricio Rodriguez. 1805-1906
Observations on the human voice. *Proc. roy. Soc. (Lond.)*, 1854-55, **7**, 399-410.
Garcia, a teacher of singing, invented the modern laryngoscope.

3330   TÜRCK, Ludwig. 1810-1868
Der Kehlkopfrachenspiegel und die Methode seines Gebrauches. *Z. k. k. Ges. Aerzte Wien*, 1858, n.F. **1**, 401-09.
Türck, at first sceptical of Garcia's laryngoscope, later adopted it and claimed from Czermak priority in its clinical employment; these two gentlemen fought one another bitterly for some years over this point.

3331   CZERMAK, Johann Nepomuk. 1828-1873
Physiologie Untersuchungen mit Garcia's Kehlkopfspiegel. *S. B. k. Akad. Wiss. Wien., math.-nat. Cl.*, 1858, **29**, 557-84.
Czermak was the first to demonstrate the utility of the laryngoscope invented by Garcia. He substituted artificial light for sunlight and made other improvements.

3332   ——. Ueber die Inspektion des Cavum pharyngo-nasale und der Nasenhöhle durch Choanen vermittelst kleiner Spiegel. *Wien. med. Wschr.*, 1859, **9**, 518-20; 1860, **10**, 257-61.
Czermak's method of exploring the nose and nasopharynx with small mirrors.

3333   TÜRCK, Ludwig. 1810-1868
Praktische Anleitung zur Laryngoscopie. Wien, *W. Braumüller*, 1860.

3334   MACKENZIE, *Sir* Morell. 1837-1892
The use of the laryngoscope in diseases of the throat; with an appendix on rhinoscopy. London, *R. Hardwicke*, 1865.

3335   KIRSTEIN, Alfred. 1863-1922
Autoskopie des Larynx und der Trachea. (Laryngoscopia directa, Euthyskopie, Besichtigung ohne Spiegel.) *Arch. Laryng. Rhin. (Berl.)*, 1895, **3**, 156-64.
First direct-vision laryngoscope.

3336   KILLIAN, Gustav. 1860-1921
       Ueber directe Bronchoskopie. *Münch. med. Wschr.*, 1898, **45**, 844-47.
       Introduction of direct bronchoscopy.

3337   JACKSON, Chevalier. 1865-1958
       Tracheo-bronchoscopy, esophagoscopy and gastroscopy. St. Louis,
       Laryngoscope Company, 1907.
       First textbook on endoscopy.

3338   KILLIAN, Gustav. 1860-1921
       Die Schwebelaryngoscopie. *Arch. Laryng. Rhin. (Berl.),* 1912, **26**, 277-317.
       Introduction of suspension laryngoscopy. English translation in 1914.

3338.1 JACKSON, Chevalier. 1865-1958, & JACKSON, Chevalier L. 1900-1961
       Diseases of the air and food passages of foreign body origin. Philadelphia,
       W.B. Saunders, 1937.
       One of the most comprehensive treatises on the subject ever published,
       with a 636-page appendix describing, and in most cases illustrating, 3266
       foreign bodies and how they were removed.

History of Laryngology and Rhinology

3339   CHAUVEAU, Claude.
       Histoire des maladies du pharynx. 5 vols. Paris, *J. B. Baillière,* 1901-06.

3340   KASSEL, Karl.
       Geschichte der Nasenheilkunde von ihren Anfängen bis zum 18.
       Jahrhundert. Vol. 1. Würzburg, *C. Kabitsch,* 1914.
       Continued through 18th and part of 19th century in articles in *Z. Laryngol.,*
       vols. 7, 8, 9, 11, 1914-23. Reprinted, 2 vols., Hildesheim, *G. Olms,* 1967, with
       title *Geschichte der Nasenheilkunde ... bis zum 19 Jahrhundert.*

3341   WRIGHT, Jonathan. 1860-1928
       A history of laryngology and rhinology. 2nd ed. Philadelphia, *Lea & Febiger,*
       1914.

3342   STEVENSON, Robert Scott. 1889-1967, & GUTHRIE, Douglas James. 1885-
       1975
       A history of oto-laryngology. Edinburgh., *E. & S. Livingstone,* 1949.
       From antiquity to the beginning of the 20th century. Reprinted, San
       Francisco, *Norman Publishing,* 1991.

3342.1 WILLEMOT, Jacques.
       Naissance et développement de l'oto-rhino-laryngologie dans l'histoire de
       la médecine. *Acta oto-rhino-laryng. belg.,* 1981, **35**, Suppl. II-.

OTOLOGY: AUDIOLOGY

3343   MERCURIALI, GIROLAMO. 1530-1606
De compositione medicamentorum; De morbis oculorum, & aurium....
Venetiis, *Apud Juntas*, 1590.

    The *De oculorum et aurium* represents the first "clinical" manual on diseases of the ear. Mercuriali was primarily concerned with treatment.

3343.1   CAPIVACCIO, GIROLAMO. ?-1589
Opera omnia quinque sectionibus comprehensa. Francofurti, *E. Paltheniana curante I. Rhodio*, 1603.

    Demonstration (Cap. I, p. 587-91) that some people who cannot hear by air conduction can do so by bone conduction.

3344   BONIFACIO, GIOVANNI.
L'arte de' cenni, con quale, formandosi favella visible, si tratta della muta eloquenza. Vicenza, *F. Grossi*, 1616.

    Bonifacio's sign-language for the deaf and dumb employed almost every part of the body for conversational purposes.

3345   BONET, JUAN PABLO. 1579-1633
Reduction de las letras, y arte para enseñar a ablar los mudos. Madrid, *F. Abarca de Angulo*, 1620.

    Bonet put into practice the "combined" system of teaching the deaf to speak and the dumb to communicate with others. He showed how the deaf could be taught to speak by reducing the letters to their phonetic value, and he advocated the use of finger-spelling. It is probable that he learned his system from Pedro Ponce de León (1510-84), another Spaniard, whose writings have been lost. English translation of the book, 1890.

3346   BULWER, JOHN. *fl.* 1654
Chironomia: or, the art of manuall rhetorique. London, *T. Harper*, 1644.

3347   ——. Chirologia; or the naturall language of the hand. Composed of the speaking motions, and discoursing gestures thereof. Whereunto is added Chironomia: or, the art of manuall rhetoricke. London, *T. Harper for H. Twyford*, 1644.

    Bulwer was the first Englishman to write about the teaching of deaf-mutes.

3348   WALLIS, JOHN. 1616-1703
Grammatica linguae anglicae. Cui praefigitur, de loquela sive sonorum formatione tractatus grammatico-physicus. Oxoniae, *excud. L. Lichfield, veneunt apud T. Robinson*, 1653.

    Wallis, a prominent teacher of deaf-mutes, classified the various sounds of the human voice. He taught by writing and gesture. He was Savilian Professor of Mathematics at Oxford.

3349   HOLDER, WILLIAM. 1616-1698
Elements of speech, an essay of inquiry into the natural production of letters; with an appendix concerning persons deaf and dumb. London, *T.N. for J. Martyn*, 1669.

    Includes a section on the education of deaf-mutes. Paracusis is described in the Appendix, p. 166.

3350　　DALGARNO, GEORGE. ?1626-1687
Didascalocophus or the deaf and dumb mans tutor, to which is added a discourse of the nature and number of double consonants: both which tracts being the first (for what the author knows) that have been published upon either of the subjects. Oxford, *T. Halton*, 1680.

　　Dalgarno considered that the deaf had an advantage over the blind in opportunities of learning languages. He invented an alphabet for the use of deaf-mutes.

3351　　DU VERNEY, GUICHARD JOSEPH. 1648-1730
Traité de l'organe de l'ouïe; contenant la structure, les usages et les maladies de toutes les parties de l'oreille. Paris, *E. Michallet*, 1683.
　　See No. 1545.

3352　　AMMAN, JOHANN KONRAAD. 1663-1730
Surdus loquens; seu, methodus, quâ qui surdus natus est loqui descere possit. Amstelaedami, 1692.

　　English translation, 1694, by John Wallis (*see* No. 3348).

3353　　——. Dissertatio de loquela, qua non solum vox humana, & loquendi artificium ex originibus suis erruunter. Amstelaedami, *J. Wolters*, 1700.

　　Amman's method of instructing deaf-mutes. He was one of the most successful of all teachers in this sphere. English translation, London, 1873.

3354　　GUYOT, EDMÉ GILLES. 1706-1786
[Instrument pour seringuer la trompe d'Eustache par la bouche.] *Hist. Acad. roy. Sci.*, 1724, Paris, 1726, 37.

　　Guyot, postmaster at Versailles, was the first to attempt catheterization of the Eustachian tube. This he did by way of the mouth.

3355　　CLELAND, ARCHIBALD.
Instruments proposed to remedy some kinds of deafness proceeding from obstructions in the external and internal auditory passages. *Phil. Trans.*, 1744, **41**, 848-51.

　　Cleland, an army surgeon, devised the method of catheterization of the Eustachian tube by way of the nose; he designed the instruments necessary for the operation.

3356　　WATHEN, JONATHAN.
A method proposed to restore the hearing, when injured from an obstruction of the tuba Eustachiana. *Phil. Trans.*, 1756, **49**, 213-22.

　　Wathen condemned Guyot's method of Eustachian catheterization and himself suggested a method of relieving catarrhal deafness by means of injections into the Eustachian tube through a catheter passed into the nose. Wathen was a surgeon practising in London.

3357　　PETIT, JEAN LOUIS. 1674-1750
Traité des maladies chirurgicales et des opérations qui leur conviennent. 3 vols., Paris, *P. F. Didot le jeune*, 1774.

　　Records (Vol, 1, pp.153, 160) the first successful operation for mastoiditis, performed by Petit in 1736. *See also* No. 3577.

3358   L'ÉPÉE, CHARLES MICHEL DE, *Abbé*. 1712-1789
Institution des sourds et muets, par la voie des signes méthodiques. Paris, *Nyon l'aîné*, 1776.

     Includes a reprint of the author's *Institution des sourds et muets; ou, recueil des exercices*. Paris, 1774.

3359   ——. La véritable manière d'instruire les sourds et muets. Paris, *Nyon l'aîné*, 1784.

     The Abbé de L'Épée met two deaf girls, decided to educate them, and soon had a class of 60 devoted pupils, whom he supported and amongst whom he lived. He based his methods on those of Bonet and Amman, and was the first to attach great importance to signs. This is l'Épée's most definitive work. It contains a reprint of No. 3358.

3360   GREEN, FRANCIS.
Vox oculis. A dissertation on the ... art of imparting speech to the naturally deaf; with a particular account of the academy of Messrs. Braidwood ... By a parent [F. Green]. London, 1783.

     Thomas Braidwood (1715-1806) founded the first British school for the deaf and dumb, in Edinburgh. His method consisted of a combination of lip-reading and signs.

3361   COOPER, *Sir* ASTLEY PASTON, *Bart*. 1768-1841
Farther observations on the effects which take place from the destruction of the membrana tympani of the ear; with an account of an operation for the removal of a particular species of deafness. *Phil. Trans.*, 1801, **91**, 435-50.

     Sir Astley Cooper reported three cases of Eustachian obstruction deafness relieved by perforation of the membrana tympani (myringotomy), an operation first performed by Eli, a quack, in 1760. Cooper's earlier paper on the subject appeared in vol. 90 of the *Phil. Trans.* He also demonstrated air and bone conduction by watch (precursor of Rinne's test). For this work he received the Copley Medal.

3362   SAUNDERS, JOHN CUNNINGHAM. 1773-1810
The anatomy of the human ear ... with a treatise on the diseases of the organ. London, *R. Phillips*, 1806.

     Saunders was the first to advise paracentesis in acute middle-ear suppuration.

3364   ITARD, JEAN MARIE GASPARD. 1774-1838
Traité des maladies de l'oreille et de l'audition. 2 vols. Paris, *Méquignon Marvis*, 1821.

     First of the modern textbooks on diseases of the ear, this work did much to establish otology on a firm basis. Itard described startle tests for the hearing of children and malingerers, and he developed an acumeter.

3365   SAISSY, JEAN ANTOINE. 1756-1822
Essai sur les maladies de l'oreille interne. Paris, *Baillière*, 1829.

     Saissy described a Eustachian bougie; he was probably the first to use this instrument. Besides dealing with the labyrinth, his book discusses diseases of the tympanum and Eustachian tube. English translation, Baltimore, 1829.

3366   KRAMER, WILHELM. 1801-1875
Erfahrungen über die Erkenntniss und Heilung der langwierigen
Schwerhörigkeit. Berlin, *Nicolai*, 1833.
    Kramer's first and best work. English translation, 1837.

3367   ——. Die Erkenntniss und Heilung der Ohrenkrankheiten. Berlin, *Nicolai*,
1835.
    Kramer was a pioneer German otologist.

3368   WEBER, ERNST HEINRICH. 1795-1878
De pulsu, resorptione, auditu et tactu. Lipsiae, *C. F. Koehler*, 1834.
    Weber's hearing test (p. 41).

3368.1   SCHMALZ, EDUARD. 1801-1871
Erfahrungen über die Krankheiten des Gehöres und ihre Heilung. Leipzig,
B. G. Teubner, 1846.
    Schmalz demonstrated the clinical significance of Weber's hearing test
(*see* No. 3368). He was a student of Weber.

3368.2   ——. Mémoire sur l'emploi de la fourchette tonique ou du diapason, pour
distinguer une dureté d'ouïe nerveuse de celle que est causée par une
obstruction. Bruxelles, *N. J. Gregoir*, 1849.
    Schwabach's hearing test (*see* No. 3389) was earlier employed by
Schmalz.

3369   WILDE, *Sir* WILLIAM ROBERT WILLS. 1815-1876
Practical observations on aural surgery and the nature and treatment of
diseases of the ear. London, *J. Churchill*, 1853.
    This work did more to place British otology on a scientific basis than
anything previously published. In his own words, Wilde "laboured to
rescue the treatment of ear diseases from empiricism and found it upon the
well-established laws of modern pathology, practical surgery, and rea-
sonable therapeutics". He showed the middle ear to be the site of origin of
most of the diseases of the ear. He is remembered for his method of treating
acute mastoiditis, using "Wilde's incision". The book was bitterly attacked
by Kramer – see especially *Lancet*, 1853, **2**, 446 – and also by Thomas
Wakley, editor of that journal. Wilde was the father of Oscar Wilde.

3370   RINNE, FRIEDRICH HEINRICH. 1819-1868
Beiträge zur Physiologie des menschlichen Ohres. *Vjschr. prakt. Heilk.*, 1855,
45, 71-123; **46**, 45-72.
    Rinne's test.

3371   FORGET, AMÉDÉE. 1811-1869
De la trépanation de l'apophyse mastoïde et des lésions morbides qui
rendent cette opération nécessaire. *Union méd.*, 1860, n.s. **6**, 193-200.
    Operative treatment of acute otitis by drainage through the antrum.

3372   MENIÈRE, PROSPER. 1799-1862
Mémoire sur des lésions de l'oreille interne donnant lieu à des symptomes
de congestion cérébrale apoplectiforme.
Gaz. méd. Paris, 1861, **16**, 88-89, 239-40, 379-80, 597-601.
    First description of aural vertigo ("Menière's syndrome"). First appeared
in summary form in *Bull. Acad. imp. Méd.*, 1860-61, **26**, 241, and in *Gaz.*

méd. Paris, 1861, **16**, 29, with title: Sur une forme de surdité grave dépendant d'une lésion de l'oreille interne. Menière's case was a symptomatic form of the disorder.

3373   TOYNBEE, JOSEPH. 1815-1866
The diseases of the ear; their nature, diagnosis, and treatment. London, *J. Churchill*, 1860.
    The foundation of aural pathology. In this book Toynbee described the method of removing the temporal bone and discussed the post mortem appearances in relation to the symptoms observed during life. He made over 2,000 dissections of the ear. His son, Arnold Toynbee, was the great social worker after whom the university settlement, Toynbee Hall, is named.

3374   TRÖLTSCH, ANTON FRIEDRICH VON. 1829-1890
Die Untersuchung des Gehörgangs und Trommelfells. Ihre Bedeutung. Kritik der bisherigen Untersuchungsmethoden und Angabe einer neuen. *Dtsch. Klinik*, 1860, **12**, 113-15, 121-23, 131-35, 143-46. 151-55.
    Invention of the modern otoscope.

3375   ———. Ein Fall von Anbohrung des Warzenfortsatzes bei Otitis interna mit Bemerkungen über diese Operation. *Virchows Arch. path. Anat.*, 1861, **21**, 295-314.
    The first modern mastoid operation was devised by von Tröltsch.

3376   ———. Die Krankheiten des Ohres. Würzburg, *Stahel*, 1862.
    Tröltsch was Professor of Otology as Würzburg. He was the founder of the *Archiv für Ohrenheilkunde*. English translation, 1874.

3377   POLITZER, ADAM. 1835-1920
Ueber ein neues Heilverfahren gegen Schwerhörigkeit in Folge von Unwegsamkeit der Eustachischen Ohrtrompete. *Wien. med. Wschr.*, 1863, **13**, 84-87, 102-04, 117-19, 148-52.
    Politzer's method of effecting permeability of the Eustachian tube.

3378   ———. Die Beleuchtungsbilder des Trommelfells im gesunden und kranken Zustande. Wien. *W. Braumüller*, 1865.
    Politzer was the first to obtain pictures of the membrana tympani by means of illumination. English translation, New York, 1869.

3378.1 BRUNTON, JOHN. 1836-1899
A new otoscope or speculum auris. *Lancet*, 1865, **2**, 617-18.
    Brunton's otoscope.

3378.2 LUCAE, AUGUST. 1835-1911
Ueber eine neue Methode zur Untersuchung des Gehörorgans zu physiologischen und diagnostischen Zwecken mit Hülfe des Interferenz Otoscopes. *Arch. Ohrenheilk.*, 1867, **3**, 186-229.
    Lucae described an interference otoscope, precursor of auditory impedance devices.

3379   VOLTOLINI, FRIEDRICH EDUARD RUDOLPH. 1819-1889
Die akute Entzündung des heutigen Labyrinthes, gewöhnlich für Meningitis cerebro-spinalis gehalten. *Mschr. Ohrenheilk.*, 1867, **1**, 9-14.

First description of "Voltolini's disease" – an acute painful inflammation of the internal ear, followed by fever, delirium, and loss of consciousness. Voltolini was the founder of the *Monatsschrift*.

3380   WREDEN, ROBERT ROBERTOVICH. 1837-1893
Sechs Fälle von Myringomykosis (Aspergillus glaucus Lk.). *Arch. Ohrenheilk.*, 1867, **3**, 1-21.
Wreden, otologist to the Czar, was the first to call special attention to otomycosis.

3381   LUCAE, AUGUST. 1835-1911
Die Schalleitung durch die Kopfknochen und ihre Bedeutung für die Diagnostik der Ohrenkrankheiten. *Würzburg, Stahel,* 1870.
Lucae was the first to study the transmission of sounds through the cranial bones for the purpose of diagnosing diseases of the ear.

3382   SCHWARTZE, HERMANN HUGO RUDOLF. 1837-1910, & EYSELL, ADOLPH. 1846-?
Ueber die künstliche Eröffnung des Warzenfortsatzes. *Arch. Ohrenheilk.*, 1873, n.F. **1**, 157-87.
These workers helped to revive the mastoid operation (which had fallen into disuse), placing it on a modern basis. They described the method of opening the ear by chiselling, "Schwartze's operation".

3383   CHARCOT, JEAN MARTIN. 1825-1893
Vertiges ab aure laesa (maladie de Menière). *Gaz. Hôp. (Paris)*, 1874, **47**, 73-74.
Charcot completed the description of the syndrome first described by Menière.

3384   HINTON, JAMES. 1822-1875
Atlas of the membrana tympani. London, *H. S. King.*, 1874.

3385   ——. The questions of aural surgery. London, *H. S. King*, 1874.
Hinton was one of the most eminent aural surgeons in England during the latter half of the 19th century, and the first Aural Surgeon to Guy's Hospital. In 1868 he performed the first operation for mastoiditis in England. He proved that aural polypus originated within the tympanum and that cholesteatomata might prove fatal by eroding the bone.

3386   BEZOLD, FRIEDRICH. 1842-1908
Erkrankungen des Warzentheiles. *Arch. Ohrenheilk.*, 1877, **13**, 26-68.
First clear description of mastoiditis.

3387   POLITZER, ADAM. 1835-1920
Lehrbuch der Ohrenheilkunde. 2 pts. Stuttgart, *F. Enke*, 1878-82.
Politzer was one of the greatest of all otologists. He was the first Professor of Otology in Vienna and his textbook was for many years the standard authority on the subject. English translation, 1883.

3387.1   ——. Ueber einen einheitlichen Hörmesser. *Arch. Ohrenheilk.*, 1877, **12**, 104-09.
Politzer described an acumeter.

3387.2 HARTMANN, ARTHUR. 1849-1931
Ueber eine neue Methode der Hörprüfung mit Hülfe elektrischer Ströme.
Arch. Anat. Physiol., Physiol. Abt., 1878, 155-57.
First audiometer.

3387.3 GELLÉ, MARIE ERNEST. 1834-1923
Les lésions nerveuses dans la surdité. *Trans. 7th int. med. Congr.*, London,
1881, **3**, 370-72.
Gellé described a test for determination of ossicular fixation.

3388 ZAUFAL, EMANUEL. 1833-1910
Sinusthrombose in Folge von Otitis media. [Trepanation des Proc. mastoid
mit Hammer und Meissel.] *Prag. med. Wschr.*, 1884, **9**, 474-75.
Improvement of the mastoid operation devised by Schwartze and
Eysell.

3389 SCHWABACH, DAGOBERT. 1846-1920
Ueber den Werth des Rinne'schen Versuches für die Diagnostik der
Gehörkrankheiten. *Z. Ohrenheilk.*, 1885, **14**, 61-148.
Schwabach's hearing test.

3389.1 HÖGYES, ENDRE. 1847-1906
Ueber Nystagmus und associierte Augenbewegungsversuche bei Hystero-
Epileptischen. *Pest. med.-chir. Presse*, 1886, **22**, 765, 787, 807, 827.
Rotational nystagmus described. First published in Magyar in *Orvosi
Hetilap*, 1886, **30**, 857, 889.

3390 ARNOLD, THOMAS. 1823-1900
Education of deaf-mutes. London, *Wertheimer, Lea & Co.*, 1888.
Includes a history of the subject.

3391 BERGMANN, ERNST VON. 1836-1907
Krankenvorstellung: Geheilter Hirnabscess. *Berl. klin. Wschr.*, 1888, **25**,
1054-56.
Radical mastoidectomy. (*See* No. 3392.)

3392 KÜSTER, ERNST GEORG FERDINAND VON. 1839-1930
Ueber die Gründsätze der Behandlung von Eiterungen in starrwandigen
Höhlen, mit besonderer Berücksichtigung des Empyems der Pleura.
Dtsch. med. Wschr., 1889, **15**, 254-57.
Küster and von Bergmann developed the operation of radical
mastoidectomy.

3393 STACKE, LUDWIG. 1859-1918
Indicationen, betreffend die Excision von Hammer und Amboss. *Verh. X.
int. med. Congr. Berlin*, 1890, **4**, xi Abt., 43-46.
Stacke introduced the operation of excision of the ossicles.

3394 ——. Weitere Mittheilungen über die operative Freilegung der
Mittelohrräume nach Ablösung der Ohrmuschel. *Berl. klin. Wschr.*, 1892,
29, 68-71.
Stacke did much to improve the surgery of the middle ear. He made
important modifications in the radical mastoidectomy operation of Küster
and von Bergmann.

3394.1   GRADENIGO, GIUSEPPE. 1859-1926
Sui caratteri clinici offerti dalle lesioni del nervo acustico. *Gazz. Osp. Clin.*,
1892, **13**, 1126.
    Gradenigo's test for tone decay. Translation in *Arch. Otol. (N.Y.)*, 1893,
22, 213-15.

3394.2   LANE, *Sir* WILLIAM ARBUTHNOT. 1856-1943
Antrectomy as a treatment for chronic purulent otitis media. *Arch. Otol.
(N.Y.)*, 1892, **21**, 118-24.
    Mastoidectomy for the efficient drainage of the results of middle ear
suppuration.

3395   POLITZER, ADAM. 1835-1920
On a peculiar affection of the labyrinthine capsule as a frequent cause of
deafness. *Trans. 1st Panamer, med. Congr.*, (1893), 1895, pt. 3, 1607-08.
    First report of otosclerosis as a separate clinical entity.

3396   BEZOLD, FRIEDRICH. 1842-1908
Ueber die funktionelle Prüfung des menschlichen Gehörorgans. 3 vols.
Wiesbaden, *J. F. Bergmann*, 1897-1909.
    Bezold introduced important tests for audition.

3397   PASSOW, ADOLF. 1859-1926
Verh. dtsch. otol. Ges., 1897, **6**, 143.
    First attempt at improving hearing by fenestration. No title; forms part
of a paper by R. Passe.

3398   GRADENIGO, GIUSEPPE. 1859-1926
Sulla leptomeningite circonscritta e sulla paralisi dell abducente di origine
otitica. *G. roy. Accad. Med. Torino*, 1904, 4 ser., **10**, 59-64, 361-67.
    "Gradenigo's syndrome" – acute otitis media followed by abductor
paralysis. Translation of the paper is in the German *Arch. Ohrenheilk.*, 1904,
62, 255-70.

3399   KELLER, HELEN ADAMS. 1880-1968
The story of my life. New York, *Grosset & Dunlap*, 1905.
    Helen Keller became blind and deaf at the age of 19 months, as the result
of an illness. Her education was a triumph of patience and skill on the part
of her teacher, Anne M. Sullivan, and a demonstration of the great
possibilities in the teaching of the blind-deaf. Keller studied French,
German, Latin, Greek, arithmetic, algebra, geometry, history, poetry, and
literature.

3400   BÁRÁNY, ROBERT. 1876-1936
Ueber die vom Ohrlabyrinth ausgelöste Gegenrollung der Augen bei
Normalhörenden. *Arch. Ohrenheilk.*, 1906, **68**, 1-30.
    Bárány's caloric test for labyrinthine function.

3401   ——. Untersuchungen über den vom Vestibularapparat des Ohres
reflektorisch ausgelösten Rhythmischen und seine Begleiterscheinungen.
Mschr. Ohrenheilk., 1906, **40**, 193-297; **41**, 477-526.
    Bárány's pointing test for the localization of circumscribed cerebellar
lesions. Republished in book form, Berlin, 1906. He was awarded the
Nobel Prize in 1914 for his work on the vestibular apparatus. Bárány's *Die*

Geschichte der Physiologie des Vestibular Apparates seit 1850 published in Politzer's *Geschichte der Ohrenheilkunde*, Vol. 2 (*see* No. 3413) was translated into English with extensive commentary by D. G. Pappas, *Ann. Otol. Rhin. Larygngol.*, 1984, **93**, Suppl. 110.

3402 ———. Vestibularapparat und Zentralnervensystem. *Med. Klin.*, 1911, **7**, 1818-21.
 "Bárány's syndrome" – unilateral deafness, vertigo, and pain in the occipital region.

3402.1 LOMBARD, ETIENNE. 1868-
 Contribution à la seméiologie de la surdité; un nouveau signe pour en dévoiler la simulation. *Bull. Acad. Méd. (Paris)*, 1910, 3 sér., **64**, 127-30.
 Lombard's test for simulated unilateral deafness.

3403 JENKINS, GEORGE JOHN. -1939
 Otosclerosis: certain clinical features and experimental operative procedures. *17th Int. Congr. Med.*, London, 1913, Sect. **16**, 609-18.
 Jenkins suggested the modern fenestration operation of otosclerosis.

3403.1 BALLANCE, *Sir* CHARLES ALFRED. 1856-1926, & GREEN, CHARLES DAVID. 1862-1937
 Essays on the surgery of the temporal bone. 2 vols. London, *Macmillan*, 1919.
 Includes history of the development of temporal bone surgery.

3404 HOLMGREN, GUNNAR. 1875-1954
 Some experiences in the surgery of otosclerosis. *Acta. oto-laryng. (Stockh.)*, 1923, **5**, 460-66.
 Holmgren's fenestration operation.

3405 GRAY, ALBERT ALEXANDER. 1869-1936
 Atlas of otology illustrating the normal and pathological anatomy of the temporal bone. 2 vols. Glasgow, *Maclehose (Jackson)*, 1924-33.

3405.1 POHLMAN, AUGUSTUS GROTE. 1879-, & KRANZ, FREDERICK WILLIAM. 1887-
 Binaural minimum audition in a subject with ranges of deficient acuity. *Proc. Soc. exp. Biol. (N.Y.)*, 1924, **21**, 335-37.
 First demonstration of the phenomenon of loudness recruitment.

3406 DANDY, WALTER EDWARD. 1886-1946
 Menière's disease; its diagnosis and a method of treatment. *Arch. Surg. (Chicago)*, 1928, **16**, 1127-52.
 Dandy's operation for relief of Menière's syndrome.

3407 MAYER, ERNST GEORG. 1893-
 Otologische Röntgendiagnostik. Wien, *J. Springer*, 1930.
 Includes a brief history of the subject.

3408 SOURDILLE, MAURICE LOUIS JOSEPH MARIE. 1885-1961
 New technique in the surgical treatment of severe and progressive deafness from otosclerosis. *Bull. N.Y. Acad. Med.*, 1937, **13**, 673-91.
 First successful attempt to restore hearing in otosclerosis by fenestration.

3409   HALLPIKE, Charles Skinner. 1900-1979, & CAIRNS, Sir Hugh William Bell. 1896-1952
        Observations on the pathology of Menière's syndrome. *Proc. roy. Soc. Med.*, 1938, **31**, 1317-36.
            Hallpike and Cairns were first to describe the characteristic histological changes in Menière's disease. Also published in *J. Laryng. Otol.*, 1938, **53**, 625-55.

3410   LEMPERT, Julius. 1890-
        Improvement of hearing in cases of otosclerosis: a new, one-stage surgical technic. *Arch. Otolaryng. (Chicago)*, 1938, **28**, 42-97.
            Lempert's fenestration operation.

3411   KOPETZKY, Samuel Joseph. 1876-1950
        History and present status of operations on the labyrinthine capsule for otosclerosis. *Surg. Gynec. Obstet.*, 1941, **72**, 466-89.
            Kopetzky improved the technique of the fenestration operation. The above has a useful history of the development of this operation. See also his earlier papers in *Ann. Otol. (St. Louis)*, 1930, **39**, 996; 1931, **40**, 157.

3412   SHAMBAUGH, George Elmer. 1903-
        The surgical treatment of deafness. *Illinois med. J.*, 1942, **81**, 104-08.
            Shambaugh improved the technique of the fenestration operation. See also *Ann. Otol. (St. Louis)*, 1942, **51**, 817-25.

3412.1 EWING, Irene Rosetta. 1883-1959, & EWING, Sir Alexander William Gordon. 1896-1980
        The ascertainment of deafness in infancy and early childhood. *J. Laryng. Otol.*, 1944, **59**, 309-33.
            Tests of hearing in children.

3412.2 METZ, Otto. 1905-
        The acoustic impedance measured on normal and pathological ears. Orientating studies on the applicability of impedance measurement. *Acta oto-laryng. (Stockh.)*, 1946, Suppl. 63.
            The modern impedance test was developed by Metz.

3412.3 BÉKÉSY, Georg von. 1899-1972
        A new audiometer. *Acta oto-laryng. (Stockh.)*, 1947, **35**, 411-22.
            Semi-automatic (Békésy) audiometer.

3412.4 DAGGETT, William Ingledew. 1900-1980
        Operative treatment of chronic suppurative otitis media. *J. Laryng. Otol.*, 1949, **63**, 635-46.
            Tympanoplasty.

3412.5 ROSEN, Samuel. 1897-
        Mobilization of the stapes to restore hearing in otosclerosis. *New York St. J. Med.*, 1953, **53**, 2650-53.
            Transmeatal exposure of the middle ear.

3412.6 BOCCA, Ettore. 1914- , *et al.*
        A new method for testing hearing in temporal lobe tumours. Preliminary report. *Acta oto-laryng. (Stockh.)*, 1954, **44**, 219-21.

The first tests for disorders of central auditory function were developed by Bocca, C. Calearo, and V. Cassinari.

3412.7   SHEA, John Joseph. 1924-
Fenestration of the oval window. *Ann. Otol. (St. Louis)*, 1958, **67**, 932-51.
Stapedectomy.

History of Otology

3413   POLITZER, Adam. 1835-1920
Geschichte der Ohrenheilkunde. 2 vols. Stuttgart, *F. Enke*, 1907-13.

It is fitting that Politzer should have been the greatest historian of otology. He was Professor of Otology in Vienna and his teaching had great influence upon the advancement of the subject. The *Geschichte* is a masterpiece of historical research. Reprinted, Hildesheim, 1967. English translation of vol. 1, Phoenix, *Columnella Press*, 1981.

3415   STEVENSON, Robert Scott. 1889-1967, & GUTHRIE, Douglas James. 1885-1975
A history of oto-laryngology. Edinburgh, *E. & S. Livingstone*, 1949. Reprinted, with new introduction by D. Pappas, San Francisco, *Norman Publishing*, 1991.

3415.1   BENDER, Ruth Elaine.
The conquest of deafness: a history of the long struggle to make possible normal living to those handicapped by lack of normal hearing. Cleveland, *Western Reserve University Press*, 1960.
Education for the deaf.

3415.2   FELDMANN, Harald. 1926-
Die geschichtliche Entwicklung der Hörprüfungsmethoden. Kurze Darstellung und Bibliographie von den Anfängen bis zur Gegenwart. Stuttgart, *G. Thieme*, 1960.
English translation, 1970.

3415.21   BERGER, Kenneth W.
The hearing aid: its operations and development. Third edition. Detroit, *National Hearing Aid Society*, 1984.
Includes a comprehensive listing of manufacturers and the models each produced.

3415.22   GUERRIER, Yves, & MOUNIER-KUHN, Pierre.
Histoire des maladies de l'oreille, du nez et de la gorge. Les grandes étapes de l'oto-rhino-laryngologie. Paris, *Roger Dacosta*, [1980].

3415.3   WILLEMOT, Jacques, *et al.*
Naissance et développement de l'oto-rhino-laryngologie dans l'histoire de la médecine. *Acta-oto-rhino-laryng. belg.*, 1981, **35**, Suppl. II-.

DISEASES OF THE DIGESTIVE SYSTEM

3416   JOHN *of Arderne*. 1307-1370
Treatise of the fistulae in the fundament, and other places *in* Francisco Arceo,
A most excellent and compendious method of curing woundes in the head,
and in other partes of the body...London, *Thomas East*, 1588.
   John of Arderne's most important contribution to surgery was his
operation for the cure of anal fistula. This was written about 1376. At one
time John of Arderne practised at Newark-on-Trent; he moved to London
in 1370. See the edition by Sir D'Arcy Power, *Treatises of fistula in ano,
haemorrhoids, and clysters*, London, *Kegan Paul*, 1910. *See also* No. 5557.

3417   DONATI, Marcello. 1538-1602
De medica historia mirabili. Mantuae, *per Fr. Osanam*, 1586.
   Lib. IV, Cap. iii, page 196: First recorded case of gastric ulcer. *See* Nos.
4011.2 & 6377.

3418   LITTRÉ, Alexis. 1658-1726
Diverses observations anatomiques. *Hist. Acad. roy. Sci. (Paris)*, (1710),
1732, 36-37.
   Littré was first to suggest colostomy in intestinal obstruction – "Littré's
operation".

3419   BLAIR, Patrick. 166?-1728
An account of the dissection of a child. *Phil. Trans.*, 1717, **30**, 631-32.
   First description of congenital hypertrophic pyloric stenosis. Reprinted
in M. M. Ravitch, The story of pyloric stenosis. *Surgery*, 1960, **48**, 1117-1143.

3420   RAWLINSON, Christopher.
A preternatural perforation found in the upper part of the stomach, with the
symptoms it produced. *Phil. Trans.*, 1727, **35**, 361-62.
   First reported case of perforating gastric ulcer.

3421   STAHL, Georg Ernst. 1660-1734
De motus hemorrhoidalis, et fluxus hemorrhoidum. Paris, *Horth-hemels*,
1730.
   A classic work on haemorrhoids.

3422   CALDER, James.
Two examples of children born with preternatural conformations of the
guts. *Med. Essays Obs. Edinb.*, 1733, **1**, 203-06.
   First description of congenital atresia of the ileum.

3423   VELSE, Cornelius Henrik.
De mutuo intestinorum ingressu. Lugduni Batavorum, *J. Luzac*, 1742.
   First recorded successful operation for intussusception in an adult. The
paper is also included in Haller's Disputationes, vol. 1.

3424   HAMBURGER, Georg Erhard. 1697-1755
De ruptura intestini duodeni. Jenae, *Lit Ritterianis*, [1746].
   First description of duodenal ulcer.

3424.1   KALTSCHMIED, CARL FRIEDRICH. 1706-1769
De tumore scirrhoso trium cum quadrante librarum glandulae parotidis
extirpato. Jenae, *Lit. Tennemannianis*, 1752.
First description of parotid tumour.

3424.2   POTT, PERCIVALL. 1714-1788
Remarks on the disease commonly called a fistula in ano. London,
Hawes..., 1765.
Probably the greatest English classic of colon–rectal surgery. Pott
recommended the practice of simple division rather than the newer, more
complicated methods proposed by Cheselden and Le Dran, and audaciously
pointed out that there were lessons regular practitioners might learn from
quacks apropos of this subject.

3425   ARMSTRONG, GEORGE. 1719-1789
An account of the diseases most incident to children, from their birth till the
age of puberty. London, *T. Cadell*, 1777.
Page 49: Important description of congenital hypertrophic pyloric
stenosis.

3426   BEARDSLEY, HEZEKIAH. 1748-1790
Case of a scirrhus in the pylorus of an infant. *Cases Obs. med. Soc. New
Haven Co.*, 1788, 81-84.
First American case report on congenital hypertrophic pyloric stenosis.
*Cases and observations by the Medical Society of New Haven County...*was
the first American medical periodical. Only one volume was published.
Beardsley's paper was reprinted in *Arch. Pediat.*, 1903, **20**, 355-57. and
also in M.M. Ravitch, The story of pyloric stenosis, *Surgery*, 1960, **48**, 1117-
1143.

3427   BAILLIE, MATTHEW. 1761-1823
The morbid anatomy of some of the most important parts of the human
body. London, *J. Johnson & G. Nicol*, 1793.
Page 87: First clear description of the morbid anatomy and symptoms
of gastric ulcer. *See also* Nos. 2281, 2736, 3167.1, 3218.

3428   PENADA, JACOPO. 1748-1828
Saggio d'osservazioni, e memoire sopra alcuni case singolari riscontrati
nell'esercizio della medicina, e della anatomia pratica. Padova, *Penada*,
1793.
Includes (pp. 33-56) an account of perforating duodenal ulcer.

3428.1   BAYFORD, DAVID. 1739-1790
An account of a singular case of obstructed deglutition. *Mem. med. Soc.
Lond.*, 1794, **2**, 275-86.
Dysphagia lusoria first reported. See the account by N. Asherson in
Ann. roy. Coll. Surg. Eng., 1979, **61**, 63-67.

3429   DURET, PIERRE. ?1745-1851
Observation sur un enfant né sans anus, et auquel il a été fait une ouverture
pour y suppléer. *Rec. périod. Soc. Méd. Paris*, 1798, **4**, 45-50.
First successful construction of artificial anus, for congenital atresia,
Oct. 20, 1793.

3430   FINE, Pierre. 1760-1814
        Mémoire et observation sur l'entérotomie. *Ann. Soc. Méd. prat. Montpellier,*
        1805, **6**, 34-54.
            The first recorded colostomy for intestinal obstruction was performed
        by Fine in 1797. The patient survived 3.5 months.

3430.1 SMITH, Thomas. 1785-1831
        An essay on wounds of the intestines. Philadelphia, *Thomas T. Stiles,* 1805.
            The first serious attempt at repairing intestinal injuries in America, and
        the first use of dogs for experimental surgery in America.

3431   MERREM, Daniel Carl Theodor. 1790-1859
        Animadversiones quaedam chirurgicae experimentis in animalibus factis
        illustratae. Giessiae, *Tasché et Mueller,* 1810.
            Experimental excision of the pylorus.

3432   PHYSICK, Philip Syng. 1768-1837
        Account of a new mode of extracting poisonous substances from the
        stomach. *Eclectic Repert.,* 1812-13, **3**, 111, 381.
            Physick was the first, in 1805, to use a stomach tube for gastric lavage
        in a case of poisoning. He acknowledged the priority of Monro *secundus*
        in the invention of a similar instrument in 1767. For history of the stomach
        tube, see R. H. Major, *Ann. med. Hist.,* 1934, n.s. **6**, 500-09.

3433   TRAVERS, Benjamin. 1783-1858
        An inquiry into the process of nature in repairing injuries of the intestines.
        London, *Longman,* 1812.
            Travers's researches on intestinal sutures recorded the first accurate
        knowledge on this subject.

3433.1 DAVIDGE, John Beale. 1768-1829
        Extirpation of the parotid gland. *Baltimore phil. J. & Rev.,* 1823, **1**, 165-183.
            Although Béclard and possibly others may have extirpated the parotid
        before Davidge, this was the first published case.

3434   BÉCLARD, Pierre Augustin. 1785-1825
        Extirpation de la parotide. *Arch. gén. Méd.,* 1824, **4**, 60-66.
            First excision of the parotid, 1823.

3435   LEMBERT, Antoine. 1802-1851
        Mémoire sur l'entéroraphie avec la description d'un procédé nouveau
        pour pratiquer cette opération chirurgicale. *Rep. gén. Anat. Physiol. path.,*
        1826, **2**, 100-07.
            Description of what is now known as Lembert's suture, which ensures
        that serous surface is applied to serous surface in suturing intestine – the
        foundation of all modern gastric and intestinal surgery. Dieffenbach (*see*
        No. 3441) was the first successfully to employ Lembert's method.

3436   PHYSICK, Philip Syng. 1768-1837
        Extracts from an account of a case in which a new and peculiar operation
        for artificial anus was performed. *Philad. J. med. phys. Sci.,* 1826, **13**, 199-
        202.
            Physick's operation for artificial anus – colocutaneous fistula formed as
        a result of mortification from a strangulated hernia.

3437   DUPUYTREN, GUILLAUME, *le baron*. 1777-1835
Mémoire sur une méthode nouvelle pour traiter les anus accidentels. *Mém. Acad. roy. Méd. (Paris)*, 1828, Sect. Méd., **1**, 259-316.
Dupuytren invented an enterotome to perform his operation for artificial anus.

3438   ———. Abcès développé dans le petit bassin. *Rev. méd. franç. étrang.*, 1829, **1**, 367-68.
"Dupuytren's abscess" of the right iliac fossa.

3439   JOBERT DE LAMBALLE, ANTOINE JOSEPH. 1799-1867
Traité théorique et pratique des maladies chirurgicales du canal intestinal. 2 vols. Paris, *Mme. Auger-Méquignon*, 1829.
Jobert, famous French surgeon, made his reputation on this book. He was at one time Consulting Physician to Louis XVIII.

3440   BRODIE, *Sir* BENJAMIN COLLINS, *Bart*. 1783-1862
Lectures on diseases of the rectum. III. Preternatural contraction of the sphincter ani. *Lond. med. Gaz.*, 1835, **16**, 26-31.
"Brodie's pile". Reprinted in *Med. Classics*, 1938, **2**, 929-40.

3440.1 WILSON, JOHN R.W.
A case of introsussception in which an operation was successfully resorted to...in December, 1831. *Transylvania J. Med. Assoc. Sci.*, 1835, **18**, 362 (only).
First operation for intussusception in the United States, performed in Rutherford County, Tennessee. The patient was a negro slave; the operation was a complete success. Reported by Wilson's pupil, W.W. Thompson.

3441   DIEFFENBACH, JOHANN FRIEDRICH. 1792-1847
Glückliche Heilung nach Ausscheidung eines Theiles des Darms und Netzes. *Wschr. ges. Heilk.*, 1836, 401-13.
First account of a resection in which Lembert's suture was successfully employed.

3441.1 BUSHE, GEORGE MACARTNEY. 1793-1836
A treatise on the malformations, injuries and diseases of the rectum and anus. Text and atlas. New York, *French & Adlard*, 1837.
The first American treatise on colon–rectal surgery.

3442   AMUSSAT, JEAN ZULÉMA. 1796-1856
Mémoire sur la possibilité d'établir un anus artificiel dans la région lombaire sans pénétrer dans le péritoine. Paris, *G. Baillière*, 1839.
In 1839 Amussat performed the first lumbar colostomy for obstruction of the colon ("Amussat's operation"). His work established lumbar colostomy as the method of choice. Translated in *Dis. Colon. Rect.*, 1983, **26**, 483-87. *See* No. 3443.

3443   PILLORE, H.
Opération d'anus artificiel, par la méthode de Littre, sur un homme adulte qui a survécu vingt-huit jours. In: Amussat, J. Z., *Mémoire sur la possibilité d'établir un anus artificiel*, Paris, 1839, pp. 85-88.

Pillore performed caecostomy in 1776, the patient surviving 28 days. Amussat went to considerable trouble to find the document describing the operation. *See* No. 3442.

3444   BÉRARD, AUGUSTE. 1802-1846
Maladies de la glande parotide et de la région parotidienne. Paris, *Germer-Baillière*, 1841.
First important treatise on parotid tumours.

3445   CURLING, THOMAS BLIZARD. 1811-1888
On acute ulceration of the duodenum, in cases of burn. *Med.-chir. Trans.*, 1842, **25**, 260-81.
"Curling's ulcer". Although not first to report duodenal ulcers as a complication of burns, Curling correlated the work of previous writers on the subject and directed attention to it.

3446   GROSS, SAMUEL DAVID. 1805-1884
An experimental and critical inquiry into the nature and treatment of wounds of the intestines. Louisville, *Prentice & Weissinger*, 1843.
Reports of a series of experiments upon dogs to determine the best way to treat intestinal wounds. First published in *West. J. Med. Surg,*, 1843. **7**, 1-50, [81]-141, [161]-224.

3447   REYBARD, JEAN FRANÇOIS. 1790-1863
Mémoire sur une tumeur cancéreuse affectant l'iliaque du colon; ablation de la tumeur et de l'intestin; réunion directe et immédiate des deux bouts de cet organe. Guérison. *Bull. Acad. roy. Méd. (Paris)*, 1844, **9**, 1031-43.
First intestinal resection for cancer.

3448   WATSON, JOHN. 1807-1863
Practical observations on organic obstruction of the oesophagus; preceded by a case which called for oesophagotomy and subsequent opening of the trachea. *Amer. J. med. Sci.*, 1844, n.s. **8**, 309-31.
First oesophagotomy for relief of stricture of the oesophagus.

3449   BIRD, GOLDING. 1814-1854, & HILTON, JOHN. 1804-1878
Case of internal strangulation of intestine relieved by operation. *Med.-chir. Trans.*, 1847, **30**, 51-67.
Records the first operation for intestinal strangulation of the small intestine by Hilton at Guy's Hospital. No anaesthetic was used; the patient died nine hours afterwards.

3450   LEIDY, JOSEPH. 1823-1891
On the existence of Entophyta in healthy animals, as a natural condition. *Proc. Acad. nat. Sci. (Philad.)*, 1848-49, **4**, 225-33.
Discovery of the bacterial flora of the intestines.

3451   SEDILLOT, CHARLES EMMANUEL. 1804-1883
Opération de gastrostomie pratiquée pour la première fois le 13 novembre 1849. *Gaz. méd. Strasbourg*, 1849, **9**, 366-77.
First gastrostomy.

3452   FENGER, Carl Emil. 1814-1884
        Ueber Anlegung einer künstlichen Magenöffnung am Menschen durch
        Gastrotomie. *Virchows Arch. path. Anat.*, 1854, **6**, 350-84.
        Fenger's operation.

3453   BERGERON, Etienne Jules. 1817-1900
        Note sur l'emploi du chlorate de potasse dans le traitement de la stomatite
        ulcéreuse. *Rec. Mém. Méd. mil.*, 1855, 2 sér., **16**, 1-46.
        Classic description of ulcero-membranous stomatitis and its treatment.

3454   BRINTON, William. 1823-1867
        On the pathology, symptoms, and treatment of ulcer of the stomach.
        London, *J. Churchill*, 1857.
        A comprehensive account of peptic ulcer; includes a review of the
        results of more than 7,000 post mortems.

3455   MALMSTEN, Pehr Henrik. 1811-1883
        Infusorier, sasom intestinaldjur hos menniskan. *Hygiea (Stockh.)*, 1857, **19**,
        491-501.
        Discovery of *Balantidium coli*, the first parasitic protozoon to be dis-
        covered and recognized as such. German translation in *Virchows Arch.
        path. Anat.*, 1857, **12**, 302-09. English translation in Kean *et al.* (No. 2268.1).

3456   MIDDELDORPF, Albrecht Theodor. 1824-1868
        De polypis oesophagi atque de tumore ejus generis primo prospere
        exstirpato. Vratislavae, *apud Max & Soc.*, 1857.
        First operation for tumour of the oesophagus.

3457   FORSTER, John Cooper. 1824-1896
        Description of the operation of gastrotomy. *Guy's Hosp. Rep.*, 1858, 3 ser.,
        4, 13-18.
        First gastrostomy in Britain.

3458   BRINTON, William. 1823-1867
        The diseases of the stomach. London, *J. Churchill*, 1859.
        Includes (pp. 310-31) original description of linitis plastica ("Brinton's
        disease"). Brinton lectured on physiology and forensic medicine at St.
        Thomas's Hospital.

3459   MIDDELDORPF, Albrecht Theodor. 1824-1868
        Commentatio de fistulis ventriculi externis et chirurgica earum sanatione.
        Vratislaviae, *apud Max & Soc.*, 1859.
        First operation for gastric fistula.

3459.1 BODENHAMER, William. 1808-1905
        A practical treatise on the etiology, pathology, and treatment of the
        congenital malformations of the rectum and anus. New York, *S. & W. Wood*,
        1860.
        The first systematic treatise on the subject, and a landmark in paediatric
        surgery. Includes an early account of colostomy and one of the earliest
        histories of that procedure.

3460   LUSCHKA, HUBERT VON. 1820-1875
        Ueber polypöse Vegetationen der gesammten Dickdarmschleimhaut.
        Virchows Arch. path. Anat., 1861, **20**, 133-42.
        First authentic description of polyposis of the colon.

3461   KRAUSS, JULIUS. 1841-
        Das perforirende Geschwür im Duodenum. Berlin, *A. Hirschwald*, 1865.
        First comprehensive study of duodenal ulcer.

3462   BRINTON, WILLIAM. 1823-1867
        Intestinal obstruction. London, *J. Churchill*, 1867.

3463   KUSSMAUL, ADOLF. 1822-1902
        Ueber die Behandlung der Magenerweiterung durch eine neue Methode
        (mittelst der Magenpumpe). *Dtsch. Arch. klin. Med.*, 1869, **6**, 455-500.
        In 1867 Kussmaul used the stomach pump for gastric dilatation due to
        pyloric obstruction. Although his advocacy of gastric lavage established
        this method of treatment in medical practice, the instrument had already
        been used many years previously.

3463.1 ANNANDALE, THOMAS. 1839-1908
        Case in which an intestinal obstruction was removed by the operation of
        gastrotomy. *Edinb. med. J.*, 1870-71, **16**, 700-04.

3464   MAURY, FRANK FONTAINE. 1840-1879
        Case of stricture of the oesophagus in which gastrotomy was performed.
        Amer. J. med. Sci., 1870, **59**, 365-71.
        First gastrostomy for obstruction of the oesophagus performed in
        America.

3465   BILLROTH, CHRISTIAN ALBERT THEODOR. 1829-1894
        Ueber die Resection des Oesophagus. *Arch. klin. Chir.*, 1872, **13**, 65-69.
        First resection of the oesophagus.

3466   HUTCHINSON, *Sir* JONATHAN. 1828-1913
        A successful case of abdominal section for intussusception. *Med.-chir.
        Trans.*, 1874, **57**, 31-75.
        In 1871 Hutchinson was the first successfully to operate on a case of
        intussusception in a two year-old infant. Preliminary account in *Med. chir.
        Trans.*, 1876, **41** (2nd ser.), 99-102.

3467   JONES, SYDNEY. 1831-1913
        Gastrostomy for stricture (cancerous?) of oesophagus; death from bronchitis
        forty days after operation. *Lancet*, 1875, **1**, 678-79.
        Successful human gastrostomy by the older (Sédillot's) method. Reported
        by S. Osborne.

3467.1 GUSSENBAUER, CARL. 1842-1903, & WINIWARTER, ALEXANDER. 1848-1916
        Die partielle Magenresektion; eine experimentelle operative Studie. *Arch.
        klin. Chir.*, 1876, **19**, 347-80.
        A practical method for excision of the pylorus, as demonstrated in
        dogs, was published by these two assistants of Billroth.

3468   VERNEUIL, ARISTIDE AUGUST STANISLAS. 1823-1895
        Observation de gastro-stomie pratiquée avec succès pour un rétrécissement
        cicatriciel infranchissable de l'oesophage. *Bull. Acad. Méd. (Paris)*, 1876,
        2 sér., **5**, 1023-38.
        Verneuil's gastrostomy operation, a modification of Sédillot's method.

3469   LINDSTEDT, ADOLF FREDRIK. 1847-1915, & WALDENSTRÖM, JOHAN ANTON.
        1839-1879
        Volvulus flexurae sigmoideae coli – Laparo-colotomia – Helsa. *Upsala
        LäkFören. Förh.*, 1878-79, **14**, 513-27.
        First recorded operation for volvulus.

3470   VOLKMANN, RICHARD VON. 1830-1889
        Ueber den Mastdarmkrebs und die Extirpatio recti. *Samml. klin. Vortr.*, 1878,
        Nr. 131 (Chir., Nr. 42), 1113-28.
        First excision of the rectum for cancer.

3471   EWALD, CARL ANTON. 1845-1915
        Klinik der Verdauungskrankheiten. 3 vols. Berlin, *A. Hirschwald*, 1879-1902.
        An important work on disorders of digestion. With Boas, Ewald devised
        the test breakfast and he utilized intubation for exploring the contents of
        the stomach. English translation of vols. 1-2, 1891-92.

3472   PÉAN, JULES EMILE. 1830-1898
        De l'ablation des tumeurs de l'estomac par la gastrectomie. *Gaz. Hôp.
        (Paris)*, 1879, **52**, 473-75.
        First gastrectomy for carcinoma; unsuccessful.

3473   KOCHER, EMIL THEODOR. 1841-1917
        Ueber Radicalheilung des Krebses. *Dtsch. Z. Chir.*, 1880, **13**, 134-66.
        Kocher's operation of radical extirpation of the tongue for carcinoma.

3473.1 RYDYGIER, LUDWIK. 1850-1920
        Wyçiecie raka odźwiernika zoládkowego, śmierć w 12 godzinach. *Przegl.
        lek.*, 1880, **19**, 637-39.
        First extirpation of carcinomatous pylorus. Death after 12 hours. Ger-
        man translation in *Dtsch. Z. Chir.*, 1881, **14**, 252-60.

3474   BILLROTH, CHRISTIAN ALBERT THEODOR. 1829-1894
        Offenes Schreiben an Herrn Dr. L. Wittelshöfer. *Wien. med. Wschr.*, 1881,
        31, 161-65, 1427.
        First successful resection of the pylorus for cancer, the Billroth I
        operation.

3475   MIKULICZ-RADECKI, JOHANN VON. 1850-1905
        Ueber Gastroskopie und Oesophagoskopie. *Wien. med. Presse*, 1881, **22**,
        1405-08, 1437-43, 1473-75, 1505-07, 1537-41, 1573-77, 1629-31.
        Mikulicz was the first to use the electric oesophagoscope invented by
        Leiter in 1880. He was among the most distinguished of Billroth's pupils
        and contributed much to cancer surgery.

3476   WÖLFLER, ANTON. 1850-1917
        Gastro-Enterostomie. *Zbl. Chir.*, 1881, **8**, 705-08.
        Wölfler perfected the operation of gastro-enterostomy.

3477   LORETA, PIETRO. 1831-1889
Intorno alla divulsione digitale del pilore; osservazione cliniche. *Mem. reale. Accad. Sci. Ist. Bologna,* 1882, 4 ser., **4**, 353-75.
    First pyloroplasty, 1882. Abstract in English in *Brit. med. J.,* 1885, **1**, 372-74.

3478   REICHMANN, MIKOLAJ. 1851-1918
Przypadek chorobowo wzmożonego wydzielania soku żołądkowego. *Gaz. Lek.,* 1882, 2 ser., **2**, 516-22.
    First description of gastrosuccorrhoea ("Reichmann's disease"). German translation in *Berl. klin. Wschr.,* 1882, **19**, 606.

3479   CLARK, HENRY EDWARD. 1845-1909
On a case of obstruction of the bowels due to volvulus, treated by abdominal section; recovery. *Lancet,* 1881, **2**, 678-80.
    First successful operation in Britain for treatment of volvulus, performed 20 February, 1883.

3480   HAUER, ERNST.
Darmresektion und Enterorhaphieen, 1878-83. *Z. Heilk.,* 1884, **5**, 83-108.
    Billroth was a pioneer in visceral surgery. Above is an account of many intestinal resections and enterorrhaphies carried out by him.

3481   FINKLER, DITTMAR. 1852-1912, & PRIOR, J.
Untersuchungen über Cholera nostras. *Dtsch. med. Wschr.,* 1884, **10**, 579-82.
    Finkler and Prior isolated *Vibrio proteus* from stools in a case of acute gastro-enteritis.

3482   TREVES, *Sir* FREDERICK, *Bart.* 1853-1923
Intestinal obstruction. London, *Cassell & Co.,* 1884.
    Jacksonian Prize essay.

3482.1   BODENHAMER, WILLIAM. 1808-1905
A theoretical and practical treatise on the hemorrhoidal disease, givings its history, nature, cases, pathology, diagnosis, and treatment. New York, *William Wood,* 1884.
    An encyclopaedic work containing considerable history and a comprehensive bibliography.

3482.2   ALLCHIN, *Sir* WILLIAM HENRY. 1846-1912
Case of acute extensive ulceration of the colon. *Trans. path. Soc. Lond.,* 1885, **36**, 199-202.
    First detailed description of ulcerative colitis.

3482.3   GREVES, EDWIN HYLA. 1856-1932
On a case of acute intestinal obstruction in a boy, with remarks upon the treatment of acute obstruction. *Liverpool med.-chir. J.,* 1885, **5**, 118-30.
    Abdominal section and ileostomy for intestinal obstruction; surgeon's report on pp. 130-35.

3483   HACKER, VIKTOR VON. 1852-1933
Zur Casuistik und Statistik der Magenresectionen und Gastro-enterostomieen. *Verh. dtsch. Ges. Chir.,* 1885, **14**, Pt. II, 62-71.

Billroth II pylorectomy, reported by von Hacker. Also published in *Arch. klin. Chir.*, 1885, **32**, 616-25.

3484   GLÉNARD, Frantz. 1848-1920
Application de la méthode naturelle à l'analyse de la dyspepsie nerveuse.
– Détermination d'une espèce. *Lyon méd.*, 1885, **48**, 449-64, 492-505, 523-43, 563-83; **49**, 8-28.
Important description of enteroptosis and gastroptosis.

3485   ——. Neurasthénie et enteroptose. *Sem. méd. (Paris)*, 1886, **6**, 211-12.
Splanchnoptosis ("Glénard's disease").

3486   HACKER, Viktor von. 1852-1933
Ueber die Verwendung des Musculus rectus abdominis zum Verschlusse der künstlichen Magenfistel. *Wien. med. Wschr.*, 1886, **36**, 1073-77, 1110-14.
Von Hacker's method of gastrostomy.

3487   MIKULICZ-RADECKI, Johann von. 1850-1905
Ein Fall von Resection des carcinomatösen Oesophagus mit plastischem Ersatz des excidierten Stückes. *Prag. med. Wschr.*, 1886, **11**, 93-94.
Von Mikulicz was the first to make a plastic reconstruction of the oesophagus after the resection of its cervical portion for carcinoma.

3488   HALSTED, William Stewart. 1852-1922
Circular suture of the intestines; an experimental study. *Amer. J. med. Sci.*, 1887, **94**, 436-61.
Halsted set down some of the fundamental rules regarding intestinal anastomosis.

3489   HIRSCHSPRUNG, Harald. 1830-1916
Stuhlträgheit Neuegeborener in Folge von Dilatation und Hypertrophie des Colons. *Jb. Kinderheilk.*, 1887-88, n.F. **27**, 1-7.
Hirschsprung's diseases (congenital megacolon).

3489.1   ——. Fälle von angeborener Pylorusstenose, beobachtet bei Säuglingen. *Jb. Kinderheilk.*, 1888, **28**, 61-68.
Hirschsprung first made the medical world aware of congenital hypertrophic pyloric stenosis as a distinct clinical entity. In this paper he made no suggestions concerning therapy.

3490   KRASKE, Paul. 1851-1930
Die sacrale Methode der Exstirpation von Mastdarmkrebsen und die Resectio recti. *Berl. klin. Wschr.*, 1887, **24**, 899-904.
Kraske introduced the sacral method of resection of the rectum for carcinoma.

3491   GEE, Samuel Jones. 1839-1911
On the coeliac affection. *St. Barth. Hosp. Rep.*, 1888, **24**, 17-20.
Coeliac disease (non-tropical sprue, idiopathic steatorrhoea) was first described by Gee. Later Thaysen (No. 3550) studied the disease, which acquired the eponym "Gee–Thaysen disease".

3492   MAYDL, KAREL. 1853-1913
Zur Technik der Kolotomie. *Zbl. Chir.*, 1888, **15**, 433-39.
First successful colostomy.

3492.1   MENETRIER, PIERRE EUGENE. 1859-1935
Des polyadénomes gastriques et de leurs rapports avec le cancer de l'estomac. *Arch. Physiol. norm. path.*, 1888, **20**, 32-55, 236-62.
"Menetrier's disease" – giant hypertrophic gastritis.

3493   MIKULICZ-RADECKI, JOHANN VON. 1850-1905
Zur operativen Behandlung des Prolapsus recti et coli invaginati. *Verh. dtsch. Ges. Chir.*, 1888, **17**, 294-317.
Description of Mikulicz's important operation for complete prolapse of the rectum.

3494   SENN, NICHOLAS. 1844-1908
Rectal insufflation of hydrogen gas an infallible test in the diagnosis of visceral injury of the gastro-intestinal canal in penetrating wounds of the abdomen. *J. Amer. med. Assoc.*, 1888, **10**, 767-77.
Senn's method of detecting intestinal perforation by insufflation with hydrogen.

3495   EINHORN, MAX. 1862-1953
Die Gastrodiaphanie. *Med. Mschr. N.Y.*, 1889, **1**, 559.
Einhorn devised the method of exploration of the stomach by means of a tube – gastrodiaphany.

3496   BOAS, ISMAR ISIDOR. 1858-1938
Ueber Darmsaftgewinnung beim Menschen. (Vorläufige Mittheilung.) *Zbl. klin. Med.*, 1889, **10**, 97-99.
Duodenal aspiration.

3497   ——. Diagnostik und Therapie der Magenkrankheiten. 2 pts. Leipzig, *G. Thieme*, 1890-93.
Boas, who devised the test breakfast, became the foremost gastro-enterologist in Europe. He founded the *Archiv für Verdauungskrankheiten*, the first journal devoted to the subject of gastro-enterology.

3498   CHIARI, HANS. 1851-1916
Ueber Magensyphilis. *Int. Beitr. wiss. Med.*, Festschr. R. Virchow, Berlin, 1891, **2**, 295-321.
Important study of gastric syphilis.

3499   PAUL, FRANK THOMAS. 1851-1941
A method of performing inguinal colotomy, with cases. *Brit. med. J.*, 1891, **2**, 118.
Paul's tube introduced.

3500   SAHLI, HERMANN. 1856-1933
Ueber eine neue Untersuchungsmethode der Verdauungsorgane und einige Resultate derselben. *KorrespBl. schweiz. Aerzte*, 1891, **21**, 65-74.
Sahli's test for estimating the functional activity of the stomach.

3501   ABBE, ROBERT. 1851-1928
Intestinal anastomosis and suturing. *Med. Rec. (N.Y.)*, 1892, **41**, 365-70.
Abbe, a New York surgeon, introduced catgut rings for intestinal
suturing. See also *Med. News (Phila.)*, 1889, **54**, 589-92.

3502   BLOCH, OSCAR THORVALD. 1847-1926
Om extra-abdominal Behandlung af cancer intestinalis (rectum derfra
undtaget) med en Fremstilling af de for denne Sygdom foretagne
Operationer og deres Resultater. *Nord. med. Ark.*, 1892, N.F. **2**, 1 Heft, 1-
76; 2 Heft, 1-10.
Bloch was first to employ the two-stage (Mikulicz) operation for cancer
of the colon. *See also* No. 3527.

3503   EINHORN, MAX. 1862-1953
On achylia gastrica. *Med. Rec. (N.Y.)*, 1892, **41**, 650-54.
Einhorn introduced the concept of achylia gastrica, to indicate a
primary nervous functional disorder of the gastric secretion.

3504   JABOULAY, MATHIEU. 1860-1913
De la gastro-duodénostomie. *Arch. prov. Chir. (Paris)*, 1892, **1**, 551-54.
Introduction of gastroduodenostomy.

3505   KRIEGE, HERMANN.
Ein Fall von einem frei in die Bauchhöhle perforirten Magengeschwür;
Laparotomie; Naht der Perforationsstelle; Heilung. *Berl. klin. Wschr.*, 1892,
29, 1244-47, 1280-84.
In 1892 Ludwig Heusner (1846-1916) successfully sutured a perforated
gastric ulcer, the first successful case on record. It was reported by H.
Kriege.

3506   MIKULICZ-RADECKI, JOHANN VON. 1850-1905
Ueber eine eigenartige symmetrische Erkrankung der Thränen- und
Mundspeicheldrüsen. In: *Beiträge zur Chirurgie. Festschrift gewid. T.
Billroth*, Stuttgart, 1892, 610-30.
First description of the syndrome of symmetrical inflammation of the
lacrymal and salivary glands ("Mikulicz's disease"). English translation in
Medical Classics, 1937, **2**, 165-86.

3507   MURPHY, JOHN BENJAMIN. 1857-1916
Cholecysto-intestinal, gastro-intestinal, entero-intestinal anastomosis, and
approximation without sutures. *Med. Rec. (N.Y.)*, 1892, **42**, 665-76.
"Murphy's button" introduced.

3508   FRANK, RUDOLF. 1862-1913
Eine neue Methode der Gastrostomie bei Carcinoma oesophagi. *Wien. klin.
Wschr.*, 1893, **6**, 231-34.
See No. 3512.

3509   PÉNIÈRES, L.
De la gastrostomie par la méthode de la valvule ou du plissement de la
muqueuse stomacale. *Arch. prov. Chir. (Paris)*, 1893, **2**, 284-93.
Pénières of Toulouse conceived the idea of the valvular method of
gastrostomy.

3510   PERRY, Sir EDWIN COOPER. 1856-1938, & SHAW, LAURISTON ELGIE. 1859-1923
On diseases of the duodenum. *Guy's Hosp. Rep.*, 1893, **50**, 171-308.
A careful examination of the records of post mortems carried out at Guy's Hospital, 1826-92, was made by Perry and Shaw, who showed that of 70 reports of duodenal ulcer, ten occurred in cases of severe burns.

3511   SENN, NICHOLAS. 1844-1908
Enterorrhaphy; its history, technique and present status. *J. Amer. med. Assoc.*, 1893, **21**, 215-35.
Senn, Professor of Surgery at Chicago, was one of the first to investigate experimentally the subject of gastro-intestinal anastomosis.

3512   SSABANEJEW, J. F.
Über die Anlegung einer röhrenformigen Magenfistel bei Verengerungen der Speiseröhre. *Zbl. Chir.*, 1893, **20**, 862.
Ssabanejew and Frank independently developed a new method of gastrostomy, the Ssabanejew–Frank operation. The above is an abstract of the original, which appeared in *Khirurgitscheski Vestnik*, June 1893.

3513   TOEPFER, GUSTAV.
Eine Methode zur titrimetrischen Bestimmung der hauptsächlichsten Factoren der Magenacidität. *Hoppe-Seyl. Z. physiol. Chem.*, 1894, **19**, 104-22.
Toepfer's test for hydrochloric acid in gastric juice.

3514   BATTLE, WILLIAM HENRY. 1855-1936
Modified incision for removal of the vermiform appendix. *Brit. med. J.*, 1895, **2**, 1360.
"Battle's incision".

3515   PAUL, FRANK THOMAS. 1851-1941
Colectomy. *Brit. med. J.*, 1895, **1**, 1136-39.
Paul's operation of extra-abdominal resection of the colon.

3516   BECHER, WOLF. 1862-1906
Zur Anwendung des Röntgenschen Verfahrens in der Medicin. *Dtsch. med. Wschr.*, 1896, **22**, 202-03.
Becher introduced a solution of lead into the stomach of a guinea-pig, making it opaque to *x* rays; he thus showed the possibility of radiological diagnosis of gastric disease.

3516.1   ROSENHEIM, THEODOR.
Ueber Gastroskopie. *Berl. klin. Wschr.*, 1896, **33**, 275-78, 298-301, 325-27.
Rosenheim's gastroscope.

3517   SCHLATTER, CARL. 1864-1934
Ueber Ernährung und Verdauung nach vollständiger Entfernung des Magens, Oesophagoenterostomie, beim Menschen. *Beitr. klin. Chir.*, 1897, **19**, 757-76; 1899, **23**, 589-94.
First successful total gastrectomy.

3518   BALDY, JOHN MONTGOMERY. 1860-1934
First removal of the stomach in America. *Amer. J. Surg. Gynec.*, 1897-98, **109**, 157-58.

Operation performed by Baldy in 1893. He refers to a claim in *J. Amer. med. Ass.*, 1898, **30**, 341-44 giving credit for the first excision of the stomach in America to A. C. Bernays (1854-1907). While Baldy probably deserves priority, the point is moot since neither Baldy's nor Bernays' operations were successful.

3519   CANNON, WALTER BRADFORD. 1871-1945
The movements of the stomach studied by means of the Roentgen rays. *Amer. J. Physiol.*, 1898, **1**, 359-82.
     Cannon introduced the bismuth meal. He showed that bismuth, opaque to *x* rays, could be of great use in conjunction with roentgenology in the investigation of the digestive tract. *See* No. 1029.

3520   GRASER, ERNST. 1860-1929
Ueber multiple falsche Darmdivertikel in der Flexura sigmoidea. *Münch. med. Wschr.*, 1899, **46**, 721-23.
     A false diverticulum of the sigmoid flexure, described by Graser, has been given the eponym "Graser's diverticulum".

3521   KILLIAN, GUSTAV. 1860-1921
Ueber Magenspiegelung. *Dtsch. Z. Chir.*, 1900-01, **58**, 500-07.
     Describes the first clinical use of the oesophagoscope by Kussmaul in 1867-68. The latter made only brief mention of it himself in his paper on the stomach pump, *Dtsch. Arch. klin. Med.*, 1869, **6**, 456.

3522   MAYO, WILLIAM JAMES. 1861-1939
Malignant diseases of the stomach and pylorus. *Trans. Amer. surg. Ass.*, 1900, **18**, 97-123.
     Mayo's operation of partial gastrectomy.

3523   DEPAGE, ANTOINE. 1862-1925
Nouveau procédé pour la gastrostomie. *J. Chir. (Brux.)*, 1901, **1**, 715-18.
     Depage used a tube formed from the anterior wall of the stomach, lined with mucous membrane, in his gastrostomy operation.

3524   ROBSON, *Sir* ARTHUR WILLIAM MAYO. 1853-1933, & MOYNIHAN, BERKELEY GEORGE ANDREW, 1*st Baron Moynihan of Leeds.* 1865-1936
Diseases of the stomach and their surgical treatment. London, *Baillière, Tindall & Cox*, 1901.

3525   WEIR, ROBERT FULTON. 1838-1927
A new use for the useless appendix, in the surgical treatment of obstinate colitis. *Med. Rec. (N.Y.)*, 1902, **62**, 201-02.
     Weir's appendicostomy operation.

3526   KELLY, HOWARD ATWOOD. 1858-1943
Instruments for use through cylindrical rectal specula, with the patients in the knee–chest posture. *Ann. Surg.*, 1903, **37**, 924-27.
     Various rectal and vesical specula were designed by Kelly.

3527   MIKULICZ-RADECKI, JOHANN VON. 1850-1905
Chirurgische Erfahrungen über das Darmcarcinom. *Arch. klin. Chir.*, 1903, **69**, 28-47.

Development of Bloch's two-stage operation for resection of tumours of the rectum. English translation in *Medical Classics*, 1937, **2**, 210-29.

3528   HERTER, CHRISTIAN ARCHIBALD. 1865-1910
On infantilism from chronic intestinal infection; characterized by the overgrowth and persistence of flora of the nursling period. New York, *Macmillan & Co.*, 1908.
"Herter's infantilism". Called also "Gee–Herter disease" (No. 3491).

3528.1   MILES, WILLIAM ERNEST. 1869-1947
A method of performing abdomino-perineal excision for carcinoma of the rectum and of the terminal portion of the pelvic colon. *Lancet*, 1908, **2**, 1812-13.
Miles devised the operation of abdomino-perineal resection.

3529   STUMPF, R.
Beitrag zur Magenchirurgie. *Beitr. klin. Clin.*, 1908, **59**, 551-641.
Report of Hofmeister's modification of the Billroth II gastro-enterostomy.

3530   GUISEZ, JEAN. 1872- , & BARCAT, JEAN JULES. 1875-
Essais de traitement de quelques cas d'épithélioma de l'oesophage par les applications locales directes de radium. *Bull. Soc. méd. Hôp. Paris*, 1909, **27**, 717-22.
Radium therapy by means of the oesophagoscope.

3531   LANE, *Sir* WILLIAM ARBUTHNOT, *Bart.* 1856-1943
The operative treatment of chronic constipation. London, *J. Nisbet,* 1909.
Lane's operation for chronic intestinal stasis ("Lane's kink") consisted in short-circuiting the intestine.

3532   BALFOUR, DONALD CHURCH. 1882-1963
A method of anastomosis between sigmoid and rectum. *Ann. Surg.*, 1910, **51**, 239-41.
Balfour's operation for resection of the sigmoid colon.

3533   HAUDEK, MARTIN. 1880-1931
Zur röntgenologischen Diagnose der Ulzerationen in der Pars media des Magens. *Münch. med. Wschr.*, 1910, **57**, 1587-91.
First demonstration of the characteristic niche in gastric ulcer.

3534   MAYO, WILLIAM JAMES. 1861-1939
Removal of the rectum for cancer: statistical report of 120 cases. *Ann. Surg.*, 1910, **51**, 854-62.
Mayo's radical operation for carcinoma of the rectum.

3535   MOYNIHAN, BERKELEY GEORGE ANDREW, 1*st Baron Moynihan of Leeds.* 1865-1936
Duodenal ulcer. Philadelphia, *W. B. Saunders Co.*, 1910.
Moynihan greatly advanced our knowledge of duodenal ulcer. He developed the concept of the so-called ulcer sequence, pain-food-ease, and he stressed the well-ordered sequence of symptoms. More than any other he established treatment of duodenal ulcer on a sound basis.

3535.1   ELSNER, HANS. 1874-
Die Gastroskopie. Berlin, *G. Thieme*, 1911.
Elsner designed a straight gastroscope with a rubber tip and an optical system to be pushed into the outer tube, which had a lamp at its tip.

3536   FOCKENS, P.
Ein operativ geheilter Fall von kongenitaler Dünndarmatresie. *Zbl. Chir.*, 1911, **38**, 532-35.
Treatment of congenital atresia of ileum by lateral anastomosis.

3537   PÓLYA, EUGEN [JENÖ] ALEXANDER. 1876-?1944
Zur Stumpversorgung nach Magenresektion. *Zbl. Chir.*, 1911, **38**, 892-94.
Pólya's modification of the Billroth II operation. Pólya is believed to have been murdered by a Nazi group during the siege of Budapest by the Russians in December, 1944, although his body was never recovered.

3538   HERTZ, ARTHUR FREDERICK [*afterwards* HURST]. 1879-1944
The cause and treatment of certain unfavourable after-effects of gastroenterostomy. *Proc. roy. Soc. Med.*, 1913, **6**, Surg. Sect., 155-63.
First description of the "dumping syndrome", so named by C. L. Mix, *Surg. Clin. N. Amer.*, 1922, **2**, 617-22.

3539   RAMMSTEDT, WILHELM CONRAD. 1867-1963
Zur Operation der angeborenen Pylorusstenose. *Med. Klin.*, 1912, **8**, 1702-05.
"Rammstedt's operation" for congenital pyloric stenosis. In 1920 Rammstedt discovered that the family name had originally been spelt Ramstedt; he therefore reverted to the original spelling for the rest of his life (see *Lancet*, 1963, **1**, 674).

3540   TOREK, FRANZ. 1861-1938
The first successful case of resection of the thoracic portion of the oesophagus for carcinoma. *Surg. Gynec. Obstet.*, 1913, **16**, 614-17.
See also *Arch. Surg. (Chicago)*, 1925, **10**, 353-60, which reported that the patient was still living.

3541   SIPPY, BERTRAM WELTON. 1866-1924
Gastric and duodenal ulcer; medical cure by an efficient removal of gastric juice corrosion. *J. Amer. med. Assoc.*, 1915, **64**, 1625-30.
"Sippy diet" for the treatment of peptic ulcer.

3542   ANDREWES, *Sir* FREDERICK WILLIAM. 1859-1932
Dysentery bacilli: the differentiation of the true dysentery bacilli from allied species. *Lancet*, 1918, **1**, 560-63.
Shigella alkalescens described.

3543   FINSTERER, HANS. 1877-1955
Ausgedehnte Magenresektion bei Ulcus duodeni statt der einfachen Duodenalresektion bzw. Pylorusausschaltung. *Zbl. Chir.*, 1918, **45**, 434-35.
Hofmeister–Finsterer gastro-enterostomy (*see* No. 3529).

3544   RYLE, JOHN ALFRED. 1889-1950
Studies in gastric secretion. Introduction. *Guy's Hosp. Rep.*, 1921, **71**, 42-44.
Ryle's tube, for obtaining specimens of gastric juice.

3545   SCHINDLER, Rudolf. 1888-1968
Probleme und Technik der Gastroskopie, mit der Beschreibung eines
neuen Gastroskops. *Arch. VerdauKr.*, 1922, **30**, 133-66.
Schindler made gastroscopy a "method". See also his paper in the
Münch. med. Wschr., 1922, **69**, 535-37.

3546   KONJETZNY, Georg Ernst. 1880-?
Die Entzündungen des Magens. In F. Henke & O. Lubarsch: *Handbuch der
speziellen pathologischen Anatomie und Histologie*, 1928, **4**, Heft 2, 768-
1116.
Konjetzny has suggested that peptic ulceration is the sequel to a specific
form of gastritis.

3547   HURST, *Sir* Arthur Frederick. 1879-1944, & STEWART, Matthew John. 1885-
1956
Gastric and duodenal ulcer. London, *Humphrey Milford*, 1929.

3548   PORGES, Otto. 1879-?
Ueber Gastrophotographie. *Wien. klin. Wschr.*, 1929, **42**, 89, 889.
Introduction of gastrophotography.

3549   SPIVACK, Julius Leo. 1889-1956
Eine neue Methode der Gastrostomie. *Beitr. klin. Chir.*, 1929, **147**, 308-18.
Introduction of tubo-valvular gastrostomy.

3550   THAYSEN, Thorald Einar Hess. 1883-1936
The "coeliac affection" – idiopathic steatorrhoeas. *Lancet*, 1929, **1**, 1086-
89.
Idiopathic steatorrhoea, first described by Gee (No. 3491) was extensively studied by Thaysen, in so far as it occurs in adults and adolescents
in non-tropical countries. It also bears the name "Gee–Thaysen disease".

3551   CROHN, Burrill Bernard. 1884-1983, *et al.*
Regional ileitis. A pathologic and clinical entity. *J. Amer. med. Assoc.*, 1932,
99, 1323-29.
"Crohn's disease" – regional ileitis. With L. Ginzburg and G. D.
Oppenheimer.

3552   CUSHING, Harvey Williams. 1869-1939
Papers relating to the pituitary body, hypothalamus, and para-sympathetic
nervous system. Springfield, *C. C. Thomas*, 1932.
Cushing advanced the theory that the hypothalamus is responsible for
the development of peptic ulcer (see p. 175 *et seq.*). This work contains his
four principal contributions to pituitary-hypothalamic interrelationships,
including a reprint of his description of pituitary basphilism (No. 3904).

3553   SCHINDLER, Rudolf. 1888-1968
Ein völlig ungefährliches, flexibles Gastroskop. *Münch. med. Wschr.*, 1932,
79, 1268-69.
Introduction of the flexible gastroscope.

3554   WANGENSTEEN, Owen Harding. 1898-1981
        The early diagnosis of acute intestinal obstruction with comments on
        pathology and treatment. With a report of successful decompression of
        three cases of mechanical bowel obstruction by nasal catheter suction
        siphonage. *West. J. Surg. Obstet. Gynec.*, 1932, **40**, 1-17.
        Wangensteen's apparatus for relief of acute intestinal obstruction.

3555   MEULENGRACHT, Einar. 1887-
        Treatment of hematemesis and melaena with food. *Acta med. Scand.*, 1934,
        Suppl. **59**, 375-85.
        Meulengracht diet.

3556   LEVEN, N. Logan. 1902-
        Congenital atresia of the esophagus with tracheoesophageal fistula. Report
        of successful extrapleural ligation of fistulous communication and cervical
        esophagostomy. *J. thorac. Surg.*, 1941, **10**, 648-57.

3557   DRAGSTEDT, Lester Reynold. 1893-1975, & OWENS, Frederick Mitchum.
        1913-
        Supra-diaphragmatic section of the vagus nerves in treatment of duodenal
        ulcer. *Proc. Soc. exp. Biol. (N.Y.)*, 1943, **53**, 152-54.
        Vagotomy for peptic ulcer.

3558   JUDD, James R.
        Atresia of the ileum. First successful case cured by enterostomy alone. *J.
        Pediat.*, 1947, **30**, 679-85.

3558.1 HOPKINS, Harold Horace. 1918- , & KAPANY, N. S.
        A flexible fibrescope, using static scanning. *Nature (Lond.)*, 1954, **173**, 39-
        41.

3558.2 ZOLLINGER, Robert Milton. 1903- , & ELLISON, Edwin Homer. 1918-
        Primary peptic ulcerations of the jejunum associated with islet cell tumors
        of the pancreas. *Ann. Surg.*, 1955, **142**, 709-28.
        Zollinger–Ellison syndrome.

3558.3 HIRSCHCOWITZ, Basil I.
        Demonstration of the new gastroscope, the "fiberscope". *Gastroenterol-
        ogy*, 1958, **35**, 50-53.

APPENDICITIS

3559   AMYAND, Claudius. 168-?-1740
        Of an inguinal rupture, with a pin in the appendix caeci, incrusted with
        stone; and some observations on wounds in the guts. *Phil. Trans.*, 1736,
        39, 329-42.
        First recorded successful appendicectomy. Amyand was Serjeant-
        Surgeon to George II and first principal surgeon to Westminster Hospital.
        See also the paper in *Surg. Gynec. Obstet.*, 1953, **97**, 643-52, which re-
        produces part of the text.

3560   PARKINSON, JOHN WILLIAM KEYS. 1785-1838
        Case of diseased appendix vermiformis. *Med.-chir. Trans.*, 1812, **3**, 57-58.
            First case of appendicitis reported in English, and the first in which
        perforation was recognized as the cause of death. John Parkinson was the
        son of James Parkinson (No. 4690).

3561   LOUYER-VILLERMAY, JEAN BAPTISTE. 1776-1837
        Observations pour servir à l'histoire des inflammations de l'appendice du
        caecum. *Arch. gén. Méd.*, 1824, **5**, 246-50.
            Report of two cases of fatal peritonitis due to perforation of the
        appendix. Of this paper, H. A. Kelly says, "It at once established a definite
        place for lesions of the appendix in the category of recognized diseases".

3562   MÉLIER, FRANÇOIS. 1798-1866
        Mémoire et observations sur quelques maladies de l'appendice cécale. *J.
        gén. Méd.*, 1827, **100**, 317-45.
            Mélier was the first to show the existence of chronic appendicitis; he
        recognized the causal relationship between the chronic affection and
        abscesses of the right iliac fossa and was first to suggest operative
        intervention.

3563   HANCOCK, HENRY. 1809-1880
        Disease of the appendix caeci cured by operation. *Lond. med. Gaz.*, 1848,
        n.s. **7**, 547-50.
            First recorded successful operation for peritonitis due to abscess in the
        appendix. Hancock was surgeon to Charing Cross Hospital, London.

3564   PARKER, WILLARD. 1800-1884
        An operation for abscess of the appendix vermiformis caeci. *Med. Rec. (N.Y.)*,
        1867, **2**, 25-27.
            Parker was the first American to operate for appendicitis. In this paper
        he described a case from 1864, but mentioned a case he had operated on
        as early as 1843. He advocated the opening of the appendicular abscesses
        at an early stage; until his time such abscesses had been opened only when
        they pointed on the surface.

3565   SANDS, HENRY BARTON. 1830-1888
        On perityphlitis. *Ann. surg. anat. Soc. (Brooklyn)*, 1880, **2**, 249-70.
            Sands published an account of 26 cases, in which he had operated
        successfully in all but two. His later publications show that he recognized
        the early signs of perforation of the appendix, and he advocated and
        practised early operation.

3566   FENWICK, SAMUEL. 1821-1902
        Clinical lectures on cases of difficult diagnosis; perforation of the appendix
        vermiformis. *Lancet*, 1884, **2**, 987-90, 1039-42.
            In 1884 Fenwick advocated tying off and removal of the perforated
        appendix.

3567   FITZ, REGINALD HEBER. 1843-1913
        Perforating inflammation of the vermiform appendix, with special refer-
        ence to its early diagnosis and treatment. *Trans. Ass. Amer. Phys.*, 1886, **1**,
        107-44.

A conclusive demonstration of the pathology and symptoms of disease of the vermiform appendix. Fitz invented the term "appendicitis"; his paper, which records 25 cases collected by himself, convinced physicians of the need to remove the appendix immediately if threatening symptoms did not subside within 24 hours. Reprinted in *Med. Classics*, 1938, **2**, 459-91.

3568   HALL, RICHARD JOHN. 1856-1897
Suppurative peritonitis due to ulceration and suppuration of the vermiform appendix; laparotomy; resection of the vermiform appendix; toilette of the peritonaeum; drainage; recovery. *N.Y. med. J.*, 1886, **43**, 662-63.
This is believed to be the first reported case of survival after removal of a perforated appendix. Hall worked with William Halsted during the 1880s and participated in Halsted's experiments with cocaine as a local anaesthetic. Like Halsted, Hall became addicted to cocaine. It caused his premature death.

3569   WOODBURY, FRANK. 1848-
Cases of exploratory laparotomy followed by appropriate remedial operation. *Trans. Coll. Phys. Philad.*, 1887, **9**, 183.
Thomas George Morton (1835-1903) was one of the first deliberately to operate for and remove the inflamed appendix after correct diagnosis, April 1887. The patient survived. Case reported by Woodbury.

3570   McBURNEY, CHARLES. 1845-1913
Experience with early operative interference in cases of disease of the vermiform appendix. *N.Y. med. J.*, 1889, **50**, 676-84.
Describes (p. 678) "McBurney's point": "The seat of greatest pain, *determined by the pressure of one finger,* has been very exactly between an inch and a half and two inches from the anterior spinous process of the ilium on a straight line drawn from that process to the umbilicus". McBurney also includes a description of some successful cases of early operation for perforative appendicitis. Reprinted in *Med. Classics*, 1938, **2**, 506-31.

3570.1   TAIT, ROBERT LAWSON. 1845-1899
Surgical treatment of typhlitis. *Bgham. med. Rev.*, 1890, **27**, 26-34, 76-89.
Lawson Tait was the first British surgeon to diagnose acute appendicitis and to treat it by removal of the appendix (May 1880). See J. A. Shepherd, *Lawson Tait. The rebellious surgeon.* Lawrence, Kansas, *Coronado Press,* 1980.

3571   KELLY, HOWARD ATWOOD. 1858-1943, & HURDON, ELIZABETH. 1869-1941
The vermiform appendix and its diseases. Philadelphia, *W. B. Saunders,* 1905.

3572   ASCHOFF, KARL ALBERT LUDWIG. 1866-1942
Die Wurmfortsatzentzündung. Jena, *G. Fischer,* 1908.
Aschoff's theory of the enterogenous origin of appendicitis.

3573   FRANCO, PIERRE. 1500-1561
Petit traité contenant une des parties principalles de chirurgie, laquelle les chirurgiens hernières excercent. Lyon, *Antoine Vincent,* 1556.

Includes the first recorded description of an operation for strangulated hernia. Franco, in 1556, was the first to perform suprapubic cystotomy. Poor, and largely self-taught, he greatly improved the technique of herniotomy. *See* No. 4279.

3573.1   STROMAYR, Caspar. *fl.* 16th cent.
Die Handschrift des Schnitt-und Augenarztes...in der Lindauer Handschrift...von 4. Juli 1559...Einführung...von Dr. med. Walter von Brunn.... Berlin, *Idra*, [1925].
Stromayr was advanced in his concept of hernia. His work is known only from this exceptionally beautiful surgical manuscript with 186 large coloured scenes of practice and instruments, probably drawn by Stromayr himself. The manuscript discovered in Lindau in 1909 also contains some drawings of eye operations in the style of Bartisch. *See* No. 5816.1.

3574   FRANCO, Pierre. 1500-1561
Traité des hernies. Lyon, *T. Payan*, 1561.

3575   LITTRE, Alexis. 1658-1726
Observation sur une nouvelle espèce de hernie. *Hist. Acad. roy. Sci. (Paris), (1700), 1719*, Mém., 300-10.
"Littre's hernia" – so named from his description of diverticulum hernia. Later Richter (No. 3578) described this condition more fully.

3576   POTT, Percivall. 1714-1788
A treatise on ruptures. London, *C. Hitch & L. Hawes*, 1756
Pott was surgeon to St. Bartholomew's Hospital. Through a fall in the street he was confined to bed for many days, and during that period wrote his classic book on hernia. He refuted many of the old theories concerning its causation and methods of treatment based on these theories. The book includes the first description of congenital hernia.

3577   PETIT, Jean Louis. 1674-1750
Traité des maladies chirurgicales, et des opérations qui leur conviennent. 3 vols., Paris, *T. F. Didot jeune*, 1774.
"Petit's hernia" and "triangle" described (vol. 2, pp. 256-58). (*See also* No. 3357.) A lumbar hernia had previously been described by R. J. C. de Garengeot, *Traité des opérations de chirurgie*, 1731, **1**, 369-71.

3578   RICHTER, August Gottlieb. 1742-1812
Abhandlung von den Brüchen. Göttingen, *J. C. Dieterich*, 1778-79.
Richter, lecturer on surgery at Göttingen, in his classic treatise on hernia, first described partial enterocele, or "Richter's hernia" (Chap. 24).

3579   GIMBERNAT ARBOS, *Don* Antonio de. 1734-1816
Nuevo método de operar en la hernia crural. Madrid, *vda. Ibarra*, 1793.
Description of Gimbernat's operation for strangulated femoral hernia. In the same work he also described the ligament in the crural arch named after him. Gimbernat was a pioneer in ophthalmology, vascular surgery, and urology. English translation of the book, by T. Beddoes, London, 1795. For biographical note, see N. M. Matheson, *Brit. med. Bull.*, 1945, **3**, 238-39.

3580   CAMPER, PIETER. 1722-1789
        Icones herniarum. Editae a S. T. Soemmerring. Francofurti ad Moenum, *Varrentrapp & Wenner*, 1801.
        Camper illustrated his own work, and was in fact one of the greatest anatomical artists. His illustrations of herniae are of great value.

3581   COOPER, *Sir* ASTLEY PASTON, *Bart.* 1768-1841
        The anatomy and surgical treatment of inguinal and congenital hernia. London, *Cox*, 1804. The anatomy and surgical treatment of crural and umbilical hernia. London, *Longman*, 1807.
        Cooper's first book, luxuriously produced, in which he described for the first time the transversalis fascia, with full appreciation of its importance in hernia, as well as the superior pubic ligament with bears his name. Cooper made a study of femoral hernia and described "Cooper's ligament". He also studied diaphragmatic hernia. The second edition of 1827, entitled *The anatomy and surgical treatment of abdominal hernia* included his description of "Cooper's hernia" (hernia femoralis fasciae superficialis).

3582   HESSELBACH, FRANZ KASPAR. 1759-1816
        Anatomisch-chirurgische Abhandlung über den Ursprung der Leistenbrüche. Würzburg, *Baumgärtner*, 1806.
        Includes description of "Hesselbach's hernia" and "triangle". He wrote a further volume on the subject in 1814.

3583   SCARPA, ANTONIO. 1752-1832
        Sull'ernie. Memorie anatomico-chirurgiche. Milano, *d. reale Stamperia*, 1809.
        This splendidly illustrated work with life-size plates includes the description of "Scarpa's fascia" (creasteric fascia) and Scarpa's triangle of the thigh.

3584   ——. Sull'ernia del perineo. Pavia, *P. Bizzoni*, 1821.
        Scarpa's work on perineal hernia included a classic description of sliding hernia, or hernia of the large bowel. His contribution to the subject of hernia ranks with that of Cooper, and he did much toward modernizing the knowledge of this specialty.

3585   CLOQUET, JULES GERMAIN. 1790-1883
        Recherches anatomiques sur les hernies de l'abdomen. Paris, *Méquignon-Marvis*, 1817.
        This is Cloquet's medical thesis. It was followed by his thesis in competition for head of the anatomy section of the Paris Faculty: *Recherches sur les causes et l'anatomie des hernies abdominales.* Paris, *Méquignon-Marvis*, 1819. Marcy (No. 3601) considered Cloquet's work to be in the class of Cooper and Scarpa. The lithographed plates in the work of 1819 were drawn on stone by Cloquet himself, and are among the earliest lithographed medical illustrations. *See* No. 409.

3586   KEY, CHARLES ANTON. 1793-1849
        A memoir on the advantages and practicability of dividing the stricture in strangulated hernia on the outside of the sac. London, *Longman*, 1833.
        Introduction of the principle of dividing a stricture outside the sac in cases of strangulated hernia.

3587 LAWRENCE, *Sir* WILLIAM. 1783-1867
Treatise on ruptures. 5th ed. London, *John Churchill*, 1838.
 This was the standard text for many years. It first appeared in 1807 as *Treatise on hernia*.

3588 LUKE, JAMES. 1798-1881
Operation for strangulated hernia. *Lond. med. Gaz.*, 1841, **28**, 863-66.
 Luke's operation for femoral hernia.

3589 TEALE, THOMAS PRIDGIN, *Snr*. 1801-1868
A practical treatise on abdominal hernia. *Longman*, 1846.

3590 RIEUX, LÉON.
Considérations sur l'étranglement de l'intestin dans la cavité abdominale et sur un mode d'étranglement non décrit par les auteurs. Paris, *Thèse No.* 128, 1853.
 Retrocaecal hernia ("Rieux's hernia") first described.

3591 TREITZ, WENZEL. 1819-1872
Hernia retroperitonealis. Ein Beitrag zur Geschichte innerer Hernien. Prag, *F. A. Crednar*, 1857.
 Treitz described retroperitoneal hernia through the duodeno-jejunal recess – "Treitz's hernia".

3592 GRUBER, WENZEL LEOPOLD. 1814-1890
Ueber einen Fall nicht incarcerierter, aber mit Incarceration des Ileum durch das Omentum complicirter Hernia interna mesogastrica. *Oest. Z. prakt. Heilk.*, 1863, **9**, 325-30, 341-45.
 "Gruber's hernia" – internal mesogastric hernia.

3592.1 MARCY, HENRY ORLANDO. 1837-1924
A new use of carbolized catgut ligatures. *Bost. med. surg. J.*, 1871, **85**, 315-317.
 Marcy was the first to stress the importance of reconstruction of the internal ring following reduction of the sac.

3593 CZERNY, VINCENZ. 1842-1916
Studien zur Radikalbehandlung der Hernien. *Wien. med. Wschr.*, 1877, **27**, 497-500, 527-30, 553-56, 578-81.

3594 MARCY, HENRY ORLANDO. 1837-1924
The radical cure of hernia by the antiseptic use of the carbolized catgut ligature. *Trans. Amer. med. Ass.*, 1878, **29**, 295-305.
 Marcy introduced antiseptic ligatures in the radical cure of hernia. *See also* No. 3601.

3594.1 WARREN, JOSEPH H. 1831-1891
Hernia, strangulated and reducible, with cure by subcutaneous injections. London, *Sampson, Low*, 1880.
 The injection method of treating hernia remained a frequently utilized procedure until the 1930s.

3595   EVE, *Sir* FREDERIC SAMUEL. 1853-1916
A case of strangulated hernia into the fossa intersigmoidea. *Brit. med. J.*, 1885, **1**, 1195-97.
First definitely authenticated case of intersigmoid hernia.

3596   MACEWEN, *Sir* WILLIAM. 1848-1924
On the radical cure of oblique inguinal hernia by internal abdominal peritoneal pad, and the restoration of the valved form of the inguinal canal. *Ann. Surg.*, 1886, **4**, 89-119.
     Macewen's method for the radical cure of oblique inguinal hernia. The sac was folded into a pad and used as a plug at the internal ring, the ring being closed in layers. Reprinted in *Brit. med. J.*, 1887, **2**, 1263-71.

3597   LUCAS-CHAMPIONNIÈRE, JUST MARIE MARCELLIN. 1843-1913
Cure radicale des hernies. Paris, *A. Delahaye et E. Lecrosnier*, 1887.

3598   BASSINI, EDOARDO. 1844-1924
Nuovo metodo per la cura radicale dell' ernia inguinale. *Atti Congr. Ass. Med. Ital.*, (1887), Pavia, 1889, **2**, 179-82.
     Bassini's operation for the radical cure of inguinal hernia. His first account was unillustrated. Translation in *J. Hist. Med.*, 1966, **21**, 401-07. Bassini expanded his paper into an illustrated book with the same title, Pavia, 1889. This book was translated into German in *Arch. f. klin. Chir.*, 1890, **40**, 429-76.

3599   HALSTED, WILLIAM STEWART. 1852-1922
The radical cure of hernia. *Johns Hopk. Hosp. Bull.*, 1889, **1**, 12-13, 112.
     Simultaneously with Bassini, Halsted devised the modern operation for the radical cure of inguinal hernia. This is known as the Halsted I repair. Later his technique differed much from that of Bassini. See also his later paper on the subject in the same journal, 1893, **4**, 17-24, which is reprinted in *Med. Classics*, 1938, **3**, 412-40.

3600   KOCHER, EMIL THEODOR. 1841-1917
Zur Radicalcur der Hernien. *KorrespBl. schweiz. Aerzte*, 1892, **22**, 561-76.
Kocher's hernia operation.

3601   MARCY, HENRY ORLANDO. 1837-1924
The anatomy and surgical treatment of hernia. New York, *D. Appleton & Co.*, 1892.
     Marcy wrote a great deal on hernia, describing high ligation of the sac, transplantion of the spermatic cord, and careful reconstruction of the inguinal canal. This work, illustrated with 66 full-page plates, is one of the most spectacular of 19th century American surgical monographs. *See* No. 3594.

3602   BASSINI, EDOARDO. 1844-1924
Nuovo metodo operativo per la cura radicale dell' ernia crurale. Padova, *Draghi*, 1893.
Bassini's operation for femoral hernia.

3603   FRANKS, *Sir* KENDAL. 1851-1920
Resection of the intestine and immediate suture in gangrenous hernia. *Brit. med. J.*, 1893, **1**, 696.

Franks finally demonstrated the advantages of primary resection for gangrenous gut in strangulated hernia.

3604   LOCKWOOD, CHARLES BARRETT. 1856-1914
The radical cure of femoral and inguinal hernia. *Lancet*, London, 1893, **2**, 1297-1302.
Lockwood's operation for femoral hernia.

3604.1   ANDREWS, EDWARD WYLLYS. 1856-1927
Imbrication or lap joint method; a plastic operation for hernia. *Chicago. med. Rec.*, 1895, **9**, 67-77.
Described imbrication of flaps in hernia repairs.

3604.2   BLOODGOOD, JOSEPH COLT. 1867-1935
The transplantation of the rectus muscle in certain cases of inguinal hernia in which the conjoined tendon is obliterated. *Johns. Hopk. Hosp. Bull.*, 1898, **29**, 96-100.
Bloodgood's operation for inguinal hernia. *See also Ann. Surg.*, 1919, **70**, 81-88.

3605   LOTHEISSEN, GEORG. 1868-?
Zur Radikaloperation der Schenkelhernien. *Zbl. Chir.*, 1898, **25**, 548-50.
Lotheissen's operation for femoral hernia.

3606   BATTLE, WILLIAM HENRY. 1855-1936
Abstract of a clinical lecture on femoral hernia. *Lancet*, 1901, **1**, 302-05.
Battle's operation for femoral hernia.

3607   MAYO, WILLIAM JAMES. 1861-1939
An operation for the radical cure of umbilical hernia. *Ann. Surg.*, 1901, **34**, 276-80.
Mayo's operation for umbilical hernia.

3608.1   FERGUSON, ALEXANDER HUGH. 1853-1912
The technic of modern operations for hernia. Chicago, *Cleveland Press*, 1907.
Includes description of the Ferguson operation.

3608.2   LAROQUE, G. PAUL. 1876-1934
The permanent cure of inguinal and femoral hernia. A modification of the standard operative procedures. *Surg. Gyn. Obst.*, 1919, **29**, 507-11.
Laroque combined a superior transperitoneal gridiron incision with a Bassini repair.

3608.3   CHEATLE, *Sir* GEORGE LENTHAL. 1865-1951
An operation for the radical cure of inguinal and femoral hernia. *Brit. med. J.*, 1920, **2**, 68-69.
First preperitoneal approach to hernia repair.

3609   GALLIE, WILLIAM EDWARD. 1882-1959, & LeMESURIER, ARTHUR BAKER. 1889-
Living sutures in the treatment of hernia. *Canad. med. Ass. J.*, 1923, **13**, 469-80.
Gallie and LeMesurier used fascial sutures in their operation for inguinal hernia.

3611 HENRY, ARNOLD KIRKPATRICK. 1886-1962
Operation for femoral hernia by a midline extraperitoneal approach; with
a preliminary note on the use of this route for reducible inguinal hernia.
Lancet, 1936, **1**, 531-33.
 Henry's operation for femoral hernia.

3611.1 TANNER, NORMAN CECIL. 1906-1982
A 'slide' operation for inguinal and femoral hernia. *Brit. J. Surg.*, 1942, **29**,
285-89.
 The Tanner slide operation as a relaxing incision.

3611.2 McVAY, CHESTER B. 1911-1987
Inguinal and femoral hernioplasty: anatomic repair. *Arch. Surg.*, 1948, **57**,
524-30.
 The McVay or Cooper ligament repair.

3611.3 SHEARBURN, EDWIN W. 1913- , & MYERS, RICHARD N. 1929- .
Shouldice repair for inguinal hernia. *Surgery*, 1969, **66**, 450-59.
 The Canadian or Shouldice repair.

3611.4 LICHTENSTEIN, IRVING. 1920-
Hernia repair without disability. St. Louis, *C.V. Mosby*, 1970.
 First monograph on ambulatory hernia surgery.

LIVER: GALL-BLADDER: PANCREAS

For DIABETES MELLITUS, *see* 3925-3979.2; for WEIL'S DISEASE, *see* 5330-5336.

3612 ARETAEUS, *the Cappadocian*. A.D. 81-138?
On jaundice, or icterus. In his *Extant works*, London, 1856, 324-28.

3613 BROWNE, JOHN. 1642-170-?
A remarkable account of a liver, appearing glandulous to the eye. *Phil.
Trans.*, 1685, **15**, 1266-68.
 First description of cirrhosis of the liver.

3614 LAENNEC, RENÉ THÉOPHILE HYACINTHE. 1781-1826
De l'auscultation médiate. 2 vols. Paris, *J. A. Brosson & J. S. Chaudé*, 1819.
 "Laennec's cirrhosis" – chronic interstitial hepatitis – is described on p.
368 of Vol. 1.

3615 BRIGHT, RICHARD. 1789-1858
Cases and observations connected with disease of the pancreas and
duodenum. *Med.-chir. Trans.*, 1832, **18**, 1-56.

3616 STANLEY, EDWARD. 1793-1862
Abscess of the liver, with hydatids. – Operation. *Lancet*, 1833, **1**, 189-90.
 Diagnostic liver puncture.

3617 BRIGHT, RICHARD. 1789-1858
Observations on jaundice. *Guy's Hosp. Rep.*, 1836, **1**, 604-37.
 Original description of acute yellow atrophy of the liver.

3618 ROKITANSKY, CARL, *Freiherr von*. 1804-1878
Handbuch der pathologischen Anatomie. 3 vols. Wien, *Braumüller u. Seidel*, 1842-46.
Vol. 3 (1842), p. 313: Rokitansky's classic description of the pathological picture of acute yellow atrophy of the liver. Rokitansky named the disease; it has also been called "Rokitansky's disease". English translation, 4 vols., London, 1849-54. *See* No. 2293.

3619 BUDD, GEORGE. 1808-1882
On diseases of the liver. London, *J. Churchill*, 1845.
Budd was Professor of Medicine at King's College, London. Section III of the above book includes a description of that form of cirrhosis to which the name "Budd's disease" has been applied. In the second edition, 1852, p. 484, *Fasciolopsis buski*, the fluke causing fasciolopsiasis, is described. George Busk (1807-1886) found specimens in the liver at necropsy and drew Budd's attention to them.

3620 FRERICHS, FRIEDRICH THEODOR. 1819-1885
Klinik der Leberkrankheiten. 2 vols. and atlas. Braunschweig, *F. Vieweg u. Sohn*, 1858-61.
Frerichs's classic monograph on diseases of the liver summarized the existing knowledge and included his own important work on the subject. He discovered leucine and tyrosine in the liver in acute yellow atrophy (*Dtsch. Klin.*, 1855, **7**, 341-43), a condition to which he devoted much study. Frerichs was Professor of Pathology at Berlin and enjoyed a great reputation; more than any other man he was responsible for the development of scientific teaching in Germany. English translation, London, 1860.

3621 BOBBS, JOHN STOUGH. 1809-1870
Case of lithotomy of the gall-bladder. *Trans. med. Soc. Indiana*, 1868, 68-73.
First cholecystotomy for the removal of gall-stones.

3622 MURCHISON, CHARLES. 1830-1879
Clinical lectures on diseases of the liver. London, *Longmans Green & Co.*, 1868.

3623 HAYEM, GEORGES. 1841-1933
Contribution à l'étude de l'hépatite interstitielle chronique avec hypertrophie (sclérose ou cirrhose hypertrophique du foie). *Arch. Physiol. norm. path.*, 1874, 2 sér., **1**, 126-57.
Classic description of chronic interstitial hepatitis.

3624 HANOT, VICTOR CHARLES. 1844-1896
Étude sur une forme de cirrhose hypertrophique du foie (cirrhose hypertrophique avec ictère chronique). Paris, *Thèse No.* 465, 1875.
"Hanot's disease". First description of hypertrophic cirrhosis of the liver with icterus. Published in book form, Paris, 1876.

3625 SIMS, JAMES MARION. 1813-1883
Remarks on cholecystotomy in dropsy of the gall-bladder. *Brit. med. J.*, 1878, **1**, 811-15.
Sims' operation of cholecystotomy.

3626   BALSER, W.
Ueber Fettnekrose, eine zuweilen tödliche Krankheit des Menschen. *Virchows Arch. path. Anat.*, 1882, **90**, 520-35.
First description of pancreatic necrosis, "Balser's fat necrosis".

3627   LANGENBUCH, CARL JOHANN AUGUST. 1846-1901
Ein Fall von Exstirpation der Gallenblase wegen chronischer Cholelithiasis; Heilung. *Berl. klin. Wschr.*, 1882, **19**, 725-27.
First successful removal of the gall-bladder.

3628   LÜRMAN, A.
Eine Icterusepidemie. *Berl. klin. Wschr.*, 1885, **22**, 20-23.
    Dr. Lürman, a general practitioner in Bremen, was first to report homologous serum hepatitis. English translation in *Human viral hepatitis*, by A. J. Zuckerman, 2nd ed., New York, 1972, pp. 4-10.

3629   SENN, NICHOLAS. 1844-1908
The surgery of the pancreas, as based upon experiments and clinical researches. *Trans. Amer. surg. Ass.*, 1886, **4**, 99-232.
    In this review of the world literature and a report of animal experimentation, Senn concluded that complete extirpation of the pancreas was invariably followed by death, but that partial excision was feasible and justifiable.

3630   BARD, LOUIS. 1857-1930, & PIC, ADRIEN. 1862-?
Contribution à l'étude clinique et anatomo-pathologique du cancer primitif du pancréas. *Rev. Méd.*, 1888, **8**, 257-82, 363-405.
"Bard–Pic syndrome" first described.

3631   RIEDEL, BERNHARD MORITZ CARL LUDWIG. 1846-1916
Ueber den zungenförmigen Fortsatz des rechten Leberlappens und seine pathognostiche Bedeutung für die Erkrankung der Gallenblase nebst Bemerkungen über Gallensteinoperationen. *Berl. klin. Wschr.*, 1888, **25**, 577-81, 602-07.
"Riedel's lobe", a form of constriction lobe of the liver.

3632   FITZ, REGINALD HEBER. 1843-1913
Acute pancreatitis; a consideration of pancreatic hemorrhage, hemorrhagic suppurative, and gangrenous pancreatitis, and of disseminated fat necrosis. *Boston. med. surg. J.*, 1889, **120**, 181-87, 205-07, 229-35.
    Fitz described three forms of acute pancreatitis, and made the earliest suggestion that disseminated fat necrosis is the result of a pathologic process in the pancreas.

3633   STADELMANN, ERNST. 1853-1941
Der Icterus und seine verschiedenen Formen. Stuttgart, *F. Enke*, 1891.

3634   NAUNYN, BERNHARD. 1839-1925
Klinik der Cholelithiasis. Leipzig, *F. C. W. Vogel*, 1892.
    Naunyn produced a classic monograph on gall-stones, devising an accurate chemical classification. He was one of Frerichs's best pupils and became Professor of Clinical Medicine successively at Dorpat, Berne, Königsberg, and Strasburg. English translation, London, 1896.

3635   LUCATELLO, LUIGI. 1863-1926
Sulla puntura del fegato a scopo diagnostico. *Lav. Congr. Med. interna, Milano*, 1895, **6**, 327-29.
Liver puncture biopsy.

3636   CHAPPUIS, J., & CHAUVEL, H.
Calculs du rein. Calculs de la vésicule biliaire. *Bull. Acad. Méd. (Paris)*, 1896, **35**, 410-11.
Chappuis and Chauvel were the first to study biliary concretions by means of Roentgen rays.

3637   BOBROFF, ALEXANDER ALEXIEVICH. 1850-1904
Ueber ein neues Operationsverfahren zur Entfernung von Echinococcus in der Leber und anderen parenchymatösen Bauchorganen. *Arch. klin. Chir.*, 1898, **56**, 819-26.
Important work on surgical treatment of hydatids of the liver. Originally appeared in Russian in *Khirurgiya*, 1898, **3**, 3-9.

3638   BUXBAUM, A.
Ueber die Photographie von Gallensteinen in vivo. *Wien. med. Presse*, 1898, **39**, col. 534-38.
First *x*-ray demonstration of gall-stones.

3639   TALMA, SAPE. 1847-1918
Chirurgische Oeffnung neuer Seitenbahnen für das Blut der Vena portae. *Berl. klin. Wschr.*, 1898, **35**, 833-36; 1900, **37**, 677-81; 1904, **41**, 893-97.
Talma's operation for the relief of ascites in cirrhosis of the liver.

3639.1   HALSTED, WILLIAM STEWART. 1852-1922
Contribution to the surgery of the bile passages, especially of the common bile-duct. *Bost. med. surg. J.*, 1899, **141**, 645-54.
"Among Halsted's many outstanding surgical accomplishments those related to surgery of the biliary tract are lesser known. However, he is commonly credited with performing the first succesful operation for a primary cancer of the ampulla of Vater" (Rutkow).

3640   HEKTOEN, LUDVIG. 1863-1951
Experimental bacillary cirrhosis of the liver. *J. Path. Bact.*, 1900-01, **7**, 214-20.
Hektoen produced experimental cirrhosis of the liver. His notable work in pathology includes the foundation of the *Archives of Pathology*.

3641   OPIE, EUGENE LINDSAY. 1873-1971
Disease of the pancreas; its cause and nature. Philadelphia, *J. B. Lippincott*, 1903.

3642   CAMMIDGE, PERCY JOHN. 1872-1956
The chemistry of the urine in diseases of the pancreas. *Lancet*, 1904, **1**, 782-87.
Test for diseases of the pancreas.

3643   BAUER, RICHARD.
Ueber die Assimilation von Galaktose und Milchzucker Beim Gesunden und Kranken. *Wien. med. Wschr.*, 1906, **56**, 20-23.
Galactose tolerance test.

3644   LOEWI, OTTO. 1873-1961
Ueber eine neue Funktion des Pankreas und ihre Beziehung zum Diabetes mellitus. *Arch. exp. path. Pharmak.*, 1908, **59**, 83-94.
Loewi's pancreatic function test.

3645   ASCHOFF, KARL ALBERT LUDWIG. 1866-1942, & BACMEISTER, ADOLF. 1882-1945.
Die Cholelithiasis. Jena, *G. Fischer*, 1909.

3646   WOHLGEMUTH, JULIUS. 1874-1948
Beitrag zur funktionellen Diagnostik des Pankreas. *Berl. klin. Wschr.*, 1910, **47**, 92-95.
Wohlgemuth's pancreatic function test.

3647   HIJMANS VAN DEN BERGH, ALBERT ABRAHAM. 1869-1943, & SNAPPER, J.
Die Farbstoffe des Blutserums. 1. Eine quantitative Bestimmung des Bilirubins im Blutserum. *Dtsch. Arch. klin. Med.*, 1913, **110**, 540-61.
The van den Bergh test.

3648   McNEE, *Sir* JOHN WILLIAM. 1887-1984
Experiments on haemolytic icterus. *J. Path. Bact.*, 1913-14, **18**, 325-42.
McNee showed that bile pigment formation is not a function of the liver cells alone, but can take place in other tissues. He thus disproved the theory propounded by Minkowski and Naunyn in 1886.

3649   MELTZER, SAMUEL JAMES. 1851-1920
The disturbance of the law of contrary innervation as a pathogenetic factor in the diseases of the bile ducts and the gall-bladder. *Amer. J. med. Sci.*, 1917, **153**, 469-77.
Non-surgical drainage of the gall-bladder was first suggested by Meltzer. *See also* No. 3651.

3650   REICH, ADOLPH. 1864-?
Accidental injection of bile ducts with petrolatum and bismuth paste. Preliminary report on a new method. *J. Amer. med. Assoc.*, 1918, **71**, 1555.
Reich was the first to obtain cholangiograms.

3651   LYON, BETHUEL BOYD VINCENT. 1880-?
Diagnosis and treatment of diseases of the gall-bladder and bilary ducts. Preliminary report on a new method. *J. Amer. med. Assoc.*, 1919, **73**, 980-82.
See No. 3649.

3652   GRAHAM, EVARTS AMBROSE. 1883-1957, & COLE, WARREN HENRY. 1898-
Roentgenologic examination of the gallbladder. *J. Amer. med. Assoc.*, 1924, **82**, 613-14.
Introduction of cholecystography.

3653   ROSENTHAL, SANFORD MORRIS. 1897- , & WHITE, EDWIN CLAY. 1888-
Studies in hepatic function. VI. A. The pharmacological behavior of certain
dyes. B. The value of selected phthalein compounds in the estimation of
hepatic function. *J. Pharmacol.*, 1924, 24, 265-88.
Bromsulphthalein test for liver function.

3654   TAKATA, MAKI. 1892- , & ARA, KIYOSHI. 1894-
Ueber eine neue kolloidchemische Liquorreaktion und ihre praktischen
Ergebnisse. *Trans. 6th Congr. Far East. Ass. trop. Med.*, 1925, 1, 667-71.
Takata–Ara reaction for the diagnosis of liver disease.

3655   EILBOTT, WILHELM. 1900-
Funktionsprüfung der Leber mittels Bilirubinbelastung. *Z. klin. Med.*, 1927,
106, 529-60.
Bilirubin excretion test of liver function. See also his thesis, published
in 1925.

3656   GIERKE, EDGAR OTTO KONRAD VON. 1877-1945
Hepato-nephromegalia glykogenika (Glykogenspeicherkrankheit der
Leber und Nieren). *Beitr. path. Anat.*, 1929, 82, 497-513.
"Von Gierke's disease", glycogen disease of hepatomegalic type. See
also the review by S. van Creveld, *Medicine*, 1939, 18, 1-128.

3657   ROLLESTON, *Sir* HUMPHRY DAVY, *Bart.* 1862-1944, & McNEE, *Sir* JOHN WILLIAM.
1887-1984.
Diseases of the liver, gall-bladder, and bile ducts. 3rd edition. London,
Macmillan & Co., 1929.

3658   BREUER, BELA.
Über ein neues Röntgensymptom der Gallensteinkrankheit. *Röntgenpraxis*,
1931, 3, 879-81.
Gas in gall-stones.

3659   QUICK, ARMAND JAMES. 1894-1977
The synthesis of hippuric acid: a new test of liver function. *Amer. J. med.
Sci.*, 1933, 185, 630-35.
Quick's liver-function test.

3659.1 WHIPPLE, ALLEN OLDFATHER. 1881-1963, *et al.*
Treatment of carcinoma of the ampulla of Vater. *Ann. Surg.*, 1935, 102, 763-
79.
Pancreaticoduodenectomy for cancer of pancreas. With W. B. Parsons
and C. R. Mullins.

3659.2 FANCONI, GUIDO. 1892-1979, *et al.*
Das Coeliakiesyndrom bei angeborener zystischer Pankreasfibromatose
und Bronchiektasien. *Wien. med. Wschr.*, 1936, 86, 753-56.
Cystic fibrosis (mucoviscidosis) described. With E. Uehlinger and C.
Knauer.

3660   BRUNSCHWIG, ALEXANDER. 1901-1969
Resection of head of pancreas and duodenum for carcinoma –
pancreatoduodenectomy. *Surg. Gynec. Obstet.*, 1937, 65, 681-84.
See also the same journal, 1943, 77, 581-84.

3661   PATEK, ARTHUR JACKSON. 1904-
Treatment of alcoholic cirrhosis of the liver with high vitamin therapy.
Proc. Soc. exp. Biol. (N.Y.), 1937, **37**, 329-30.
A pioneer paper on the dietary treatment of cirrhosis.

3662   HANGER, FRANKLIN McCUE. 1894-1971
The flocculation of cephalin-cholesterol emulsions by pathological sera.
Trans. Ass. Amer. Phys., 1938, **53**, 148-51.
Cephalin-cholesterol liver-function test.

3663   QUICK, ARMAND JAMES. 1894-1977, *et al.*
Synthesis of hippuric acid in man following intravenous injection of
sodium benzoate. *Proc. Soc. exp. Biol. (N.Y.)*, 1938, **38**, 77-78.
Intravenous hippuric acid test for liver function. With H. N. Ottenstein
and H. Weltchek. See also *Amer. J. Dis.*, 1939, **6**, 716-17.

3664   IVERSON, POUL. 1889- , & ROHOLM, KAJ.
On aspiration biopsy of the liver, with remarks on its diagnostic significance.
Acta med. Scand., 1939, **102**, 1-16.
Modern method of liver puncture.

3664.1   VOEGT, H.
Zur Aetiologie der Hepatitis epidemica. *Münch. med. Wschr.*, 1942, **89**, 76-
79.
Transmission of infective hepatitis agent.

3664.2   MacCALLUM, FREDERIC OGDEN, & BRADLEY, W.H.
Transmission of infective hepatitis to human volunteers. *Lancet,* 1944, **2**,
228 (only).
MacCallum and Bradley finally proved the nature of both serum and
infective hepatitis.

3664.3   ———. & BAUER, DENIS JOHN. 1914-
Homologous serum jaundice. Transmission experiments with human
volunteers. *Lancet,* 1944, **1**, 622-7.

3665   MACLAGAN, NOEL FRANCIS. 1904-
The serum colloidal gold reactions as a liver function test. *Brit. J. exp. Path.*,
1944, **25**, 15-20.

3666   ———. The thymol turbidity test as an indicator of liver dysfunction. *Brit. J.
exp. Path.*, 1944, **25**, 234-41.

3666.1   WELCH, CHARLES STUART. 1909-
A note on transplantation of the whole liver in dogs. *Transplant. Bull.*, 1955,
2, 54-55.
Placement of auxiliary whole liver.

3666.2   MOORE, FRANCIS DANIELS. 1913- , *et al.*
One-stage homotransplantation of the liver following total hepatectomy in
dogs. *Transplant. Bull.*, 1959, **6**, 103-07.
With nine co-authors.

3666.3　STARZL, THOMAS EARL. 1926- , *et al.*
Homotransplantation of the liver in humans. *Surg. Gynec. Obstet.*, 1963, **117**, 659-76.
　　First human liver transplant (three patients; one died during operation, the second after 7.5 days, and the third after 22 days). With five co-authors.

3666.4　BLUMBERG, BARUCH SAMUEL. 1925- , *et al.*
A "new" antigen in leukemia sera. *J. Amer. med. Assoc.*, 1965, **191**, 541-46.
　　Discovery of Australia antigen, hepatitis B antigen. With H. J. Alter and S. Visnich. Blumberg shared the Nobel Prize with D. C. Gajdusek in 1976 for work on infectious diseases.

3666.5　KRUGMAN, SAUL. 1911- , *et al.*
Infectious hepatitis. Evidence for two distinctive clinical, epidemiological, and immunological types of infection. *J. Amer. med. Assoc.*, 1967, **200**, 365-73.
　　With J. P. Giles and J. Hammond.

History of Gastroenterology

3666.6　MANI, NIKOLAUS.
Die historischen Grundlagen der Leberforschung. 2 vols. Basel, *B. Schwabe*, 1959-67.

3666.7　FRANKEN, FRANZ HERMANN.
Die Leber und ihre Krankheiten. Zweihundert Jahre Hepatologie. Stuttgart, *F. Enke*, 1968.
　　Contains short biographies and an excellent bibliography.

3666.8　COCHETON, JEAN-JACQUES, GUERRE, JEAN, & PEQUIGNOT, HENRI.
Histoire illustrée de l'hépato-gastro-entérologie de l'antiquité à nos jours. Paris, *Roger Dacosta,* [1987].

DENTISTRY: ORTHODONTICS: ORAL SURGERY

3666.81　CELSUS, AULUS AURELIUS CORNELIUS. 25 B.C.-A.D. 50
De medicina. Florentiae, *Nicolaus [Laurentius],* 1478.
　　Celsus contains numerous important contributions to dentistry, including some of the earliest Western accounts of the treatment of toothache, oral surgery, tooth extraction, and fractures of the jaw. *See* No. 20.

3666.82　ABUL QASIM [Albucasis]. 936-1013
Cyrurgia Albucasis cum cauteriis & Aliis instrumentis. (Issued with Guy de Chauliac, Chyrurgia parva,) [Venice, *Bonetus Locatellus*, 1500/01].
　　"Of great importance for the development of practical dentistry" (Hoffmann-Axthelm). Chapter 28 discusses excision of epulis. Chapter 29 deals with calculus. Albucasis understood that calculus on the teeth is a major cause of periodontal disease and gave explicit instructions for scaling the teeth, describing the instruments which he invented for this purpose. Chapter 30 covers tooth extraction, and Chapter 33 contains one of the earliest discussions of tooth prostheses, and describes some oral surgery procedures. The work contains some of the earliest illustrations of dental instruments. *See* No. 5550.

3666.83   GUY DE CHAULIAC. ?1298-1368
La pratique en chirurgie du maistre Guidon de Chauliac. Lyons, *Barthelemy Buyer*, 1478.
Chauliac discussed the anatomy of the teeth and their eruption. He also listed the maladies to which the teeth are subject, and their cures, including hygienic rules which for the most part remain true today. He described the double-lever pelican and its method of use. He also records how surgeons were using botanic medicines to prevent their patients from feeling pain during operations. *See* No. 5556.

3666.84   ARCOLANI, GIOVANNI. d.1460 or 1484
Cirurgia practica. Venice, *Stagninus*, 1493.
Includes the first documentation for the use of gold for filling diseased teeth.

3667   ARTZNEY BUCHLEIN.
Artzney Buchlein, wider allerlei Kranckeyten und Gebrachen der Tzeen. [Leipzig, *Michael Blum*,] 1530.
The first book on dentistry. The unidentified writer confined himself to extracts from the works of recent writers on the subject; the book was intended for the general public. It attained 11 editions in 45 years. Reproduced in facsimile, Berlin, *Meusser*, 1921.

3667.1   RYFF, WALTHER HERMANN. (d. before 1562)
Nützlicher bericht wie man die Augen und das Gesicht wo das selbig magelhafft blöde dunckel oder befinstert. Scherpfen gesundt erhalten stercken und bekrefftigen soll...Mit weitterer unterrichtung. Wie man den Mundt die Zän und Biller...Würzburg, *Johann Myller*, [1548].
This popular guide to health includes the first monograph on dentistry for the layman, encouraging the practice of oral hygiene and simple dental care. The first part of the book deals with the eyes, the second with the teeth proper, and the third with the primary dentition.

3668   EUSTACHI, BARTOLOMEO [EUSTACHIUS]. *circa* 1510/20-1574
Libellus de dentibus. In his *Opuscula anatomica*, Venetiis, *Vincentius Luchinus*, [1563]-64.
Basing his work on the dissection of foetuses and newborn children, Eustachi was the first to study the teeth in any considerable detail. He provided an important description of the first and second dentitions and described the hard outer tissue and soft inner structure of the teeth. He also attempted an explanation of the problem of the sensitivity of the tooth's hard structure. The *Libellus* has a separate title page dated 1563. It was reprinted with German translation, Wien, *Urban & Schwarzenberg*, 1951. Eustachi's illustrations of the teeth were first published in his *Tabulae anatomicae*, edited by Giovanni Maria Lancisi (No. 391).

3668.1   PARÉ, AMBROISE. 1510-1590
Dix livres de la chirurgie, avec le magasin des instrumens nécessaires à icelle. Paris, *Jean Le Royer*, 1564.
Paré had an extensive dental practice and his books contain much information on the subject. He designed several instruments for extracting teeth, including an extraction forceps for breaking and pulling the teeth, sponge obturators, and an obturator with screw closure and special forceps for placement. He described a variety of pelican which he called

a *daviet*. He also described and illustrated artificial teeth made of bone which he attached by silver wire. English translation, Athens, Georgia, 1969. *See* No. 5564.

3668.2   MARTINEZ, FRANCISCO. 1518-88
Colloquio breve y copedioso. Sobre la materi de la detadura, y marauilloso obra de la boca. Valladolid, *Sebastian Martinez*, 1557.
    First Spanish book on dentistry. Second edition, Madrid, 1570.

3668.3   HÉMARD, URBAIN. 1548-1616
Recherche de la vraye anathomie des dents, nature et propriété d'icelles. Lyon, *Benoist Rigaud*, 1582.
    First French book on dentistry.

3669   GUILLEMEAU, JACQUES. 1550-1613
La chirurgie françoise recueillie des antiens medecins et chirurgiens. Paris, *N. Gilles*, 1594.
    This work contains a good deal about dentistry; it describes pyorrhoea alveolaris for the first time and is also the first work to refer to inorganic materials for tooth fillings and for the construction of artificial teeth. English translation, Dordrecht, 1597.

3669.1   SCHULTES, JOHANN [SCULTETUS]. 1595-1645
Χειροπλοθήκη seu armamentarium chirurgicum. Ulmae Suevorum, *B. Kühnen*, 1655.
    Scultetus describes and illustrates stomatological operations and includes fine illustrations of extraction instruments. English translation, London, 1674.

3669.3   BORELLI, GIOVANNI ALFONSO. 1608-1679
De motu animalium. 2 pts. Romae, *ex typ. A. Bernabo,* 1680-81.
    Borelli's experiments included what are probably the first measurements of masticatory force. *See* No. 762.

3669.4   LEEUWENHOEK, ANTHONY VAN. 1632-1723
An abstract of a letter...Sep. 17, 1683. containing some microscopical observations, about animals in the scurf of the teeth. *Phil. Trans.*, 1684, **14**, 568-74.
    Records discovery of bacteria in the mouth, with the first illustrations of the basic types – cocci, bacteria and spiral forms. Although Leeuwenhoek had observed bacteria earlier, this paper has usually been considered to be the first memoir on bacteria.

3670   ALLEN, CHARLES. *fl.* 1685
The operator for the teeth. York, *John White*, 1685.
    First British book on dentistry. Editions were published in Dublin, 1686, and London, 1687. The 1685 edition was reprinted London, *Dawson*, 1969, and the Dublin edition was reprinted by the British Dental Association, 1924.

3670.1   COWPER, WILLIAM. 1666-1709
Of the nose. In James Drake: *Anthropologia nova*, London, 1707, vol. 2, pp. 526-49.

Cowper pioneered the surgical treatment of diseases of the maxillary sinus. "In order to empty Highmore's antrum of deposits and to be able to carry out the necessary irrigations, he extracted in most cases the first permanent molar, and then penetrated through its aveolus into the sinus with a pointed instrument" (Guerini).

3671   FAUCHARD, Pierre. 1678-1761
Le chirurgien dentiste, ou traité des dents. 2 vols. Paris, *J. Mariette*, 1728.
     Pierre Fauchard has been called the "Father of Dentistry"; his comprehensive and scientific account of all that concerned dentistry in the 18th century is one of the greatest books in the history of the subject. The second edition, published in 1746, contains a good description (vol. 1, pp. 275-77) of pyorrhoea alveolaris; it was reprinted, Paris, 1961, and was translated into English by Lilian Lindsay and published by the British Dental Association in 1946 (reprinted Pound Ridge, N.Y., *Milford House*, 1969).

3672   HURLOCK, Joseph.
A practical treatise upon dentition; or, the breeding of teeth in children. London, *C. Rimington & S. Austen, J. Hodges*, 1742.
     The first English book on children's teeth. Reprinted, *Dawson*, 1966.

3672.1   BUNON, Robert. 1702-1748
Essai sur les maladies des dents. Paris, *Briasson*, 1743.
     The first book incorporating specialized odontological research. Bunon investigated the genesis of enamel hypoplasia.

3672.2   MOUTON, Claude. *d.* 1786.
Essai d'odontotechnie, ou dissertation sur les dents artificielles. Paris, *Boudel*, 1746.
     The first specialized book on dental prosthetics.

3673   PFAFF, Philipp. 1716-1780
Abhandlung von den Zähnen des menschlichen Körpers und deren Krankheiten. Berlin, *Haude & Spener*, 1756.
     The first important German manual of dentistry. Pfaff, dentist to Frederick the Great, was the first to describe the taking of dental impressions and the casting of models for false teeth. This book ranks in importance with the work of Fauchard and Hunter. Reprinted Hildesheim, *G. Olms*, 1966.

3673.1   BOURDET, Etienne. 1722-89
Recherches et observations sur toutes les parties de l'art du dentiste. 2 vols., Paris, *Jean Thomas Hérissant*,1757.
     "Probably the most significant [French dental] author after Fauchard" (Hoffmann-Axthelm). Bourdet's greatest contributions were to dental prosthetics. He also described severe periodontoclasia and his treatment of the condition – similar to modern gingivectomy.

3674   BERDMORE, Thomas. 1740-1785
A treatise on the disorders and deformities of the teeth and gums. London, *B. White*, 1768.
     Earliest English dental textbook. Berdmore was the first to mention the use of the microscope for the study of the minute structure of teeth.

3675   HUNTER, JOHN. 1728-1793
The natural history of the human teeth. London, *J. Johnson*, 1771.

This is a detailed study of the mouth, jaws and teeth with exceptionally accurate plates. Hunter correctly understood the growth and development of the jaws and their relation to the muscles of mastication. He coined the terms cuspids, bicuspids, molars and incisors.

3676   ——. A practical treatise on the diseases of the teeth, intended as a supplement to the natural history of those parts. London, *J. Johnson*, 1778.

This and *The natural history of the human teeth* revolutionized the practice of dentistry and provided a basis for later dental research. Hunter devised appliances for the correction of malocclusion. He described the various stages of inflammation of affected teeth, and gave an accurate description of periodontal disease. In the above work he includes instructions with regard to the operation of tooth transplantation from one living person directly to the jaw of another. Hunter's outstanding reputation made this highly dubious procedure more widely accepted than it should have been.

3676.1   JOURDAIN, ANSELME LOUIS BERNARD BERCHILLET. 1734-1816
Traité des maladies et des opérations réellement chirurgicales de la bouche. 2 vols., Paris, *Valleyre*, 1778.

The first specialist book on oral surgery. The first volume deals with diseases of the maxilla; and the second, with diseases of the mandible. Jourdain was particularly expert in diseases of the maxillary sinus and describes all forms of inflammation, and cystic and tumourous alterations of the sinuses. The appendix to Volume one deals with specific problems exclusive to oral surgery and quotes for the first time case histories of other physicians. English translations, Baltimore, 1849 and Philadelphia, 1851.

3676.2   WOOFENDALE, ROBERT. 1742-1828
Practical observations on the human teeth. London, *J. Johnson*, 1783.

Woofendale was the first professional dentist to travel to the American colonies (1766) and to set up practice there. During his two years of practice in America he may have made the first set of artificial teeth contructed in what is now the United States. He returned to England in 1769. The above work was "the most important [English] dental text of the time after Berdmore's" (Ring).

3677   DUBOIS DE CHE:MANT, NICOLAS. 1753-1824
Dissertation sur les avantages des nouvelles dents, et rateliers artificiels, incorruptibles et sans odeur. Paris, Chez l'auteur, 1788.

Dubois de Chémant was the first dentist to manufacture porcelain teeth by a process modified from that originally invented by an apothecary named Alexis Duchâteau in 1776.

3677.1   GARDETTE, JACQUES. 1756-1831
Remarks on the diseases of the teeth. American Museum, *Universal Magazine*, 1790.

The first scientific paper on dentistry to appear in an American periodical. Trained in France, Gardette accepted a commission as a surgeon in the French navy and went to America in 1778 when France sent her ships to defend the cause of the American Revolution.

3678   SKINNER, RICHARD CORTLAND. *d.c.* 1834
A treatise on the human teeth, concisely explaining their structure and cause of disease and decay. New York, *Johnson & Stryker*, 1801.

First American book on the teeth, a pamphlet of 26pp. It was intended for the lay public and listed sound rules of oral hygiene, explained the nature of dental diseases and their treatment, and stressed preventive maintenance of the teeth. In 1792 Skinner founded at the New York Dispensary the first in-hospital dental clinic in the United States. He also offered his services free of charge to the Hospital and Alms House of New York City, establishing the first dental clinic for the poor in America. Reprinted New York, *Argosy*, 1967.

3678.1   SERRE, JOHANN JACOB JOSEPH. 1759-1830
Praktische Darstellung aller Operationen der Zahnheilkunst. Berlin, *La Garde*, 1803.

This work contains one of the earliest histories of dentistry.

3679   FOX, JOSEPH. 1775-1816
The natural history of the human teeth. London, *T. Cox.*, 1803.

Fox's classic treatise on the teeth is the first to include explicit directions for correcting dental irregularities. It is the first work on orthodontics.

3679.1   ——. The history and treatment of diseases of the teeth, the gums, and the alveolar processes, etc. London, *T. Cox*, 1806.

Fox was a surgeon practising dentistry. By some of the authorities his book is considered more valuable than Hunter's (No. 3676). This is the first book to illustrate diseases of the teeth.

3679.2   FONZI, GIUSEPPANGELO. 1768-1840
Rapport sur les dents artificielles terro-métalliques. Paris, 1808.

Fonzi produced the first sets of individual porcelain teeth mounted on a base and also discovered a means of partially imitating the semitransparent tint peculiar to natural teeth.

3679.3   JAMES, BENJAMIN.
A treatise on the management of the teeth. Boston, *Callender*, 1814.

The first full-length book on dentistry published in the United States, and the first with a dental illustration.

3679.4   DELABARRE, CHRISTOPHE FRANÇOIS. 1777-1862
Odontologie. Paris, *chez l'Auteur*, 1815.
Delabarre was one of the first to systematize occlusal anomalies through description and illustration of individual kinds. He also developed some of the earliest orthodontic appliances using bands.

3679.5   ——. Traité de la partie mécanique de l'art du chirugien-dentiste. 2 vols., Paris, *chez l'Auteur*, 1820.
The first scientifically written textbook of dental prosthetics.

3679.6   MAURY, [J.C.] F.
Traité complet de l'art du dentiste. Paris, *Gabon*, 1828.

Maury probably invented the dental probe. His book also shows one of the earliest illustrations of a dental mouth mirror. English translation, Philadelphia, 1843.

3679.7   SPOONER, SHEARJASHUB. 1809-1859
Guide to sound teeth or a popular treatise on the teeth. New York, *Wiley & Long*, 1836.
John Roach Spooner, an American dentist living in Montreal, was the first to use arsenous acid to devitalize the pulp. This discovery was first published in the above work by his brother.

3679.8   KNEISEL, FRIEDRICH CHRISTOPH. 1797-1883?
Der Schiefstand der Zähne. Berlin, *Ernst Siegfried Mittler*, 1836.
The first specialized orthodontic work, on anomalous positions of the teeth. A French translation was issued simultaneously by the same publisher.

3680   HARRIS, CHAPIN AARON. 1806-1860
The dental art, a practical treatise on dental surgery. Baltimore, *Armstrong & Berry*, 1839.
One of the most popular books on the subject ever published. It underwent 13 editions during the next 74 years! Harris was instrumental in founding the first dental college in the world, the Baltimore College of Dental Surgery, as well as the first national association of dentists in the U.S., and the first authoritative dental periodical, the *American Journal of Dental Science*.

3681   NASMYTH, ALEXANDER. ?-1848
On the structure, physiology, and pathology of the persistent capsular investments and pulp of the tooth. *Med.-chir. Trans.*, 1839, **22**, 310-328.
"Nasmyth's membrane", or persistent dental capsule.

3681.1   OWEN, *Sir* RICHARD. 1804-1892
Odontography, or, a treatise on the comparative anatomy of the teeth. 2 vols., London, *H. Baillière*, 1840-45.
Owen's first large-scale original work covered the whole range of the toothed vertebrates, living and fossil, and discussed in detail the micrsocopic structure of the teeth and the physiology of dentition. Includes 168 plates.

3681.2   DESIRABODE, MALAGOU ANTOINE. 1781-185-?
Nouveaux éléments complets de la science et de l'art du dentiste. Suivis d'une notice historique et chronologique des travaux imprimés sur l'art du dentiste. 2 vols., Paris, *Labé*, 1843.
Desirabode may have been the first to discuss the use of fluoride compounds for caries prevention. *See* No. 3692.1. English translation of 2nd ed., Baltimore, 1847.

3682   CARABELLI, GEORG, *Edler von Lunkaszprie*. 1787-1842
Systematisches Handbuch der Zahnheilkunde. Bd. 2. Anatomie des Mundes. Wien, *Braumüller & Seidel*, 1844.
Original description (p. 107) of "Carabelli's cusp", tuberculus anomalus, sometimes found on the lingual surface of the upper permanent molars. It was illustrated on Tab. XI, Fig. 4e, and Tab. XIV, Fig. 4, of *Kupfertafeln zu v. Carabelli's Anatomie des Mundes*, Wien, 1842.

3683   TOMES, *Sir* JOHN. 1815-1895
A course of lectures on dental physiology and surgery. London, *John W. Parker*, 1848.

Tomes invented a set of anatomically correct forceps for tooth extraction, thereby elevating this device, which had been previously neglected, to dentistry's most important extraction instrument. Tomes persuaded the Royal College of Surgeons to grant a Licence, was a co-founder of the Odontological Society in 1856, and founded the (Royal) Dental Hospital in 1858. He played a leading part in the movement which led to the passing of the Dentists Act, 1878.

3683.1   ——. On the presence of fibrils of soft tissue in the dentinal tubes. *Phil. Trans.*, 1856, **146**, 515-522.

Tomes described and drew the protoplasmic processes from the odontoblasts which are known as "Tomes's fibrils". These had been previously seen by Johannes Müller and others.

3684   GAINE, CHARLES.

On certain irregularities of the teeth with cases illustrative of a novel method of successful treatment. Bath, *C. W. Oliver*, 1858.

First work devoted exclusively to irregularities of the teeth.

3684.1   GARRETSON, JAMES EDWARD. 1828-1895

A treatise on the diseases and surgery of the mouth, jaws, and associated parts. Philadelphia, *J.B. Lippincott*, 1869.

The first modern textbook of oral surgery. Garretson received the first official hospital appointment as "oral surgeon". He helped to establish oral surgery as a specialty.

3685   RIGGS, JOHN M. 1810-1885

Suppurative inflammation of the gums, and absorption of the gums and alveolar process. *Penn. J. dent. Sci.*, 1876, **3**, 99-104.

"Riggs's disease" – pyorrhoea alveolaris. Treatment of the disease by scraping was introduced by Riggs.

3685.01   WITZEL, ADOLF.

Pathologie und Therapie der Pulpakrankheiten des Zahnes. Hagen, *H. Risel*, 1886.

Witzel used histological methods to analyse pulp diseases, and applied antiseptic principles to their treatment.

3685.1   KINGSLEY, NORMAN WILLIAM. 1829-1913

A treatise on oral deformities. New York, *D. Appleton*, 1880.

First book on the scientific treatment of irregularities of the teeth. Kingsley made the first attempt at systematizing the treatment of occlusal abnormalities.

3686   ANGLE, EDWARD HARTLEY. 1855-1930

Notes on orthodontia, with a new system of regulation and retention. *Trans. 9th Int. Congr. Med.*, 1887, **5**, 565-72.

The specialty of orthodontics received a new impetus with the work of Angle. He organized and classified the various abnormalities of the teeth and jaws and devised many methods of treating them. Through a series of books and pamphlets he standardized appliances, inventing the systems now widely used, with modifications.

3687   MILLER, WILLOUGHBY DAYTON. 1853-1907

The micro-organisms of the human mouth. Philadelphia, *S. S. White Dental Mfg. Co.*, 1890.

In 1884 Miller became professor of dentistry at the University of Berlin, the first foreigner ever to receive a professorial appointment at a German University. Inspired by study of bacteriology under Robert Koch, Miller argued that "carbohydrates trapped around the teeth were fermented by bacterial components of the normal oral flora and the resulting acids decalcified the tooth enamel; other bacteria then entered the tooth through the initial defect and destroyed the underlying dentine" (Ring). His book first appeared in a German edition in 1889. Reprint of English edition, Basel, *Karger*, 1973.

3688   HARRISON, Frank.
The "x" rays in the practice of dental surgery. *J. Brit. dent. Ass.*, 1896, **17**, 624-28.
    Harrison was the first to describe a method of making dental radiographs.

3689   MORTON, William James. 1846-1920
The x-ray and its application to dentistry. *Dental Cosmos*, 1896, **38**, 478-86.
    First dental radiography in America.

3689.1   TAGGART, William Henry.
A new and accurate method of making gold inlays. *Dent. Cosmos*, 1907, **49**, 1117-1121.
    Taggart invented the modern method of making gold inlays.

3689.2   BLACK, Greene Vardiman, 1836-1915
A work on operative dentistry. 2 vols., Chicago, *Chicago Medical Dental Publishing Co.*, 1908.
    Black established a system of cavity preparation from which modern techniques have been derived. He constructed a "gnathodynamometer" with which the pressure exerted on the human tooth and therefore on the filling material could be measured. Through experimentation he established an ideal metal mixture which was stable and did not discolour. Publication of his results led to standardization of the alloys.

3690   THOMA, Kurt Hermann. 1883-
Oral roentgenology. Boston, *Ritter & Co.*, 1917.

3690.1   STILLMAN, Paul Roscoe. 1871-1945 & McCALL, John Oppie. 1879-
A textbook of clinical periodontia. New York, *Macmillan*, 1922.
    "The first authoritative book in the field" (Ring).

3691   McINTOSH, James, *et al.*
An investigation into the aetiology of dental caries. *Brit. J. exp. Path.*, London, 1922, **3**, 138-45; 1924, **5**, 175-84.
    Isolation of *L. odontolyticus I* and *II* from carious teeth; this organism is suspected of causing dental caries. With W. W. James and P. Lazarus-Barlow.

3691.1   GREGORY, William King. 1897-1970
The origin and evolution of the human dentition. Baltimore, *Williams & Wilkins*, 1922.
    Reprinted with revisions and new index from *J. dent. Res.*, 1920, **2**, 89-175, 215-426, 604-717; 1921, **3**, 87-228.

3692   RAPER, HOWARD RILEY.
A new kind of x-ray examination for preventive dentistry. *Int. J. Orthodont.*, 1925, **11**, 275-79, 370-74, 470-77.
Original description of technique of making "bite-wing" radiographs.

3692.1   DEAN, HENRY TRENDLEY. -1962, *et al.*
Studies on mass control of dental caries through fluoridation of the public water supply. *Publ. Hlth. Rep. (Wash.)*, 1950, **65**, 1403-08.
It has not been conclusively demonstrated whether fluoride serves a specific physiological role, but fluoridation of public water supplies was followed by a reduction in the incidence of dental caries. One of the first studies on mass control of dental caries was that published by Dean, F. A. Arnold, P. Jay, and J. W. Knutson. *See* No. 3681.2.

History of Dentistry

3693   HILL, ALFRED. 1826-1922
The history of the reform movement in the dental profession in Great Britain during the last twenty years. London, *Trübner & Co.*, 1877.
The history of the beginnings of an organized dental profession in Britain.

3694   CROWLEY, C. GEORGE.
Dental bibliography: a standard reference list of books on dentistry published throughout the world from 1536 to 1885. Philadelphia, *S. S. White Dental Mfg. Co.*, 1885.
Reprinted Amsterdam, 1968.

3694.1   DAVID, THÉOPHILE.
Bibliographie français de l'art dentaire. Paris, *Félix Alcan*, 1889.
Reprinted Amsterdam, 1970.

3695   GUERINI, VINCENZO. 1859-1955
A history of dentistry from the most ancient times until the end of the eighteenth century. Philadelphia, *Lea & Febiger*, 1909.
Reprinted Amsterdam, 1967.

3696   PROSKAUER, CURT. 1887-1972
Kulturgeschichte der Zahnheilkunde. 4 vols. Berlin, *H. Meusser*, 1913-26.

3697   SUDHOFF, KARL FRIEDRICH JAKOB. 1853-1938
Geschichte der Zahnheilkunde. Leipzig, *J. A. Barth*, 1921.
Second edition, 1926 (reprinted 1964).

3698   Index to the periodical dental literature in the English language. Chicago, 1921-
In progress. Retrospective from 1839. Now known as *Index to dental literature.*

3699   WEINBERGER, BERNHARD WOLF. 1885-1960
Orthodontics; an historical review of its origin and evolution, including an extensive bibliography of orthodontic literature up to the time of specialization. 2 vols. St. Louis, *C. V. Mosby*, 1926.

3699.1 ———. Dental bibliography. 2 vols., New York, *First District Dental Society*, [1929]-1932.
Catalogue, without annotations, of the dental collections of the New York Academy of Medicine.

3699.2 POLETTI, GIOVANNI BAPTISTA
De re dentaria apud veteres, sive repertorium bibliographicum. Bologna, *L. Cappelli*, 1935.
An annotated bibliography in Italian of dental books printed before 1800, and of books on general medicine with significant contributions to dentistry.

3700 STRÖMGREN, HEDVIG LIDFORSS. 1877-
Die Zahnheilkunde im achtzehnten Jahrhundert. Kopenhagen, *Levin & Munksgaard*, 1935.

3701 ———. Die Zahnheilkunde im neunzehnten Jahrhundert. Kopenhagen, *Levin & Munksgaard*, 1945.

3702 LUFKIN, ARTHUR WARD. 1889-
A history of dentistry. 2nd edition. Philadelphia, *Lea & Febiger*, 1948.

3703 WEINBERGER, BERNHARD WOLF. 1885-1960
An introduction to the history of dentistry. 2 vols. St. Louis, *C. V. Mosby Co.*, 1948.
The first volume covers the history to 1800; the second deals solely with the history of dentistry in America.

3704 CAMPBELL, JOHN MENZIES. 1887-1974
A dental bibliography: British and American, 1692-1880. London, *David Low*, 1949.

3705 COLYER, *Sir* FRANK. 1866-1954
Old instruments used for extracting teeth. London, *Staples Press*, 1952.

3705.01 FASTLICHT, SAMUEL.
Bibliografia odontologica Mexicana. Mexico, La Prensa Medica Mexicana, 1954.

3705.02 PROSKAUER, CURT. 1887-1972, & WITT, FRITZ H.
Pictorial history of dentistry. Cologne, *Dumont Schauberg*, 1962.

3705.03 GULLETT, D.W.
A history of dentistry in Canada. Toronto, *University of Toronto Press for Canadian Dental Assoc.*, [1971].

3705.04 ASBELL, MILTON B.
A bibliography of dentistry in America, 1790-1840. Cherry Hill, N.J., *Sussex House*, 1973.
Covers monographs and periodical literature.

3705.05 FASTLICHT, SAMUEL.
Tooth mutilations and dentistry in pre-Columbian Mexico. Chicago, *Quintessence*, 1976.

3705.1   DECHAUME, MICHEL. 1897- , *et al.*
         Histoire illustrée de l'art dentaire: stomatologie et odontologie. Paris, *R. Dacosta*, [1977].
         With P. Huard and M. J. Imbault-Huart.

3705.2   NAKAHARA, KEN. *et al*
         Manners and customs of dentistry in Ukiyoe. Tokyo, *Ishiyaku*, 1980.

3705.3   HOFFMANN-AXTHELM, WALTER. 1908-
         History of dentistry. Translated by H. M. Koehler. Chicago, *Quintessence Books*, 1981.
         The author does not consider this a simple translation of his *Geschichte der Zahnheilkunde* (1973), as in the sections devoted to the 19th and early 20th centuries it has been so substantially revised as to be "almost a different book". This is the best history of dentistry from the bibliographic point of view. Second edition in German, 1985.

3705.4   RING, MALVIN E.
         Dentistry: an illustrated history. St. Louis, *C.V. Mosby Co.*, [1985].

3705.5   BENNION, ELISABETH.
         Antique dental instruments. London, *Sotheby's Publications*, [1986].

DEFICIENCY DISEASES

See also 1042-1092, NUTRITION: VITAMINS

3706   STEPP, WILHELM OTTO. 1882-1963, & GYÖRGY, PAUL. 1893-1976
         Avitaminosen und verwandte Krankheitszustände. Berlin, *J. Springer*, 1927.

3707   SEBRELL, WILLIAM HENRY. 1901- , & BUTLER, ROY EDWIN. 1902-
         Riboflavin deficiency in man; a preliminary note. *Publ. Hlth. Rep. (Wash.)*, 1938, **53**, 2282-84.
         Ariboflavinosis.

3708   WANG, Y. L., & HARRIS, LESLIE JULIUS. 1898-1973
         Methods for assessing the level of nutrition of the human subject: estimation of vitamin B_1 in urine by the thiochrome test. *Biochem. J.*, 1939, **33**, 1356-69.
         Wang's test for avitaminosis.

3709   BICKNELL, FRANKLIN. 1906-
         The vitamins in medicine. 4th ed., edited by Riam M. Barker and David A. Bender. 2 vols., London, *W. Heinemann*, 1980.

Scurvy

3710   RONSSEUS, BALDUINUS [RONSSE, (BOUDEWIJN)]. 1525-1597
         De magnis Hippocratis lienibus, Pliniique stomacace, ac sceletyrbe, seu vulgo dicto scorbuto, libellus. Antverpiae, *apud viduam Martini Nutii*, 1564.
         Jean de Joinville was probably the first, about 1250, to describe scurvy; Vasco da Gama noted its occurrence at sea, and Jacques Cartier mentions

it. Ronsseus gave an early medical account describing how sailors cured themselves by eating oranges and lemons as soon as they reached the coast of Spain.

3711   WOODALL, JOHN. 1570-1643
The surgions mate. London, *E. Griffin*, 1617.
Woodall knew the value of limes, lemons, and oranges, and gave them a prominent place in his account of the treatment of scurvy. He was surgeon to St. Bartholomew's Hospital and a contemporary of Harvey. Facsimile edition, Bath, 1978. *See* No. 2144.

3712   ABREU, ALEXO DE. 1568-1630
Tratado de las siete enfermedades, de la inflammacion universal del higado, zirbo, pyloron, y riñones, y de la obstruction, de la satiriasi, de la terciana y febre maligna, y passion hipocondriaca. Lleva otros tres tratados, del mal de Loanda, del guzano, y de las fuentes y sedales. Lisboa, *P. Craesbeeck*, 1623.
Includes a precise clinical description of scurvy (fol. 150v. to 193). Abreu treated the disease with fresh milk and antiscorbutic syrups, particularly rose syrup – a rich natural source of ascorbic acid.

3713   LIND, JAMES. 1716-1794
A treatise of the scurvy. Edinburgh, *Sands, Murray & Cochran*, 1753.
Lind, founder of naval hygiene in England, wrote a classic treatise on scurvy, in which he described many important experiments he made on the disease. These experiments have been called "the first deliberately planned controlled therapeutic trial ever undertaken". Lind showed that in preserved form citrus juices could be carried for long periods on board ship, and that, if administered properly, they would prevent the disease. The application of this knowledge by naval surgeons who followed Lind led to the eventual elimination of the disease from the British Navy. Reprinted, with notes, Edinburgh, 1953.

3714   COOK, JAMES. 1728-1779
The method taken for preserving the health of the crew of H.M.S. the Resolution during her late voyage round the world. *In:* Sir John Pringle, A discourse upon some late improvements in the means for preserving the health of mariners. London, *Royal Society*, 1776.
Following the scurvy-preventing suggestions of James Lind, Cook lost only one man to disease on his second voyage from 1768-1771. Reprinted in *Phil. Trans.*, 1776, **66**, 402-06. *See* No. 2156.

3715   BLANE, *Sir* GILBERT. 1749-1834
Observations on the diseases incident to seamen. London, *J. Cooper*, 1785.
Although Blane added nothing to the knowledge on scurvy, he demonstrated the value of fresh lemons, limes, and oranges; through his influence the issue of lemon juice in the British Navy was ordered in 1795, after which scurvy soon disappeared. Blane's extreme coldness of manner earned him the nickname "Chilblain".

3716   TROTTER, THOMAS. 1761-1832
Observations on the scurvy. Edinburgh, *C. Eliot & G. G. J. & J. Robinson*, 1786.

3717   KREBEL, RUDOLPH.
        Der Scorbut in geschichtlich-literarischer, pathologischer, prophylactischer
        und therapeutischer Beziehung. Leipzig, *E. Wartig*, 1836.

3718   MÖLLER, JULIUS OTTO LUDWIG. 1819-1887
        Ueber akute Rachitis. *Königsb. med. Jb.*, 1859, **1**, 377-79.
            Möller was the first to describe the acute form of rickets combined with
        scurvy now associated with the name of Barlow (No. 3720).

3719   CHEADLE, WALTER BUTLER. 1836-1910
        Three cases of scurvy supervening on rickets in young children. *Lancet*, 1878,
        2, 685-87.
            Infantile scurvy was confused with rickets until Cheadle differentiated
        between the two conditions.

3720   BARLOW, *Sir* THOMAS. 1845-1945
        On cases described as "acute rickets" which are probably a combination of
        scurvy and rickets, the scurvy being an essential, and the rickets a variable,
        element. *Med.-chir. Trans.*, 1883, **66**, 159-219.
            Classic description of infantile scurvy ("Barlow's disease"), which
        includes the pathology of the condition. See also his earlier paper in *Trans.
        int. med. Congr.*, 1881, **4**, 116-28. Reprinted, but without the coloured
        lithographs and detailed list of cases included in the original, in *Arch. Dis.
        Childh.*, 1935, **10**, 223-52.

3721   HOLST, AXEL. 1861-1931
        Experimental studies relating to "ship-beri-beri" and scurvy. *J. Hyg. (Lond.)*,
        1907, **7**, 619-33.
            Experimental production of scurvy in guinea-pigs. Holst published
        further papers on the subject in the same journal, 1907, **7**, 634-71, and in
        Z. Hyg., 1912, **72**, 1-120, both with Theodor Froelich. Their work made it
        possible to employ guinea-pigs for assessing the relative values of
        antiscorbutic foods.

3722   ASCHOFF, KARL ALBERT LUDWIG. 1866-1942, & KOCH, WALTER KARL. 1880-
        Der Skorbut. Jena, *G. Fischer*, 1919.

3723   HESS, ALFRED FABIAN. 1875-1933
        Scurvy, past and present. Philadelphia, *J. B. Lippincott*, (1920).
            Includes a history and bibliography.

3724   BOAS, MARGARET AVERIL.
        The effect of desiccation upon the nutritive properties of egg-white.
        Biochem. J., 1927, **21**, 712-24.
            Demonstration of the effect of deprivation of biotin.

3725   PARSONS, *Sir* LEONARD GREGORY. 1879-1950
        Scurvy treated with ascorbic acid. *Proc. roy. Soc. Med.*, 1933, **26**, 1533.
            First case of infantile scurvy cured by the administration of ascorbic
        acid.

3726   CARPENTER, KENNETH JOHN. 1923-
        The history of scurvy and vitamin C. Cambridge, *Cambridge University Press*, [1986].

Rickets

3727   WHISTLER, DANIEL. 1619-1684
        Disputatio medica inauguralis, de morbo puerili Anglorum, quem patrio idiomate indigenae vocant The Rickets. Lugduni Batavorum, *ex. off. W. C. Boxii*, 1645.
        In his 26th year Whistler published his graduation thesis at Leiden; this was the first description of rickets as a definite disease manifesting itself by a more or less constant association of symptoms. Still (No. 6356) gives an interesting account of Whistler, with abstracts from the above work. The book attracted little attention, and the credit for the first description is usually given to Glisson. English translation by G.T. Smerdon, *J. Hist. Med.*, 1950, **5**, 397-415.

3728   BOATE, ARNOLD [BOOTIUS]. ?1600-?1653
        Observationes medicae de affectibus omissis. London, *T. Whitaker*, 1649.
        Boate who spent many years in Ireland, included a full first-hand account of rickets in Chapter 12 of the above book ("De tabe pectorea"). He showed how widespread the disease was at that time. Reprinted in *Opuscula Selecta Neerlandicorum*, Fasc. 5, pp. 260-73, Amsterdam, 1926.

3729   GLISSON, FRANCIS. 1597-1677
        De rachitide sive morbo puerili, qui vulgo The Rickets dicitur. Londini, *typ. G. Du-gardi*, 1650.
        Although anticipated by Whistler and others in the description of infantile rickets, Glisson's account was the fullest that had till then appeared. He was first (Chap. 22) to describe infantile scurvy. Glisson's book on rickets was one of the earliest instances of collaborative medical research in England, combining the observations of Glisson and seven other contributors. G.Bate and A. Regemorter are credited as co-authors. An English translation appeared in 1651. *See* No. 4297.91.

3730   SCHÜTTE, D.
        Beobachtungen Über den Nutzen des Berger Leberthrans (Oleum jecoris Aselli, von Gadus asellus L.). *Arch. med. Erfahr.*, 1824, **2**, 79-92.
        First report of the value of cod-liver oil in the treatment of rickets.

3731   POMMER, GUSTAV. 1851-1935
        Untersuchungen über Osteomalacie und Rachitis. Leipzig, *F. C. W. Vogel*, 1885.
        Hess considered this the foremost contribution to the subject during the 19th century.

3732   HULDSCHINSKY, KURT. 1883-1941
        Heilung von Rachitis durch künstliche Höhensonne. *Dtsch. med. Wschr.*, Berlin, 1919,m **45**, 712-13.
        Rickets cured by ultra-violet irradiation.

3733   MELLANBY, *Sir* EDWARD. 1884-1955
The part played by an "accessory factor" in the production of experimental rickets. *J. Physiol. (Lond.)*, 1918-19, **52**, xi-xii, liii-liv.
First convincing experimental evidence that rickets is a deficiency disease, curable by correct diet.

3734   ———. An experimental investigation on rickets. *Lancet*, 1919, **1**, 407-12.
In his important experiments on rickets, Mellanby both induced and controlled the disease by diet.

3735   HESS, ALFRED FABIAN. 1875-1933
Rickets, including osteomalacia and tetany. Philadelphia, *Lea & Febiger*, 1929.
Hess made numerous clinical observations on rickets and scurvy and discovered that antirachitic properties could be imparted to certain oils and to food by exposing them to ultra-violet rays. His book includes an important history and bibliography of the subject.

Beri-beri

3736   BONDT, JACOB DE [BONTIUS]. 1592-1631
De paralyseos quadam specie, quam indigenae beriberii vocant. In his: *De medicina Indorum*. Lugduni Batavorum, 1642, 115-20.
Beri-beri, the deficiency disease endemic to Eastern and Southern Asia (sporadic elsewhere), results from a thiamine deficiency caused by too great a dependence on polished rice in the diet. (See No. 3740). It was mentioned in Chinese literature before the Christian era. The first modern scientific description was given by Bondt, who saw cases of it in the East Indies. *See* No. 2263.

3737   TULP, NICOLAAS. 1593-1674
Observationes medicae. Amstelodami, *apud L. Elzevirium*, 1652.
One of the earliest accounts of beri-beri is on pp. 300-05 of this work. Tulp, notable as the demonstrator in Rembrandt's "Anatomy Lesson", was among the first, in the same book, to describe the ileo-caecal valve ("Tulp's valve"). The first edition was published in 1641.

3738   MALCOLMSON, JOHN GRANT. ?-1844
A practical essay on the history and treatment of beriberi. Madras, *Govt. Press*, 1835.
A classic account, in which the author brought together all that was known about the disease in his day.

3739   BAELZ, ERWIN OTTO EDUARD VON. 1849-1933
Kakke (Beriberi). *Mitt. deutsch. Ges. Nat. u. Völkerk. Ostasiens*, 1880-84, **3**, 301-19.
In his important account of beri-beri, Baelz dealt with the Tokyo outbreak of 1881.

3740   TAKAKI, KANEHIRO, *Baron*. 1849-1915
On the cause and prevention of kakke. *Trans. Sei.-I-Kwai*, Tokyo, 1885, **4**, 29-37.

Takaki was the first conclusively to show the dietary origin of beri-beri. Measures introduced by him resulted in its eradication from the Japanese Navy, where it had previously been a serious problem.

3741   EIJKMAN, CHRISTIAAN. 1858-1930
Polyneuritis bij hoenders. *Geneesk. T. nederl. Indië*, 1890, **30**, 295; 1893, **32**, 353; 1896, **36**, 214.
Eijkman produced beri-beri experimentally in fowls; from this he was led to conclude that a diet of over-milled rice was the chief cause, both in fowls and humans. Thus his work was of great importance in determining the aetiology of beri-beri, and he further has the distinction of being the first to produce experimentally a disease of dietary deficiency origin. He shared a Nobel Prize with F. G. Hopkins in 1929. German translation in *Virchows Arch. path. Anat.*, 1897, **148**, 523-32.

3742   GRIJNS, GERRIT. 1865-1944
Over polyneuritis gallinarum. *Geneesk. T. nederl. Indië*, 1901, **41**, 3-110.
Grijns succeeded Eijkman as director of the Research Laboratory for Pathological Anatomy and Bacteriology in Batavia. He was the first to adopt the view that beri-beri was simply a "deficiency disease", since he found it to be due to the lack of an unknown substance in the diet. English translation of this and related papers in Grijns, *Researches on vitamins 1900-1911*, Gorinchem, 1935.

3743   FRASER, HENRY. 1873-1930, & STANTON, *Sir* AMBROSE THOMAS. 1875-1938
An inquiry concerning the etiology of beri-beri. Singapore, *Kelly & Walsh*, 1909.
Studies from the Institute for Medical Research, F. M. S., No. 10. Careful and long-continued experiments on the aetiology of beri-beri were carried out by Fraser and Stanton in Malaya.

3744   FUNK, CASIMIR. 1884-1967
On the chemical nature of the substance which cures polyneuritis in birds induced by a diet of polished rice. *J. Physiol. (Lond.)*, 1911, **43**, 395-400.
Funk determined the chemical nature of the substance in rice polishings which could cure beri-beri.

3745   VEDDER, EDWARD BRIGHT. 1878-1952
Beriberi. New York, *W. Wood & Co.*, 1913.
Important studies of beri-beri are recorded in this book. After its publication the author made many additional contributions to the literature on the subject.

3746   JANSEN, BAREND COENRAAD PETRUS. 1884-1962, & DONATH, WILLEM FREDERIK. 1889-1957
Antineuritische Vitamine. *Chem. Weekbl.*, 1926, **23**, 1387-1409.
Isolation of vitamin B_1 (aneurine, thiamine), lack of which is a cause of beri-beri.

3747   WENCKEBACH, KAREL FREDERIK. 1864-1940
Das Beriberi-Herz. Berlin, *J. Springer*, 1934.
Wenckebach wrote a classic account of the heart in beri-beri.

3748   WILLIAMS, ROBERT RUNNELS. 1886- , & CLINE, JOSEPH KALMAN. 1908-
Synthesis of vitamin B_1. *J. Amer. Chem. Soc.*, 1936, **58**, 1504-05.

Pellagra

3749 THIÉRRY, François [Thiéry]. 1719
Description d'une maladie appelée mal de la rosa. *J. Méd. Chir. Pharm.*, 1755, **2**, 337-46.
 Thiérry wrote an account of pellagra from what he had seen or heard of Casal's cases. His work antedates that of Casal in date of publication but is not a first-hand description. English translation in No. 2241.

3750 CASAL Y JULIAN, Gaspar. 1679-1759
Historia natural, y medica de el Principado de Asturias. Madrid, *M. Martin*, 1762.
 The first recognizable description of pellagra is included on pp. 327-60 of this book, which was written in 1735 but not published until 1762, after the writer's death. He called the disease *mal de la rosa*. See No. 3752. Reprinted, Oviedo, 1900.

3751 FRAPOLLI, Francesco ? –1773?
Animadversiones in morbum, vulgo pellagram. [Mediolani, *apud J. Galcatium*], 1771.
 In Frapolli's careful description of pellagra, the disease was first given its present name. This book is also the first Italian account of the malady. Partial English translation in No. 2241.

3752 STRAMBIO, Gaetano. 1752-1831
De pellagra. 3 vols. Mediolani. *J. B. Bianchi*, [1786]-89.
 By 1776, pellagra had attained serious proportions in Italy; Strambio was placed in charge of a hospital for the treatment of pellagrins, and he left an important account of the disease. He and Casal y Julian (No. 3750) first pointed out that pellagra might occur without the cutaneous lesions, till then regarded as characteristic.

3753 ROUSSEL, Jean Baptiste Victor Théophile. 1816-1903
Traité de la pellagre et des pseudo-pellagres. Paris, *J. B. Baillière*, 1866.
 Roussel was awarded a prize of 5,000 francs for this work.

3754 LOMBROSO, Cesare. 1836-1909
Studii clinici ed esperimentali sulla natura, causa e terapia della pellagra. Bologna, *F. E. Garagnani*, 1869.
 Lombroso upheld the maize theory of the origin of pellagra. He believed that the symptoms were caused by a toxin which developed in deteriorated maize. Reprinted from *Riv. clin. Bologna*, 1869, **8**, 289-314, 321-44.

3755 GOLDBERGER, Joseph. 1874-1929, *et al.*
The treatment and prevention of pellagra. *U. S. publ. Hlth. Serv. Rep.*, 1914, **29**, 2821-25.
 With C. H. Waring and D. G. Willets. A collection of Goldberger's most important papers with a list of his publications appeared in 1964.

3756 HARRIS, Henry Fauntleroy. 1867-1926
Pellagra. New York, *Macmillan & Co.*, 1919.

3757 GOLDBERGER, JOSEPH. 1874-1929, & WHEELER, GEORGE ALEXANDER. 1885-
The experimental production of pellagra in human subjects by means of
diet. *U. S. Publ. Hlth. Serv. Lab. Bull.*, No. 120, 1920, 7-116.

Goldberger was born in Central Europe in poor circumstances. He
migrated to America, and following attendance at a lecture by Austin Flint,
decided to study medicine. He entered the U. S. Public Health Service in
1899. He was a pioneer in the study and treatment of pellagra, demonstrating
its experimental production and its prevention by proper diet.

3758 ———. A further study of butter, fresh beef, and yeast as pellagra preventatives,
with consideration of the relation of factor P-P of pellagra (and black
tongue of dogs) to vitamin B. *Publ. Hlth. Rep. (Wash.)*, 1926, **41**, 297-318.

Anti-pellagra vitamin. With G. A. Wheeler, R. D. Lillie, and L. M. Rogers.

3759 WILLIAMS, CICELY DELPHINE. 1893-
Kwashiorkor. A nutritional disease of children associated with a maize diet.
Lancet, 1935, **2**, 1151-52.

First accurate description. "Kwashiorkor" was the local name in Ghana
for a nutritional disease of children, associated with a maize diet. The first
modern account was probably that of L. Normet in *Bull. Soc. Path. exot.*,
1926, **19**, 207-13.

3760 ELVEHJEM, CONRAD ARNOLD. 1901-1962, *et al.*
The isolation and identification of the anti-black tongue factor. *J. biol. Chem.*,
1938, **123**, 137-49.

Isolation of nicotinic acid, the pellagra-preventing factor. With R. J.
Madden, F. N. Strong, and D. W. Woolley.

SPLEEN: LYMPHATICS

3761 ZAMBECCARI, GIUSEPPE. 1665-1728
Esperienze del Dottor Giuseppe Zambeccari intorno a diverse viscere
tagliate a diversi animali viventi. Firenze, *F. Onofri*, 1680.

Proof that the spleen is not essential to life. For a translation and notes
on the book, see *Bull. Hist. Med.*, 1941, **9**, 144-76, 311-31 (S. Jarcho).

3762 HODGKIN, THOMAS. 1798-1866
On some morbid appearances of the absorbent glands and spleen. *Med.-
chir. Trans.*, 1832, **17**, 68-114.

First full description of lymphadenoma, which Wilks in 1865 referred to
as "Hodgkin's disease". In 1666 Malpighi had vaguely outlined the condition. Hodgkin was pathologist at Guy's Hospital. The paper is reproduced
in *Med. Classics*, 1937, **1**, 741-70.

3763 QUITTENBAUM, CARL FRIEDRICH. 1793-1852
Commentatio de splenis hypertrophia et historia extirpationis splenis
hypertrophici cum fortuna adversa. Rostochii, *typ. Adlerianis*, [1836].

While most people in Germany still considered splenectomy beyond
the bounds of possibility, Quittenbaum performed the operation in 1829,
establishing it as a surgical procedure.

3764   WILKS, *Sir* SAMUEL, *Bart.* 1824-1911
Cases of a peculiar enlargement of the lymphatic glands frequently associated with disease of the spleen. *Guy's Hosp. Rep.*, 1856, 3 ser., **2**, 114-32; 1865, 3 ser., **11**, 56-67.
    Wilks really put Hodgkin's disease "on the map"; the second paper for the first time attached Hodgkin's name to the disease.

3765   SIMON, GUSTAV. 1824-1876
Die Exstirpation der Milz am Menschen. Giessen, *Heyer,* 1857.

3766   GRIESINGER, WILHELM. 1817-1868
Ein Fall von Anaemia splenica bei einem Kinde. *Berl. klin. Wschr.*, 1866, **3**, 212-14.
    First reported case of (infantile) splenic anaemia.

3766.1   VANLAIR, CONSTANT. 1839-1914, & MASIUS, JEAN BAPTISTE NICOLAS VOLTAIRE. 1836-1912
De la microcythémie. *Bull. Acad. roy. Méd. Belg.*, 1871, 3 sér., **5**, 515-613.
    Vanlair and Masius were the first to suggest the concept of hereditary haemolytic anaemia. Their paper was republished in book form, Brussels, 1871.

3767   LANGHANS, THEODOR. 1839-1915
Das maligne Lymphosarkom (Pseudoleukämie). *Virchows Arch. path. Anat.*, 1872, **54**, 509-37.
    Langhans noted the presence of giant cells in the lesions of Hodgkin's disease.

3768   GREENFIELD, WILLIAM SMITH. 1846-1919
Specimens illustrative of the pathology of lymphadenoma and leucocythemia. *Trans. path. Soc. Lond.*, 1878, **29**, 272-304.
    Greenfield also drew attention to the giant cells in lymphadenoma, which later became known as "Dorothy Reed's giant cells" (*see* No. 3780).

3769   GAUCHER, PHILIPPE CHARLES ERNEST. 1854-1918
De l'épithélioma primitif de la rate, hypertrophie idiopathique de la rate sans leucémie. Paris, *Thèse,* 1882.
    Familial splenic anaemia ("Gaucher's disease").

3770   PEL, PIETER KLAZES. 1852-1919
Zur Symptomatologie der sog. Pseudo-Leukämie. *Berl. klin. Wschr.*, 1885, **22**, 3-7.
    "Pel–Ebstein disease", a remittant pyrexia occurring in Hodgkin's disease (*see also* No. 3771).

3771   EBSTEIN, WILHELM. 1836-1912
Das chronische Rückfallsfieber, eine neue Infektionskrankheit. *Berl. klin. Wschr.*, 1887, **24**, 565-68.

3772   DRESCHFELD, JULIUS. 1845-1907
Clinical lecture on acute Hodgkin's disease. *Brit. med. J.*, 1892, **1**, 893-96.
    Dreschfeld preceded Kundrat in differentiating Hodgkin's disease and lymphosarcoma.

3773   KUNDRAT, Hans. 1845-1893
Ueber Lympho-Sarkomatosis. *Wien. klin. Wschr.*, 1893, **6**, 211-13, 234-39.
Kundrat separated lymphosarcoma ("Kundrat's disease") from other malignant tumours involving the lymphatic system.

3774   BANTI, Guido. 1852-1925
La splenomegalia con cirrosi del fegato. *Sperimentale*, 1894, **48**, Com. e riv., 447-52; Sez. biol., 407-32.
"Banti's syndrome", splenomegalic anaemia. Reprinted with translation in *Med. Classics*, 1937, **1**, 901-27. (For his earlier work on the subject, *see* No. 3126.)

3775   PALTAUF, Richard. 1858-1924
Lymphosarkom (Lymphosarkomatose, Pseudoleukämie, Myelom, Chlorom). *Ergebn. allg. Path. path. Anat.,* (1896), 1897, **3**, 1 Heft, 652-91.
"Paltauf–Sternberg disease" (*see also* No. 3776). On the European Continent the name "Hodgkin–Paltauf–Sternberg disease" is in use.

3776   STERNBERG, Carl. 1872-1935
Ueber eine eigenartige, unter dem Bilde der Pseudoleukämie verlaufende Tuberkulose des lymphatischen Apparates. *Z. Heilk.*, 1898, **19**, 21-90.
In his classic description of lymphadenoma, Sternberg separated it from aleukaemic leukaemia, with which it had hitherto been included.

3777   HAYEM, Georges. 1841-1933
Sur une variété particulière d'ictère chronique splénomégalique. *J. Méd. intern.*, 1898, **2**, 116-18.
"Hayem–Widal disease" – acquired haemolytic anaemia (*see also* No. 3783).

3779   MINKOWSKI, Oscar. 1858-1931.
Ueber eine hereditäre, unter dem Bilde eines chronischen Icterus mit Urobilinurie Splenomegalie, und Nierensiderosis verlaufende Affection. *Verh. Kongr. inn. Med.*, 1900, **18**, 316-21.
"Minkowski–Chauffard disease", familial haemolytic jaundice. *See also* No. 3781.

3780   REED, Dorothy, *Mrs. Mendenhall.*
On the pathological changes in Hodgkin's disease, with especial reference to its relation to tuberculosis. *Johns Hopk. Hosp. Rep.*, 1902, **10**, 133-96.
Dorothy Reed's classic work on Hodgkin's disease included a study of the histological picture. She described the proliferation of the endothelial and reticular cells, and the formation of lymphadenoma cells – "Dorothy Reed's giant cells".

3781   CHAUFFARD, Anatole Marie Emile. 1855-1932
Pathogénie de l'ictère de l'adulte. *Semaine méd.*, 1907, **27**, 25-29.
"Minkowski–Chauffard disease" (*see* No. 3779).

3782   WHIPPLE, George Hoyt. 1878-1976
A hitherto undescribed disease characterized anatomically by deposits of fat and fatty acids in the intestinal and mesenteric lymphatic tissues. *Johns Hopk. Hosp. Bull.*, 1907, **18**, 382-91.
"Whipple's disease". Whipple suggested the name "intestinal lipodystrophy" for this condition, now attributed to bacilliform bodies.

3783   WIDAL, Georges Fernand Isidor. 1862-1929, & ABRAMI, Pierre. 1879-1945
        Ictères hémolytiques non congénitaux avec anémie. *Presse méd.*, 1907, **15**,
        749.
        "Widal–Abrami disease" (Hayem–Widal disease), acquired haemolytic
        anaemia. (*See also* No. 3777.)

3784   NIEMANN, Albert. 1880-1921
        Ein unbekanntes Krankheitsbild. *Jb. Kinderheilk*, 1914, 79, 1-10.
        First description of that form of xanthomatosis which Pick described
        more fully in 1926 (No. 3785) and to which the eponym "Niemann–Pick
        disease" has been applied.

3785   PICK, Ludwig. 1868-1935
        Der Morbus Gaucher und die ihm ähnlichen Erkrankungen. (Die
        lipoidzellige Splenohepatomegalie Typus Niemann und die diabetische
        Lipoidzellenhyperplasie der Milz.) *Ergebn. inn Med. Kinderheilk.*, 1926,
        29, 519-627.
        "Niemann–Pick disease" – a form of xanthomatosis to which attention
        was first drawn by Niemann (No. 3784) in 1914. Pick's account is of greater
        importance.

3786   BRILL, Nathan Edwin. 1860-1925, *et al.*
        Generalized giant lymph follicle hyperplasia of lymph nodes and spleen;
        a hitherto undescribed type. *J. Amer. med. Assoc.*, 1925, **84**, 668-71.
        See No. 3787. With G. Baehr and N. Rosenthal.

3787   SYMMERS, Douglas. 1879-1952
        Follicular lymphadenopathy with splenomegaly: a newly recognized
        disease of the lymphatic system. *Arch. Path. Lab. Med.*, 1927, **3**, 816-20.
        "Brill–Symmers disease" (*see* No. 3786).

3787.1 DAMESHEK, William. 1900-1969, & SCHWARTS, Steven Otto. 1911-
        Hemolysins as the cause of clinical and experimental hemolytic anemias.
        Amer. J. med. Sci., 1938, **196**, 769-92.
        Acquired haemolytic anaemia was the first condition to be recognized
        as an auto-immune disease.

3787.2 GILBERT, René.
        Radiotherapy in Hodgkin's disease (malignant granulomatosis). Anatomic
        and clinical foundations; governing principles; results. *Amer. J. Roentgenol.*,
        1939, **41**, 198-241.
        Gilbert was among the first to achieve durable responses to radiotherapy
        in Hodgkin's disease.

3788   GILMAN, Alfred. 1908- , & PHILIPS, Frederick Stanley. 1916-
        The biological actions and therapeutic applications of the ß-chloroethyl
        amines and sulfides. *Science*, 1946, **103**, 409-15.
        Introduction of nitrogen mustard in treatment of Hodgkin's disease.

3788.1 RHOADS, Cornelius Packard. 1898-1959, *et al.*
        Triethylene melamine in the treatment of Hodgkin's disease and allied
        neoplasms. *Trans. Ass. Amer. Phycns.*, 1950, **63**, 136-46.
        TEM. With D. A. Karnofsky, J. H. Burchenal, and L. F. Craver.

3788.2   JOHNSON, IRVING STANLEY. 1925- , *et al.*
The *Vinca* alkaloids: a new class of oncolytic agents. *Cancer Res.*, 1963,
23, 1390-1427.
Clinical use of vinblastine (for Hodgkin's disease and other lymphomas)
and vincristine (for acute leukaemias of childhood). With J. G. Armstrong,
M. Gorman, and J. P. Burnett. Preliminary communication in *J. Lab. clin.
Med.*, 1959, **54**, 830.

ENDOCRINE DISORDERS

3789   PLATTER, FELIX [PLATERUS]. 1536-1614
Observationum in hominis affectibus. Basileae, *L. König*, 1614.
First known report of a case of death from hypertrophy of the thymus,
in an infant, is reported on p. 172; it is reproduced on p. 239 of J. Ruhräh's
Pediatrics of the past, New York, 1925.

3790   HUTCHINSON, *Sir* JONATHAN. 1828-1913
Congenital absence of hair and mammary glands with atrophic condition
of the skin and its appendages in a boy whose mother had been almost
wholly bald from alopecia areata from the age of six. *Med.-chir. Trans.*, 1886,
69, 473-77.
First description of progeria.

3791   MARCHAND, FELIX JACOB. 1846-1928
Ueber eine Geschwulst der sogen. Glandula carotica oder des Nodulus
caroticus. In *Festschrift Rudolf Virchow*, Berlin, *A. Hirschwald*, 1891, **1**, 547-
54.
First account of the pathology of carotid body tumours.

3792   GILFORD, HASTINGS. 1861-1941
On a condition of mixed premature and immature development. *Med.-chir.
Trans.*, 1897, **80**, 17-45.
Hastings Gilford gave progeria its name; it was first fully reported by
him in *Practitioner*, 1904, **73**, 188-217.

3793   SAJOUS, CHARLES EUCHARISTE DE MEDICIS. 1852-1929
The internal secretions and the principles of medicine. 2 vols. Philadelphia,
F. A. Davis, 1903-07.
Sajous, pioneer American endocrinologist, wrote the first treatise on the
subject. In this work he regarded the adrenal, pituitary, and thyroid glands
as controlling the immunizing mechanism of the body.

3794   BIEDL, ARTUR. 1869-1933
Innere Sekretion. Berlin, Wien, *Urban & Schwarzenberg*, 1910.
Biedl's classic work shows the rapid development of the knowledge
concerning endocrinology. In 1890 there were few publications dealing
with internal secretion, but Biedl, in the second edition of his book, 1913,
was able to include a bibliography of 8,500 items.

3795   FALTA, WILHELM. 1875-1950
Die Erkrankungen der Blutdrüsen. Berlin, *J. Springer*, 1913.
First attempt to systematize the endocrine disorders. English translation,
1915.

3796   STEINACH, Eugen. 1861-1944
Verjüngung durch experimentelle Neubelebung der alternden Pubertätsdrüse. Berlin, *J. Springer*, 1920.
Steinach rejuvenation operation, ligation of the vas deferens.

3797   VORONOFF, Serge. 1866-1951
Greffes testiculaires. Paris, *O. Doin*, 1923.
Voronoff first reported his controversial experimental rejuvenation by means of testicular transplants in 1919.

3798   BARKER, Lewellys Franklin. 1867-1943
Endocrinology and metabolism presented in their scientific and practical clinical aspects by ninety-eight contributors. Edited by L. F. Barker. 5 vols. New York, *D. Appleton & Co.*, 1922-24.

3799   DODDS, *Sir* Edward Charles. 1899-1973, *et al.*
The oestrogenic activity of certain synthetic compounds. *Nature (Lond.)*, 1938, **141**, 247-48.
Introduction of stilboestrol, the first synthetic oestrogen. With L. Golberg, W. Lawson, and R. Robinson.

3800   ———. Oestrogenic activity of alkylated stilboestrols. *Nature (Lond.)*, 1938. **142**, 34.
Introduction of dienoestrol. With L. Golberg, W. Lawson, and R. Robinson.

3801   CAMPBELL, N. R., *et al.*
Oestrogenic activity of anol; a highly active phenol isolated from the by-products. *Nature (Lond.)*, 1938, **142**, 1121.
Isolation of hexoestrol. With E. C. Dodds and W. Lawson.

3801.1   TURNER, Henry Hubert. 1892-1970
A syndrome of infantilism, congenital webbed neck, and cubitus valgus. *Endocrinology*, 1938, **23**, 566-74.
"Turner's syndrome".

3802   GOLDZIEHER, Maximilian A. 1883-1969
The endocrine glands. New York, *Appleton-Century*, 1939.
Goldzieher dealt very fully with the history, theory, and practice of endocrinology.

3803   MACPHERSON, Archibald Ian Stewart, & ROBERTSON, Edwin Moody. 1902-
Clinical use of triphenylchlorethylene. *Lancet*, 1939, **2**, 1362-66.

3804   KLINEFELTER, Harry Fitch. 1912- , *et al.*
Syndrome characterized by gynecomastia, aspermatogenesis without A-Leydigism, and increased excretion of follicle-stimulating hormone. *J. clin. Endocr.*, 1942, **2**, 615-27.
Klinefelter syndrome. With E. C. Reifenstein and F. Albright.

3805 PARACELSUS [BOMBASTUS VON HOHENHEIM, THEOPHRASTUS PHILIPPUS AUREOLUS].
1493-1541
De generatione stultorum. In his *Opera*, Strassburg, 1603, **2**, 174-82.
Paracelsus was the first to note the coincidence of cretinism and
endemic goitre. It was not until the 19th century that the possibility of the
occurrence of cretinism in adults was entertained. Partial English translation
in No. 2241.

3806 DU LAURENS, ANDRÉ [LAURENTIUS]. 1558-1609.
De mirabili strumas sanandi. Parisiis, *M. Orry*, 1609.
An early historical record of goitre which du Laurens maintained was
contagious. Du Laurens was at one time physician to Henri IV.

3807 PROSSER, THOMAS.
An account and method of cure of the bronchocele or Derby neck. London,
W. Owen, 1769.
Prosser gave the prescription of a powder containing calcined sponge,
to be taken for the cure of goitre. This is probably the first recorded use of
an iodine preparation in England.

3808 WILMER, BRADFORD.
Cases and remarks in surgery: to which is subjoined an appendix containing
the method of curing the bronchocele in Coventry. London, *T. Longman*,
1779.
The "Coventry treatment" for goitre, which introduced the burnt sponge
remedy into England, is mentioned on pp. 251-54.

3809 MALACARNE, MICHAELE VINCENZO GIACINTO. 1744-1816
Sui gozzi e sulla stupiditá ec. dei cretini. Torino, 1789.
Hirsch considered this the first important work on cretinism and goitre.
See also Malacarne's *Lettre*, in J. P. Frank: *Delectus opusculorum medicorum*,
1789, **6**, 241-58.

3810 FODÉRÉ, FRANÇOIS EMMANUEL. 1764-1835.
Essai sur le goitre et le crétinage. Turin, 1792.
Fodéré considered cretinism to be due to the concentrated air in deep
valleys, rather than to water. He also drew attention to the skeletal changes.

3811 FLAJANI, GIUSEPPE. 1741-1808
Sopra un tumor freddo nell'anterior parte del collo detto broncocele. In his
Collezione d'osservazione e riflessioni di chirurgia, Roma, 1802, **3**, 270-73.
One of the earliest accounts of exophthalmic goitre. The author noted
cardiac disturbances in thyroid enlargement.

3812 COINDET, JEAN FRANÇOIS. 1774-1834
Découverte d'un nouveau remède contre le goitre. *Bibliothèque universelle*,
1820, **14**, 190-98; also in *Ann. Chim. Phys.*, 1820, **15**, 49-59.
Coindet is usually regarded as the first to administer iodine in cases of
goitre, with beneficial results. It had previously been prepared from
seaweed by B. Courtois in 1812 (Ann. Chim. (Paris), 1813, **88**, 304-10), and
both Ampère and Humphry Davy were interested in it. W. Prout, however,
in his *Chemistry, meteorology, etc.*, London, 1834, p. 113, claimed that he

had recommended it to John Elliotson, who had used it in 1819 at St. Thomas's Hospital. There is an English translation of his paper in *Lond. med. Phys. J.*, 1820, **44**, 486-89.

3813   PARRY, CALEB HILLIER. 1755-1822
Enlargement of the thyroid gland in connection with enlargement or palpitation of the heart. In: *Collections from the unpublished medical writings of C. H. Parry*, London, 1825, **2**, 111-29.
A classic account of exophthalmic goitre. Although Graves and Basedow have both been credited with the first description of the condition, giving their names to it, Osler called attention to the priority of Parry's claim, and it is now sometimes referred to as "Parry's disease". Garrison says that Parry first noted the condition in 1786; he briefly reported it in his *Elements of pathology and therapeutics*, 1815. Reprinted in *Med. Classics*, 1940, **5**, 8-30. *See* No. 2210.

3814   GREEN, JOSEPH HENRY. 1791-1863
Removal of the right lobe of the thyroid gland. *Lancet*, 1828-29, **2**, 351-52.
To Green, of St. Thomas's Hospital, London, is accredited the first thyroidectomy, the patient succumbing 15 days later from sepsis.

3815   GRAVES, ROBERT JAMES. 1796-1853
[Palpitation of the heart with enlargement of the thyroid gland.] *Lond. med. surg. J. (Renshaw)*, 1835, **7**, 516-17.
This is considered the first accurate account of exophthalmic goitre, later known as "Parry's disease", "Graves's disease", and "Basedow's disease". An interesting fact about the *London Medical & Surgical Journal* is that after the first five volumes had been published by Renshaw and edited by M. Ryan, these two separated, each continuing to publish a separate edition of the same journal. Graves's paper appeared in the series published by Renshaw. Reprinted in *Med. Classics*, 1940, **5**, 33-36.

3816   BASEDOW, CARL ADOLPH VON. 1799-1854
Exophthalmos durch Hypertrophie des Zellgewebes in der Augenhöhle. *Wschr. ges. Heilk.*, 1840, **6**, 197-204, 220-28.
In Europe, outside the British Isles, exophthalmic goitre, or Graves's disease, is known as "Basedow's disease". His accurate description of four cases in which he described exophthalmos, goitre and palpitation led to the phrase "Merseburg triad", associating these conditions with the name of his own town. He also mentioned emaciation, excessive perspiration, and nervousness as additional symptoms and anticipated later methods of treatment by his advocacy of mineral waters containing iodide and bromide of sodium. Partial English translation in No. 2241.

3817   CHATIN, GASPARD ADOLPH. 1813-1901
Existence de l'iode dans les plantes d'eau douce. Conséquences de ce fait pour la géognosie, la physiologie végétale, la thérapeutique et peut-être pour l'industrie. *C. R. Acad. Sci. (Paris)*, 1850, **30**, 352-54.
Chatin showed that iodine could prevent endemic goitre and cretinism.

3818   CURLING, THOMAS BLIZARD. 1811-1888
Two cases of absence of the thyroid body and symmetrical swellings of fat tissue at the sides of the neck, connected with defective cerebral development. *Med.-chir. Trans.*, 1850, **33**, 303-06.

Curling, of the London Hospital, was the first accurately to note the clinical picture of cretinism, which Ord was later to name "myxoedema". Curling was also the first to suggest deficiency of the thyroid as a case of cretinism.

3819   SCHIFF, MORITZ. 1823-1896
Untersuchungen über die Zuckerbildung in der Leber und den Einfluss des Nervensystems auf die Erzeugung des Diabetes. *Schweiz. Mschr. prakt. Med.*, 1859, **4**, 267-75.

This paper includes Schiff's reports on his experimental thyroidectomies, which were attended with fatal results. Schiff also wrote a 159-page book with the same title, (Würzburg, *Stahel*, 1859). Subsequently (*Arch. exp. Path. Pharmak.*, 1884, **18**, 25) he showed that intra-abdominal transplantation of the gland would obviate fatal results in thyroidectomy.

3820   GRAEFE, FRIEDRICH WILHELM ERNST ALBRECHT VON. 1828-1870
Ueber Basedow'sche Krankheit. *Dtsch. Klinik*, 1864, **16**, 158-59.

"Graefe's sign" – the discovery by von Graefe of the failure of the eyelid to follow the eye when it is rolled downward – diagnostic of exophthalmic goitre. Partial English translation in No. 2241.

3821   SICK, PAUL AUGUSTE. 1836-1900
Ueber die totale Exstirpation einer kropfig entarteten Schilddrüse, und über die Rückwirkung dieser Operation auf die Circulationsverhältnisse im Kopfe. *Med. CorrespBl. württemb. ärztl. Vereins*, 1867, **37**, 199-205.

Sick is credited with being the first to notice symptoms of loss of thyroid function following thyroidectomy. According to Halsted, the above is the first report of total thyroidectomy and "the first report of the condition which we now recognize as *status thyreoprivus*".

3822   FAGGE, CHARLES HILTON. 1838-1883
On sporadic cretinism. *Med.-chir. Trans.*, 1871, **54**, 155-70.

In this paper Fagge, nephew of John Hilton of Guy's Hospital, described sporadic cretinism as distinct from the endemic variety.

3823   GULL, *Sir* WILLIAM WITHEY. 1816-1890
On a cretinoid state supervening in adult life in women. *Trans. clin. Soc. Lond.*, 1873-74, **7**, 180-85.

Gull was among the first to point out the cause of myxoedema, of which the above paper gives a classic description. Gull was associated with Guy's Hospital, London, for most of his life.

3824   WATSON, *Sir* PATRICK HERON. 1832-1907
Excision of the thyroid gland. *Edinb. med. J.*, 1874, **19**, 252-55.

Watson was a pioneer of thyroidectomy in the treatment of goitre, although Green (No. 3814) was the first to perform the operation. Also in *Brit. med. J.*, 1875, **2**, 386-88.

3825   ORD, WILLIAM MILLER. 1834-1902
On myxoedema. *Med.-chir. Trans.*, 1878, **61**, 57-78.

Ord coined the term "myxoedema" for the condition noted earlier by Curling and Gull.

3826   KOCHER, EMIL THEODOR. 1841-1917
Exstirpation einer Struma retrooesophagea. *KorrespBl. schweiz. Aerzte*, 1878, **8**, 702-05.

Kocher, a pupil of Billroth, was a pioneer of thyroidectomy for goitre. Before his time the operation was seldom performed. Garrison says that he performed this difficult operation 2,000 times, with a mortality rate of only 4.5 per cent. Kocher received the Nobel Prize in 1909.

3827   ——. Ueber Kropfexstirpation und ihre Folgen. *Arch. klin. Chir.*, 1883, **29**, 254-337.

Kocher coined the term "cachexia strumipriva" to describe the myxoedema following total extirpation of the thyroid. His work on the subject led to a better understanding of the cause of myxoedema.

3828   REVERDIN, JACQUES LOUIS. 1842-1929
Accidents consécutifs à l'ablation totale du goitre. *Rev. méd. Suisse rom.*, 1882, **2**, 539.

Reverdin produced myxoedema by removal of the thyroid as a whole or in part. This confirmed the earlier work of Schiff, of which Reverdin had probably not heard. *See also* No. 3836.

3829   ——. Note sur vingt-deux opérations de goitre. *Rev. méd. Suisse rom.*, 1883, **3**, 169-98, 233-78, 309-64.

3830   MARIE, PIERRE. 1853-1940
Sur la nature et sur quelques-uns des symptomes de la maladie de Basedow. *Arch. Neurol. (Paris)*, 1883, **6**, 79-85.

The fourth cardinal sign in exophthalmic goitre – tremor – was first mentioned by Pierre Marie.

3831   SEMON, *Sir* FELIX. 1849-1921
A typical case of myxoedema. *Brit. med. J.*, 1883, **2**, 1072.

Semon argued that cachexia strumipriva, myxoedema, and cretinism were all due to loss of function of the thyroid. His contention, at first criticized, was later fully endorsed by the report of a committee set up by the Clinical Society of London to investigate the subject of myxoedema.

3832   WÖLFLER, ANTON. 1850-1917
Ueber die Entwickelung und den Bau des Kropfes. *Arch. klin. Chir.*, 1883, **29**, 1-97.

Important classification of thyroid tumours; foetal adenoma is described on p. 40.

3833   REHN, LUDWIG. 1849-1930
Ueber die Exstirpation des Kropfs bei Morbus basedowii. *Berl. klin. Wschr.*, 1884, **21**, 163-66.

First thyroidectomy for exophthalmic goitre. The operation reported was performed in 1880.

3834   HORSLEY, *Sir* VICTOR ALEXANDER HADEN. 1857-1916
A recent specimen of artificial myxoedema in a monkey. *Lancet*, 1884, **2**, 827.

By experimental removal of the thyroid Horsley produced artificial myxoedema, confirming previous work by Reverdin and others. At the time his results were regarded as proof that total thyroidectomy produces operative myxoedema, but some of the symptoms he described are now known to have been due to removal of the parathyroids.

3835 ———. Functional nervous disorders due to the loss of thyroid gland and pituitary body. *Lancet,* 1886, **1**, 5.

3836 REVERDIN, Jacques Louis. 1842-1929
Contribution à l'étude du myxoedème consécutif à l'extirpation totale ou partielle du corps thyroïde. *Rev. méd. Suisse rom.,* 1887, **7**, 275-91, 318-30.

3837 LANNELONGUE, Odilon Marc. 1840-1911
Transplantation du corps thyroïde sur l'homme. *Bull. méd.,* 1890, **4**, 225.
First thyroid transplantation (for treatment of cretinism).

3838 MURRAY, George Redmayne. 1865-1939
Note on the treatment of myxoedema by hypodermic injections of an extract of the thyroid gland of a sheep. *Brit. med. J.,* 1891, **2**, 796-97.
Murray injected thyroid extract subcutaneously in the treatment of myxoedema with highly successful results.

3839 MÜLLER, Friedrich von. 1858-1941
Beiträge zur Kenntniss der Basedow'schen Krankheit. *Dtsch. Arch. klin. Med.,* 1893, **51**, 335-412.
Müller demonstrated that an increased metabolism accompanies exophthalmic goitre.

3840 MAGNUS-LEVY, Adolf. 1865-1955
Ueber den respiratorischen Gaswechsel unter dem Einfluss der Thyreoidea sowie unter verschiedenen pathologischen Zuständen. *Berl. klin. Wschr.,* 1895, **32**, 650-52.
Magnus-Levy demonstrated the increased metabolic rate in toxic goitre, confirming the work of Müller. His experimental investigations laid the foundation for the modern conception of thyroid function. See also *Z. klin. Med.,* 1897, **33**, 269-314.

3840.1 PENDRED, Vaughan. 1869-1946
Deaf-mutism and goitre. *Lancet,* 1896, **2**, 532.
Pendred drew attention to the association of goitre with deaf-mutism.

3841 RIEDEL, Bernhard Moritz Karl Ludwig. 1846-1916
Die chronische, zur Bildung eisenharter Tumoren führende Entzündung der Schilddrüse. *Verh. dtsch. Ges. Chir.,* 1896, **25**, 101-05.
Riedel described a type of chronic inflammation of the thyroid ("Riedel's disease").

3842 PINELES, Friedrich. 1868-1936
Ueber Thyreoaplasie (kongenitales Myxoedem und infantiles Myxoedem). *Wien. klin. Wschr.,* 1902, **15**, 1129-36.
Pineles differentiated endemic (familial) cretinism associated with goitre from sporadic cretinism.

3843   BRISSAUD, EDOUARD. 1852-1909
        L'infantilisme vrai. *N. Iconogr. Salpêt.*, 1907, **20**, 1-17.
        Brissaud described thyroid infantilism.

3844   MARINE, DAVID. 1880-1976, & WILLIAMS, WILLIAM WHITRIDGE. 1875-
        The relation of iodin to the structure of the thyroid gland. *Arch. intern. Med.*,
        1908, **1**, 349-84.
        Marks the beginning of Marine's lifelong study of the thyroid.

3845   HASHIMOTO, HAKARU. 1881-1934
        Zur Kenntniss der lymphomatösen Veränderung der Schilddrüse (Struma
        lymphomatosa). *Arch. klin. Chir.*, 1912, **97**, 219-48.
        "Hashimoto's disease", struma lymphomatosa, lymphoid infiltration of
        the thyroid.

3846   WAGNER VON JAUREGG, JULIUS. 1857-1940
        Myxödem und Kretinismus. Leipzig, *F. Deuticke*, 1912.

3847   McCARRISON, *Sir* ROBERT. 1878-1960
        The pathogenesis of experimentally produced goitre. *Indian J. med. Res.*,
        1914, **2**, 183-213.

3848   CANNON, WALTER BRADFORD. 1871-1945, *et al.*
        Experimental hyperthyroidism. *Amer. J. Physiol.*, 1915, **36**, 363-64.
        First successful experimental production of exophthalmic goitre. With
        C. A. L. Binger and R. Fitz.

3849   ZONDEK, HERMANN. 1887-1979
        Das Myxödemherz. *Münch. med. Wschr.*, 1918, **65**, 1180-82.
        First systematic study of the characteristic changes of the heart in
        myxoedema.

3849.1 DUNHILL, *Sir* THOMAS PEEL. 1876-1957
        Some considerations on the operation for exophthalmic goitre. *Brit. J. Surg.*,
        1919, **7**, 195-210.
        Dunhill's operation of exophthalmic goitre is described above. He was
        a pioneer in thyroid surgery.

3850   GOETSCH, EMIL. 1883-1963
        Epinephrin hypersensitiveness test in the diagnosis of hyperthyroidism.
        Penn. med. J., 1919-20, **23**, 431-37.
        Goetsch devised a skin reaction for use in the diagnosis of
        hyperthyroidism.

3851   PLUMMER, HENRY STANLEY. 1874-1937, & BOOTHBY, WALTER MEREDITH.
        1880-1953
        The value of iodine in exophthalmic goitre. *J. Iowa med. Soc.*, 1924, **14**, 66-73.
        Plummer and Boothby recommended the pre-operative administration
        of iodine in exophthalmic goitre.

3852   JOLL, CECIL AUGUSTUS. 1885-1945
        Diseases of the thyroid gland, with special reference to thyrotoxicosis.
        London, *W. Heinemann*, 1932.
        Second edition, 1951. Joll was a pioneer in the treatment of thyrotoxicosis
        by means of subtotal thyroidectomy.

3853   HERTZ, Saul. 1905- , & ROBERTS. A.
Application of radioactive iodine in therapy of Graves's disease. *J. clin. Invest.*, 1942, **21**, 624.

3854   ASTWOOD, Edwin Bennett. 1909-1976
Treatment of hyperthyroidism with thiourea and thiouracil. *J. Amer. med. Assoc.*, 1943, **122**, 78-81.
Astwood was the first to treat human cases of hyperthyroidism with thiourea and thiouracil.

3855   ——. Some observations on the use of thiobarbital as an antithyroid agent in the treatment of Graves's disease. *J. clin. Endocr.*, 1945, **5**, 345-52.
Clinical introduction of thiobarbital.

3855.1   JONES, Reuben G., *et al.*
Imidazoles. IV. The synthesis and antithyroid activity of some 1-substituted-2-mercaptoimidazoles. *J. Amer. chem. Soc.*, 1949, **71**, 4000-02.
Synthesis of methimazole ("mercazole"), an antithyroid drug more potent than methylthiouracil. With E. C. Kornfeld, K. C. McLaughlin, and R. C. Anderson.

3855.2   LAWSON, Alexander, *et al.*
Antithyroid activity of 2-carbethoxythio-1-methylglyoxaline. *Lancet*, 1951, **2**, 619-20.
Synthesis of carbimazole. With C. Rimington and C. E. Searle. For clinical application see *Lancet*, 1951, **2**, 621.

3855.3   WITEBSKY, Ernest. 1901-1969, & ROSE, Noel Richard. 1927-
Studies on organ specificity. IV. Production of rabbit thyroid antibodies in the rabbit. *J. Immunol.*, 1956, **76**, 408-16.
Autoimmune thyroiditis.

For history, see No. 3911.

PARATHYROID GLANDS

See also 4825-4838, Tetany

3856   EISELSBERG, Anton von. 1860-1939
Ueber erfolgreiche Einheilung der Katzenschilddrüse in die Bauchdecke und Auftreten von Tetanie nach deren Exstirpation. *Wien. klin. Wschr.*, 1892, **5**, 81-85.
Experimental production of tetany by excision of the thyroid of a cat, previously successfully transplanted into the abdomen.

3857   VASSALE, Giulio. 1862-1912, & GENERALI, Francesco.
Sugli effeti dell' estirpazione delle ghiandole paratiroidee. *Riv. Patol. nerv. ment.*, 1896, **1**, 95-99.
Demonstration that tetany follows removal of the parathyroids. A French translation of the paper is in *Arch. ital. Biol.*, 1896, **25**, 459-64.

3858   ASKANAZY, Max. 1865-1940
Ueber Ostitis deformans ohne osteoides Gewebe. *Arb. path.-anat. Inst. Tübingen*, 1904, **4**, 398-422.
Askanazy was the first to associate osteitis fibrosa cystica with parathyroid tumours.

3859   MacCALLUM, William George. 1874-1944, & VOEGTLIN, Carl. 1879-1960
On the relation of tetany to the parathyroid glands and to calcium metabolism. *J. exp. Med.*, 1909, **11**, 118-51.
Proof that the parathyroids control calcium metabolism. MacCallum and Voegtlin were able to demonstrate the removal of post-parathyroidectomy tetany by administration of calcium.

3860   HALSTED, William Stewart. 1852-1922
Auto- and isotransplantation, in dogs, of the parathyroid glandules. *J. exp. Med.*, 1909, **11**, 175-99.

3861   COLLIP, James Bertram. 1892-1965
The extraction of a parathyroid hormone which will prevent or control parathyroid tetany and which regulates the level of blood calcium. *J. biol. Chem.*, 1925, **63**, 395-438.
Collip's "parathormone". He showed that it raises the calcium level in para-thyroidectomized dogs.

3862   ——. & LEITCH, Douglas Burrows. 1888-?
A case of tetany treated with parathyrin. *Canad. med. Ass. J.*, 1925, **15**, 59-60.
First use of parathyroid hormone in treatment of tetany.

3863   MANDL, Felix. 1892-1957
Therapeutischer Versuch bei Ostitis fibrosa generalisata mittels Exstirpation eines Epithelkörperchentumors. *Wien. klin. Wschr.*, 1925, **38**, 1343-44.
Mandl was the first successfully to treat generalized osteitis fibrosa by extirpation of a parathyroid tumour.

ADRENALS

3864   ADDISON, Thomas. 1793-1860
On the constitutional and local effects of disease of the supra-renal capsules. London, *S. Highley*, 1855.
Addison was the first to draw attention to the importance of the adrenals in clinical medicine. The above work first appeared in the *Lond. med. Gaz.*, 1849, **43**, 517-18, and was later expanded into book form. It described the conditions, which later became known as "Addison's disease" and pernicious anaemia, which was later renamed "Addisonian anaemia" by Trousseau. Text reprinted in *Med. Classics*, 1937, **2**, 244-77. Facsimile edition, London, *Dawson*, 1968.

3865   FRÄNKEL, Felix.
Ein Fall von doppelseitigem, völlig latent verlaufenen Nebennieren-tumor und gleichzeitiger Nephritis mit Veränderungen am Circulationsapparat und Retinitis. *Virchows Arch. path. Anat.*, 1886, **103**, 244-63.
Phaeochromocytoma first described. Republished in book form.

3866   PEPPER, WILLIAM. 1874-1947
A study of congenital sarcoma of the liver and suprarenal. With report of
a case. *Amer. J. med. Sci.*, 1901, **121**, 287-99.
> Pepper's type of adrenal medullary tumour.

3867   BULLOCH, WILLIAM. 1868-1941, & SEQUEIRA, JAMES HARRY. 1865-1948
On the relation of the suprarenal capsules to the sex organs. *Trans. path.
Soc. Lond.*, 1905, **56**, 189-208.
> First recognition of the "adrenogenital syndrome". This paper showed
> a relationship to exist between the adrenals and the sex organs.

3868   HUTCHISON, *Sir* ROBERT. 1871-1960
On suprarenal sarcoma in children with metastases in the skull. *Quart. J.
Med.*, 1907, **1**, 33-38.
> Hutchison's tumours.

3869   ROTH, GRACE M., & KVALE, WALTER FREDERICK. 1907-
A tentative test for pheochromocytoma. *Amer. J. med. Sci.*, 1945, **210**, 653-
60.
> The Roth–Kvale histamine test for the diagnosis of phaeochromocytoma.

3870   ACHARD, EMILE CHARLES. 1860-1944, & THIERS, JOSEPH.
La virilisme pilaire et son association à l'insuffisance glycolytique (Diabète
des femmes à barbe). *Bull. Acad. Méd.*, 1921, 3 sér., **86**, 51-66.
> "Achard–Thiers syndrome". These writers established as a definite
> syndrome the combination of hirsutism with diabetes.

3871   LABBE, ERNEST MARCEL. 1870-1939, *et al.*
Crises solaires et hypertension paroxystique en rapport avec une tumeur
surrénale. *Bull. Soc. méd. Hôp. Paris*, 1922, 3 sér., **46**, 982-90.
> First full description of chromaffin cell tumours of the adrenal medulla.
> With J. Tinel and E. Doumer.

3872   HOLMES, *Sir* GORDON MORGAN. 1876-1965
A case of virilism associated with a suprarenal tumour: recovery after its
removal. *Quart. J. Med.*, 1925, **18**, 143-52.
> Records the first removal (by P. Sargent) of an adrenal cortical tumour.
> This was followed by disappearance of the heterosexual symptoms, thus
> establishing the relationship of sexual abnormality and adrenal tumours.

3873   ROGOFF, JULIUS MOSES. 1883-1966, & STEWART, GEORGE NEIL. 1860-1930
Suprarenal cortical extracts in suprarenal insufficiency (Addison's disease).
J. Amer. med. Assoc., 1929, **92**, 1569-71.
> Rogoff and Stewart were the first to use adrenal cortical extract ("inter-
> renalin") in the treatment of adrenal insufficiency. *See also* No. 1148.

3874   SWINGLE, WILBUR WILLIS. 1891- , & PFIFFNER, JOSEPH JOHN. 1903-1975
The adrenal cortical hormone. *Medicine*, 1932, **11**, 371-433.
> The cortical hormone prepared by Swingle and Pfiffner ("eschatin")
> was found to be very effective in the treatment of Addison's disease. Their
> first paper on the subject appeared in *Science*, 1930, **71**, 321.

3875 BROSTER, Lennox Ross. 1889-1965, & VINES, Howard William Copland. 1893-
The adrenal cortex; a surgical and pathological study. London, *H. K. Lewis*, 1933.
Includes the demonstration, by Vines, of virilism with the aid of a new stain; cortical cells of the adrenals removed at operation stained an abnormal (red) colour – the so-called Ponceau fuchsin stain.

3876 YOUNG, Hugh Hampton. 1870-1945, *et al.*
Genital abnormalities, hermaphroditism and related adrenal diseases. Baltimore, *Williams & Wilkins*, 1937.

3877 THORN, George Widmer. 1906- , *et al.*
Treatment of adrenal insufficiency by means of subcutaneous implants of pellets of desoxycorticosterone acetate (a synthetic adrenal cortical hormone). *Bull. Johns Hopk. Hosp.*, 1939, **64**, 155-66.
With L. L. Engel and H. Eisenberg. For treatment of Addison's disease by the same method, see the same journal, pp. 339-65.

3877.1 CONN, Jerome W. 1907-
Primary aldosteronism, a new clinical syndrome. *J. Lab. clin. Med.*, 1955, **45**, 661-64.
Primary aldosteronism ("Conn's syndrome").

PITUITARY GLAND

3878 HAEN, Anton de. 1704-1776
De cranii ustione. In his: *Ratio medendi*, Viennae Austriae, 1759, **6**, 264-72.
Haen mentioned amenorrhoea in connection with a pituitary tumour.

3879 FRANK, Johann Peter. 1745-1821
De curandis hominum morbis epitome. Liber V. Mannheim, *C. F. Schwann & C. G. Goetz*, 1794.
Frank was the first to define diabetes insipidus (pp. 38-67).

3880 SAUCEROTTE, Nicolas. 1741-1812
Accroissement singulier en grosseur des os d'un homme âgé de 39 ans. In his *Mélanges de chirurgie*, Paris, 1801, 407-11.
Saucerotte described before the Académie de Chirurgie in 1772 a case of what is now known to have been acromegaly. This is the first known clinical description of the disease, and is one of the five cases included in Pierre Marie's classic account (No. 3884).

3881 RAYER, Pierre François Olive. 1793-1867
Observations sur les maladies de l'appendice sus-sphenoïdal (glande pituitaire) du cerveau. *Arch. gén. Méd.*, 1823, **3**, 350-67.
Includes description of pituitary obesity.

3882 MOHR, Bernhard. 1809-1848
Hypertrophie der Hypophysis cerebri und dadurch bedingter Druck auf die Hirngrundfläche, insbesondere auf die Sehnerven, das Chiasma derselben und den linkseitigen Hirnschenkel. *Wschr. ges. Heilk.*, 1840, **6**, 565-71.

The first case of pituitary obesity with infantilism (Fröhlich's syndrome) was reported by Mohr. Coincidentally, this appears in the same volume of the *Wochenschrift* as does Basedow's classic description of exophthalmic goitre.

3883   FANEAU DE LA COUR, FERDINAND VALÈRE.
Du féminisme et de l'infantilisme chez les tuberculeux. Paris, *Thèse No.* 1, 1871.
        In a letter prefaced to Faneau de La Cour's thesis, Paul Joseph Lorain (1827-1875) described the idiopathic arrest of growth now known as "Lorain's type". It was subsequently ascribed to hypopituitarism. The word "infantilism" first appeared in this work.

3884   MARIE, PIERRE. 1853-1940
Sur deux cas d'acromégalie. Hypertrophie singulière non congénitale des extrémités supérieures, inférieures et céphalique. *Rev. Méd.*, 1886, **6**, 297-333.
        In this, the first complete clinical description of the condition, Marie suggested the name "acromegaly". The paper excited much interest and was translated into English and published by the New Sydenham Society, 1891.

3885   MINKOWSKI, OSCAR. 1858-1931
Ueber einen Fall von Akromegalie. *Berl. klin. Wschr.*, 1887, **24**, 371-74.
        Minkowski called attention to the constancy of pituitary enlargement on acromegaly; he was the first definitely to note this relationship.

3886   CATON, RICHARD. 1842-1926, & PAUL, FRANK THOMAS. 1851-1941
Notes on a case of acromegaly treated by operation. *Brit. med, J.*, 1893, **2**, 1421-23.
        First attempt (unsuccessful) to treat acromegaly operatively. Decompression was performed to relieve cranial pressure.

3887   BABINSKI, JOSEPH FRANÇOIS FÉLIX. 1857-1932
Tumeur du corps pituitaire sans acromégalie et avec arrêt de développement des organes génitaux. *Rev. neurol. (Paris)*, 1900, **8**, 531-33.
        Babinski preceded Fröhlich in describing dystrophia adiposo-genitalis.

3888   BENDA, CARL. 1857-1933
Beiträge zur normalen und pathologischen Histologie der menschlichen Hypophysis cerebri. *Berl. klin. Wschr.*, 1900, **37**, 1205-10.
        Benda showed that the pituitary tumour in acromegaly consists of chromophil cells.

3889   FRÖHLICH, ALFRED. 1871-1953
Ein Fall von Tumor der Hypophysis cerebri ohne Akromegalie. *Wien. klin. Rdsch.*, 1901, **15**, 883-86, 906-08.
        Fröhlich's classic description of dystrophia adiposogenitalis, pituitary tumour, with obesity and sexual infantilism ("Fröhlich's syndrome"). Reprinted (in German) in Research Publications, Association for Nervous and Mental Disease, XX: *The hypothalamus*, Baltimore, 1940, pp. xvi-xxviii. Partial English translation in No. 2241.

3890   CUSHING, HARVEY WILLIAMS. 1869-1939
Sexual infantilism with optic atrophy in cases of tumor affecting the
hypophysis cerebri. *J. nerv. ment. Dis.*, 1906, **33**, 704-16.

3891   SCHLOFFER, HERMANN. 1868-1937
Zur Frage der Operationen an der Hypophyse. *Beitr. klin. Chir.*, 1906, **50**,
767-817.
       Schloffer's operation for acromegaly. He was the first successfully to
operate upon a pituitary tumour in man (*see* No. 3892).

3892   ——. Erfolgreiche Operation eines hypophysen Tumors auf nasalem
Wege. *Wien. klin. Wschr.*, 1907, **20**, 621-24, 670-71, 1075-78.
       Schloffer's operation by the nasal route.

3893   RENON, LOUIS. 1863-1922, & DELILLE, ARTHUR. 1876-
Insuffisance thyro-ovarienne et hyperactivité hypophysaire (troubles
acromégaliques). *Bull. Soc. méd. Hôp. Paris*, 1908, 3 sér., **25**, 973-79.
       Rénon–Delille syndrome – dyspituitarism manifested by lowered blood-
pressure, tachycardia, oliguria, insomnia, hyperhidrosis, and intolerance
to heat.

3894   CROWE, SAMUEL JAMES. 1883-1955, *et al.*
Experimental hypophysectomy. *Johns Hopk. Hosp. Bull.*, 1910, **21**, 127-69.
       Demonstration that hypophysectomy causes genital atrophy. With
Harvey Cushing and J. Homans.

3895   HIRSCH, OSKAR. 1877-
Ueber endonasale Operationsmethoden bei Hypophysis-Tumoren. *Berl.
klin. Wschr.*, 1911, **48**, 1933-35.
       Hirsch's endonasal method.

3896   CUSHING, HARVEY WILLIAMS. 1869-1939
The pituitary body and its disorders. Philadelphia, *J. B. Lippincott*, 1912.
       The first clinical monograph on the hypophysis. Cushing, outstanding
neurological surgeon of the present century, added much to our knowledge of the pituitary body and its disorders. The above work includes a
description of his own method of operating on the pituitary. He assumed
that in diabetes insipidus the pituitary was involved. *See* Nos. 1161 & 4883.1.

3897   FRANK, ALFRED ERICH. 1884-1957
Ueber Beziehungen der Hypophyse zum Diabetes insipidus. *Berl. klin.,
Wschr.*, 1912, **49**, 393-97.
       Frank was the first definitely to connect the posterior lobe of the
pituitary with diabetes insipidus.

3898   MARK, LEONARD PORTAL. 1855-1930
Acromegaly: a personal experience. London, *Baillière, Tindall & Cox*, 1912.
       Mark, a medical practitioner, suffered from acromegaly from the age of
24. The condition was obvious to his friends, but Mark was 50 before he
realized the cause of the symptoms of which he had kept a record for many
years. He left an interesting account of his personal experience and also
drew attention to several sculptural and pictorial representations of
acromegalics.

3899   SOUQUES, ACHILLE ALEXANDRE. 1860-1944, & CHAUVET, STEPHEN. 1885-1950
Infantilism hypophysaire. *Nouv. Iconogr. Salpêt.*, 1913, **26**, 69-80.
Classic account of pituitary infantilism.

3900   GLIŃSKI, LEON KONRAD. 1870-1918
Z kazuistyki zmian anatomo-patholigicznych w przysadce mózgowej.
Przegl. Lek., 1913, **4**, 13-14.
Glinski preceded Simmonds in this important description of post-partum necrosis of the anterior pituitary. Abstract in *Dtsch med. Wschr.*, 1913, **39**, 473.

3901   SIMMONDS, MORRIS. 1855-1925
Ueber Hypophysisschwund mit tödlichem Ausgang. *Dtsch. med. Wschr.*, 1914, **40**, 322-23.
"Simmonds's disease" – pituitary cachexia. See also *Virchows Arch. path. Anat.*, 1914, **217**, 226-39.

3902   ERDHEIM, JAKOB. 1874-1937
Nanosomia pituitaria. *Beitr. path. Anat.*, 1916, **62**, 302-77.
Erdheim made important studies on the pathology of the pituitary. He gave the name "nanosomia pituitaria" to describe pituitary dwarfism. See also his paper in *Ergebn. allg. Path*, 1926, **21**, 482.

3903   ATKINSON, FREDERICK RICHARD BREEKS. 1867-1939
Acromegaly. London, *John Bale*, 1932.
An extensive analytical tabulation of acromegaly; 1,319 cases are reported.

3904   CUSHING, HARVEY WILLIAMS. 1869-1939
The basophil adenomas of the pituitary body and their clinical manifestations (pituitary basophilism). *Bull. Johns Hopk. Hosp.*, 1932, **50**, 137-95.
"Cushing's syndrome".

3905   INGRAM, WALTER ROBINSON. 1905-1978, *et al.*
Experimental diabetes insipidus in the monkey. *Arch. intern. Med.*, 1936, **57**, 1067-80.
With C. Fisher and S. W. Ransom.

3907   BIGGART, *Sir* JOHN HENRY. 1905-1979, & ALEXANDER, GEORGE LIONEL.
Experimental diabetes insipidus. *J. Path. Bact.*, 1939, **48**, 405-25.
Production of diabetes insipidus in dogs by injury to the hypothalamus.

3907.1   SHEEHAN, HAROLD LEEMING. 1900-1988
Post-partum necrosis of the anterior pituitary. *J. Path. Bact.*, 1937, **45**, 189-214.
Sheehan's syndrome – panhypopituitarism due to pituitary necrosis following post-partum haemorrhage.

3908   KINSELL, LAURANCE WILKIE. 1907-1968, *et al.*
Studies in growth. I. Interrelationship between pituitary growth factor and growth-promoting androgens in acromegaly and gigantism. II. Quantitative evaluation of bone and soft tissue growth in acromegaly and gigantism. *J. clin. Endocr.*, 1948, **8**, 1013-36.
L. W. Kinsell, G. D. Michaels, C. H. Li, and W. E. Larsen showed that there is an increase in growth hormone in plasma in acromegaly.

3908.1   LUFT, Rolf, & OLIVECRONA, Herbert. 1891-1980
Experience with hypophysectomy in man. *J. Neurosurg.*, 1953, **10**, 301-16.
Demonstration of the beneficial effect of hypophysectomy in cancer of the breast and of the testis.

History of Endocrinology

3909   ROLLESTON, *Sir* Humphry Davy, *Bart.* 1862-1944
The endocrine organs in health and disease. With an historical review. London, *Oxford Univ. Press*, 1936.
As a history of the subject, this work is unsurpassed in detail and accuracy.

3910   MEDVEI, Victor Cornelius.
A history of endocrinology. Lancaster, *MTP Press*, 1982.
A detailed illustrated history, tracing the development of knowledge from ancient times to the present. Includes biographical notes on the important pioneers in the field and chronological tables.

3911   MERKE, F.
Geschichte und Ikonographie des endemischen Kropfes und Kretinismus. Bern, *Hans Huber*, 1971.
A superbly produced and illustrated work, with tipped-in colour plates. English translation. Lancaster, *MTP Press*, 1984.

3911.1   MEITES, Joseph. 1913- , DONOVAN, B.T., & McCANN, S.M.
Pioneers in neuroendocrinology. 2 vols., New York, *Plenum*, 1975-78.

3911.2   McCANN, Samuel McDonald. 1925-
Endocrinology: people and ideas. Bethesda, *American Physiological Society*, [1988].
Thematic historical essays written by pioneers in the field, edited by McCann.

METABOLIC DISORDERS

3912   MARCET, Alexander John Gaspard. 1770-1822
Account of a singular variety of urine, which turned black soon after being discharged; with some particulars respecting its chemical properties. *Med.-chir. Trans.*, 1822-23, **12**, 37-45.
Alkaptonuria described.

3912.1   GARROD, *Sir* Alfred Baring. 1819-1907
Several specimens of cystine exhibited, with the particulars of two cases in which this deposit occurred in the urine. *Trans. path. Soc. Lond.*, 1846-8, **1**, 126-29.
Cystinuria described.

3913   BOEDEKER, CARL WILHELM. 1815-1895
Ueber das Alcapton; ein neuer Beitrag zur Frage: welche Stoffe des Harns
können Kupferreduction bewirken? *Z. rat. Med.*, 1859, 3 R., **7**, 130-45.
Excretion of homogentisic acid (in alkaptonuria) first described.

3914   BANTING, WILLIAM. 1779-1878
Letter on corpulence; address to the public. London, *Harrison & Sons*, 1863.
Banting devised a diet low in saccharine, farinaceous, and oily matter,
for the treatment of obesity. This became known as "Bantingism" or the
"Banting diet". This book is probably the first of the endless stream of best-
selling books by physicians on how to lose weight.

3914.1   THUDICHUM, JOHANN LUDWIG WILHELM. 1829-1901
On researches intended to promote an improved chemical identification
of diseases. 10*th Rep. Med. Offr. Privy Council.* With appendix, 1867.
London, 1868, pp. 152-294.
Discovery of the first porphyrin, haematoporphyrin (p. 227).

3915   TROUSSEAU, ARMAND. 1801-1867
Glycosurie, diabète sucré. In his *Clinique médicale de l'Hôtel-Dieu*, 2me.
éd., Paris, 1865, **2**, 663-98.
First description of haemochromatosis.

3916   RECKLINGHAUSEN, FRIEDRICH DANIEL VON. 1833-1910
Ueber Haemochromatose. *Berl. klin. Wschr.*, 1889, **26**, 925.
Recklinghausen gave to haemochromatosis its present name.

3917   DERCUM, FRANCIS XAVIER. 1856-1931
A subcutaneous connective tissue dystrophy of the arms and back, associated with symptoms resembling myxoedema. *Univ. med. Mag. (Philad.)*,
1888-89, **1**, 140-50.
First description of adiposis dolorosa ("Dercum's disease").

3918   SALKOWSKI, ERNST LEOPOLD. 1844-1923
Ueber die Pentosurie, eine neue Anomalie des Stoffwechsels. *Berl. klin.
Wschr.*, 1895, **32**, 364-68.
Pentosuria first described.

3919   NOORDEN, CARL HARKO VON. 1858-1944
Sammlung klinischer Abhandlungen über Pathologie und Therapie der
Stoffwechsel- und Ernährungsstörungen. 9 pts. Berlin, 1900-10.
Noorden succeeded Nothnagel at Vienna. He made important studies
of metabolism and its disorders.

3920   ABDERHALDEN, EMIL. 1877-1950
Familiäre Cystindiathese. *Hoppe-Seyl. Z. physiol. Chem.*, 1903, **38**, 557-61.
Cystinosis described.

3921   GARROD, *Sir* ARCHIBALD EDWARD. 1857-1936
Inborn errors of metabolism. London, *H. Frowde,* 1909.
The influence of the individual's constitution on the incidence of
disease has long been recognized. Garrod showed that constitutional
variation in function, as well as in structure, can give rise to what he termed

"chemical malformations" – alkaptonuria, cystinuria, pentosuria, etc. The book was based on his Croonian Lectures, published in *Lancet*, 1908, **2**, 1-7, 142-8, 173-9, 214-20. A second edition appeared in 1923. It was reprinted with supplement by H. Harris, London, 1963. Garrod's first paper on the subject dealt with alkaptonuria (*Lancet*, 1901, **2**, 1484-6). *See* No. 244.1.

3921.1   GÖPPERT, Friedrich. 1870-1927
Galaktosurie nach Milchzuckergabe bei angeborenen, familiärem, chronischem Leberleiden. *Berl. klin. Wschr.*, 1917, **54**, 473-77.
First clear account of galactosaemia (although A. von. Reuss may have been describing a case in *Wien. med. Wschr.*, 1908, **58**, 799).

3922   FOLIN, Otto Knut Olof. 1867-1934, & WU, Hsien. 1893-1959
A system of blood analysis. *J. biol. Chem.*, 1919, **38**, 81-110.
Folin–Wu test for blood sugar.

3923   BENEDICT, Stanley Rossiter. 1884-1936
The analysis of whole-blood. II. The determination of sugar and of saccharoids (non-fermentable copper-reducing substances). *J. biol. Chem.*, 1931, **92**, 141-59.
Benedict's test for blood-sugar.

3923.1   MEDES, Grace. 1886-1967
A new error of tyrosine metabolism: tyrosinosis, intermediary metabolism of tyrosine and phenylalanine. *Biochem. J.*, 1932, **26**, 917-40.

3924   FØLLING, Ivar Asbjorn. 1888-1973
Utskillelse av fenylpyrodruesyre i urinen som stoffskifteanomali i forbindelse med imbecilletet, *Nord. med. T.*, 1934, **8**, 1054-59.
Phenylketonuria first described. This was the first hereditary metabolic disorder shown to be responsible for mental retardation. German translation in *Hoppe-Seyl. Z. physiol. Chem.*, 1934, **227**, 169-76. English translation in Boyer (ed.), *Papers on human genetics*, Englewood Cliffs, N.J., *Prentice-Hall*, 1963.

3924.1   WALDENSTRÖM, Jan Gösta. 1906-
Incipient myelomatosis or "essential" hyperglobulinemia with fibrinogenopenia – a new syndrome? *Acta. med. scand.*, 1944, **117**, 216-47.
"Waldenström's macroglobulinaemia".

3924.2   REFSUM, Sigvald.
Heredopathia atactica polyneuritiformis; a familial syndrome not hitherto described. *Acta psychiat. scand.*, 1946, Suppl. 38.
"Refsum's syndrome", an inherited disorder of lipid metabolism.

3924.3   MENKES, John H. 1928- , *et al.*
A new syndrome: progressive familial infantile cerebral dysfunction associated with unusual urinary substance. *Pediatrics*, 1954, **14**, 462-6.
Maple syrup urine disease described. With P. L. Hurst and J. M. Craig.

3924.4   GUTHRIE, Robert. 1916- , & SUSI, Ada.
A simple phenylalanine method for detecting phenylketonuria in large populations of newborn infants. *Pediatrics*, 1963, **32**, 338-43.
Bacterial inhibition test for phenylketonuria.

3925   ARETAEUS, *the Cappadocian*. A.D. 81-138?
On diabetes. In his *Extant works*, ed. F. ADAMS. London, 1856, 338-40, 485-86.

The first accurate account of diabetes, to which Aretaeus gave its present name; he insisted on the part which thirst plays in the symptomatology.

3926   WILLIS, THOMAS. 1621-1675
Pharmaceutice rationalis sive diatriba de medicamentorum operationibus in humano corpore. 2 vols. Londini, *R. Scott*, 1674-75.

Willis noted the sweetness of the urine in diabetes mellitus; he differentiated between this condition and diabetes insipidus. (Sect IV, Chap. 3.) English translation, 1679.

3927   BRUNNER, JOHANN CONRAD À. 1653-1727
Experimenta nova circa pancreas. Amstelaedami, *apud. H. Wetstenium*, 1683.

Brunner came near to discovering pancreatic diabetes. His experiments on the dog represent pioneer work on internal secretion. Following excision of the pancreas, he recorded extreme thirst and polyuria. Translated in *Ann. med. Hist.*, 1941, **3**, 91-100.

3928   DOBSON, MATTHEW. 1731?-1784
Experiments and observations on the urine in diabetes. *Med. Obs. Inqu.*, 1776, **5**, 298-316.

Dobson proved that the sweetish taste of diabetic urine was produced by sugar, an observation following on Willis's discovery of the sweetness of diabetic urine. He also discovered hyperglycaemia.

3929   CAWLEY, THOMAS.
A singular case of diabetes, consisting entirely in the quality of the urine; with an inquiry into the different theories of that disease. *Lond. med. J.*, 1788, **9**, 286-308.

Cawley was the first to suggest a relationship between the pancreas and diabetes, observing that the disease may follow injury to that organ.

3930   ROLLO, JOHN. ?-1809
An account of two cases of the diabetes mellitus, with remarks as they arose during the progress of the cure. London, *C. Dilly*, 1797.

Rollo reported the success of a meat diet in the treatment of diabetes. He was a pioneer in the systematic treatment of diabetes by restricted diet.

3931   CHEVREUL, MICHEL EUGÈNE. 1786-1889
Note sur le sucre de diabètes. *Ann. Chim. (Paris)*, 1815, **95**, 319-20.
Chevreul proved that the sugar in diabetic urine is glucose.

3932   TROMMER, CARL AUGUST. 1806-1879
Unterscheidung von Gummi, Dextrin, Traubenzucker, und Rohrzucker. *Ann. Chem. (Heidelberg)*, 1841, **39**, 360-62.
Trommer's test for glucose in urine.

3933   BERNARD, CLAUDE. 1813-1878
       Chiens rendus diabétiques. *C. R. Soc. Biol. (Paris)*, (1849), 1850, **1**, 60.
       By experimental puncture (piqûre) of the fourth ventricle of the brain,
       Claude Bernard produced temporary glycosuria.

3934   SCHIFF, MORITZ. 1823-1896
       Bericht über einige Versuche, um den Ursprung des Harnzuckers bei
       künstlichem Diabetes zu ermitteln. *Nachr. Georg-Aug. Univ. k. Ges. Wiss.
       Göttingen*, 1856, 243-47.
       Schiff's important experiments on the production of artificial diabetes.

3935   PETTERS, WILHELM.
       Untersuchungen über die Honigharnruhr. *Vjschr. prakt. Heilk.*, 1857, **55**,
       81-94.
       Petters discovered acetone in diabetic urine.

3936   PAVY, FREDERICK WILLIAM. 1829-1911
       Researches on the nature and treatment of diabetes. London, *J. Churchill*,
       1862.
       Pavy devoted many years to the study of diabetes. He concluded that
       there was a definite relationship between the degree of hyperglycaemia
       and glycosuria.

3937   GERHARDT, CARL ADOLPH CHRISTIAN JACOB. 1833-1902
       Diabetes mellitus und Aceton. *Wien. med. Presse*, 1865, **6**, 672.
       Gerhard's iron-chloride reaction for aceto-acetic acid in acetonaemic
       urine.

3938   NOYES, HENRY DEWEY. 1832-1900
       Retinitis in glycosuria. *Trans. Amer. ophthal. Soc.*, (1867-68), 1869, 71-75.
       First investigation of retinitis accompanying glycosuria.

3939   KUSSMAUL, ADOLF. 1822-1902
       Zur Lehre vom diabetes mellitus. *Dtsch. Arch. klin. Med.*, 1874, **14**, 1-46.
       Kussmaul explained diabetic coma as being due to acetonaemia. He
       described the air-hunger ("Kussmaul's respiration") present in this condition.
       Partial English translation in No. 2241.

3940   BOUCHARDAT, APOLLINAIRE. 1806-1886
       De la glycosurie ou diabète sucré; son traitement hygiénique. Paris,
       Germer-Ballière, 1875.
       Bouchardat used the fermentation test, polariscope and copper solu-
       tions for the detection of diabetes; he substituted fresh fats for carbohydrates,
       advised the avoidance of milk and alcohol, invented gluten bread and
       advocated the use of green vegetables. In fact, he devised the most rational
       method of treatment of diabetes up to his time.

3941   LEBER, THEODOR. 1840-1917
       Ueber die Erkrankungen des Auges bei Diabetes mellitus. *v. Graefe's Arch.
       Ophthal.*, 1875, **21**, Abt. iii, 206-337.
       A record of Leber's important studies on the disorders of the eye in
       diabetes.

3942   BERNARD, Claude. 1813-1878
Leçons sur le diabète et la glycogenèse animale. Paris, *J. B. Baillière,* 1877.
      Bernard showed that in diabetes there is primarily glycaemia followed by glycosuria.

3943   LANCEREAUX, Etienne. 1829-1910
Notes et reflexions à propos de 2 cas de diabète sucré avec altération du pancreas. *Bull. Acad. Méd. (Paris),* 1877, 2 *sér.,* **6**, 1215-40.
      Lancereaux was the first definitely to claim a causal relationship between lesions of the pancreas and diabetes.

3944   EBSTEIN, Wilhelm. 1836-1912
Ueber Drüsenepithelnekrosen beim Diabetes mellitus mit besonderer Berücksichtigung des diabetischen Coma. *Dtsch. Arch. klin. Med.,* 1881, **28**, 143-242.
      "Ebstein's disease", hyaline degeneration and necrosis of the epithelial cells of the renal tubules, sometimes seen in diabetes mellitus.

3945   STADELMANN, Ernst. 1853-1941
Ueber die Ursachen der pathologischen Ammoniakausscheidung beim Diabetes mellitus und des Coma diabeticum. *Arch. exp. Path. Pharmak.,* 1883, **17**, 419-44.
      Stadelmann studied ammonia excretion in diabetes and noted an acid substance in the urine, which Minkowski (No. 3947) showed to be ß-oxybutyric acid. Stadelmann recognized that diabetic coma was the result of the increased formation and accumulation of acids.

3946   ARNOZAN, Charles Louis Xavier.1852-1928, & VAILLARD, Louis. 1850-1935
Contribution à l'étude du pancreas du lapin. Lésions provoquées par la ligature du canal de Wirsung. *Arch. Physiol. norm. path.,* 1884, 3 *sér.,* **3**, 287-316.
      Arnozan and Vaillard showed that blockage of the pancreatic ducts caused atrophy of the pancreas but not diabetes.

3947   MINKOWSKI, Oscar. 1858-1931
Ueber das Vorkommen von Oxybuttersäure im Harn bei Diabetes mellitus. *Arch. exp. Path. Pharmak.,* 1884, **18**, 35-48.
      Discovery of ß-oxybutyric acid in diabetic urine.

3948   JAKSCH, Rudolf von, *Ritter von Wartenborst.* 1855-1947
Ueber Acetonurie und Diaceturie. Berlin, *A. Hirschwald,* 1885.
      An important investigation concerning acetone in diabetic urine.

3949   MERING, Joseph von. 1849-1908
Ueber experimentellen Diabetes. *Verh. Congr. inn. Med.,* 1886, **5**, 185-89.
      Mering was able to produce experimental diabetes by means of phloridzin.

3950   ——. & MINKOWSKI, Oscar. 1858-1931
Diabetes mellitus nach Pankreasextirpation. *Arch. exp. Path. Pharmak.,* 1890, **26**, 371-87.

Minkowski produced experimental diabetes by removing the pancreas of a dog. This proof of the role of the pancreas in diabetes was of the first importance; previous experiments on similar lines had attracted attention. Partial English translation in No. 2241.

3951   NOORDEN, CARL HARKO VON. 1858-1944
Die Zuckerkrankheit und ihre Behandlung. Berlin, A. Hirschwald, 1895.
Noorden's extensive studies on diabetes greatly advanced our knowledge of the subject. He made many observations regarding metabolism in diabetes.

3952   NAUNYN, BERNARD. 1839-1925
Der Diabetes mellitus. Wien, A. Hölder, 1898.
Naunyn devoted his life to the study of metabolism in diabetes and in diseases of the liver and pancreas, the above book being his most important work. He was a co-founder of the Archiv für experimentelle Pathologie.

3953   MAGNUS-LEVY, ADOLF. 1865-1955
Die Oxybuttersäure und ihre Beziehungen zum Coma diabeticum. Arch. exp. Path. Pharmak., 1899, 42, 149-237.

3954   ——. Untersuchungen über die Acidosis im Diabetes melitus und die Säureintoxication im Coma diabeticum. Arch. exp. Path. Pharmak., 1901, 45, 389-434.
Magnus-Levy studied the relationship of ß-oxybutyric acid and diabetic coma.

3955   OPIE, EUGENE LINDSAY. 1873-1971
On the relation of chronic interstitial pancreatitis to the islands of Langerhans and to diabetes mellitus. J. exp. Med., 1900-01, 5, 397-428.

3956   ——. The relation of diabetes mellitus to lesions of the pancreas. Hyaline degeneration of the islands of Langerhans. J. exp. Med., 1900-01, 5, 527-40.
Mering and Minkowski had focused attention upon the pancreas as the seat of diabetes, Opie's work was another important step forward; he established the association between failure of the islets of Langerhans and the occurrence of diabetes.

3957   SOBOLEW, LEONID WASSILYEVITCH [SOBOLEFF]. 1876-1919
Zur normalen und pathologischen Morphologie der inneren Secretion der Bauchspeicheldrüse. (Die Bedeutung der Langerhans'-schen Inseln. Virchows Arch. path. Anat., 1902, 168, 91-128.
Sobolew found that ligation of the pancreatic excretory ducts led to atrophy of the acinous tissue, the islets of Langerhans remaining intact.

3958   FROMMER, VIKTOR.
Neue Reaktion zum Nachweis von Aceton, samt Vemerkungen über Acetonurie. Berl. klin. Wschr., 1905, 42, 1008-10.
Frommer's test for acetone in urine.

3959   DE WITT, Lydia Maria. 1859-1928
        Morphology and physiology of areas of Langerhans in some vertebrates.
        J. exp. Med., 1906, **8**, 193-239.
            Lydia De Witt ligated the pancreatic ducts and obtained extracts from
        the islets of Langerhans in cats, noting their glycolytic qualities.

3960   ROTHERA, Arthur Cecil Hamel. 1880-1915
        Note on the sodium nitro-prusside reaction for acetone. *J. Physiol. (Lond.)*,
        1908, **37**, 491-94.
            Test for acetone bodies in urine.

3961   ZUELZER, Georg Ludwig. 1870-1949
        Ueber Versuche einer specifischen Fermenttherapie des Diabetes. *Z. exp.
        Path. Therap.*, 1908, **5**, 307-18.
            Zuelzer succeeded in isolating the pancreatic extract which contained
        what we now know as insulin; serious hypoglycaemic reactions sometimes
        followed its use, however, and led to its abandonment. Preliminary paper
        in *Berl. klin. Wschr.*, 1907, **44**, 474-75.

3962   MacCALLUM William George. 1874-1944
        On the relation of the islands of Langerhans to glycosuria. *Johns Hopk. Hosp.
        Bull.*, 1909, **20**, 265-68.
            MacCallum suggested a relationship between lesions of the islands of
        Langerhans and the glycosuria of diabetes.

3963   MAGNUS-LEVY, Adolph. 1865-1955
        Das Coma diabeticum und seine Behandlung. *Samml. zwangl. Abhandl.
        Geb. Verdauungs-u. Stoffwechs.*, Halle, 1909, **1**, 1-54.
            Magnus-Levy is remembered for his work on the treatment of diabetic
        coma.

3964   BARRON, Moses. 1883-
        The relation of the islets of Langerhans to diabetes with special refer-
        ence to cases of pancreatic lithiasis. *Surg. Gynec. Obstet.*, 1920, **31**, 437-
        48.
            Barron confirmed the experimental work of Sobolew. It was whilst
        reading the above paper that Banting first formulated the hypothesis upon
        which he based his successful experiments.

3965   PAULESCO, Nicolas Constantin. 1869-1931
        Recherches sur le rôle du pancréas dans l'assimilation nutritive. *Arch. int.
        Physiol.*, 1921, **17**, 85-109.
            Paulesco isolated the anti-diabetic hormone of the pancreas before
        Banting and Best. He named it "pancréine".

3966   BANTING, *Sir* Frederick Grant. 1891-1941, *et al.*
        The internal secretion of the pancreas. *Amer. J. Physiol.*, 1922, **59**, 479.
            A preliminary communication regarding the isolation of insulin, made
        to a meeting of the American Physiological Society in December 1921. With
        C. H. Best and J. J. R. Macleod. Banting and Macleod were awarded the
        Nobel Prize in 1923.

3967   ——. & BEST. Charles Herbert. 1899-1978
The internal secretion of the pancreas. *J. Lab. clin. Med.*, 1922, **7**, 251-66.
    This paper reports the isolation of insulin. An extract from the pancreas of a dog, removed after ligation of the excretory duct, was found to exercise a reducing influence on the percentage of sugar in the blood. This extract was called "insulin" and was crystallized by Abel in 1926.

3968   ——. Pancreatic extracts in the treatment of diabetes mellitus. *Canad. med. Ass. J.*, 1922, **12**, 141-46.
    First clinical application of insulin in the treatment of diabetes. Written in conjunction with C. H. Best, J. B. Collip, W. R. Campbell, and A. A. Fletcher.

3969   COLLIP, JAMES BERTRAM. 1892-1965
The original method as used for the isolation of insulin in semipure form for the treatment of the first clinical cases. *J. biol. Chem.*, 1923, **55**, xl-xli.
    Collip improved insulin.

3970   BANTING, *Sir* FREDERICK GRANT. 1891-1941
Insulin. *Int. Clin.*, 1924, 34 ser., **4**, 109-16.

3971   ABEL, JOHN JACOB. 1857-1938
Crystalline insulin. *Proc. nat. Acad. Sci.(Wash.)*, 1926, **12**, 132-36.
    Crystallization of insulin.

3972   WILDER, RUSSELL MORSE. 1885-1959, *et al.*
Carcinoma of the islands of the pancreas; hyperinsulinism and hypoglycemia. *J. Amer. med. Assoc.*, 1927, **89**, 348-55.
    R. M. Wilder, F. N. Allan, M. H. Power, and H. E. Robertson reported the occurrence of carcinoma with hyperinsulinism.

3973   RUIZ, CELESTINO L. 1904- , *et al.*
Contribución al estudio sobre la composición quimica de la insulina. Estudio de algunos cuerpos sintéticos solfurados con acción hipoglucemiante. *Rev. Soc. argent Biol.*, 1930, **6**, 134-41.
    Discovery of the hypoglycaemic effect of certain sulphonamide derivatives. With L. L. Silva and L. Libenson.

3974   HAGEDORN, HANS CHRISTIAN. 1888-1971, *et al.*
Protamine insulinate. *J. Amer. med. Ass.*, 1936, **106**, 177-80.
    H. C. Hagedorn, B. N. Jensen, N. B. Krarup, and I. Wodstrup introduced insulin combined with protamine to delay the absorption rate.

3975   KERR, ROBERT BEWS. 1908- , *et al.*
Protamine insulin. *Canad. med. Ass. J.*, 1936, **34**, 400-01.
    R. B. Kerr, C. H. Best, W. R. Campbell, and A. A. Fletcher advocated the combination of zinc with insulin to delay its absorption rate. Later this was combined with protamine to form protamine zinc insulin.

3976   YOUNG, *Sir* FRANK GEORGE. 1908-1988
Permanent experimental diabetes produced by pituitary (anterior lobe) injections. *Lancet*, 1937, **2**, 372-74.
    Anterior pituitary diabetogenic hormone.

3976.1   LOUBATIÈRES, Auguste. 1912-1977
Analyse du mécanisme de l'action hypoglycémiante de *p*-aminobenzène-sulfamido-isopropylthiodiazol (2254 RP). *C. R. Soc. Biol. (Paris)*, 1944, **138**, 766-7.
> Loubatières initiated work on the hypoglycaemic sulphonamides. See his historical account in *Ann. N.Y. Acad. Sci.*, 1957, **71**, 4-11.

3977   DOHAN, Francis Curtis. 1907- , & LUKENS, Francis Dring Wetherill. 1899- Experimental diabetes produced by the administration of glucose. *Endocrinology*, 1948, **42**, 244-62.
> Experimental diabetes produced by artificially-induced hyperglycaemia.

3978   HALLAS-MØLLER, Knud. 1914- , *et al.*
Kliniske undersøgelser med nye retarderet virkende insulin-praeparater. *Ugeskr. Laeg.*, 1951, **113**, 1767-71.
> First clinical trials of lente, ultralente, and semilente insulin zinc suspension. See also *Science*, 1952, **116**, 394-98; and *J. Amer. med. Assoc.*, 1952, **150**, 1667. With M. Jersild, K. Peterson, and J. Schlichtkrull.

3978.1   FRANKE, Hans. 1909-1955, & FUCHS, J.
Ein neues antidiabetisches Prinzip. Ergebnisse klinischer Untersuchungen. *Dtsch. med. Wschr.*, 1955, **80**, 1449-52.
> Introduction of carbutamide (BZ55), the first of the sulphonylureas. It was followed by tolbutamide and chlorpropamide.

3978.2   MASKE, Helmut. 1921-
Über die orale Behandlung des Diabetes mellitus mit N-(4-Methyl-Benzolsulfonyl)-N'Butyl-Harnstoff (D 860). *Dtsch. med. Wschr.*, 1956, **81**, 823-46.
> A symposium on tolbutamide, introduced by H. Maske.

3978.3   UNGAR, Georges. 1906- , *et al.*
Pharmacological studies of a new oral hypoglycemic drug. *Proc. Soc. exp. Biol. (N.Y.)*, 1957, **95**, 190-92.
> Phenformin, a biguanide used in diabetes. With L. Freedman and S. L. Shapiro. Clinical report on pp. 193-4.

3978.4   SCHUMACHER, Joseph. 1902-
Index zum Diabetes mellitus. Eine internationale Bibliographie. München, *Urban & Schwarzenberg,* 1961.

History of Diabetes

3978.5   WRENSHALL, Gerald Alfred, *et al.*
The story of insulin: forty years of success against diabetes. London, *Bodley Head*, 1962.
> With G. Hetenyi and W. R. Feasby.

3979   PAPASPYROS, Nikos S.
The history of diabetes mellitus. 2nd ed. Stuttgart, *G. Thieme*, 1964.

3979.1   BLISS, Michael.
The discovery of insulin. Chicago, *University of Chicago Press*, 1982.

3979.2   PEUMERY, Jean-Jacques.
Histoire illustrée du diabète de l'antiquité à nos jours. Paris, *Roger Dacosta*,
[1987].

DERMATOLOGY

3980   MERCURIALI, Girolamo. 1530-1606
De morbis cutaneis, et omnibus corporis humani excrementis tractatus.
Venetiis, *apud. P. & A. Meietos*, 1572.
The first systematic textbook on diseases of the skin. English translation
by R. L. Sutton Jr, Kansas City, Missouri, *Lowell Press*, 1986. Mercuriali enjoyed
a great reputation in his day; he wrote on many medical subjects, including
medical gymnastics. *See* No. 1986.1.

3981   TURNER, Daniel. 1667-1742
De morbis cutaneis. A treatise of diseases incident to the skin. London, *R.
Bonwicke*, 1714.
Turner may be regarded as the founder of British dermatology. His
book, the first English text on the subject, gives a good idea of contemporary
knowledge of skin diseases. Turner began his career as a barber surgeon,
but eventually bought his way out of the guild. He obtained membership
in the College of Physicians without an official medical degree. Yale
College conferred an honorary MD on Turner in 1723, for donating a
collection of books to the school's library. This was the first medical degree
awarded in English-speaking America. Its circumstances led one wit of the
period to suggest that the letters on Turner's diploma actually stood for
Multum Donavit.

3982   PLENCK, Joseph Jacob von. 1738-1807
Doctrina de morbis cutaneis. Viennae, *R. Graeffer*, 1776.
A classification of skin diseases upon the basis of their clinical appearance.
Until the time of Willan, von Plenck's book was the greatest authority on
dermatology. He mentioned 115 different skin diseases, all that were
known at that time, and divided them into 14 classes.

3983   LORRY, Anne Charles de. 1726-1783
Tractatus e morbis cutaneis. Parisiis, *P. G. Cavelier*, 1777.
Lorry is regarded as the founder of French dermatology. A pupil of Jean
Astruc, his most important work is his *Tractatus*, in which he attempted the
classification of diseases on the basis of essential relations, their physi-
ological, pathological, and etiological similarities. It is the first modern text
on the subject, and the last major work on dermatology to be published in
Latin.

3984   JACKSON, Seguin Henry. 1750-1816
Dermato-pathologia; or practical observations, from some new thoughts
on the pathology and proximate cause of diseases of the true skin. London,
H. Reynell, 1792.
An attempt to classify skin diseases upon the basis of their pathology.

3985   WILLAN, ROBERT. 1757-1812
On cutaneous diseases. Vol. 1 [All published]. London, *J. Johnson*, [1796]-1808.

     Modern dermatology may be said to start with Willan. His classification of skin diseases gained him the Fothergillian Medal of the Medical Society of London in 1790. He established a standard nomenclature which is still more or less in use today. He was also a clinician of great ability who made numerous original observations. His book was issued in four parts under the title "Description and treatment of cutaneous diseases", from 1798 to 1808, and only vol. 1 had been completed when Willan died. The first three parts exist in revised versions. Copies of the book may contain varying states of the parts. See F. Sutherland, Willan's Cutaneous diseases, *J. Hist. Med.*, 1958, **13**, 92-94, supplementing T. Beswick, Robert Willan, *J. Hist. Med.*, 1957, **12**, 349-65. The above work and that of Alibert (No. 3986) are the first dermatological works with coloured plates. *See* No. 4018.

3986   ALIBERT, JEAN LOUIS MARC, *le baron*. 1768-1837
Description des maladies de la peau observées à l'hôpital Saint Louis. Paris, *Barrois*, 1806.

     The largest and most spectacular of the early classics of dermatology, with hand-coloured illustrations unsurpassed for their quality of execution. The illustrations are also the first on the subject in a French book. This book also contains the original description of mycosis fungoides. *See* No. 4019.

3987   ———. Précis théorique et pratique sur les maladies de la peau. 2 vols. Paris, *Caille & Ravier*, 1810-18.

3988   BATEMAN, THOMAS. 1778-1821
Delineations of cutaneous diseases exhibiting the characteristic appearances of the principal genera and species comprised in the classification of the late Dr. Willan; and completing the series of engravings begun by that author. London, *Longman*, 1817.

     Bateman, the pupil of Willan, continued his teacher's classification of skin diseases. The above work is notable for its 72 coloured plates. Strictly speaking it is the first atlas of dermatology, as Willan's work falls more into the category of illustrated treatise. This book includes numerous original contributions by Bateman. Originally issued in 12 fasciculi from 1814-1817. Unchanged reprint, 1828. *See* No. 4022.

3989   RAYER, PIERRE FRANÇOIS OLIVE. 1793-1867
Traité théorique et pratique des maladies de la peau. 2 vols. and atlas. Paris, *J. B. Baillière*, 1826-27.

     A classic summary of dermatological literature of the period. Rayer first described adenoma sebaceum and xanthoma multiplex. He was the first to differentiate between acute and chronic eczema. The second edition, Paris, *Baillière*, 1835 includes an entirely new third volume of text and a much enlarged atlas of coloured plates. English translation, 1883.

3990   CAZENAVE, PIERRE LOUIS ALPHÉE. 1795-1877, & SCHEDEL, HENRY EDWARD. ?-1856
Abrégé pratique des maladies de la peau. Paris, *Bechet jeune*, 1828.

     This book codified and published the lectures, doctrines and observations of Laurent Biett (1781-1840), the leading clinical teacher in dermatology of the early 19th century, who published very little himself.

Cazenave was a master clinician who founded the first scientific periodical devoted exclusively to dermatology. The *Abrégé* improves upon Bateman, especially in the section on the cutaneous manifestions of syphilis. "Continually revised and translated into all of the important languages of the Western World, the *Abrégé* became the most influential text of the time and remained so for 30 years" (Crissey & Parish). English translations 1829, 1832, 1842.

3990.1   ALIBERT, JEAN LOUIS MARC, *le baron*. 1768-1837
Monographie des dermatoses. Paris, *Daynac*, 1832.
This includes the first published illustration of Alibert's famous "family tree" for the classification of skin diseases, a concept which Alibert borrowed freely from Torti (No. 5231). This classification was never widely adopted. The book contains an important description of dermatolysis.

3991   HEBRA, FERDINAND VON. 1816-1880
Versuch einer auf pathologische Anatomie gegründeten Eintheilung der Hautkrankheiten. *Z. k. k. Ges. Aerzte Wien*, 1845, **2**, 34-52, 143-155, 211-31.
Hebra's classification of skin diseases was based upon their pathological anatomy.

3991.1   WORCESTER, NOAH. 1812-1847
A synopsis of the symptoms, diagnosis, and treatment of the more common and important diseases of the skin. Philadelphia, *T. Cowperthwait & Co.*, 1845.
First comprehensive American work on dermatology.

3992   HEBRA, FERDINAND VON. 1816-1880
Atlas der Hautkrankheiten. 10 parts. Wien, *k.k. Hof- und Staatsdr.*, 1856-76.

3992.1   CAZENAVE, PIERRE LOUIS ALPHÉE. 1795-1877
Leçons sur les maladies de la peau. Paris, *Labé*, 1856.
Cazenave was among the first to classify skin diseases on an anatomical basis. He founded the first journal devoted entirely to dermatology (*Annales des maladies de la peau et de la syphilis*). This large folio atlas is the most visually impressive of all his books. From publication in fascicules, 1845-56.

3993   ANDERSON, *Sir* THOMAS M'CALL. 1836-1908
On the parasitic affections of the skin. London, *J. Churchill*, 1861.
Anderson was Professor of Clinical Medicine at Glasgow.

3994   WILSON, *Sir* WILLIAM JAMES ERASMUS. 1809-1884
Lectures on dermatology. 4 vols. London, *J. & A. Churchill*, 1871-78.
Erasmus Wilson gave the original descriptions of several cutaneous diseases, and made a fine collection of dermatological preparations. He classified skin diseases on an anatomical basis. The above book consists of his lectures at the Royal College of Surgeons, at which institution he founded a chair of dermatology.

3995   KAPOSI, [KOHN], MORIZ. 1837-1902
Pathologie und Therapie der Hautkrankheiten. Wien & Leipzig, *Urban & Schwarzenberg*, 1880.
One of the most important books in dermatology. English translation by J. C. Johnston in 1895.

3996   FOX, GEORGE HENRY. 1846-1937
Photographic illustrations of skin diseases. New York, *E. B. Treat*, 1880.
Fox, who was Professor of Dermatology in New York, produced a valuable atlas of skin diseases.

3997   HEBRA, HANS VON. 1847-1902
Die krankhaften Veränderungen der Haut. Braunschweig, *F. Wreden*, 1884.
Hans von Hebra was the son of Ferdinand, whose work he continued. His textbook correlated skin diseases to diseases of the entire organism.

3998   CROCKER, HENRY RADCLIFFE. 1845-1909
Diseases of the skin. London, *H. K. Lewis*, 1888.

3999   SABOURAUD, RAYMOND JACQUES ADRIEN. 1864-1938
Les tricophyties humaines. Paris, 1894, *Thèse No*. 227.
In his extensive studies of the role of fungi in skin diseases, Sabouraud revived and elaborated the discoveries of Gruby (Nos. 4030, 4034-36), which had remained neglected for half a century. *See also* No. 4116.

4000   UNNA, PAUL GERSON. 1850-1929
Die Histopathologie der Hautkrankheiten. Berlin, *A. Hirschwald*, 1894.
This monumental work is a landmark in dermatological history. Sir Norman Walker translated it into English in 1896. Unna, short in stature but a giant among dermatologists, initiated the study of the skin by means of diascopy and gave several original descriptions of affections of the skin. The acne bacillus is for the first time described on p. 357.

4001   KAPOSI, [KOHN], MORIZ. 1837-1902
Handatlas der Hautkrankheiten. 3 pts. Wien & Leipzig, *W. Braumüller*, 1898-1900.
An extensive and valuable collection of illustrations in dermatology.

4002   FINSEN, NIELS RYBERG. 1860-1904
La photothérapie. Les rayons chimiques et la variole. La lumière comme agent d'excitabilité. Traitement du lupus vulgaire par des rayons chimiques concentrés. Paris, *G. Carré & C. Naud*, 1899.
Finsen was a pioneer in the treatment of lupus by means of light. English translation, 1901.

4003   DANLOS, HENRI ALEXANDRE. 1844-1912, & BLOCH, P.
Note sur le traitement du lupus érythémateux par des applications de radium. *Bull. Soc. franç. Derm. Syph.*, 1901, **12**, 438-40.
First application of radium in the treatment of lupus.

4004   SABOURAUD, RAYMOND JACQUES ADRIEN. 1864-1938
Sur la radiothérapie des teignes. *Ann. Derm. Syph.* (*Paris*), 1904, 4 sér., **5**, 577-87.
Sabouraud's method of radiological treatment of ringworm.

4005   DARIER, JEAN. 1856-1938
Précis de dermatologie. Paris, *Masson & Cie.*, 1909.

4006   JADASSOHN, Josef. 1863-1936
Handbuch der Haut- und Geschlechtskrankheiten. Hrsg ... von J. JADASSOHN.
24 vols. [in 42]. Berlin, *J. Springer*, 1927-37.

4007   CHAOUL, Henri. 1887- , & ADAM, Albert.
Die Röntgen-Nahbestrahlung maligner Tumoren. *Strahlentherapie*, 1933,
48, 31-50.
> Chaoul therapy.

4008   COCKAYNE, Edward Alfred. 1880-1956
Inherited abnormalities of the skin and its appendages. London, *H. Milford*,
1933.

4009   DARIER, Jean. 1856-1938, *et al.*
Nouvelle pratique dermatologique. 8 vols. Paris, *Masson & Cie.*, 1936.

4010   CHARPY, Jacques. 1900-
Technique de traitement du lupus tuberculeux. *Ann. Derm. Syph.* (*Paris*),
1943, 8 sér., **3**, 331.
> Introduction of calciferol in the treatment of lupus. A more extensive
report, "Le traitement des tuberculoses cutanées par la vitamine D_2 à hautes
doses", appeared in the same journal, 1946, 8 sér., **6**, 310-46.

4011   DOWLING, Geoffrey Barrow. 1891-1976, & THOMAS, Ebenezer William
Prosser.
Lupus vulgaris treated with calciferol. *Proc. roy. Soc. Med.*, 1945, **39**, 96-99.
> Dowling and Prosser Thomas introduced calciferol in the treatment of
lupus independently of Charpy (no. 4010) whose work was unknown to
them owing to the wartime isolation of France.

4011.1   GENTLES, James Clark.
Experimental ringworm in guinea pigs: oral treatment with griseofulvin.
Nature (*Lond.*), 1958, **182**, 476-77.
> Use of griseofulvin in the treatment of ringworm.

ORIGINAL OR IMPORTANT ACCOUNTS OF DERMATOSES

4011.2   DONATI, Marcello. 1538-1602
De medica historia mirabili. Mantuae, *per Fr. Osanam*, 1586.
> Lib. VI. cap. iii. First description of angioneurotic oedema (Quincke's
oedema, No. 4081). *See* Nos. 3417 & 6377.

4012   BONOMO, Giovanni Cosimo. 1666-1696. & CESTONI, Giacinto (1637-1718).
Osservazioni intorno a' pellicelli del corpo umano. Firenze, *Piero Matini*,
1687.
> First clinical and experimental proof of infection by a microparasite.
Bonomo observed *Sarcoptes scabiei*, the scabies mite. This gave researchers grounds to think in terms of objective, exogenous pathogenic
agents as the cause of disease. This pamphlet is in part translated by
Richard Mead in *Phil. Trans.*, (1702-03), 1703, **23**, 1296-99; it is reproduced
in facsimile, with Mead's translation, in *Arch. Derm. Syph.* (Chicago), 1928,
18, 1-25. *See* 2529.1.

4013   MACHIN, John. ?-1751
An uncommon case of a distempered skin. *Phil. Trans.*, (1731-32), 1733, **37**, 299-301.
First known description of ichthyosis hystrix. Machin's observations referred to the Lambert family and were followed through successive generations of the family by Baker (*Phil. Trans.*, 1755, **49**, 21-24) and by Tilesius (*Ausführliche Beschreibung . . . der beiden sog. Stachelschweinmenschen*, Altenburg, 1802).

4014   CRUSIO, Carlo [Curzio].
An account of an extraordinary disease of the skin and its cure. Extracted from the Italian of Carlo Crusio, with a letter of the Abbé Nollet to Mr. William Watson by Robert Watson. *Phil. Trans.*, 1754, **48**, 579-87.
The early history of scleroderma is confused with that of leprosy, ichthyosis, and keloid. Crusio appears to be the first to differentiate it. Gintrac in 1847 coined the term "scleroderma". It is now included among the connective tissue diseases.

4015   UNDERWOOD, Michael. 1737-1820
Treatise on the diseases of children. London, *J. Mathews*, 1784.
First description (p. 76) of sclerema neonatorum ("Underwood's disease").

4015.1 AKENSIDE, Mark. 1721-1770
Observations on cancers. *Med. Trans. Coll. Phys. Lond.*, 1786, **1**, 64-92.
An early description of multiple neurofibromatosis.

4016   WICHMANN, Johann Ernst. 1740-1802
Aetiologie der Krätze. Hannover, *Gebr. Helwing*, 1786.
Wichmann definitely established the parasitic aetiology of scabies.

4017   HOME, *Sir* Everard. 1756-1832
Observations on certain horny excrescences of the human body. *Phil. Trans.*, 1791, **81**, 95-105.
Original description of cornu cutaneum.

4018   WILLAN, Robert. 1757-1812
On cutaneous diseases. Vol. 1. London, *J. Johnson*, [1796]-1808.
Includes (pp. 73-76) original description of prurigo mitis; under the name "ichthyosis cornea" Willan quoted Crusio's case of scleroderma (see pp. 197-212); Willan also established psoriasis as a separate skin disease (pp. 152-88). *See* No. 3985.

4019   ALIBERT, Jean Louis Marc, *le baron*. 1768-1837
Description des maladies de la peau. Paris, 1806, p. 157; pl. xxxvi.
First description of mycosis fungoides (pian fungoide, framboesia mycoides), one of several conditions to which the name of Alibert has been attached.

4020   STOKES, Whitley. 1763-1845
On an eruptive disease of children. *Dublin med. phys. Essays*, 1807-08, **1**, 146-53.
First description of ecthyma terebrans, "pemphigus gangrenosa".

4021   BATEMAN, THOMAS. 1778-1821
         A practical synopsis of cutaneous diseases according to the arrangement
         of Dr. Willan. London, *Longman*, 1813.
         This was the most influential textbook of dermatology of the 19th
         century, and the work which conveyed Willan's system to most of the
         medical world. Included in the book was material by Willan which
         remained unpublished from his unfinished *On cutaneous diseases*. The
         Synopsis also "contained material original to Bateman himself...and it also
         provided insights into the origins of the morphologic system and an
         appreciation of its limitations not to be found in the work it was designed
         to complete" (Crissey & Parish). Description of lichen urticatus appears on
         p. 13.

4021.1   WILLAN, ROBERT. 1757-1812
         Practical treatise on porrigo, or scald head, and on impetigo, the humid or
         running teter. Edited by Ashby Smith. London, *E. Cox*, 1814.
         This treatise on infantile eczema is the only fascicule of the second
         volume of Willan's *On cutaneous diseases* (No. 4018) that ever appeared
         in print.

4022   BATEMAN, THOMAS. 1778-1821
         Delineations of cutaneous diseases. London, *Longman*, 1817.
         Includes (pl. lii) important description of herpes iris (erythema iris), and
         of the eczema due to external irritation (pl. lv-lviii, eczema solare,
         impetiginoides, rubrum mercuriale). Pl. lxi represents the first description
         of molluscum contagiosum, but according to Paterson (No. 4032) the
         disease was probably noticed by Tilesius about 1793. Bateman refers to
         Tilesius but calls his case molluscum pendulum. *See* No. 3988.

4023   ALIBERT, JEAN LOUIS MARC, *le baron*. 1768-1837
         Note sur la keloide. *J. univ. Sci. méd.*, 1816, **2**, 207-16.
         First accurate description of keloid ("Alibert's keloid"), although it was
         mentioned by Retz in 1790.

4024   ———. Description des maladies de la peau. 2me. édition. 2 vols. Paris, *A.*
         Wahlen, 1825.
         Contains (vol. 2, p. 214) first description of sycosis barbae ("Alibert's
         mentagra").

4025   JACOB, ARTHUR. 1790-1874
         Observations respecting an ulcer of peculiar character, which attacks the
         eyelids and other parts of the face. *Dublin Hosp. Rep.*, 1827, **4**, 232-39.
         Arthur Jacob, Professor of Anatomy and physiology in Dublin, described
         "Jacob's ulcer", rodent ulcer attacking the face, especially the eyelid.

4027   RENUCCI, SIMON FRANÇOIS.
         Sur la découverte de l'insecte qui produit la contagion de la gale, du prurigo
         et du phlyzacia. Paris, *Thèse No.* 83, 1835.
         Demonstration of the human itch-mite, *Sarcoptes scabiei*. It was due to
         Renucci that the *Sarcoptes* was recognized as the one cause of scabies and
         its parasitic nature finally accepted.

4028   CAZENAVE, PIERRE LOUIS ALPHÉE. 1795-1877, & SCHEDEL, HENRY EDWARD. - 1856
        Abrégé pratique des maladies de la peau. 3me. éd. Paris, *Bechet jeune*, 1838.
            Laurent Théodore Biett (1781-1840), was a pupil of Alibert, Willan, and Bateman. His classic description of lupus erythematoides migrans ("Biett's disease") occurs on pp. 11 and 415 of the above work.

4029   SCHÖNLEIN, JOHANN LUCAS. 1793-1864
        Zur Pathogenie der Impetigines. *Arch. Anat. Physiol. wiss. Med.*, 1839, 82.
            The discovery of a fungus as the cause of favus (*Achorion schönleinii*). Schönlein communicated this important discovery in a letter of less than 200 words and one illustration. It represents the first conspicuous step in the attribution of disease to the action of minute parasites. Schönlein was the founder of modern clinical teaching in Germany.

4030   GRUBY, DAVID. 1810-1898
        Mémoire sur une végétation qui constitue la vraie teigne. *C.R. Acad. Sci. (Paris)*, 1841, **13**, 72-75.
            Independently of Schönlein (No. 4029) Gruby discovered the achorion of favus, describing it definitely as the cause of the disease, a point about which Schönlein was in doubt.

4031   HENDERSON, WILLIAM. 1810-1872
        Notice of the molluscum contagiosum. *Edinb. med. surg. J.*, 1841, **56**, 213-18.
            See No. 4032.

4032   PATERSON, ROBERT. 1814-1889
        Cases and observations on the molluscum contagiosum of Bateman, with an account of the minute structure of the tumours. *Edinb. med. J.*, 1841, **56**, 279-88.
            Henderson and Paterson described the inclusion body of molluscum contagiosum, "Henderson–Paterson body".

4033   BOECK, CARL WILHELM. 1808-1875
        Om den spedalske sygdom. Elephantiasis graecorum. *Norsk. Mag. Laegevid.*, 1842, **4**, 1-73; 127-216.
            Boeck, eminent Norwegian dermatologist and syphilologist, was the first to describe Norwegian itch, scabies crustosa ("Boeck's scabies").

4034   GRUBY, DAVID. 1810-1898
        Sur une espèce de mentagre contagieuse résultant du développement d'un nouveau cryptogame dans la racine des poils de la barbe de l'homme. *C. R. Acad. Sci. (Paris)*, 1842, **15**, 512-15.
            First accurate description of *Trichophyton mentagrophytes*, the fungus responsible for sycosis barbae. English translation of this and Gruby's other five papers read to l'Académie des Sciences in Zakon & Benedek, David Gruby and the centenary of medical mycology, 1841-1941, *Bull. Hist. Med.*, 1944, **16**, 155-68.

4035   ——. Recherches sur la nature, le siège et le développement du Porrigo decalvans ou phytoalopécie. *C. R. Acad. Sci. (Paris)*, 1843, **17**, 301-03.
            First accurate description of *Microsporon audouini*, the fungus of Willan's porrigo decalvans, tinea tonsurans, "Gruby's disease".

4036 ——. Recherches sur les cryptogames qui constituent la maladie contagieuse du cuir chevelu décrite sous le nom de Teigne tondante (Mahon). Herpes tonsurans (Cazenave). *C. R. Acad. Sci.* (*Paris*), 1844, **18**, 583-85.

Gruby discovered a fungus, *Trichophyton tonsurans*, in ringworm of the scalp.

4037 CAZENAVE, PIERRE LOUIS ALPHÉE. 1795-1877
Pemphigus chronique, générale; forme rare de pemphigus foliacé; mort: autopsie; altération du foie. *Ann. Mal. Peau*, 1844, **1**, 208-10.

First description of pemphigus foliaceus, "Cazenave's disease". The article is unsigned.

4038 EICHSTEDT, CARL FERDINAND. 1816-1892
Ueber die Krätzmilben des Menschen, ihre Entwicklung und ihr Verhältniss zur Krätze. *N. Notiz. Geb. Nat. Heilk.*, 1846, **38**, col. 105-10; **39**, col. 265-70.

4039 ——. Pilzbildung in der Pityriasis versicolor. *N. Notiz. Geb. Nat. Heilk.*, 1846, **39**, col. 270-71.

Eichstedt discovered *Pityrosporum orbiculare*, fungus of pityriasis versicolor ("Eichstedt's disease").

4040 CAZENAVE, PIERRE LOUIS ALPHÉE. 1795-1877
Des principales formes du lupus et de son traitement. *Gaz. Hôp.* (*Paris*), 1850, 3 sér., **2**, 383.

Lupus erythematosus – "Cazenave's disease".

4041 ADDISON, THOMAS. 1793-1860, & GULL, Sir WILLIAM WITHEY. 1816-1890
On a certain affection of the skin, vitiligoidea: α Plana, ß tuberosa. *Guy's Hosp. Rep.*, 1851, 2 ser., **7**, 265-76.

In their classic account of xanthoma multiplex, Addison and Gull believed they were describing a new disease, but Rayer had been the first to mention it. (*See* No. 3989; see also the later paper by Gull, *Guy's Hosp. Rep.*, 1852, 2 ser., **8**, 149.)

4042 ——. On the keloid of Alibert, and on true keloid. *Med.-chir. Trans.*, 1854, **37**, 27-47.

Addison described two forms of keloid, that described by Alibert, and the "true keloid" (the skin disease morphoea, "Addison's keloid").

4043 BÄRENSPRUNG, FRIEDRICH WILHELM FELIX VON. 1822-1864
Ueber die Folge und den Verlauf epidermischer Krankheiten. Halles, *H. W. Schmidt*, 1854.

First description of tinea cruris (eczema marginatum, "Bärensprung's disease").

4044 DEVERGIE, MARIE GUILLAUME ALPHONSE. 1798-1879
Pityriasis pilaris, maladie de peau non décrite par les dermatologistes. *Gaz. hebd. Méd.*, 1856, **3**, 197-201.

Devergie is remembered for his clear description of pityriasis rubra pilaris, ("Devergie's disease"). He was the first to demonstrate the presence of a fungus in eczema marginatum.

4045   HEBRA, FERDINAND VON. 1816-1880
Lichen exsudativus ruber. *Allg. Wien. med. Ztg.*, 1857, **2**, 75-76.
First description of this condition ("Hebra's pityriasis").

4046   LE ROY DE MÉRICOURT, ALFRED. 1825-1901
Sur la coloration partielle en noir ou en bleu de la peau chez les femmes.
Bull. Acad. Méd. (Paris), 1857-58, **23**, 1141-44; 1860-61, **26**, 773-75.
Chromidrosis first described.

4047   CARTER, HENRY VANDYKE. 1831-1897
On a new and striking form of fungus disease, principally affecting the foot,
and prevailing endemically in many parts of India. *Trans. med. phys. Soc.
Bombay*, (1860), 1861, n.s. **6**, 104-42.
First modern description of mycetoma of the foot – "Madura foot",
"Carter's mycetoma". It was mentioned by E. Kaempfer in his *Amoenitates
exoticae*, Lemgo, 1712, p. 561. Colebrook at the Madura Dispensary is said
to have given it the name "Madura foot" in 1846. *See also* No. 4066.

4048   GIBERT, CAMILLE MELCHIOR. 1797-1866
Traité pratique des maladies de la peau. 3 éd., 2 vols. Paris, *H. Plon*, 1860.
Gibert's name is associated with pityriasis rosea, which he first established as a definite clinical entity. His complete and accurate description of
this condition is on page 402 of vol. 1 of the above work.

4049   HEBRA, FERDINAND VON. 1816-1880
Das umschriebene Eczem. Eczema marginatum. In Virchow's *Handbuch
der spec. Path. u. Therap.*, Erlangen, 1860, **3**, 1 Abt., 361-63.
Complete description of tinea cruris (eczema marginatum), first described
by Bärensprung in 1854.

4050   LUTZ, HENRI CHARLES.
De l'hypertrophie générale du système sébacé. Paris, *Thèse No.* 65, 1860.
First description of keratosis follicularis.

4051   BAZIN, PIERRE ANTOINE ERNEST. 1807-1878
Leçons sur la scrofule, *etc.* 2me édition. Paris, 1861, p. 145, 501.
Erythema induratum scrophulosorum ("Bazin's disease") first described.

4052   WILKS, *Sir* SAMUEL, *Bart.* 1824-1911
A peculiar atrophy of the skin (Lineae atrophicae). *Guy's Hosp. Rep.*, 1861,
3 ser., **7**, 197-301.
First description of lineae atrophicae.

4053   ——. Disease of the skin produced by post mortem examinations, or
verruca necrogenica. *Guy's Hosp. Rep.*, 1862, 3 ser., **8**, 263-65.
Description of dissecting-room warts (verrucae necrogenicae), the
cutaneous tuberculosis of Laennec, sometimes called "Wilks's disease".

4054   WAGNER, ERNST LEBERECHT. 1829-1888
Fall einer selten Muskelkrankheit. *Arch. Heilk.*, 1863, **4**, 282-83.
First recorded case of dermatomyositis, now regarded as a connective
tissue disease.

4055   FOX, WILLIAM TILBURY. 1836-1879
On impetigo contagiosa, or porrigo. *Brit. med. J.*, 1864, **1**, 78-79, 467-68, 495-96, 553-55, 607-09.
"Impetigo of Tilbury Fox", impetigo contagiosa, first described.

4056   WAGNER, ERNST LEBERECHT. 1829-1888
Das Colloid-Milium der Haut. *Arch. Heilk.*, 1866, **7**, 463-64.
Colloid degeneration of the skin ("Wagner's disease") was first described by Wagner who gave it the name "Colloid milium".

4056.1   ROTHMUND, AUGUST. 1830-1906
Ueber Cataracten in Verbindung mit einer eigenthümlichen Haut-degeneration. *Graefe's Arch. Ophthal.*, 1868, **14**, 159-82.
Poikiloderma congenitale (Rothmund).

4057   NETTLESHIP, EDWARD. 1845-1913
Chronic urticaria leaving brown stains: nearly two years' duration. *Brit. med. J.*, 1869, **2**, 323.
Urticaria pigmentosa, described by Nettleship, is named eponymically "Nettleship's disease".

4058   PAXTON, FRANCIS VALENTINE. ?-1924
On a diseased condition of the hairs of the axilla, probably of parasitic origin. *J. cutan. Med.*, 1869, **3**, 133-36.
Tinea nodosa (trichorrhexis nodosa, "Paxton's disease") first described.

4059   TURNER, GEORGE ALEXANDER. 1845-1900
Lafa Tokelau, or Tokelau ringworm. *Glasg. med. J.*, 1869-70, **2**, 510-12.
First description, tinea imbricata.

4060   RITTERSHAIN, GOTTFRIED VON, *Ritter.* 1820-1883
Dermatitis erysipelatosa; Gangraena; Enkephalitis. *Öst. Jb. Pädiat.*, 1870, **1**, 23-24.
First description of dermatitis exfoliativa neonatorum ("Rittershain's disease").

4061   WILSON, *Sir* WILLIAM JAMES ERASMUS. 1809-1884
On dermatitis exfoliativa. *Med. Times Gaz.*, 1870, **1**, 118-20.
Although Hippocrates mentioned this condition, Erasmus Wilson first named it and described it as we know it today. It has been called "Wilson's disease"; an eponym discarded since its use to describe the progressive lenticular degeneration of Kinnier Wilson.

4062   HEBRA, FERDINAND VON. 1816-1880
Ueber einzelne während der Schwangerschaft, dem Wochenbette und bei Uterinalkrankheiten der Frauen zu beobachtende Hautkrankheiten. *Wien. med. Wschr.*, 1872, **22**, 1197-1201.
Hebra was the first to describe impetigo herpetiformis, more fully dealt with by Kaposi, his son-in-law.

4063 KAPOSI [KOHN], MORIZ. 1837-1902
Idiopathisches multiples Pigmentsarkom der Haut. *Arch. Derm. Syph.* (*Prag.*), 1872, **4**, 265-73.
First description of "Kaposi's sarcoma" – multiple idiopathic haemorrhagic sarcoma. English translation in *CA*, 1982, **32**, 342-47.

4064 BAKER, WILLIAM MORRANT. 1839-1896
Erythema serpens. *St. Barth. Hosp. Rep.*, 1873, **9**, 198-211.
First description of erythema serpens, usually called "erysipeloid of Rosenbach", following the latter's paper in *Arch. klin. Chir.*, 1887, **36**, 346.

4065 FOX, WILLIAM TILBURY. 1836-1879
On dysidrosis (an undescribed eruption). *Brit. med. J.*, 1873, **2**, 365-66.
Original description of dysidrosis (pompholyx).

4066 CARTER, HENRY VANDYKE. 1831-1897
On mycetoma, or the fungus disease of India. London, *J. & A. Churchill*, 1874.
See No. 4047.

4067 HUTCHINSON, *Sir* JONATHAN. 1828-1913
Illustrations of clinical surgery. Vol. 1. London, *J. Churchill*, 1875-1878.
Pp. 49-52: Hutchinson's classic description of cheiropompholyx, dysidrosis ("Hutchinson's disease"). The first description and illustration of sarcoidosis is on p. 42.

4068 NEUMANN, ISIDOR, *Edler von Heilwart*. 1832-1906
Ueber eine noch wenig gekannte Hautkrankeit (Dermatitis circumscripta herpetiformis). *Vjschr. Derm.*, 1875, **2**, 41-52.
First description of porokeratosis (Mibelli).

4069 TAYLOR, ROBERT WILLIAM. 1842-1906
On a rare case of idiopathic localized or partial atrophy of the skin. *Arch. Derm.* (*N.Y.*), 1875-76, **2**, 114-21.
First description of the condition called by Herxheimer and Hartmann in 1902 "acrodermatitis chronica atrophicans", and known eponymically as "Taylor's disease".

4070 MILTON, JOHN LAWS. 1820-1898
On giant urticaria. *Edinb. med. J.*, 1876-77, **22**, 513-26.
Although Quincke described angioneurotic oedema with great precision and has given his name to it ("Quincke's disease", "Quincke's oedema"), Milton first noted it, calling it "giant urticaria".

4070.1. KOEBNER, HEINRICH. 1838-1904
Zur Aetiologie der Psoriasis. *Viertelj. Dermatol. Syph.*, 1876, **8**, 559-561.
"Koebner phenomenon" – appearance at points of injury of any skin lesion that is not an ordinary manifestation or complication of the injury.

4071 COTTLE, WYNDHAM. ?-1919.
Warty growths. *St. George's Hosp. Rep.*, (1877-1878), 1879, **9**, 753-62.
Original description of angiokeratoma ("Mibelli's disease" – so named from the latter's description of it in 1891; *see* No. 4105).

4073   FOX, WILLIAM TILBURY. 1836-1879, & CROCKER, HENRY RADCLIFFE. 1845-1909
        The minute anatomy of dysidrosis. *Trans. path. Soc. Lond.*, 1877-78, **29**, 264-68.

4074   HUTCHINSON, *Sir* JONATHAN. 1828-1913
        Summer prurigo, prurigo aestivalis, seu prurigo adolescentium, seu acne-prurigo. *Med. Times Gaz.*, 1878, **1**, 161-63.
        Hutchinson's summer prurigo.

4075   ———. Lectures on clinical surgery. Pt. 2. London, *J. & A. Churchill*, 1879.
        On p. 298 is the first description of hydradenitis destruens suppurativa, later named "Pollitzer's disease" from the latter's important description of it in *J. cutan. gen.-urin. Dis.*, 1892, **10**, 9-24.

4075.1 SQUIRE, ALEXANDER JOHN BALMANNO. *d.* 1908
        On the treatment of psoriasis by an ointment of chrysophanic acid. London, *J. & A. Churchill*, 1878.
        Introduction of chrysarobin in dermatology.

4076   HARDAWAY, WILLIAM AUGUSTUS. 1850-1923
        A case of multiple tumors of the skin accompanied by intense pruritis. *Arch. Derm. (Philad.)*, 1879, **5**, 385; 1880, **6**, 129-32.
        First description of prurigo nodularis. In 1909 J. N. Hyde (*Diseases of the skin*, Philadelphia, p. 174) was responsible for its present name and for the eponym "Hyde's disease".

4077   FOX, WILLIAM TILBURY. 1836-1879
        Notes on unusual or rare forms of skin disease. Congenital ulceration of skin (two cases) with pemphigus eruption and arrest of development generally. *Lancet*, 1879, **1**, 766-67.
        First description of epidermolysis bullosa.

4078   ———. A clinical study of hydroa. *Arch. Derm. (Philad.)*, 1880, **6**, 16-52.
        First description of dermatitis herpetiformis ("Duhring's disease"; *see* No. 4083).

4079   MAFFUCCI, ANGELO. 1845-1903
        Di un caso di encondroma et angioma multiplo. Contribuzione alla genesi embrionale dei tumori. *Movimento med.-chir.*, 1881, **3**, 399-412.
        "Maffucci's syndrome" – cavernous haemangioma with enchondromas of skeleton, producing deformities.

4080   KAPOSI [KOHN], MORIZ. 1837-1902
        Xeroderma pigmentosum. *Med. Jb.*, 1882, 619-33.
        Excellent pathological study of this condition ("Kaposi's disease"), which he first described in Virchow's *Handbuch der speziellen Pathologie und Therapie*, 1876, **2**, 182.

4081   QUINCKE, HEINRICH IRENAEUS. 1842-1922
        Ueber akutes umschriebenes Hautödem. *Mh. prakt. Derm.*, 1882, **1**, 129-31.
        Angioneurotic oedema is also known as Quincke's oedema, from the latter's excellent description of it, but he was preceded by several other writers, including Donati (No. 4011.2) and Milton (No. 4070). It is also called "Bannister's disease". English translation in No. 2241.

4082   RECKLINGHAUSEN, FRIEDRICH DANIEL VON. 1833-1910
Ueber die multiplen Fibrome der Haut und ihre Beziehung zu den
multiplen Neuromen. Berlin, *Hirschwald*, 1882.

         One of Virchow's distinguished pupils, von Recklinghausen gave a
classic description of neurofibromatosis, adding much to the knowledge
of the condition, which later became known as "Recklinghausen's disease". The article first appeared as a contribution to the Virchow Festschrift,
also published in 1882. *See* No. 4566.

4082.1   BALZER, FÉLIX. 1849-1929
Recherches sur les caractères anatomiques du xanthélasma. *Arch. Physiol.
norm. Path.*, 1884, 3 ser., **4**, 65-80.

         First description of skin changes and necropsy findings in
pseudoxanthoma elasticum. *See* No. 4096.1 and *Trans. St. John's Hosp.
Derm. Soc.*, 1972, **58**, 235-50 (F.M. Pope).

4083   DUHRING, LOUIS ADOLPHUS. 1845-1913
Dermatitis herpetiformis. *J. Amer. med. Assoc.*, 1884, **3**, 225-29.

         Duhring's best work in dermatology. He brought together, under the
name of "dermatitis herpetiformis" ("Duhring's disease") the group of
eruptions which morphologically lay between urticaria and the toxic
erythemas on the one hand and pemphigus on the other. Duhring wrote
the first American textbook on dermatology.

4084   ROBINSON, ANDREW ROSE. 1845-1924
Hidrocystoma. *Trans. Amer. derm. Ass.*, 1884, 14-16; *J. cutan. gen.-urin.
Dis.*, 1893, **11**, 293-303.

         Robinson wrote an excellent textbook on dermatology in 1884, the year
in which he published the first description of hydrocystoma ("Robinson's
disease").

4085   KAPOSI [KOHN], MORIZ. 1837-1902
Ueber eine neue Form von Hautkrankheit, "Lymphodermia perniciosa".
Med. Jb., 1885, 129-47.

         First description of lymphoderma perniciosa, premycotic or leukaemic
erythrodermia.

4086   ——. Lichen ruber monileformis – Korallen schnurartiger Lichen ruber.
Vjschr. Derm., 1886, **13**, 571-82.

         Kaposi is credited with the first description of this condition, sometimes
called "Kaposi's disease", and probably a rare variety of lichen planus.

4087   NEUMANN, ISIDOR, *Edler von Heilwart*. 1832-1906
Ueber Pemphigus vegetans (frambösioides). *Vjschr. Derm.*, 1886, **13**, 157-
78.

         "Neumann's disease" – pemphigus vegetans. This was first described
by Alibert. English translation (New Sydenham Society), 1897.

4088   VIDAL, JEAN BAPTISTE EMILE. 1825-1893
Du lichen (lichen, prurigo, strophulus). *Ann. Derm. Syph. (Paris)*, 1886, 2
sér., **7**, 133-54.

         "Vidal's disease" – neurodermatitis.

4089   BOCKHART, Max.
Ueber die Aetiologie und Therapie der Impetigo, des Furunkels und der Sykosis. *Mh. prakt. Derm.*, 1887, **6**, 450-71.
First description of impetigo circumpilaris infantilis ("Bockhart's impetigo").

4090   GIOVANNINI, Sebastiano. 1851-1920
Ueber die normale Entwicklung und über einige Veränderungen der menschlichen Haare. *Vjschr. Derm. Syph.*, 1887, **14**, 1049-75.
"Giovanni's disease". He described the developmental defect of hair follicles known as pili multigemini.

4091   KAPOSI [Kohn], Moriz. 1837-1902
Impetigo herpetiformis. *Vjschr. Derm.*, 1887, **14**, 273-96.
Although not the first to describe this condition, Kaposi established its status.

4092   UNNA, Paul Gerson. 1850-1929
Das seborrhoische Ekzem. *Mh. prakt. Derm.*, 1887, **6**, 827-46.
Unna's seborrhoeic eczema.

4093   WHITE, James Clarke. 1833-1916
Dermatitis venenata: An account of the action of external irritants upon the skin. Boston, *Cupples & Hurd*, 1887.
White, a pupil of Hebra, was an outstanding personality in American dermatology; he held the first chair in that subject in the U.S.A. The eponym "White's disease" refers to his description of keratosis follicularis in *J. cutan. gen.-urin. Dis.*, 1889, **7**, 201-09, a condition described earlier by Lutz and later by Darier.

4094   QUINQUAUD, Charles Eugène. 1841-1894
Folliculite épilante décalvante. *Réunions clin. Hôp. St. Louis, C. R. (Paris)*, 1888-89, **9**, 17.
Folliculitis decalvans of Quinquaud first described. At about the same time, P. A. Robert described it independently in his thesis, Paris, 1889.

4095   BESNIER, Ernest. 1831-1909
Lupus pernio de la face; synovites fongueuses (scrofulo-tuberculeuses) symétriques des extrémités supérieures. *Ann. Derm. Syph. (Paris)*, 1889, 2 sér., **10**, 333-36.
Besnier–Boeck–Schaumann disease, Boeck's sarcoid. Boeck (No. 4128) wrote a classic paper on the subject and later Schaumann's paper (No. 4149) resulted in a triple eponym. (*See* No. 4067).

4096   BURY, Judson Sykes. 1852-1944
A case of erythema with remarkable nodular thickening and induration of skin, associated with intermittent albuminuria. *Illustr. med. News*, 1889, **3**, 145-48.
Erythema elevatum diutinum ("Bury's disease").

4096.1   CHAUFFARD, Anatole Marie Emile. 1855-1932
Xanthélasma disséminé et symétrique, sans insuffance hépatique. *Bull. Mém. Soc. méd. Hôp. Paris*, 1889, 3 sér., **6**, 412-19.

In 1889 Chauffard gave an important description of pseudoxanthoma elasticum. Further reports on his patient were published by Besnier and Doyon, Darier, and Hallopeau and Laffitte, the last in *Ann. Derm. Syph. (Paris)*, 1903, **4**, 595.

4097   DARIER, JEAN. 1856-1938
De la psorospermose folliculaire végétante. *Ann. Derm. Syph. (Paris)*, 1889, **10**, 597-612.

Dyskeratosis follicularis was so well described by Darier that it is universally known as "Darier's disease". J. C. White also described it (*see* No. 4093) and the first description is accredited to H.C. Lutz (No. 4050).

4098   HUTCHINSON, *Sir* JONATHAN. 1828-1913
A rare form of lupus (marginatus). *Arch. Surg. (Lond.)*, 1889-1890, **1**, Plates 13-14.

"Hilliard's lupus". Hutchinson made an innovation in terminology when he named the disease after the patient instead of the physician describing it. The *Archives*, which ran to 11 volumes, were written entirely by Hutchinson. See also *Polyclinic*, 1900, **2**, 104-09, for a fuller description of this patient.

4099   JACQUET, LUCIEN. 1860-1915
Des érythèmes papuleux fessiers post-érosifs. *Rev. Mal. Enf.*, 1889, **4**, 208-18.

"Jacquet's disease", "Jacquet's dermatitis", papulo-lenticular erythema of the napkin area.

4100   TAENZER, PAUL. 1858-1919
Ueber das Ulerythema ophryogenes, eine noch nicht beschriebene Hautkrankheit. *Mh. prakt. Derm.*, 1889, **8**, 197-208.

Ulerythema ophryogenes ("Taenzer's disease") first described.

4101   HALLOPEAU, FRANÇOIS HENRI. 1842-1919
Sur une nouvelle forme de dermatite pustuleuse chronique en foyer à progression excentrique. *Congr. int. Derm. Syph., C. R.*, 1889, Paris, 1890, 344.

Pyodermite végétante. Hallopeau described a suppurative form of Neumann's pemphigus vegetans.

4102   POLLITZER, SIGMUND. 1859-1937, & JANOVSKY, VIKTOR. 1847-1925
Acanthosis nigricans. In: *Int. Atlas seltener Hautkrankheiten*, Hamburg, 1890, Heft 4, plates x-xi.

First description of acanthosis nigricans.

4103   PRINGLE, JOHN JAMES. 1855-1922
Ueber einen Fall von kongenitalem Adenoma sebaceum. *Mh. prakt. Derm.*, 1890, **10**, 197-211.

Sebaceous adenoma, type Pringle.

4104   HUTCHINSON, *Sir* JONATHAN. 1828-1913
Infective angeioma or naevus-lupus. *Arch. Surg. (Lond.)*, 1891-92, **3**, 166-68.

Angioma serpiginosum.

4105   MIBELLI, VITTORIO. 1860-1910
        L'angiocheratoma. *G. ital. Mal. vener.*, 1891, **26**, 159-80, 260-76.
        Mibelli gave the name to angiokeratoma although it had already been
        described by Cottle in 1877. It is also called "Mibelli's disease".

4106   NONNE, MAX. 1860-1910
        Vier Fälle von Elephantiasis congenita hereditaria. *Virchow's Arch. path.
        Anat.*, 1891, **125**, 189-96.
        First description of hereditary oedema of the legs, generally known as
        "Milroy's disease" or as "Meige's disease" (No. 4129).

4107   BESNIER, ERNEST. 1831-1909
        Première note et observations préliminaires pour servir d'introduction à
        l'étude des prurigos diathésiques (dermites multiformes prurigineuses
        chroniques exacerbantes et paroxystiques, du type du prurigo de Hebra).
        Ann. Derm. Syph. (Paris), 1892, 3 sér., **3**, 634-48.
        "Besnier's prurigo".

4108   JADASSOHN, JOSEF. 1863-1936
        Ueber eine eigenartige Form von Atrophia maculosa cutis. *Verh. dtsch. derm.
        Ges.*, 1890-92, **2-3**, 342-58.
        "Jadassohn's disease" – maculo-papular erythrodermia; Anetoderma
        erythematosum of Jadassohn.

4109   MILROY, WILLIAM FORSYTH. 1855-1942
        An undescribed variety of hereditary oedema. *N.Y. med. J.*, 1892, **56**, 505-
        08.
        Independently of Nonne (No. 4106) Milroy described congenital oedema
        of the legs; it has been given the eponym "Milroy's disease".

4110   UNNA, PAUL GERSON. 1850-1929
        Drei Favusarten. *Mh. prakt. Derm.*, 1892, **14**, 1-16.
        Unna described the different fungi of favus. He founded the above-
        mentioned journal, and he is one of the most eminent figures in modern
        dermatology.

4113   DARIER, JEAN. 1856-1938
        Dystrophie papillaire et pigmentaire. *Ann. Derm. Syph. (Paris)*, 1893, 3
        sér., **4**, 865-75.
        Acanthosis nigricans.

4114   MIBELLI, VITTORIO. 1860-1910
        Contributo allo studio della ipercheratosi dei canali sudoriferi
        (porokeratosis). *G. ital. Mal. vener.*, 1893, **28**, 313-55.
        Mibelli is sometimes credited with the original description of
        porokeratosis ("Mibélli's disease"), but Neumann described it in 1875
        under the name of "dermatitis circumscripta herpetiformis". *See* No. 4068.

4115   RESPIGHI, EMILIO.
        Di una ipercheratosi non ancora descritta. *G. ital. Mal. vener.*, 1893, **28**, 356-
        86.
        First description of hyperkeratosis excentrica, porokeratosis.

4116   SABOURAUD, RAYMOND JACQUES ADRIEN. 1864-1938
         La teigne trichophytique et la teigne spéciale de Gruby. Paris, *Rueff et Cie.*,
         1894.

4117   VINCENT, JEAN HYACINTHE. 1862-1950
         Étude sur le parasite du "pied de Madura". *Ann. Inst. Pasteur,* 1894, **8**, 129-
         51.
              Isolation of *Streptothrix (Actinomyces) madurae.*

4120   KAPOSI [KOHN], MORIZ. 1837-1902
         Lichen ruber acuminatus und Lichen ruber planus. *Arch. Derm. Syph.*
         (*Wien*), 1895, **31**, 1-32.

4121   OSLER, *Sir* WILLIAM, *Bart.* 1849-1919
         On the visceral complication of erythema exudativum multiforme. *Amer.
         J. med. Sci.,* 1895, **110**, 629-46.

4122   DARIER, JEAN. 1856-1938
         Des "tubercules" cutanées. *Ann. Derm. Syph.* (*Paris*), 1896, 3 sér., **7**, 1431-
         36.
              Darier grouped together, under the heading "tuberculides", the skin
         eruptions associated with tuberculosis.

4123   FORDYCE, JOHN ADDISON. 1858-1925
         A peculiar affection of the mucous membrane of the lips and the oral cavity.
         J. cutan. gen.-urin. Dis., 1896, **14**, 413-19.
              Fordyce, remembered for the description of "Fox–Fordyce disease",
         also described a pseudocolloid of the buccal mucosa, which is known as
         "Fordyce's disease".

4125   MAJOCCHI, DOMENICO. 1849-1929
         Sopra una dermatosi telangettode non ancora descritta "Purpura annularis"
         "Telangectasia follicularis annulata" studio clinico. *G. ital. Mal. vener.,*
         1896, **31**, 242-43.
              Purpura annularis telangiectodes (Majocchi) first described.

4126   SABOURAUD, RAYMOND JACQUES ADRIEN. 1864-1938
         La séborrhée grasse et la pelade. *Ann. Inst. Pasteur,* 1897, **11**, 134-59.
              Acne bacillus first cultivated.

4127   SCHENCK, BENJAMIN ROBINSON. 1873-1920
         On refractory subcutaneous abscesses caused by a fungus possibly related
         to the sporotricha. *Johns Hopk. Hosp. Bull.,* 1898, **9**, 286-90.
              Schenck first described a form of sporotrichosis, due to a pathogenic
         fungus, which later became known as *Sporotrichum beurmanni,* after more
         thorough studies upon it by de Beurmann in 1903.

4128   BOECK, CAESAR PETER MOELLER. 1845-1917
         Multipelt benignt hud-sarcoid. *Norsk Mag. Laegevid,* 1899, 4 R., **14**, 1321-34.
              The syndrome of benign sarcoid ("Boeck's sarcoid") was first estab-
         lished by Boeck. English translation in *J. cutan. gen.-urin. Dis.,* 1899, **17**,
         543-50. In 1940 Danbolt (*Schweiz. med. Wschr.,* 1947, **77**, 1149-50) re-
         examined Boeck's original patient, then aged 80.

4129   MEIGE, Henri. 1866-1940
Le trophoedème chronique héréditaire. *N. Iconogr. Salpêtr.*, 1899, **12**, 453-80; 1901, **14**, 465-72.
"Meige's disease" – first described by Nonne (No. 4106).

4130   BUSCHKE, Abraham. 1868-1943
Ueber Scleroedem. *Berl. klin. Wschr.*, 1902, **39**, 955-7. *Arch. Derm. Syph.* (*Wien*), 1900, **53**, 383-6.
Scleroedema adultorum syndrome of Buschke.

4131   KLIPPEL, Maurice. 1858-1942, & TRENAUNAY, Paul. 1875-
Du naevus variqueux ostéo-hypertrophique. *Arch. gén. Méd.*, 1900, **185**, 641-672.
"Klippel–Trenaunay syndrome".

4131.1   SEEBER, Guillermo Rudolfo.
Un nuevo esporozoario parasíto del hombre. Dos casos encontrados en pólipos nasales. *Tesis*, Univ. Nac. de Buenos Aires, 1900.
Rhinosporidiosis first described.

4132   EHLERS, Edvard. 1863-1937
Cutis laxa. Neigung zu Haemorrhagien in der Haut, Lockerung mehrerer Artikulationen. *Derm. Z.*, 1901, **8**, 173-74.
Description of the syndrome to which the name "Ehlers–Danlos syndrome" was later attached (*see also* No. 4144), earlier described by Tschernogubow: Cutis laxa, *Mb. prakt. Derm.*, 1892, **14**, 76.

4133   JADASSOHN, Josef. 1863-1936
Ueber eine eigenartige Erkrankung der Nasenhaut bei Kindern ("Granulosis rubra nasi"). *Arch. Derm. Syph.* (*Wien*), 1901, **58**, 145-158.
In his important paper on granulosis rubra nasi, Jadassohn gave the condition its present name. Previously Pringle, 1894, and Luithlen, 1900, had described probable cases.

4134   SCHAMBERG, Jay Frank. 1870-1934
A peculiar progressive pigmentary disease of the skin. *Brit. J. Derm.*, 1901, **13**, 1-5.
Schamberg's progressive pigmentary dermatosis; first description.

4135   BROCQ, Louis Anne Jean. 1856-1928
Les parapsoriasis. *Ann. Derm. Syph.* (*Paris*), 1902, 4 sér., **3**, 313-15, 433-68.
"Brocq's disease"; he proposed the term "parapsoriasis" for the condition which had previously been described under various names and often mistaken for other dermatoses.

4137   FOX, George Henry. 1846-1937, & FORDYCE, John Addison. 1858-1925.
Two cases of a rare papular disease affecting the axillary region. *J. cutan. gen.-urin. Dis.*, 1902, **20**, 1-5.
"Fox–Fordyce disease". These writers described a papular, itchy eruption, confined to the axillae, nipples and pubes, and considered to be due to a dysfunction of the apocrine glands.

4138   HERXHEIMER, KARL. 1861-1944, & HARTMANN, KUNO.
Ueber Acrodermatitis chronica atrophicans. *Arch. Derm. Syph.*, (*Wien*),
1902, **61**, 57-76.
Taylor described the condition in 1876 (No. 4069) and Herxheimer and
Hartmann named it, separating it from other atrophies which had been
called by a number of different names.

4139   SABOURAUD, RAYMOND JACQUES ADRIEN. 1864-1938
Pityriasis et alopécies pelliculaires. Paris, *Masson et Cie.*, 1904.
Classic account of the different varieties of *Trichophyton.*

4140   JULIUSBERG, MAX. 1874-?
Zur Kenntnis des Virus des Molluscum contagiosum des Menschen. *Dtsch.*
med. Wschr., 1905, **31**, 1598-99.
Juliusberg showed that the virus of molluscum contagiosum passed a
Chamberland filter.

4141   JACOBI, EDUARD. 1862-1915
Fall zur Diagnose (Poikiloderma vascularis atrophicans). *Verh. dtsch. derm.*
Ges., (1906), Berlin, 1907, **9**, 321-23.
First description.

4142   CIUFFO, GIUSEPPE.
Innesto positivo con filtrato de verruca volgare. *G. ital. Mal. vener.*, 1907,
42, 12-17.
Ciuffo showed the aetiological agent in common warts to be filterable.

4143   PINKUS, FELIX. 1868-1947
Ueber eine neue knötchenförmige Hauteruption; Lichen nitidus. *Arch.*
Derm. Syph. (*Wien*), 1907, **85**, 11-36.
Original description of lichen nitidus, "Pinkus's disease". Pinkus first
showed a case before the Berlin Dermatological Society on 3 Dec, 1901,
and himself gave the name "lichen nitidus".

4144   DANLOS, HENRI ALEXANDRE. 1844-1937
Un cas de cutis laxa avec tumeurs par contusion chronique des coudes et
des genoux. *Bull. Soc. franç. Derm. Syph.*, 1908, **19**, 70-72.
Ehlers-Danlos syndrome (*see also* No. 4132). Danlos noted the subcutaneous tumours that may occur in this condition.

4145   LEINER, KARL. 1871-1930
Ueber Erythrodermia desquamativa, eine eigenartige universelle Dermatose
der Brustkinder. *Arch. Derm. Syph.* (*Wien*), 1908, **89**, 65-76, 163-90.
Desquamative erythroderma of nurslings (Leiner); apparently a toxic
eruption peculiar to breast-fed children suffering from enteritis.

4145.1 HEERFORDT, CHRISTIAN FREDERIK. 1872-1953
Ueber eine "Febris uveo-parotidea subchronica", an der Glandula parotis
und der Uvea des Auges lokalisiert und häufig mit Paresen cerebrospinaler
Nerven kompliziert. *v. Graefes Arch. Ophthal.*, 1909, **70**, 254-73.
"Heerfordt's syndrome", uveo-parotid fever, a form of sarcoidosis.

4146   QUEYRAT, Auguste. 1872-?
Érythroplasie du gland. *Bull. Soc. franç. Derm. Syph.*, 1911, **22**, 378-382.
Erythroplasia of Queyrat, a condition similar to the precancerous dermatosis described by Bowen (No. 4148).

4147   BEURMANN, Charles Lucien de. 1851-1923, & GOUGEROT, Henri. 1881-1955
Les sporotrichoses. Paris, *F. Alcan*, 1912.
First complete description of sporotrichosis ("de Beurmann–Gougerot disease").

4148   BOWEN, John Templeton. 1857-1940
Precancerous dermatosis. A study of two cases of chronic atypical epithelial proliferation. *J. cutan. gen.-urin. Dis.*, 1912, **30**, 241-55.
Bowen, a Boston dermatologist, first described a precancerous dermatosis ("Bowen's disease"), which is now considered to be a variant of an intra-epidermal basal cell epithelioma.

4149   SCHAUMANN, Jörgen Nilsen. 1879-1953
Étude sur le lupus pernio et ses rapports avec les sarcoïdes et la tuberculose. *Ann. Derm. Syph. (Paris)*, 1917, 5 sér., **6**, 357-73.
"Besnier–Boeck–Schaumann disease" (*see also* Nos. 4095, 4128). Through Schaumann's paper the systemic nature of sarcoidosis came to be recognized.

4150   STEVENS, Albert Mason. 1884-1945, & JOHNSON, Frank Chambliss. 1894-1934
A new eruptive fever associated with stomatitis and ophthalmia; report of two cases in children. *Amer. J. Dis. Child.*, 1922, **24**, 526-33.
"Stevens-Johnson syndrome", a generalized eruption, continued fever, inflamed buccal mucosa, and severe purulent conjunctivitis. B.A. Thomas (*Brit. med. J.*, 1950, **1**, 1393) believes this to be merely a severe form of Hebra's erythema multiforme exudativum (No. 4049, p. 198).

4150.1 MENDES DA COSTA, Samuel. 1862-?
Erythro- et keratodermia variabilis in a mother and daughter. *Acta dermatovener. (Stockh.)*, 1925, **6**, 255-61.
"Mendes Da Costa's syndrome" – erythrokeratoderma variabilis.

4151   WEBER, Frederick Parkes. 1863-1962
A case of relapsing non-suppurative nodular panniculitis, showing phagocytosis of subcutaneous fat-cells by macrophages. *Brit. J. Derm.*, 1925, **37**, 301-11.
Weber–Christian disease (*see* No. 4152).

4151.1 ABRIKOSOV, Aleksi Ivanovitch. 1875-1955
Über Myome, ausgehend von der quergestreiften willkürlichen Muskulatur. *Virchows Arch. path. Anat.*, 1926, **260**, 215-33.
"Abrikosov's tumour", granular-cell myoblastoma.

4151.2 SENEAR, Francis Eugene. 1889- , & USHER, Barney David. 1899-
An unusual type of pemphigus, combining features of lupus erythematosus. *Arch. Derm. Syph. (Chicago)*, 1926, **13**, 761-81.
Pemphigus erythematodes. "Senear–Usher syndrome".

4152   CHRISTIAN, Henry Asbury. 1876-1951
Relapsing febrile nodular nonsuppurative panniculitis. *Arch. intern. Med.*,
1928, **42**, 338-51.
See No. 4151.

4152.1   HAILEY, William Howard. 1898- , & HAILEY, Hugh Edward. 1909-
Familial benign chronic pemphigus. *Arch. Derm.* (*Chicago*), 1939, **39**, 679-85.
"Hailey–Hailey disease", earlier described by H. Gougerot, *Arch. derm.-
syph. Clin. St Louis*, 1933, **5**, 255-57.

4153   KVEIM, Morten Ansgar. 1892-
En ny og spesifikk kutan-reaksjon ved Boecks sarcoid. En foreløbig
meddelelse. *Nord. Med.*, 1941, **9**, 169-72.
Kveim's test for sarcoidosis.

4154   DEGOS, Robert. 1904- , *et al.*
Dermatite papulo-squameuse atrophiante. *Bull. Soc. franç. Derm. Syph.*,
1942, **49**, 148-50, 281.
"Degos's disease", malignant atrophic papulosis. With J. Delort and R.
Tricot. Earlier described by W. Köhlmeier, *Frankf. Z. Path.*, 1940, **54**, 413.

4154.1   SPITZ, Sophie. 1910-
Melanomas of childhood. *Amer. J. Path.*, 1948, **24**, 591-609.
Spitz first defined the histologic criteria for the diagnosis of juvenile
melanoma.

4154.2   BECKER, Samuel William. 1924-
Concurrent melanosis and hypertrichosis in distribution of nevus unius
lateris. *Arch. Derm.* (*Chicago*), 1949, **60**, 155-60.
"Becker's naevus", pigmented hairy epidermal naevus.

4154.3   ZOON, Johannes Jacobus. 1902-
Balanitis circumscripta chronica met plasmacellen-infiltraat. *Ned. T.
Geneesk.*, 1950, **94**, 1529-30.
Zoon's plasma cell balanitis.

4154.4   WAARDENBURG, Petrus Johannes. 1886-1979
A new syndrome combining developmental anomalies of the eyelids,
eyebrows and nose root with pigmentary defects of the iris and head hair
with congenital deafness. *Amer. J. hum. Genet.*, 1951, **3**, 195-253.
"Waardenburg's syndrome".

4154.5   PINKUS, Hermann. 1905-
Alopecia mucinosa. Inflammatory plaques with alopecia characterized by
root-sheath mucinosis. *Arch. Derm.* (*Chicago*), 1957, **76**, 419-26.
Follicular mucinosis.

4154.6   NETHERTON, Earl Weldon. 1893-
A unique case of trichorrhexis nodosa – "bamboo hairs". *Arch. Derm.*
(*Chicago*), 1958, **78**, 483-7.
"Netherton's syndrome".

4154.7   DENTON, James Fred. 1914- , *et al.*
Isolation of *Blastomyces dermatitidis* from soil. *Science*, 1961, **133**, 1126-7.
With E.S. McDonough, L. Ajello and R.J. Ausherman.

4154.8   WELLS, ROBERT STUART, & KERR, CHARLES BALDWIN.
         Genetic classification of ichthyosis. *Arch. Derm. (Chicago)*, 1965, **92**, 1-
         6.
             Sex-linked recessive ichthyosis shown to be an important but not
         uncommon entity. See also Kerr & Wells: Sex-linked ichthyosis. *Ann. hum.
         Genet.*, 1965, **29**, 33-50.

History of Dermatology

4155   RICHTER, PAUL CAESAR. 1865-1938
         Geschichte der Dermatologie. In: J. JADASSOHN'S *Handbuch der Haut- und
         Geschlechtskrankheiten*, Berlin, **14**, pt. 2, pp. 1-252, 1928.

4156   PUSEY, WILLIAM ALLEN. 1865-1940
         The history of dermatology. Springfield, *C. C. Thomas*, 1933.
             Reprinted, New York, 1976.

4158   SHELLEY, WALTER BROWN. 1917- , & CRISSEY, JOHN THORNE. 1924-
         Classics in clinical dermatology. With biographical sketches. Springfield,
         C. C. Thomas, 1953.
             Contains 143 classic descriptions of cutaneous diseases by 93 writers.
         Many portraits are also included.

4158.1   SCHOENFELD, WALTHER. 1888-1977
         Kurze Geschichte der Dermatologie und Venereologie und ihre
         kulturgeschichtliche Spiegelung. Hannover, *T. Oppermann*, 1954.

4158.2   CRISSEY, JOHN THORNE. 1924-, & PARISH, LAWRENCE CHARLES.
         The dermatology and syphilology of the nineteenth century. New York,
         Praeger, 1981.
             A scholarly work written in a particularly entertaining style.

4158.3   AINSWORTH, GEOFFREY CLOUGH. 1905-
         Introduction to the history of medical and veterinary mycology. Cam-
         bridge, *Cambridge University Press*, [1986].
             Authoritative and well-illustrated history with excellent chronological
         bibliography.

DISEASES OF THE
GENITO-URINARY SYSTEM

See also 5195-5227.1, SEXUALLY TRANSMITTED DISEASES; 6008-6135, GYNAECOLOGY.

4159   LAGUNA, ANDRÉS [LACUNA]. 1499-1560
         Methodus cognoscendi, extirpandique excrescentes in vesicae collo
         carunculas. [1551.]
             Laguna, "the Spanish Galen", wrote several important books, among
         them the above, a method of excising vesical caruncles. Laguna was
         among the first to suggest this method.

4160 DIAZ, FRANCISCO. *fl.* 1580
Tratado de todas las enfermedades de los riñones, vexiga, y carnosidades de la verga, y urina. Madrid, *Fr. Sanchez*, 1588.
First treatise on diseases of the urinary tract. Also describes the high operation for stone. Diaz is sometimes called the "Father of Urology".

4160.1 BRIAN, THOMAS. *fl.* 1637
The pisse-prophet; or, certaine pisse-pot lectures. Wherein are newly discovered the old fallacies, deceit, and jugling of the pisse-pot science, used by all those... who pretend knowledge of diseases, by the urine.... London, *E.P. for R. Thrale*, 1637.
Brian attacked the "pisse-mongers" and "pisse-prognosticators" hoping to eliminate the frauds of uromancy. He warned patients against diagnosis "prescribed only by the sight of the Urine", and argued that uroscopy should be performed by "University trained physicians".

4161 DEKKERS, FREDERIK [DECKERS]. 1648-1720
Exercitationes medicae practicae circa medendi methodum. Lugduni Batavorum et Amstelodami, *apud D. Abrahamum et Adrianum à Gaesbeck*, 1673.
Albuminuria was first described by Dekkers (Chapter V). A translation of this chapter is in Major, *Classic descriptions of disease*, 3rd ed., 1945, p. 528. *See* No. 4204.1.

4162 BELLINI, LORENZO. 1643-1704
De urinis et pulsibus., de missione sanguinis., de febribus., de morbis capitis, et pectoris. *Bononiae, Ex typographia Antonii Pisarii*, 1683.
Bellini realized the value of the urine as an aid to diagnosis and insisted on its chemical analysis in pathological conditions. *See* No. 762.1.

4163 LA PEYRONIE, FRANÇOIS DE. 1678-1747
Mémoire sur quelques obstacles qui s'opposent à l'éjaculation naturelle de la semence. *Mém. Acad. roy. Chir. (Paris)*, 1743, **1**, 425-34.
"Peyronie's disease", plastic induration of the penis.

4164 POTT, PERCIVALL. 1714-1788
Practical remarks on the hydrocele or watry rupture. London, *C. Hitch & L. Hawes*, 1762.
Classic description of hydrocele.

4165 ——. Chirurgical observations relative to the cataract, the polypus of the nose, the cancer of the scrotum, *etc.* London, *Hawes, Clarke & Collins*, 1775.
Includes the first description of occupational cancer. By describing chimney sweeps' cancer of the scrotum, Pott was the first to trace the origin of a type of cancer to a specific external cause. The above work also includes his description of senile gangrene, sometimes referred to as "Pott's gangrene".

4165.01 CHOPART, FRANÇOIS. 1743-1795
Traité des maladies des voies urinaires. 2 vols. Paris, *J.B. Baillière*, 1791-92.
Chopart and Desault were the founders of urological surgery, both emphasizing the importance of considering the urinary tract as a whole. "They were close friends and were both able clinicians, surgeons and

teachers. Desault was a brilliant lecturer who wrote little while Chopart, a poor speaker, published an outstanding textbook on urology" (Desnos, transl. Murphy).

4165.02   DESAULT, PIERRE JOSEPH. 1744-1795
Œuvres chirurgicales. 3 vols. Paris, *C. Ve. Desault*, an VI [1798]-1803.
    Vol. 3, edited by P.J. ROUX, concerns urological diseases. With Chopart Desault founded urological surgery, and was one of the first to have a clear understanding of urological disease. *See* No. 5580.

4165.1   SÉGALAS, PIERRE SALOMAN. 1792-1875
Un moyen d'éclairer l'urètre et la vessie de manière à voir dans l'intérieur de ces organes. *Rev. méd. franç. étrang.*, 1827, **1**, 157-8.
    Urethro-cystic speculum (endoscope).

4166   COOPER, *Sir* ASTLEY PASTON, *Bart.* 1768-1841
Observations on the structure and diseases of the testis. London, *Longmans*, 1830.

4167   GUTHRIE, GEORGE JAMES. 1785-1856
On the anatomy and diseases of the neck of the bladder, and of the urethra. London, *Burgess & Hill,* 1834.
    Guthrie was the first to describe non-prostatic obstruction at the neck of the bladder. On p. 252 of the above work is an account of Guthrie's prostatic catheter for use in trans-urethral prostatectomy.

4168   MAISONNEUVE, JACQUES GILLES THOMAS. 1809-1877
Mémoire sur un moyen très simple et très sur de pratiquer le cathétérisme dans les cas même les plus difficiles. *C. R. Acad. Sci.* (*Paris*), 1845, **20**, 70-72.
    Maisonneuve introduced a hair catheter.

4168.1   MERCIER, LOUIS AUGUSTE. 1811-1882
Sur les cathéters coudés, sur la manière de les introduire et sur les avantages qu'on peut rétirer de leur emploi. *Gaz. Hôp. Paris*, 1845, 2 sér., **7**, 13-15.
    Mercier introduced the coudé catheter in 1836 and the bicoudé about 1841.

4169   PARKER, WILLARD. 1800-1884
Cystitis; lateral operation on the bladder, death; tuberculous kidney. *N.Y. J. Med.*, 1851, n.s. **7**, 83-86.
    First cystotomy for inflammation and rupture of the bladder.

4169.1   SIMON, *Sir* JOHN. 1816-1904
Ectropia vesicae (absence of the anterior walls of the bladder and pubic abdominal parietes); operation for directing the orifices of the ureters into the rectum; temporary success; subsequent death; autopsy. *Lancet*, 1852, **2**, 568-70.
    First uretero-intestinal anastomosis.

4169.2   DRESSLER, Lucas Anton. 1815-1896.
Ein Fall von intermittirender Albumenurie und Chromaturie. *Virchows Arch. path. Anat.*, 1854, **6**, 264-66.
Paroxysmal cold haemoglobinuria described. English translation in No. 2241.

4170   PANCOAST, Joseph. 1805-1882
[Plastic operation for exstrophy of the bladder in the male; reported by S. D. Gross.] *N. Amer. med.-chir. Rev.*, 1859, **3**, 710-11.
Pancoast performed the first successful operation for exstrophy of the bladder (ectopia vesicae).

4171   HARLEY, George. 1829-1896
On intermittent haematuria; with remarks upon its pathology and treatment. *Med.-chir. Trans.*, 1865, **48**, 161-73.
Harley's classic description of paroxysmal haemoglobinuria, "Harley's disease".

4172   DESORMEAUX, Antonin Jean. ?-1894
De l'endoscope et de ses applications au diagnostic et au traitement des affections de l'urèthre et de la vessie. Paris, *J. B. Baillière*, 1865.
Desormeaux was a pioneer of endoscopy.

4173   THOMPSON, *Sir* Henry, *Bart.* 1820-1904
Clinical lectures on diseases of the urinary organs. London, *J. Churchill*, 1868.
Thompson was Professor of Clinical Surgery at University College, London, and an eminent genito-urinary surgeon. He performed the operation of lithotrity upon Leopold I and Napoleon III; he also developed the two-glass urine test in gonorrhoea. *The versatile Victorian*, a biography of Thompson, was published by Sir Zachary Cope in 1951.

4174   GUSSENBAUER, Carl. 1842-1903
Exstirpation eines Harnblasenmyoms nach vorausgehendem tiefen und hohen Blasenschnitt. Heilung. *Arch. klin. Chir.*, 1875, **18**, 411-423.
First abdominal resection of a tumour of the bladder. The operation was performed by Billroth.

4174.1   GRÜNFELD, Joseph. 1840-1910
Sondirung des Harnleiters mit Hilfe des Endoskops. *Wien. med. Presse,* 1876, **17**, 919, 949.
Successful catheterization of the ureter under vision.

4175   NITZE, Max. 1848-1906
Eine neue Beobachtungs- und Untersuchungsmethode für Harnröhre, Harnblase und Rectum. *Wien. med. Wschr.*, 1879, **29**, 649-52, 688-90, 713-16, 776-82, 806-10.
Nitze devised an electrically lighted cystoscope in 1877, which made possible great improvements in the surgery of the bladder.

4176   FLEISCHER, Richard. 1848-
Ueber eine neue Form von Haemoglobinurie beim Menschen. *Berl. klin. Wschr.*, 1881, **18**, 691-94.

First description of "march haemoglobinuria" – the condition in which physical exertion gives rise to the passage of red urine containing haemoglobin in solution.

4177   GUYON, JEAN CASIMIR FÉLIX. 1831-1920
        Leçons cliniques sur les maladies des voies urinaires. Paris, *J. B. Baillière*, 1881.
        Guyon was the outstanding French urologist of his day, an operator of great skill and a brilliant lithotomist.

4177.1 ROBERTS, *Sir* WILLIAM. 1830-1899
        On the occurrence of micro-organisms in fresh urine. *Brit. med. J.*, 1881, **2**, 623-5.
        Roberts reported a relationship between the finding of bacteria in the urine and the development of cystitis after catheterization.

4178   SENATOR, HERMANN. 1834-1911
        Die Albuminurie im gesunden und kranken Zustande. Berlin, *A. Hirschwald*, 1882.

4179   OTIS, FESSENDEN NOTT. 1825-1900
        The hydrochlorate of cocaine in genito-urinary procedures. *N.Y. med. J.*, 1884, **40**, 635-37.
        Local anaesthesia first employed in urology.

4180   THOMPSON, *Sir* HENRY, *Bart*. 1820-1904
        On tumours of the bladder. London, *J. & A. Churchill*, 1884.
        Includes description of Thompson's operation for tumours of the bladder.

4181   PAVY, FREDERICK WILLIAM. 1829-1911
        On cyclic albuminuria (albuminuria in the apparently healthy). *Brit. med. J.*, 1885, **2**, 789-91.
        "Pavy's disease" – recurrent albuminuria.

4182   MacCORMAC, *Sir* WILLIAM. 1836-1901
        Some observations on rupture of the urinary bladder, with an account of two cases of intra-peritoneal rupture successfully treated by abdominal section and subsequent suture of the vesical rent. *Lancet*, 1886, **2**, 1118-22.
        MacCormac introduced an operation for the treatment of intraperitoneal rupture of the bladder.

4183   GUYON, JEAN CASIMIR FÉLIX. 1831-1920
        Leçons cliniques sur les affections chirurgicales de la vessie et de la prostate. Paris, *J. B. Baillière*, 1888.
        Guyon was Professor of Genito-urinary Surgery at Paris, and a great teacher (*see also* No. 4177).

4183.1 MIKULICZ-RADECKI, JOHANN VON. 1850-1905
        Zur Operation der angeborenen Blasenspalte. *Zbl. Chir.*, 1889, **26**, 641-3.
        First enterocystoplasty.

4184   NITZE, MAX. 1848-1906
Lehrbuch der Kystoskopie. Wiesbaden, *J. F. Bergmann*, 1889.
    Nitze introduced the cystoscope in 1877 (*see* No. 4175) and in 1889
published his important monograph on cystoscopy.

4184.1   PAWLIK, KAREL. 1849-1914
Über Blasenekstirpation. *Wien. med. Wschr.*, 1891, **41**, 1814-6.
    First successful total cystectomy.

4185   ALBARRAN Y DOMINGUEZ, JOAQUIN MARIA. 1860-1912
Les tumeurs de la vessie. Paris, *G. Steinheil*, 1891.
    Includes description of "Albarran's glands", subtrigonal glands in the
bladder. He introduced a classification based on embryological origin. *See
also* No. 4195.

4185.1   BROWN, JAMES. 1854-1895
Catheterization of the male ureters. A preliminary report. *Johns Hopk. Hosp.
Bull.*, 1893, **4**, 73-74.
    First catheterization of male ureters.

4186   VAN HOOK, WELLER. 1862-1933
The surgery of the ureters. A clinical, literary, and experimental research.
J. Amer. med. Assoc., 1893, **21**, 911-16, 965-73.
    Uretero-ureterostomy. Van Hook originated modern methods of ureteral
repair.

4187   KELLY, HOWARD ATWOOD. 1858-1943
The examination of the female bladder and the catheterization of the
ureters under direct inspection. *Johns Hopk. Hosp. Bull.*, 1893, **4**, 101-02.
    Kelly introduced aeroscopic examination of the bladder and catheteri-
zation of the ureters. See also *Ann. Surg.*, 1898, **27**, 475-86.

4188   ——. Uretero-ureteral anastomosis; uretero-ureterostomy. *Ann. Surg.*, 1894,
19, 70-77.
    Kelly's method of uretero-ureteral anastomosis included the use of the
catheter as a temporary ureteral splint.

4188.1   MAYDL, KAREL. 1853-1913
Ueber die Radikaltherapie der Ektopia vesicae urinariae. *Wien. med. Wschr.*,
1894, **44**, 1113-5, 1169-72, 1209-10, 1256-8, 1297-1301.
    Maydl's operation, uretero-intestinal anastomosis.

4189   PÉAN, JULES ÉMILE. 1830-1898
Vessie et urètre surnuméraires. *Bull. Acad. Méd. (Paris)*, 1895, 3 sér., **33**,
542-45.
    Péan was first to operate on diverticula of the bladder.

4190   NITZE, MAX. 1848-1906
Eine neue Modifikation des Harnleiterkatheters. *Zbl. Krankh. Harn-u* .
SexOrg., 1897, **8**, 8-13.
    With Nitze's operative cystoscope it became possible to excise bladder
tumours *in situ*.

4191   BEVAN, ARTHUR DEAN. 1860-1943
Operation for undescended testicle and congenital inguinal hernia. *J. Amer. med. Assoc.*, 1899, **33**, 773-77.
Bevan's operation for undescended testicle.

4191.1   TUFFIER, THÉODORE. 1857-1929
Sonde urétérale opaque. In *Traité de chirurgie*, 2e ed. S. Duplay & P. Reclus, vol. 7, p. 414. Paris, *Masson*, 1899.
Tuffier made the first pioneer attempt to visualize the urinary tract by the combination of an opaque ureteral styletted catheter and radiography.

4191.2   KRAUSE, FEDOR. 1856-1937
Extirpation einer Harnblase mit Einpflanzung der Ureteren in die Flexura iliaca. *Dtsch. med. Wschr.*, 1903, **29**, Ver.-Beil., 76 (only).
Total cystectomy and bilateral ureterosigmoidostomy.

4191.3   WITTEK, ARNOLD.
Zur Technik der Röntgenphotographie (Lendenwirbel, Blasensteine). *Fortschr. Röntgenstr.*, 1903, **7**, 26-7.
Cystography. Wittek filled the bladder with air and was able to demonstrate vertebrae and urinary calculus.

4191.4   WULLF, P.
Verwendbarkeit der X-Strahlen für die Diagnose der Blasendifformitäten. *Fortschr. Röntgenstr.*, 1904-5, **8**, 193-4.
Wulff outlined the bladder with a suspension of bismuth subnitrate.

4192   VOELCKER, FRIEDRICH. 1872-1955, & LICHTENBERG, ALEXANDER VON. 1880-1949
Die Gestalt der menschlichen Harnblase im Röntgenbilde. *Münch. med. Wschr.*, 1905, **52**, 1576-78.
First cystograms.

4194   HAGNER, FRANCIS RANDALL. 1873-1940
The operative treatment of acute gonorrheal epididymitis. *Med. Rec. (N.Y.)*, 1906, **70**, 944-46.
Hagner devised the open operation for the relief of acute epididymitis.

4194.1   GRAY, ALFRED LEFTWICH. 1873-1932
The treatment of malignant diseases of the bladder through suprapubic incision, with report of a case. *Amer. Quart. Roentgenol.*, 1906-07, **1**, 53-56.
Radiotherapy for carcinoma of bladder.

4195   ALBARRAN Y DOMINGUEZ, JOAQUIN MARIA. 1860-1912
Médecine opératoire des voies urinaires. Paris, *Masson & Cie.*, 1909.
Albarran, a Cuban, became a teacher of the highest rank and attained a professorship at Paris in 1892. He was the first surgeon in France to perform perineal prostatectomy.

4195.1   BUERGER, LEO. 1879-1943
A new direct irrigating observation and double catheterizing cystoscope. *Ann. Surg.*, 1909, **49**, 225-37.
Brown–Buerger cystoscope.

4196 TOREK, FRANZ. 1861-1938
The technique of orcheopexy. *N.Y. med. J.*, 1909, **90**, 948-53.
Torek's operation for undescended testicle.

4196.1 CUNNINGHAM, JOHN HENRY. 1877-
The diagnosis of stricture of the urethra by the roentgen rays. *Trans. Amer. Ass. gen.-urin. Surg.*, 1910, **5**, 369-71.
Urethrography.

4196.2 COFFEY, ROBERT CALVIN. 1869-1933
Physiologic implantation of the severed ureter or common bile-duct into the intestine. *J. Amer. med. Assoc.*, 1911, **56**, 397-403.
The modern method of uretero-intestinal anastomosis followed the experimental work of Coffey.

4197 KAPPIS, MAX. 1881-1938
Ueber Leitungsanästhesie bei Nierenoperationen und Thorakoplastiken überhaupt bei Operationen am Rumpf. *Zbl. Chir.*, 1912, **39**, 249-52.
Paravertebral anaesthesia in urology.

4198 YOUNG, HUGH HAMPTON, 1870-1945, & WATERS, CHARLES ALEXANDER. 1885-
X-ray studies of the seminal vesicles and vasa deferentia after urethroscopic injection of the ejaculatory ducts with thorium – a new diagnostic method. *Amer. J. Roentgenol.*, 1920, n.s. **7**, 16-22.
Vesiculography first demonstrated.

4198.1 McCARTHY, JOSEPH FRANCIS. 1874-1965
A new type of observation and operating cysto-urethroscope. *J. Urol.*, 1923, **10**, 519-23.
McCarthy foroblique pan-endoscope.

4199 OSBORNE, EARL DORLAND. 1895-1960, *et al.*
Roentgenography of the urinary tract during excretion of sodium iodide. *J. Amer. med. Assoc.*, 1923, **80**, 368-73.
Sodium iodide was first used in uretero-pyelography by E. D. Osborne, C. G. Sutherland, A. J. Scholl, and L. G. Rowntree.

4200 SWICK, MOSES. 1900-
Darstellung der Niere und Harnwege im Röntgenbild durch intravenöse Einbringung eines neuen Kontraststoffes, des Uroselectans. *Klin. Wschr.*, 1929, **8**, 2087-89.
Introduction of Uroselectan. In a following paper (pp. 2089-91), A. von Lichtenberg and M. Swick used it in human excretion urography.

4201 ——. Excretion urography by means of the intravenous and oral administration of sodium ortho-iodohippurate: with some physiological considerations. *Surg. Gybec, Obstet.*, 1933, **56**, 62-65.
Introduction of Hippuran.

4202 ROSENHEIM, MAX LEONARD, *Lord Rosenheim*. 1908-1972
Mandelic acid in the treatment of urinary infections. *Lancet*, 1935, **1**, 1032-37.
Introduction of mandelic acid in the treatment of urinary infections.

4203 DE NICOLA, Rocco Robert. 1916-
Permanent artificial (silicone) urethra. *J. Urol.*, 1950, **63**, 168-72.
First implantation of silicone rubber tube to replace urethra.

4203.1 COUVELAIRE, Roger. 1903-
Le réservoir iléal de substitution après la cystectomie totale chez l'homme. *J. Urol. méd. chir.*, 1951, **57**, 408-17.
Artificial bladder.

4203.90 HIPPOCRATES. 460-375 B.C.
Aphorisms, Section VII, number 34. In his *Works.* Ed. W.H.S. Jones and E.T. Withington, London, 1927.
The first description of the association of proteinuria and chronic renal disease.

4204 SALICETO, Gulielmus de [Salicetti; William of Salicet]. *circa* 1210-1280
Liber in scientia medicinali. [Placentiae, *Johannes Petrus de Ferratis*, 1476.]
Contains (Cap. cxl) his classic account of renal dropsy: De duritie in renibus, an English translation of which is in Major, *Classic descriptions of disease*, 3rd ed., 1945, p. 527.

4204.1 DEKKERS, Frederik [Deckers]. 1648-1720
Exercitationes medicae practicae circa medendi methodum. Lugduni Batavorum et Amstelodami, *apud D. Abrahamum et Adrianum à Gaesbeck*, 1673.
This work contains the first clear description of proteinuria, noting precipitation of urine with heat or acetic acid. *See* No. 4161.

4204.2 COTUGNO, Domenico [cotunnius]. 1736-1822
De ischiade nervosa commentarius. Neapoli, *apud Frat. Simonios,* 1764.
This classic work on sciatica includes the first clear description of the association of oedema with proteinuria. *See* Nos. 1382 & 4515.

4205 WELLS, William Charles. 1757-1817
On the presence of the red matter and serum of blood in the urine of dropsy, which has not originated from scarlet fever. *Trans. Soc. Improve. med. chir. Knowl.*, 1812, **3**, 194-240.
Wells was the first to notice the presence of blood and albumin in dropsical urine. He also established the fact that the dropsy occurred in the upper parts of the body, and he described the uraemic seizures to which such cases are liable.

4206 BRIGHT, Richard. 1789-1858
Reports of medical cases selected with a view of illustrating the symptoms and cure of diseases by a reference to morbid anatomy. 2 vols. London, *Longman*, 1827-31.
Bright's classic description of chronic nephritis has led to its designation as "Bright's disease", one of the best known and most permanent of medical eponyms. Bright distinguished renal from cardiac dropsy. He was the first clearly to recognize the association of dropsy, coagulable urine, and disease of the kidney. *See* No. 2285.

4207 ———. Cases and observations, illustrative of renal disease accompanied with the secretion of albuminous urine. *Guy's Hosp. Rep.*, 1836, **1**, 338-400; 1840, **5**, 101-161.

As a result of greater experience on renal disease, Bright rounded off his work on the subject with the above paper, wherein he recorded his extended observations; by this time he had come to more definite conclusions, expecially with regard to the treatment of the condition. Bright's papers on the subject were reprinted, London, 1937, edited by A. A. Osman.

4208 RAYER, PIERRE FRANÇOIS OLIVE. 1793-1867
Traité des maladies des reins. 3 vols. and atlas. Paris, *J. B. Baillière*, 1839-41.

Rayer insisted on the exhaustive analysis of the urine as an aid to the diagnosis of lesions. He classified "albuminuric nephritis" into six distinct forms and distinguished these from other forms of nephritis associated with infection, gout, rheumatism, and toxins. He noticed the existence of albuminuria in diabetes mellitus and also described the existence of renal vein thrombosis. His treatise on diseases of the kidney includes a spectacular colour-plate atlas.

4209 FRERICHS, FRIEDRICH THEODOR. 1819-1885
Die Bright'sche Nierenkrankheit. Braunschweig, *F. Vieweg u. Sohn*, 1851.

Frerichs divided the progression of renal disease into three stages: initial hyperaemia, fatty infiltration and exudation, and organization leading to fibrosis and atrophy. This is one of the earliest works on kidney disease to incorporate histological appearances. However, Frerichs did not recognize the primary involvement of the glomerulus in what later became known as glomerulonephritis. *See* No. 4212.

4210 STODDARD, CHARLES L.
Case of encephaloid disease of the kidney; removal, etc. *Med. Surg. Reporter (Philad.)*, 1861, **7**, 126-27.

Erastus Bradley Wolcott (1804-1880) was first to excise the kidney (for renal tumour). The preoperative diagnosis had been tumour of the liver. Only after the operation did the surgeons realize that they had removed the kidney. The patient lived 15 days after the operation. The operation was recorded by Stoddard.

4211 DIETL, JOSEF. 1804-1878
Wandernde Nieren und deren Einklemmung. *Wien. med. Wschr.*, 1864, **14**, 563-66, 579-81, 593-95.

"Dietl's crisis". Dietl described the sudden severe attacks of nephralgic or gastric pain, chills, fever, nausea and vomiting, and general collapse, ascribing them to partial turning of the kidney upon its pedicle. First published in *Przeglad Lekarski*, 1864, **3**, 225, 233, 241.

4211.1 HILLIER, THOMAS. 1831-1868
Hydronephrosis in a boy four years old, repeatedly tapped; recovery. *Proc. Roy. Med. Chir. Soc.*, 1865, **5**, 59-60.

Hillier performed the first therapeutic percutaneous nephrostomy.

4212 KLEBS, THEODOR ALBRECHT EDWIN. 1834-1913
Handbuch der pathologischen Anatomie. I. Abt. Berlin, *A. Hirschwald*, 1870.

A classic description of glomerulonephritis ("Klebs's disease") is on pp. 644-48.

4213 SIMON, Gustav. 1824-1876
Exstirpation einer Niere am Menschen. *Dtsch. Klin.* 1870, **22**, 137-138.
First successful planned nephrectomy for urinary tract fistula. A more detailed, illustrated account of the case appears in No. 4214.

4214 ———. Chirurgie der Nieren. Theil 1-2. Erlangen, *F. Enke*, 1871-76.
Simon was Professor of Surgery at Rostock and Heidelberg. The work was projected as 3 vols., but Simon died before it was completed.

4215 GULL, *Sir* William Withey. 1816-1890, & SUTTON, Henry Gawen. 1837-1891
On the pathology of the morbid state commonly called chronic Bright's disease with contracted kidney ("arterio-capillary fibrosis"). *Med.-chir. Trans.*, 1872, **55**, 273-326.
First clear description of arteriosclerotic atrophy of the kidney ("Gull–Sutton disease"), and probably the first description of hypertensive nephrosclerosis.

4215.1 JOHNSON, George. 1818-1896
Lectures on Bright's disease: with special reference to pathology, diagnosis, and treatment. London, *Smith, Elder*, 1873.
Johnson showed that fatty infiltrations of the renal tubules are reflected by the presence of fatty casts and droplets in the urine, thus introducing the concept of lipoid nephrosis associated with nephrotic syndrome.

4216 GOWERS, *Sir* William Richard. 1845-1915
The state of the arteries in Bright's disease. *Brit. med. J.*, 1876, **2**, 743-45.
Gowers's important account of the changes in the retinal vessels in Bright's disease is reproduced in Willius & Keys, *Cardiac classics*, 1941, pp. 605-11.

4216.1 LANGENBUCH, Carl Johann August. 1846-1901
Eine eigenthümliche Nierenexstirpation. *Berl. klin. Wschr.*, 1877, **14**, 337-40.
First nephrectomy for malignant disease.

4216.2 CHARCOT, Jean Martin. 1825-1893
Leçons sur les maladies du foie, des voies biliaires et des reins. Paris: *Progrés Médical & Adrien Delahaye*, 1877.
Charcot defined "scarlatinous nephritis" and "amyloid kidney" as distinct pathological entities. English translation, New York, 1878.

4217 WEIGERT, Carl. 1845-1904
Die Bright'sche Nierenkrankung vom pathologisch-anatomischen Standpunkte. *Samml. klin. Vortr.*, 1879, Nr. 162-63 (Inn. Med., Nr. 55), 1411-60.
Classic study of the pathological anatomy of Bright's disease.

4218 HAHN, Eugen. 1841-1902
Die operative Behandlung der beweglichen Niere durch Fixation. *Zbl. Chir.*, 1881, **8**, 449-52.
Hahn devised the operation of nephropexy (nephrorrhaphy) for the relief of movable kidney.

4219   BASSINI, EDOARDO. 1844-1924
Un caso di rene mobile fissato col mezzo dell'operazione cruenta. *Ann. Univ. Med. (Milano)*, 1882, **261**, 281-86.
Important modification of Hahn's operation of nephropexy.

4220   GRAWITZ, PAUL ALBERT. 1850-1932
Die Entstehung von Nierentumoren aus Nebennierengewebe. *Verh. dtsch. Ges. Chir.*, 1884, **13**, pt. 2, 28-38.
An important investigation of the origin of hypernephroma ("Grawitz tumour"). See also *Arch. klin. Chir.*, 1884, **30**, 824-34.

4221   BOZEMAN, NATHAN. 1825-1905
Chronic pyelitis, successfully treated by kolpo-uretero-cystotomy. *Amer. J. med. Sci.*, 1888, **95**, 255-65, 368-76.
Bozeman treated vesical and faecal fistulae in women, dealing with the complication of pyelitis by catheterization of the ureter through a vesico-vaginal opening.

4222   TRENDELENBURG, FRIEDRICH. 1844-1924
Ueber Blasenscheidenfisteloperationen und über Beckenhochlagerung bei Operationen in der Bauchhöhle. *Samml. klin. Vortr.*, 1890, Nr. 355 (Chir., Nr. 109), 3373-92.
Includes an account of his attempt, 1886, to cure hydronephrosis by a plastic operation – the first recorded surgical intervention for the relief of this condition.

4223   KÜSTER, ERNST GEORG FERDINAND VON. 1839-1930
Ein Fall von Resektion des Harnleiters. *Zbl. Chir.*, 1892, **19**, Suppl., 110-11.
First successful plastic operation for the relief of hydronephrosis.

4224   EDEBOHLS, GEORGE MICHAEL. 1853-1908
Movable kidney; with a report of twelve cases treated by nephrorrhaphy. *Amer. J. med. Sci.*, 1893, **105**, 247-59, 417-32.
In his nephropexy operation Edebohls utilized flaps of the capsule of the kidney. He believed that decapsulation improved the renal blood supply.

4225   FENGER, CHRISTIAN. 1840-1902
Operation for the relief of valve formation and stricture of the ureter in hydro- or pyo-nephrosis. *J. Amer. med. Assoc.*, 1894, **22**, 335-43.
Fenger's operation for stenosis of the uretero-pelvic junction.

4226   KORÁNYI, SANDOR, *Baron*. 1866-1944
A vizelet fagypontjának diagnostikus érteke. [The diagnostic value of the freezing point of urine.] *Budapesti k. orvosegy*, 1894-iki évokönyve, 1895, 74-75.
Korányi established cryoscopy of the urine as a kidney function test. See also his later papers in *Z. klin. Med.*, 1897, **33**, 1-54; 1898, **34**, 1-52. Previously H. Dreser had made experiments on this subject; for these see *Arch. exp. Path.*, 1892, **29**, 303-19.

4226.1   ALBARRAN Y DOMINGUEZ, JOAQUIN MARIA. 1860-1912
Sur un série de quarante opérations pratiquées sur la rein. *Rev. Chir.*, 1896, **16**, 882-4.
First planned nephrostomy.

4227   WILMS, MAX. 1867-1918
Die Mischgeschwülste. I. Die Mischgeschwülste der Niere. Leipzig, *A. Georgi*, 1899.
Embryoma of the kidney ("Wilms's tumour"). For the history of the operation for Wilms's tumour see B. Thomasson and M.M. Ravitch, Wilms Tumor, *Urol. Surg.*, 1961, **11**, 83-100.

4228   EDEBOHLS, GEORGE MICHAEL. 1853-1908
Chronic nephritis affecting a movable kidney as an indication for nephropexy. *Med. News (N.Y.)*, 1899, **74**, 481-83.
First operation on the kidneys for the relief of Bright's disease.

4229   ——. The cure of chronic Bright's disease by operation. *Med. Rec. (N.Y.)*, 1901, **60**, 961-70.
Edebohls introduced the operation of renal decortication for the treatment of chronic nephritis.

4229.1 ULLMANN, EMERICH. 1861-1937
Experimentelle Nierentransplantation. Vorläufige Mittheilung. *Wien. klin. Wschr.*, 1902, **15**, 281-2.
Successful autotransplantation of kidneys in dogs.

4230   VOELCKER, FRIEDRICH. 1872-1955, & JOSEPH, EUGEN. 1879-?
Funktionelle Nierendiagnostik ohne Ureterenkatheter. *Münch. med. Wschr.*, 1903, **50**, 2081-89.
Voelcker's kidney-function test.

4231   ——. & LICHTENBERG, ALEXANDER VON. 1880-1949
Pyelographie (Roentgenographie des Nierenbeckens nach Kollargolfüllung). *Münch. med. Wschr.*, 1906, **53**, 105-07.
Introduction of pyelography.

4232   ALBARRAN Y DOMINGUEZ, JOAQUIN MARIA. 1860-1912
Exploration des fonctions rénales. Paris, *Masson & Cie.*, 1905.
Albarran's polyuria test for renal inadequacy.

4233   ——. Technique de la néphropexie. *Presse méd.*, 1906, **14**, 253-56.
"Albarran's operation" – nephropexy.

4234   LÖHLEIN, MAX HERMANN FRIEDRICH. 1877-1921
Ueber die entzündlichen Veränderungen der Glomeruli der menschlichen Nieren und ihre Bedeutung für die Nephritis. Leipzig, *S. Hirzel*, 1907.
"Focal nephritis". Löhlein established the importance of the initial inflammatory reaction in the glomerular capillaries in glomerulonephritis. Forms part 4 of *Arb. path. Inst. Leipzig*.

4235   CARREL, ALEXIS. 1873-1944
Transplantation in mass of the kidneys. *J. exp. Med.*, 1908, **10**, 98-140.
Carrel, Nobel Prize winner in 1912, revolutionized vascular surgery. He transplanted the kidney from one animal to another, an operation later carried out successfully in man. For his earlier work on vascular anastomosis and transplantation of viscera, *see* No. 2909.

4236   ROWNTREE, LEONARD GEORGE. 1883-1959, & GERAGHTY, JOHN TIMOTHY. 1876-1924
        An experimental and clinical study of the functional activity of the kidneys by means of phenolsulphonephthalein. *J. Pharmacol.*, 1910, **1**, 579-661.
        The phenolsulphonephthalein kidney-function test.

4237   MUNK, FRITZ. 1879-
        Klinische Diagnostik der degenerativen Nierenerkrankungen. *Z. klin. Med.*, 1913, **78**, 1-52.
        Munk introduced the term "lipoid nephrosis". He found that urine in such cases contained anisotropic lipoid droplets.

4238   VOLHARD, FRANZ. 1872-1950, & FAHR, KARL THEODOR. 1877-1945
        Die Brightsche Nierenkrankheit. Berlin, *J. Springer*, 1914.
        First full description of pure nephrosis, relating clinical features to morbid anatomy.

4238.1 HINMAN, FRANK. 1880-1961
        Experimental hydronephrosis; repair following ureterocysto-neostomy in white rats with complete ureteral obstruction. *Trans. Sect. Genito-urin. Dis. Amer. med. Ass.*, 1918, **69**, 103-17; *J. Urol.*, 1919, **3**, 147-74.
        Commencement of Hinman's classic work on treatment of hydronephrosis.

4239   LEATHES, JOHN BERESFORD. 1864-1956
        Renal efficiency tests in nephritis, and the reaction of the urine. *Brit. med. J.*, 1919, **2**, 165-67.
        Alkaline tide of urine.

4240   MacLEAN, HUGH. 1879-1957, & DE WESSELOW, OWEN LAMBERT VAUGHAN. 1883-1959
        On the testing of renal efficiency, with observations on the "urea coefficient". *Brit. J. exp. Path.*, 1920, **1**, 53-65.
        Urea concentration test.

4241   CARELLI, HUMBERTO HORATIO. 1882-1962, & SORDELLI, ALFREDO. 1891-1967
        Un nuevo procedimiento para explorar al riñón. *Rev. Asoc. méd. argent.*, 1921, **34**, 424.
        Perirenal insufflation of oxygen, for the roentgenological study of the kidney.

4242   GANTER, G.
        Ueber die Beseitigung giftiger Stoffe aus dem Blute durch Dialyse. *Münch. med. Wschr.*, 1923, **70**, 1478-80.
        First description of the experimental use of peritoneal dialysis in uraemia.

4243   MINAMI, SEIGO.
        Ueber Nierenveränderungen nach Verschüttung. *Virchows Arch. path. Anat.*, 1923, **245**, 247-67.
        Crush syndrome.

4244   ANDREWES, *Sir* CHRISTOPHER HOWARD. 1896-1988
        An unexplained diazo-colour-reaction in uraemic sera. *Lancet*, 1924, **1**, 590-91.
        Diazo-colour test of renal function.

4246   MÖLLER, EGGERT HUGO HEIBERG, *et al.*
        Studies of urea excretion. *J. clin. Invest.*, 1928-29, **6**, 427-504.
        Blood urea clearance test. With J. F. McIntosh and D. D. Van Slyke.

4248   FANCONI, GUIDO. 1892-1979
        Die nicht diabetischen Glykosurien und Hyperglykämien des älteren Kindes. *Jb. Kinderheilk.*, 1931, **133**, 257-300.
        "Fanconi's syndrome", dysfunction of the renal tubules with hypophosphataemia, renal glycosuria, and metabolic disturbances.

4249   MASUGI, MATAZO.
        Über das Wesen der spezifischen Veränderungen der Niere und der Leber durch das Nephrotoxin bzw. das Hepatotoxin. *Beitr. path. Anat.*, 1933, **91**, 82-112.
        Experimental production of acute glomerulonephritis. For Masugi's later work, see the same journal, 1933-34, **92**, 429, and *Klin. Wschr.*, 1935, **14**, 373.

4250   KIMMELSTIEL, PAUL. 1900-1970, & WILSON, CLIFFORD. 1906-
        Intercapillary lesions in the glomeruli of the kidney. *Amer. J. Path.*, 1936, **12**, 83-98.
        "Kimmelstiel–Wilson syndrome". First description of nodular intercapillary glomerulosclerosis, the only known morphological alteration specific, or almost so, for diabetes mellitus.

4250.1 FOLEY, FREDERIC EUGENE BASIL. 1891-1966
        A new plastic operation for stricture at the uretero-pelvic junction: report of 20 operations. *J. Urol.*, 1937, **38**, 643-72.
        Foley's operation for hydronephrosis.

4250.2 OLIVER, JEAN REDMAN. 1889-1976.
        Architecture of the kidney in chronic Bright's disease. New York, *Paul Hoeber*, 1939.
        A description of the morphological changes in the nephrons of diseased kidneys. Hypertrophic, atrophic and aglomerular units are described.

4251   ALVING, ALF SVEN. 1902- , & MILLER, BENJAMIN FRANK. 1907-
        A practical method for the measurement of glomerular filtration rate (inulin clearance) with an evaluation of the clinical significance of this determination. *Arch. intern. Med.*, 1940, **66**, 306-18.
        Inulin clearance test.

4252   BYWATERS, ERIC GEORGE LAPTHORNE. 1910- , & BEALL, DESMOND.
        Crush injuries with impairment of renal function. *Brit. med. J.*, 1941, **1**, 427-32.
        Bywaters and Beall encountered cases of the "crush syndrome" among victims of the London air-raids of 1940-41.

4253   WILSON, CLIFFORD. 1906- , & BYROM, FRANK BURNET.
The vicious circle in chronic Bright's disease. Experimental evidence from the hypertensive rat. *Quart. J. Med.*, 1941, **10**, 65-93.

4254   ELLIS, *Sir* ARTHUR WILLIAM MICKLE. 1883-1966
Natural history of Bright's disease. Clinical, histological and experimental observations. *Lancet*, 1942, **1**, 1-7, 34-36, 72-76.
Ellis's classification of nephritis.

4255   KOLFF, WILLEM JOHAN. 1911- , *et al.*
The artificial kidney: dialyser with great area. *Acta med. scand.*, 1944, **117**, 121-34.
The Kolff artificial kidney. With H. T. J. Berk and others. *See also* No. 1976.

4256   FINE, JACOB. 1900- , *et al.*
The treatment of acute renal failure by peritoneal irrigation. *Ann. Surg.*, 1946, **124**, 857-78.
With H. A. Frank and A. M. Seligman.

4256.1   LAWLER, RICHARD H. 1895-1982, *et al.*
Homotransplantation of the kidney in human; preliminary report. *J. Amer. med. Assoc.*, 1950, **144**, 844-5.
Report of first human patient to survive a kidney transplant. The operation was on June 17, 1950, and the patient was discharged on August 26. With four co-authors. *See* No. 4257.

4256.11   OLIVER, JEAN. 1889-1976, MACDOWELL, M., & TRACY, A.
The pathogenesis of acute renal failure associated with traumatic and toxic injury. Renal ischemia, nephrotoxic damage and the ischemuric episode. *J. clin. Inves.*, 1951, **30**, 1305-1439.
Oliver's work on the structural lesions associated with acute renal failure in which he differentiated between the two types of damage: nephrotoxic, due to toxic substances, and tubulorhexic, due to ischaemia, established our present understanding of the morphological basis for this condition.

4256.2   EVANS, JOHN ARTHUR. 1909- , *et al.*
Nephrotomography. A preliminary report. *Amer. J. Roentgenol.*, 1954, **71**, 213-23.
With W. Dubilier and J. C. Monteith.

4256.3   HUME, DAVID MILFORD. 1917-1973, *et al.*
Experiences with renal homotransplantation in the human. Report of nine cases. *J. clin. Invest.*, 1955, **34**, 327-82.
With J. P. Merrill, B. F. Miller and G. W. Thorn.

4257   MERRILL, JOHN PUTNAM. 1917-1986, *et al.*
Successful homotransplantation of the human kidney between identical twins. *J. Amer. med. Assoc.*, 1956, **160**, 277-82.
This was the first successful kidney transplant. The patient, both of whose own kidneys had been removed, was alive 11 months after the transplant. With J. E. Murray, J. H. Harrison, and W. R. Guild. See No. 4256.1.

4257.1　　KOLFF, WILLEM JOHAN. 1911- , & WATSCHINGER, B.
　　　　　Further developments of a coil kidney. Disposable artificial kidney. *J. Lab.*
　　　　　clin. Med., 1956, **47**, 969-77.
　　　　　　　Disposable twin coil kidney.

4257.2　　QUINTON, WAYNE E., *et al.*
　　　　　Cannulation of blood vessels for prolonged hemodialysis. *Trans. Amer.*
　　　　　Soc. artif. intern. Organs, 1960, **6**, 104-13.
　　　　　　　Quinton, D. Dillard and B. H. Scribner made repeated dialysis possible
　　　　　by their development of indwelling Teflon–Silastic arteriovenous shunts.

PROSTATE

4258　　　LANGSTAFF, GEORGE. 1780-1846
　　　　　Cases of Fungus haematodes, with observations. *Med.-chir. Trans.*, 1817,
　　　　　8, 272-305.
　　　　　　　Prostatic carcinoma first reported (p. 279).

4259　　　STAFFORD, RICHARD ANTHONY. 1801-1854
　　　　　A case of enlargement from melanoid tumour of the prostate gland, in a
　　　　　child of five years of age. *Med.-chir. Trans.*, 1839, **22**, 218-21.
　　　　　　　Sarcoma of the prostate was first recorded by Stafford.

4259.1　　MERCIER, LOUIS AUGUSTE. 1811-1882
　　　　　Recherches anatomiques, pathologiques et thérapeutiques sur les mala-
　　　　　dies des organes urinaires et génitaux considerés specialement chez les
　　　　　hommes agés. Paris, *Bechet jeune et Labé*, 1841.
　　　　　　　Mercier emphasized the importance of the muscle fibres around the
　　　　　bladder neck, "Mercier's bar", in prostatism.

4260　　　ADAMS, JOHN. 1806-1877
　　　　　The anatomy and diseases of the prostate gland. London, *Longman*, 1851.
　　　　　　　Adams was the first to distinguish between hypertrophy and carcinoma
　　　　　of the prostate.

4261　　　BOTTINI, ENRICO. 1837-1903
　　　　　Di un nuovo cauterizzatore ed incisore termo-galvanico contro le iscurie
　　　　　da ipertrofia prostatica. *Galvani (Bologna)*, 1874, **2**, 437-52.
　　　　　　　Bottini's galvano-cautery for relief of prostatic obstruction.

4262　　　——. Ueber radicale Behandlung der auf Hypertrophie der Prostata
　　　　　beruhenden Ischurie. *Verb. X. int. med. Congr.*, 1890, Berlin, 1891, **3**, 7Abt.,
　　　　　90-97.
　　　　　　　Bottini's operation for hypertrophy of the prostate.

4262.1　　McGILL, ARTHUR FERGUSON. 1846-1890
　　　　　On supra-pubic prostatectomy, with three cases in which the operation
　　　　　was successfully performed for chronic prostatic hypertrophy. *Trans. clin.*
　　　　　Soc. Lond., 1888, **21**, 52-57.
　　　　　　　McGill pioneered the operation of suprapubic prostatectomy, first
　　　　　performed by him in March 1887.

4263   FULLER, Eugene. 1858-1930
        Six successful and successive cases of prostatectomy. *J. cutan. gen.-urin. Dis.*, 1895, **13**, 229-39.
        Fuller was the first to accomplish the removal of both intra-vesical and intra-urethral enlargements of the prostate by the process of suprapubic enucleation.

4264   FREYER, *Sir* Peter Johnston. 1851-1921
        A clinical lecture on total extirpation of the prostate for radical cure of enlargement of that organ with four successful cases. *Brit. med. J.*, 1901, **2**, 125-29.
        Freyer claimed priority over Fuller (No. 4263) in originating the recto-vesical method of prostatectomy. Although mistaken in this claim, Freyer certainly popularized the operation. Regarding the controversy, see *Brit. med. J.*, 1907, **1**, 551.

4265   YOUNG, Hugh Hampton. 1870-1945
        Conservative perineal prostatectomy. *J. Amer. med. Assoc.*, 1903, **41**, 999-1009.
        Young's operation of perineal prostatectomy.

4265.1 GOODFELLOW, George. 1856-1910
        Median perineal prostatectomy. *J. Amer. med. Assoc.*, 1904, **43**, 194-7.
        Complete perineal prostatectomy, September 1891.

4266   WATSON, Francis Sedgwick. 1853-1942
        Some anatomical points connected with the performance of prostatectomy. With remarks upon the operative treatment of prostatic hypertrophy. *Ann. Surg.*, 1905, **41**, 507-19.
        Watson first performed median perineal prostatectomy in 1889.

4266.1 YOUNG, Hugh Hampton. 1870-1945
        The early diagnosis and radical cure of carcinoma of the prostate. Being a study of 40 cases and presentation of a radical operation which was carried out in four cases. *Johns Hopk. Hosp. Bull.*, 1905, **16**, 315-21.
        First radical prostatectomy for carcinoma.

4267   BRIGGS, James Emmons. 1869-1942
        A method of controlling the bleeding after suprapubic prostatectomy. *New Engl. med. Gaz.*, 1906, **41**, 391-93.
        The distensible bag for controlling haemorrhage after suprapubic prostatectomy was introduced by Briggs in 1905.

4268   BEER, Edwin. 1876-1938
        Removal of neoplasms of the urinary bladder. A new method of employing high-frequency (Oudin) current through a catheterizing cystoscope. *J. Amer. med. Assoc.*, 1910, **54**, 1768-69.
        Beer's method of transurethral fulguration of bladder tumours, from which arose the operation of transurethral prostatectomy.

4269   SQUIER, John Bentley. 1873-1948
        Suprapubic intra-urethral enucleation of the prostate. *Boston med. surg. J.*, 1911, **164**, 911-17.
        Squier modified the operation of total suprapubic prostatectomy.

4270   YOUNG, HUGH HAMPTON. 1870-1945
A new procedure (punch operation) for small prostatic bars and contracture of the prostatic orifice. *J. Amer. med. Assoc.*, 1913, **60**, 253-57.
      Young's punch prostatectomy operation.

4271   CAULK, JOHN ROBERTS. 1881-1938
Infiltration anesthesia of the internal vesical orifice for the removal of minor obstructions: presentation of a cautery punch. *J. Urol. (Baltimore)*, 1920, **4**, 399-408.
      Caulk's cautery punch.

4272   GERAGHTY, JOHN TIMOTHY. 1876-1924
A new method of perineal prostatectomy which insures more perfect functional results. *J. Urol. (Baltimore)*, 1922, **7**, 339-51.
      Geraghty's modification of Young's perineal prostatectomy.

4273   STERN, MAXIMILIAN. 1877-
Minor surgery of the prostate gland; a new cystoscopic instrument employing a cutting current capable of operation in a water medium. *Int. J. Med. Surg.*, 1926, **39**, 72-77.
      Stern's resectoscope.

4274   RANDALL, ALEXANDER. 1883-1951
Surgical pathology of prostatic obstructions. Baltimore, *Williams & Wilkins*, 1931.

4275   HARRIS, SAMUEL HARRY. 1880-1936
Suprapubic prostatectomy with closure. *Aust. N.Z. J. Surg.*, 1934-35, **4**, 226-44.
      Harris's operation, first described by him on 26 March, 1927, and briefly reported in *Med. J. Aust.*, 1927, **1**, 460.

4276   HUGGINS, CHARLES BRENTON. 1901- , & HODGES, CLARENCE VERNARD. 1914-
Studies on prostatic cancer. I. The effect of castration, of estrogen, and of androgen injection on serum phosphatases in metastatic carcinoma of the prostate. *Cancer Res.*, 1941, **1**, 293-97.
      Treatment of prostatic cancer with stilboestrol. For his work on hormone-dependent tumours Huggins shared the Nobel Prize with F. Peyton Rous (No. 2637) in 1966.

4276.1   ———. & SCOTT, WILLIAM WALLACE. 1913-
Bilateral adrenalectomy in prostatic cancer; clinical features and urinary excretion of 17-ketosteroids and estrogen. *Ann. Surg.*, 1945, **122**, 1031-41.
      Adrenalectomy for carcinoma of the prostate.

4277   MILLIN, TERENCE JOHN. 1903-1980
Retropubic prostatectomy. A new extravesical technique. *Lancet*, 1945, **2**, 693-96.
      Retropubic prostatectomy.

4278   SANTO, MARIANO. 1488-1577
De lapide renum curiosum opusculum nuperrime in lucem aeditum.
[Venetiis, *per Petrum de Nicolinis* de Sabio], 1535.
        Marianus Sanctus Barolitanus popularized the operation of lithotomy
introduced by the father of Giovanni Vigo of Rapallo. This method passed
on to Giovanni di Romani and from him to Marianus. It became known as
the "Marian operation" and was the forerunner of the more modern lateral
lithotomy.

4279   FRANCO, PIERRE. 1500-1561
Petit traité contenant une des parties principalles de chirurgie, laquelle les
chirurgiens hernieres exercent. Lyon, *Antoine Vincent*, 1556.
        Clifford Allbutt considered Franco the best lithotomist of the 16th
century. His skill in extracting the stone by the perineal route was of a high
order; in 1556 he introduced the operation of suprapubic cystotomy in
operating for stone, which is recorded in the above. *See* No. 3573.

4279.1 ALGHISI, TOMMASO. 1669-1713
Litotomia...Florence, *Manni*, 1707.
        A renowned specialist and pupil of Bellini, Alghisi was probably the first
to use an indwelling urethral catheter to drain urine away from the wound
after lithotomy. The inclined position of the patient with the head raised
during the operation was also adopted from him. Illustrated with fine
copperplates.

4280   GROENVELDT, JAN [GREENFIELD, JOHN]. ?1647-1710
A compleat treatise of the stone and gravel. London, *R. Smith*, 1710.
        Groenveldt was a famous lithotomist, using the suprapubic technique.
He also enjoyed a rather unsavoury reputation as a quack for his determi-
nation to promote the use of cantharides. He changed his name to
Greenfield when he came to England from Holland. See his earlier work
on the same subject, London, 1677.

4281   DOUGLAS, JOHN. ?-1759
Lithotomia Douglassiana; or, an account of a new method of making the
high operation, in order to extract the stone out of the bladder. London, *T.
Woodward*, 1720.
        Douglas accused Cheselden of plagiarizing his work, although the
latter had acknowledged his indebtedness to Douglas. It is possible that
this was the reason which prompted Cheselden to drop the high operation
in favour of lateral lithotomy.

4282   CHESELDEN, WILLIAM. 1688-1752
A treatise on the high operation for the stone. London, *J. Osborn*, 1723.
        Cheselden was surgeon to St. Thomas's Hospital and an outstanding
figure in British surgery in the first half of the 18th century. The above work
describes his method of performing suprapubic lithotomy, a method
which he abandoned in 1727 for the lateral operation. Includes an English
translation of Rousset on suprapubic lithotomy, from his book on caesarean
section (No. 6236). Rousset laid out the basic principles of the operation
although he did not perform it on a living subject. Biography of Cheselden
by Sir Zachary Cope, 1953.

4282.1   COLOT, François. 1630-1706
Traité de l'opération de la taille. Paris, *J. Vincent*, 1727.
    François Colot was the last and best-known member of the Colot family, itinerant lithotomists.

4283   LE DRAN, Henri François. 1685-1770
Parallèle des différentes manières de tirer la pierre hors de la vessie. Paris, *C. Osmont*, 1730.
    Le Dran, famous French lithotomist, improved the operation of lithotomy. Murphy credits him for originating the lateral lithotomy usually attributed to Cheselden, whose method he discusses. Le Dran was one of Haller's teachers.

4284   REID, Alexander.
A remarkable case of a person cut for the stone in the new way, commonly called the lateral; by William Cheselden. *Phil. Trans.*, (1746), 1748, **44**, 33-35.
    Cheselden's lateral lithotomy first described.

4285   BASEILHAC, Jean, *Frère Côme*. 1703-1781
Nouvelle méthode d'extraire la pierre de la vessie urinaire. Paris, *D. Houry*, 1779.
    Frère Côme devised several new instruments for use in suprapubic lithotomy. This operation, placed in retirement when Cheselden adopted the lateral approach, was once more brought to the fore by Frère Côme.

4286   CAMPER, Pieter. 1722-1789
Observationes circa mutationes quas subeunt calculi in vesica. Pestini, *sumpt. J. M. Weingand*, 1784.

4287   WOLLASTON, William Hyde. 1766-1828
On gouty and urinary concretions. *Phil. Trans.*, 1797, **87**, 386-400.
    Wollaston showed that, in addition to stones consisting of uric acid, renal calculi might also consist of calcium phosphate, magnesium, ammonium phosphate, and calcium oxalate, or a mixture of these.

4288   CARPUE, Joseph Constantine. 1764-1846
A history of the high operation for the stone, by incision above the pubis; with observations on the advantages attending it; and an account of the various methods of lithotomy, from the earliest periods to the present time. London, *Longman*, 1819.
    Carpue popularized suprapubic lithotomy, a procedure not often previously carried out.

4289   CIVIALE, Jean. 1792-1867
Sur la lithotritie ou broiement de la pierre dans la vessie. *Arch. gén. Méd.*, 1826, **10**, 393-419.
    Civiale invented a *lithotriteur* for crushing stones inside the bladder and was responsible for putting the operation of lithotrity upon a sound basis. His claim to have introduced the operation was opposed by Leroy d'Etoilles and other contemporaries.

4290   HEURTELOUP, CHARLES LOUIS STANISLAS, *le baron.* 1793-1864
Lithotripsie. Mémoires sur la lithotripsie par percussion. Paris, *Béchet*, 1833.
    Heurteloup designed the best lithotrite of the time. He was one of several claimants to the distinction of having introduced modern lithotrity. See *Lancet*, 1831-32, **2**, 567-70.

4290.1   DUPUYTREN, GUILLAUME, *le baron.* 1777-1835
Mémoire sur une manière nouvelle de pratiquer l'opération de la pierre...
Terminé et publié par J.L. Sanson et par L.J. Bégin...Paris, *Baillière*, 1836.
    Posthumously published by Sanson, whose method of rectovesical lithotomy is considered here along with the controversial method of lithotrity. Dupuytren tried both but dropped them in favour of continuing the method of bilateral lithotomy. which he invented in 1812, and which was adopted as the normal procedure, with later modifications.

4291   HELLER, JOHANN FLORIAN. 1813-1871
Die Harnconcretionen. Wien, *Tendler u. Comp.*, 1860.
    Heller introduced several urine tests and wrote (above) an important work on urinary calculi.

4292   BIGELOW, HENRY JACOB. 1818-1890
Lithotrity by a single operation. *Amer. J. med. Sci.*, 1878, **75**, 117-34.
    Introduction of litholapaxy at one sitting.

4292.1   MORRIS, *Sir* HENRY. 1844-1926
A case of nephro-lithotomy; or the extraction of a calculus from an undilated kidney. *Trans. clin. Soc. Lond.*, 1880-81, **14**, 30-44.
    Nephrolithotomy; removal of a renal calculus by a lumbar incision.

4293   MACINTYRE, JOHN. 1857-1928
Roentgen rays. Photography of renal calculus. *Lancet,* 1896, **2**, 118.
    First radiogram of renal calculus.

4294   ILLYÉS, GÉZA VON. 1870-
Uretercatheterezés és radiographia. *Orvosi hetilap*, 1901, **45**, 659-62.
    Géza von Illyés showed that ureteral calculi could be accurately demonstrated by x rays with the help of an indwelling opaque catheter. German translation in *Dtsch. Z. Chir.*, 1901, **62**, 132-40.

4295   KELLY, HOWARD ATWOOD. 1858-1943
Scratch-marks on the wax-tipped catheter as a means of determining the presence of stone in the kidney and in the ureter. *Amer. J. Obstet. Dis. Wom.*, 1901, **44**, 441-54.
    Kelly tipped the catheter with wax, so that it registered clearly any pressure from sharp stones. This became an important means of diagnosing calculi.

4296   McCARRISON, *Sir* ROBERT. 1878-1960
The experimental production of stone-in-the-bladder. *Indian J. med. Res.*, 1927, **14**, 895-99; 1927-28, **15**, 197-205, 485-88, 801-06.
    McCarrison's experiments showed that urinary calculi could follow a diet probably deficient in vitamin A.

History of Urology

4296.50   VIELLARD, CAMILLE.
L'urologie et les médecins urologues dans la médicine ancienne. Paris, *Rudeval*, 1903.
Reproduces rare documents and illustrations, with texts by Gilles de Corbeil and de Cuba.

4297   BALLENGER, EDGAR GARRISON. 1877-1945
History of urology. Prepared under the auspices of the American Urological Association. Editorial committee: Edgar G. Ballenger, William A. Frontz, Homer G. Hamer, and Bransford Lewis. 2 vols. Baltimore, *Williams & Wilkins*, 1933.
Every aspect of the subject is covered exhaustively by the various contributors to this collective work; valuable bibliographies are included.

4297.1   ELLIS, HAROLD. 1926-
A history of bladder stone. Oxford, *Blackwell*, 1970.

4297.2   MURPHY, LEONARD JAMES THOMAS. 1914-
The history of urology. Springfield, *C. C. Thomas*, 1971.
A scholarly, detailed work. Part 1 is an adapted translation of E. Desnos: Histoire de l'urologie, in *Encyclopédie française d'urologie*, eds. A. Pousson & E. Desnos, 1914, **1**, 1-294.

4297.3   BLEKER, JOHANNA.
Die Geschichte der Nierenkrankheiten. Mannheim, *Boehringer,* 1972.

DISEASES OF BONES AND JOINTS: ORTHOPAEDICS

See also 4730-4771.1, MYOPATHIES; 6253-6266, PELVIC ANOMALIES.

4297.9   PLATTER, FELIX [PLATERUS]. 1536-1614
Observationum in hominis affectibus. Basileae, *L. König*, 1614.
Platter first described flexion contracture deformity of the fingers ("Dupuytren's contracture") in Liber I, 140. *See* No. 4317.

4297.91   GLISSON, FRANCIS. 1597-1677
De rachitide sive morbo puerili, qui vulgo The Rickets dicitur. Londini, *typ. G. Du-gardi*, 1650.
This monograph on the biomechanics of deformities included an early study of the pathologic anatomy of scoliosis. English translation, London, 1651. See No. 3729.

4298   CONNOR [O'CONNOR], BERNARD. 1666-1698
Lettre écrite à Monsieur le Chevalier Guillaume de Waldegrave . . . contenant une dissertation physique sur la continuité de plusieurs os, à l'occasion d'une fabrique surprenante d'un tronc de squelette humain, où les vertebres, les côtes, l'os sacrum, & les os des iles, qui naturellement sont

distincts & separés, ne font qu'un seul os continu & inseparable. Paris, *Jean Cusson*, [1693?].

First description of ankylosing spondylitis. The British Museum copy of the title page of this work has been mutilated, apparently deliberately, in two places; the author's surname may originally have appeared as "O'Connor", and the last part of the date has been cut away and appears as MDCXCI; other authorities give 1693 as date. The copy presented to the Royal Society of London is also mutilated to read "Connor". Connor graduated MD in Rheims in 1693. Partial translation by B. S. and J. L. Blumberg, *J. Hist. Med.*, 1958, **13**, 349-66.

4299   MALPIGHI, MARCELLO. 1628-1694
        Opera posthuma. Amstelodami, *G. Gallet*, 1700.
        Page 68: first description of leontiasis ossea.

4300   PETIT, JEAN LOUIS. 1674-1750
        L'art de guérir les maladies des os. Paris, *L. d'Houry*, 1705.
        Petit was the first director of the Académie de Chirurgie, Paris. He is particularly remembered for his work on bone diseases. He invented the screw tourniquet, gave the first account of osteomalacia, and was first to open the mastoid process. New edition entitled *Traité des maladies des os*, 2 vols., 1723; English translation of latter, 1726. *See* Nos. 3357 & 3577.

4301   ANDRY, NICHOLAS. 1658-1742
        L'orthopédie ou l'art de prévenir et de corriger dans les enfans, les difformités du corps. 2 vols. Paris, *la veuve Alix*, 1741.
        The first book on orthopaedics, which term Andry himself introduced. He advised attention to proper posture in the prevention and correction of spinal curvature; he had a practical knowledge of body mechanics. This is also the first book on diseases of children to include mention of chlorosis. English translation, 2 vols., 1743, reproduced in facsimile, Philadelphia, 1961. German translation, Berlin, 1744.

4302   PLATNER, JOHANN ZACHARIAS. 1694-1747
        De iis, qui ex tuberculis gibberosi fiunt. Lipsiae, *ex. off. Langenhemiana*, 1744.
        Platner affirmed the tuberculous nature of humpback, which had earlier been surmised by Hippocrates and confirmed by Galen.

4302.1 ROUSSELOT. *d.* 1772.
        Nouvelles observations, ou méthode certaine sur le traitement des cors. La Haye & Paris, *Alex. le Prieur*, 1762.
        The first "book" (45pp.) on podiatry or chiropody. In the above work Rousselot urged that podiatry become a specialty of surgery.

4302.2 MORAND, SAUVEUR-FRANÇOIS. 1697-1773
        Sur un enfant auquel il manquoit les deux clavicules, le sternum et les cartilages, qui dans l'état naturel l'attachent aux côtes. *Hist. Acad. roy. Sci. (Paris)*, (1760), 1766, 47-48.
        First description of cleido-cranial dysostosis.

4303   DAVID, JEAN PIERRE. 1737-1784
        Dissertation sur les effets du mouvement et du repos dans les maladies chirurgicales. Paris, *Vve. Vallet-La-Chapelle*, 1779.

Includes a description of Pott's disease, with post-mortem findings, better than Pott's own account. This is an important early work on the effect of movement and of rest in the treatment of joint conditions. English translation, 1790.

4304   POTT, PERCIVALL. 1714-1788
Remarks on that kind of palsy of the lower limbs, which is frequently found to accompany a curvature of the spine. London, *J. Johnson*, 1779.
    "Pott's disease". Percival Pott, surgeon to St. Bartholomew's Hospital for more than 40 years, left a classic description of spinal curvature due to tuberculous caries and causing paralysis of the lower limbs. He did not, however, recognize its tuberculous nature. Pott published a further book on the subject in 1782. Reprinted in *Med. Classics*, 1936, **1**, 281-328.

4304.1 EKMAN, OLAUS JACOB.
Dissertatio medica descriptionem et casus aliquot osteomalaciae sistens. Upsaliae, *J. Edman*, [1788].
    In his doctoral thesis Ekman gave an account of osteogenesis imperfecta in three generations. For extensive translation *see* No. 4404.1. K.S. Seedorff, *Osteogenesis imperfecta*, Copenhagen, 1949.

4305   VENEL, JEAN ANDRÉ. 1740-1791
Description de plusieurs nouveaux moyens mécaniques propres à prevénir, borner et même corriger dans certains cas les courbures latérales et la torsion de l'épine du dos. *Mém. Soc. Sci. phys. Lausanne*, 1789, **2**, 66- , 197- .
    Venel stressed the necessity for prolonged periods of recumbency, rather than exercise, in the correction of spinal curvature. He invented a corset and extension bed for treating spinal deformities. His extension bed gave an entirely new direction to treatment and was widely adopted. In 1790 he founded at Orbe, Switzerland, the first orthopaedic hospital.

4305.1 CAMPER, PIETER. 1722-1789
Dissertation sur la meilleure forme des souliers. [No place, 1781.]
    Classic discussion of childhood shoe-induced deformities. Dutch edition, 1781. English translation in Dowie, *The foot and its covering*, London, 1861.

4306   SOEMMERRING, SAMUEL THOMAS. 1755-1830
Abbildungen und Beschreibungen einiger Misgeburten. Mainz, *Universitätsbuchhandlung*, 1791.
    Achondroplasia is first described on page 30 and pictured on plate 11. English translation in No. 2241.

4307   RUSSELL, JAMES. 1755-1836
A practical essay on a certain disease of the bones termed necrosis. Edinburgh, *Bell & Bradfute*, 1794.
    One of the first attempts at a complete and detailed description of necrosis. Russell was the first Professor of Clinical Surgery at Edinburgh.

4308   SCARPA, ANTONIO. 1752-1832
Memoria chirurgica sui piedi torti congenita dei fanciulli. Pavia, *G. Comini*, 1803.
    First accurate description of the pathological anatomy of congenital club-foot. English translation, Edinburgh, 1818.

4308.1   HEY, WILLIAM. 1736-1819
Practical observations in surgery. London, *T. Cadell, jun., & W. Davies,* 1803.
Hey described subacute osteomyelitis of the tibia before Brodie (No. 4311). He may have become interested in the knee after banging his own knee while getting out of a bath in 1773. He remained lame for the rest of his life. Hey coined the phrase, "internal derangement of the knee", and described injuries to the meniscal cartilages. He also devised a type of amputation of the foot ("Hey's amputation"). His book includes a description of the falciform ligament of the saphenous opening, "Hey's ligament". See No. 5582.

4309   BAYNTON, THOMAS. 1761-1820
An account of a successful method of treating diseases of the spine. London, *Longman,* 1813.
By his advocacy of absolute rest in the horizontal position without the aid of caustics and setons, Baynton can be said to have introduced the modern treatment of spinal caries in England. The book is dedicated to Edward Jenner.

4310   ROMBERG, MORITZ HEINRICH. 1795-1873
De rachitide congenita. Berolini, *typ. C. A. Plateni,* 1817.
Classic description of achondroplasia. Romberg's graduation thesis. English translation (Sydenham Society), 1853.

4311   BRODIE, *Sir* BENJAMIN COLLINS, *Bart.* 1783-1862
Pathological and surgical observations on the diseases of the joints. London, *Longman,* 1818.
Brodie's best work. It includes his description of hysterical pseudo-fracture of the spine and the first clinical description of ankylosing spondylitis. The fifth edition, 1850, gives (p. 77) a description of "Brodie's disease" – chronic synovitis with a pulpy degeneration of the affected parts.

4312   DELPECH, JACQUES MATHIEU. 1777-1832
Considérations sur la difformité appelée pied-bots. In his *Chirurgie clinique de Montpellier,* Paris, 1823, **1**, 147-231.
Delpech described (pp. 184-92) the beneficial effect of section of the tendo Achillis for club-foot; he performed the operation on May 9, 1816, and although not first to do so, he was the first to demonstrate the value of tenotomy in the correction of contracture deformities of the extremities.

4313   SMITH, NATHAN. 1762-1829
Observations on the pathology and treatment of necrosis. *Philad. month. J. Med.,* 1827, **1**, 11-19, 66-75.
Classic early account of osteomyelitis. Smith trephined for bone necrosis. Reproduced in *Med. Classics,* 1937, **1**, 820-38.

4314   BRODIE, *Sir* BENJAMIN COLLINS, *Bart.* 1783-1862
On trephining the tibia. *Lond. med. Gaz.,* 1828, **2**, 70-74.
"Brodie's abscess". The patient was first seen in 1824. Brodie published an account of some further cases in *Med.-chir. Trans.,* 1832, **17**, 239-49, which paper is reprinted in *Med. Classics,* 1938, **2**, 900-06.

4315   DELPECH, JACQUES MATHIEU. 1777-1832
De l'orthomorphie. 2 vols. and atlas. Paris, *Gabon*, 1828.

Delpech, Professor of Surgery at Montpellier, published a comprehensive treatise on deformities of the bones and joints. He established the tuberculous nature of Pott's disease. Delpech did more than any other man toward the development of orthopaedics in France.

4316   RANDOLPH, JACOB. 1796-1848
Some remarks on morbus coxarius, with an account of Dr. P. S. Physick's method of treating this disease. *Amer. J. med. Sci.*, 1830, **7**, 299-308.

Randolph was the son-in-law of Philip Syng Physick. Physick's method "consisted in the application of a carved splint, which would keep the limb strictly at rest, and prevent the least possible motion of the joint; and also in the prosecution of a course of active and long continued purging".

4316.1   GROSS, SAMUEL DAVID. 1805-1884
The anatomy, physiology, and diseases of the bones and joints. Philadelphia, *John Grigg*, 1830.

The first American treatise on orthopaedics. In his autobiography Gross wrote that, "The title was unfortunate; it should have been *A practical treatise on fractures and dislocations, with an account of the diseases of the bones and joints*".

4317   DUPUYTREN, GUILLAUME, *le baron*. 1777-1835
De la rétraction des doigts par suite d'une affection de l'aponévrose palmaire, opération chirurgicale qui convient dans ce cas. *J. univ. hebd. Méd. Chir. prat.*, 1831, 2 sér., **5**, 352-65.

Dupuytren devised an operation for the treatment of contracture of the palmar fascia ("Dupuytren's contracture"). Reprinted, with translation, in *Med. Classics*, 1939, **4**, 127-50. The condition was first mentioned by Platter, No. 4297.9.

4318   LOBSTEIN, JEAN GEORGES CHRÉTIEN FRÉDÉRIC MARTIN. 1777-1835
De la fragilité des os, ou de l'ostéopsathyrose. In his *Traité de l'anatomie pathologique*, Paris, 1833, **2**, 204-12.

Osteopsathyrosis ("Lobstein's disease"), osteogenesis imperfecta, earlier described by Ekman (No. 4304.1).

4319   RUST, JOHANN NEPOMUK. 1775-1840
Aufsätze und Abhandlungen aus dem Gebiete der Medizin, Chirurgie und Staatsarzneikunde. Berlin, *T. C. F. Enslin*, 1834, **1**, 196.

First description of "Rust's disease" – tuberculous spondylitis of the cervical vertebrae.

4320   STROMEYER, GEORG FRIEDRICH LUDWIG. 1804-1876
Die Durchschneidung der Achillessehne, als Heilmethode des Klumpfusses, durch zwei Fälle erläutert. *Mag. ges. Heilk.*, 1833, **39**, 195-218.

Successful tenotomy for club-foot established the reputation of Stromeyer as an orthopaedic surgeon.

4321   ——. Beiträge zur operativen Orthopädik. Hannover, *Helwing*, 1838.
Stromeyer is the founder of modern surgery of the locomotor system. He advocated and practised subcutaneous tenotomy for all deformities of the body arising from muscular defects.

4322   DUPUYTREN, GUILLAUME, *le baron*. 1777-1835
Leçons orales de clinique chirurgicale. 2me. éd. Tom. 3. Paris, *Germer-Baillière*, 1839.
    Pp. 455-61: Dupuytren was the first to treat wry neck by subcutaneous section of the sternomastoid muscle. This he did on 16 Jan, 1822. The operation was first reported in C. Averill: *Short treatise on operative surgery*, London, 1823, 61-64. *See* No. 5590.

4322.1   LITTLE, WILLIAM JOHN. 1810-1894
On the nature of club-foot and analogous distortions. London, *Jeffs*, 1839.
    Little suffered from club-foot himself. This is the greatest English classic on the subject. *See* No. 4329.

4322.2   BROWN, JOHN BALL. 1784-1862
Operations on club-feet. *Boston med. surg. J.*, 1839, **21**, 153-59.
    Brown was the first surgeon in the United States to specialize in orthopaedics, founding the Orthopedic Infirmary of the City of Boston (soon renamed the Boston Orthopedic Institution) in 1838. Brown was also the first in New England to popularize tenotomies for club–feet.

4323   DIEFFENBACH, JOHANN FRIEDRICH. 1792-1847
Ueber die Durchschneidung der Sehnen und Muskeln. Berlin, *A. Förster*, 1841.
    Report on 140 cases of tenotomy for treatment of club-foot.

4323.1   FERGUSSON, *Sir* WILLIAM. 1808-1877
Excision of a portion of the scapula. *Lancet*, 1842-43, **1**, 917-18.
    First description of operation for partial excision of scapula.

4324   BUCK, GURDON. 1807-1877
The knee-joint anchylosed at a right angle – restored nearly to a straight position after the excision of a wedge-shaped portion of bone, consisting of the patella, condyles and articular surface of the tibia. *Amer. J. med. Sci.*, 1845, n.s. **10**, 277-84.
    Buck's operation, "one of the more spectacular surgical feats by an American surgeon in the first half of the nineteenth century" (Rutkow). The paper is reprinted in *Med. Classics*, 1939, **3**, 791-99.

4325   DURLACHER, LEWIS. 1792-1864
A treatise on corns, bunions, the diseases of nails, and the general management of the feet. London, *Simpkin, Marshall & Co.*, 1845.
    Durlacher, surgeon chiropodist to Queen Victoria, gave the first description of anterior metatarsalgia (p. 52), to which the name "Morton's metatarsalgia" has been given (*see* No. 4341).

4325.1   DALRYMPLE, JOHN. 1804-1852
On the microscopical character of mollities ossium. *Dublin Quart. J. med. Sci.*, 1846, **2**, 85-95.
    Report of the histological examination of bone material containing multiple myeloma from the patient described by Macintyre (No. 4327).

4326   JONES, HENRY BENCE. 1814-1873
On a new substance occurring in the urine of a patient with mollities ossium. *Phil. Trans.*, 1848, **138**, 55-62.

Bence Jones described the myelopathic albumosuria (Bence Jones proteinuria) seen in Macintyre's patient (No. 4327). Preliminary notes in *Lancet*, 1847, **2**, 88, and *Proc. roy. Soc. Lond.*, 1847, **5**, 673.

4326.1   LANGENBECK, BERNHARD RUDOLPH CONRAD VON. 1810-1887
Grosses Enchondrom (Gallertknorpel-Geschwulst) des Schulterblattes; Exstirpation des ganzen Schulterblattes mit Ausnahme des *Processus coracoides* am 6 Febr.; Tod am 7 Febr. *Dtsch. Klinik*, 1850, **2**, 73-76.

Complete excision of the scapula.

4327   MACINTYRE, WILLIAM.
Case of mollities and fragilitas ossium. *Med.-chir. Trans.*, 1850, **33**, 211-32.

Multiple myeloma first described.

4328   MATHIJSEN, ANTONIUS. 1805-1878
Nieuwe wijze van aanwending van het gips-verband bij beenbreuken. Eene bijdrage tot de militaire chirurgie. Haarlem, *van Loghem*, 1852.

Introduction of the modern plaster of Paris bandage. Two different French translations of the above work were published in journals in 1852-53. In 1854 Mathijsen published two separate expanded French versions, of which that published in Liège was illustrated. The original edition plus the Liège version were reprinted with an introduction and bibliography, by G.J. Bremer, Nieuwkoop, 1962. English translation in Bick, *Classics of orthopaedics*, 66-71.

4329   LITTLE, WILLIAM JOHN. 1810-1894
On the nature and treatment of the deformities of the human frame. London, *Longman,* 1853.

Little was the first eminent orthopaedic surgeon in the British Isles. He studied under Stromeyer and, in 1838, he founded the Orthopaedic Institution, now the (Royal) National Orthopaedic Hospital, London. The above work is an elaboration of lectures delivered in 1843. *See* No. 4735.

4330   BREITHAUPT.
Zur Pathologie des menschlichen Fusses. *Med. Zeitung*, 1855, **24**, 169, 175.

First description of osteoperiostitis of the metatarsal bones, named "Busquet's disease" after the latter's description of it in *Rev. Chir.* (*Paris*), 1897, **17**, 1065.

4331   SAYRE, LEWIS ALBERT. 1820-1900
Exsection of the head of the femur and removal of the upper rim of the acetabulum, for morbus coxarius, with perfect recovery. *N.Y.J. Med.*, 1855, n.s. **14**, 70-82.

Resection of the hip for ankylosis.

4332   EULENBURG, MORITZ MICHAEL. 1811-1877
Hochgradige Dislocation der Scapula. *Arch. klin. Chir.*, 1863, **4**, 304-11.

First description of congenital high-scapula "Sprengel's deformity"; *see also* No. 4359.

4333 HENKE, Philipp Jakob Wilhelm. 1834-1896
Contractur des Metatarsus. *Z. rat. Med.*, 1863, 3 R., **17**, 188-94.
Congenital metatarsus varus described.

4334 BAUER, Louis. 1814-1898
Lectures on orthopaedic surgery. Philadelphia, *Lindsay & Blakiston*, 1864.
Before emigrating to America, Bauer studied under Stromeyer. Hugh
Owen Thomas considered him "the first exponent of American orthopae-
dics". This is the first comprehensive American textbook of orthopaedics.
First published in *Phila. med. surg. Rep.*, 1862.

4335 ENGEL, Gerhard.
Ueber einen Fall von cystoider Entartung des ganzen Skelettes. Giessen, *F.
C. Pietsch*, 1864.
First description of osteitis fibrosa cystica – hyperparathyroid bone
disease, also known as "von Recklinghausen's disease of bone".

4336 PRICE, Peter Charles. 1832-1864
A description of the diseased conditions of the knee-joint which require
amputation of the limb, and those conditions which are favourable to
excision of the joint. London, *J. Churchill*, 1865.
A valuable contribution to the knowledge and surgical treatment of
diseases of the knee-joint.

4336.1 OLLIER, Louis Xavier Edouard Leopold. 1830-1900
Traité experimentale et clinique de la régénération des os. Paris, *Victor
Masson*, 1867.
Ollier pioneered research in bone allografting.

4337 CHARCOT, Jean Martin. 1825-1893
Sur quelques arthropathies qui paraissent dépendre d'une lésion du
cerveau ou de la moëlle épinière. *Arch. Physiol. norm. path.*, 1868, **1**, 161-78.
Charcot called attention to tabetic arthropathy, a condition which has
since borne his name, while the tabetic joints he so well described are now
known as "Charcot's joints".

4338 WILKS, *Sir* Samuel, *Bart*. 1824-1911
Case of osteoporosis, or spongy hypertrophy of the bones (calvaria,
clavicle, os femoris, and rib). *Trans. path. Soc. Lond.*, 1868-69, **20**, 273-77.
A classic account of osteitis deformans. Wilks was associated with Guy's
Hospital all his life. A kindly, charming man, he was described by Osler as
one of the handsomest men in London in his time, even until the age of 70.

4339 WEGNER, Friedrich Rudolph Georg. 1843-1917
Ueber hereditäre Knochensyphilis bei jungen Kindern. *Virchows Arch. path.
Anat.*, 1870, **50**, 305-22.
"Wegner's disease" – osteochondritic separation of the epiphyses in
congenital syphilis.

4339.1 HOOD, Wharton Peter. 1833-1916
On bone setting (so-called), and its relation to the treatment of joints
crippled by injury, rheumatism, inflammation, etc. London, *Macmillan &
Co.*, 1871.
First work on manipulation written by a physician.

4339.2　　DUPLAY, SIMON. 1836-1924
De la périarthrite scapulo-humérale et des raideurs de l'épaule qui en sont la conséquence. *Arch. gén. Méd.*, 1872, **20**, 513-42.
"Frozen shoulder" syndrome described.

4340　　THOMAS, HUGH OWEN. 1834-1891
Diseases of the hip, knee and ankle joints, with their deformities, treated by a new and efficient method. Liverpool, *T. Dobb & Co.*, 1875.
Thomas splint. Enlarged second edition, 1876. *See* No. 4348.

4341　　MORTON, THOMAS GEORGE. 1835-1903
A peculiar and painful affection of the fourth metatarso-phalangeal articulation. *Amer. J. med. Sci.*, Philadelphia, 1876, **71**, 37-45.
First complete description of anterior metatarsalgia ("Morton's disease"). *See also* No. 4325.

4342　　BAKER, WILLIAM MORRANT. 1839-1896
On the formation of synovial cysts in the leg in connection with disease of the knee joint. *St. Barth. Hosp. Rep.*, 1877, **13**, 245-61; 1885, **21**, 177-90.
"Baker's cysts" of the knee-joint. Reprinted in *Med. Classics*, 1941, **5**, 785-820.

4342.1　　SAYRE, LEWIS ALBERT. 1820-1900
Lectures on orthopaedic surgery and diseases of the joints. New York, *D. Appleton*, 1876.
See Nos. 4344 & 4344.1.

4343　　PAGET, *Sir* JAMES, *Bart.* 1814-1899
On a form of chronic inflammation of bones (osteitis deformans). *Med.-chir. Trans.*, 1877, **60**, 37-64; 1882, **65**, 225-36.
Paget was at one time Serjeant Surgeon to Queen Victoria. His classic description of osteitis deformans led that condition to be called "Paget's disease". Reprinted in *Med. Classics*, 1936, **1**, 29-71.

4344　　SAYRE, LEWIS ALBERT. 1820-1900
Report on Pott's disease, or caries of the spine; treated by extension, and the plaster of Paris bandage. *Trans. Amer. med. Ass.*, 1876, **27**, 573-629.
Sayre was the first to use plaster of Paris as a support for the spinal column in scoliosis and Pott's disease. His name is eponymically linked with Sayre's jacket, a plaster of Paris jacket applied while the patient is suspended by the head and axillae, and with Sayre's suspension apparatus, a tripod derrick with rope and pulley for head traction during the application of a plaster of Paris jacket.

4344.1　　——. Spinal disease and spinal curvature, their treatment by suspension and the use of the plaster of Paris bandage. London, *Smith, Elder*, 1877.
Sayre's monograph on his methods of treating tuberculosis of the spine and scolosis is the first American surgical textbook to contain actual mounted photographs, some of which are remarkable for their artistic qualities. The book was first published in London while Sayre was a delegate to the British Medical Congress. The virtually identical American edition was published in Philadelphia by Lippincott, also in 1877.

4345   MADELUNG, OTTO WILHELM. 1846-1926
Die spontane Subluxation der Hand nach vorne. *Verh. dtsch. Ges. Chir.*, 1878, **7**, pt. 2, 259-76.
"Madelung's deformity" of the wrist. Madelung regarded the condition as a defect of growth of the wrist joint.

4346   GROSS, SAMUEL WEISSEL. 1837-1889
Sarcoma of the long bones; based upon a study of one hundred and sixty-five cases. *Amer. J. med. Sci.*, 1879, n.s. **78**, 17-57, 338-77.
First comprehensive work on bone sarcoma.

4346.1   HELFERICH, HEINRICH. 1851-1945
Ein Fall von sogenannter Myositis ossificans progressiver. *Aerztl. Intelligenz-Bl.*, 1879, **26**, 485-89.
Helferich described the association of microdactyly with myositis ossificans progressiva.

4346.2   MACEWEN, *Sir* WILLIAM. 1848-1924
Observations concerning transplantation of bone. Illustrated by a case of inter-human osseous transplantation, whereby over two-thirds of the shaft of a humerus was restored. *Proc. R. Soc. (Lond).*, 1881, **32**, 232-47.
First allograft transplantation of bone in humans.

4347   ALBERT, EDUARD. 1841-1900
Einige Fälle von kunstlicher Ankylosenbildung an paralytischen Gliedmassen. *Wien. med. Presse,* 1882, **23**, 725-28.
Albert introduced the concept of joint arthrodesis into orthopaedic surgery. This is the first description of arthrodesis of an ankle for paralytic foot. English translation in Bick, *Classics of orthopaedics*, 52-54.

4348   THOMAS, HUGH OWEN. 1834-1891
Contributions to surgery and medicine. 8 pts. London, *H. K. Lewis,* 1883-90.
Thomas was the veritable founder of modern orthopaedics in the British Isles. The conservative methods introduced by him were developed by Sir Robert Jones. Thomas is remembered eponymically by the "Thomas splint".

4349   STRÜMPELL, ERNST ADOLPH GUSTAV GOTTFRIED. 1853-1925
Lehrbuch der speciellen Pathologie und Therapie der innern Krankheiten. Bd. 2, ii. Leipzig, *F. C. W. Vogel,* 1884.
Strümpell gave an excellent description of ankylosing spondylitis ("Strümpell's disease", the "spondylose rhizomélique" of Pierre Marie, No. 4368) on p. 152 of his *Lehrbuch. See* No. 2229. He published an important paper on the subject in *Dtsch. Z. Nervenheilk.*, 1897, **11**, 338-42, which was translated into English in Bick, *Classics of orthopaedics*, 345-47.

4350   KÖNIG, FRANZ. 1832-1910
Ueber freie Körper in den Gelenken. *Dtsch. Z. Chir.*, 1888, **27**, 90-109.
König of Göttingen was the first to use the term "osteochondritis dissecans".

4351   KAHLER, Otto. 1849-1893
Zur Symptomatologie des multiplen Myeloms. *Prag. med. Wschr.*, 1889,
14, 33-35, 44-49.
"Kahler's disease" – multiple myeloma.

4352   OLLIER, Louis Xavier Edouard Leopold. 1830-1900
Exostoses multiples. *Mém. C. R. Soc. Sci. méd. Lyon*, (1889), 1890, **29**, 2,
12.
"Ollier's disease". He described a form of dyschondroplasia.

4353   BRADFORD, Edward Hickling. 1848-1926, & LOVETT, Robert Williamson.
1859-1924
Treatise on orthopedic surgery. New York, *W. Wood & Co.*, 1890.
Includes a description of the "Bradford frame", used in the treatment of
spinal disorders.

4354   MARIE, Pierre. 1853-1940
De l'ostéo-arthropathie hypertrophiante pneumonique. *Rev. Méd.*, 1890,
10, 1-36.
Original description of hypertrophic osteoarthropathy, sometimes called
"Bamberger–Marie disease".

4355   HOFFA, Albert. 1859-1908
Zur operativen Behandlung der angeborenen Hüftgelenksverrenkungen.
Verh. dtsch. Ges. Chir., 1890, **19**, 44-53.
Hoffa's method of operative treatment of congenital dislocation of the
hip-joint.

4356   ——. Lehrbuch der orthopädischen Chirurgie. Stuttgart, *F. Enke,* 1891.
Hoffa, a leading German orthopaedist, made important contributions
to the subject and founded the *Zeitschrift für orthopädische Chirurgie.*

4357   KÜMMELL, Hermann. 1852-1937
Traumatische rarefizierende Ostitis. *Verh. Ges. Dtsch. Naturf. Aerzte,* (1891),
1892, 282-85.
"Kümmell's disease". He described a form of traumatic spondylitis.

4358   RECKLINGHAUSEN, Friedrich Daniel von. 1833-1910
Die fibröse oder deformirende Ostitis, die Osteomalacie und die
osteoplastische Carcinose in ihren gegenseitigen Beziehungen. In *Festschrift
R. Virchow,* Berlin, *G. Reimer,* 1891.
Recklinghausen gave an important description of generalized osteitis
fibrosa. His reference to the earlier case reported by Engel (*see* No. 4335)
has led to this condition being sometimes referred to as "Engel–
Recklinghausen disease" or "von Recklinghausen's disease of bone".

4359   SPRENGEL, Otto Gerhard Karl. 1852-1915
Die angeborene Verschiebung des Schulterblattes nach oben. *Arch. klin.
Chir.*, 1891, **42**, 545-49.
Classic description of "Sprengel's deformity", a congenital upward
displacement of the scapula (*see also* No. 4332).

4359.1   HADRA, BERTHOLD ERNEST. 1842-1903.
Wiring of the vertebrae as a means of immobilization in fracture and Pott's disease. *Med. Times Reg.*, 1891, **22**, 423-425.
"In a case of fracture-dislocation of the cervical spine (C 6-7) he [Hadra] performed open reduction, twisting metal wires around the spinous processes to stabilize the injured sector" (Bick). This is the first report of any type of spinal surgical immobilization being planned and successfully carried out.

4359.2   ——. Wiring the spinal processes in Pott's disease. *Trans. Amer. Orthop. Ass.*, 1891, **4**, 206-08.
First spinal fusion.

4360   BECHTEREV, VLADIMIR MICHAILOVICH [BEKHTEREV]. 1857-1927
Oderevenielost pozvonochnika s iskrivleniyem yevo, kak osobaya forma zabolievaniya. [Ankylosis of the spine with curvature as a special form of disease.] *Vrach*, 1892, **13**, 899-903.
Bechterev's disease – ankylosing spondylitis, previously described by Strümpell. A German translation of the paper is in *Neurol. Zbl.*, 1893, **12**, 426-34.

4361   KAUFMANN, EDUARD. 1860-1931
Untersuchungen über die sogenannte foetale Rachitis (Chondrodystrophia foetalis). Berlin, *Reimer*, 1892.
First study of the cartilage changes in achondroplasia.

4362   KLIPPEL, MAURICE. 1858-1942
De la pseudo-paralysie générale arthritique. *Rev. Méd.*, 1892, **12**, 280-85.
First description of "Klippel's disease", arthritic general pseudo-paralysis.

4363   PARRISH, B. F.
A new operation for paralytic talipes valgus, and the enunciation of a new surgical principle. *N.Y. med. J.*, 1892, **56**, 402-03.
First successful tendon transplantation.

4364   ALBERT, EDUARD. 1841-1900
Achillodynie. *Wien. med. Presse*, 1893, **34**, 41-43.
Tendo Achilles bursitis, "Albert's disease".

4364.1   PÉAN, JULES ÉMILE. 1830-1898
Des moyens prothétiques destinés à obtenir la réparation des parties osseuses. *Gaz. Hôp. (Paris)*, 1894, **67**, 289-92.
Total prosthetic replacement of shoulder (p. 291) using an artificial joint made of hardened rubber and platinum. English translation in Bick, *Classics of orthopaedics*, 443-46.

4365   LORENZ, ADOLF. 1854-1946
The operative treatment of congenital dislocation of the hip-joint. *Trans. Amer. orthop. Ass.*, (1894), (1895), **7**, 99-103.
Lorenz suggested a bloodless method for closed reduction of congenital dislocation of the hip-joint – the "Hoffa–Lorenz" method.

4365.1   MARFAN, Bernard Jean Antonin. 1858-1942
Un cas de déformation congénitale des quatre membres, plus prononcée aux extrémités, charactérisée par l'allongement des os avec un certain degré d'amincissement. *Bull. Mém. Soc. méd. Hôp. Paris*, 1896, 3 sér., **13**, 220-26.
"Marfan syndrome". Marfan described only the skeletal deformities. He called the condition *dolichostenomelia*. Later writers recorded bilateral ectopia lentis and cardiovascular complications in this syndrome.

4366   TUBBY, Alfred Herbert. 1862-1930
Deformities; a treatise on orthopaedic surgery. London, *Macmillan & Co.*, 1896.
Includes a valuable discussion of congenital anomalies of the bones and joints from the orthopaedic point of view. Greatly expanded second edition, 2 vols., London, 1912.

4367   BRUCK, Alfred. 1865-?
Ueber eine seltene Form von Erkrankung der Knochen und Gelenke. *Dtsch. med. Wschr.*, 1897, **23**, 152-55.
"Bruck's disease" – deformity of bones, multiple fractures, ankylosis of joints, and muscular atrophy.

4368   MARIE, Pierre. 1853-1940
Sur la spondylose rhizomélique. *Rev. Méd.*, 1898, **18**, 285-315.
Marie described as "spondylose rhizomélique" the ankylosing spondylitis or spondylitis deformans originally reported by Strümpell and called variously "Strümpell's disease", "Bechterev's disease", "Marie's disease".

4369   ———. & SAINTON, Paul. 1868-1958
Sur la dysostose cléido-crânienne héréditaire. *Rev. neurol. (Paris)*, 1898, **6**, 835-38.
In their important description of cleido-cranial dysostosis, Marie and Sainton gave to it its present name. It was first described by Morand (No. 4302.1) in 1760. English translation in Bick, *Classics of orthopaedics*, 230-32.

4370   KIENBÖCK, Robert. 1871-1953
Ueber acute Knochenatrophie bei Entzündungsprocessen an den Extremitäten (fälschlich sogenannte Inactivitätsatrophie der Knochen) und ihre Diagnose nach dem Röntgen-Bilde. *Wien. med. Wschr.*, 1901, **51**, 1346-48.
"Kienböck's atrophy" – acute atrophy of bone in inflammatory conditions of the extremities.

4371   MOSETIG-MOORHOF, Albert von. 1838-1907
Die Jodoformknochenplombe. *Zbl. Chir.*, 1903, **30**, 433-38.
Use of iodoform to plug bone defects.

4372   ALBERS-SCHÖNBERG, Heinrich Ernst. 1865-1921
Projektions-Röntgenbilder einer seltenen Knochenerkrankung. *Fortschr. Röntgenstr.*, 1903-04, **7**, 158-59.
First description of osteosclerosis fragilis, marble bones ("Albers-Schönberg disease").

4373   OSGOOD, ROBERT BAYLEY. 1873-1956
Lesions of the tibial tubercle occurring during adolescence. *Boston med. surg. J.*, 1903, **148**, 114-17.
Osgood was the first to draw attention to a condition of the tibial tuberosity; this is now referred to as "Osgood–Schlatter disease" (*see also* No. 4374).

4374   SCHLATTER, CARL. 1864-1934
Verletzungen des schnabelförmigen Fortsatzes der oberen Tibia-epiphyse. *Beitr. klin. Chir.*, 1903, **38**, 874-87.
"Osgood–Schlatter disease". A further description of the painful affection of the tibial tuberosity first noted by Osgood.

4375   NAU, PIERRE.
Les scolioses congénitales. Paris, *Thèse No.* 446, 1904.
First description of platyspondylia.

4375.1 CODIVILLA, ALESSANDRO. 1861-1912
On the means of lengthening in the lower limbs, the muscles and tissues which are shortened through deformity. *Amer. J. orthop. Surg.*, 1905, **2**, 353-69.
First attempt at surgical lengthening of limbs.

4376   BÜDINGER, KONRAD. 1867-?
Ueber Ablösung von Gelenkteilen und verwandte Prozesse. *Dtsch. Z. Chir.*, 1906, **84**, 311-65.
Büdinger was the first to describe pathological fracture of the cartilage of the patella. See also his later paper in the same journal, 1908, **92**, 510-36. Later descriptions by Karl Ludloff, *Verh. dtsch. Ges. Chir.*, 1910, 223-25, and by Arthur Laewen, *Beitr. klin. Chir.*, 1925, **134**, 265-307, led to the eponym "Büdinger–Ludloff–Laewen disease".

4376.1 LOOSER, EMILE.
Ueber Osteogenesis imperfecta tarda. *Verh. Dtsch. path. Ges.*, (1905), 1906, 239-42.
Looser's syndrome.

4377   KÖHLER, ALBAN. 1874-1947
Ueber eine häufige, bisher anscheinend unbekannte Erkrankung einzelner kindlicher Knochen. *Münch. med. Wschr.*, 1908, **55**, 1923-25.
"Köhler's disease" of the scaphoid bone of the foot in children. *See* No. 4387.

4377.1 LEXER, ERICH. 1867-1937
Ueber Gelenktransplantation. *Med. Klin.*, 1908, **4**, 817-20.
First osteoarticular joint transplant. English translation in *Clin. orthop.*, 1985, **197**, 1-10. See also his paper, Substitution of whole or half joints from freshly amputated extremities by free plastic operation. *Surg. Gynec. Obstet.*, 1908, **6**, 601-07.

4378   KIRSCHNER, MARTIN. 1879-1942
        Ueber Nagelextension. *Beitr. klin. Chir.*, 1909, **64**, 266-79.
        Kirschner wire, for skeletal traction, and for stabilization of bone fragments or joint immobilization.

4379   KIENBÖCK, ROBERT. 1871-1953
        Über Luxationen im Bereiche der Handwurzel. *Fortschr. Röntgenstr.*, 1910-11, **16**, 103-15.
        First description of a slowly progressive osteonecrosis of the lunate bone of the wrist; carpal lunate malacia. ("Kienböck's disease").

4380   LEGG, ARTHUR THORNTON. 1874-1939
        An obscure affection of the hip-joint. *Boston med. surg. J.*, 1910, **162**, 202-04.
        Juvenile osteochondritis deformans ("Calvé–Legg–Perthes disease"; *see also* Nos. 4381 and 4382.). Previously described by H. Waldenström, *Z. orthop. Chir.*, 1909, **24**, 486.

4381   CALVÉ, JACQUES. 1875-1954
        Sur une forme particulière de pseudo-coxalgie greffée sur des déformations caractéristiques de l'extrémité supérieure du fémur. *Rev. Chir.(Paris)*, 1910, **42**, 54-84. *See* No. 4380.

4382   PERTHES, GEORG CLEMENS. 1869-1927
        Ueber Arthritis deformans juvenilis. *Dtsch. Z. Chir.*, 1910, **107**, 111-59. *See* No. 4380.

4383   GOLDTHWAIT, JOEL ERNEST. 1866-1961
        The lumbo-sacral articulation. An explanation of many cases of "lumbago", "sciatica" and paraplegia. *Boston med. surg. J.*, 1911, **164**, 365-72.
        Goldthwait suggested that lumbago and sciatica might be due to intervertebral disc injury.

4383.1 HIBBS, RUSSELL AUBRA. 1869-1932
        An operation for progressive spinal deformities. *N.Y. med. J.*, 1911, **93**, 1013-16.
        Spinal fusion first used for the treatment of scoliosis.

4384   MIDDLETON, GEORGE STEVENSON. 1854-1928, & TEACHER, JOHN HAMMOND. 1869-1930
        Injury of the spinal cord due to rupture of an intervertebral disc during muscular effort. *Glasg. med. J.*, 1911, **76**, 1-6.
        Report of a case of "sciatica" due to rupture of an intervertebral disc.

4384.1 ALBEE, FRED HOUDLETT. 1876-1945
        Transplantation of a portion of the tibia into the spine for Pott's disease. A preliminary report. *J. Amer. med. Ass.*, 1911, **57**, 885-86.
        The beginning of bone graft surgery as a planned, carefully designed procedure. Albee was the first to employ living bone grafts as internal splints. *See* No. 5757.

4385   CROUZON, Octave. 1874-1938
Dysostose cranio-faciale héréditaire. *Bull. Soc. méd. Hôp. Paris*, 1912, 3 sér., **33**, 545-55.
First description of cranio-facial dysostosis, hypertelorism.

4386   KLIPPEL, Maurice. 1858-1942, & FEIL, André. 1884-
Un cas d'absence des vertèbres cervicales avec cage thoracique remontant jusqu'à la base du crâne (cage thoracique cervicale). *Nouv. Iconogr. Salpêtr.*, 1912, **25**, 223-50.
"Klippel–Feil syndrome" – absence or incomplete development of cervical vertebrae. English translation in Bick, *Classics of orthopaedics*, 511-16.

4386.01   KANAVEL, Allen Buchner. 1874-1938
Infections of the hand: a guide to the surgical treatment of acute and chronic suppurative processes in the fingers, hand, and forearm. Philadelphia, *Lea & Febiger*, 1912.
The first comprehensive treatise on hand surgery, and the classic work on tendon and bursal hand spaces relevant to management of hand infections. Kanavel's book "did more to awaken the surgical conscience to the anatomic intricacies of hand surgery than did almost any other single contribution" (Bick).

4386.02   DARRACH, William. 1876-1948
Anterior dislocation of the head of the ulna. *Ann. Surg.*, 1912, **56**, 802-03.
Darrach procedure for problems of the distal ulna.

4386.1   ALBERS-SCHÖNBERG, Heinrich Ernst. 1869-1921
Eine seltene, bisher nicht bekannte Strukturanomalie des Skelettes. *Fortschr. Röntgenstr.*, 1915, **23**, 174-75.
First definitive description of osteopoikilosis.

4386.2   FROMENT, Jules. 1876-1946
La préhension dans les paralysies du nerf cubital et le signe du pouce. *Presse Méd.*, 1915, **23**, 409.
"Froment's sign" of ulnar nerve paralysis.

4386.3   MAYER, Leo. 1884-1972
The physiological method of tendon transplanation. *Surg. Gynecol. Obstet.*, 1916, **22**, 182-97.
Mayer's method of tendon transfer, using tendon sheaths to preserve the gliding surfaces.

4387   KÖHLER, Alban. 1874-1947
Eine typische Erkrankung des 2. Metatarsophalangealgelenkes. *Münch. med. Wschr.*, 1920, **67**, 1289-90.
"Köhler's second disease" – juvenile deforming metatarsophalangeal osteochondritis. English translation in *Amer. J. Roentgenol.*, 1923, **10**, 705-10. Also known as "Freiberg's infraction" or "Freiberg–Köhler disease".

4388   EWING, James. 1866-1943
Diffuse endothelioma of bone. *Proc. N.Y. path. Soc.*, 1921, n.s. **21**, 17-24.
Ewing described a form of bone sarcoma ("Ewing's sarcoma"), usually involving the shaft of long bones.

4388.1   LÉRI, ANDRÉ. 1875-1930
Une maladie congénitale et héréditaire de l'ossification: la pléonostéose familiale. *Bull. Mém. Soc. méd. Hôp. Paris*, 1921, 3 sér., **45**, 1228-30.
"Léri's pleonosteosis" first described.

4388.2   BIRCHER, EUGEN.
Die Arthroendoskopie. *Zentralbl. Chir.*, 1921, **48**, 1460-61.
First published account of the use of the laparoscope for arthroscopy.

4389   SCHEUERMANN, HOLGER WERFEL. 1877-1960
Kyphosis dorsalis juvenilis. *Z. orthop. Chir.*, 1921, **41**, 305-17.
"Scheuermann's disease" – necrosis of the epiphyses of the vertebrae, causing kyphosis.

4390   APERT, EUGÈNE. 1868-1940, *et al.*
Nouvelle observation d'acrocéphalosyndactylie. *Bull. Soc. méd. Hôp. Paris*, 1923, 3 sér., **47**, 1672-75.
"Apert's syndrome". With Tixier, Huc, and Kermorgant.

4391   JONES, *Sir* ROBERT. 1858-1933, & LOVETT, ROBERT WILLIAMSON. 1859-1924
Orthopaedic surgery. London, *H. Frowde,* 1923.
Jones was a pupil of Hugh Owen Thomas and a pioneer of active surgical intervention in orthopaedics. He advocated tendon transplantation, bone grafting, and other reconstructive and restorative procedures. He did much valuable work during the war of 1914-18, and he is one of the greatest figures in British orthopaedics.

4392   GREIG, DAVID MIDDLETON. 1864-1936
Hypertelorism. A hitherto undifferentiated congenital cranio-facial deformity. *Edinb. med. J.*, 1924, **31**, 560-93.
First description of hypertelorism as a separate entity.

4392.1   WHITMAN, ROYAL. 1857-1946
The reconstruction operation for arthritis deformans of the hip-joint. *Ann. Surg.*, 1924, **80**, 779-785.
The first sustained attempt to relieve osteoarthrosis of the hip by surgical means other than fusion.

4393   CODMAN, ERNEST AMORY. 1869-1940
Bone sarcoma, an interpretation of the nomenclature used by the Committee on the Registry of Bone Sarcoma of the American College of Surgeons. New York, *P. B. Hoeber,* 1925.

4394   KOLODNY, ANATOLE. 1892-
Bone sarcoma. The primary malignant tumors of bone and the giant cell tumor. *Surg. Gynec. Obstet.*, 1927, **44**, Suppl., 1-214.
Based on material collected by the Registry of Bone Sacrcoma in Boston since its foundation in 1921.

4395   JANSEN, MURK. 1863-1935
Dissociation of bone growth. (Exostoses and enchondromata, of Ollier's dyschondroplasia and associated phenomena.) In *The Robert Jones Birthday Volume*, London, *Oxford Univ. Press,* 1928, 43-72.
Jansen's theory of dissociation of bone growth.

4395.1   ENGELMANN, GUIDO. 1876-
          Ein Fall von Osteopathia hyperostotica (sclerotisans) multiplex infantilis.
          Fortschr. Röntgenstr., 1929, **39**, 1101-06.
          "Engelmann's disease", a rare bone dystrophy causing osteosclerosis.

4396   MAXWELL, JOHN PRESTON. 1871-1961
          Further studies in osteomalacia. *Proc. roy. Soc. Med.*, 1929-30, **23**, 639-52.
          Maxwell showed osteomalacia to be due to lack of vitamin D.

4397   MORQUIO, LUIS. 1867-1935
          Sur une forme de dystrophie osseuse familiale. *Arch. Méd. Enf.*, 1929, **32**,
          129-40; *Bull. Soc. Pédiat. Paris*, 1929, **27**, 145-52.
          "Morquio's disease", eccentro-osteochondrodysplasia.

4397.1   BRAILSFORD, JAMES FREDERICK. 1888-1961
          Chondro-osteo-dystrophy. Roentgenographic and clinical features of a
          child with dislocation of vertebrae. *Amer. J. Surg.*, 1929, **7**, 404-10.
          Morquio–Brailsford disease (*see* No. 4397).

4398   MILKMAN, LOUIS ARTHUR. 1895-1951
          Pseudofractures (hunger osteopathy, late rickets, osteomalacia): report of
          a case. *Amer. J. Roentgenol.*, 1930, **24**, 29-37.
          "Milkman's syndrome".

4399   BAER, WILLIAM STEVENSON. 1872-1931
          The treatment of chronic osteomyelitis with the maggot (larva of the blow
          fly). *J. Bone Jt. Surg.*, 1931, **13**, 438-75.
              Larrey observed the therapeutic effect of maggots on wounds; W. S.
          Baer inaugurated the method of treating osteomyelitis by this means ("Baer
          therapy").

4400   GESCHICKTER, CHARLES FREEBORN. 1901- , & COPELAND, MURRAY MARCUS.
          1902-1981
          Tumors of bone. New York, *Amer. J. Cancer*, 1931.

4400.1   BURMAN, MICHAEL S.
          Arthroscopy or the direct visualization of joints: An experimental cadaver
          study. *J. Bone Jt. Surg.*, 1931, **13**, 669-95.
              The first description of arthroscopic appearance of joints other than the
          knee, and a classic on the fundamental principles of the procedure.
          Follow-up paper by Burman, H. Finkelstein, & L. Mayer: Arthroscopy of the
          knee joint. *J. Bone Jt. Surg.*, 1934, **16**, 255-68.

4400.2   PHELPS, WINTHROP MORGAN. 1894-
          Cerebral birth injuries: Their orthopaedic classification and subsequent
          treatment. *J. Bone Jt. Surg,,* 1932, **14**, 773-82.
              Phelps established the modern classification and approach to these
          injuries.

4400.3   PHEMISTER, DALLAS B. 1882-1951
          Operative arrestment of longitudinal growth of bones in the treatment of
          deformities. *J. Bone Joint Surg.*, 1933, **15**, 1-15.
              Epiphysiodesis to inhibit bone growth of a longer leg.

4400.4   CODMAN, ERNEST AMORY. 1869-1940
The shoulder. Boston, *Privately printed*, 1934.
     Definitive study of the rotator cuff, written in Codman's idiosyncratic and iconoclastic style. Reprint, Malabar, Fl., *Krieger*, 1965.

4400.5   PAUWELS, FRIEDRICH. 1885-1980
Der Schenkelhalsbruch, Ein mechanische Problem. Stuttgart, *F. Enkes*, 1935.
     Pioneering study of the biomechanics of the hip joint.

4401   ALBRIGHT, FULLER. 1900-1969, *et al.*
Syndrome characterized by osteitis fibrosa disseminata, areas of pigmentation and endocrine dysfunction, with precocious puberty in females. Report of five cases. *New Engl. J. Med.* 1937, **216**, 727-46.
     "Albright's syndrome". With A. M. Butler, A. O. Hampton, and P. Smith.

4402   VENABLE, CHARLES SCOTT. 1877-, *et al.*
The effects on bone of the presence of metals; based upon electrolysis. An experimental study. *Ann. Surg.*, 1937, **105**, 917-38.
     Introduction of vitallium. With W. Stuck and A. Beach.

4403   SMITH-PETERSEN, MARIUS NYGAARD. 1886-1953
Arthroplasty of the hip. A new method. *J. Bone Jt Surg.*, 1939, **21**, 269-88.
     Vitallium cup arthroplasty.

4403.1   KITE, JOSEPH HIRAM. 1891-
Principles involved in the treatment of congenital clubfoot. *J. Bone Jt. Surg.*, 1939, **21**, 595-606.
     Kite's method involving "a series of plaster casts and wedgings, without the use of anesthetics, forcible manipulations, or operative procedures", became standard practice.

4403.2   CAMPBELL, WILLIS C. 1880-1941
Operative orthopedics. St. Louis, *C.V. Mosby*, 1939.
     The most influential American textbook of orthopaedics in the twentieth century.

4403.3   STEINDLER, ARTHUR. 1878-1959
Tendon transplanation in the upper extremity. *Am. J. Surg.*, 1939, **44**, 260-71.
     Correction to this article in *Am. J. Surg.*, 1939, **44**, 534.

4404   MORCH, ERNST TRIER. 1908-
Chondrodystrophic dwarfs in Denmark (supplemented with investigations from Sweden and Norway) with special reference to the inheritance of chondrodystrophy. Copenhagen, *E. Munksgaard*, 1941.
     Morch established the fact that chondrodystrophy may be inherited.

4404.01   INCLAN, ALBERTO FRANCIS. 1916-
The use of preserved bone grafts in orthopaedic surgery. *J. Bone Jt. Surg.*, 1942, **24**, 81-96.
     These studies form the basis of the modern use of bone preserved by refrigeration.

4404.02   BUNNELL, STERLING. 1882-1957
Surgery of the hand. Philadelphia, *J.B. Lippincott*, 1944.
Bunnell originated hand surgery as a specialty.

4404.1   SEEDORFF, KNUD STAKEMANN.
Osteogenesis imperfecta. A study of clinical features and heredity based on 55 Danish families comprising 180 affected members. Århus, *Universitetsforlaget*, 1949.
Includes a translation of Ekman's thesis (No. 4304.1). Also gives a case reported in 1678.

4404.2   BLOUNT, WALTER P. 1900- & CLARKE, GEORGE R.
Control of bone growth by epiphyseal stapling: A preliminary report. *J. Bone Jt. Surg.*, 1949, **31-A**, 464-78.
"Blount staple". Unlike previous processes, epiphyseal stapling permitted subsequent correction.

4405   JUDET, JEAN. 1905- , & JUDET, ROBERT LOUIS. 1909-
The use of an artificial femoral head for arthroplasty of the hip joint. *J. Bone Jt Surg.*, 1950, **32B**, 166-73.
Judet acrylic prosthesis.

4405.01   WATANABE, MASAKI.
Atlas of arthroscopy. Tokyo, *Igaku Shoin*, 1957.
The first atlas of arthroscopy, a major step in gaining wide acceptance of this operating technique. The colour illustrations were prepared by an artist as available arthroscopes did not permit colour photography. Watanabe was a pupil of Kenji Takagi (1888-1963) who in 1920 designed the first specialised arthroscope. Takagi was the first to use the arthroscope for operations on the inside of knee. However, he did not publish on the subject until 1932. See *Clin. Ortho.*, 1982, **167**, 6-8. Watanabe refined and developed the arthroscope. This atlas was co-authored with S. Takeda and H. Ikeuchi. Revised and enlarged second edition with colour photographs through the arthroscope, Tokyo, *Igaku Shoin*, [1969].

4405.02   BRANNON, EARL W. & KLEIN, GEROLD.
Experiences with a finger-joint prosthesis. *J. Bone Jt. Surg.*, 1959, **41-A**, 87-102.
First prosthetic device for replacement of destroyed finger-joints.

4405.1   CHARNLEY, *Sir* JOHN. 1911-1982
Arthroplasty of the hip: a new operation. *Lancet*, 1961, **1**, 1129-32.
Total hip replacement; Charnley arthroplasty.

4405.2   HARRINGTON, PAUL R.
Treatment of scoliosis: Correction and internal fixation by spine instrumentation. *J. Bone Jt. Surg.*, 1962, **44-A**, 591-610.
The "Harrington rod" system for scoliosis and spine fracture surgery.

4405.3   MALT, RONALD A. 1931- & McKHANN, CHARLES FREEMONT. 1930-
Replantation of severed arms. *J. Amer. med. Ass.*, 1964, **189**, 716-722.
First successful reattachment of a completely amputated human limb.

4405.4   SWANSON, A. B.
A flexible implant for replacement of arthritic or destroyed joints in the hand. *N.Y. Univ. Post-Grad. Med. Sch. Inter-Clinic Information Bull.*, 1966, **6**, 16-19.

"Swanson prosthesis" – flexible silicone rubber finger-joint prosthesis.

4405.5   GUNSTON, FRANK H. 1933-
Polycentric knee arthoplasty: Prosthetic simulation of normal knee movement. *J. Bone Jt. Surg.*, 1971, **53-B**, 272-277.

Total knee replacement (replacing diseased articular surfaces of both femur and tibia), holding the metal and plastic components in place with acrylic cement.

FRACTURES AND DISLOCATIONS

4406   HIPPOCRATES. 460-375 B.C.
Fractures, joints, instruments of reduction. In [Works] with an English translation by E.T. WITHINGTON, London, *W. Heinemann*, 1927, **3**, 83-449.

4406.1   GUIDI, GUIDO [VIDIUS]. 1508-69
Chirurgia e graeco in latinum conversa. Paris, *Petrus Galterius*, 1544.

Guidi translated an illustrated Byzantine manuscript containing surgical works of Hippocrates, Galen and Oribasius, adding commentaries of his own. Much of the work concerns fractures and dislocations. The magnificent woodcut illustrations for this book were probably redrawn by the Mannerist, Primaticcio, but perhaps also with the participation of other Italian masters.

4407   WHITE, CHARLES. 1728-1813
An account of a new method of reducing shoulders (without the use of an ambe) which have been several months dislocated, in cases where the common methods have proved inefficient. *Med. Obs. Inqu.*, 1762, **2**, 373-81.

White's method of reducing shoulder dislocations by means of suspending the patient from the affected arm. This method either reduced the dislocation entirely, or moved the head of the humerus into a position where it could be reduced by traditional methods such as applying the surgeon's heel to the axilla.

4408   POTT, PERCIVALL. 1714-1788
Some few general remarks on fractures and dislocations. London, *L. Hawes, W. Clarke, R. Collins*, 1767.

The methods outlined by Pott in his classic work on fractures and dislocations were eventually adopted all over the world. He described (pp. 57-64) "Pott's fracture" in this book, and he stressed the necessity for the immediate setting of a fracture and the need for relaxation of the muscles in order that the setting should be carried out successfully. Reprinted in *Med. Classics*, 1936, **1**, 332-37.

4409   CAMPER, PIETER. 1722-1789
Dissertatio de fractura patellae et olecrani. Hagae Comitum, *I. van Cleef*, 1789.

4409.1   PHYSICK, PHILIP SYNG. 1768-1837
A case of fracture of the os humeri, in which the broken ends of the bone not uniting the usual manner, a cure was effected by means of a seton. *Med. Repos.*(2nd Ser.), 1804, **1**, 122-24.

The first paper on orthopaedic surgery published in the United States. Physick introduced the use of the seton in the treatment of ununited fractures.

4410   COLLES, ABRAHAM. 1773-1843
On the fracture of the carpal extremity of the radius. *Edinb. med. surg. J.*, 1814, **10**, 182-86.

Colles's description of fracture of the carpal end of the radius led that type of fracture to be named "Colles's fracture". He was Professor of Surgery at Dublin for more than 30 years. Reprinted in *Med. Classics*, 1940, **4**, 1038-42.

4411   DUPUYTREN, GUILLAUME, *le baron.* 1777-1835
Mémoire sur la fracture de l'extrémité inférieure du péroné, les luxations et les accidens qui en sont la suite. *Ann. méd.-chir. Hôp. Paris*, 1819, **1**, 1-212.

"Dupuytren's fracture", of the ankle, described in a learned 212-page review of ankle fractures, and of the normal anatomy and function of the ankle joint. "Of especial interest is the description of experimental fractures produced in cadavers to elucidate the mechanism of injury" (Peltier).

4411.1   BARTON, JOHN RHEA. 1794-1871
Remarks on certain injuries of the bones in children. *Amer. Med. Rec.*, 1821, **4**, 9-20.

On bending fractures in children.

4412.1   COOPER, *Sir* ASTLEY PASTON. 1768-1841
A treatise on dislocations, and on fractures of the joints. London, *Longman*, 1822.

Through this and numerous subsequent editions this was the principal reference work on the subject in England and America for 30 years. "Many later clinical modifications were developed from Cooper's methods" (Bick).

4413   DUPUYTREN, GUILLAUME, *le baron.* 1777-1835
Mémoire sur un déplacement originel ou congénital de la tête des fémurs. *Répert. gén. Anat. Physiol. path.*, 1826, **2**, 82-93.

First clear pathological description of congenital dislocation of the hip-joint. Dupuytren distinguished this syndrome caused by failure of foetal development of the acetabulum from deformities due to tuberculosis and pyarthrotic disease of the hip joint.

4414   RODGERS, JOHN KEARNEY. 1793-1851
Case of un-united fracture of the os brachii, successfully treated. *N.Y. med. phys. J.*, 1827, **6**, 521-23.

Successful wiring of ununited fracture of humerus.

4414.1   RICHTER, Adolph Leopold. 1798-1876
          Theoretisch-praktische Handbuch der Lehre von den Bruchen und
          Verrenkungen der Knochen. 1 vol. and atlas. Berlin, *Enslin*, 1828.
          The remarkable atlas accompanying this work illustrates in remarkable
          detail all of the various types of dressings, splints and apparatus used in the
          treatment of fractures at the time.

4415   BARTON, John Rhea. 1794-1871
          Views and treatment of an important injury of the wrist. *Med. Examiner*, 1838,
          1, 365-68.
          "Barton's fracture" of the radius.

4416   HEINE, Jacob von. 1799-1879
          Ueber spontane und congenitale Luxationen. Stuttgart, *Ebner & Seubert*,
          1842.

4417   MALGAIGNE, Joseph François. 1806-1865
          Traité des fractures et des luxations. 2 vols. and atlas. Paris, *Chez l'auteur,
          J.B. Baillière*, 1847-55.
          This was Malgaigne's greatest work. His description of bilateral vertical
          fracture of the pelvis ("Malgaigne's fracture") is in vol. 1, pp. 650-56.
          English translation of the first volume on fractures, Philadelphia, 1859. The
          second volume on luxations has not been translated.

4417.1   SMITH, Robert William. 1807-1873
          A treatise on fractures in the vicinity of joints and on certain forms of
          accidental and congenital dislocations. Dublin, *Hodges & Smith*, 1847.
          The first important work on fractures by an Irish author. It includes the
          description of "Smith's fracture". In his chapter "On fractures of the bones
          of the forearm in the vicinity of the wrist joint" Smith corrected Colles's
          original description (No. 4410) by placing the site of the fracture more
          distally. "It was Smith who firmly attached Colles's eponym to the fracture
          that Colles described" (Peltier).

4418   REID, William Wharry. 1799-1866
          Dislocation of the femur on the dorsum ilii, reducible without pulleys, or any
          other mechanical power, three cases. *Buffalo med. J.*, 1851-52, **7**, 129-43.
          Reduction of dislocation without manipulation. Reid demonstrated the
          futility of attempting to reduce a dorsal dislocation of the hip by forcible
          longitudinal traction with pulleys.

4418.1   BRAINARD, Daniel. 1812-1866
          Essay on a new method of treating ununited fractures and certain deformities
          of the osseous system. New York, *Godwin*, 1854.
          Experimenting on animals and cadavers, Brainard developed a special
          bone drill or "perforator" introduced subcutaneously to perforate the bone
          ends, simulating a recent fracture, and thus stimulating callus formation.

4419   BUCK, Gurdon. 1807-1877
          [New treatment for fractures of the femur]. *Bull. N.Y. Acad. Med.*, 1860-62,
          1, 181-88.
          Buck's extension apparatus, an improved method of treating fractures
          of the femur. Reprinted in *Med. Classics*, 1939, **3**, 764-82.

4420   HAMILTON, FRANK HASTINGS. 1813-1886
        A practical treatise on fractures and dislocations. Philadelphia, *Blanchard
        & Lea*, 1860.
        The first complete work in English on the subject. *See* No. 1742.

4421   PERRIN, MAURICE. 1826-1889
        Luxation traumatique suivie de luxation volontaire du fémur droit. *Bull. Soc.
        Chir. Paris,* (1859), 1860, **10**, 12-21.
        "Perrin–Ferraton disease" of the hip, later more fully dealt with by L.
        Ferraton, *Rev. Orthop. (Paris)*, 1905, 2 sér., **6**, 45-51.

4422   SMITH, NATHAN RYNO. 1797-1877.
        A new instrument for the treatment of fractures of the lower extremity.
        Maryland & Virginia med. surg. J., 1860, **14**, 1-5, 177-181.
        Smith devised an anterior or suspensatory splint for use in the treatment
        of fractures of the femur. The apparatus was heavily used during the U.S.
        Civil War and was especially valuable in treating compound fractures.

4422.1 GURLT, ERNST JULIUS. 1825-1899
        Handbuch der Lehre von den Knochenbruchen. 2 vols., Hamm, *G. Grote*,
        1862-65.
        Gurlt, the celebrated historian of surgery (*see* No. 5800), wrote an ex-
        haustive and detailed review of the literature on fractures. As a source of
        obscure and arcane information it is unsurpassed.

4423   SMITH, NATHAN RYNO. 1797-1877
        Treatment of fractures of the lower extremity, by use of the anterior
        suspensory apparatus. Baltimore, *Kelly & Piet,* 1867.

4423.1 LISTER, JOSEPH, 1st *Baron Lister.* 1827-1912
        On a new method of treating compound fracture, abscess, etc., with
        observations on the conditions of suppuration. *Lancet.*, 1867, **1**, 326-29,
        357-59, 387-89, 507-09; **2**, 95-96.
        Lister's work on the antiseptic principle in surgery. *See* No. 5634.

4424   BIGELOW, HENRY JACOB. 1818-1890
        The mechanism of dislocation and fracture of the hip. With the reduction
        of the dislocations by the flexion method. Philadelphia, *H. C. Lea*, 1869.
        Bigelow was the first to describe in detail the mechanism of the ilio-
        femoral (Bigelow's) ligament, and to show its importance in the reduction
        of dislocation by the flexion method.

4425   KOCHER, EMIL THEODOR. 1841-1917
        Eine neue Reductionsmethode für Schulterverrenkung. *Berl. klin. Wschr.*,
        1870, **7**, 101-05.
        Kocher was Professor of Surgery at Berne, and among the greatest
        surgeons of his day. He is remembered, among other things, for his method
        of reduction of subluxation of the shoulder-joint.

4425.1 BERENGER-FÉRAUD, LAURENT JEAN BAPTISTE. 1832-1900
        Traité de l'immobilisation directe des fragments osseux dans les fractures.
        Paris, *Adrien Delahaye*, 1870.
        First book devoted to the treatment of fractures by internal fixation.

4426   BENNETT, Edward Hallaran. 1837-1907
Fractures of the metacarpal bones. *Dublin J. med. Sci.*, 1882, **73**, 72-75.
"Bennett's fracture" of the first metacarpal. He was Professor of Surgery at Trinity College, Dublin.

4426.1   ANNANDALE, Thomas. 1839-1908
An operation for displaced semilunar cartilage. *Brit. med. J.*, 1885, **1**, 779.
The first deliberate and planned operation for the relief of internal derangement of the knee-joint caused by a displaced cartilage. Annandale succeeded Lister as Professor of Clinical Surgery at Edinburgh in 1877.

4427   SPRENGEL, Otto Gerhard Karl. 1852-1915
Die angeborene Verschiebung des Schulterblattes nach oben. *Arch. klin. Chir.*, 1891, **42**, 545-49.
"Sprengel's deformity" – congenital elevation of the scapula.

4428   TRENDELENBURG, Friedrich. 1844-1924
Ueber den Gang bei angeborener Hüftgelenksluxation. *Dtsch. med. Wschr.*, 1895, **21**, 21-24.
"Trendelenburg's sign" of congenital dislocation of the hip-joint.

4429   LANE, *Sir* William Arbuthnot. 1856-1943
A method of treating simple oblique fractures of the tibia and fibula more efficient than those in common use. *Trans. clin. Soc. Lond.*, 1894, **27**, 167-75.
Lane's method of "osteo-synthesis" in the treatment of fractures – the perfect re-apposition of the affected parts by means of operative intervention.

4429.1   POLAND, John. 1855-1937
Traumatic separation of the epiphyses. London, *Smith, Elder*, 1898.
Definitive and exhaustive study of growth plate fractures in children. Poland also published the series of *x* rays included in the above work as a separate atlas: *Skiagraphic atlas showing the development of the bones of the wrist and hand*, London, *Smith, Elder*, 1898.

4429.2   PARKHILL, Clayton. 1860-1902
Further observations regarding the use of the bone-clamp in ununited fractures, fractures with malunion, and recent fractures with a tendency to displacement. *Ann. Surg.*, 1898, **27**, 553-570.
Parkhill introduced external fixation for the treatment of fractures.

4430   LANE, *Sir* William Arbuthnot. 1856-1943.
Clinical remarks on the operative treatment of fractures. *Brit. med. J.*, 1907, **1**, 1037-38.
Lane's plates and screws for union of fractures.

4431   STEINMANN, Fritz. 1872-1932
Eine neue Extensionsmethode in der Frakturenbehandlung. *Zbl. Chir.*, 1907, **34**, 938-42.
Steinmann nail or pin, for insertion through a distal fragment and controlled by direct skeletal traction. English translation in Bick, *Classics of orthopaedics.*

4431.1   LAMBOTTE, ALBIN. 1866-1956
L'intervention opératoire dans les fractures. Brussels, *Edit. Lambertin*, 1907.
    Lambotte developed an external fracture fixation device using pins on either side of the fracture, connected by a solid rod.

4432   BANKART, ARTHUR SYDNEY BLUNDELL. 1879-1951
Recurrent or habitual dislocation of the shoulder-joint. *Brit. med. J.*, 1923, **2**, 1132-33.
    Blundell Bankart's operation.

4433   BÖHLER, LORENZ. 1885-1973
Technik der Knochenbruchbehandlung. Wien, *W. Maudrich*, 1929.
    Böhler introduced several new methods and devised new apparatus for the treatment of fractures. His clinic in Vienna became world-famous. 12-13th ed., 1951.

4433.1   ORR, HIRAM WINNETT. 1877-1956
Osteomyelitis and compound fractures and other infected wounds: Treatment by the method of drainage and rest. St. Louis, *C.V. Mosby Co.*, 1929.
    Orr developed a treatment for open fractures "consisting of thorough debridement, reduction of the fracture, and usually, maintenance of the reduction by the technique of pins transfixing the fragments and incorporated into the plaster" (Peltier).

4434   SMITH-PETERSEN, MARIUS NYGAARD. 1886-1953, *et al.*
Intracapsular fractures of the neck of the femur. Treatment by internal fixation. *Arch. Surg. (Chicago)*, 1931, **23**, 715-59.
    Smith-Petersen nail, a three-flanged nail which prevented rotation of the femoral head. With E. F. Cave and G. W. Van Gorder.

4435   MIXTER, WILLIAM JASON. 1880-1958, & BARR, JOSEPH SEATON. 1901-1963
Rupture of the intervertebral disc with involvement of the spinal canal. *New Engl. J. Med.*, 1934, **211**, 210-15.
    Demonstration of the causal role of intervertebral disc herniation in sciatica.

4435.01   HOFFMANN, RAOUL.
"Rotules à os" pour la réduction dirigée, non sanglante, des fractures ("ostéotaxis"). *Helvetica med. Acta*, 1938, **5**, 844-50.
    Hoffmann, a Swiss general surgeon with a doctorate in theology and unusual skill in carpentry, developed the versatile Hoffmann system of external fixation devices.

4435.1   TRUETA, JOSEP. 1897-1977
El tratamiento de la fractura de guerra. Barcelona, *Biblioteca Médica de Cataluña*, 1938.
    During the Spanish Civil War (1935-38) Trueta adopted as standard treatment for gunshot wounds and compound fractures the closed plaster method originated by H. Winnett Orr. Trueta called this the biological treatment of wounds. The treatment consisted of débridement and wound excision followed by packing the wound open and immobilizing the limb in a plaster dressing. English translation, London, 1939. *See* No. 5632.

4435.2 RUSH, LESLIE V. 1905- , & RUSH, H. LOWRY. 1897-1965
Evolution of medullary fixation of fractures by the longitudinal pin. *Amer. J. Surg.*, 1949, **78**, 324-33.
"Rush pins", made of specially hardened type 316 stainless steel, for fractures of the long bones.

4435.3 CHARNLEY, *Sir* JOHN. 1911-1982
The closed treatment of common fractures. Edinburgh, *Livingstone*, 1950.
"A classic exposition of the non-operative approach" (Peltier).

4435.4 YASUDA, IWAO. 1909-
Fundamental aspects of fracture treatment. [In Japanese] *J. Kyoto med. Soc.*, 1953, **4**, 395-406.
First electrically-induced osteogenesis. Yasuda demonstrated that small amounts of electric current applied to bone stimulated osteogenesis at the cathode. He was also the first to describe stress generated potentials in bone. Abridged English translation in *Clin. orthop.*,1977, **124**, 5-8.

4435.5 HOLDSWORTH, *Sir* FRANK WILD. 1904-1969
Fractures, dislocations and fracture-dislocations of the spine. *J. Bone Jt. Surg.*, 1963, **45B**, 6-20.
Holdsworth classification of spinal injuries.

4435.6 SALTER, ROBERT BRUCE. 1924- & HARRIS, W. ROBERT.
Injuries involving the epiphyseal plate. *J. Bone Jt. Surg.*, 1963, **45A**, 587-622.
Standard classification of growth plate fractures in children.

4436 YONGE, JAMES. 1646-1721
Currus triumphalis, è terebinthô . . . wherein also, the common methods, and medicaments, used to restrain hemorrhagies, are examined. London, *J. Martyn*, 1679.
Includes an account of the first flap amputation.

4437 WHITE, CHARLES. 1728-1813
An account of a case in which the upper head of the os humeri was sawed off, a large portion of the bone afterwards exfoliated, and yet the entire motion of the limb was preserved. *Phil. Trans.*, (1769), 1770, **59**, 39-46.
First recorded excision of the head of the humerus.

4438 PARK, HENRY. 1744-1831
An account of a new method of treating diseases of the joints of the knee and elbow. London. *J. Johnson*, 1733 [1783].
This was originally a letter to Pott. Park became famous for his operation of excision and arthrodesis as a treatment for destructive joint disease. The title page is misprinted "MDCCXXXIII"; the letter is dated 1783. The second edition of this work, Glasgow, 1806, contains the English translation of No. 4440.

4439   FOURCROY, ANTOINE FRANÇOIS. 1755-1809
        La médecine éclairée par les sciences physiques. 4 vols., Paris, *chez Buisson*, 1791-92.
            This work edited by Fourcroy contains in vol. 4 (pp. 85-88) the first description of Chopart's method of partial amputation of the foot. This is in the form of a note by Lafiteau: "Observation sur une amputation partielle du pied". Lafiteau also named "Chopart's joint", the astragaloscaphoid and calcaneo-cuboid articulation. François Chopart was born in 1743 and died in 1795.

4440   MOREAU, P. F.
        Observations pratiques relatives à la résection des articulations affectées de carie. Paris, *Farge*, an XI [1803].
            Excision and arthrodesis in joint disease. Moreau was the first to excise the elbow. English translation, Glasgow, 1806. *See* No. 4438.

4441   WACHTER, GEORG HEINRICH. 1790-1864
        Diss. de articulis exstirpandis, imprimis de genu exstirpato. Groningae, *T. Spoormaker,* [1810].

4442   LARREY, DOMINIQUE JEAN, *le baron.* 1766-1842
        Mémoires de chirurgie militaire. Paris, *J. Smith*, 1812, **2**, 180-95.
            Successful amputation at the hip-joint. Larrey was one of the first to perform this operation, with at least two successful cases. *See* No. 2160.

4443   LISFRANC, JACQUES. 1790-1847
        Nouvelle méthode opératoire pour l'amputation partielle du pied dans son articulation tarso-métatarsienne. Paris, *Gabon*, 1815.
            "Lisfranc's amputation" of the foot.

4444   DUPUYTREN, GUILLAUME, *le baron.* 1777-1835
        Observation sur une résection de la mâchoire inférieure. *J. univ. Sci. méd.*, 1820, **19**, 77-98.
            Dupuytren was the first successfully to excise the lower jaw, in 1812, as recorded in his *Leçons orales*, 1829, **2**, 421-53. The above paper deals with a later operation of the same type.

4445   GUTHRIE, GEORGE JAMES. 1785-1856
        A treatise on gun-shot wounds. 2nd. ed. London, *Longman*, 1820, 332-40.
            Successful amputation at the hip-joint, after the battle of Waterloo, 7 July, 1815.

4446   JAMESON, HORATIO GATES. 1788-1855
        Case of tumour of the superior jaw. *Amer. med. Recorder*, 1821, **4**, 222-30.
            First excision of the superior maxilla, 11 Nov, 1820.

4447   MOTT, VALENTINE. 1785-1865
        Case of osteo-sarcoma in which the right side of the lower jaw was removed successfully after tying the carotid artery. N.Y. med. phys. J., 1822, 1, 385-93.
            Mott resected the entire half of the bone, necessitating a disarticulation at the temporo-mandibular joint.

4448   DEADERICK, WILLIAM HARVEY. 1773-1858
Case of removal of a portion of the lower maxillary bone. *Amer. Med. Recorder*, 1823, **6**, 516-17.
Deaderick resected a portion of the jaw in 1810. He wrote this paper to obtain priority over Mott (No. 4447).

4449   ROGERS, DAVID L. 1799-1877
Case of osteo-sarcoma of the superior maxillary bone, with the operation for its removal. *N.Y. med. phys. J.,* 1824, **3**, 301-03.
Rogers removed nearly all of the upper jaw. Operation performed in 1810.

4450   SMITH, NATHAN. 1762-1829
On the amputation of the knee-joint. *Amer. med. Rev.* , 1825, **2**, 370-71.
Smith amputated the knee-joint in 1824, being the first in America to do so.

4451   BARTON, JOHN RHEA. 1794-1871
On the treatment of anchylosis, by the formation of artificial joints. *N. Amer. med. surg. J.,* 1827, **3**, 279-92.
Barton performed a femoral osteotomy between the greater and lesser trochanters to secure motion in an ankylosed hip. This has been called the first successful arthroplasty. Reprinted in *Clin. Orthop.*, 1984, **182**, 4-13.

4451.1   MOTT, VALENTINE. 1785-1865
Successful amputation at the hip-joint. *Phila. J. med. phys. Sci.*, 1827, **14**, 101-05.
This is "the first reported amputation at the hip joint found in the American medical literature" (Rutkow). *See* No. 4462.

4452   ———. An account of a case of osteo-sarcoma of the left clavicle, in which exsection of that bone was successfully performed. *Amer. J. med. Sci.,* 1828, **3**, 100-08.
Valentine Mott was an outstanding figure in American surgery during the first half of the 19th century. A pupil of Astley Cooper, he particularly distinguished himself in vascular surgery and in operations involving the bones and joints. *See* No. 4463.

4453   SYME, JAMES. 1799-1870
Case of osteo-sarcoma of the lower jaw. *Edinb. med. surg. J.,* 1828, **30**, 286-90.
Syme's operation of excision of the lower jaw for osteosarcoma.

4454   ———. Three cases in which the elbow-joint was successfully excised. *Edinb. med. surg. J.,* 1829, **31**, 256-66.

4455   HUTCHINSON, ALEXANDER COPLAND.
Removal of the arm, scapula and clavicle. *Lond. med. Gaz.*, 1829-30, **5**, 273.
Records the first interscapulo-thoracic amputation, performed by Ralph Cuming (d. 1808), a naval surgeon, in 1808.

4456   ROUX, PHILIBERT JOSEPH. 1780-1854
Résection des os. *Rev. Méd. franç. étrang.*, 1830, **37**, 8-13.
    Among the French surgeons of the 19th century, Roux was second in importance only to Dupuytren. He performed staphylorrhaphy in 1819 and sutured the ruptured female peritoneum in 1832; he is also remembered on account of his method of resection of bone.

4457   SYME, JAMES. 1799-1870
Treatise on the excision of diseased joints. Edinburgh, *A. Black,* 1831.
    Syme, teacher and father-in-law of Lister, was one of the greatest of the Scottish surgeons. He is remembered for his method of amputation at the ankle (*see* No. 4459), for his speedy adoption of anaesthesia and antisepsis, and for the above book, which showed that excision of joints is usually preferable to amputation – a principle soon generally adopted.

4458   WHITE, ANTHONY. 1782-1849
[Excision of the head of the femur for disease of the hip-joint.] In S. COOPER: *A dictionary of practical surgery.* 7th ed. London, 1838, 272-73.
    White was the first to perform this operation, April 1821.

4459   SYME, JAMES. 1799-1870
Amputation at the ankle-joint. *Lond. Edinb. month. J. med. Sci.*, 1843, **3**, 93-96.
    "Syme's amputation" at the ankle joint, an operation first successfully performed by him on 8 Sept, 1842.

4460   MACKENZIE, RICHARD JAMES. 1821-1854
On amputation at the ankle-joint by internal lateral flap. *Monthly J. med. Sci.*, 1849, **9**, 951-54.
    "Mackenzie's operation", a modification of Syme's amputation (No. 4459). Mackenzie volunteered for service in the Crimean War and died of Asiatic cholera near Sebastopol.

4461   BIGELOW, HENRY JACOB. 1818-1890
Resection of the head of the femur. *Amer. J. med. Sci.*, 1852, **24**, 90.
    First excision of the hip-joint in America. Unfortunately the one-page article provides no details.

4462   BRASHEAR, WALTER. 1776-1860
Amputations. *Trans. Kentucky med. Soc.* , 1853, **2**, 264-68.
    The first successful amputation of the hip-joint was performed by Brashear in 1806 at Bardstown, Kentucky; he first amputated the thigh through its middle third, and tied off the bleeding vessels; then he made a long incision on the outside of the limb, exposing the remainder of the bone, which was disarticulated at its socket. This article is part of a study on surgery in Kentucky authored by Samuel D. Gross, who wrote that Brashear was "alternately or successively, doctor, merchant, legislator, lawyer, and naturalist. For some years he served his adopted State in the Senate of the United States". *See* No. 4451.1.

4463   McCREARY, CHARLES. 1785-1826
Exsection of the clavicle. *Trans. Kentucky med. Soc.* (1852), 1853, **2**, 276-77.

J. H. Johnson (*New Orleans med. surg. J.*, 1850, **6**, 474-76) stated that McCreary performed the first resection of the clavicle in the United States on 4 May, 1811. Valentine Mott reported the operation in 1828. *See* No. 4452.

4464   HEYFELDER, JOHANN FERDINAND MARTIN. 1798-1869
Ueber Resectionen und Amputationen. Breslau, Bonn, *E. Weber,* 1854.

4465   PIROGOV, NIKOLAI IVANOVICH. 1810-1881
Kostno-plasticheskoye udlineniye kostei goleni pri vilushtshenii stopi. [Osteoplastic elongation of the bones of the leg in amputation of the foot.] *Voyenno-med. J.*, 1854, **63**, 2 sect., 83-100.
Pirogov's method of complete osteoplastic amputation of the foot. German translation, Leipzig, 1854.

4466   GRITTI, ROCCO. 1828-1920
Dell'amputazione del femore al terzo inferiore e della disarticulazione del ginocchio. *Ann. univ. Med. (Milano)*, 1857, **161**, 5-32.
Gritti's amputation of the thigh was later improved by Stokes (*see* No. 4470).

4467   TEALE, THOMAS PRIDGIN, *Snr.* 1801-1868
On amputation by a long and a short rectangular flap. London, *J. Churchill,* 1858.
Teale's method of amputation.

4468   CARDEN, HENRY DOUGLAS. ?-1872
On amputation by a single flap. *Brit. med. J.*, 1864, **1**, 416-21.
Carden devised a single flap operation, cutting through the femur just above the knee-joint. He published a book on the subject in 1864.

4469   LISTER, JOSEPH, *1st Baron Lister.* 1827-1912
On excision of the wrist for caries. *Lancet*, 1865, **1**, 308-12, 335-38, 362-64.

4470   STOKES, *Sir* WILLIAM. 1839-1900
On supra-condyloid amputation of the thigh. *Med.-chir. Trans.*, 1870, **53**, 175-86.
Gritti–Stokes amputation (*see also* No. 4466).

4471   BERGER, PAUL. 1845-1908
Amputation du membre supérieur dans la contiguïté du tronc (désarticulation de l'omoplate). *Bull. Soc. Chir. Paris*, 1883, **9**, 656.
"Berger's operation", interscapulothoracic amputation. See also his monograph, Paris, *Masson*, 1887.

4472   JABOULAY, MATHIEU. 1860-1913.
La désarticulation interilio-abdominale. *Lyon méd.*, 1894, **75**, 507-10.
Interilio-abdominal amputation first described.

4473   GIRARD, CHARLES. 1850-1916
Désarticulation de l'os iliaque pour sarcome. *Congr. franç. Chir.*, 1895, **9**, 823-27.
First successful hind-quarter amputation.

4474   VANGHETTI, GIULIANO. 1861-1940
        Amputazione, disarticulazione et protesi. Firenze, 1898.
        Vanghetti was the first to suggest the use of the musculature remaining
        above the amputation stump to form a motor unit for artificial limbs –
        "kinematization of stumps".

4475   CECI, ANTONIO. 1852-1920
        Tecnica generale della amputazioni mucosi. Amputazioni plastico-
        ortopediche con metodo proprio secundo la proposta del Vanghetti.
        Dimonstrazioni pratiche. *Arch. Atti Soc. ital. Chir.*, 1906, **18**.
        Ceci was the first to operate on the lines suggested by Vanghetti.

4476   KRUKENBERG, HERMANN. 1863-
        Eine neue osteoplastische Amputationsmethode des Oberschenkels. *Zbl.
        Chir.*, 1917, **44**, 578.

4477   PUTTI, VITTORIO. 1880-1940
        The utilization of the muscles of a stump to actuate artificial limbs:
        cinematic amputations. *Brit. med. J.*, 1918, **1**, 635-38.
        Putti developed and improved kineplastic surgery.

4478   GORDON-TAYLOR, *Sir* GORDON. 1878-1960, & WILES, PHILIP. 1899-1967
        Interinnomino-abdominal (hind-quarter) amputation. *Brit. J. Surg.*, 1935,
        22, 671-95.
        One-stage operation.

SPORTS MEDICINE

4478.99   MENDEZ, CHRISTOBAL. *b. circa* 1500
           Libro de exercicio corporal...[Seville, *Gregorio de la Torre*,] 1553.
           The first separate book on exercise by a physician. Facsimile with
           English translation by Francisco Guerra, New Haven, 1960.

4478.100   MERCURIALI, GIROLAMO. 1530-1606
           Artis gymnasticae apud antiquos celeberrimae, nostris temporibus ignoratae.
           Venetiis, *apud Iuntas*, 1569.
           A history of the attitudes and practices of the Greeks and Romans
           concerning diet, hygiene, bathing, and exercise. This is one of the earliest
           books to discuss the therapeutic value of gymnastics and sports generally
           for the cure of disease and disability. The second edition, *De arte gymnastica
           libri sex*, Venice, Juntas, 1573, is the first illustrated book on gymnastics. It
           contains 20 woodcuts by Coriolan. Partial English translation of 2nd ed. in
           The muscles and their story... including the whole text of Mercurialis.... by
           J.W.F. Blundell, London, 1864. *See* No. 1986.1.

4478.101   RAMAZZINI, BERNARDINO. 1633-1714
           De morbis artificum diatriba. Mutinae, *A. Capponi*, 1700.
           Ramazzini wrote the first comprehensive and systematic treatise on
           occupational diseases. He included a study of the diseases of athletes. It
           was translated into English in 1705; a new English translation by Wilmer
           Cave Wright appeared in 1940. *See* No. 2121.

4478.102   FULLER, FRANCIS. 1670-1706
Medicina gymnastica; or, a treatise concerning the power of exercise.
London, *Knaplock,* 1705.
    The first English book on the power of exercise in treating disease.
Fuller also recommended exercise for aid in the recovery from psychological
and emotional disorders. In this he preceded Cheyne (No. 4840).

4478.103   TISSOT, CLEMENT JOSEPH. 1750-1826
Gymnastique médicinale et chirurgicale, ou essai sur l'utilité du mouvement,
ou des différens exercices du corps, et du repos dans la cure des maladies.
Paris, *Bastien,* 1780.
    The first book on therapeutic exercise as the term is understood today.
English translation, with reduced facsimiles of 18th century translations
into German, Italian and Swedish, New Haven, 1964.

4478.104   LING, PER HENRIK. 1776-1839
Gymnastikens allmänna grunder. Upsala, *Palmblad & Co.,* 1834; *Leffler & Sebell,* 1840.
    The foundation of modern gymnastics and therapeutic massage. Ling
established the Swedish school of physiotherapy with his institute for
training gymnastics teachers in Stockholm in 1813. He developed the
ancient Greek art of calisthenics into a science based on sound anatomical
and physiological principles. "After Ling, scientific body building by
rational calisthenics became a recognized procedure not only for the weak
child or adult, but, of even greater consequence, as an integral part of the
plans for preventative medicine which were taking form in the schools and
gymnasia of all civilized nations" (Bick).

4478.105   DARLING, EUGENE A.
The effects of training. A study of the Harvard University Crews. *A Boston
med. surg. J.,* 1899, **141**, 205-09, 229-33.
    Pioneering study of the physiological effects of training.

4478.106   WEISSBEIN, SIEGFRIED. 1876-
Hygiene des Sport... Heraugegeben von Siegfried Weissebein. 2 vols.,
Leipzig, *Greuthlein,* 1910.
    First comprehensive work on sports medicine.

4478.107   HEALD, CHARLES BREHMER. 1879-
Injuries and sport. A general guide for the practitioner. London, *Oxford Univ.
Press,* 1931.
    The first English treatise on sports medicine.

4478.108   MEANWELL, WALTER ERNEST. 1884-1953 & ROCKNE, KNUTE KENNETH. 1888-1931
Training, conditioning, and the care of injuries. Madison, Wisc., *W.E.
Meanwell,* 1931.
    The first American book on sports medicine, co-authored by the
legendary football coach, Knute Rockne.

4478.109   STEVENS, MARVIN ALLEN & PHELPS, WINTHROP MORGAN. 1894-
The control of football injuries. New York, *A.S. Barnes,* 1933.
    Apparently the first book on the prevention and treatment of injuries in
a single sport, written after fifty players were killed in the 1931 American

football season. Stevens was a surgeon who became head football coach at Yale University. Phelps was professor of orthopaedics at Yale.

4478.110   PALMER, IVOR.
On the injuries to the ligaments of the knee joint: A clinical study. *Acta. chir. Scand.*, 1938, **81**, Suppl. 53.
Classic study of knee ligament injuries.

4478.111   GUTTMANN, *Sir* LUDWIG. 1899-1980
Textbook of sports for the disabled. Aylesbury, *H.M.&M. Publishers*, 1976.
Pioneer treatise on sports for the handicapped by the physician who first introduced archery competition as a therapeutic measure for paraplegic war veterans in 1948.

History of Orthopaedic Surgery

4479   KEITH, *Sir* ARTHUR. 1866-1955
Menders of the maimed. London, *H. Frowde*, 1919.
Gives details of the work of John Hunter, John Hilton, Hugh Owen Thomas, Little, Stromeyer, Marshall Hall, Arbuthnot Lane, Syme, Julius Wolff, etc., in the development of modern orthopaedics. Second edition, 1925. Facsimile reprint of first edition, 1952. Reprinted, Malabar, Fl., *Krieger*, 1975.

4480   OSGOOD, ROBERT BAYLEY. 1873-1956
The evolution of orthopaedic surgery. St. Louis, *C. V. Mosby*, [1925].

4481   BLENCKE, AUGUST. 1869-1937, & GOCHT, HERMANN. 1869-1938.
Die orthopädische Weltliteratur 1903-30. Herausg. von A. BLENCKE und H. GOCHT. (Ergänzungsband 1931-35, hrsg, von E. WITTE.) 3 vols. Stuttgart, *F. Enke*, 1936-38.

4482   BICK, EDGAR MILTON. 1902-1978
Source book of orthopaedics. 2nd ed. Baltimore, *Williams & Wilkins*, 1948.
A concise, thematic history of orthopaedic surgery from the earliest times. Includes a useful bibliography. Reprinted 1968.

4483   ORR, HIRAM WINNETT. 1877-1956
On the contributions of Hugh Owen Thomas of Liverpool, Sir Robert Jones of Liverpool and London, John Ridlon, M.D., of New York and Chicago, to modern orthopedic surgery. Springfield, *C. C. Thomas*, 1949.

4483.1   VALENTIN, BRUNO. 1885-1969
Geschichte der Orthopädie. Stuttgart, *Georg Thieme*, 1961.

4483.2   RANG, MERCER CHARLES.
Anthology of orthopaedics. Edinburgh, *E. & S. Livingstone*, 1966.
Selections (often abridged) from classic primary sources, arranged thematically, with commentary.

4483.3   BICK, EDGAR MILTON. 1902-1978
Classics of orthopaedics. Philadelphia, *Lippincott*, 1976.

Eighty classic papers and sections from books, reprinted from the series of articles in *Clinical Orthopaedics and Related Research*.

4483.4   SHANDS, Alfred Rives, Jr. 1899-
The early orthopaedic surgeons of America. St. Louis, *C.V. Mosby*, 1970.

4483.5   BOYES, Joseph H.
On the shoulders of giants. Notable names in hand surgery. Philadelphia, *Lippincott*, [1976].
A history of hand surgery.

4483.6   PELTIER, Leonard F. 1920-
Fractures: a history and iconography of their treatment. San Francisco, *Norman Publishing*, 1990.

RHEUMATISM AND GOUT

4484   ARETAEUS, *the Cappadocian*. A.D. 81-?138
On arthritis and sciatica. In his *Extant works,* transl. by F. Adams, London, 1856, 362-65, 492-93.

4484.1   BURGAUER, Dominicus. *fl.* 1534
Ob das Podagra möglich zu generen oder nit. Nutzlich zu wissen allen denen, die damit behafft. Straszburg, *M. Apiarius*, 1534.
First known medical monograph on gout. Abridged English translation by W. S. C. Copeman and M. Winder in *Med. Hist.*, 1969, **13**, 288-93.

4485   BAILLOU, Guillaume de [Ballonius]. 1538-1616
Liber de rheumatismo et pleuritide dorsale. Parisiis, *J. Quesnel*, 1642.
De Baillou introduced the term "rheumatism". He was court physician in Paris at the time of Henri IV. His book, the first on rheumatism, was translated into English by C. C. Barnard in *Brit. J. Rheum.*, London, 1940, **2**, 141-62.

4485.1   LA MARTINIÈRE, Pierre Martin de. 1634-1690
Traité de la maladie vénérienne, de ses causes et des accidens provenans du mercure, ou vif-argent. Paris, *L'autheur*, 1664.
First to describe gonococcal arthritis.

4486   SYDENHAM, Thomas. 1624-1689
Tractatus de podagra et hydrope. Londini, *G. Kettilby*, 1683.
Of the many great works of Sydenham, this is considered his masterpiece. He clearly differentiated gout from rheumatism. For an English translation, see his *Works*, published by the Sydenham Society, 1850, **2**, 123-84.

4487   CHEYNE, George. 1671-1743
Observations concerning the nature and due method of treating the gout. London, *G. Strahan, W. Mears*, 1720.

4488   SWIETEN, Gerard L. B. van. 1700-1772
Podagra. In his *Commentaria in Hermanni Boerhaave aphorismos de cognoscendis et curandis morbis.* Lugduni Batavorum, *J. & H. Verbeek,* 1764, **4**, 287-393.

4489   CADOGAN, William. 1711-1797
A dissertation on the gout, and all chronic diseases, jointly considered, as proceeding from the same causes; what those causes are; and a rational and natural method of cure proposed. London, *J. Dodsley,* 1771.
        This book excited great attention and ran through eight editions in one year. Cadogan's advice on moderate exercise and moderation in drinking as a cure for gout caused much criticism. Indirectly through this work Cadogan became a friend of David Garrick, at whose death he was present. A reprint of the 10th edition of this essay appears in *Ann. med. Hist.,* 1925, **7**, 67-90.

4490   LANDRÉ-BEAUVAIS, Augustin Jacob. 1772-1840
Doit-on admettre une nouvelle espèce de goutte sous la dénomination de goutte asthénique primitive? Paris, *J. Brosson,* an VIII [1800].
        Landré-Beauvais gave the first reasonably accurate description of rheumatoid arthritis.

4491   HEBERDEN, William, *Snr.* 1710-1801
De nodis digitorum. In his *Commentarii de morborum historia.* Londini, *T. Payne,* 1802, p. 130.
        Heberden described a form of rheumatic gout in which nodules ("Heberden's nodes") appeared at the interphalangeal joints of the fingers.

4492   HAYGARTH, John. 1740-1827
A clinical history of diseases. Part first: being 1. A clinical history of the acute rheumatism. 2. A clinical history of the nodosity of the joints. London, *Cadell & Davies,* 1805.
        Haygarth was a pioneer epidemiologist in England. He demonstrated the uselessness of Elisha Perkins's metallic tractors by obtaining the same results with wooden ones. This is the first monograph on acute rheumatism.

4493   MITCHELL, John Kearsley. 1793-1858
On a new practice in acute and chronic rheumatism. *Amer. J. med. Sci.,* 1831, **8**, 55-64.
        First description of the neurotic spinal arthropathies.

4494   BOUILLAUD, Jean Baptiste. 1796-1881.
Traité clinique du rhumatisme articulaire. Paris, *J. B. Baillière,* 1840.
        Extension of Bouillaud's work on the coincidence of heart disease and acute rheumatism. He regarded fever as the effect of endocarditis (*see also* No. 2749).

4495   GARROD, *Sir* Alfred Baring. 1819-1907
Observations on certain pathological conditions of the blood and urine in gout, rheumatism and Bright's disease. *Med.-chir. Trans.,* 1848, **31**, 83-97; 1854, **37**, 49-59.
        The "thread test" in gout was introduced by Garrod. Later he wrote more fully on gout and rheumatism (*see* No. 4497).

4496   ADAMS, ROBERT. 1791-1875
A treatise on rheumatic gout, or chronic rheumatic arthritis, of all the joints.
London, *J. Churchill*, 1857.
    An excellent description of chronic rheumatic arthritis. Adams also
published *Illustrations of the effects of rheumatic gout*, London, 1857.

4497   GARROD, *Sir* ALFRED BARING. 1819-1907
The nature and treatment of gout and rheumatic gout. London, *Walton &*
Maberly, 1859.
    Garrod was the leading authority of his time on gout, which he
separated from other forms of arthritis by his discovery of excess of uric
acid in the blood of gouty sufferers. He gave to rheumatoid arthritis its
present name.

4498   CHARCOT, JEAN MARTIN. 1825-1893, & CORNIL, ANDRÉ VICTOR. 1837-1898
Contributions à l'étude des altérations anatomiques de la goutte. *C. R. Soc.*
Biol. (Mémoires), (1863), 1864, 3 sér., **5**, 139-63.
    Charcot and Cornil gave an important description of the renal lesions in
gout.

4499   CORNIL, ANDRÉ VICTOR. 1837-1898
Mémoire sur les coincidences pathologiques du rhumatisme articulaire
chronique. *C. R. Soc. Biol. (Paris), (Mémoires),* 1864, 4 sér., **1**, 3-25.
    First description of chronic arthritis in childhood.

4499.1   MEYNET, PAUL. 1831-1892
Rhumatisme articulaire subaigu avec production de tumeurs multiples
dans les tissus fibreux périarticulaires et sur le périoste d'un grand nombre
d'os. *Lyon méd.,* 1875, **20**, 495-99.
    Meynet was the first to draw special attention to the subcutaneous
fibroid nodules in rheumatism.

4500   BESNIER, ERNEST. 1831-1909
Rhumatisme. *Dict. encyclopéd. Sci. méd.,* Paris, 1876, 3 sér., **4**, 446-819.
    Besnier wrote an important description of rheumatism.

4501   MACLAGAN, THOMAS JOHN. 1838-1903
The treatment of acute rheumatism by salicin. *Lancet,* 1876, **1**, 342-43, 383-84.
    Introduction of salicylates in the treatment of rheumatism.

4501.1   FOWLER, *Sir* JAMES KINGSTON. 1852-1934
On the association of affections of the throat with acute rheumatism.
Lancet, 1880, **2**, 933-34.
    Fowler drew attention to the association of throat infections with acute
rheumatism.

4502   EBSTEIN, WILHELM. 1836-1912
Das Regimen bei der Gicht. Wiesbaden, *J. F. Bergmann,* 1885.
    A pupil of Frerichs, Virchow, and Romberg, Ebstein became Professor
of Medicine at Göttingen.

4502.1   HÖCK, HEINRICH.
Ein Beitrag zur Arthritis blennorrhoica. *Wien. klin. Wschr.,* 1893, **6**, 736-38.
    Gonococci isolated from an arthritic joint.

4503   STILL, *Sir* GEORGE FREDERIC. 1868-1941
        On a form of chronic joint disease in children. *Med.-chir. Trans.*, 1896-97,
        80, 47-59.
            "Still's disease", chronic articular rheumatism in children. *See also* Nos.
        4499 and 6356.

4504   PONCET, ANTONIN. 1849-1913
        Polyarthrite tuberculeuse simulant des lésions rhumatismales chroniques
        déformantes. *Gaz. Hôp.* (*Paris*), 1897, **70**, 1219.
            Tuberculous rheumatism ("Poncet's disease"). See also his later paper
        in *Bull. Acad. Méd.* (*Paris*), 1902, 3 sér., **48**, 97-114.

4504.1 TRIBOULET, HENRI. 1864-1920, & COYON, AMAND. 1871-1928
        Bactériologie du rhumatisme articulaire. Endocardite végétante mitrale
        provoquée chez le lapin par inoculation intra-veineuse d'un cocco-bacille
        en points doubles extraits du sang du rhumatisme articulaire aigu de
        l'homme. *C. R. Soc. Biol.*, 1898, **50**, 124-28.
            Isolation of streptococci from patients with acute rheumatism reported.

4505   POYNTON, FREDERICK JOHN. 1869-1943, & PAINE, ALEXANDER.
        The etiology of rheumatic fever. *Lancet*, 1900, **2**, 861-69, 932-35.
            After extensive bacteriological researches, Poynton and Paine considered
        that a diplococcus was the cause of rheumatic fever.

4505.1 NICOLAIER, ARTHUR. 1862-?, & DOHRN, MAX.
        Ueber die Wirkung von Chinolincarbonsäuren und ihrer Derivate auf die
        Ausscheidung der Harnsäure. *Dtsch. Arch. klin. Med.*, 1908, **93**, 331-55.
            Introduction of cinchophen in the treatment of gout.

4506   FELTY, AUGUSTUS ROI. 1895-
        Chronic arthritis in the adult, associated with splenomegaly and leucopenia.
        Johns Hopk. Hosp. Bull., 1924, **35**, 16-20.
            "Felty syndrome".

4506.1 FORESTIER, JACQUES. 1890-
        L'aurothérapie dans les rhumatismes chroniques. *Bull. Soc. méd. Hôp.
        Paris*, 1929, 323-27.
            Introduction of gold therapy.

4507   SCHLESINGER, BERNARD. 1896-1984
        The relationship of throat infection to acute rheumatism in childhood.
        Arch. Dis. Childh., 1930, **5**, 411-30.
            Schlesinger showed that haemolytic streptococcal infection was a
        cause of acute rheumatism in children.

4508   HENCH, PHILIP SHOWALTER. 1896-1965, *et al.*
        The effects of a hormone of the adrenal cortex (17-hydroxy-11-
        dehydrocorticosterone: compound E) and of pituitary adrenocorticotropic
        hormone on rheumatoid arthritis. *Proc. Mayo Clin.*, 1949, **24**, 181-97.
            Introduction of cortisone and A.C.T.H. in treatment of rheumatoid
        arthritis. With E. C. Kendall, C. H. Slocumb, and H. F. Polley. Hench and
        Kendall shared a Nobel Prize with T. Reichstein (No. 1153) in 1950.

4509   ——. The effects of the adrenal cortical hormone 17-hydroxy-11-dehydrocorticosterone (compound E) on the acute phase of rheumatic fever: preliminary report. *Proc. Mayo Clin.*, 1949, **24**, 277-97.

Compound E (cortisone) introduced in the treatment of rheumatic fever. With C. H. Slocumb, A. R. Barnes, H. L. Smith, H. F. Polley, and E. C. Kendall.

4509.1   COPEMAN, William Sydney Charles. 1900-1970
A short history of the gout and the rheumatic diseases. Berkeley, *University of California Press*, 1964.

DISEASES OF THE NERVOUS SYSTEM

4510   ARETAEUS, *the Cappadocian*. A.D. 81-?138
On paralysis. In his *Extant works,* transl. by F. Adams, London, 1856, 305-09.

4511   GALEN. A.D. 130-200
De tremore, palpitatione, convulsione, et rigore. In *Opera omnia*, ed. cur. C. G. Kühn, Lipsiae, C. *Cnobloch*, 1824, **7**, 584-642.

Complete English translation by D.Sider and M. McVaugh in *Trans. stud. Coll. Phys. Phila.*, 1979, **1**, 183-210.

4511.01   ALBERTI, Johannes Michael
De omnibus ingeniis augede memorie. Bologna, *Franciscus (Plato) de Benedictis*, 1491.

An early work on memory disorders and aids to memory.

4511.02   PRATENSIS, Jason. 1486-1558
De cerebri morbis...Basileae, *Per Henrichum Petri*, [1549].

The first book devoted entirely to brain disorders, including tremor, tetanus, vertigo, epilepsy and hemicrania.

4511.1   PLATTER, Felix [Plater]. 1536-1614
Observationum in hominis affectibus. Basileae, *L. König*, 1614.

On p. 13 is recorded an account of a meningioma.

4511.2   WEPFER, Johann Jacob. 1620-1695
Observationes anatomicae, ex cadaveribus eorum, quos sustulit apoplexia. Schaffhusii, *J. C. Suteri*, 1658.

Wepfer showed apoplexy to be a result of haemorrhage into the brain. He described four cases, with clinical and post mortem findings. He preceded Willis (No. 1378) in describing the "circle of Willis". Partial English translation in Ruskin, *Classics in arterial hypertension* (1956).

4512   FEHR, Johannes Michael. 1610-1688, & SCHMIDT, Elias.
Naturae genius, medicorum Celsus, Jason Argonautarum, Bauschius occubuit. *Misc. Cur. med.-phys. Acad. nat. cur.*, Jenae, 1671, **2**.

First authentic case of trigeminal neuralgia. It concerned J. L. Bausch, who died from the condition in 1665. The account is to be found in the unpaged part of the volume, starting at sig. *d* 3 and occupying the two following pages.

4513   WILLIS, Thomas. 1621-1675
        De anima brutorum. Oxonii, *imp. R. Davis*, 1672.
        Part 2, Cap. I, deals with headache.

4514   SYDENHAM, Thomas. 1624-1689
        Schedula monitoria de novae febris ingressu. Londini, *G. Kettilby*, 1686.
        Includes (pp. 25-28) his classic description of chorea minor ("Sydenham's chorea"). Reprinted in *Med. Classics*, 1939, **4**, 327-53. In the Sydenham Society translation (*see* No. 64) the passage occurs in vol. 2, pp. 198-99.

4515   COTUGNO, Domenico. 1736-1822
        De ischiade nervosa commentarius. Neapoli, *apud frat. Simonios,* 1764.
        Cotugno published a classic description of sciatica, which is useful even today. He recognized two types – arthritic and nervous; the latter has been called "Cotugno's disease", and his book is confined to that type. The book, which also describes a case of acute nephritis, appeared in English in 1775. *See* Nos. 1382 & 4204.2.

4516   FOTHERGILL, John. 1712-1780
        Of a painful affection of the face. *Med. Obs. Inqu.*, 1776, **5**, 129-42.
        Original description of facial neuralgia. Reprinted in *Med. Classics*, 1940, **5**, 100-06.

4517   ——. Remarks on that complaint commonly known under the name of the sick head-ach. *Med. Obs. & Inqu.*, London, 1777-84, **6**, 103-37.
        First accurate description of migraine.

4518   FRANK, Johann Peter. 1745-1821
        De vertebralis columnae in morbis dignitate. In his *Delectus opusculorum medicorum*, Ticini, 1792, **11**, 1-50.
        Frank, best remembered for his great services to public health, was the first physician to emphasize the gravity of diseases of the spinal cord.

4519   FRIEDREICH, Nicolaus Anton 1761-1836
        De paralysi musculorum faciei rheumatici. Wirceburgi, 1797.
        Facial paralysis first described.

4519.1 CHEYNE, John. 1777-1836
        Cases of apoplexy and lethargy: with observations upon the comatose diseases. London, *Thomas Underwood*, 1812.
        Cheyne believed that cerebral anaemia might be the cause of apoplexy, and described pathological cases of cerebral infarction and of cerebral haemorrhage. The work contains the first illustration of a subarachnoid haemorrhage.

4519.2 COOKE, John. 1756-1838
        A treatise on nervous diseases. 2 vols., London, *Longman*, 1820-23.
        "The earliest separate work on clinical neurology" (McHenry). Includes the Croonian lecture (1819) on apoplexy, and sections on palsy and epilepsy. The work includes the first history of neurological thought.

4520   BELL, *Sir* CHARLES. 1774-1842
        On the nerves; giving an account of some experiments on their structure
        and functions, which lead to a new arrangement of the system. *Phil. Trans.*,
        1821, **111**, 398-424.
        "Bell's palsy". The facial paralysis ensuing upon lesion of the motor
        nerve of the face is here for the first time described. See also his later paper,
        with more detailed description, in the same journal, 1829, **119**, 317-30.
        Reprinted in *Med. Classics*, 1936, **1**, 152-69.

4521   JACKSON, JAMES. 1777-1867
        On a peculiar disease resulting from the use of ardent spirits. *New Engl. J.
        Med. Surg.*, 1822, **2**, 351-53.
        Jackson drew attention to alcoholic neuritis – arthrodynia *a potu*.
        Jackson was professor at Boston Medical School.

4522   PARRY, CALEB HILLIER. 1755-1822
        Facial hemiatrophy. In *Collections from the unpublished writings...* Lon-
        don, 1825, **1**, 478-80.
        Parry was the first to record cases of facial hemiatrophy.

4523   WOOD, WILLIAM. 1774-1857
        Observations on neuroma. *Trans. med.-chir. Soc. Edinb.*, 1828-29, **3**, 367-433.
        Neuroma first described.

4524   ADDISON, THOMAS. 1793-1860
        On the influence of electricity, as a remedy in certain convulsive and
        spasmodic diseases. *Guy's Hosp. Rep.*, 1837, **2**, 493-507.
        First therapeutic employment of static electricity.

4525   STANLEY, EDWARD. 1793-1862
        A case of disease in the posterior columns of the spinal cord. *Med.-chir.
        Trans.*, 1839-40, **23**, 80-84.
        Stanley was the first to describe disease of the posterior columns of the
        spinal cord.

4526   VALLEIX, FRANÇOIS LOUIS ISIDORE. 1807-1855
        Traité des névralgies ou affections douloureuses des nerfs. Paris, *J. B.
        Baillière*, 1841.
        Includes (p. 40 *et seq.*) description of "Valleix's points", tender points on
        the course of certain nerves in neuralgia.

4527   ROMBERG, MORITZ HEINRICH. 1795-1873
        Klinische Ergebnisse. Berlin, *A. Förstner*, 1846.
        Includes (p. 75) a classic description of facial hemiatrophy – "Romberg's
        disease".

4528   ———. Lehrbuch der Nervenkrankheiten des Menschen. Bd. 1. Berlin, *A.
        Duncker*, 1846.
        Romberg inaugurated the modern era in the study of diseases of the
        nervous system. His *Lehrbuch* is the first formal treatise in this field. On p.
        795 is to be found the original description of "Romberg's sign",
        pathognomonic of tabes dorsalis. English translation, 1853.

4529   SMITH, ROBERT WILLIAM. 1807-1873.
A treatise on the pathology, diagnosis, and treatment of neuroma. Dublin, *Hodges & Smith*, 1849.
Includes a full description of generalized neurofibromatosis ("Recklinghausen's disease"; *see* No. 4566).

4530   BROWN-SÉQUARD, CHARLES ÉDOUARD. 1817-1894
De la transmission croisée des impressions sensitives par la moëlle épinière. *C. R. Soc. Biol. (Paris)*, (1850), 1851, **2**, 33-34.
"Brown-Séquard's paralysis". Lesion of one lateral half of the spinal cord causes paralysis of motion on one side and of sensation on the other. See also the writer's later paper on pp. 70-73 of the same volume.

4531   GUBLER, ADOLPHE. 1821-1897
De l'hémiplégie alterne envisagée comme signe de lésion de la protrubérance annulaire et comme preuve de la décussation des nerfs faciaux. *Gaz. hebd. Méd. Chir.*, 1856, **3**, 749-54, 789-92, 811-16.
"Gubler's paralysis" – crossed hemiplegia. English translation in Wolf, *The classical brain stem syndromes*, Springfield, *Thomas*, 1971.

4532   GULL, *Sir* WILLIAM WITHEY. 1816-1890
Cases of paraplegia [with autopsies of ataxic cases, showing lesions in the posterior columns of the spinal cord]. *Guy's Hosp. Rep.*, 1856, 3 ser., **2**, 143-90; 1858, 3 ser., **4**, 169-216.
Gull showed the lesions of tabes dorsalis to be located in the posterior columns of the spinal cord.

4533   FOVILLE, ACHILLE LOUIS FRANÇOIS. 1799-1878
Note sur une paralysie peu connue de certains muscles de l'oeil, et sa liaison avec quelques points de l'anatomie et la physiologie de la protubérance annulaire. *Bull. Soc. Anat. Paris*, 1858, **33**, 393-414.
"Foville's syndrome" – crossed paralysis of the limbs on one side of the body and of the face on the other side, together with loss of ability to rotate the eyes to that side. English translation in Wolf, *The classical brain stem syndromes*, Springfield, *Thomas*, 1971.

4534   REMAK, ROBERT. 1815-1865
Galvanotherapie der Nerven- und Muskelkrankheiten. Berlin, *A. Hirschwald*, 1858.
Remak was a pioneer of galvanotherapy, and this was a leading German language textbook on the subject.

4535   BOUCHUT, EUGÈNE. 1818-1891
De l'état nerveux aigu et chronique ou nervosisme. Paris, *J. B. Baillière*, 1860.
First adequate description of neurasthenia.

4536   GRAEFE, FRIEDRICH WILHELM ERNST ALBRECHT VON. 1828-1870
Ueber Complication von Sehnervenentzündung mit Gehirnkrankheiten. *v. Graefes Arch. Ophthal.*, 1860, **7**, 2 Abt., 58-71.
Graefe showed that most cases of blindness and impaired vision connected with cerebral disorders can be traced to optic neuritis rather than paralysis of the optic nerve.

4537   JACKSON, JOHN HUGHLINGS. 1835-1911
        Observations on defects of sight in brain disease. *Ophthal. Hosp. Rep.*, 1863-65, **4**, 10-19, 389-446; 1865-66, **5**, 51-78, 251-306.
        In this work Jackson showed the importance of the ophthalmoscope in the investigation of diseases of the nervous system. Reprinted in *Med. Classics*, 1939, **3**, 918-26.

4538   WEBER, *Sir* HERMANN DAVID. 1823-1918
        A contribution to the pathology of the crura cerebri. *Med.-chir. Trans.*, 1863, **46**, 121-39.
        "Weber's syndrome" or "Weber–Gubler syndrome" – hemiplegia associated with disease of the crura cerebri; first described by Gubler (No. 4531).

4538.1 ERICHSEN, Sir JOHN ERIC. 1818-1896
        On railway and other injuries of the nervous system. London, *Walton & Maberly*, 1866.
        The first book to discuss the injuries now widely known as whiplash, which first appeared as the by-product of the increased speed of railway travel.

4539   WILKS, *Sir* SAMUEL, *Bart*. 1824-1911
        Drunkard's or alcoholic paraplegia. *Med. Times Gaz.*, 1868, **2**, 470.
        Classic account of alcoholic paraplegia.

4540   ROBERTSON, DOUGLAS MORAY COOPER LAMB ARGYLL. 1837-1909
        On an interesting series of eye symptoms in a case of spinal disease, with remarks on the action of belladonna on the iris. *Edinb. med. J.*, 1869, **14**, 696-708.
        "Argyll Robertson pupil" first described. See also his later paper in the same journal, 1869, **15**, 487-93. Reprinted in *Med. Classics*, 1937, **1**, 851-76.

4541   BRUNS, PAUL VON. 1846-1916
        Das Rankenneurom. Tübingen, *H. Laupp*, 1870.
        Original description of plexiform neurofibroma.

4542   HAMMOND, WILLIAM ALEXANDER. 1828-1900
        Treatise on diseases of the nervous system. New York, *D. Appleton & Co.*, 1871.
        The first American treatise on neurology. The original description of athetosis, sometimes called "Hammond's disease", appears on pp. 654-62. During his tenure as Surgeon General of the Army during the U.S. Civil War, Hammond established the U.S. Army Hospital for Diseases of the Nervous System.

4543   DUCHENNE DE BOULOGNE, GUILLAUME BENJAMIN AMAND. 1806-1875.
        De l'électrisation localisée et de son application à la pathologie et à la thérapeutique. 3me. éd. Paris, *J. B. Baillière*, 1872.
        Early description, page 357, of partial brachial plexus paralysis, upper type ("Duchenne-Erb palsy": *see* No. 4548). An English translation of the 3rd ed., by H. Tibbitts, actually appeared in Philadelphia in 1871, one year before the French edition. The translator states that he prepared the translation from sheets of the 3rd edition, the publication of which was delayed by the German occupation of Paris.

4544   MITCHELL, SILAS WEIR. 1829-1914
Injuries of nerves and their consequences. Philadelphia, *J. B. Lippincott & Co.*, 1872.
Includes the first description of ascending neuritis, and also of the treatment of neuritis by cold and splint rests. The book was written as a result of Mitchell's experiences in the American Civil War. *See* No. 2167.

4545   ——. Clinical lecture on certain painful affections of the feet. *Philad. med. Times*, 1872, **3**, 81-82, 113-115.
Mitchell suggested the name "erythromelalgia" for this condition, which is also known as "Mitchell's disease". He records four earlier writers on the subject, the first being Graves in 1848. See also his paper in *Amer. J. med. Sci.*, 1878, **76**, 17-36.

4546   CHARCOT, JEAN MARTIN. 1825-1893
Leçons sur les maladies du système nerveux faites à La Salpêtrière. 3 vols. Paris, *A. Delahaye,* 1872-87.
An excellent idea of Charcot's work is gained by perusal of his *Leçons*, dealing with his teaching on nervous disorders. In the second volume, pp. 1-72, is a classic account of the anomalies of tabes dorsalis. Charcot became one of the greatest of all neurologists. English translation, 1877-89.

4547   JACKSON, JOHN HUGHLINGS. 1835-1911
On a case of paralysis of the tongue from haemorrhage in the medulla oblongata. *Lancet*, 1872, **2**, 770-73.
Jackson here described the syndrome consisting of paralysis of half the tongue, the same half of the palate, and of one vocal cord – "Jackson's syndrome".

4548   ERB, WILHELM HEINRICH. 1840-1921
Ueber eine eigenthümliche Localisation von Lähmungen im Plexus brachialis. *Verh. nat.-med. Vereins. Heidelb.*, 1873-77, n.F. **1**, 130-36.
"Erb's palsy", first described by Smellie in 1763 and later by Duchenne (No. 4543).

4549   LIVEING, EDWARD. 1832-1919
On megrim, sick-headache, and some allied disorders. London, *J. & A. Churchill*, 1873.
Liveing's classic account of migraine showed the close association of this condition with tetany, asthma, and false angina pectoris, with epilepsy, and the alternation of all these conditions in the same subject or the transference permanently from one to another.

4550   LEYDEN, ERNST VON. 1832-1910
Klinik der Rückenmarks-Krankheiten. 2 vols. Berlin, *A. Hirschwald,* 1874-75.
One of Leyden's best works. He was Professor of Medicine at Berlin, Königsberg, and Strassburg. In vol. 2, p. 65, of the above is given an account of "Leyden's paralysis", a form of hemiplegia probably first described in 1856 by Gubler (*see* No. 4531).

4551   MITCHELL, SILAS WEIR. 1829-1914
Headaches, from heat-stroke, from fevers, after meningitis, from overuse of brain, from eyestrain. *Med. surg. Reporter*, 1874, **31**, 67-71.
Mitchell drew attention to the importance of eyestrain as a cause of headache.

4552   ———. Post-paralytic chorea. *Amer. J. med. Sci.*, 1874, **68**, 342-52.
            First description.

4553   ———. On rest in the treatment of nervous disease. New York, *G. P. Putnam's Sons*, 1875.
            First account of the "Weir Mitchell treatment".

4554   ———. Fat and blood and how to make them. Philadelphia, *J. B. Lippincott & Co.*, 1877.
            Includes full account of Weir Mitchell's rest cure for nervous disorders.

4555   ———. The relation of pain to weather, being a study of the natural history of a case of traumatic neuralgia. *Amer. J. med. Sci.*, 1877, **73**, 305-29.
            First study of the subject.

4556   ERB, WILHELM HEINRICH. 1840-1921.
            Ueber einen wenig bekannten spinalen Symptomencomplex. *Berl. klin. Wschr.*, 1875, **12**, 357-59.
            "Erb–Charcot disease" (spastic spinal paralysis).

4557   ———. Handbuch der Krankheiten des Nervensystems. 2 vols. Leipzig, *F. C. W. Vogel*, 1876-78.
            Erb was Professor of Neurology at Heidelberg. He gave the original descriptions of several nervous disorders, especially the muscular dystrophies, and was a pioneer in the use of electrotherapy.

4558   CHARCOT, JEAN MARTIN. 1825-1893
            Leçons sur les localisations dans les maladies du cerveau. 2 vols. Paris, *Progrès médical & V. A. Delahaye*, 1876-80.
            Charcot is especially notable for his important study of the localization of functions in diseases of the brain. Volume two is entitled *Leçons sur les localisations dans les maladies du cerveau et de la moëlle épinière...* English translation (New Sydenham Society), 1883.

4558.1   BOURNEVILLE, DÉSIRÉ MAGLOIRE (1840-1909) and REGNARD, PAUL (1850-1927).
            Iconographie photographique de la Salpêtrière. Service de M. Charcot. 3 vols. Paris, *Bureaux du Progrès Médical; V. Adrien Delahaye & Cie. [Vol. III: V. Adrien Delahaye et Lecroisnier]*, 1876-80.
            A photographic atlas devoted to cases of hysteria and epilepsy, with case histories; the third volume includes discussions of hypnotism, somnambulism and magnetism. Bourneville was Charcot's assistant at the Salpêtrière from 1870-79. See No. 4575.

4559   BERNHARDT, MARTIN. 1844-1915
            Neuropathologische Beobachtungen. *Dtsch. Arch. klin. Med.*, 1878, **22**, 362-93.
            Bernhardt drew attention to meralgia paraesthetica in the leg ("Bernhardt's disease") due to disease of the external cutaneous nerve of the thigh.

4560   NOTHNAGEL, CARL WILHELM HERMANN. 1841-1905
            Topische Diagnostik der Gehirnkrankheiten. Berlin, *A. Hirschwald*, 1879.
            On p. 220 is the description of unilateral oculomotor paralysis combined with cerebellar ataxia, "Nothnagel's syndrome".

4560.1   STURGE, WILLIAM ALLEN. 1850-1919
A case of partial epilepsy, apparently due to a lesion of one of the vasomotor centres of the brain. *Trans. clin. Soc. Lond.*, 1879, **12**, 162-67.
"Sturge–Weber syndrome" – association of a port-wine naevus in the skin of the face with a vascular abnormality of the meninges on the same side. *See* No. 4605.2.

4561   GÉLINEAU, JEAN BAPTISTE EDOUARD. 1859-
De la narcolepsie. *Gaz. Hôp.* (*Paris*), 1880, **53**, 626-28, 635-37.
Narcolepsy first fully described.

4562   GOWERS, *Sir* WILLIAM RICHARD. 1845-1915
The diagnosis of diseases of the spinal cord. London, *J. & A. Churchill*, 1880.
Gowers demonstrated the dorsal spinocerebellar tract, "Gowers's tract", and introduced the terms *myotatic* and *knee-jerk,* which he elicited with the rubber edge of his stethoscope or a percussion hammer.

4563   FORST, J. J.
Contribution à l'étude clinique de la sciatique. Paris, *Thèse No.* 33, 1881.
"Lasègue's sign" in sciatica. Although discovered by E. C. Lasègue, it was first reported by his pupil Forst.

4564   FRIEDREICH, NIKOLAUS. 1825-1882
Paramyoklonus multiplex. *Virchows Arch. path. Anat.*, 1881, **86**, 421-30.
First description of paramyoclonus multiplex, "Friedreich's disease".

4565   BRAMWELL, *Sir* BYROM. 1847-1931
The diseases of the spinal cord. Edinburgh, *Maclachlan & Stewart*, 1882.

4566   RECKLINGHAUSEN, FRIEDRICH DANIEL VON. 1833-1910
Ueber die multiplen Fibrome der Haut und ihre Beziehung zu den multiplen Neuromen. Berlin, *Hirschwald,* 1882.
"Recklinghausen's disease" (*see* No. 4082).

4566.1   CLELAND, JOHN. 1835-1925
Contribution to the study of spina bifida, encephalocele, and anencephalus. *J. Anat. Physiol.* (*London*), 1883, **17**, 257-91.
Early description of the Arnold–Chiari malformation (*see* Nos. 4577.1, 4581.1).

4567   MÖBIUS, PAUL JULIUS. 1853-1907
Ueber periodisch wiederkehrende Oculomotoriuslähmung. *Berl. klin. Wschr.*, 1884, **21**, 604-08.
"Möbius's disease" – ophthalmoplegic migraine.

4568   GOWERS, *Sir* WILLIAM RICHARD. 1845-1915
Lectures on the diagnosis of diseases of the brain. London, *J. & A. Churchill,* 1885.

4569   ——. A manual of diseases of the nervous system. 2 vols. London, *J. & A. Churchill,* 1886-88.
Gowers was physician and Professor of Clinical Medicine at University College, London. He especially distinguished himself in the field of neurology, and the above book is his greatest work. Gowers was interested

in stenography, advised his students to take down his lectures in short-hand, and founded the Society of Medical Phonographers. *See* No. 4751. Biography by Macdonald Critchley, London, 1949.

4570   BASTIAN, HENRY CHARLTON. 1837-1915
Paralyses, cerebral, bulbar and spinal. London, *H. K. Lewis*, 1886.
Bastian was one of the founders of English neurology. He is remembered for "Bastian's law" (*see* No. 4577).

4571   MACKENZIE, *Sir* STEPHEN. 1844-1909
Two cases of associated paralysis of the tongue, soft palate, and vocal cord on the same side. *Trans. clin. Soc. Lond.*, 1886, **19**, 317-19.
"Mackenzie's syndrome".

4572   PANAS, PHOTINOS. 1832-1903
D'un nouveau procédé opératoire applicable au ptosis congénital et au ptosis paralytique. *Arch. Ophthal.*, 1886, **6**, 1-14.
An operation for congenital and paralytic ptosis was introduced by Panas.

4573   BLOCQ, PAUL. 1860-1896
Sur une affection caractérisée par de l'astasie et de l'abasie. *Arch. Neurol.* (*Paris*), 1888, **15**, 24-51, 187-211.
"Blocq's disease" – astasia–abasia.

4574   BRAMWELL, *Sir* BYROM. 1847-1931
Intracranial tumours. Edinburgh, *Y. J. Pentland*, 1888.

4575   NOUVELLE ICONOGRAPHIE DE LA SALPÊTRIÈRE.
28 vols. Paris, 1888-1918.
Henry Meige, Richer, and other pupils of Charcot published many valuable studies of the constitutional aspects of nervous diseases in the above work, an album unique in the history of medicine and of great value for the study of nervous diseases. This journal is the successor to No. 4558.1.

4576   BENEDIKT, MORITZ. 1835-1920
Tremblement avec paralysie croisée du moteur oculaire commun. *Bull. méd.* (*Paris*), 1889, **3**, 547-48.
"Benedikt's syndrome" – paralysis of the oculomotor nerve on one side with intensive trembling of the other side. English translation in Wolf, *The classical brain stem syndromes*, Springfield, *Thomas*, 1971.

4577   BASTIAN, HENRY CHARLTON. 1837-1915
On the symptomatology of total transverse lesions of the spinal cord, with special reference to the condition of the various reflexes. *Med.-chir. Trans.*, 1890, **73**, 151-217.
"Bastian's law", transverse lesion of the cord above the lumbar enlargement results in the abolition of the tendon reflexes of the lower extremities.

4577.1   CHIARI, HANS. 1851-1916
Ueber Veränderungen des Kleinhirns infolge von Hydrocephalus des Grosshirns. *Dtsch. med. Wschr.*, 1891, **17**, 1172-75.
See No. 4581.1. See also *Denkschr. Akad. Wiss. Wien*, 1896, **63**, 71-116.

4578   SCHMIDT, ADOLF. 1865-1918
         Casuistische Beiträge zur Nervenpathologie. II. Doppelseitige Access-
         oriuslähmung bei Syringomyelie. *Dtsch. med. Wschr.*, 1892, **18**, 606-08.
             "Schmidt's syndrome" – a hemiplegia affecting the vocal cord, palate,
         trapezius, and sternocleidomastoid muscles, due to lesion of the nucleus
         ambiguus and nucleus accessorius.

4579   WESTPHAL, CARL FRIEDRICH OTTO. 1833-1890
         Gesammelte Abhandlungen. 2 vols. Berlin, 1892.

4580   DEJERINE, JOSEPH JULES. 1849-1917, & SOTTAS, JULES. 1866-?
         Sur la névrite interstitielle hypertrophique et progressive de l'enfance. *C.
         R. Soc. Biol. (Paris)*, 1893, **45**, 63-96.
             First description of hypertrophic progressive interstitial neuritis.
         "Dejerine–Sottas disease".

4581   HEAD, *Sir* HENRY. 1861-1940
         On disturbances of sensation with especial reference to the pain of visceral
         disease. *Brain,* 1893, **16**, 1-133; 1894, **17**, 339-480; 1896, **19**, 153-276.
             "Head's areas", zones of hyperalgesia of skin, associated with visceral
         disease.

4581.1   ARNOLD, JULIUS. 1835-1915
         Myelocyste, Transposition von Gewebskeimen und Sympodie. *Beitr. path.
         Anat.*, 1894, **16**, 1-28.
             Arnold–Chiari malformation (*see* No. 4577.1).

4582   OPPENHEIM, HERMANN. 1858-1919
         Lehrbuch der Nervenkrankheiten. Berlin, *S. Karger,* 1894.
             The best edition is the English translation of the 5th German edn., 2
         vols., London, 1911.

4583   BABINSKI, JOSEPH FRANÇOIS FÉLIX. 1857-1932
         Sur le réflexe cutané plantaire dans certaines affections organiques du
         système nerveux central. *C. R. Soc. Biol. (Paris)*, 1896, **48**, 207-08.
             "Babinski's reflex".

4584   BARKER, LEWELLYS FRANKLIN. 1867-1943
         A case of circumscribed unilateral, and elective sensory paralysis. *J. exp.
         Med.*, 1896, **1**, 348-60.

4585   HILL, *Sir* LEONARD ERSKINE. 1866-1952
         The physiology and pathology of the cerebral circulation. London, *J. & A.
         Churchill,* 1896.

4586   JACKSON, JOHN HUGHLINGS. 1835-1911
         Remarks on the relations of different divisions of the central nervous system
         to one another and to parts of the body. *Brit. med. J.*, 1898, **1**, 65-69.

4586.1   MILLS, CHARLES KARSNER. 1845-1931
         The nervous system and its diseases. Philadelphia, *J.B. Lippincott,* 1898.
             "The foremost American neurology book of the Nineteenth Century"
         (McHenry), and the only text of the period to contain a section on the
         chemistry of the nervous system.

4587   REMAK, ERNST JULIUS. 1848-1911, & FLATAU, EDWARD. 1869-1932
Neuritis und Polyneuritis. 2 pts. Wien, *A. Hölder*, 1899-1900.
In Nothnagel's *Handbuch der speziellen Pathologie und Therapie*, XI,
Bd. 3, Abt. 3-4.

4588   LIEPMANN, HUGO KARL. 1863-1925
Das Krankheitsbild der Apraxie (motorischen Asymbolie) auf Grund eines
Falles von einseitiger Apraxie. *Mschr. Psychiat. Neurol.*, 1900, **8**, 15-44, 102-
32, 182-97.
First adequate description of apraxia.

4589   BABINSKI, JOSEPH FRANÇOIS FÉLIX. 1857-1932, & NAGEOTTE, JEAN. 1866-1948
Hémiasynergie, latéropulsion et myosis bulbaires avec hémianesthésie et
hémiplégie croisées. *Rev. neurol. (Paris)*, 1902, **10**, 358-65.
"Babinski–Nageotte syndrome".

4590   DEJERINE, JOSEPH JULES. 1849-1917, & THOMAS, ANDRÉ. 1867-1963
Traité des maladies de la moëlle épinière. Paris, *J. B. Baillière,* 1902.

4591   KIENBÖCK, ROBERT. 1871-1953
Kritik der sogenannten "traumatischen Syringomyelie". *Jb. Psychiat.*, 1902,
21, 50-210.
Traumatic cavity formation in the spinal cord, so well described by
Kienböck, is known as "Kienböck's disease".

4592   CESTAN, RAYMOND. 1872-1934, & CHENAIS, LOUIS JEAN. 1872-
Du myosis dans certaines lésions bulbaires en foyer (hémiplégie du type
Avellis associée au syndrome oculaire sympathique). *Gaz. Hôp. (Paris)*,
1903, **76**, 1229-33.
"Cestan–Chenais syndrome".

4593   VERGER, HENRI. 1873-1930
Essai de classification de quelques névralgies faciales par les injections de
cocaine loco dolenti. *Rev. Médecine*, 1904, **24**, 34-63, 134-64.
Classification of the neuralgias.

4594   GARCIA TAPIA, ANTONIO. 1875-1950
Un caso de parálisis del lado derecho de la laringe y de la lengua, con
parálisis del esterno-cleido-mastoidea y trapecio del mismo lado;
accompañado de hemiplejia total temporal del lado izquierdo del cuerpo.
Siglo méd., 1905, **52**, 211-13.
"Tapia's syndrome" – palato-pharyngo-laryngeal hemiplegia.

4594.1   FRIEDMANN, MAX.
Ueber die nicht epileptischen Absencen oder kurzen narkoleptischen
Anfälle. *Dtsch. Z. Nervenheilk.*, 1906, **30**, 462-92.
First description of pyknolepsy.

4595   SLUDER, GREENFIELD. 1865-1928
The syndrome of sphenopalatine-ganglion neurosis. *Amer. J. med. Sci.*,
1910, **140**, 868-78.
"Sluder's neuralgia" first described.

4596   MESTREZAT, WILLIAM. 1883-1928
Le liquide céphalo-rachidien normal et pathologique, valeur clinique de l'examen chimique. Montpellier, *Thèse No.* 17, 1911.
    Mestrezat gave the first exact description of the chemical constitution of the cerebrospinal fluid. Also published at Paris, *Maloine*, 1912.

4596.1   SCHÜLLER, ARTUR. 1874-1958
Röntgen-diagnostik der Erkrankungen des Kopfes. Wien, Leipzig, *A. Hölder*, 1912.
    A fundamental work on radiological examination of the skull. English translation, St. Louis, 1918.

4596.2   BABINSKI, JOSEPH FRANÇOIS FÉLIX. 1857-1932
Contribution à l'étude des troubles mentaux dans l'hémiplégie organique cérébrale (anosognosie). *Rev. neurol.*, 1914, **22**, 845-48.
    Babinski drew attention to anosognosia, a name he gave to unconcern or denial of striking neurological disorders.

4597   DANDY, WALTER EDWARD. 1886-1946, & BLACKFAN, KENNETH DANIEL. 1883-1941
Internal hydrocephalus. *Amer. J. Dis. Child.*, 1914, **8**, 406-82; 1917, **14**, 424-43.
    Experimental production of hydrocephalus.

4598   DEJERINE, JOSEPH JULES. 1849-1917
Sémiologie des affections du système nerveux. Paris, *Masson & Cie.*, 1914.

4599   JELLIFFE, SMITH ELY. 1866-1945, & WHITE, WILLIAM ALANSON. 1870-1937
Diseases of the nervous system. Philadelphia, *Lea & Febiger*, 1915.
    Sixth edition, 1935.

4600   QUECKENSTEDT, HANS HEINRICH GEORG. 1876-1918
Zur Diagnose der Rückenmarkskompression. *Dtsch. Z. Nervenheilk.*, 1916, **55**, 325-33.
    "Queckenstedt's test" for determining patency of the spinal subarachnoid space.

4601   CUSHING, HARVEY WILLIAMS. 1869-1939
Tumors of the nervus acusticus and the syndrome of the cerebello-pontile angle. Philadelphia, *W. B. Saunders*, 1917.
    Reprinted 1963.

4602   DANDY, WALTER EDWARD. 1886-1946
Ventriculography following the injection of air into the cerebral ventricles. *Ann. Surg.*, 1918, **68**, 5-11; also *Amer. J. Roentgenol.*, 1919, n.s. **6**, 26-36.
    Dandy was responsible for the introduction of ventriculography.

4603   ——. Röntgenography of the brain after the injection of air into the spinal canal. *Ann. Surg.*, 1919, **70**, 397-403.
    Introduction of pneumoencephalography.

4604 FOERSTER, OTFRID. 1873-1941
Zur Analyse und Pathophysiologie der striären Bewegungsstörungen. *Z. ges. Neurol. Psychiat.*, 1921, **73**, 1-169.
Foerster made a most important contribution to the literature on extrapyramidal diseases.

4605 SICARD, JEAN ATHANASE. 1872-1929, & FORESTIER, JACQUES. 1890-
Méthode radiographique d'exploration de la cavité épidurale par la lipiodol. *Rev. neurol. (Paris)*, 1921, **28**, 1264-66.
Positive contrast myelography with iodised oil (lipiodol).

4605.1 WIDERÖE, SOFUS 1880-?
Über die diagnostische Bedeutung der intraspinalen Luftinjektionen bei Rückenmarksleiden, besonders bei Geschwülsten. *Zbl. Chir.*, 1921, **48**, 394-97.
Myelography by air injection into spinal subarachnoid space.

4605.2 WEBER, FREDERICK PARKES. 1863-1962
Right-sided hemi-hypertrophy resulting from right-sided congenital spastic hemiplegia, with a morbid condition of the left side of the brain, revealed by radiograms. *J. Neurol. Psychopath.*, 1922, **3**, 134-39.
Sturge–Weber syndrome (*see* No. 4560.1).

·4605.3 GERSTMANN, JOSEF. 1887-?
Fingeragnosie. Eine umschriebene Störung der Orientierung am eigenen Körper. *Wien. klin. Wschr.*, 1924, **37**, 1010-12.
Gerstmann's syndrome, due to cerebral lesion. Translation in *Arch. Neurol. Psychiat.*, 1971, **24**, 475-76.

4606 WILSON, SAMUEL ALEXANDER KINNIER. 1878-1937
Some problems in neurology. No. 2. Pathological laughing and crying. *J. Neurol. Psychopath.*, 1924, **4**, 299-333.
An important paper on the pathology of facial movements.

4607 ADIE, WILLIAM JOHN. 1886-1935
Idiopathic narcolepsy: a disease sui generis; with remarks on the mechanism of sleep. *Brain*, 1926, **49**, 257-306.
Adie's description of narcolepsy is called "maladie d'Adie" by some French writers.

4608 BAILEY, PERCIVAL. 1892-1973, & CUSHING, HARVEY WILLIAMS. 1869-1939
A classification of the tumors of the glioma group on a histogenetic basis with a correlated study of prognosis. Philadelphia, *J. B. Lippincott*, 1926.
German translation, 1930.

4609 SCHAFFER, KAROLY. 1864-1939
Über das morphologische Wesen und die Histopathologie der hereditaersystematischen Nervenkrankheiten. Berlin, *J. Springer*, 1926.
Schaffer was a pioneer Hungarian neuropathologist. He laid down a triad of criteria for judging whether or not a neurological disease is hereditary.

4610   EGAS MONIZ, ANTONIO CAETANO DE. 1874-1955
        L'encéphalographie artérielle, son importance dans la localisation des
        tumeurs cérébrales. *Rev. neurol.*, (*Paris*), 1927, **34**, **II**, 72-90.
            Introduction of cerebral arteriography. See also *Presse méd.*, 1928, **36**,
        689-93. English translation in *J. Neurosurg.*, 1964, **21**, 145-56.

4610.1 ———. Injections intracarotidiennes et substances injectables opaques aux
        rayons X. *Presse méd.*, 1927, **35**, 969-71.
            Carotid arteriography.

4611   ADIE, WILLIAM JOHN. 1886-1935
        Pseudo-Argyll Robertson pupils with absent tendon reflexes; a benign
        disorder simulating tabes dorsalis. *Brit. med. J.*, 1931, **1**, 928-30.
            "Adie's syndrome"; see also his later paper in *Brain*, 1932, **55**, 98-113.
        It was earlier reported by J. Strasberger, by A. Saenger and by M. Nonne in
        Neurol. Zbl., 1902, **21**, 738, 837, and 1000. *See also* No. 5950.

4611.1 LYSHOLM, ERIK. 1891-1947
        Apparatus and technique for roentgen examination of the skull. *Acta radiol.
        Stockh.*, 1931, Suppl. 12.
            Lysholm–Schönander skull table, allowing precise radiography of the
        skull.

4611.2 NYLÉN, CARL OLOF. 1892-
        A clinical study on positional nystagmus in cases of brain tumour. *Acta oto-
        laryng.*, 1931, Suppl. 15.

4611.3 DAVIDOFF, LEO MAX. 1898-1975, & DYKE, CORNELIUS G.
        An improved method of encephalography. *Bull. neurol. Inst. N.Y.*, 1932,
        2, 75-94.
            Lumbar encephalography.

4612   CUSHING, HARVEY WILLIAMS. 1869-1939, & EISENHARDT, LOUISE CHARLOTTE.
        1891-1967
        Meningiomas. Their classification, regional behavior, life history, and
        surgical end results. Springfield, *C. C. Thomas*, 1938.

4613   BUMKE, OSWALD. 1877-1950, & FOERSTER, OTFRID. 1873-1941
        Handbuch der Neurologie. 17 vols. [in 18]. Berlin, *J. Springer*, 1935-37.
            For its era, the definitive encyclopaedia of neurology.

4614   WILSON, SAMUEL ALEXANDER KINNIER. 1878-1937
        Neurology. Edited by A. N. BRUCE. 2 pts. London, *E. Arnold & Co.*, (1940).
            Wilson died before this monumental work was completed and it was
        edited by A. N. Bruce. It includes a vast amount of history and hundreds
        of references. Second edition, 1954.

4614.1 ROBERTSON, EDWARD GRAEME. 1903-
        Encephalography. Melbourne, *Macmillan*, 1941.
            Robertson improved the accuracy and reliability of encephalography
        and reduced its discomforts.

4614.2   THÉVENARD, ANDRÉ. 1898-
L'acropathie ulcéro-mutilante familiale. *Rev. neurol.*, 1942, **74**, 193-212.
"Thévenard's disease" – hereditary sensory neuropathy, earlier reported by Auguste Nélaton: Affection singulière des os du pied. *Gaz. Hôp. Paris*, 1852, **4**, 13.

4615   STEINHAUSEN, THEODORE BEHN. 1914- , *et al.*
Iodinated organic compounds as contrast media for radiographic diagnoses. III. Experimental and clinical myelography with ethyl iodophenylundecylate (pantopaque). *Radiology*, 1944, **43**, 230-35.
Introduction of "pantopaque" for diagnosis of cerebral tumours. With C. E. Dungan, J. B. Furst, J. T. Plati, S. W. Smith, A. P. Darling, and E. C. Wolcott.

4615.1   MOORE, GEORGE EUGENE. 1922-
Fluorescein as an agent in the differentiation of normal and malignant tissues. *Science*, 1947, **106**, 130-31.
Radioactive isotopes used in neuroradiology. See also *Science*, 1948, **107**, 569-71.

4615.2   ———. The clinical use of fluorescein in neurosurgery; localization of brain tumors. *J. Neurosurg.*, 1948, **5**, 392-98.
Tumour localization by radio-isotopes. With W. T. Peyton, L. A. French, and W. W. Walker. Preliminary reports in *Science*, 1947, **106**, 130-31; 1948, **107**, 569-71.

4615.3   CRITCHLEY, MACDONALD. 1900-
The parietal lobes. London, *Edward Arnold*, [1953].
Defines for the first time the various functions of the parietal lobes.

APHASIA, ETC.

4616   LINNÉ, CARL [LINNAEUS]. 1707-1778
Glömska af alla substantiva och i synnerhet namn. *K. Swenska Wetensk. Acad. Handl.*, 1745, **6**, 116-17.
Aphasia first described. Facsimile reproduction and English translation by H. R. Viets, *Bull. Hist. Med.*, 1943, **13**, 328-33.

4617   BUXTORF, JOHANN LUDWIG.
Lethargus cum impotentia loquelae, tandem convulsivus et lethalis. *Acta helv.*, 1758, **3**, 397-400.

4618   BOUILLAUD, JEAN BAPTISTE. 1796-1881
Recherches cliniques propres à démontrer que la perte de la parole correspond à la lésion des lobules antérieurs du cerveau. *Arch. gén. Méd.*, 1825, **8**, 25-45.
Classic account of aphasia. Bouillaud was the first to suggest that injuries of the frontal lobe were a cause of aphasia.

4619   BROCA, PIERRE PAUL. 1824-1880
Perte de la parole; ramollissement chronique et destruction partielle du lobe antérieur gauche du cerveau. *Bull. Soc. Anthrop. Paris*, 1861, **2**, 235-38.
Broca localized the speech centre in the left frontal lobe. He asserted that aphasia was associated with a lesion on the left third frontal con-

volution of the brain – "Broca's centre". He was preceded in this discovery by Marc Dax, a student who recorded in his unpublished thesis submitted to the Faculty of Medicine in Montpellier in 1836 his observations that the left hemisphere was usually found damaged in aphasics. English translation in *J. Neurosurg.*, 1964, **21**, 426-27. The standard biography is *Paul Broca, founder of French anthropology, explorer of the brain* by F. Schiller. Berkeley, *University of California Press*, [1979]. *See also* No. 1400.

4620   JACKSON, JOHN HUGHLINGS. 1835-1911.
Loss of speech: its association with valvular disease of the heart, and with hemiplegia on the right side. Defects of smell. Defects of speech in chorea. Arterial regions in epilepsy. *Clin. Lect. Rep. Lond. Hosp.*, 1864, **1**, 388-471.
Jackson studied aphasia for 30 years. He emphasized its psychological aspects and laid the foundation for present knowledge of the condition, but he was ahead of his time and the value of his work was not recognized for many years.

4621   ——. Notes on the physiology and pathology of language. *Med. Times. Gaz.*, 1866, **1**, 659-62.

4621.1   FALRET, JULES. 1824-1902
Aphasie, aphémie, alalie. *Dict. encycl. Sci. méd.*, Paris, 1866, **5**, 605-644.
Includes a history of aphasia.

4622   BASTIAN, HENRY CHARLTON. 1837-1915
On the various forms of loss of speech in cerebral disease. *Brit. for. med.-chir. Rev.*, 1869, **43**, 209-36.
Bastian's first important paper on aphasia. His axiom "We think in words" explains his whole work on the subject. See also his later paper on pp. 470-92 of the same volume.

4623   WERNICKE, CARL. 1848-1905
Der aphasische Symptomencomplex. Breslau, *M. Cohn & Weigert*, 1874.
Sensory aphasia ("Wernicke's aphasia"). Wernicke did important work on the localization of aphasia; he included in his book accounts of alexia and agraphia.

4624   KUSSMAUL, ADOLF. 1822-1902
Die Störungen der Sprache. Leipzig, *F. C. W. Vogel*, 1877.
Kussmaul's best work. He termed aphasia "word-blindness". The book was issued as a supplement to vol. 12 of Ziemssen's *Handbuch der speciellen Pathologie und Therapie*. English translation in Ziemssen's *Cyclopedia of the practice of medicine*, Vol. 14, New York, 1877.

4625   PITRES, JEAN ALBERT. 1848-1928
Considérations sur l'agraphie à propos d'une observation nouvelle d'agraphie motrice pure. *Rev. Médecine*, 1884, **4**, 855-73.
Classic account of agraphia.

4626   LICHTHEIM, LUDWIG. 1845-1928
Ueber Aphasie. *Dtsch. Arch. klin. Med.*, 1885, **36**, 204-68.
"Lichtheim's disease" – subcortical sensory aphasia. Lichtheim noted that although the patient could not speak, he was able to indicate with his fingers the number of syllables in the word of which he was thinking ("Lichtheim's sign"). The paper is translated into English in *Brain*, 1885, **7**, 433-84.

4627 BERLIN, Rudolf. 1833-1897
    Eine besondere Art der Wortblindheit. Wiesbaden, *J. F. Bergmann,* 1887.
     Berlin first suggested the term "dyslexia".

4627.1 FREUD, Sigmund. 1856-1939
    Zur Auffassung der Aphasien. Leipzig & Vienna, *Deuticke,* 1891.
     Freud refuted the Wernicke–Lichtheim doctrine (Nos. 4623 & 4626) that the losses of function in aphasia were due to lesions to anatomically circumscribed centres corresponding to the various functions involved in language. He distinguished between defects in naming objects, which he called asymbolic aphasia, and defects in recognizing objects, for which he introduced the term "agnosia". English translation, London, 1953.

4628 PITRES, Jean Albert. 1848-1928
    Étude sur l'aphasie chez les polyglottes. *Rev. Médecine,* 1895, **15**, 873-99.
     Important account of paraphrasia.

4629 BASTIAN, Henry Charlton. 1837-1915
    A treatise on aphasia and other speech defects. London, *H. K. Lewis,* 1898.
     Bastian localized the auditory and visual centres, and he described word-blindness and word-deafness. (*See also* No. 4622.)

4630 MARIE, Pierre. 1853-1940
    Revision de la question de l'aphasie; la troisième circonvolution frontale gauche ne joue aucun rôle spécial dans la fonction du langage. *Sem. méd.* (*Paris*), 1906, **26**, 241-47.
     Marie disputed Broca's claim that the third left frontal convolution of the brain is the speech centre. He classified aphasia into three groups: anarthria (defects of articulation), Broca's (motor) aphasia, and Wernicke's (sensory) aphasia.

4631 HINSELWOOD, James. 1859-1919
    Congenital word-blindness. London, *H. K. Lewis,* 1917.

4632 HENSCHEN, Salomon Eberhard. 1847-1930
    Klinische und anatomische Beiträge zur Pathologie des Gehirns. 8 pts. in 10 vols. Upsala, *Almquist & Wiksell* (vols.1-4); *Nordiska* (vols.5-6); *the author* (vols.7-8), 1890-1930.
     An important summary of the knowledge concerning aphasia appears in vols.5-7.

4633 HEAD, *Sir* Henry. 1861-1940
    Aphasia and kindred disorders of speech. 2 vols. Cambridge, *Univ. Press,* 1926.
     The most important work on the subject in the English language. Head's theory of aphasia conceived the condition as being "a disorder of symbolic formulation and expression". Reprinted 1963.

For history, see Nos. 4621.1, 5019.7

4634   WHYTT, ROBERT. 1714-1766
        Observations on the dropsy in the brain. Edinburgh, *J. Balfour*, 1768.
        First account of the clinical course of tuberculous meningitis in chil-
        dren. This work is notable for its fullness of detail and its accuracy. Whytt
        divided the disease into three stages, according to the character of the
        pulse, and he attributed its various manifestations to the presence of a
        serous exudate in the brain.

4635   CHEYNE, JOHN. 1777-1836
        An essay on hydrocephalus acutus, or dropsy in the brain. Edinburgh,
        Mundell, Doig & Stevenson, 1808.
        Acute hydrocephalus first described.

4636   GERHARD, WILLIAM WOOD. 1809-1872
        Cerebral affections of children. *Amer. J. med. Sci.*, 1834, **13**, 313-59; **14**, 99-
        111.
        Accurate clinical description of tuberculous meningitis.

4637   DUBINI, ANGELO. 1813-1902
        Primi cenni sulla corea elettrica. *Ann. univ. Med. (Milano)*, 1846, **117**, 5-50.
        First description of electric chorea, "Dubini's chorea", the myoclonic
        form of epidemic encephalitis.

4638   LEBERT, HERMANN. 1813-1878
        Ueber Gehirnabscesse. *Virchows Arch. path. Anat.*, 1856, **10**, 78-109, 352-
        400, 426-48.
        First systematic account of brain abscess.

4639   LANDRY, JEAN BAPTISTE OCTAVE. 1826-1865
        Note sur la paralysie ascendante aiguë. *Gaz. hebd. Méd. Chir.*, 1859, **6**, 472-
        74, 486-88.
        "Landry's paralysis" – acute infective polyneuritis. It is difficult to assess
        the claim of Landry as first to record this condition, since Adolf Kussmaul
        reported two cases in the same year (*Zwei Fälle von Paraplegie*, Erlangen).

4640   BÄRENSPRUNG, FRIEDRICH WILHELM FELIX VON. 1822-1864
        Die Gürtelkrankheit. *Ann. Charité-Krankenh. Berlin*, 1861, **9**, 2 Heft, 40-
        128; 1862, **10**, 1 Heft, 37-53; 1863, **11**, 2 Heft, 96-116.
        Herpes zoster first ascribed to a lesion of the spinal ganglia.

4641   GAYET, CHARLES JULES ALPHONSE. 1833-1904
        Affection encéphalique (encéphalite diffuse probable) localisée aux étages
        supérieurs des pédoncules cérébraux et aux couches optiques. *Arch.
        Physiol. norm. path.*, 1875, 2 sér., **2**, 341-51.
        First description of acute superior haemorrhagic polioencephalitis.
        Called also "Wernicke's encephalopathy", following the latter's descrip-
        tion in his *Lehrbuch der Gehirnkrankheiten*, Kassel, 1881, **2**, 229-42.

4642   LANDOUZY, LOUIS THÉOPHILE JOSEPH. 1845-1917
        Fièvre zoster et exanthèmes zostériformes. *J. Conn. méd. prat. Pharm.*, 1884,
        3 sér., **6**, 19, 26, 37, 44, 52.
        Landouzy first suggested the infective nature of herpes.

4643 STRÜMPELL, ERNST ADOLF GUSTAV GOTTFRIED. 1853-1925
Ueber die akute Encephalitis der Kinder (Polioencephalitis acuta, cerebrale Kinderlähmung). *Jb. Kinderheilk.*, 1885, **22**, 173-78.
"Strümpell's disease" – polioencephalomyelitis.

4644 HEAD, *Sir* HENRY. 1861-1940, & CAMPBELL, ALFRED WALTER. 1868-1937
The pathology of herpes zoster and its bearing on sensory localisation. *Brain,* 1900, **23**, 353-523.
Head and Campbell showed herpes zoster to be a haemorrhagic inflammation of the posterior nerve roots and the homologous spinal ganglia.

4645 FROIN, GEORGES. 1874-
Inflammations meningées avec réactions chromatique, fibrineuse et cytologique du liquide cephalo-rachidien. *Gaz. Hôp.* (*Paris*), 1903, **76**, 1005-06.
"Froin's syndrome" – a coagulation of the cerebrospinal fluid.

4646 SCHILDER, PAUL FERDINAND. 1886-1940
Zur Kenntnis der sogenannten diffusen Sklerose (über Encephalitis periaxialis diffusa). *Z. ges. Neurol.*, 1912, **10**, Orig., 1-60.
"Schilder's disease" – encephalitis periaxialis diffusa.

4647 GUILLAIN, GEORGES. 1876-1961, *et al.*
Sur un syndrome de radiculo-névrite avec hyperalbuminose du liquide céphalo-rachidien sans réaction cellulaire. Remarques sur les caractères cliniques et graphiques des réflexes tendineux. *Bull. Soc. méd. Hôp. Paris,* 1916, **40**, 1462-70.
"Guillain–Barré syndrome", acute infective polyneuritis. With J. A. Barré and A. Strohl.

4648 CLELAND, *Sir* JOHN BURTON. 1878-1971, & CAMPBELL, ALFRED WALTER. 1868-1937
The Australian epidemics of an acute polio-encephalomyelitis (X disease). *Rep. Director-Gen. publ. Hlth., New S. Wales,* 1917, 150-280.
Murray Valley encephalitis (Australian X disease). Cleland and Campbell isolated a virus from the cerebral tissue of three patients.

4649 CRUCHET, JEAN RENÉ. 1875-1959, *et al.*
Quarante cas d'encéphalo-myélite subaiguë. *Bull. Soc. méd. Hôp. Paris,* 1917, 3 sér., **41**, 614-16.
Cruchet's account of epidemic encephalitis was given on 27 April 1917, preceding that of Economo by 13 days. With Moutier and Calmettes.

4650 ECONOMO, CONSTANTIN, *Freiherr von San Serff.* 1876-1931.
Encephalitis lethargica. *Wien. klin. Wschr.*, 1917, **30**, 581-85.
Economo's classic description of epidemic encephalitis ("von Economo's disease") was published on 10 May 1917; *see* No. 4649.

4651 LOEWE, LEO. 1896- , & STRAUSS, ISRAEL. 1873-?
Etiology of epidemic (lethargic) encephalitis. Preliminary note. *J. Amer. med. Assoc.*, Chicago, 1919, **73**, 1056-57.
Experimental transmission of encephalitis lethargica.

4652   KUNDRATITZ, KARL.
        Experimentelle Übertragung von Herpes zoster auf den Menschen und die
        Beziehungen von Herpes zoster zu Varicellen. *Mschr. Kinderheilk.*, 1925,
        29, 516-23.
        First demonstration of the infectivity of herpes.

4653   BALÓ, JÓSZEF. 1896-
        A leukoenkephalitis periaxialis concentricaról. *Magy. orv. Arch.*, 1927, **28**,
        108-24.
        "Baló's disease" – encephalitis periaxialis concentrica. Translation in
        Arch. Neurol. Psychiat. (Chicago), 1928, **19**, 242-64.

4654   KANEKO, RENJIRO. 1886-, & AOKI, Y.
        Ueber die Encephalitis epidemica in Japan. *Ergebn. inn. Med. Kinderheilk.*,
        1928, **34**, 342-456.
        Japanese encephalitis distinguished from encephalitis lethargica.

4656   MUCKENFUSS, RALPH S., *et al.*
        Encephalitis: studies on experimental transmission. *Publ. Hlth. Rep. (Wash.)*,
        1933, **48**, 1341-43.
        Isolation of the St. Louis encephalitis virus. With C. Armstrong and H.
        A. McCordock.

4657   HAYASHI, MICHITOMO.
        Übertragung des Virus von Encephalitis epidemica auf Affen. *Proc. imp.
        Acad. Japan*, 1934, **10**, 41-44.
        Experimental transmission of Japanese B encephalitis.

4658   SABIN, ALBERT BRUCE. 1906- , & WRIGHT, ARTHUR M.
        Acute ascending myelitis following a monkey bite, with the isolation of a
        virus capable of reproducing the disease. *J. exp. Med.*, 1934, **59**, 115-36.
        Herpesvirus simiae (B virus) infection; isolation of the virus.

4659   TANIGUCHI, TENJI. 1889-1961, *et al.*
        A virus isolated in 1935 epidemic of summer encephalitis in Japan. *Jap. J.
        exp. Med.*, 1936, **14**, 185-96.
        T. Taniguchi, M. Hosokawa, and S. Kuga established a virus aetiology
        for Japanese B encephalitis.

4659.1 FOTHERGILL, LEROY DRYDEN. 1901-1967, *et al.*
        Human encephalitis caused by the virus of the Eastern variety of equine
        encephalomyelitis. *New Engl. J. med.*, 1938, **219**, 411.
        Isolation of the virus of Eastern equine encephalitis from man. With J.
        H. Dingle, S. Farber, and M. L. Connerley.

4660   HOWITT, BEATRICE FAY. 1891-
        Recovery of the virus of equine encephalomyelitis from the brain of a child.
        Science, 1938, **88**, 455-56.
        Western equine encephalitis virus recovered from man.

4660.1 ZIL'BER, L. A.
        Vesennij (vesenne-letnij) endemiceskij klescevoj encefalit. [Vernal (verno-
        aestival) endemic tick-borne encephalitis.] *Arkh. biol. Nauk.*, 1939, **56**, No.
        2, 9-37.
        Isolation of the virus of spring–summer (Russian Far East) encephalitis.

4661   DURAND, Paul. 1895-1961
Virus filtrant pathogène pour l'homme et les animaux de laboratoire, et à affinité meningée et pulmonaire. *Arch. Inst. Pasteur Tunis,* 1940, **29**, 179-227.
     "Durand's disease" – D virus infection. Durand isolated the virus from his own blood. See also the paper by G. M. Findlay, *Trans. roy. Soc. trop. Med.,* 1942, **35**, 303-18.

4661.1   JUNGEBLUT, Claus W. 1897- , & SANDERS, Murray. 1910-
Studies of a murine strain of poliomyelitis virus in cotton rats and white mice. *J. exp. Med.,* 1940, **72**, 407-36.
     Isolation of encephalomyocarditis virus.

4661.2   LUMSDEN, Leslie Leon. 1875-1946
St. Louis encephalitis in 1933; observations on epidemiological features. *Publ. Hlth. Rep. (Wash.),* 1958, **73**, 340-53.
     In a report to the Surgeon General in 1933, Lumsden concluded that the *Culex* mosquito was the vector of the St. Louis encephalitis virus. His report was not published until 1958.

Poliomyelitis

4662   UNDERWOOD, Michael. 1737-1820
Debility of the lower extremities. In his *Treatise on the diseases of children.* New ed., London, *J. Mathews,* 1789, **2**, 53-57.
     Underwood was the first to consider poliomyelitis as an entity.

4663   BADHAM, John. 1807-1840
Paralysis in childhood. Four remarkable cases of suddenly induced paralysis in the extremities, occurring in children, without any apparent cerebral or cerebro-spinal lesion. *Lond. med. Gaz.* 1835, **17**, 215-18.
     Important clinical description.

4664   HEINE, Jacob von. 1799-1879
Beobachtungen über Lähmungszustände der untern Extremitäten und deren Behandlung. Stuttgart, *F. H. Köhler,* 1840.
     First description of acute anterior poliomyelitis, which Heine separated from other forms of paralysis; he described the deformities arising from the disease. He also called attention to congenital spastic paraplegia, which, following Little's classic description (No. 4691.1), was termed "Little's disease".

4665   CHARCOT, Jean Martin. 1825-1893, & JOFFROY, Alex. 1844-1908
Une observation de paralysie infantile s'accompagnant d'une altération des cornes antérieures de la substance grise de la moëlle. *C. R. Soc. Biol. (Paris),* (1869), 1870, 5 sér., **1**, 312-15.
     First demonstration of the atrophy of the anterior horns of the spinal cord in infantile paralysis, confirming earlier suggestions of von Heine and Duchenne.

4665.1   ERB, WILHELM HEINRICH. 1840-1921
Ueber acute Spinallähmung (Poliomyelitis anterior acuta) bei Erwachsenen und über verwandte spinale Erkrankungen. *Arch. Psychiat. Nervenkr.*, 1875, **5**, 758-91.
    Erb was first to use the term "acute anterior poliomyelitis".

4666   LEYDEN, ERNST VON. 1832-1910
Ueber Poliomyelitis und Neuritis. *Z. klin. Med.*, 1879-80, **1**, 387-434.
    Leyden enjoyed a great reputation as a neurologist and his paper on poliomyelitis and neuritis is one of his best works. He was one of the founders of the journal in which it appeared.

4667   MEDIN, OSKAR. 1847-1927
En epidemi af infantil paralysi. *Hygiea*, Stockholm, 1890, **52**, 657-68.
    The epidemic character of poliomyelitis was first noted by Medin. The disease is also known as "Heine–Medin disease" from the descriptions given by these two writers (*see also* No. 4664). German version in *Verh. X. Int. Med. Kongr.*, 1890, **2**, Abt. 6, 37-47, 1891. English translation in Bick, *Classics of orthopaedics*, 116-23.

4668   WICKMAN, OTTO IVAR. 1872-1914
Studien über Poliomyelitis acuta. *Arb. path. Inst. Univ. Helsingfors*, 1905, **1**, 109-293.
    Wickman was the first to produce evidence confirming the infectious nature of poliomyelitis.

4669   LANDSTEINER, KARL. 1868-1943, & POPPER, ERWIN.
Uebertragung der Poliomyelitis acuta auf Affen. *Z. ImmunForsch.*, 1909, **2**, 1 Teil, 377-90.
    Landsteiner and Popper were the first to transmit poliomyelitis to monkeys.

4670   FLEXNER, SIMON. 1863-1946, & LEWIS, PAUL A. 1879-1929
Experimental poliomyelitis in monkeys: active immunization and passive serum protection. *J. Amer. med. Assoc.*, 1910, **54**, 1780-82.
    Demonstration of antibodies in convalescent serum in monkeys.

4670.1   GAY, FREDERICK PARKER. 1874-1939, & LUCAS, WILLIAM PALMER. 1880-1960
Anterior poliomyelitis. Methods of diagnosis from spinal fluid and blood in monkeys and in human beings. *Arch. intern. Med.*, 1910, **6**, 330-38.
    Gay and Lucas were the first to make accurate cell counts of the spinal fluid in poliomyelitis.

4670.2   NETTER, ARNOLD. 1855-1936, & LEVADITI, CONSTANTIN. 1874-1953
Action microbicide exercée sur la virus de la poliomyélite aiguë dans le sérum des sujets antérieurement atteints de paralysie infantile. Sa constatation dans le sérum d'un sujet qui a présenté une forme abortive. *C. R. Soc. Biol.* (*Paris*), 1910, **68**, 855-57.
    Antibodies discovered in human convalescent serum. *See also* No. 4670.3.

4670.3   LEVADITI, CONSTANTIN. 1874-1953, & LANDSTEINER, KARL. 1868-1943
La poliomyélite experimental. *C. R. Soc. Biol.* (*Paris*), 1910, **68**, 311-13.
    Serum from a monkey that had recovered from experimental poliomyelitis was mixed with an emulsion containing active polio virus; it failed to produce paralytic disease when injected into fresh monkeys.

4670.4   KLING, Carl. 1887-1967, et al.
Experimental and pathological investigation. *In* Investigations on epidemic infantile paralysis, report from the State Medical Institute of Sweden to the XVth International Congress on Hygiene and Demography. Washington, 1912.
Kling, A. Pettersson, and W. Wernstedt recovered the poliomyelitis virus from the intestinal wall and contents, disproving the contention of Flexner that it was exclusively neurotropic.

4670.5   BURNET, *Sir* Frank Macfarlane. 1899-1985, & MACNAMARA, *Dame* Jean
Immunological differences between strains of poliomyelitis virus. *Brit. J. exp. Path.*, 1931, **12**, 57-61.

4670.6   SABIN, Albert Bruce. 1906- , & OLITSKY, Peter Kosciusko. 1886-1964
Cultivation of poliomyelitis virus *in vitro* in human embryonic nervous tissue. *Proc. Soc. exp. Biol. (N.Y.)*, 1936, **34**, 357-59.
Isolation and propagation of the poliomyelitis virus in pure culture.

4671   KENNY, Elizabeth. 1886-1952
Infantile paralysis and cerebral diplegia: methods used for the restoration of function. Sydney, *Angus & Robertson,* 1937.

4671.1   ENDERS, John Franklin. 1897-1985, et al.
Cultivation of the Lansing strain of poliomyelitis virus in cultures of various human embryonic tissues. *Science*, 1949, **109**, 85-87.
J. F. Enders, T. H. Weller, and F. C. Robbins grew the poliomyelitis virus in cultures of different tissues. Their method proved of great value in virus research, and removed the final obstacles to vaccine production. They received the Nobel Prize in 1954.

4671.2   ARMSTRONG, Charles. 1886-1967
Successful transfer of the Lansing strain of poliomyelitis virus from the cotton rat to the white mouse. *Publ. Hlth. Rep. (Wash.)*, 1939, **54**, 2302-05.
Armstrong adapted the Lansing strain of poliomyelitis to the cotton rat and then to the mouse, greatly facilitating experimental work on the disease.

4672   HAMMON, William McDowell. 1904- , et al.
Evaluation of Red Cross gamma globulin as a prophylactic agent for poliomyelitis. *J. Amer. med. Assoc.*, 1952, **150**, 739-60.
Trial of gamma globulin in the prophylaxis of poliomyelitis. With L. L. Coriell, J. Stokes, P. F. Wehrle, and C. R. Klimt.

4672.1   KOPROWSKI, Hilary. 1916- , et al.
Immune responses in human volunteers upon oral administration of a rodent-adapted strain of poliomyelitis virus. *Amer. J. Hyg.*, 1952, **55**, 108-26.
Successful immunization against poliomyelitis with a living attenuated virus vaccine. With G. A. Jervis and T. W. Norton.

4672.2   SALK, Jonas Edward. 1914- , et al.
Studies in human subjects on active immunization against poliomyelitis. 1. A preliminary report of experiments in progress. *J. Amer. med. Assoc.*, 1953, **151**, 1081-98.
Killed-virus vaccine. With four co-authors.

4672.3   SABIN, ALBERT BRUCE. 1906-
Characteristics and genetic potentialities of experimentally produced and
naturally occurring variants of poliomyelitis virus. *Ann. N.Y. Acad. Sci.*, 1955,
61, 924-38.
    Sabin's live attenuated poliomyelitis virus vaccine.

4672.4   FISHBEIN, MORRIS. 1889-1976, *et al.*
A bibliography of infantile paralysis 1789-1949. With selected abstracts and
annotations. Edited by M. Fishbein and Ella M. Salmonsen, with L. Hektoen.
2nd edition. Philadelphia, *Lippincott,* 1951.
    An exhaustive list of books and papers.

4672.5   PAUL, JOHN RODMAN. 1893-1971
A history of poliomyelitis. New Haven, *Yale University Press*, 1971.

Cerebrospinal Meningitis

4673   WILLIS, THOMAS. 1621-1675
A description of an epidemical feaver. . .1661. In his *Practice of physick,*
London, *T. Dring,* 1684, Treatise VIII, pp. 46-54.
    Willis was probably the first to report an epidemic of cerebrospinal
fever.

4674   VIEUSSEUX, GASPARD. 1746-1814
Mémoire sur la maladie qui a régné à Genève au printemps de 1805. *J. Méd.
Chir. Pharm.*, 1805, **11**, 163-82.
    First definite description of cerebrospinal meningitis. Partial English
translation in No. 2241.

4675   STRONG, NATHAN. 1781-1837
An inaugural dissertation on the disease termed petechial, or spotted fever.
Hartford, *P. B. Gleason,* 1810.
    This graduation dissertation was the first published brochure on
cerebrospinal meningitis.

4676   NORTH, ELISHA. 1771-1843
A treatise on a malignant epidemic, commonly called spotted fever. New
York, *T. & J. Swords,* 1811.
    First book on cerebrospinal meningitis; in it North recommended the
use of the clinical thermometer, not in general use until the time of
Wunderlich. For more information on this book, see the article by F. L.
Pleadwell in *Ann. med. Hist.*, 1924, **6**, 245-57.

4677   KERNIG, VLADIMIR MIKHAILOVICH. 1840-1917
Ein Krankheitssymptom der acuten Meningitis. *St. Petersb. med. Wschr.*,
1882, **7**, 398.
    Kernig drew attention to a flexor contracture of the leg on attempting
to extend it on the thigh ("Kernig's sign"), almost always present in
cerebrospinal meningitis and an important diagnostic sign. A fuller description is in *Z. klin. Med.*, 1907, **64**, 19-69.

4678   WEICHSELBAUM, ANTON. 1845-1920
Ueber die Aetiologie der akuten Meningitis cerebro-spinalis. *Fortschr. Med.*,
1887, **5**, 573-83, 620-26.
     Weichselbaum discovered the meningococcus, *Neisseria meningitidis,*
causative agent of cerebrospinal meningitis.

4679   VOELCKER, ARTHUR FRANCIS. 1861-1946
Middx. Hosp. Rep. med. surg. path. Registrars, (1894), 1895, 278.
     First description of the Waterhouse–Friderichsen syndrome (Nos. 4685-
86). Abstract of post mortem report, no title.

4680   HEUBNER, JOHANN OTTO LEONHARD. 1843-1926
Beobachtungen und Versuche über den Meningokokkus intracellularis
(Weichselbaum–Jaeger). *Jb. Kinderheilk.*, 1896, **43**, 1-22.
     Heubner was the first to isolate meningococci from the cerebrospinal
fluid of living beings.

4681   SLAWYK.
Ein Fall von Allgemeininfection mit Influenzabacillen. *Z. Hyg. InfektKr.*,
1899, **32**, 443-48.
     First description of influenzal meningitis.

4682   JOCHMANN, GEORG. 1874-1915
Versuche zur Serodiagnostik und Serotherapie der epidemischen
Genickstarre. *Dtsch. med. Wschr.*, 1906, **32**, 788-93.
     First attempts at the serum treatment of cerebrospinal meningitis.

4683   FLEXNER, SIMON. 1863-1946
Concerning a serum therapy for experimental infection with Diplococcus
intracellularis. *J. exp. Med.*, 1907, **9**, 168-85.
     Flexner prepared an antiserum for use in cerebrospinal meningitis.

4684   ———. & JOBLING, JAMES WESLEY. 1876-
Serum treatment of epidemic cerebrospinal meningitis. *J. exp. Med.*, 1908,
10, 141-203.

4685   WATERHOUSE, RUPERT. 1873-1958
A case of suprarenal apoplexy. *Lancet*, 1911, **1**, 577-78.
     Waterhouse–Friderichsen syndrome (*see also* Nos. 4679, 4686).

4686   FRIDERICHSEN, CARL. 1886-
Nebennierenapoplexie bei kleinen Kindern. *Jb. Kinderheilk.*, 1918, **87**, 109-
25.
     See No. 4685.

4687   WALLGREN, ARVID JOHAN. 1889-1973
Une nouvelle maladie infectieuse du système nerveux central? *Acta paediat.*
(*Stockh.*), 1924, **4**, 158-82.
     Acute lymphocytic choriomeningitis (aseptic meningitis syndrome)
first described.

4688   ARMSTRONG, CHARLES. 1886-1967, & LILLIE, RALPH DOUGALL. 1896-
Experimental lymphocytic choriomeningitis of monkeys and mice produced by a virus encountered in studies of the 1933 St. Louis encephalitis
epidemic. *Publ. Hlth. Rep.* (*Wash.*), 1934, **49**, 1019-27.
Isolation of the virus of benign lymphocytic choriomeningits.

4689   SCHWENTKER, FRANCIS FREDERIC. 1904-1954, *et al.*
The treatment of meningococcic meningitis with sulfanilamide. *J. Amer.
med. Assoc.*, 1937, **108**, 1407-08.
With S. Gelman and P. H. Long.

4689.1   ROSENBERG, DAVID HARRY. 1903- , & ARLING, PHILIP ARTHUR. 1908-
Penicillin in the treatment of meningitis. *J. Amer. med. Assoc.*, 1944, **125**,
1011-17.

DEGENERATIVE DISORDERS

4690   PARKINSON, JAMES. 1755-1824
An essay on the shaking palsy. London, *Whittingham & Rowland*, 1817.
"Parkinson's disease" – paralysis agitans. Reprinted in *Med. Classics*, 1938,
2, 946-97. Facsimile reproduction, 1959. Facsimile edition, with biography
of Parkinson by Macdonald Critchley, London, 1955.

4691   DUNGLISON, ROBLEY. 1798-1869
Practice of medicine. Vol. 2. Philadelphia, *Lea & Blanchard*, 1842.
A case of chronic hereditary chorea in adults ("Huntington's chorea",
see No. 4699) is described on pp. 321-23. This is in the form of a letter from
Charles Oscar Waters (1816-1892).

4691.1   LITTLE, WILLIAM JOHN. 1810-1894.
Course of lectures on the deformities of the human frame. Lecture IX.
Lancet, 1843-44, **1**, 350-54.
Little's description of congenital cerebral spastic diplegia resulted in the
condition being named "Little's disease". *See also* No. 4735.

4692   FRERICHS, FRIEDRICH THEODOR. 1819-1885
Ueber Hirnsklerose. *Arch. ges. Med.*, 1849, **10**, 334-50.
First important account of multiple sclerosis. Carswell (No. 2291) and
Cruveilhier (No. 2286) both gave illustrations of the disease; the latter is
also accredited with the first description.

4693   ——. Klinik der Leberkrankheiten. Bd. 2.Braunschweig, *F. Vieweg u. Sohn*,
1861.
Pp. 62-64: First description of progressive familial hepatolenticular
degeneration ("Kinnier Wilson's disease"; *see* No. 4717).

4695   GULL, *Sir* WILLIAM WITHEY. 1816-1890
Case of progressive atrophy of the muscles of the hands: enlargement of
the ventricle of the cord in the cervical region, with atrophy of the gray
matter. *Guy's Hosp. Rep.*, 1862, **8**, 244-50.
First description of syringomyelia.

4696   FRIEDREICH, NIKOLAUS. 1825-1882
       Ueber degenerative Atrophie der spinalen Hinterstränge. *Virchows Arch.*
       path. Anat., 1863, **26**, 391-419, 433-59; **27**, 1-26; 1876, **68**, 145-245; 1877,
       70, 140-52.
         Friedreich was the first to describe a form of ataxia ("Friedreich's
       ataxia"), hereditary, attended with impairment of speech, lateral curvature
       of the spine, and with paralysis of the muscles of the lower limbs. The titles
       of the last two papers vary.

4697   CLARKE, JACOB AUGUSTUS LOCKHART. 1817-1880, & JACKSON, JOHN HUGHLINGS.
       1835-1911
       On a case of muscular atrophy, with disease of the spinal cord and medulla
       oblongata. *Med.-chir. Trans.*, 1867, **50**, 489-96.
         First important account of syringomyelia.

4698   CHARCOT, JEAN MARTIN. 1825-1893
       Histologie de la sclérose en plaques. *Gaz. Hôp.* (*Paris*), 1868, **41**, 554-55,
       557-58, 566.
         An important description of multiple sclerosis.

4699   HUNTINGTON, GEORGE. 1850-1916
       On chorea. *Med. surg. Reporter*, 1872, **26**, 317-21.
         The classic description by Huntington of the chronic degenerative
       hereditary type of chorea led to the eponym "Huntington's chorea". Earlier
       accounts of the disease were given by John Elliotson (*Lancet*, 1832, **1**, 163),
       Waters (*see* No. 4691), and I. W. Lyon (*Amer. med. Times*, 1863, **7**, 289-90).
       For historical note see D. L. Stevens, *J. roy. Coll. Phycns.*, 1972, **6**, 271-82.
       For bibliography *see* No. 5019.12.

4700   BOURNEVILLE, DÉSIRÉ MAGLOIRE. 1840-1909
       Contribution à l'étude de l'idiotie. *Arch. Neurol.* (*Paris*), 1880, **1**, 69-91.
         "Bourneville's disease", tuberous sclerosis, epiloia (p. 81).

4701   MORVAN, AUGUSTIN MARIE. 1819-1897
       De la parésie analgésique à panaris des extrémités supérieures ou paréso-
       analgésie des extrémités supérieures. *Gaz. hebd. Méd.*, 1883, n.s. **20**, 580-
       83, 590-94, 624-26, 721-22.
         First description of "Morvan's disease" – a form of syringomyelia.

4702   WESTPHAL, CARL FRIEDRICH OTTO. 1833-1890
       Ueber eine dem Bilde der cerebrospinalen grauen Degeneration ähnliche
       Erkrankung des centralen Nervensystems ohne anatomischen Befund,
       nebst einigen Bemerkungen über paradoxe Contraction. *Arch. Psychiat.*
       Nervenkr., 1883, **14**, 87-134.
         "Westphal's pseudosclerosis". Later Strümpell's description of this
       condition (No. 4709) led to the eponym "Westphal–Strümpell disease".

4703   PELIZAEUS, FRIEDRICH. 1850-1917
       Über eine eigentümliche Form spastischer Lähmung mit Cerebraler-
       scheinungen auf hereditärer Grundlage. (Multiple Sklerose.) *Arch. Psychiat.*
       Nervenkr., 1885, **16**, 698-710.
         "Pelizaeus–Merzbacher disease" (*see* No. 4715).

4704   STRÜMPELL, ERNST ADOLF GUSTAV GOTTFRIED. 1853-1925
Ueber eine bestimmte Form der primären combinirten Systemerkrankungen
des Rückenmarks. *Arch. Psychiat. Nervenkr.*, 1886, **17**, 217-38.
"Strümpell's disease" – hereditary spastic spinal paralysis, previously
described by Erb and by Charcot.

4705   SACHS, BERNARD. 1858-1944
On arrested cerebral development, with special reference to its cortical
pathology. *J. nerv. ment. Dis.*, 1887, **14**, 541-53.
Sachs described the cerebral changes in amaurotic familial idiocy.
Earlier, Tay (No. 5918) had recorded the ocular manifestations of this
condition, which became known as "Tay–Sachs's disease". Two further
papers on the subject by Sachs are in the same journal, 1892, **17**, 603-07;
1896, **21**, 475-79.

4706   KAHLER, OTTO. 1849-1893
Ueber die Diagnose der Syringomyelie. *Prag. med. Wschr.* 1888, **13**, 45, 63.
First complete description of syringomyelia.

4706.1   LEYDEN, ERNST VON. 1832-1910
Ueber acute Ataxie. *Z. klin. Med.*, 1891, **18**, 576-87.
"Leyden's (acute) ataxia".

4707   PICK, ARNOLD. 1851-1924
Ueber die Beziehungen der senilen Hirnatrophie zur Aphasie. *Prag. med.
Wschr.*, 1892, **17**, 165-67.
"Pick's disease" – circumscribed atrophy of the brain with the develop-
ment of aphasia and presenile dementia.

4708   PUTNAM, JAMES WRIGHT. 1860-1938
A case of complete athetosis with post-mortem. *J. nerv. ment. Dis.*, 1892,
n.s. **17**, 124-26.
One of the earliest accounts of bilateral athetosis ("Vogt syndrome", No.
4720).

4708.1   MARIE, PIERRE. 1853-1940
Sur l'hérédo-ataxie cérébelleuse. *Sem. méd.* (*Paris*), 1893, **13**, 444-47.
Original description of hereditary cerebellar ataxia.

4708.2   FREUD, SIGMUND. 1856-1939
Die infantile Cerebrallähmung. Wien, *A. Hölder*, 1897.
Freud gave an excellent description of the various forms of cerebral
palsy, with precise classification of the different spastic symptoms; he also
mentioned the extra-pyramidal symptoms. Forms Bd. IX, II Theil, II Abt. of
H. Nothnagel's *Specielle Pathologie und Therapie.* English translation, New
York, 1968.

4709   STRÜMPELL, ERNST ADOLF GUSTAV GOTTFRIED. 1853-1925
Ueber die Westphal'sche Pseudosklerose und über diffuse Hirnsklerose,
insbesondere bei Kindern. *Dtsch. Z. Nervenheilk.*, 1898, **12**, 115-49.
"Westphal-Strümpell disease" – pseudosclerosis of the brain. (*See also*
No. 4702.) Probably cases of Kinnier Wilson's disease.

4710   RUSSELL, JAMES SAMUEL RISIEN. 1863-1939, *et al.*
Subacute combined degeneration of the spinal cord. *Brain*, 1900, **23**, 39-110.
First full description. With F. E. Batten and J. S. Collier.

4711   MILLS, CHARLES KARSNER. 1845-1931
A case of unilateral progressive ascending paralysis, probably representing a new form of degenerative disease. *J. nerv. ment. Dis.*, 1900, **27**, 195-200.
First description of unilateral progressive ascending paralysis ("Mills's disease").

4712   BATTEN, FREDERICK EUSTACE. 1865-1918
Cerebral degeneration with symmetrical changes in the maculae in two members of a family. *Trans. ophthal. Soc. U.K.*, 1903, **23**, 386-90.
See No. 4713.

4713   MAYOU, MARMADUKE STEPHEN. 1876-1934
Cerebral degeneration, with symmetrical changes in the maculae, in three members of a family. *Trans. ophthal. Soc. U.K.*, 1904, **24**, 142-45.
"Batten-Mayou disease", juvenile amaurotic idiocy (*see also* No. 4712).

4713.1   VOGT, HEINRICH. 1875-
Über familiäre amaurotische Idiotie und verwandte Krankheitsbilder. *Mschr. Psych. Neurol.*, 1905, **18**, 161-71, 310-57.
Spielmayer-Vogt disease, the juvenile form of cerebromacular degeneration.

4714   MILLS, CHARLES KARSNER. 1845-1931
Unilateral ascending paralysis and unilateral descending paralysis. *J. Amer. med. Assoc.*, 1906, **47**, 1638-45.
First description of unilateral descending paralysis.

4714.1   SPIELMAYER, WALTHER. 1879-
Klinische und anatomische Untersuchungen über eine besondere Form von familiärer amaurotische Idiotie. Freiburg i. Br., *Gotha*, 1907.
See No. 4713.1. Reprinted in *Histologische und Histopathologische Arbeiten über die Grosshirnrinde* (Nissl), 1908, **2**, 193-213.

4715   MERZBACHER, LUDWIG. 1875-
Weitere Mitteilungen über eine eigenartige hereditär-familiäre Erkrankung des Zentralnervensystems. *Med. Klin.*, 1908, **4**, 1952-55.
"Pelizaeus-Merzbacher disease", familial centrolobar sclerosis (*see also* No. 4703).

4716   SCHWALBE, MARCUS WALTER. 1883-
Eine eigentümliche tonische Krampfform mit hysterischen Symptomen. *Inaug. Diss.*, Berlin, 1907.
First description of torsion-spasm, dystonia musculorum deformans; also called "Ziehen–Oppenheim disease" following reports of cases by these writers in *Neurol. Zbl.*, 1911, **30**, 109, 1090.

4716.1   DEJERINE, JOSEPH JULES. 1849-1917, & THOMAS, ANDRÉ. 1867-1963
L'atrophie olivo-ponto-cérébelleuse. *Nouv. Iconogr. Salpêtr.*, 1912, **25**, 223-50.
     Olivo-ponto-cerebellar atrophy. English translation in Rottenberg & Hochberg, No. 5019.14, pp. 219-51.

4717   WILSON, SAMUEL ALEXANDER KINNIER. 1878-1937
Progressive lenticular degeneration, a familial nervous disease associated with cirrhosis of the liver. *Brain*, 1912, **34**, 295-509.
     Classic description of progressive familial hepatolenticular degeneration ("Wilson's disease"), first described by Frerichs in 1861 (*see* No. 4693), now considered to be a disorder of copper and ceruloplasmin metabolism.

4718   DAWSON, JAMES WALKER. 1870-1927
The histology of disseminated sclerosis. *Trans. roy. Soc. Edinb.* (1913-14), 1916, **50**, 517-740.
     A classic monograph on the pathology of multiple sclerosis.

4719   VILLARET, MAURICE. 1877-1946
Le syndrome nerveux de l'espace rétro-parotidien postérieur. *Rev. neurol. (Paris)*, 1916, **23**, pt. 1, 188-90.
     "Villaret's syndrome".

4719.1   CREUTZFELD, HANS GERHARD. 1885-1964
Ueber eine eigenartige herdförmige Erkrankung des Zentralnervensystems. *Z. ges. Neurol. Psychiat.*, 1920, **57**, 1-18.
     Creutzfeld-Jakob disease (*see* No. 4722). English translation in No. 5019.14, pp. 97-112.

4720   VOGT, CÉCILE. 1875-1962, & VOGT, OSKAR. 1870-1959
Zur Lehre der Erkrankungen des striären Systems. *J. Psychol. Neurol. (Lpz.)*, 1920, **25**, Ergänzht. iii, 627-846.
     "Vogt syndrome", disease of the corpora striata.

4721   FOIX, CHARLES. 1882-1927
Les lésions anatomiques de la maladie de Parkinson. *Rev. neurol. (Paris)*, 1921, **28**, 593-600.
     Foix and his colleagues showed that the specific lesion in Parkinson's disease is in the substantia nigra of the mid-brain.

4722   JAKOB, ALFONS MARIA. 1884-1931
Ueber eigenartige Erkrankungen der Zentralnervensystems mit bemerkenswertem anatomischem Befunde. *Z. ges. Neurol. Psychiat.*, 1921, **64**, Orig., 147-228.
     "Creutzfeld–Jakob disease", spastic pseudosclerosis. *See also* No. 4719.1.

4723   SOUQUES, ACHILLE ALEXANDRE. 1860-1944.
Rapport sur les syndromes parkinsoniens. *Rev. neurol. (Paris)*, 1921, **28**, 534-73.
     Souques recognized the importance of encephalitis lethargica as a cause of Parkinsonism; more than any other neurologist he was responsible for unifying its diverse manifestations.

4724   HALLERVORDEN, JULIUS. 1882-1965, & SPATZ, HUGO. 1888-1969
Eigenartige Erkrankung in extrapyramidalen System mit besonderer
Beteiligung des Globus pallidus und der Substantia nigra. *Z. ges. Neurol.
Psychiat.*, 1922, **79**, 254-302.
    The (extrapyramidal) syndrome of Hallervorden and Spatz.

4725   VINCENT, CLOVIS. 1879-1947, & BOGAERT, LUDO VAN. 1897-
Contribution à l'étude des syndromes du globe pâle. La dégénérescence
progressive du globe pâle et de la portion réticulée de la substance noire
(maladie d'Hallervorden–Spatz). *Rev. neurol. (Paris)*, 1936, **65**, 921-59.
    Clovis Vincent, a pioneer French neurosurgeon, contributed a valuable
study of Hallervorden–Spatz disease.

4726   GRÜNTHAL, ERNST.
Ueber Parpanit, einen neuen estrapyramidal-motorische Störungen
beeinflussenden Stoff. *Schweitz. med. Wschr.*, 1946, **76**, 1286-89.
    Introduction of caramiphen ("parpanit") in the treatment of Parkinson's
disease.

4727   SIGWALD, JEAN. 1903- , *et al.*
Le traitement de la maladie de Parkinson par le chlorhydrate de
diéthylaminoéthyl-N-thiodiphénylamine (2987 R.P.). Premiers résultats.
Rev. neurol. (Paris), 1946, **78**, 581-84.
    Introduction of "diparcol" in the treatment of Parkinson's disease. With
D. Boyet and G. Dumont.

4728   ——. Un nouveau médicament symptomatique des syndromes
parkinsoniens: le chlorhydrate de [(diéthylamino-2'-méthyl-2') éthyl-1-']
N-dibenzoparathiazine. *Presse méd.*, 1949, **57**, 819-20.
    Introduction of ethopropazine ("lysivane") in the treatment of Parkinson's
disease.

4729   CORBIN, KENDALL BROOKS. 1907-
Trihexyphenidyl. Evaluation of the new agent in the treatment of
parkinsonism. *J. Amer. med. Assoc.*, 1949, **141**, 377-82.
    Clinical introduction of benzhexol ("artane") in Parkinson's disease.

4729.1   GAJDUSEK, DANIEL CARLETON. 1923- , & ZIGAS, V.
Degenerative disease of the central nervous system in New Guinea. The
endemic occurrence of "kuru" in the native population. *New Engl. J. Med.*,
1957, **257**, 974-78.
    First description of kuru, a disease occurring in natives of New Guinea.
Gajdusek shared the Nobel Prize with B. S. Blumberg in 1976 for his work
on infectious diseases.

4729.2   ——. & GIBBS, CLARENCE J.
Transmission of two subacute spongiform encephalopathies of man (kuru
and Creutzfeldt–Jakob disease) to New World monkeys. *Nature (London)*,
1971, **230**, 588-91.
    Transmission of kuru and Creutzfeldt–Jakob disease to primates. Simi-
larity in the clinical course of the diseases and in the cellular pathology of
brain material suggested similar causative agents.

Myopathies

4730   WILLIS, THOMAS. 1621-1675
De anima brutorum. Oxonii, *imp. R. Davis*, 1672.
    A probable description of myasthenia gravis is given in Pars. 2, Cap. IX.

4731   FREKE, JOHN. 1688-1756
A case of extraordinary exostoses on the back of a boy. *Phil. Trans.*, 1740,
41, 369-70.
    Probably the earliest description of myositis ossificans progressiva.
Freke was a friend of Fielding, who mentioned him in *Tom Jones*.

4732   DUCHENNE DE BOULOGNE, GUILLAUME BENJAMIN AMAND. 1806-1875
Recherches faites à l'aide du galvanisme sur l'état de la contractilité et de
la sensibilité électro-musculaires dans les paralysies des membres
supérieures. *C. R. Acad. Sci.* (*Paris*), 1849, **29**, 667-70.
    "Aran–Duchenne disease", progressive muscular atrophy, with which
the name of Cruveilhier is also associated. A fuller account is included in
Duchenne's *Électrisation localisée*, 1861, 437-547.

4733   ARAN, FRANÇOIS AMILCAR. 1817-1861
Recherches sur une maladie non encore décrite du système musculaire.
(Atrophie musculaire progressive). *Arch. gén. Méd.*, 1850, 4 sér., **24**, 4-35,
172-214.
    "Aran–Duchenne disease" (*see* No. 4732)

4734   CRUVEILHIER, JEAN. 1791-1874
Sur la paralysie musculaire, progressive, atrophique. *Bull. Acad. Méd.*
(*Paris*), 1852-53, **18**, 490-502, 546-83.
    "Cruveilhier's palsy", the progressive muscular atrophy already de-
scribed by Duchenne and Aran. The slimness of the anterior roots was first
noticed by Cruveilhier and was thought to be the essential lesion until Luys
(No. 4737) reported degeneration of the anterior horn cells.

4734.1   MERYON, EDWARD. 1809-1880
On granular and fatty degeneration of the voluntary muscles. *Med.-chir.
Trans.*, 1852, **35**, 73-84.
    "Duchenne's muscular dystrophy" (No. 4739) described.

4735   LITTLE, WILLIAM JOHN. 1810-1894
On the nature and treatment of the deformities of the human frame.
London, *Longman*, 1853.
    Early description of progressive muscular dystrophy (p. 14). *See* No. 4329.

4736   DUCHENNE DE BOULOGNE, GUILLAUME BENJAMIN AMAND. 1806-1875
Paralysie musculaire progressive de la langue, du voile du palais et des
lèvres; affection non encore décrite comme espèce morbide distincte.
Arch. gén. Méd., 1860, 5 sér., **16**, 283-96, 431-45.
    First description of chronic progressive bulbar paralysis ("Duchenne's
paralysis").

4737   LUYS, JULES BERNARD. 1828-1897
Atrophie musculaire progressive. Lésions histologiques de la substance grise de la moëlle épinière. *Gaz. méd. Paris*, 1860, 3 sér., **15**, 505.
Luys was the first to note the degeneration of the anterior horn cells in progressive muscular atrophy.

4738   GRIESINGER, WILHELM. 1817-1868
Ueber Muskelhypertrophie. *Arch. Heilk.*, 1865, **6**, 1-13.
Progressive muscular dystrophy with pseudo-hypertrophy. From the description given later by Duchenne (No. 4739) the condition has been named "Duchenne-Griesinger disease".

4739   DUCHENNE DE BOULOGNE, GUILLAUME BENJAMIN AMAND. 1806-1875
Recherches sur la paralysie musculaire pseudo-hypertrophique, ou paralysie myo-sclérosique. *Arch. gén. Méd.*, 1868, 6 sér., **11**, 5-25, 179-209, 305-21, 421-43, 552-88.
"Duchenne muscular dystrophy". English translation of first portion in Bick, *Classics of orthopaedics*, 72-75.

4740   CHARCOT, JEAN MARTIN. 1825-1893, & JOFFROY, ALEX. 1844-1908
Deux cas d'atrophie musculaire progressive avec lésions de la substance grise et des faisceaux antéro-latéraux de la moëlle épinière. *Arch. Physiol. norm. path.*, 1869, **2**, 744-60.
Description of the lesions of the spinal cord in muscular atrophy.

4741   MÜNCHMEYER, ERNST. 1846-1880
Ueber Myositis ossificans progressiva. *Z. rat. Med.*, 1869, 3 R., **34**, 9-41.
Münchmeyer described a form of progressive ossifying myositis ("Münchmeyer's disease").

4742   CHARCOT, JEAN MARTIN. 1825-1893
Des amyotrophies spinales chroniques. *Progr. méd.*, 1874, **2**, 573-74.
Charcot differentiated between the ordinary (Aran–Duchenne) type of muscular atrophy and the rarer amyotrophic lateral sclerosis, at one time called "Charcot's disease".

4743   LEYDEN, ERNST VON. 1832-1910
Klinik der Rückenmarks-Krankheiten. Bd. 2, pt.2. Berlin, *A. Hirschwald*, 1875-76.
First description of myotonia congenita occurs on p. 550.

4744   THOMSEN, ASMUS JULIUS THOMAS. 1815-1896
Tonische Krämpfe in willkürlich beweglichen Muskeln in Folge von ererbter psychischer Disposition (Ataxia muscularis?). *Arch. Psychiat. Nervenkr.*, 1876, **6**, 702-18.
Thomsen, himself a sufferer from myotonia congenita, gave the first full description of the condition, which later became known as "Thomsen's disease".

4745   WILKS, *Sir* SAMUEL, *Bart.* 1824-1911
On cerebritis, hysteria, and bulbar paralysis, as illustrative of arrest of function of the cerebro-spinal centres. *Guy's Hosp. Rep.*, 1877, 3 ser., **22**, 7-55.
The case of "bulbar paralysis" (pp. 45-55) is believed to be the first definite record of myasthenia gravis.

4746　　　ERB, WILHELM HEINRICH. 1840-1921
Ueber einen eigenthümlichen bulbären (?) Symptomenkomplex. *Arch. Psychiat. Nervenkr.*, 1879, **9**, 172-73.
　　　Myasthenia gravis ("Erb–Goldflam disease"; *see also* No. 4757). A further paper on the subject by Erb appears in the above volume, pp. 325-50.

4747　　　——. Ueber die juvenile Form der progressiven Muskelatrophie und ihre Beziehungen zur sogenannten Pseudohypertrophie der Muskeln. *Dtsch. Arch. klin. Med.*, 1884, **34**, 467-519.
　　　Progressive muscular dystrophy ("Erb's muscular atrophy"). Erb did much to establish the modern conception of the muscular dystrophies.

4748　　　DEJERINE-KLUMPKE, AUGUSTA. 1859-1927
Contribution à l'étude des paralysies radiculaires du plexus brachial. *Rev. Méd.*, 1885, **5**, 591-616, 739-90.
　　　First description of atrophic paralysis of the muscles of the hand following lesion of the brachial plexus and eighth cervical and first dorsal nerves ("Klumpke's paralysis").

4749　　　CHARCOT, JEAN MARTIN. 1825-1893, & MARIE, PIERRE. 1853-1940
Sur une forme particulière d'atrophie musculaire progressive souvent familiale débutant par les pieds et les jambes et atteignant plus tard les mains. *Rev. Méd.*, 1886, **6**, 97-138.
　　　First description of the peroneal form of muscular atrophy, the so-called Charcot–Marie–Tooth type.

4750　　　TOOTH, HOWARD HENRY. 1856-1925
The peroneal type of progressive muscular atrophy. London, *H. K. Lewis*, 1886.
　　　Tooth described peroneal muscular atrophy independently of, and in the same year as, Charcot and Marie.

4751　　　GOWERS, *Sir* WILLIAM RICHARD. 1845-1915
A manual of diseases of the nervous system. Vol. 1. London, *J. & A. Churchill*, 1886.
　　　Page 365: first description of local panatrophy. *See also Rev. Neurol. Psychiat.* (*Edinb.*), 1903, **1**, 3-4. *See also* No. 4569.

4752　　　LANDOUZY, LOUIS THÉOPHILE JOSEPH. 1845-1917, & DEJERINE, JOSEPH JULES. 1849-1917
Contribution à l'étude de la myopathie atrophique progressive (myopathie atrophique progressive, à type scapulo-huméral). *C. R. Soc. Biol.* (*Paris*), 1886, 8 sér., **3**, 478-81.
　　　"Landouzy–Dejerine type" of progressive muscular dystrophy.

4753　　　DANA, CHARLES LOOMIS. 1852-1935
An atypical case of Thomsen's disease (myotonia congenita). *Med. Rec.* (*N.Y.*), 1888, **33**, 433-35.
　　　Dana described a combination of myotonia and muscular atrophy.

4754   DÉLÉAGE, Francisque. 1862-
        Étude clinique sur la maladie de Thomsen (myotonie congénitale). Paris,
        Thèse No. 385, 1890; *O. Doin,* 1890.
        First description of dystrophia myotonica ("Déléage's disease").

4755   WERDNIG, Guido. 1862-
        Zwei frühinfantile hereditäre Fälle von progressiver Muskelatrophie unter
        dem Bilde der Dystrophie, aber auf neurotischer Grundlage. *Arch. Psychiat.*
        Nervenkr., 1891, **22,** 437-80.
        "Werdnig-Hoffmann muscular atrophy", an infantile familial form of
        progressive muscular atrophy. Hoffmann independently described it (*see*
        No. 4756).

4756   HOFFMANN, Johann. 1857-1919
        Ueber chronische spinale Muskelatrophie im Kindesalter, auf familiärer
        Basis. *Dtsch. Z. Nervenheilk.,* 1891, **1,** 95-120; 1893, **3,** 427-70.
        "Hoffmann's muscular atrophy" – independently described by Werdnig
        (No. 4755).

4757   GOLDFLAM, Samuel Vulfovich. 1852-1932
        Ueber einen scheinbar heilbaren bulbärparalytischen Symptomen-complex
        mit Betheiligung der Extremitäten. *Dtsch. Z. Nervenheilk.,* 1893, **4,** 312-52.
        Myasthenia pseudoparalytica (Erb–Goldflam symptom complex). *See*
        No. 4746.

4758   CHARCOT, Jean Baptiste Auguste Étienne. 1867-1936
        Contribution à l'étude de l'atrophie musculaire progressive type Duchenne–
        Aran. Paris, *Thèse No.* 313, 1895.

4759   MARIE, Pierre. 1853-1940
        Existe-t-il une atrophie musculaire progressive Aran-Duchenne? *Rev. neurol.*
        (*Paris*), 1897, **5,** 686-90.
        Marie disbelieved in the Aran–Duchenne type of muscular progressive
        atrophy.

4760   OPPENHEIM, Hermann. 1858-1919
        Ueber allgemeine und localisierte Atonie der Muskulatur (Myatonie) im
        frühen Kindesalter. *Mschr. Psychiat. Neurol.,* 1900, **8,** 232-33.
        First description of "Oppenheim's disease" – amyotonia congenita.

4761   WEIGERT, Carl. 1845-1904
        Pathologisch-anatomischer Beitrag zur Erb'schen Krankheit (Myasthenia
        gravis). *Neurol. Zbl.,* 1901, **20,** 597-601.
        Weigert noted the connection of myasthenia gravis with hypertrophy of
        the thymus.

4762   GOWERS, *Sir* William Richard. 1845-1915
        On myopathy and a distal form. *Brit. med. J.,* 1902, **2,** 89-92.
        "Distal myopathy of Gowers", a form of progressive muscular dystrophy.

4763   CRUCHET, Jean René. 1875-1959
        Traité des torticolis spasmodiques. Paris, *Masson,* 1907.
        In this classic monograph, 357 cases of torticollis are recorded.

4764   SAUERBRUCH, ERNST FERDINAND. 1875-1951
        Thymektomie bei einem Fall von Morbus Basedowi mit Myasthenie. *Mitt. Grenzgeb. Med. Chir.*, 1912-13, **25**, 746-65.
        Thymectomy for myasthenia gravis. Reported by C. H. Schumacher and – . Roth.

4765   EDGEWORTH, HARRIET ISABEL. 1892-
        A report of progress on the use of ephedrine in a case of myasthenia gravis. *J. Amer. med. Assoc.*, 1930, **94**, 1136.
        Harriet Edgeworth discovered by accident the beneficial effect of ephedrine in myasthenia gravis.

4766   BOOTHBY, WALTER MEREDITH. 1880-1953
        Myasthenia gravis: a preliminary report on the effect of treatment with glycine. *Proc. Mayo Clin.*, 1932, **7**, 557-62.
        Introduction of glycine (glycocoll) in the treatment of myasthenia gravis.

4767   REMEN, LAZAR. 1907-
        Zur Pathogenese und Therapie der Myasthenie gravis pseudoparalytica. *Dtsch. Z. Nervenheilk.*, 1932, **128**, 66-78.
        Introduction of neostigmine in the treatment of myasthenia gravis.

4768   WALKER, MARY BROADFOOT. 1888-1974
        Treatment of myasthenia gravis with physostigmine. *Lancet*, 1934, **1**, 1200-01.
        Introduction of physostigmine in treatment of myasthenia gravis. She replaced this with neostigmine in 1935 (*Proc. roy. Soc. Med.*, **28**, 759-61).

4769   LAURENT, LOUIS PHILIPPE EUGENE, & WALTHER, WILLIAM WERNER.
        The influence of large doses of potassium chloride on myasthenia gravis. *Lancet*, 1935, **1**, 1434-35.
        Potassium salts first used in treatment of myasthenia gravis.

4770   MINOT, ANN STONE. 1894- , *et al.*
        The response of the myasthenic state to guanidine hydrochloride. *Science*, 1938, **87**, 348-50.
        Guanidine first used in treatment of myasthenia gravis. With K. Dodd and S. S. Riven.

4771   BLALOCK, ALFRED. 1899-1964, *et al.*
        Myasthenia gravis and tumors of the thymic region. Report of a case in which the tumor was removed. *Ann. Surg.*, 1939, **110**, 544-61.
        First deliberate treatment of myasthenia gravis by thymectomy. with M. F. Mason, H. J. Morgan, and S. S. Riven.

4771.1 BECKER, P. E., & KEINER, F.
        Eine neue *x*-chromosomale Muskeldystrophie. *Arch. Psychiat. Nervenkr.*, 1955, **193**, 427-48.
        Becker-type muscular dystrophy.

NEUROSYPHILIS

4772   LOEWENHARDT, Sigismund Eduard. 1796-1875
De myelophthisi chronica vera et notha. Berolini, *typ. Haynianis,* [1817].
First important account of tabes dorsalis.

4773   HORN, Wilhelm von. 1803-1871
De tabe dorsuali praelusio. Berolini, *formis Krausianis,* [1827].
Gives the views of his father, Ernst Horn (1744-1848), on tabes.

4774   DUCHENNE DE BOULOGNE, Guillaume Benjamin Amand. 1806-1875
De l'ataxie locomotrice progressive. *Arch. gén. Méd.,* 1858, 5 sér., **12**, 641-52; 1859, **13**, 36-62, 158-81, 417-51.
Although far from being the first to describe tabes dorsalis, Duchenne gave a classic account of the condition, earning the eponym "Duchenne's disease".

4775   CHARCOT, Jean Martin. 1825-1893, & BOUCHARD, Abel. 1833-1899
Douleurs fulgurantes de l'ataxie sans incoordination des mouvements; sclérose commençante des cordons postérieurs de la moëlle épinière. *Gaz. méd. Paris,* 1866, 3 sér., **21**, 122-24.
First clinical description of the electric pains in tabes.

4776   DELAMARRE, Georges.
Des troubles gastriques dans l'ataxie locomotrice progressive. Paris, *Thèse No.* 250, 1866.
Tabetic gastric crises first described.

4777   CHARCOT, Jean Martin. 1825-1893
Sur quelques arthropathies qui paraissent dépendre d'une lésion du cerveau ou de la moëlle épinière. *Arch. Physiol. norm. path.,* 1868, **1**, 161-78.
Charcot called attention to tabetic arthropathy, which has since then borne his name, while the tabetic joints he so well described are known as "Charcot's joints".

4778   ALLBUTT, *Sir* Thomas Clifford. 1836-1925
Case of cerebral disease in a syphilitic patient. *St. George's Hosp. Rep.,* 1868, **3**, 55-65.
Syphilitic endarteritis of cerebral arteries described.

4779   ————. Remarks on a case of locomotor ataxy with hydrarthrosis. *St. George's Hosp. Rep.,* 1869, **4**, 259-60.
An early description of the joint symptoms in tabes dorsalis.

4780   ERB, Wilhelm Heinrich. 1840-1921
Ueber Sehnenreflexe bei Gesunden und bei Rückenmarkskranken. *Arch. Psychiat. Nervenkr.,* 1875, **5**, 792-802.
Knee-jerk first used as diagnostic measure in tabes dorsalis.

4781   WESTPHAL, Carl Friedrich Otto. 1833-1890
Ueber einige durch mechanische Einwirkung auf Sehnen und Muskeln hervorgebrachte Bewegungs-Erscheinungen. *Arch. Psychiat. Nervenkr.,* 1875, **5**, 803-34.
Westphal discovered the diagnostic value of the knee-jerk simultaneously with Erb.

4782   FOURNIER, JEAN ALFRED. 1832-1914
De l'ataxie locomotrice d'origine syphilitique. Paris, *G. Masson*, 1876.
Fournier advanced the doctrine of the syphilitic origin of tabes, a hypothesis which was opposed for a time.

4783   LEICHTENSTERN, OTTO MICHAEL. 1845-1900
Ueber progressive perniciöse Anämie bei Tabeskranken. *Dtsch. med. Wschr.*, 1884, **10**, 849.
First description of subacute combined degeneration of the spinal cord.

4784   DEJERINE, JOSEPH JULES. 1849-1917
Sur un cas de paraplégie par névrites périphériques, chez un ataxique morphiomane. *C. R. Soc. Biol. (Paris)*, 1887, 8 sér., **4**, 137-43.
First description of peripheral neuritis, "Dejerine's neurotabes".

4785   ———. Sur l'atrophie musculaire des ataxiques. Paris, *F. Alcan*, 1889.
Dejerine ranks high in French neurology. He became clinical chief at the Salpêtrière. He separated peripheral from medullary tabes, wrote on the tabetic muscular atrophies, on the parietal lobe syndrome, and made many other contributions to neurological literature.

4786   FRENKEL, HEINRICH. 1860-1931
Die Therapie atactischer Bewegungsstörungen. *Münch. med. Wschr.*, 1890, **37**, 917-20.
Frenkel devised certain muscular exercises for use in the treatment of tabes dorsalis.

4788   ERB, WILHELM HEINRICH. 1840-1921
Ueber syphilitische Spinalparalyse. *Neurol. Zbl.*, 1892, **11**, 161-68.
Erb's classic description of syphilitic spinal paralysis, sometimes called "Erb's disease".

4789   ———. Die Aetiologie der Tabes. *Samml. klin. Vortr.*, 1892, N.F., Nr. 53. (Inn. Med. Nr. 18), 515-42.
English translation, 1900.

4791   PEL, PIETER KLUZES. 1852-1919
Augenkrisen bei Tabes dorsalis. *Berl. klin. Wschr.*, 1898, **35**, 25-27.
"Pel's crises" – the ocular crises in tabes.

4792   NONNE, MAX. 1861-1959
Syphilis und Nervensystem. Berlin, *S. Karger*, 1902.

General Paralysis

4793   WILLIS, THOMAS. 1621-1675
De anima brutorum. Oxonii, *R. Davis*, 1672.
Two Oxford editions were published in 1672: the first, in quarto, in which a description of general paralysis appears on pp. 392-432, and the second, in octavo, in which it appears on pp. 278-307. In his *Practice of Physick* (1684) the translation of this section appears on pp. 161-78.

4794 HASLAM, JOHN. 1764-1844
Observations on insanity. *F. & C. Rivington*, 1798.
Haslam was among the first to describe general paralysis; he recorded three cases (pp. 64, 67, 92, 120).

4795 BAYLE, ANTOINE LAURENT JESSÉ. 1799-1858
Recherches sur l'arachnitis chronique. Paris, *Thèse No.* 247, 1822.
Bayle was a most distinguished physician and pathologist. His classic description of dementia paralytica, the first clear delineation, led to the eponym "Bayle's disease". Commercial issue: Paris, *Didot le Jeune*, 1822. Partial English translation in *Arch. Neurol. Psychiat. (Chicago)*, 1934, **32**, 808-829.

4796 DELAYE, J. B.
Considérations sur une espèce de paralysie qui affecte particulièrement les aliénés. Paris, *Thèse No.* 224, 1824.
Delaye, a pupil of Esquirol, selected for his thesis the subject of "incomplete general paralysis of the insane", which he differentiated from other forms of paralysis. He recorded the early signs of the disease, emphasizing the speech disturbance.

4797 CALMEIL, LOUIS FLORENTIN. 1798-1895
De la paralysie considérée chez les aliénés. Paris, *J. B. Baillière*, 1826.
Classic description of general paralysis. Calmeil's work complements Bayle's earlier delineation of general paralysis (No. 4795). Between the two of them they established the clinical picture of general paralysis of the insane, associating it with chronic inflammation of the brain. This was the first breakthrough in neuro-psychiatric research, and it gave psychiatry the spur to precise and systematic clinical, pathological, and statistical innovation on its own terms.

4798 ESQUIROL, JEAN ETIENNE DOMINIQUE. 1772-1840
Des maladies mentales. Tom. 2. Paris, *J. B. Baillière*, 1838.
Contains, p. 264, a classic description of paresis. Esquirol regarded general paralysis as a complication of various forms of mental disorder.

4799 CLOUSTON, *Sir* THOMAS SMITH. 1841-1915
A case of general paralysis at the age of sixteen. *J. ment. Sci.*, 1877, **23**, 419-20.
Clouston, eminent English psychiatrist, was the first definitely to recognize the relationship between paresis and congenital syphilis and to report a case. This paper is also of interest as being the only recorded case of juvenile paresis at the time Ibsen wrote *Ghosts*, with its excellent portrayal of the condition in the person of Oswald Alving.

4800 FOURNIER, JEAN ALFRED. 1832-1914
Les affections parasyphilitiques. Paris, *Rueff & Cie.*, 1894.
Fournier, great French venereologist, introduced the concept of "parasyphilis". He showed statistically the causal relationship of syphilis to paresis and tabes.

4801   RAECKE, JULIUS. 1872-1930
Paralyse und Tabes bei Eheleuten. Ein Beitrag zur Aetiologie beider
Krankheiten. *Mschr. Psychiat. Neurol.*, 1899, **6**, 266-86.

4802   STORCH, ERNST. 1866-
Ueber einige Fälle atypischer progressiver Paralyse. Nach einem
hinterlassenen Manuscript Dr. H. Lissauer's. *Mschr. Psychiat. Neurol.*, 1901,
9, 401-34.
    "Lissauer's atypical general paralysis" first described. Heinrich Lissauer
was born in 1861 and died in 1891.

4803   NISSL, FRANZ. 1860-1919
Histologische und histopathologische Arbeiten über die Grosshirnrinde.
Vol. 1. Jena, *G. Fischer,* 1904.
    Pages 315-494 contain Nissl's classic account of the histopathology of
general paresis.

4804   WASSERMANN, AUGUST VON. 1866-1925, & PLAUT, FELIX. 1877-
Ueber das Vorhandensein syphilitischer Antistoffe in der
Cerebrospinalflüssigkeit von Paralytikern. *Dtsch. med. Wschr.,* 1906, **32**,
1769-72.
    Wassermann applied his test (No. 2402) to the cerebrospinal fluid and,
in paretics, obtained positive results in over 90 per cent of cases. The test
greatly facilitated the diagnosis of general paralysis.

4805   NOGUCHI, HIDEYO. 1876-1928, & MOORE, JOSEPH WALDRON. 1879-
A demonstration of Treponema pallidum in the brain in cases of general
paralysis. *J. exp. Med.*, 1913, **17**, 232-38.
    A pure culture of *Trep. pallidum* was obtained from a case of dementia
paralytica.

4806   WAGNER VON JAUREGG, JULIUS. 1857-1940
Ueber die Einwirkung der Malaria auf die progressive Paralyse. *Psychiat.-
neurol. Wschr.*, 1918-19, **20**, 132-34, 251-55.
    In 1917 Wagner von Jauregg returned to the idea of the inoculation of
paretics with malaria to induce pyrexia, first proposed by him in 1887
(Ueber die Einwirkung fieberhafter Erkrankungen auf Psychosen, *Jb.
Psychiat.*, **7**, 94-131). He was awarded the Nobel Prize in 1927.

EPILEPSY

4807   HIPPOCRATES. 460-375 B.C.
The sacred disease. In [Works]. . .edited with an English translation by W.
H. S. JONES. London, *W. Heinemann*, 1923, **2**, 127-83.
    This includes the first mention of epilepsy in children. Hippocrates
grouped all convulsive attacks together as ἱερα νοῦσος, the sacred disease.
He did not employ the word ἐπίληψις, (which seems first to have been
used in the 10th century by Avicenna) but the terms 'ιρόν νίσημα, παθος
παίδειον and νοσημα   παιδειον. The standard Greek edition is *Die
hippokratische Schrift Über die heilige Krankheit.* Herausgegeben, übersetzt
und erläutert von H. Grensemann, Berlin, 1968.

4808   ARETAEUS, *the Cappadocian. circa* A.D. 81-138
On epilepsy. In his *Extant works,* translated by F. ADAMS, London, 1856, 243, 296, 399, 468.

    Aretaeus was well acquainted with hemi-epilepsy from local injury in the opposite half of the brain; partly from this knowledge he formulated the "decussation in the form of the letter X" of the motor path. He first described epilepsy resulting from a depressed fracture of the skull. In his excellent description he made the first mention of the aura.

4808.1   CAELIUS AURELIANUS. *fl.* A.D. 500
Tardarum passionum libri V. Basileae, *Henricus Petrus,* 1529.

    Garrison describes Caelius as a 5th century neurologist who gave one of the best early descriptions of epilepsy, including its convulsive and comatose forms, and the tendency of victims of vertigo to become epileptic. Caelius also distinguished between sensory and motor impairment, and between spastic and flaccid paralysis. English translation, Chicago, 1950. *See* No. 4915.1.

4809   PRICHARD, JAMES COWLES. 1786-1848
A treatise on diseases of the nervous system. London, *T. & G. Underwood,* 1822.

    Includes the best early account of epilepsy after Willis.

4810   BRAVAIS, LOUIS FRANÇOIS. ?-1842
Recherches sur les symptômes et le traitement de l'épilepsie hémiplégique. Paris, *Thèse No.* 118, 1827.

    First description of hemiplegic epilepsy so well depicted by Jackson (No. 4816) and referred to by Charcot as "Bravais–Jacksonian épilepsie".

4811   BRIGHT, RICHARD. 1789-1858
Fatal epilepsy, from suppuration between the dura mater and arachnoid, in consequence of blood having been effused in that situation. *Guy's Hosp. Rep.,* 1836, **1,** 36-40.

    Bright was the first to describe unilateral ("Jacksonian") epilepsy.

4812   HALL, MARSHALL. 1790-1857
Synopsis of cerebral and spinal seizures of inorganic origin and of paroxysmal form as a class; and of their pathology as involved in the structures and actions of the neck. London, *J. Mallett,* [1851].

    Hall was the first to suggest that the paroxysmal nervous discharges in epilepsy were produced by the spinal nervous system, first to notice the connection of anaemia with epilepsy, and first to deduce that epilepsy was produced by anaemia of the medulla.

4813   BROWN-SÉQUARD, CHARLES ÉDOUARD. 1817-1894
Recherches expérimentales sur la production d'une affection convulsive épileptiforme, à la suite de lésions de la moëlle épinière. *Arch. gén. Méd.,* 1856, 5 sér., **7,** 143-49.

    Experimental epilepsy (section of sciatic nerve). See also *Arch. Physiol. norm. path.,* 1869, **2,** 211-20, 422-38, 496-503; 1870, **3,** 153-60.

4813.1   LOCOCK, *Sir* CHARLES, *Bart*. 1799-1875
[Contribution to discussion on paper by E. H. Sieveking.] *Lancet*, 1857, **1**, 528.
    Locock, physician accoucheur to Queen Victoria, recommended bro-
mide of potassium in the treatment of epilepsy.

4814   O'CONNOR, WILLIAM.   ?-1880
Cases of epilepsy, associated with amenorrhoea and vicarious menstruation,
successfully treated with the iodide of potassium. *Lancet*, 1857, **1**, 525.
    O'Connor was apparently the first to use potassium bromide for the
treatment of epilepsy.

4815   SCHROEDER VAN DER KOLK, JACOB LUDWIG CONRAD. 1797-1862
Bau und Functionen der Medulla spinalis und oblongata, und nächste
Ursache und rationelle Behandlung der Epilepsie. Braunschweig, *F. Vieweg
u. Sohn*, 1859.
    The work of Schroeder van der Kolk brought histological examination
to the forefront in connection with theories on the localization of function.
His careful microscopical studies confirmed the medulla as being the
ultimate seat of epilepsy. The book was translated into English for the New
Sydenham Society in the same year.

4816   JACKSON, JOHN HUGHLINGS. 1835-1911
Unilateral epileptiform seizures, attended by temporary defect of sight.
Med. Times Gaz., 1863, **1**, 588-89.
    "Jacksonian epilepsy" is so called from the excellent account of unilateral
epilepsy with spasm given by Jackson. Actually, Bravais (No. 4810) was
first to note the condition.

4817   ——. Case of hemikinesis. *Brit. Med. J.*, 1875, **1**, 773.

4818   GOWERS, *Sir* WILLIAM RICHARD. 1845-1915
Epilepsy and other chronic convulsive diseases. London, *J. & A. Churchill*,
1881.
    Gowers left a classic account of epilepsy, a book which today is still one
of the most important on the subject. He was first to note the tetanic nature
of the epileptic convulsion.

4819   UNVERRICHT, HEINRICH. 1853-1912
Die Myoclonie. Wien, *F. Deuticke*, 1891.
    First description of "Unverricht's disease" – familial myoclonus epilepsy.

4820   KOŽEVNIKOV, ALEKSEI YAKOVLEVIČ. 1836-1902
Osobyj vid kortikal'noj epilepsii. *Med. Obozrenie*, 1894, **42**, 9-118.
    "Koževnikov's epilepsy", an atypical form of cortical origin. German
translation by H. Heintel and H. Müller-Dietz, Hamburg, 1974.

4821   GOWERS, *Sir* WILLIAM RICHARD. 1845-1915
The border-land of epilepsy. Faints, vagal attacks, vertigo, migraine, sleep
symptoms, and their treatment. London, *J. & A. Churchill*, 1907.

4822   DAVENPORT, CHARLES BENEDICT. 1866-1944, & WEEKS, DAVID FAIRCHILD.
1874-1929
A first study of inheritance of epilepsy. *J. nerv. ment. Dis.*, 1911, **38**, 641-70.
    Davenport and Weeks produced strong evidence in support of the
hereditary origin of epilepsy.

4823   HAUPTMANN, ALFRED. 1881-1948
        Luminal bei Epilepsie. *Münch. med. Wschr.*, 1912, **59**, 1907-09.
        Introduction of phenobarbitone in the treatment of epilepsy.

4824   GOLLA, FREDERICK LUCIEN. 1878-1968, *et al.*
        The electro-encephalogram in epilepsy. *J. ment. Sci.*, 1937, **83,** 137-55.
        Demonstration of the changes in the electro-encephalogram in epilepsy. With S. Graham and W. Grey Walter.

4824.1 MERRITT, HIRAM HOUSTON. 1902-1979, & PUTNAM, TRACY J.
        Sodium diphenyl hydantoinate in the treatment of convulsive disorders. *J. Amer. med. Assoc.*, 1938, **111**, 1068-73.
        Introduction of diphenylhydantoin.

For history, see No. 5015

See also 3856-3863, PARATHYROID GLANDS.

4825   CLARKE, JOHN. 1761-1815
        Commentaries on some of the most important diseases of children. Part the first. London, *Longman, etc.*, 1815.
        First account of infantile tetany is given on pp. 86-97.

4826   KELLIE, GEORGE. ?1770-1830
        Notes on the swelling of the tops of the hands and feet, and on a spasmodic affection of the thumbs and toes, which very commonly attends it. *Edinb. med. surg. J.*, 1816, **12**, 448-52.
        In his early account of chronic tetany, Kellie referred to carpo-pedal spasm and spasms of the glottis as part of the syndrome.

4827   STEINHEIM, SALOMON LEVI. 1789-1866
        Zwei seltene Formen von hitzigem Rheumatismus. *Litt. Ann. ges. Heilk.*, 1830, **17**, 22-30.
        German writers usually credit Steinheim with the first description of parathyroid tetany.

4828   DANCE, JEAN BAPTISTE HIPPOLYTE. 1797-1832
        Observations sur une espèce de tétanos intermittent. *Arch. gén. Méd.*, 1831, **26**, 190-205.
        Dance's important early description of parathyroid tetany followed closely on that of Steinheim.

4829   CORVISART, FRANÇOIS RÉMY LUCIEN. 1824-1882
        De la contracture des extrémités ou tétanie. Paris, *Thèse No.* 223, 1852.
        In his graduation thesis, Lucien Corvisart, nephew of the more famous Baron Corvisart (No. 2737), introduced the term "tétanie".

4830   TROUSSEAU, ARMAND. 1801-1867
        Clinique médicale de l'Hôtel-Dieu de Paris. Tom. 2. Paris, *J. B. Baillière*, 1861.
        On pp. 112-14 Trousseau describes the phenomenon in tetany which now bears his name. This is produced by pressure upon the arm sufficient

to stop the circulation; the result is a sudden contraction of the fingers and hand into the so-called "obstetrical position".

4831 KUSSMAUL, Adolf. 1822-1902
Zur Lehre von der Tetanie. *Berl. klin. Wschr.*, 1872, **9**, 441-44.
Important observations on gastric tetany were made by Kussmaul. He called attention to the convulsions sometimes accompanying dilatation of the stomach. He first mentioned "gastric tetany" in 1869 in his paper on gastric lavage (No. 3463).

4832 ERB, Wilhelm Heinrich. 1840-1921
Zur Lehre von der Tetanie nebst Bemerkungen über die Prufung der electrischen Erregbarkeit motorischer Nerven. *Arch. Psychiat. Nervenkr.*, 1873-74, **4**, 271-316.
"Erb's sign".

4833 CHVOSTEK, František. 1835-1884
Beitrag zur Tetanie. *Wien. med. Presse,* 1876, **17**, 1201-03, 1225-27, 1253-58, 1313-16.
"Chvostek's sign", a reliable diagnostic sign in latent tetany in small children.

4834 FRANKL-HOCHWART, Lothar von. 1862-1915
Die Tetanie. Berlin, *A. Hirschwald,* 1891.

4835 ESCHERICH, Theodor. 1857-1911
Die Tetanie der Kinder. Wien, *A. Hölder,* 1909.

4836 HULDSCHINSKY, Kurt. 1883-1941
Die Beeinflussung der Tetanie durch Ultraviolettlicht. *Z. Kinderheilk.*, 1920, **26**, 207-14.
Treatment of tetany with ultra-violet light.

4837 COLLIP, James Bertram. 1892-1965, & LEITCH, Douglas Burrows. 1888-
A case of tetany treated with parathyrin. *Canad. med. Ass. J.*, 1925, **15**, 59-60.
First use of parathyroid hormone in the treatment of tetany.

4838 HOLTZ, Friedrich.
Die Behandlung der postoperativen Tetanie. *Arch. klin. Chir.*, 1933, **177**, 32-34.
Introduction of A.T. 10 ("Antitetanisches Präparat Nr. 10"), dihydrotachysterol, in the treatment of tetany.

NEUROSES AND PSYCHONEUROSES

4839 WILLIS, Thomas. 1621-1675
Affectionum quae dicuntur hystericae e hypochondriacae pathologia spasmodica vindicata...London, *Jacob Allestry,* 1670.
In this treatise on hysteria and hypochondria, Willis showed that hysteria was a nervous disease and not a uterine disorder as had been traditionally believed. He compared hysteria in women to hypochondria in men. He considered the key feature of hysteria to be the "fit" or episodic

disturbance of sensation short of "universal convulsions" and classified it under convulsive diseases. This caused hysteria to be linked with epilepsy as in Charcot's hybrid, "hystero-epilepsy".

4840   CHEYNE, GEORGE. 1671-1743
The English malady; or, a treatise of nervous diseases of all kinds. London, G. Strahan, 1733.
    Cheyne attributed hypochondria ("Cheyne's disease") to the moisture of the air and variability of the weather in the British Isles. Cheyne himself suffered from this disease and the work includes a careful account of his own case history.

4841   WHYTT, ROBERT. 1714-1766
Observations on the nature, causes, and cure of those disorders which have been commonly called nervous hypochondriac, or hysteric, to which are prefixed some remarks on the sympathy of the nerves. Edinburgh, printed for T. Becket and P. Du Hondt, London, and J. Balfour, Edinburgh, 1765.
    "First important English work on neurology after Willis" (Garrison).

4842   BRIQUET, PAUL. 1796-1881
Traité clinique et thérapeutique de l'hystérie. Paris, J. B. Baillière, 1859.
    Includes, p. 297, first description of ataxia analgica hysterica ("Briquet's ataxia"), and p. 475, hysterical paralysis of the diaphragm with dyspnoea and aphonia ("Briquet's syndrome").

4843   BEARD, GEORGE MILLER. 1839-1883
Neurasthenia, or nervous exhaustion. Boston med. surg. J., 1869, **80**, 217-21.
    "Beard's disease" (neurasthenia) first described. See also No. 4846.

4844   WESTPHAL, CARL FRIEDRICH OTTO. 1833-1890
Die Agoraphobie, eine neuropathische Erscheinung. Arch. Psychiat. Nervenkr., 1871-72, **3**, 138-61.
    First description of agoraphobia.

4845   GULL, Sir WILLIAM WITHEY. 1816-1890
Anorexia nervosa (apepsia hysterica, anorexia hysterica). Trans. clin. Soc. Lond., 1874, **7**, 22-28.
    Classic description of anorexia nervosa.

4846   BEARD, GEORGE MILLER. 1839-1883
A practical treatise on nervous exhaustion (neurasthenia). New York, W. Wood & Co., 1880.

4847   ALLBUTT, Sir THOMAS CLIFFORD. 1836-1925
On visceral neuroses. London, J. & A Churchill, 1884.
    Gulstonian Lectures.

4848   GILLES DE LA TOURETTE, GEORGES. 1857-1904
Jumping, latah, myriachit. Arch. Neurol. (Paris), 1884, **8**, 68-74.
    Latah, motor incoordination associated with echolalia and coprolalia, is named "Gilles de la Tourette's disease" after his classic description of it.

4849   GANSER, SIGBERT JOSEPH MARIA. 1853-1931
Ueber einen eigenartigen hysterischen Dämmerzustand. *Arch. Psychiat. Nervenkr.*, 1898, **30**, 633-40.
"Ganser's syndrome" – an acute hallucinatory mania.

NEUROLOGICAL SURGERY

4850   EDWIN SMITH PAPYRUS.
The Edwin Smith Surgical Papyrus. Published in facsimile and hieroglyphic transliteration with translation and commentary by JAMES HENRY BREASTED. 2 vols. Chicago, *Univ. Press*, 1930.
The original text of the Edwin Smith Surgical Papyrus was written about 3000 B.C., and the present manuscript is a copy dating about 1600 B.C. It is the oldest known surgical treatise and consists entirely of case reports; it describes 47 different cases of injuries and affections of the head, nose, and mouth, together with methods of bandaging. *See* No. 5547.

4850.1   HIPPOCRATES, 460-375 B.C.
Chirurgie d'Hippocrate. 2 vols. Paris, *Imprimérie nationale*, 1877-78.
A Greek–French edition with extensive notes and commentaries by J. E. Pétrequin. Hippocrates performed trephining and paracentesis.

4850.2   BERENGARIO DA CARPI. GIACOMO. *circa* 1460-1530[?]
Tractatus de fractura calve sive cranei. [Bologna, *Hieronymus de Bendictis*, 1518.]
The first separate treatise on head wounds, and their surgical treatment. Berengario described several types of skull fractures and grouped the resulting lesions according to their symptoms, citing the relation between location and neurological effect. The book also discussed apoplexy, meningitis and paralysis.

4850.3   PARÉ, AMBROISE. 1510-1590
La méthode curative des playes, & fractures de la teste humaine. Paris, *Jean Le Royer*, 1561.
Written after the death of Paré's patient, Henri II, who was struck in the eye by the shaft of a lance at a tournament in celebration of the marriage of Philip, King of Spain, with Elizabeth of France. Paré discusses surgery of head wounds with special attention to skull fractures.

4850.4   CROCE, GIOVANNI ANDREA DELLA. 1514-1575.
Chirurgiae...libri septem...Venetiis, *Apud Jordanum Zilettum*, 1573.
Croce improved the instruments for trephination, and published classic woodcuts depicting the operation, including the first illustration of a neurological surgery operation actually taking place. The work is also important for Croce's descriptions of cranial and cerebral diseases. In hundreds of woodcuts of instruments and procedures Croce illustrated all of the instruments used before and during his own time.

4850.5   POTT, PERCIVALL. 1714-1788
Observations on the nature and consequences of wounds and contusions of the head, fractures of the skull, concussions of the brain, etc. London, *C. Hitch & L. Hawes*, 1760.

746

This book, which showed Pott's extensive knowledge of surgical literature, systematized the treatment of head injuries. It shows what a variety of injuries of the head could be sustained even before the advent of the motor-car. Includes the first description of "Pott's puffy tumour". Pott was born in Threadneedle Street, where the Bank of England now stands; he succeeded Cheselden as the greatest surgeon of his day. The book was altered and re-published under a different title in 1768.

4851   MORAND, SAUVEUR FRANÇOIS. 1697-1773
Opuscules de chirurgie. Pt. 1. Paris, *G. Desprez et P. A. Le Prieur,* 1768.
     Records, p. 161, a successful operation for temporo-sphenoidal abscess, 1752. The patient, a monk, had otorrhoea followed by a mastoid abscess, which Morand opened.

4851.1   DUDLEY, BENJAMIN WINSLOW. 1785-1870
Case reports: From injuries of the head. *Transylvania. J. Med.,* 1823, **1**, 9-40.
     Dudley was for many years the leading surgeon on the western frontier of the United States. This paper reports the first operations on the brain performed in the United States. Three of the five patients were relieved of their symptoms.

4852   NOTT, JOSIAH CLARK. 1804-1873
Exstirpation of the os coccygis for neuralgia. *New Orleans med. surg. J.,* 1844-45, **1**, 58-60.

4853   DETMOLD, WILLIAM. 1808-1894
Abscess in the substance of the brain; the lateral ventricles opened by an operation. *Amer. J. med. Sci.,* 1850, n.s. **19**, 86-95.
     Lateral ventricles of the brain first opened for the treatment of cerebral abscess.

4854   CARNOCHAN, JOHN MURRAY. 1817-1887
Exsection of the trunk of the second branch of the fifth pair of nerves, beyond the ganglion of Meckel, for severe neuralgia of the face; with three cases. *Amer. J. med. Sci.,* 1858, n.s. **35**, 134-43.
     First excision of the superior maxillary nerve for the treatment of facial neuralgia.

4855   PANCOAST, JOSEPH. 1805-1882
New operation for the relief of persistent facial neuralgia. *Philad. med. Times,* 1871-72, **2**, 285-87.
     Pancoast devised the operative procedure of sectioning the second and third branches of the fifth pair of nerves as they emerge from the base of the brain. Reported by F. Woodbury.

4856   MACEWEN, *Sir* WILLIAM. 1848-1924
Tumour of the dura mater – convulsions – removal of tumour by trephining – recovery. *Glasg. med. J.,* 1879, **12**, 210-13.

4857   MEARS, JAMES EWING. 1838-1919
Study of the pathological changes occurring in trifacial neuralgia, with the report of a case in which three inches of the inferior dental nerve were excised. *Med. News (Philad.),* 1884, **45**, 58-63.
     Mears first suggested Gasserian ganglionectomy for trigeminal neuralgia.

4858   BENNETT, ALEXANDER HUGHES. 1848-1901, & GODLEE, *Sir* RICKMAN JOHN. 1849-1925
Case of cerebral tumour. *Med.-chir. Trans.*, 1885, **68**, 243-75.
First instance of diagnosis, accurate clinical localization, and operative removal of a tumour of the brain, 25 November, 1884. The patient survived for one month. Preliminary report in *Lancet,* 1884, **2**, 1090-91.

4859   BERGMANN, ERNST VON. 1836-1907
Die chirurgische Behandlung von Hirnkrankheiten. Berlin, *A. Hirschwald,* 1888.
Bergmann greatly improved the surgical treatment of diseases of the brain.

4860   GOWERS, *Sir* WILLIAM RICHARD. 1845-1915, & HORSLEY, *Sir* VICTOR ALEX-ANDER HADEN. 1857-1916
A case of tumour of the spinal cord. Removal; recovery. *Med.-chir. Trans.*, 1888, **71**, 377-430.
Horsley was the founder of neurosurgery in England. The above paper records the first successful operation for the removal of an extramedullary tumour of the spinal cord.

4860.1   ABBE, ROBERT. 1851-1928
A contribution to the surgery of the spine. *Med. Rec.*, 1889, **35**, 149-52.
Posterior rhizotomy.

4861   ALEXANDER, WILLIAM. 1844-1919
The treatment of epilepsy. Edinburgh, *Y. J. Pentland,* 1889.
Alexander was the first to attempt the treatment of epilepsy by surgical means. He removed the superior cervical sympathetic ganglia.

4861.1   BENNETT, *Sir* WILLIAM HENRY. 1852-1931
A case in which acute spasmodic pain in the left lower extremity was completely relieved by sub-dural division of the posterior roots of certain spinal nerves, all other treatment having proved useless. Death from sudden collapse and cerebral haemorrhage on the twelfth day after the operation, at the commencement of apparent convalescence. *Med.-chir. Trans.*, 1889, **72**, 329-48.
Posterior rhizotomy.

4862   WAGNER, WILHELM. 1848-1900
Die temporäre Resektion der Schädeldaches an Stelle der Trepanation. *Zbl. Chir.*, 1889, **16**, 833-38.
Osteoplastic flap operation. Wagner's method of opening the skull made a large area of the brain more easily accessible than by trephining. Translation in *J. Neurosurg.*, 1962, **19**, 1099.

4863   ROSE, WILLIAM. 1847-1910
Removal of the gasserian ganglion for severe neuralgia. *Lancet,* 1890, **2**, 914-15.
Gasserian ganglionectomy for trigeminal neuralgia; the patient lived for at least two years.

4864   BURCKHARDT, G.
Ueber Rindenexcisionen, als Beitrag zur operativen Therapie der Psychosen. *Allg. Z. Psychiat.*, 1891, **47**, 463-548.
Burckhardt, physician at a Swiss mental hospital, performed frontal lobotomy on four patients in 1890, with good results in some cases.

4865   HORSLEY, *Sir* Victor Alexander Haden. 1857-1916, *et al.*
Remarks on the various surgical procedures devised for the relief or cure of trigeminal neuralgia (tic douloureux). *Brit. med. J.*, 1891, **2**, 1139-43, 1191-93, 1249-52.
Horsley, with J. Taylor and W. S. Coleman, devised an operation for treatment of trigeminal neuralgia in which the Gasserian ganglion was removed by a temporal approach.

4866   KEEN, William Williams. 1837-1932
Linear craniotomy (miscalled craniectomy) for microcephalus. *Am. J. med. Sci.*, 1891, **101**, 549-55.
Keen was a pioneer in linear craniotomy and one of the first successfully to operate for meningioma. He was Professor of Surgery at Jefferson Medical College.

4867   ———. A new operation for spasmodic wry neck, namely, division or exsection of the nerves supplying the posterior rotator muscles of the head. *Ann. Surg.*, 1891, **13**, 44-47.
Spastic torticollis treated by division of spinal accessory nerve and posterior roots of first, second, and third spinal nerves.

4868   WYNTER, Walter Essex. 1860-1945
Four cases of tubercular meningitis in which paracentesis of the theca vertebralis was performed for the relief of fluid pressure. *Lancet*, 1891, **1**, 981-82.
Lumbar puncture. Reprinted in *Middx. Hosp. J.*, 1951, **51**, 147.

4869   QUINCKE, Heinrich Irenaeus. 1842-1922
Die Lumbalpunction des Hydrocephalus. *Berl. klin. Wschr.*, 1891, **28**, 929-33, 965-68.
Quincke popularized lumbar puncture, which he had introduced independently of Wynter and others. He used it both for diagnostic and therapeutic purposes. He first presented his method at the German Congress of Internal Medicine (*Verh. Congr. inn. Med.*, 1891, **10**, 321-31).

4870   HARTLEY, Frank. 1856-1913
Intracranial neurectomy of the second and third divisions of the fifth nerve. *N.Y. med. J.*, 1892, **55**, 317-19.
Hartley originated the operation of intracranial neurectomy for facial neuralgia.

4871   KRAUSE, Fedor. 1856-1937
Resection des Trigeminus innerhalb der Schädelhöhle. *Arch. klin. Chir.*, 1892, **44**, 821-32.
Hartley–Krause operation for relief of facial neuralgia (*see also* No. 4870).

4872   MACEWEN, *Sir* WILLIAM. 1848-1924
Pyogenic infective diseases of the brain and spinal cord. Glasgow, *J. Maclehose & Sons,* 1893.
Macewen's greatest work was in connection with the surgery of the brain. In the above book he included extensive case reports of 65 patients under his care, with details of operative procedures. A biography of Macewen was written by A. K. Bowman, London, 1942. *See* No. 431.

4873   FÜRBRINGER, PAUL. 1849-1930
Zur klinischen Bedeutung der spinalen Punction. *Berl. klin. Wschr.,* 1895, **32**, 272-77.
Fürbringer demonstrated the diagnostic value of spinal puncture.

4874   GIGLI, LEONARDO. 1863-1908
Zur Technik der temporären Schädelresektion mit meiner Drahtsäge. *Zbl. Chir.,* 1898, **25**, 425-28.
Gigli's saw adapted for craniotomy. Translation in *J. Neurosurg.,* 1962, **19**, 1103.

4875   CUSHING, HARVEY WILLIAMS. 1869-1939
A method of total exstirpation of the Gasserian ganglion for trigeminal neuralgia, by a route through the temporal fossa and beneath the middle meningeal artery. *J. Amer. med. Assoc.,* 1900, **34**, 1035-41.

4876   SPILLER, WILLIAM GIBSON. 1863-1940, & FRAZIER, CHARLES HARRISON. 1870-1936
The division of the sensory root of the trigeminus for the relief of tic douloureux; an experimental, pathological, and clinical study, with a preliminary report of one surgically successful case. *Univ. Penn. med. Bull.,* 1901, **14**, 342-52.
Introduction of intracranial trigeminal neurotomy, using a modification of the techniques of Horsley (No. 4865) and Krause (No. 4871). Also published in *Philad. med. J.,* 1901, **8**, 1039-49.

4877   ABADIE, JOSEPH LOUIS IRÉNÉE JEAN. 1873-?
Névralgie faciale; présentation de malade. *Mém. Bull. Soc. Méd. Chir. Bordeaux,* (1902), 1903, 59-63.
Alcohol injection of the Gasserian ganglion for treatment of trigeminal neuralgia. See also pp. 91-96 of the same volume.

4877.1 CUSHING, HARVEY WILLIAMS. 1869-1939
Pneumatic tourniquets: With especial reference to their use in craniotomies. *Med. News,* 1904, **84**, 577-80.
First report of tourniquet with pneumatic pressure of measurable degree. This inflatable cuff was the forerunner of the modern technique used generally in surgery.

4878   ——. Concerning surgical intervention for the intracranial hemorrhages of the new-born. *Amer. J. med. Sci.,* 1905, **130**, 563-81.
Successful operative intervention in intracranial haemorrhage of the new-born.

4879   ——. The establishment of cerebral hernia as a decompressive measure for inaccessible brain tumors. *Surg. Gynec. Obstet.,* 1905, **1**, 297-314.

4879.01   BALLANCE, *Sir* CHARLES ALFRED. 1865-1936
Some points on the surgery of the brain and its membranes. London, *Macmillan*, 1907.
Ballance recognized and described chronic subdural haematoma with great accuracy, described a successful operation for it and also for subdural hydroma, discussed brain abscess fully and devoted 243pp. to brain tumours.

4879.1   HORSLEY, *Sir* VICTOR ALEXANDER HADEN. 1857-1916, & CLARKE, ROBERT HENRY. 1850-1926
The structure and functions of the cerebellum examined by a new method. *Brain*, 1908, **31**, 45-124.
The apparatus devised by Horsley and Clarke opened the way to stereotactic surgery of the brain.

4880   FOERSTER, OTFRID. 1873-1941
Ueber eine neue operative Methode der Behandlung spastischer Lähmungen mittels Resektion hinterer Rückenmarkswurzeln. *Z. orthop. Chir.*, 1908, **22**, 203-23.
Foerster's operation of rhizotomy for spastic paralysis.

4880.1   CUSHING, HARVEY WILLIAMS. 1869-1939
Surgery of the head. *In:* Surgery: its principles and practice, edited by William Williams KEEN, **3**, 17-276. Philadelphia, *W.B. Saunders*, 1908.
Cushing's first treatise on neurosurgery. "As a result of this detailed monograph, neurological surgery became almost at once recognized as a clear-cut field of surgical endeavor" (J.F. Fulton, *Harvey Cushing* [1947] 268).

4880.2   KRAUSE, FEDOR. 1856-1937
Chirurgie des Gehirns und Rückenmarks nach eigenen Erfahrungen. 2 vols., Berlin, *Urban & Schwarzenberg*, 1908-11.
With Macewen and Cushing, Krause pioneered the development of neurosurgery as a specialty. This is his most comprehensive work. English translation by H.A. Haubold and M. Thorek, 3 vols., New York, *Rebman*, [1909-12].

4881   ———. & KÜTTNER, HERMANN. 1870-1932
Ueber operative Behandlung gastrischer Krisen durch Resektion der 7-10. hinteren Dorsalwurzel. *Beitr. klin. Chir.*, 1909, **63**, 245-56.
Foerster's operation for tabes.

4882   HORSLEY, *Sir* VICTOR ALEXANDER HADEN. 1857-1916
The Linacre lecture on the function of the so-called motor area of the brain. *Brit. med. J.*, 1909, **2**, 125-32.
Horsley demonstrated that removal of the precentral area in man abolished athetosis.

4883   SPILLER, WILLIAM GIBSON. 1863-1940, & MARTIN, EDWARD. 1859-1938
The treatment of persistent pain of organic origin in the lower part of the body by division of the anterolateral column of the spinal cord. *J. Amer. med. Assoc.*, 1912, **58**, 1489-90.
Cordotomy for the relief of intractable pain.

4883.1   CUSHING, HARVEY WILLIAMS. 1869-1939
The pituitary body and its disorders. Philadelphia, *J. B. Lippincott*, 1912.
    This landmark in endocrinology also includes Cushing's pioneering method of operating on tumours of the pituitary. *See* No. 3896.

4884   LUCKETT, WILLIAM HENRY. 1872-?
Air in the ventricles of the brain, following a fracture of the skull. *Surg. Gynec. Obstet.*, 1913, **17**, 237-40.
    Luckett's finding of air in the ventricles gave Dandy (No. 4602) the idea for ventriculography.

4884.1   OPPENHEIM, HERMANN. 1858-1919, & KRAUSE, FEDOR. 1856-1937
Operative Erfolge bei Geschwülsten der Sehhügel- und Vierhügel gegend. *Berl. klin. Wschr.*, 1913, **50**, 2316-22.
    Successful removal of pineal tumour.

4885   LERICHE, RENÉ. 1879-1955
De la causalgie envisagée comme une névrite du sympathique et de son traitement par la dénudation et l'excision des plexus nerveux périartériels. *Presse méd.*, 1916, **24**, 178-80.
    Periarterial sympathectomy.

4886   MOSHER, HARRIS PEYTON. 1867-?
The wire gauze brain drain. *Surg. Gynec. Obstet.*, 1916, **23**, 740-41.
    Mosher initiated the modern method of trephining and draining inflammatory processes of the brain.

4887   TINEL, JULES. 1879-1952
Les blessures des nerfs. Paris, *Masson & Cie.*, 1916.
    A study of the effect of gunshot wounds on nerves. English translation, London, 1917.

4888   DANDY, WALTER EDWARD. 1886-1949
Extirpation of the choroid plexus of the lateral ventricles in communicating hydrocephalus. *Ann. Surg.*, 1918, **68**, 569-79.

4889   PEET, MAX MINOR. 1885-1949
Tic douloureux and its treatment, with a review of the cases operated upon at the University Hospital in 1917. *J. Mich. St. med. Ass.*, 1918, **17**, 91-99.
    Trigeminal nerve resection with conservation of the motor root, for treatment of trigeminal neuralgia.

4889.1   BALLANCE, *Sir* CHARLES ALFRED. 1856-1936, & GREEN, CHARLES DAVID.
Essays on the surgery of the temporal bone. 2 vols., London, *Macmillan*, 1919.
    Finely illustrated, and beautifully produced, with several historical chapters.

4890   AYER, JAMES BOURNE. 1882-1963
Puncture of the cisterna magna. *Arch. Neurol. Psychiat. (Chicago)*, 1920, **4**, 529-41.
    Introduction of cisternal puncture.

4891   BIANCHI, LEONARDO. 1848-1919
La meccanica del cervello e la funzione dei lobi frontale. Torino, *Bocca*, 1920.
    Bianchi showed that bilateral destruction of the frontal lobes caused character changes, a finding put to practical use by Egas Moniz and others. English translation, Edinburgh, 1922.

4892   SICARD, R., & ROBINEAU, I.
Algie vélo-pharyngée essentielle. Traitement chirurgical. *Rev. neurol.*, 1920
27, 256-57.
    Idiopathic glossopharyngeal neuralgia described and treated.

4893   HUNTER, JOHN IRVINE. 1898-1924
The influence of the sympathetic nervous system in the genesis of the rigidity of striated muscle in a spastic paralysis. *Surg. Gynec. Obstet.*, 1924, **39**, 721-43.
    Hunter believed in the sympathetic innervation of skeletal muscle and on this assumption devised the technique of sympathetic ramisection carried out by Royle (No. 4894). Biography by M.J. Blunt, Sydney, 1985.

4894   ROYLE, NORMAN DAWSON. ?-1944
A new operative procedure in the treatment of spastic paralysis and its experimental basis. *Med. J. Aust.*, 1924, **1**, 77-86.
    Sympathetic ramisection. See also *Surg. Gynec. Obstet.*, 1924, **39**, 701-20.

4895   COTTE, GASTON. 1879-1951
La sympathectomie hypogastrique a-t-elle sa place dans la thérapeutique gynécologique? *Presse méd.*, 1925, **33**, 98-99.
    Presacral neurectomy.

4896   DANDY, WALTER EDWARD. 1886-1946
Section of the sensory root of the trigeminal nerve at the pons. Preliminary report of the operative procedure. *Bull. Johns Hopk. Hosp.*, 1925, **36**, 105-06.
    Intracranial section for glossopharyngeal neuralgia. For a more detailed account see his paper in *Arch. Surg. (Chicago)*, 1929, **18**, 687-734.

4897   PUUSEPP, LYUDVIG MARTINOVICH. 1875-1942
Die Operationstechnik der Hirntumoren (nach eigenen Erfahrungen). *Folia neuropath. eston.*, 1926, **6**, 127-49.
    Puusepp was a great neurosurgeon, particularly notable for his method of removing cerebral tumours. The above journal was founded and edited by him, and vol. 16 (1935) is a *Festschrift* in his honour.

4897.1   CUSHING, HARVEY WILLIAMS. 1869-1939
Electro-surgery as an aid to the removal of intracranial tumors. With a preliminary note on a new surgical-current generator by W. T. Bovie. *Surg. Gynec. Obstet.*, 1928, **47**, 751-84.
    Introduction of electrocoagulation in neurosurgery.

4897.2   BIRLEY, JAMES LEATHAM. 1884-1934
Traumatic aneurysm of the intracranial portion of the internal carotid artery. With a note by Wilfred Trotter. *Brain*, 1928, **51**, 184-208.
    In 1924 Wilfred Trotter (1872-1939) performed the first planned operation for intracranial aneurysm diagnosed pre-operatively.

4898   DOGLIOTTI, ACHILE MARIO. 1897-1966
Traitement des syndromes douloureux de la périphérie par l'alcoolisation
sub-arachnoïdienne des racines postérieures à leur émergence de la
moelle épinière. *Presse méd.*, 1931, **39**, 1249-52.
Subarachnoid injection of alcohol for the relief of pain.

4899   BALLANCE, *Sir* CHARLES ALFRED. 1856-1936, & DUEL, ARTHUR BALDWIN. 1870-
1936
The operative treatment of facial palsy by the introduction of nerve grafts
into the Fallopian canal and by other intratemporal methods. *Arch.
Otolaryng. (Chicago)*, 1932, **15**, 1-70.
A classic paper which includes some history of the surgical treatment of
facial palsy.

4900   CUSHING, HARVEY WILLIAMS. 1869-1939
Intracranial tumours. Springfield, *C. C. Thomas*, 1932.
Cushing's operating technique reduced the mortality rate dramatically
in intracranial surgery. This was his last published report on the statistical
results of brain tumours as a whole.

4901   DOTT, NORMAN MCOMISH. 1897-1973
Intracranial aneurysms: cerebral arterioradiography: surgical treatment.
Trans. med.-chir. Soc. Edinb., 1932-33, n.s. **47**, 219-34.
First planned intracranial operation for aneurysm.

4902   LERICHE, RENÉ. 1879-1955, & FONTAINE, RENÉ.
Techniques des diverses sympathectomies lombaires. *Presse méd.*, 1933,
41, 1819-22.
Lumbar sympathectomy by the antero-lateral extraperitoneal approach.

4903   PUTNAM, TRACY JACKSON. 1894-
Treatment of hydrocephalus by endoscopic coagulation of the choroid
plexus. Description of a new instrument and preliminary report of results.
New Engl. J. Med., 1934, **210**, 1373-76.

4904   LIVINGSTON, WILLIAM KENNETH. 1892-
The clinical aspects of visceral neurology with special reference to the
surgery of the sympathetic nervous system. Springfield, *C. C. Thomas*, 1935.

4904.1 BERGSTRAND, KARL JOSEPH HILDING. 1886- , OLIVECRONA, HERBERT. 1891-
1980, & TÖNNIS, WILHELM.
Gefässmissbildungen und Gefässgeschwülste des Gehirns. Leipzig, *G.
Thieme,* 1936.
Olivecrona first successfully removed an intracranial aneurysm in 1932.

4905   EGAS MONIZ, ANTONIO CAETANO DE. 1874-1955
Essai d'un traitement chirurgical de certaines psychoses. *Bull. Acad. Méd.
(Paris)*, 1936, 3 sér., **115**, 385-92.
Prefrontal leucotomy. Translation in *J. Neurosurg.*, 1964, **21**, 1110-14.
See also his book *Tentatives opératoires dans le traitement de certaines
psychoses,* Paris, 1936. Egas Moniz shared the Nobel Prize with Hess in 1949
for his work in this field. His name was originally Antonio Caetano de
Abreu Freire, and the name of Egas Moniz, a Portuguese national hero, was
added at his baptism.

4906   FREEMAN, WALTER. 1895-1972, & WATTS, JAMES WINSTON. 1904-
Prefrontal lobotomy in agitated depression. Report of a case. *Med. Ann.
Distr. Columbia*, 1936, **5**, 326-28.

      See also the book by the same authors, *Psychosurgery: Intelligence,
emotion, and social behavior following prefrontal lobotomy for mental
disorders.* Springfield, *C.C. Thomas*, 1942.

4907   WALTER, WILLIAM GREY. 1911-1977
The location of cerebral tumours by electro-encephalography. *Lancet,*
1936, **2**, 305-08.

4908   SJÖQVIST, CARL OLOF. 1901-
Eine neue Operationsmethode bei Trigeminusneuralgie: Durchschneidung
des Tractus spinalis trigemini. *Zbl. Neurochir.*, 1937, **2**, 274-81.

      Trigeminal tractotomy. See also *Acta psychiat. neurol. (Kbh.)*, 1938,
Suppl. 17, 1-139.

4909   DOGLIOTTI, ACHILE MARIO. 1897-1966
First surgical sections, in man, of the lemniscus lateralis (pain-temperature
path) at the brain stem, for the treatment of diffused rebellious pain. *Curr.
Res. Anesth.*, 1938, **17**, 143-45.

4909.01   CUSHING, HARVEY WILLIAMS. 1869-1939, & EISENHARDT LOUISE CHARLOTTE.
1891-1967
Meningiomas. Their classification, regional behavior, life history, and
surgical end results. Springfield, *C. C. Thomas*, 1938.

      Begun in 1915, soon after the monograph on pituitary disorders, this
represents 25 years of work, and is, by common consent, regarded as
Cushing's greatest clinical monograph. Reprint, 2 vols., New York, *Hafner,*
1962.

4909.1   TORKILDSEN, ARNE.
A new palliative operation in cases of inoperable occlusion of the Sylvian
aqueduct. *Acta chir. scand.*, 1939, **82**, 117-24.

      Ventriculocisternostomy for the relief of obstructive hydrocephalus.

4910   ELSBERG, CHARLES ALBERT. 1871-1948
Surgical diseases of the spinal cord, membranes, and nerve roots. New
York, *P. B. Hoeber,* (1941).

      Elsberg, American pioneer in neurosurgery, made valuable contribu-
tions to the surgery of the spinal cord. His first book on the subject
appeared in 1916, and another on tumours of the cord in 1925.

4910.1   PENFIELD, WILDER GRAVES. 1891-1976 & ERICKSON, THEODORE
Epilepsy and cerebral localization: A study of the mechanism, treatment
and prevention of epileptic seizures. Springfield, *C.C. Thomas*, 1951.

      Penfield's most widely recognized contribution was the gradual de-
velopment of cortical excision an an accepted and valuable method of
treating medically refractory focal epilepsy. *See also* No. 4914.2.

4911   SEDDON, *Sir* HERBERT JOHN. 1903-
Three types of nerve injury. *Brain,* 1943, **66**, 237-88.

      Seddon's classification of nerve injuries.

4912   TARLOV, Isadore Max. 1905-   , & BENJAMIN, Bernard. 1903-
Plasma clot and silk suture of nerves. 1. An experimental study of comparative tissue reaction. *Surg. Gynec. Obstet.*, 1943, **76**, 366-74.
   Plasma clot nerve suture. Preliminary communication in *Science*, 1942, **95**, 258.

4912.1   SPIEGEL, Ernest Adolf. 1895-1985, *et al.*
Stereotaxic apparatus for operations on the human brain. *Science,* 1947, **106**, 349-50.
   Stereotactic surgery performed on humans. With H. T. Wycis, M. Marks, and A. J. Lee.

4914   BECK, Claude Schaeffer. 1894-1971, *et al.*
Revascularization of the brain through establishment of a cervical arteriovenous fistula. Effects in children with mental retardation and convulsive disorders. *J. Pediat.*, 1949, **35**, 317-29.
   With C. F. McKhann and W. D. Belnap.

4914.1   SCOVILLE, William Beecher. 1906-
Selective cortical undercutting as a means of modifying and studying frontal lobe function in man. Preliminary report of forty-three operative cases. *J. Neurosurg.*, 1949, **6**, 65-73.

4914.2   PENFIELD, Wilder Graves. 1891-1976, & JASPAR, Herbert.
Epilepsy and the functional anatomy of the human brain. Boston, *Little, Brown*, 1954.
   This comprehensive monograph on the mechanism and surgical treatment of epileptic seizures remains Penfield's most substantial scientific work. *See also* No. 4910.1.

4914.3   KNIGHT, Geoffrey Cureton. 1906-
Stereotactic tractotomy in the surgical treatment of mental illness. *J. Neurol. Neurosurg. Psychiat.*, 1965, **28**, 304-10.

4914.4   PLUM, Fred. 1924- & POSNER, Jerome B. 1932-
The diagnosis of stupor and coma. Philadelphia, *F.A. Davis,* 1966.
   Rationalized the diagnosis of various levels of the unconscious state, correlating these with brain lesions.

4914.5   HARDY, Jules.
Transphenoidal microsurgery of the normal and pathological pituitary. *In:* Clinical neurosurgery: Proceedings of the Congress of Neurological Surgeons...1968, 185-217. Baltimore, *Williams & Wilkins,* 1969.
   Confirmation of Cushing's idea that a micro-tumour causes Cushing's syndrome. *See* No. 3904.

4914.6   KELLY, Desmond Hamilton Wilson, *et al.*
Stereotactic limbic leucotomy: neurophysiological aspects and operative technique. *Brit. J. Psychiat.*, 1973, **123**, 133-40.
   With A. Richardson and N. Mitchell-Heggs.

4914.7 JENNETT, WILLIAM BRYAN. 1926- & TEASDALE, GRAHAM.
Aspects of coma after severe head injury. *Lancet*, 1977, **1**, 878-81.
Glasgow Coma Scale for grading brain injury following head trauma.

For history, see No. 5001 *et seq.*

PSYCHIATRY

4915 ARETAEUS, *the Cappadocian. circa* A.D. 81-138
Extant works. Edited F. ADAMS. London, *Sydenham Society,* 1856.
Aretaeus wrote important accounts of melancholy (pp. 298-300, 473-78) and madness (pp. 301-04).

4915.1 CAELIUS AURELIANUS. *fl.* A.D.500
Tardarum passionum libri V. Basileae, *Henricus Petrus* 1529.
Garrison described Caelius as a 5th century neurologist who gave the most sensible and humane treatment of insanity in antiquity. *See also* No. 4808.1. English translation, Chicago, 1950.

4916 WEYER, JOHANN [WIER]. 1515-1588
De praestigiis daemonum. Basileae, *per J. Oporinum,* 1563.
Weyer was the first European physician to take an empirical, scientific approach to the study of mental illness. At the height of the witchcraft delusion he argued that witches were mentally ill women who deserved humane treatment instead of torture and punishment. Weyer "reduced the clinical problems of psychopathology to simple terms of everyday life and everyday, human, inner experiences" (Zilboorg).

4916.1 PARACELSUS, [BOMBASTUS VON HOHENHEIM, THEOPRASTUS PHILIPPUS AUREOLUS].
1493-1541
Von den Kranckheyten so die vernunfft berauben als da sein S. Veyts Thantz...[Basel, *no publisher cited*], 1567.
In this work on the "diseases that deprive man of his reason" Paracelsus anticipated the descriptive method in psychiatry, giving a purely medical account of the clinical manifestations of epilepsy, mania, and hysteria, refuting previous theories that these diseases were caused by demonic possession or other supernatural means. He was "the first to differentiate the sexual components and the unconcious factors in the development of hysteria" (Zilboorg). English translation by G. Zilboorg in H.E. Sigerist (ed.), *Four treatises of ...Paracelsus*, Baltimore, 1941.

4916.2 LAVATER, LUDWIG. 1527-1586
De spectris...Genevae, *Anchora Crispiniana,* 1570.
This work on ghosts is one of the earliest works on psychic experiences, illusions, hallucinations, and delusions. The English translation, London, 1572, probably gave Shakespeare some pointers on the behaviour of the ghost in Hamlet.

4917 SCOT, REGINALD [SCOTT]. ?1538-1599
The discoverie of witchcraft. [London, *W. Brome*], 1584.
Scot identified as mentally ill a large group of people who had hitherto been considered to be involved in witchcraft.

4918 BRIGHT, TIMOTHY. ?1551-1616
A treatise of melancholie, containing the causes thereof. London, *T. Vautrollier,* 1586.
 First comprehensive description of depression in English. Bright also produced the first noteworthy geometrical system of shorthand, consisting of circles, half-circles, and straight lines (*Characterie,* London, 1588).

4918.1 BURTON, ROBERT. 1577-1640
The anatomy of melancholy, what it is. With all the kindes, causes, symptomes, prognostickes, and severall cures of it. Oxford, *John Lichfield...,* 1621.
 The first psychiatric encyclopaedia, citing nearly 500 medical authors, and also a literary *tour de force.* Burton was prompted write this book because of his own bouts with depression. It is one of the most popular psychiatric books ever written, appearing in over 70 editions since its original publication. It was one of Sir William Osler's favourite books.

4919 WILLIS, THOMAS. 1621-1675
De anima brutorum. Oxonii, *imp. R. Davis,* 1672.
 In Pars 2, Cap. III is an account of lethargy, and Cap. XIII gives an account of "stupidity or foolishness".

4919.1 BATTIE, WILLIAM. 1703-1776
Treatise on madness. London, *J. Whiston & B. White,* 1758.
 Battie was among the first to teach psychiatry at the bedside. His book is the first English text book on the subject. Reprinted with J. Monro's *Remarks on Dr. Battie's treatise on madness,* London, *Dawsons,* 1962.

4920 ARNOLD, THOMAS. 1742-1816
Observation on the nature, kinds, causes and prevention of insanity, lunacy, or madness. 2 vols. Leicester, *G. Ireland,* 1782-86.
 Best historical account to the time. 2nd ed., 1806.

4920.1 CULLEN, WILLIAM. 1710-1790
First lines on the practice of physic. 4th ed. Vol. 3. Edinburgh, *Charles Elliot,* 1784.
 Cullen introduced the term "neuroses" (pp. 121-23).

4920.2 CHIARUGI, VINCENZO. 1739-1820
Remarks and rules set by him *in:* Regolamento dei Regi Spedali di Santa Maria Nuova & di Bonifazio. Florence, *Gaetano Cambiagi,* 1789.
 Chiarugi's regulations for the Bonifazio mental asylum mark the first appearance in print of his landmark reforms in the humane treatment of the mentally ill. Chiarugi was the first to practise the humanitarian treatment of the insane.

4921 ———. Della pazzia in genere, e in specie. 3 vols. Firenze, *L. Carlieri,* 1793.
 Chiarugi was the first in Europe to abandon chains and fetters in a mental hospital. He required a case history for each patient, hygienic rooms with segregation of the sexes, no restraint beyond strait jacket and cotton strips, and regard for the patient as a person. He encouraged the patients to work and their attendants to practise kindness towards them. English translation by George Mora, Canton, Mass., *Watson,* 1987.

4922   PINEL, PHILIPPE. 1745-1826
Traité médico-philosophique sur l'aliénation mentale ou la manie. Paris, *Richard, Caille & Ravier*, an IX [1801].

Pinel was among the first to treat the insane humanely; he dispensed with chains and placed his patients under the care of specially selected physicians. Garrison considered the above book one of the foremost medical classics, giving as it did a great impetus to humanitarian treatment of the insane. Pinel founded the French School of Psychiatry. English translation, Sheffield, 1806. The second French edition, Paris, *Brosson*, 1809 is very substantially enlarged by Pinel.

4923   REIL, JOHANN CHRISTIAN. 1759-1813
Rhapsodieen über die Anwendung der psychischen Curmethode auf Geisteszerrüttungen. Halle, *Curt*, 1803.

The versatile Reil, physician and physiologist, was an early advocate of humane treatment for the insane. He was instrumental in the establishment of the first journal devoted to mental disease – the *Magazin für Nervenheilkund*; he was the founder of modern psychiatry.

4924   RUSH, BENJAMIN. 1745-1813
Medical inquiries and observations upon the diseases of the mind. Philadelphia, *Kimber & Richardson*, 1812.

The first American textbook on psychiatry, and, considering the state of that science in Rush's time, one of the most noteworthy. It ran to four editions.

4924.1   HASLAM, JOHN. 1764-1844
Illustrations of madness: exhibiting a singular case of insanity... with a description of the tortures experienced by bomb-bursting, lobster-cracking and lengthening the brain. London, *Rivingtons*, 1810.

The first medical book devoted to a single case of insanity, and the first illustration of an influencing machine, commonly complained of by paranoid patients.

4925   SUTTON, THOMAS. 1767-1835
Tracts on delirium tremens. London, *T. Underwood,* 1813.

Sutton named and described alcoholic delirium tremens, differentiating the condition from phrenitis.

4925.1   TUKE, SAMUEL. 1784-1857
Description of The Retreat, an institution near York, for insane persons...York, *W. Alexander*, 1813.

The pioneer work by an Englishman advocating humane treatment of the mentally ill. Tuke set out in this work the successful results of his experience with the "mild system of treatment" which had been instituted at The Retreat since its foundation. More than a multitude of learned tomes, this unpretentious work by a layman convinced both professionals and public alike of the value of humane treatment in psychiatric care.

4926   HEINROTH, JOHANN CHRISTIAN AUGUST. 1773-1843
Lehrbuch der Störungen des Seelenlebens. Leipzig, *F. C. W. Vogel*, 1818.

Heinroth drew his psychology from the Bible and maintained that mental health was maintained only by piety and that sin engendered madness; for him treatment was by repentance and a return to the fold. English translation, 2 vols., Baltimore, *Johns Hopkins Univ. Press*, 1975.

4928   PRICHARD, JAMES COWLES. 1786-1848
A treatise on insanity and other disorders affecting the mind. London, *Sherwood, Gilbert & Piper*, 1835.
    Prichard, better known for his work in the field of anthropology (No. 159), was the first to describe moral insanity. He described a syndrome he called incoherence or senile dementia. Alzheimer (No. 4956) may have described essentially the same disorder. Reprint of Philadelphia, 1837 edition, New York, *Arno Press*, 1973.

4929   ESQUIROL, JEAN ETIENNE DOMINIQUE. 1772-1840
Des maladies mentales. 2 vols. and atlas. Paris, *J. B. Baillière*, 1838.
    Esquirol succeeded Pinel at the Salpêtrière, and was the first lecturer on psychiatry. After Pinel he was a founder of the French School. This is the first modern textbook on psychiatry. It is notable for its striking illustrations of the insane. English translation, without the illustrations, Philadelphia, 1845, reprinted 1965.

4929.01   RAY, ISAAC. 1807-1881
A treatise on the medical jurisprudence of insanity. Boston, *Charles C. Little and James Brown*, 1838.
    First authoritative and comprehensive treatise in English on the relation between law and psychiatry. Ray became the most influential American writer on forensic psychiatry in the 19th century. Reprint of first edition with introduction and notes by W. Overholser, Cambridge, Mass., *Harvard Univ. Press*, 1962.

4929.1   FEUCHTERSLEBEN, ERNST, *Freiherr von*. 1806-1849
Lehrbuch der ärztlichen Seelenkunde. Wien, *C. Gerold*, 1845.
    Feuchtersleben introduced the terms psychosis, psychiatrics, and psychopathology. The book includes a short history of psychiatry. English translation, *Sydenham Society*, 1847.

4930   GRIESINGER, WILHELM. 1817-1868
Die Pathologie und Therapie der psychischen Krankheiten. Stuttgart, *A. Krabbe*, 1845.
    Griesinger put an end to the moralistic theory of insanity as advanced by Heinroth. He was the first in Germany to abandon violence in the treatment of the insane; his book remained an authority on the subject for 30 years. English translation, London, 1867.

4931   LASÈGUE, ERNEST CHARLES. 1816-1883
Du délire des persécutions. *Arch. gén. Méd.*, 1852, 4 sér., **28**, 129-50.
    "Lasègue's disease" – persecution mania.

4932   FALRET, JEAN PIERRE. 1794-1870
Mémoire sur la folie circulaire. *Bull. Acad. imp. Méd.* (*Paris*), 1853-1854, **19**, 382-400.
    Circular (manic-depressive) insanity first described.

4933 CONOLLY, JOHN. 1794-1866
The treatment of the insane without mechanical restraints. London, *Smith, Elder & Co.*, 1856.

As early as 1839, Conolly treated the insane without any form of restraint at Hanwell Asylum, now St. Bernard's Hospital. Facsimile reprint with introduction by R. Hunter and I. Macalpine, London, *Dawsons*, 1973.

4933.1 MOREL, BENEDICT AUGUSTIN. 1809-1873
Traité des dégénérescences physiques, intellectuelles et morales de l'espèce humaine. 1 vol. and atlas. Paris, *Baillière*, 1857.

The main support for the theory of mental illness as regression which dominated psychiatric practice for several decades. Morel described and illustrated the nature, causes, and signs of human degeneration. He focused on physical signs but also included various intellectual and moral deviations. This led to the classification of criminals and geniuses as types of degenerates or deviates along with the insane and neurotic. Morel emphasized the hereditary factor and his work helped bring about a de-emphasis on therapeutic work in the psychiatry of his time. The atlas reproduces by lithography some of the earliest photographs of the insane.

4934 BUCKNILL, *Sir* JOHN CHARLES. 1817-1897, & TUKE, DANIEL HACK. 1827-1895
A manual of psychological medicine. London, *J. Churchill*, 1858.

Bucknill and Tuke were both distinguished neurologists, and advocates of no restraint in the institutional treatment of mental patients. Their book was for many years the standard English work on psychological medicine. Reprinted 1968.

4936 DOWN, JOHN LANGDON HAYDON. 1828-1896
Observations on an ethnic classification of idiots. *Lond. Hosp. clin. Lect. Rep.*, 1866, **3**, 259-62.

Langdon Down suggested that the physiognomical features of certain defectives enabled them to be arranged in ethnic groups; of these he differentiated Mongolian, Ethiopian, Caucasian, and American Indian. Such an ethnic classification has been abandoned, but the term "mongolism" has been used to describe one important variety of ailment, although recently giving way to "Down's syndrome", for an explanation of which, see N. Howard-Jones, *Med. Hist.*, 1979, **23**, 102-04.

4937 SÉGUIN, ÉDOUARD. 1812-1880
Traitement moral, hygiène et education des idiots...Paris, *Baillière*, 1846.

Séguin was the first to outline a complete plan for the training of mental defectives. A pupil of Itard and Esquirol, he subsequently worked in America, where he published *Idiocy: and its treatment by the physiological method*. New York, 1866.

4938 KAHLBAUM, KARL. 1828-1899
Die Katatonie. Berlin, *A. Hirschwald*, 1874.

In 1869 Kahlbaum suggested catatonia as a separate disease entity and in 1874 his classic monograph appeared. English translation, Baltimore, 1973.

4939 LOMBROSO, CESARE. 1836-1909
L'uomo delinquente, studiato in rapporto alla antropologia, alla medicina legale ed alle discipline carcerarie. Milano, *U. Hoepli*, 1876.
See No. 174.

4940　　　　KRAFFT-EBING, RICHARD VON. 1840-1902
　　　　　　Lehrbuch der Psychiatrie auf klinischer Grundlage. Stuttgart, *F. Enke*, 1879.
　　　　　　　English translation, Philadelphia, 1905.

4941　　　　KRAEPELIN, EMIL. 1856-1926
　　　　　　Compendium der Psychiatrie. Leipzig, *A. Abel*, 1883.
　　　　　　　Later editions of this book were called *Lehrbuch*. The sixth edition is
　　　　　　notable in that in it manic-depressive psychoses were first mentioned as
　　　　　　such. Ninth edition in 1927. Kraepelin, Professor of Psychiatry successively
　　　　　　at Dorpat, Heidelberg, and Munich, was one of the greatest of all psychiatrists
　　　　　　and a pioneer of experimental psychiatry.

4942　　　　MEYNERT, THEODOR HERMANN. 1833-1892
　　　　　　Psychiatrie. Klinik der Erkrankungen der Vorderhirns. Wien, *W. Braumüller*,
　　　　　　1884.
　　　　　　　Meynert, Professor of Neurology at Vienna, is by some regarded as the
　　　　　　father of the architectonics of the brain. English translation, 1886.

4943　　　　RIBOT, THÉODULE ARMAND. 1839-1916
　　　　　　Les maladies de la personnalité. Paris, *Germer-Baillière*, 1885.

4944　　　　KRAFFT-EBING, RICHARD VON. 1840-1902
　　　　　　Psychopathia sexualis. Stuttgart, *F. Enke*, 1886.

4945　　　　KORSAKOFF, SERGEI SERGEIEVICH. 1853-1900
　　　　　　[Disturbance of psychic activity in alcoholic paralysis]. *Vestn. klin. Psichiat.
　　　　　　Neurol.*, 1887, **4**, No. 2, 1-102.
　　　　　　　"Korsakoff's psychosis" or syndrome – alcoholic polyneuritis with loss
　　　　　　and falsification of memory. A second paper on the subject in *Ezhened. klin.
　　　　　　Gaz.*, 1889, **9**, 85, 115, 136, is translated into English in *Neurology*, 1955, **5**,
　　　　　　395-406.

4946　　　　WAGNER VON JAUREGG, JULIUS. 1857-1940
　　　　　　Ueber die Einwirkung fieberhafter Erkrankungen auf Psychosen. *Jb.
　　　　　　Psychiat.*, 1887, **7**, 94-134.
　　　　　　　Wagner von Jauregg's first studies of the effect of fevers upon psychotic
　　　　　　conditions. *See also* No. 4806.

4947　　　　TUKE, DANIEL HACK. 1827-1895
　　　　　　A dictionary of psychological medicine. 2 vols. London, *J. & A. Churchill*,
　　　　　　1892.

4948　　　　WESTPHAL, CARL FRIEDRICH OTTO. 1833-1890
　　　　　　Psychiatrische Abhandlungen. Berlin, *A. Hirschwald*, 1892.
　　　　　　　Westphal was Professor of Psychiatry at Berlin. The above forms vol. 1
　　　　　　of his *Gesammelte Abhandlungen*.

4949　　　　WERNICKE, CARL. 1848-1905
　　　　　　Grundriss der Psychiatrie in klinischen Vorlesungen. Leipzig, *G. Thieme*,
　　　　　　1894-1900.
　　　　　　　Wernicke made valuable contributions to the subject of sensory aphasia,
　　　　　　mind-blindness, and apraxia. He correlated all psychic action with the
　　　　　　function of speech, each perversion being interpreted as showing a minus
　　　　　　or plus activity.

4950   KRAEPELIN, EMIL. 1856-1926
Der psychologische Versuch in der Psychiatrie. *Psychol. Arb.*, 1896, **1**, 1-91.

4951   SOMMER, ROBERT. 1864-1937
Lehrbuch der psychopathologischen Untersuchungsmethoden. Berlin, Wien, *Urban & Schwarzenberg*, 1899.
Sommer introduced new methods in psychopathological investigation.

4952   KRAEPELIN, EMIL. 1856-1926
Einführung in die psychiatrische Klinik. Leipzig, *J. A. Barth*, 1901.
Kraepelin evolved a new classification of insanity. He introduced the concepts "dementia praecox" and "manic-depressive insanity". (Regarding the latter, *see also* No. 4932.)

4953   FOREL, AUGUSTE HENRI. 1848-1931
Hygiene der Nerven und des Geistes im gesunden und kranken Zustande. Stuttgart, *E. H. Moritz,* [1903].
English translation, New York, 1907.

4954   JANET, PIERRE MARIE FÉLIX. 1859-1947
Les obsessions et la psychasthénie. Paris, *F. Alcan*, 1903.
Janet was the first to describe psychasthenia.

4955   MARCHIAFAVA, ETTORE. 1847-1935, & BIGNAMI, AMICO. 1862-1929
Sopra un' alterazione del corpo calloso osservata in soggetti alcoolisti. *Riv. Patol. nerv. ment.*, 1903, **8**, 544-49.
Marchiafava–Bignami disease – degeneration of the corpus callosum in alcoholism.

4956   ALZHEIMER, ALOIS. 1864-1915
Ueber eine eigenartige Erkrankung der Hirnrinde. *Allg. Z. Psychiat.*, 1907, **64**, 146-48.
"Alzheimer's disease" – presenile dementia. Preliminary note in *Neurol. Zbl.*, 1906, **25**, 1134. English translation in *Arch. neurol.*, 1969, **21**, 109-110, and in K. Bick (ed.) *The early story of Alzheimer's disease*, New York, *Raven Press*, [1987].

4957   BLEULER, PAUL EUGEN. 1857-1939
Dementia praecox oder die Gruppe der Schizophrenien. Leipzig, Wien, *F. Deuticke*, 1911.
Bleuler introduced the concept of schizophrenia. He showed that Kraepelin's "dementia praecox" (No. 4952) should include all the schizophrenic disorders.

4958   BROUSSEAU, KATE. ?-1938
Mongolism. A study of the physical and mental characteristics of mongolian imbeciles. Revised by H. G. Brainerd. Baltimore, *Williams & Wilkins*, 1928.

4959   SEN, GANNETH, & BOSE, KATRICK CHANDRA.
Rauwolfia serpentina, a new Indian drug for insanity and high blood pressure. *Indian med. Wld.*, 1931, **2**, 194-201.
Introduction of reserpine in the treatment of psychoses.

4960   SAKEL, MANFRED JOSHUA. 1900-1957
Schizophreniebehandlung mittels Insulin-Hypoglykämie sowie
hypoglykämischer Schocks. *Wien med. Wschr.*, 1934, **84**, 1211-14.
Insulin shock therapy of schizophrenia. Sakel wrote several subsequent
papers on this subject in the same journal. English version in *Amer. J.
Psychiat.*, 1937, **93**, 829-41.

4961   MEDUNA, LADISLAUS JOSEPH. 1896-1965
Versuche über die biologische Beeinflussung des Ablaufes der
Schizophrenie. 1. Campher- und Cardiazolkrämpfe. *Z. ges. Neurol. Psychiat.*,
1935, **152**, 235-62.
Cardiazol (metrazol) convulsion therapy of schizophrenia was intro-
duced by Meduna in 1934.

4962   CERLETTI, UGO. 1877-1963, & BINI, LUCIO. 1908-1964
Un nuovo metodo di shockterapia: "L'elettroshock". (Riassunto.) *Boll. R.
Accad. Med. Roma*, 1938, **64**, 136-38.
Introduction of electric convulsion therapy.

4962.1 PENROSE, LIONEL SHARPLES. 1898-1972
A clinical and genetic study of 1,280 cases of mental defect. *Spec. Rep. Ser.
Med. Res. Coun. (Lond.)*, 1938, No. 229.
In this exhaustive study Penrose showed (p. 36) the significance of
maternal age in the aetiology of Down's syndrome.

4962.2 ——. The biology of mental defect. London, *Sidgwick & Jackson,* 1949.

4962.3 DELAY, JEAN. 1907- , & DENIKER, PIERRE. ?-1917
Trente-huit cas de psychoses traitées par la cure prolongée et continue de
4560 R.P. *C. R. Congr. Alien. et Neurol. de Langue Franç.*, Paris, *Masson &
Cie.*, 1952.
Introduction of chlorpromazine in the treatment of psychosis.

4962.4 BERGER, FRANK MILAN. 1913-
The pharmacological properties of 2-methyl-2-*m*-propyl-1, 3-propanediol
dicarbamate (Miltown), a new interneuronal blocking agent. *J. Pharmacol.*,
1954, **112**, 413-23.
Introduction of meprobamate, later used for the treatment of anxiety.

4962.5 LEJEUNE, JEROME, *et al.*
Étude des chromosomes somatiques de neuf enfants mongoliens. *C. R.
Acad. Sci. (Paris)*, 1959, **248**, 1721-22.
Discovery of trisomy-21, cause of Down's syndrome. With M. Gautier
and R. Turpin.

For history, see Nos. 5001-5019.22

MEDICAL PSYCHOLOGY

4963   ARISTOTLE. 384-322 B.C.
De Anima. In his *Works... translated into English.* Edited by J. A. SMITH and
W. D. ROSS, Oxford, 1931, **3**, 402a-35b.
Aristotle, regarded as the founder of psychology, meant by *anima* or
psyche the living principle which characterizes living substance.

4963.1 GALEN. A.D.130-200
De propriorum animi cuiuslibet affectuum dignotione et curatione. De animi cuiuslibet peccatorum dignotione et curatione ed. W. DE BOER. Corpus Medicorum Graecorum V, 4, 1,1. Lipsiae et Berolini, *B.G. Teubner*, 1937, 1-68.

English translation by P.W. Harkins, *Galen on the passions and errors of the soul.* Columbus, Ohio, 1963.

4963.2 VIVES, JUAN LUIS. 1492-1540
De anima et vita libri tres. Basel, [*Robert Winter*, 1538.]

Vives anticipated Bacon and Descartes in developing an empirical psychology in which the mind was to be studied both through introspection and observation of others. From his exhaustive analysis of memory he developed a theory of association of ideas, which recognized the emotional origin of certain associations, as well as the link between associations, emotions and memory. He was also the first to describe the physiological effects of fear.

4964 HUARTE, JUAN DE DIOS [HUARTE DE SAN JUAN]. 1530-1591
Examen de ingenios para las ciencias. Baeza, 1575.

Huarte was a distinguished Spanish physician and psychologist. His *Examen*, which gained for him a European reputation, was the first attempt to show the connection between psychology and physiology. There were English editions in 1594, 1616, and 1698, and Lessing translated the book into German.

4965 DESCARTES, RENÉ. 1596-1650
Des passions de l'âme. Amsterdam, 1649.

Descartes believed the soul to be a definite entity, giving rise to thoughts, feelings, and acts of volition. He was one of the first to regard the brain as an organ integrating the functions of mind and body. English translation, London, 1650.

4966 WILLIS, THOMAS. 1621-1675
De anima brutorum. Oxonii, *R. Davis*, 1672.

English translation in his *Practice of physick*, London, 1684, Treatise IX.

4967 LOCKE, JOHN. 1632-1704
An essay concerning humane understanding. London, *By Eliz. Holt, for Thomas Basset*, 1690.

Locke, a physician, laid the foundation of modern psychology. For two centuries the principles laid down by him were unquestioned. The writing of the *Essay* occupied him on and off for twenty years.

4968 BONNOT DE CONDILLAC, ÉTIENNE. 1715-1780
Traité des sensations. 2 vols. Londres, Paris, 1754.

Condillac considered that we perceive only what our senses supply in the form of sensations: the "real being" of things is beyond us. English translation, London, 1930.

4969 KANT, IMMANUEL. 1724-1804
Anthropologie in pragmatischer Hinsicht abgefasst. Königsberg, *F. Nicolovius*, 1798.

Kant attempted a classification of mental diseases.

4969.1 ITARD, JEAN MARIE GASPARD. 1774-1822
De l'éducation d'un homme sauvage, ou des premier développemens physiques et moraux du jeune sauvage de l'Aveyron. Paris, *Goujon fils*, An X (1801).

A pupil of Pinel, Itard pioneered in the attempt to educate a young "wild boy" who had lived since infancy entirely apart from human contact. In adapting the methods of teaching deaf-mutes to his extraordinary pupil, Itard created a new system of pedagogy which has profoundly influenced modern educational methods. He was very optimistic in the above work issued nine months after he had started working with the boy. By his second account, *Rapport...sur les nouveaux développemens et de l'état actuel du sauvage de l'Aveyron*, Paris, 1807, Itard regretfully concluded that the boy was incapable of learning speech and that some of the effects of prolonged isolation are irreversible, especially when the isolation occurs during the crucial period of early childhood. English translation of first work, London, 1802.

4969.2 THELWALL, JOHN. 1764-1834
A letter to Henry Cline, Esq. on imperfect developments of the faculties, mental and moral...and on the treatment of impediments of speech. London, *Arch*...1810.

The first book on mental deficiency. Thelwall recognized that sensory deprivation could be a cause of apparent mental defect through his work with handicapped children. He established criteria for distinguishing between intellectual capability and performance.

4970 LOTZE, RUDOLPH HERMANN. 1817-1881
Medicinische Psychologie, oder Physiologie der Seele. Leipzig, *Weidmann*, 1852.

Lotze was a pioneer in the investigation of unconscious and subconscious states.

4972 FECHNER, GUSTAV THEODOR. 1801-1887
Elemente der Psychophysik. 2 vols. Leipzig, *Breitkopf u. Härtel*, 1860.

The first treatise on the subject. Fechner applied the laws of mathematical physics to the physiology of sensation. He discussed the functional relations of the dependence between mind and body and investigated the cutaneous and muscular senses. *See also* No. 1464.

4973 DUCHENNE DE BOULOGNE, GUILLAUME BENJAMIN AMAND. 1806-1875
Mécanisme de la physionomie humaine, ou analyse électro-physiologique de l'expression des passions applicable à la pratique des arts plastiques. Premier fascicule. [All published]. 1 vol. and atlas of photographs by Duchenne. Paris, *Vve. J. Renouard*, 1862.

Duchenne studied the mechanism of facial expression during emotion; his atlas of photographs is a most important contribution to medical photography. Darwin reproduced a number of his photographs in *The expression of the emotions* (No. 4975).

4974 DONDERS, FRANS CORNELIS. 1818-1889
Die Schnelligkeit psychischer Prozesse. *Arch. Anat. Physiol. wiss. Med.*, 1868, 657-81.

Donders was the first to measure the reaction-time of a psychical process.

4975   DARWIN, CHARLES ROBERT. 1809-1882
The expression of the emotions in man and animals. London, *John Murray*, 1872.

Darwin examined the causes, physiological and psychological, of all the fundamental emotions in man and animals. He concluded that "the chief expressive actions exhibited by man and by the lower animals are now innate or inherited", and that most of the movements of expression must have been gradually acquired. Reproduces a number of photographs from Duchenne (No. 4973), and other photographs by Reijlander. Reprinted, New York, 1955. See P. Ekman (ed.): *Darwin and facial expression. A century of research in review.* New York, 1973.

4976   WUNDT, WILHELM MAX. 1832-1920
Grundzüge der physiologischen Psychologie. 2 pts. Leipzig, *W. Engelmann,* 1873-74.

Wundt made experimental investigations of normal individual reactions, reflex responses, and general behaviour, and interpreted them in terms of neural mechanisms. He is the founder of experimental psychology, and his book remains the most important on the subject.

4976.1   JANET, PIERRE MARIE FÉLIX. 1859-1947
L'Automatisme psychologique. Paris, *Alcan,* 1889.

Janet argued that "hysterical symptoms are due to subconscious fixed ideas that have been isolated and usually forgotten. Split off from consciousness – 'dissociated' – they embody painful experiences, but become autonomous by virtue of their segregation from the main stream of consciousness" (E.L. Bliss, *Multliple personality, allied disorders, and hypnosis,* N.Y., *Oxford University Press,* 1986). This predated Breuer and Freud's announcement of their virtually identical discovery (No.4977.3) by four years.

4977.2   JAMES, WILLIAM. 1842-1910
The principles of psychology. 2 vols., New York, *Henry Holt,* 1890.

The foundation of the American school of experimental psychology. Under the influence of Wundt, James viewed psychology as an experimental science based on physiology. He founded the earliest laboratory for the study of experimental psychology in America.

4977.3   FREUD, SIGMUND. 1856-1939, & BREUER, JOSEF. 1842-1925
Über den psychischen Mechanismus hysterischer Phänomene. (Vorläufige Mittheilung.) *Neur. Centralbl.,* 1893, **12,** 4-10, 43-47.

The preliminary announcement of the results of the collaboration that was the starting point of psychoanalysis. It described work begun several years previously. *See* No. 4978.

4978   ——. Studien über Hysterie. Leipzig & Wien, *F. Deuticke,* 1895.

The foundation of psychoanalysis. Using what they called the cathartic method, in which hysterical patients were made to describe the manifestations of their symptoms in detail, with or without hypnosis, Breuer and Freud were successful in providing the patients with temporary relief from symptoms. Breuer chose not to continue research on these patients.

However, Freud, who had studied hypnosis with Charcot (No. 4995), as well as the psychotherapeutic methods of Liébault(Nos. 4994 & 4998) and Bernheim (No. 4995.1), used this work as the basis for development of the method of free association, and the essential psychoanalytic concepts of the unconscious, repression and transference. Abridged English translation, New York, 1909. First complete translation, London, *Hogarth Press*, 1956.

4980 FREUD, SIGMUND. 1856-1939
Die Traumdeutung. Leipzig & Vienna, *F. Deuticke*, 1900.
 Freud's greatest work, the influence of which has been felt far beyond the psychiatric and medical community. Here he refined his understanding of the operation of the unconscious, interpreted dreams on the basis of wish-fulfillment theory, discussed displacement, the extensive appearance of symbols for repressed thought in conscious thought, regression, and the erotic nature of dreams.

4981 ELLIS, HENRY HAVELOCK. 1859-1939
Studies in the psychology of sex. 7 vols. Philadelphia, *F. A. Davis*, 1900-28.
 Ellis has probably done more than any other person to free discussion of sex from the conspiracy of silence which once surrounded it. His *Studies* represent a lifetime devoted to the subject, at first in the face of bitter opposition.

4982 FREUD, SIGMUND. 1856-1939
Zur Psychopathologie des Alltagslebens. Berlin, *S. Karger,* 1904.
 An exposition of psychoanalytic theory for a popular audience. Includes descriptions of the well-known "Freudian slip". English translation, London, 1914.

4983 ——. Drei Abhandlungen zur Sexualtheorie. Leipzig, *F. Deuticke*, 1905.
 The work which Freud considered second in importance only to his *Die Traumdeutung*. Freud's epochal theory of infantile sexuality linked the forces motivating the development of body and mind from earliest infancy. Infantile sexuality was a fact known, Freud said, to every nursemaid, yet the above work provoked and continues to provoke controversy in both scientific and popular sectors. English translation, 1910.

4984 ADLER, ALFRED. 1870-1937
Studie über Minderwertigkeit von Organen. Berlin, Wien, *Urban & Schwarzenberg,* 1907.
 Adler, a disciple of Freud, introduced the concept of the inferiority complex and the method of compensation needed to overcome it.

4985 BINET, ALFRED. 1857-1911, & SIMON, THÉODORE. 1873-
La mesure du développement de l'intelligence chez les jeunes enfants. Paris, *A. Coneslant*, 1911.
 Binet–Simon intelligence tests. As early as 1895 Binet had published a plan for studying intelligence. English translation, 1912.

4985.1 ADLER, ALFRED. 1870-1937
Über die nervösen Charakter. Wiesbaden, *J. F. Bergmann*, 1912.

Adler seceded from Freud's psycho-analytical group and founded the school of individual psychology. English translation of above, 1917. See also his *Practice and theory of individual psychology*, 1924.

4985.2   JUNG, CARL GUSTAV. 1875-1961
Wandlungen und Symbole der Libido. Beiträge zur Entwicklungsgeschichte des Denkens. *Jb. psycho-analyst. psychopath. Forsch.*, 1911, **3**, 120-227; 1912, **4**, 162-464.
　　Reprinted in book form, Leipzig, *F. Deuticke*, 1912. Jung was among the first to support Freud's views on psycho-analysis, and was considered by Freud to be his most brilliant pupil. Jung applied psychoanalytic theory to the study of myths, developing the idea of the collective unconscious. In 1913 Jung broke away from Freud and founded the school of analytical psychology. English translation, *Psychology of the unconscious*, New York, *Moffat, Yard*, 1916.

4986   TERMAN, LEWIS MADISON. 1877-1957, *et al.*
The Stanford revision and extension of the Binet–Simon scale for measuring intelligence. Baltimore, *Warwick & York*, 1917.

4987   WATSON, JOHN BROADUS. 1878-1958
Psychology from the standpoint of a behaviorist. Philadelphia, *J. B. Lippincott*, 1919.
　　Watson was the principal exponent of behaviourist psychology.

4988   KRETSCHMER, ERNST. 1884-1964
Körperbau und Charakter. Berlin, *J. Springer*, 1921.
　　Kretschmer has attempted to correlate body build and constitution with character and mentality.

4988.1   RORSCHACH, HERMANN. 1884-1922
Psychodiagnostik. 1 vol & atlas of test cards. Bern, *Bircher*, 1921.
　　Rorschach test. 2nd ed., Bern, 1932. English translation, Bern, *Huber*, 1942. See the biography of Rorschach in *Bull. Menninger Clin.*, 1954, **18**, 173-219.

4990   JANET, PIERRE MARIE FÉLIX. 1859-1947
La médecine psychologique. Paris, *E. Flammarion*, 1923.
　　Janet's summary of his work with hypnosis, including one of the most detailed histories of hypnosis available. English translation, as *Psychological healing*, 2 vols., 1925.

4990.1   FREUD, ANNA. 1895-1982
Einführung in die Technik der Kinderanalyse. Leipzig, *Internat. Psychoanal. Verlag*, 1927.
　　Daughter of Sigmund Freud, Anna Freud made the psychoanalysis of children her own province. This is probably the most famous classic of child analysis.

4991   KÖHLER, WOLFGANG. 1887-1967
Gestalt psychology. New York, *Liveright Publ. Co.*, 1929.

4991.1   WIENER, NORBERT. 1894-1964
Cybernetics: or control and communication in the animal and the machine.
New York, *Wiley*, 1948.
The science of cybernetics was founded and named by Wiener. It
includes the study of human control functions.

Psychotherapy: Hypnotism

4992   GREATRAKES, VALENTINE [GREATOREX]. 1629-1683
A brief account of Mr Valentine Greatrakes, and divers of the strange cures
by him lately performed. Written by himself in a letter addressed to the
Honourable Robert Boyle Esq., 1666. London, *J. Starkey*, 1666.
The earliest scientific account, by a practitioner, and corroborated by
witnesses, of healing by the "laying-on of hands". Greatrakes became
known as "the Irish stroker" because of his method of healing by stroking
the affected part. He recognized the limited types of conditions which
stroking could treat, and was a sincere and well-meaning practitioner. He
wrote the above work to defend himself against charges that he was a
charlatan.

4992.1   MESMER, FRANZ ANTON. 1734-1815
Mémoire sur la découverte du magnétisme animal. Genève, Paris, *P. F. Didot
le jeune*, 1779.
Mesmer promoted his system of treatment, based on his confused
doctrine of a universal magnetic fluid influencing tides and men alike, with
books and great personal showmanship. His treatment became such a
popular health care sensation in France that it was as much a social
movement as a medical practice. The *ancien régime* considered the
leaders of the animal magnetism movement to be politically dangerous.
See R. Darnton, *Mesmerism and the ancien régime*, Cambridge, Mass., 1968.
The attention Mesmer directed toward hypnosis and suggestion in psychiatry
led eventually to its scientific investigation by Braid and others. It also led
to the more scientific development of suggestion in treatment, which has
been termed after him "mesmerism". Following an enquiry instituted by
Louis XVI, Mesmer's career came to an abrupt end. English translations by
G. Frankau, 1948, and G. J. Bloch, Los Altos, Calif., *William Kaufmann*,
1980.

4992.2   RAPPORT des commissaires chargés par le roi, de l'examen du magnétisme
animal. Paris, *l'Imprimerie Royale*, 1784.
Responding to Mesmer's growing notoriety, the Medical Faculty of Paris
became alarmed and urged the King to appoint a blue-ribbon committee
of inquiry. The committee included Benjamin Franklin, Antoine Laurent
Lavoisier, Antoine de Jussieu, etc. Finding no evidence of a magnetic fluid,
these scientists attributed the power of mesmerism to the "imagination"
and so drove Mesmer from Paris. Lavoisier may have been the author of the
report. English translation, London, 1785.

4992.3   BRAID, JAMES. 1795-1860
Satanic agency and mesmerism reviewed. Manchester, *Simms & Dinham*,
1842.

Braid's scientific investigations of mesmerism convinced him that its effects did not depend on an outside force, but were natural phenomena arising from the subject's heightened suggestibility. This pamphlet contains his first statement of these discoveries and contains the first use of the term "[neuro]hypnotism", which Braid coined to replace the unscientific "mesmerism" and "animal magnetism".

4993 ———. Neurypnology, or, the rationale of nervous sleep. London, *J. Churchill*, 1843.

Braid inaugurated modern hypnotism, the word itself being introduced by him. His theories were adopted by Broca, Charcot, Liébeault, and Bernheim; thus he founded the French School.

4994 LIÉBEAULT, Ambroise Auguste. 1823-1904
Le sommeil provoqué et les états analogues considérés sur au point du vue de l'action du moral et de physique. Paris, *Victor Masson,* 1866.

The substitution of psychotherapy for hypnotic suggestion starts with the work of Liébeault.

4995 CHARCOT, Jean Martin. 1825-1893
Leçons sur les maladies du système nerveux faites à La Salpêtrière. 3 vols. Paris, *A. Delahaye,* 1872-87.

Charcot's pioneering research on the application of hypnosis to the psychoneuroses brought this subject to the attention of the scientific community.

4995.1 BERNHEIM, Hippolyte Marie. 1840-1919
De la suggestion dans l'état hypnotique et dans l'état de veille. Paris: *Octave Doin,* 1884.

The foundation of the Nancy school of hypnosis. Like Liébeault, Bernheim studied the scientific applications of hypnotism and substituted verbal for sensory stimuli; he interpreted hypnotism and its consequent phenomena as being the result of suggestion.

4996 FOREL, Auguste Henri. 1848-1931
Der Hypnotismus und die suggestive Psychotherapie. Stuttgart, *F. Enke,* 1888.

4998 LIÉBEAULT, Ambroise Auguste. 1823-1904
Thérapeutique suggestive. Paris, *O. Doin,* 1891.

4999 FREUD, Sigmund. 1856-1939
Studien über Hysterie. Leipzig & Wien, *F. Deuticke,* 1895.

Using what they called the cathartic method, in which hysterical patients were made to describe the manifestations of their symptoms in detail, with or without hypnosis, Breuer and Freud were successful in providing the patients with temporary relief from symptoms. Breuer chose not to continue research on these patients. However, Freud, who had studied hypnosis with Charcot (No. 4995), as well as the psychotherapeutic methods of Liébault (Nos. 4994 & 4998) and Bernheim (No. 4995.1), used this work as the basis for development of the method of free association, and the essential psychoanalytic concepts of the unconscious, repression and transference. Abridged English translation, New York, 1909. First complete translation, London, *Hogarth Press*, 1956.

History of Neurology, Neurological Surgery, Psychology, and Psychiatry

5000   VIGILIIS VON CREUTZENFELD, Stephan Hieronymus de.
Bibliotheca chirurgica. 2 vols., Vindobonae, *J.T. de Trattner*, 1781.
     Fulton (No. 6785) points out that this work contains the "most complete bibliographical study of the literature of head injury that had been brought together up to that time".

5001   BUCKNILL, *Sir* John Charles. 1817-1897
The mad folk of Shakespeare. 2nd ed. London, *Macmillan*, 1867.
     First published as *The psychology of Shakespeare*, London, 1859.

5002   PREYER, Thierry Wilhelm. 1841-1897
Die Entdeckung des Hypnotismus. Berlin, *Gebrüder Paetel,* 1881.
     A history of hypnotism.

5003   TUKE, Daniel Hack. 1827-1895
Chapters in the history of the insane in the British Isles. London, *Kegan Paul,* 1882.

5003.1   ——. The insane in the United States and Canada. London, *H.K. Lewis,* 1885.
     The first history of psychiatry in the United States and Canada. Chapter 5 is the first survey of psychiatry in Canada.

5004   LAEHR, Heinrich. 1820-1905
Gedenktage der Psychiatrie. 4te. Aufl. Berlin, *G. Reimer,* 1893.
     A history of the subject, arranged in calendar form.

5005   ——. Die Literatur der Psychiatrie, Neurologie und Psychologie von 1459-1799. 3 vols. Berlin, *G. Reimer,* 1900.

5005.1   BRAMWELL, John Milne. 1852-
Hypnosis: Its history, practice and theory. London, *Grant Richards,* 1903.
     An unexcelled "scholarly, critical, and detailed analysis of hypnosis" (Bliss).

5006   HURD, Henry Mills. 1843-1927
The institutional care of the insane in the United States and Canada. 4 vols. Baltimore, *Johns Hopkins Press,* 1916-17.
     Hurd, who edited the above, was Professor of Psychiatry at Johns Hopkins University. The work includes his history of American psychiatry.

5007   KRAEPELIN, Emil. 1856-1926
Hundert Jahre Psychiatrie. *Z. ges. Neurol.* 1918, **38**, 161-275.
     English translation, New York, 1962.

5008   BALLANCE, *Sir* Charles Alfred. 1856-1936
A glimpse into the history of the surgery of the brain. London, *Macmillan & Co.,* 1922.
     Thomas Vicary Lecture. First published in *Lancet,* 1922, **1**, 111-16, 165-72.

5010   LAIGNEL-LAVASTINE, Maxime Paul Marie. 1875-1953, & VINCHON, Jean.
       Les malades de l'esprit et leurs médecins du XVIe siècle. Les étapes des
       connaissances psychiatriques de la Renaissance à Pinel. Paris, *Maloine*, 1930.

5012   SEMELAIGNE, René. 1855-1934
       Les pionniers de la psychiatrie française avant et après Pinel. 2 vols. Paris,
       Baillière, 1930.
          A history of French psychiatry from Fernel to the end of the 19th
       century, focused around the work of each pioneer. Semelaigne was the
       great grand-nephew of Pinel.

5013   ZILBOORG, Gregory. 1890-1959, & HENRY, George William. 1889-
       A history of medical psychology. New York, *W. W. Norton*, 1941.

5014   WARTENBERG, Robert. 1887-1956
       Studies in reflexes. History, psychology, synthesis and nomenclature.
       Arch. Neurol. Psychiat., 1944, **51**, 113-33, 414; **52**, 341-58, 359-82.
          Also published in book form, Chicago, 1945.

5015   TEMKIN, Owsei, 1902-
       The falling sickness: a history of epilepsy from the Greeks to the beginnings
       of modern neurology. Second edition. Baltimore, *Johns Hopkins Press*, 1945.
          Revised second edition. Baltimore, 1971.

5015.1 DEUTSCH, Albert. 1905-1961
       The mentally ill in America. A history of their care and treatment from
       colonial times. Second edition, revised and enlarged. New York, *Columbia
       University Press*, [1949].

5016   BRAZIER, Mary Agnes Burniston. 1904-
       Bibliography of electroencephalography, 1875-1948. *Electro-
       encephalography and Clinical Neurophysiology*, Suppl. No. 1, 1950.
          Covers both normal and disease states. Suppl. No. 23 (1964), ed. M.
       Fink, covers the period 1951-62.

5017   WALKER, Arthur Earl. 1907-
       A history of neurological surgery. Edited by A. Earl Walker. Baltimore,
       Williams & Wilkins, 1951.
          Includes a bibliography of nearly 2,400 references, nearly all of which
       are secondary sources.

5018   SACHS, Ernest. 1879-1958
       The history and development of neurological surgery. New York, *P. B.
       Hoeber*, 1952.

5019   KOLLE, Kurt. 1898-
       Grosse Nervenärzte. 3 vols. Stuttgart, *G. Thieme*, 1956-63.

5019.1 RIESE, Walther. 1890-1976
       A history of neurology. New York, *M. D. Publications*, [1959].

5019.2 LEIGH, ARCHIBALD DENIS. 1915-
The historical development of British psychiatry. Vol. 1-. Oxford, *Pergamon Press*, 1961- .

5019.3 HUNTER, RICHARD ALFRED, 1923-1981, & MACALPINE, IDA. 1899-1974
Three hundred years of psychiatry, 1535-1860; a history presented in selected English texts. London, *Oxford University Press*, 1963. Reprinted, Hartsdale, NY, 1982.

5019.4 KIELL, NORMAN. 1916-
Psychoanalysis, psychology and literature: a bibliography. Madison, *University of Wisconsin Press*, 1963.
Contains 4,460 references.

5019.5 WILKINS, ROBERT H.
Neurosurgical classics. Compiled by Robert H. Wilkins. New York, *Johnson Reprint Corp.*, 1965.
A collection of 52 classic contributions to neurosurgery, translated, where necessary, into English, with an appendix containing over 200 additional references related to the historical development of neurological surgery.

5019.6 ALEXANDER, FRANZ. 1891-1964, & SELESNICK, SHELDON THEODORE. 1925-
The history of psychiatry: an evaluation of psychiatric thought and practice from prehistoric times to the present. New York, *Harper & Row*, 1966.

5019.7 ELDRIDGE, MARGARET.
A history of the treatment of speech disorders. Edinburgh, *E. & S. Livingstone*, 1968.

5019.8 McHENRY, LAWRENCE C. 1929-1985
Garrison's History of neurology. Revised and enlarged with a bibliography of classical, original and standard works in neurology. Springfield, *C. C. Thomas*, 1969.
A comprehensive, well-illustrated history of the subject, considerably enlarging Garrison's work previously published in C. L. Dana's *Textbook of nervous diseases*, 1925, pp. xv-lvi.

5019.9 HAYMAKER, WEBB EDWARD. 1902- , & SCHILLER, FRANCIS.
The founders of neurology. One hundred and forty-six biographical sketches by eighty-nine authors. Compiled and edited by W. E. Haymaker and F. Schiller. 2nd edition. Springfield, *C. C. Thomas*, 1970.
Neuroanatomists, neurophysiologists, neuropathologists, clinical neurologists and neurosurgeons are included. 1st ed., 1953, had 133 biographies; 2nd ed. has 146, 34 of which have been added. Because the 2nd edition deleted certain biographies, readers should also consult the 1st edition.

5019.10 TINTEROW, MAURICE M.
Foundations of hypnosis, from Mesmer to Freud. Springfield, *C.C. Thomas*, [1970].
Readings, including translations, from classic texts, with commentary.

5019.11   WOLF, JOHN K.
The classical brain stem syndromes. Translations of the original papers with notes on the evolution of clinical neuroanatomy. Springfield, *C.C. Thomas*, [1971.]

5019.12   HUNTER, RICHARD ALFRED. 1923-1981, & MACALPINE, IDA. 1899-1974
Psychiatry for the poor. 1851 Colney Hatch Asylum: Friern Hospital 1973. A medical and social history. London, *Dawsons*, 1974.
This is in effect a history of institutional psychiatry in Britain. It reflects what was happening elsewhere over the last 100 years and what is now coming to an end.

5019.13   ANDERSON, EVELYN and HAYMAKER, WEBB EDWARD. 1902-
Breakthroughs in hypothalamic and pituitary research. *In*: Integrative hypothalamic activity, D.F. SWAAB & J.P. SCHADÉ (eds.), *Progess in brain research*, 1974, **41**, 1-60.

5019.14   ROTTENBERG, DAVID ALLAN, & HOCHBERG, FRED HARVEY.
Neurological classics in modern translation. Edited by David A. Rottenberg and Fred H. Hochberg. New York, *Hafner Press*, 1977.
Full translations of 20 classic European contributions to 19th and 20th century neurology.

5019.15   BRUYN, G. W., *et al.*
A centennial bibliography of Huntington's chorea, 1872-1972. Leuven, *University Press*; The Hague, *Nijhoff*, 1974.
Over 2,000 references to original works. Chronological arrangement. Author, geographic and other indexes. With F. Baro and N. C. Myrianthopoulos.

5019.16   DIAMOND, SOLOMON.
The roots of psychology. A sourcebook in the history of ideas, edited by Solomon Diamond. New York, *Basic Books*, [1974].

5019.17   HOWELLS, JOHN GWILYM.
World history of psychiatry. Edited by J. G. Howells, New York, Brunner/ Mazel, 1975.
Contributions by 42 authors.

5019.18   SPILLANE, JOHN DAVID. 1909-1985
The doctrine of the nerves. Chapters in the history of neurology. Oxford, *University Press*, 1981.
Deals with the structure, function, and diseases of the nervous system to the end of the 19th century.

5019.19   PIGEAUD, JACKIE.
La maladie de l'âme. Etude sur la relation de l'âme et du corps dans la tradition médico-philosophique antique. Paris, *Belles Lettres*, 1981.

5019.20   BUCY, PAUL CLANCY. 1904-
Neurosurgical giants: feet of clay and iron. New York, *Elsevier*, [1985].

Brief biographical essays by various authors, edited by Bucy. The companion volume, *Modern neurosurgical giants* (1986) includes articles on living neurosurgeons, written by colleagues. Neither volume includes bibliographies.

5019.21 CRABTREE, ADAM.
Animal magnetism, early hypnotism, and psychical research, 1766-1925. An annotated bibliography. White Plains, N.Y., *Kraus International Publications*, [1988].
Describes 1905 works, mostly with detailed annotations.

5019.22 ASHWAL, STEPHEN. 1945- .
The founders of child neurology, edited by Stephen Ashwal. San Francisco, *Norman Publishing in association with the Child Neurology Society*, 1990.
125 biographical essays, with portraits and bibliographies, documenting the history of child neurology from the 17th century to the present.

COMMUNICABLE DISEASES

ENTERIC FEVER

5020 WILLIS, THOMAS. 1621-1675
Diatribae duae medico-philosophicae, quarum prior agit de fermentatione sive de motu intestino particularum in quovis corpore, altera de febribus sive de motu earundum in sanguine animalium. Londini, *T. Roycroft*, 1659.
Includes (De febribus, cap. X, XIV) first description of epidemic typhoid. English translation in his *Practice of physick*, 1684, Treatise II, 83-98, 1111-18.

5021 ROEDERER, JOHANN GEORG. 1727-1763, & WAGLER, CARL GOTTLIEB. ?-1778
De morbo mucoso. Gottingae, *V. Bossiegel*, 1762.
An exhaustive study of typhoid, which the writers confused with dysentery and relapsing fever.

5022 SMITH, NATHAN. 1762-1829
A practical essay on typhous fever. New York, *E. Bliss & E. White*, 1824.
Nathan Smith left a classic account of typhoid; this was reprinted in *Med. Classics*, 1937, **1**, 781-819. He clearly recognized the contagious nature of the disease.

5023 LOUIS, PIERRE CHARLES ALEXANDRE. 1787-1872
Recherches anatomiques, pathologiques et thérapeutiques sur la maladie connue sous les noms de gastro-entérite; fièvre putride, adynamique, ataxique, typhoïde, etc. 2 vols. Paris, *J. B. Baillière*, 1829.
Louis introduced the term "typhoid fever" in reference to the disturbed mental condition of the patient; he first described the lenticular rose spots. His book established the pathological picture of the disease. English translation, Boston, 1836.

5023.1 PERRY, ROBERT. 1783-1848
Observations on continued fever, as it occurs in the city of Glasgow hospitals. *Edinb. med. surg. J.*, 1836, **45**, 64-70.
Perry correctly described many of the distinctions between typhus and typhoid.

5024   GERHARD, William Wood. 1809-1872
On the typhus fever which occurred at Philadelphia in the spring and summer of 1836; illustrated by clinical observations at the Philadelphia Hospital; showing the distinction between this form of disease and dothinenteritis, or the typhoid fever with alteration of the follicles of the small intestine. *Amer J. med. Sci.*, 1837, **19**, 289-322; **20**, 289-322.

Gerhard, a pupil of Louis, correctly differentiated between typhus and typhoid. Part of his paper is reproduced in R. H. Major, *Classic descriptions of disease*, 3rd ed., 1945, p. 174.

5025   STEWART, Alexander Patrick. 1813-1883
Some considerations on the nature and pathology of typhus and typhoid fever, applied to the solution of the question of the identity or non-identity of the two diseases. *Edinb. med. surg. J.*, 1840, **54**, 289-339.

Typhoid and typhus were often confused. Stewart made a careful analysis of a number of cases of both fevers and clearly demonstrated that there were in Britain two distinct fevers – typhoid and typhus.

5026   RITCHIE, Charles. 1799-1878
Practical remarks on the continued fevers of Great Britain, and on the generic distinctions between enteric fever and typhus. *Monthly J. med. Sci.*, 1846-47, **7**, 347-58.

Introduction of the term "enteric fever". Ritchie carefully differentiated the symptoms of typhus and typhoid.

5027   JENNER, *Sir* William. 1815-1898
On typhoid and typhus fevers, – an attempt to determine the question of their identity or non-identity, by an analysis of the symptoms, and of the appearances found after death in 66 fatal cases observed at the London Fever Hospital from Jan. 1847–Feb. 1849. *Monthly J. med. Sci.*, 1849, **9**, 663-80.

Despite Stewart's work there was still controversy as to the identity of typhoid and typhus. Jenner's paper demonstrated that the aetiology of the two was quite different, that one did not communicate or protect against the other, and that epidemics of the two did not prevail simultaneously.

5028   BRAND, Ernst. 1827-1897
Die Hydrotherapie des Typhus. Stettin, *T. von der Nahmer*, 1861.

Brand's cold bath treatment of typhoid fever consisted of total immersion in water at 65°F. and the pouring of cold water over the neck and shoulders. The cold bath treatment of fevers was instituted by Currie (*see* No. 1988).

5029   BUDD, William. 1811-1880
Typhoid fever; its nature, mode of spreading, and prevention. London, *Longmans, Green & Co.*, 1873.

Budd insisted that typhoid fever was spread by contagion and established the fact that infection with typhoid came from the dejecta of the patients; he strengthened the theory of water-borne infection. See also his earlier papers in *Lancet*, 1856, **2**, 617, 694; 1859, **2**, (several papers); 1860, **1**, (several papers).

5030   EBERTH, Carl Joseph. 1835-1926
Die Organismen in den Organen bei Typhus abdominalis. *Virchows Arch. path. Anat.*, 1880, **81**, 58-74.

Salmonella typhi, causal organism of typhoid, was discovered by Eberth. Some European writers refer to the disease as "Eberth's disease".

5031   KLEBS, THEODOR ALBRECHT EDWIN. 1834-1913
Der Bacillus des Abdominaltyphus und der typhöse Process. *Arch exp. Path. Pharmak.*, 1881, **13**, 381-460.
Klebs probably saw the typhoid bacillus before Eberth, reporting it later.

5032   GAFFKY, GEORG. 1850-1918
Zur Aetiologie des Abdominaltyphus. *Mitt. k. GesundhAmte*, Berlin, 1884, **2**, 372-420.
Gaffky was the first to grow pure cultures of *Salmonella typhi*; he showed it to be the true activator of the disease. English translation, *New Sydenham Society*, 1886.

5033   ANTON, BERNHARD. & FÜTTERER, GUSTAV. 1854-1922
Untersuchungen über Typhus abdominalis. *Münch med. Wschr.*, 1888, **35**, 315-18.
Salmonella typhi first demonstrated in the gall-bladder in cases of typhoid.

5034   CHANTEMESSE, ANDRÉ. 1851-1919, & WIDAL, GEORGES FERNAND ISIDOR. 1862-1929
De l'immunité contre le virus de la fièvre typhoïde conférée par des substances solubles. *Ann. Inst. Pasteur*, 1888, **2**, 54-59.
Experimental antityphoid inoculation.

5035   ACHARD, EMILE CHARLES. 1860-1941, & BENSAUDE, RAOUL.
Infections paratyphoïdiques. *Bull. Soc. méd Hôp. Paris*, 1896, 3 sér., **13**, 820-33.
Isolation of *Salmonella paratyphi B*. First use of the term "paratyphoid fever".

5036   GRUBER, MAX. 1853-1927, & DURHAM, HERBERT EDWARD. 1866-1945
Eine neue Methode zur raschen Erkennung des Choleravibrio und des Typhusbacillus. *Münch med. Wschr.*, 1896, **43**, 285-86.
The discovery of bacterial agglutination was made when Gruber and Durham found that the serum of typhoid patients had an agglutinating action on the typhoid bacillus; they realized its value as a clinical test in the identification of typhoid.

5037   WIDAL, GEORGES FERNAND ISIDOR. 1862-1929, & SICARD, ARTHUR.
Recherches de la réaction agglutinante dans le sang le sérum desséchés des typhiques et dans la sérosité des vésicatoires. *Bull. Soc. méd. Hôp. Paris*, 1896, 3 sér., **13**, 681-82.
Widal and Sicard demonstrated specific agglutinins in the blood of typhoid patients, making possible an agglutination reaction for the diagnosis of typhoid ("Gruber–Widal test").

5038   GWYN, NORMAN BEECHEY. 1875-1952
On infection with a para-colon bacillus in a case with all the clinical features of typhoid fever. *Johns Hopk. Hosp. Bull.*, 1898, **9**, 54-56.
Isolation of *Salmonella paratyphi A*.

5039   WRIGHT, *Sir* ALMROTH EDWARD. 1861-1947, & LEISHMAN, *Sir* WILLIAM BOOG. 1865-1926
Remarks on the results which have been obtained by the antityphoid inoculations. *Brit. med. J.*, 1900, **1**, 122-29.
The active inoculation of man against typhoid was first performed by Wright in 1896. For a preliminary note see *Lancet*, 1896, **2**, 807.

5040   KOCH, ROBERT. 1843-1910
Die Bekämpfung des Typhus. Berlin, *A. Hirschwald*, 1903.
The prophylactic measures for the control of typhoid suggested by Koch have been adopted almost everywhere.

5041   UHLENHUTH, PAUL THEODOR. 1870-1957, & HÜBENER, ERICH AUGUST. 1870-
Weitere Mitteilungen über Schweinepest mit besonderer Berücksichtigung der Bakteriologie der Hogcholeragruppe. *Zbl. Bakt.*, 1 Abt., 1908, **42**, Beilage, 127-38.
First description of *Salmonella paratyphi C.*

5042   RUSSELL, FREDERICK FULLER. 1870-1960
The control of typhoid in the Army by vaccination. *N.Y. State J. Med.*, 1910, **10**, 535-48.
Russell carried out important and long-continued investigations on anti-typhoid vaccination in the U.S. Army, demonstrating beyond question its value in selected groups. The war of 1914-18 confirmed the value of the work of Wright and Russell.

5043   SAXL, PAUL. 1880-1932
Ueber die Behandlung von Typhus mit Milchinjektionen. *Wien Klin. Wschr.*, 1916, **29**, 1043-45.

5044   HIRZFELD, LUDWIK MAURYCY. 1884-1954
A new generation of paratyphoid. *Lancet*, 1919, **1**, 296-97.
Hirzfeld gave an important description of *Salmonella paratyphi C.* ("Hirzfeld's bacillus").

5044.1   KAUFFMANN, FRITZ.
Der heutige Stand der Paratyphusforschung. *Zbl. ges. Hyg.*, 1931, **25**, 273-311.
Kauffmann–White classification of *Salmonella* based on antigenic structure. For historical note, including the part played by P. B. White, see *J. Hyg. (Camb.)*, 1934, **34**, 335.

5045   FELIX, ARTHUR. 1887-1956, & PITT, R. MARGARET.
A new antigen of B. typhosus. Its relation to virulence and to active and passive immunisation. *Lancet*, 1934, **2**, 186-91.
Vi antigens first described.

5045.1   ——. & PETRIE, GEORGE FORD. 1863-1955
The preparation of anti-typhoid serum in the horse for therapeutic use in man. *J. Hyg. (Camb.)*, 1938, **38**, 673-82.
Typhoid antiserum.

5046   ARETAEUS, *the Cappadocian*. A.D. 81-?138
On ulcerations about the tonsils. *In* : Extant works, ed. F. ADAMS, London, 1856, 253-55.
   Aretaeus's description of ulcerations about the tonsils, which he called "ulcera Syrica", clearly referred to diphtheria, of which it was the first unmistakable description. For his treatment of the disease, see pp. 409-10 of the same work.

5047   BAILLOU, GUILLAUME DE [BALLONIUS]. 1538-1616
Epidemiorum et ephemeridum libri duo. Paris, *J. Quensel*, 1640.
   A pupil of Fernel, de Baillou was a brilliant writer and speaker. The above work includes a description of the epidemic of diphtheria in Paris, 1576. Later de Baillou advocated tracheotomy, although there is no evidence that he performed that operation.

5048   MARTINE, GEORGE. 1702-1741
Account of the operation of bronchotome, as it was performed at St. Andrews. *Phil. Trans.*, 1730, **36**, 448-55.
   Martine was the first to perform tracheotomy for diphtheria.

5049   FOTHERGILL, JOHN. 1712-1780
An account of the sore throat attended with ulcers. London, *C. Davis*, 1748.
   First authoritative account of both diphtheria and scarlatinal angina, although the writer failed to differentiate between the two conditions. Reprinted in *Med. Classics*, 1940, **5**, 58-99.

5050   HUXHAM, JOHN. 1692-1768
A dissertation on the malignant, ulcerous sore-throat. London, *J. Hinton*, 1757.
   Huxham's reputation rests mainly on his *Essays on fevers*, but he also left an excellent account of diphtheria. Although he failed to differentiate the disease from scarlatinal angina, he was the first to observe the paralysis of the soft palate.

5051   HOME, FRANCIS. 1719-1813
An enquiry into the nature, cause, and cure of the croup. Edinburgh, *Kincaid & Bell*, 1765.
   First clear and complete clinical description of diphtheria.

5052   BARD, SAMUEL. 1742-1821
An enquiry into the nature, cause and cure of the angina suffocativa, or sore throat distemper, as it is commonly called by the inhabitants of this city and colony. New York, *S. Inslee, & A. Car*, 1771.
   One of the earliest accurate descriptions of diphtheria. Osler considered the book "an American classic of the first rank".

5053   BRETONNEAU, PIERRE FIDÈLE. 1778-1862
Des inflammations spéciales du tissu muqueux et en particulier de la diphthérite, ou inflammation pelliculaire. Paris, *Crevot*, 1826.
   Bretonneau showed that croup, malignant angina, and "scorbutic gangrene of the gums" were all the same disease, for which he suggested

the term "diphtheritis", later substituting "diphthérite". He performed (pp. 300-38) tracheotomy for croup. English translation in New Sydenham Society's *Memoirs on diphtheria*, London, 1859.

5054   TROUSSEAU, ARMAND. 1801-1867
Mémoire sur un cas de trachéotomie pratiquée dans la période extrême de croup. *J. Connaiss. méd.-chir.*, 1833, **1**, 5, 41.
Trousseau popularized tracheotomy.

5055   KLEBS, THEODOR ALBRECHT EDWIN. 1834-1913
Ueber Diphtherie. *Verh. Congr. inn. Med.*, 1883, **2**, 139-54.
First account of *Corynebacterium diphtheriae* (Klebs–Loeffler bacillus), causal organism in diphtheria, discovered by Klebs.

5056   LOEFFLER, FRIEDRICH, 1852-1915
Untersuchungen über die Bedeutung der Mikroorganismen für die Entstehung der Diphtherie beim Menschen, bei der Taube und beim Kalbe. *Mitt. k. GesundhAmte*, 1884, **2**, 421-99.
Loeffler succeeded in cultivating *C. diphtheriae*; he reproduced the characteristic membrane by swabbing the mucous membranes of various animals with pure cultures of the bacillus.

5057   O'DWYER, JOSEPH P. 1841-1898
Intubation of the larynx. *N.Y. med. J.*, 1885, **42**, 145-47.
O'Dwyer perfected the operation of laryngeal intubation in croup.

5059   ROUX, PIERRE PAUL EMILE. 1853-1933, & YERSIN, ALEXANDRE EMIL JEAN. 1863-1943
Contribution à l'étude de la diphtérie. *Ann. Inst. Pasteur*, 1888, **2**, 629-61; 1889, **3**, 273-88; 1890, **4**, 385-426.
Confirmation of the work of Loeffler and demonstration of the exotoxin. This work is the starting point of the development of an immunizing serum.

5060   BEHRING, EMIL ADOLF VON. 1854-1917, & KITASATO, SHIBASABURO, *Baron*. 1852-1931
Ueber das Zustandekommen der Diphtherie-Immunität und der Tetanus-Immunität bei Thieren. *Dtsch. med. Wschr.*, 1890, **16**, 1113-14, 1145-48.
Antitoxins and their immunizing powers were discovered when Behring and Kitasato published their paper dealing with immunity to tetanus and diphtheria. This work laid the foundation of all future treatment with antitoxins. The paper was reprinted in the same journal, 1940, **66**, 1348-49. Part 2, which deals with diphtheria, is by Behring alone.

5060.1   FRAENKEL, CARL. 1861-1915
Immunisirungsversuche bei Diphtherie. *Berl. klin. Wschr.*, 1890, **27**, 1133-35.
Artificial immunity to diphtheria produced in guinea-pigs by injection of attenuated cultures of the bacillus.

5061   WELCH, WILLIAM HENRY. 1850-1934, & FLEXNER, SIMON. 1863-1946
The histological changes in experimental diphtheria. *Johns Hopk. Hosp. Bull.*, 1891, **2**, 107-10; 1892, **3**, 17-18.
An account of the pathological changes brought about by experimental inoculation of diphtheria toxins.

5062   BEHRING, EMIL ADOLF VON. 1854-1917
        Die Behandlung der Diphtherie mit Diphtherieheilserum. *Dtsch. med. Wschr.*, 1893, **19**, 543-47; 1894, **20**, 645-46.
        In 1890 Behring and Kitasato discovered the diphtheria and tetanus antitoxins (*see* No. 5060). The above papers deal more fully with the use of the diphtheria antitoxin.

5063   ROUX, PIERRE PAUL EMILE. 1853-1933, & MARTIN, ANDRÉ LOUIS FRANÇOIS JUSTIN. 1853-1921
        Contribution à l'étude de la diphtérie (sérum thérapie). *Ann. Inst. Pasteur,* 1894, **8**, 609-39.
        Roux and Martin demonstrated the value of Behring's specific antitoxin in the treatment of human diphtheria, and showed how it could be produced on a large scale.

5064   EHRLICH, PAUL. 1854-1915
        Die Wertbestimmung des Diphtherieheilserums. *Klin. Jb.*, 1897, **6**, 299-326.
        Ehrlich improved Behring's diphtheria antitoxin through quantitative titration and established an international standard for this and other antitoxins. This was the beginning of the concept of biological standardization. The first exposition of Ehrlich's side-chain theory appeared in this paper. Abridged English translation in Bibel, *Milestones in immunology* (1988).

5065   SCHICK, BELA. 1877-1967
        Kutanreaktion bei Impfung mit Diphtherietoxin. *Münch. med. Wschr.*, 1908, **55**, 504-06.
        The Schick test for the determination of susceptibility to diphtheria.

5066   ———. Die Diphtherietoxin – Hautreaktion des Menschen als Vorprobe der prophylaktischen Diphtherieheilseruminjektion. *Münch. med. Wschr.*, 1913, **60**, 2608-10.
        Schick developed his test for use as an indication as to whether or not prophylactic injections of antitoxin are necessary in children already exposed to diphtheria. English translation in *J. Mt. Sinai Hosp.*, 1938, **5**, 26-28.

5067   BEHRING, EMIL ADOLF VON. 1854-1917
        Ueber ein neues Diphtherieschutzmittel. *Dtsch. med. Wschr.*, 1913, **39**, 873-76; 1914, **40**, 1139.
        Toxin–antitoxin for immunization against diphtheria.

5068   PARK, WILLIAM HALLOCK. 1863-1939, *et al.*
        Active immunization in diphtheria and treatment by toxin–antitoxin. *J. Amer. med. Assoc.*, 1914, **63**, 859-61.
        With A. Zingher and M. H. Serota. Park was an early advocate of diphtheria immunization with toxin–antitoxin. A second paper is in the same journal, 1915, **65**, 2216-20.

5069   KASSOWITZ, KARL ERHARD. 1886-?
        Ueber cutane Hautreaktion mittels Diphtherie-Toxin zum Nachweis der Diphtherie-Immunität. *Klin Wschr.*, 1924, **3**, 1317-18.
        The "scratch test", a cutaneous reaction for determination of susceptibility to diphtheria.

5070   RAMON, GASTON LÉON. 1886-1963
L'anatoxine diphtérique. Ses propriétés – ses applications. *Ann. Inst. Pasteur,* 1928, **42**, 959-1009.

In 1923 Ramon so modified the diphtheria toxin with formaldehyde that it lost its toxic properties while retaining its antigenic virtues. This modified "anatoxin" (toxoid) superseded toxin–antitoxin as an immunizing agent against diphtheria. Preliminary paper in *C. R. Soc. Biol. (Paris),* 1923, **89**, 2-4.

5071   GLENNY, ALEXANDER THOMAS. 1882-1965
Insoluble precipitates in diphtheria and tetanus immunization. *Brit. med. J.,* 1930, **2**, 244-45.

Alum-precipitated toxoid for active immunization.

5072   ANDERSON, JAMES STIRLING. 1891-1976, *et al.*
On the existence of two forms of diphtheria bacillus – *B. diphtheriae gravis* and *B. diphtheriae mitis. J. Path. Bact.,* 1931, **34**, 667-81.

J. S. Anderson, F. C. Happold, J. W. McLeod, and J. G. Thomson were the first to distinguish the *gravis, mitis,* and intermediate types of *C. diphtheriae.*

SCARLET FEVER

5073   INGRASSIA, Giovanni Filippo. 1510-1580
De tumoribus praeter naturam. Neapoli, 1553.

Includes (p. 194) the first known description of an epidemic disease resembling scarlet fever. This was a prevalent malady in Italy, and was commonly called *rossania* or *rossalia.*

5074   SENNERT, DANIEL. 1572-1637
De febribus libri IV. Venetiis, *F. Baba,* 1641.

Sennert gave the first scientific description of scarlet fever. He was the first to mention the scarlatinal desquamation, the early arthritis, and post-scarlatinal dropsy, but made no mention of sore throat.

5075   SYDENHAM, THOMAS. 1624-1689
Febris scarlatina. *In*: Observationes medicae, London, 1676, p. 387.

The reputation of Sydenham, "the English Hippocrates", rests today on his excellent account of diseases, of which the description of scarlet fever is one of the best. He first clearly differentiated scarlatina from measles, giving it its present name. Translation in his *Works,* London, 1850, **2**, 242.

5076   DOUGLASS, WILLIAM. 1691?-1752
The practical history of a new epidemical eruptive miliary fever, with an angina ulcusculosa, which prevailed in Boston New England in the years 1735 and 1736. Boston, N. E., *T. Fleet,* 1736.

Douglass left the first adequate clinical description of scarlet fever, which he called angina ulcusculosa, in his account of New England's first scarlet fever epidemic. He was one of the first American physicians to hold the M.D.

5077   FOTHERGILL, JOHN. 1712-1780
        An account of the sore throat attended with ulcers. London, *C. Davis*, 1748.
        First authoritative account of both diphtheria and scarlatinal angina,
        although failing to differentiate between the two conditions. Reprinted in
        Med. Classics, 1940, **5**, 58-99.

5078   PLENCIZ, MARC ANTON VON. 1705-1786
        Opera medico-physica in quatuor tractatus digesta. Viennae Austriae, *J. T.
        Trattner*, 1762.
        Plenciz was the first to grasp the significance of Leeuwenhoek's
        animalculae for the aetiology of contagious disease. Part III of the above
        is concerned with scarlatina.

5079   WITHERING, WILLIAM. 1741-1799
        An account of the scarlet fever and sore throat, or scarlatina anginosa;
        particularly as it appeared at Birmingham in the year 1778. London, *T. Cadell*,
        1779.
        Withering, best remembered for his book on the foxglove, described
        the epidemics of scarlet fever which occurred in England in 1771 and 1778.

5080   KLEIN, EDWARD EMANUEL. 1844-1925
        Report on a disease of cows prevailing at a farm from which scarlatina had
        been distributed along with the milk of cows. 15*th Ann. Rep. Local Govt.
        Bd., Suppl. containing Report of the Medical Officer for 1885*, London, 1886,
        pp. 90-110.
        Contains the first suggestion of the streptococcal origin of scarlet fever.

5080.1 BERGE, ANDRÉ.
        Sur la pathogénie de la scarlatine. *C. R. Soc. Biol. (Paris)*, 1893, **45**, 1012-
        14.
        Bergé stated all the essential facts concerning the aetiology of scarlet
        fever, and definitely attributed its cause to a streptococcus. He published
        a thesis on the subject in 1895.

5081   SCHULTZ, WERNER. 1878-1944, & CHARLTON, WILLY. 1889-?
        Serologische Beobachtungen am Scharlachexanthem. *Z. Kinderheilk.*, 1918,
        Orig., **17**, 328-33.
        Schultz–Charlton reaction.

5082   DICK, GEORGE FREDERICK. 1881-1967, & DICK, GLADYS ROWENA HENRY. 1881-
        1963
        A skin test for susceptibility to scarlet fever. *J. Amer. med. Assoc.*, 1924, **82**,
        265-66.
        The "Dick test" for the determination of individual susceptibility to
        scarlet fever.

5082.1 ——. The etiology of scarlet fever. *J. Amer. med. Assoc.*, 1924, **82**, 301-02.
        Proof that streptococcus is the cause of scarlet fever.

5083   ——. A scarlet fever antitoxin. *J. Amer. med. Assoc.*, 1924, **82**, 1246-47.
        Following their successful attempts to establish individual susceptibility
        to scarlet fever, these workers prepared an antitoxin for immunization.

5084 DOCHEZ, ALPHONSE RAYMOND. 1882-1964, & SHERMAN, LILLIAN.
The significance of Streptococcus hemolyticus in scarlet fever and the preparation of a specific anti-scarlatinal serum by immunization of the horse to Streptococcus hemolyticus-scarlatinae. *J. Amer. med. Assoc.*, 1924, **82**, 542-44.

Dochez and Sherman immunized a horse by repeated injections of scarlet fever toxin. A serum obtained from the horse blanched a scarlet fever rash and, when injected subcutaneously, caused marked amelioration of the early symptoms. They also confirmed the relation of streptococci to scarlet fever.

WHOOPING COUGH

5085 BAILLOU, GUILLAUME DE [BALLONIUS]. 1538-1616
Quinta. *In:* Epidemiorum et ephemeridum libri duo. Paris, *J. Quesnel*, 1640, p. 237.

First description of whooping cough. This was originally written in 1578. Baillou called it "tussis quintana". For translation see R. H. Major, *Classic descriptions of disease*, 3rd ed., 1945, p. 210.

5086 WILLIS, THOMAS. 1621-1675
Pharmaceutice rationalis sive diatriba de medicamentorum operationibus in humano corpore. Pars secunda. [Oxonii], *e Theatro Sheldoniano*, 1675.

Contains (p. 99) a description of "puerorum tussis convulsiva, chincough dicta" – a clear account of whooping cough (Treatise IX, pt. 2, p. 38 of his *Practice of physick*, 1684).

5086.1 WATT, ROBERT. 1774-1819
Treatise on the history, nature, and treatment of chincough: including a variety of cases and dissections. Glasgow, *J. Smith & Son*, 1813.

Probably the first book on the subject. Watt was the compiler of the monumental *Bibliotheca Britannica* (1819-24) which includes many medical items.

5087 BORDET, JULES JEAN BAPTISTE VINCENT. 1870-1961, & GENGOU, OCTAVE. 1875-1957
Le microbe de la coqueluche. *Ann. Inst. Pasteur*, 1906, **20**, 731-41; 1907, **21**, 720-26.

The cocco-bacillus *Haemophilus pertussis*, commonly regarded as the causal organism of whooping cough, was at first named "Bordet–Gengou bacillus" after its discoverers. It has recently been renamed *Bordetella pertussis*.

5087.1 LESLIE, PATRICK HOLT, & GARDNER, ARTHUR DUNCAN. 1884-
The phases of *Haemophilus pertussis. J. Hyg. (Camb.)*, 1931, **31**, 423-34.

Leslie and Gardner classified *H. pertussis* cultures into four types and established an experimental basis for the development of an effective vaccine.

5087.2 KENDRICK, PEARL L. 1890- , & ELDERING. GRACE.
A study in active immunization against pertussis. *Amer. J. Hyg.*, 1939, **29**, Sect. B, 133-53.

Pertussis vaccine.

5088   STICKER, GEORG. 1860-1960
        Der Keuchhusten. Wien, *A. Hölder*, 1896.
        An important history of whooping cough.

BACILLARY DYSENTERY

5089   ARETAEUS, *the Cappadocian*. A.D. 81-?138
        On dysentery. *In*: Extant works, ed. F. ADAMS, London, 1856, 353-57.
        Prior to Lösch's discovery of *E. histolytica*, all forms of dysentery were
        differentiated only on clinical grounds.

5090   ZIMMERMANN, JOHANN GEORG. 1728-1795
        Von der Ruhr unter dem Volke im Jahr 1765. Zürich, *Fuessli & Co.*, 1767.
        First important monograph on bacillary dysentery. English translation,
        London, 1771.

5090.1 CHANTEMESSE, ANDRÉ. 1851-1919, & WIDAL, GEORGES FERNAND ISIDOR.
        1862-1929
        Sur les microbes de la dysentérie épidémique. *Bull. Acad. Méd. (Paris)*, 1888,
        19, 522-29.
        The dysentery bacillus was isolated by Chantemesse and Widal, although
        they failed to establish its aetiological relationship to the disease.

5091   SHIGA, KIYOSHI. 1870-1957
        Ueber den Dysenteriebacillus (Bacillus dysenteriae). *Zbl. Bakt.*, 1898, 1
        Abt., **24**, 817-28, 870-74.
        Discovery of the dysentery bacillus, *Shigella*. Preliminary paper in the
        same journal, 1898, **23**, 599-600.

5092   KRUSE, WALTHER. 1864-1943
        Ueber die Ruhr als Volkskrankheit und ihren Erreger. *Dtsch. med. Wschr.*,
        1900, **26**, 637-39.
        Further work on dysentery by Kruse led to the coupling of his name
        with Shiga to designate both the "Shiga–Kruse bacillus" and "Shiga–Kruse
        disease".

5093   FLEXNER, SIMON. 1863-1946
        On the etiology of tropical dysentery. *Johns Hopk. Hosp. Bull.*, 1900, **11**, 231-
        42.
        The organism isolated by Flexner was at first thought to be identical
        with Shiga's bacillus. Later Martini and Lentz, *Z. Hyg.*, 1902, **41**, 540, showed
        it to be different; it was named *Bact. flexneri*, and later *Shigella flexneri*.

5094   SONNE, CARL OLAF. 1882-1948
        Ueber die Bakteriologie der giftarmen Dysenteriebacillen (Para-
        dysenteriebacillen). *Zbl. Bakt.*, 1915, 1 Abt., **75**, Orig., 408-56.
        Sonne's bacillus (*Shigella sonnei*) was probably described earlier by
        others, but it was Sonne who first drew serious attention to it. First
        published as inaugural dissertation, 1914.

5095   SCHMITZ, KARL EITEL FRIEDRICH. 1889-
        Eine neuer Typus aus der Gruppe der Ruhrbazillen als Erreger einer
        grösseren Epidemie. *Z. Hyg. InfektKr.*, 1917, **84**, 449-516.
            Schmitz's bacillus – *Bact. ambiguum (Shigella schmitzii)*, a cause of
        dysentery.

5096   MARSHALL, ELI KENNERLEY. 1889-1966, *et al.*
        Sulfanilylguanidine in the treatment of acute bacillary dysentery in children.
        Johns Hopk. Hosp. Bull., 1941, **68**, 94-111.
            E. K. Marshall, A. C. Bratton, L. B. Edwards, and E. L. Walker were the
        first to use sulphaguanidine in the treatment of bacillary dysentery.

BRUCELLOSIS

5097   MARSTON, JEFFERY ALLEN. 1831-1911
        Report on fever (Malta). *Army med. Dept. statist. Rep. (Lond.)*, (1861), 1863,
        3, 486-521.
            Marston wrote the first description of Malta fever as a distinct disease.
        He contracted the disease while serving in the Mediterranean area and
        described his own case.

5098   BRUCE, *Sir* DAVID. 1855-1931
        Note on the discovery of a micro-organism in Malta fever. *Practitioner*, 1887,
        39, 161-70.
            Malta fever was shown by Bruce to be due to *Micrococcus (Brucella)
        melitensis.*

5099   BANG, BERNHARD LAURITS FREDERIK. 1848-1932
        Die Aetiologie des seuchenhaften ("infectiösen") Verwerfens. *Z. Thiermed.*,
        1897, **1**, 241-78.
            Discovery of *Brucella abortus.*

5100   HUGHES, MATTHEW LOUIS. 1867-1899
        Mediterranean, Malta, or undulant fever. London, *Macmillan & Co.*, 1897.
            An authoritative summary of current knowledge of Malta fever.

5101   WRIGHT, *Sir* ALMROTH EDWARD. 1861-1947, & SMITH, FREDERICK.
        On the application of the serum test to the differential diagnosis of typhoid
        and Malta fever. *Lancet*, 1897, **1**, 656-59.
            Agglutination test for the diagnosis of undulant fever.

5102   REPORTS of the Commission appointed by the Admiralty, the War Office,
        and the Civil Government of Malta, for the investigation of Mediterranean
        fever, under the supervision of an advisory committee of the Royal Society.
        7 pts. London, *Harrison & Sons*, 1905-07.
            The important findings of the Mediterranean Fever Commission are
        summarized in Topley & Wilson's *Bacteriology*, 1975, p. 2173; probably the
        most valuable was that of T. Zammit, who showed goat's milk to be the
        main source of infection (pt. 4, p. 97).

5103   EVANS, ALICE CATHERINE. 1881-1975
        Studies on Brucella (Alkaligenes) melitensis. Washington, *Govt. Printing
        Office*, 1925.

Forms Bulletin No. 143 of the U.S. Public Health Service Hygienic Laboratory. Alice Evans showed that the causal organism of Malta fever was closely related to *Brucella abortus*, responsible for contagious abortion in cattle. See also her earlier paper in *J. infect. Dis.*, 1918, **22**, 580-93.

CHOLERA

5104   GARCIA D'ORTA. 1501-1568
Colloquios dos simples, e drogas he causas mediçinais da India. Goa, *Joannes*, 1563.
Includes a classic description of Asiatic cholera, the first account of the disease by a European in modern times (*see also* No. 1815).

5104.1   SONNERAT, PIERRE. 1749-1814
Voyage aux Indes Orientales et à la Chine, fait par ordre du Roi depuis 1774 jusqu'en 1781. 2 vols. Paris, *L'Auteur*, 1782.
Vol. 1, pp. 113-16, "No author before the time of Sonnerat gives us so distinct an account of the epidemic prevalence of cholera, so full a description of its varieties or has attributed it so positively to the physical misery of the natives of the country" (Macpherson, No. 5111.2). English translation, 1788-89.

5105   PARKIN, JOHN. 1801-1886
Suggestions respecting the cause, nature, and treatment of cholera, *Lond. med. surg. J.*, 1832, n.s. **2**, 151-53.
Parkin suggested the water-borne character of cholera and the use of charcoal filters for water purification.

5106   SNOW, JOHN. 1813-1858
On the pathology and mode of communication of the cholera. *Lond. med. Gaz.*, 1849, **44**, 730-32, 745-52, 923-29.
The water-borne character of cholera was demonstrated by Snow, who collected data regarding a large number of outbreaks and correlated them with water supplies. His book *On the mode of communication of cholera* appeared in the same year, and its second edition (1855) was in fact a new book, reporting much more elaborate and refined investigations on cholera incidence and water supply; it included the story of the Broad Street pump. It was reprinted, New York, 1936.

5106.1   PACINI, FILIPPO. 1812-1883
Osservazioni microscopiche e deduzioni patologiche sul cholera asiatico. *Gazz. med. ital. fed. tosc.*, 1854, 2 ser., **4**, 397-401, 405-12.
Pacini described vibrios seen in the intestinal contents of cholera victims. He incriminated these vibrios as the pathogen in the disease, anticipating Koch (No. 5108) by 30 years. See N. Howard-Jones. *Perspect. Biol. Med.*, 1971, **13**, 422-33.

5107   PETTENKOFER, MAX JOSEF VON. 1818-1901
Unterschungen und Beobachtungen über die Verbreitungsart der Cholera. München, *J. G. Cotta*, 1855.

Pettenkofer gave much attention to the aetiology of cholera. He postulated the theory that a specific germ, certain local conditions, certain seasonal conditions, and certain individual conditions are all necessary for an epidemic to occur (the Boden theory).

5108   KOCH, ROBERT. 1843-1910
Ueber die Cholerabakterien. *Dtsch. med. Wschr.*, 1884, **10**, 725-28.
Discovery of the cholera vibrio and of its transmission by drinking water, food, and clothing.

5109   HAFFKINE, WALDEMAR MORDECAI WOLFF. 1860-1930
Le choléra asiatique chez le cobaye. *C. R. Soc. Biol. (Paris)*, 1892, **44**, 635-37, 671.
Haffkine's vaccine against cholera was the first to meet with any success.

5110   PFEIFFER, RICHARD FRIEDRICH JOHANNES. 1858-1945, & ISAYEV, VASILY ISAYEVICH. 1854-1911
Ueber die specifische Bedeutung der Choleraimmunität (Bakteriolyse). *Z. Hyg. InfektKr.*, 1894, **17**, 355-400; **18**, 1-16.
Pfeiffer and Isayev recorded the occurrence of bacteriolysis in cholera vibrios under certain conditions ("Pfeiffer's phenomenon").

5111   KOLLE, WILHELM. 1868-1935
Zur aktiven Immunisierung des Menschen gegen Cholera. *Zbl. Bakt.*, Abt. I, 1896, **19**, 97-104.
Kolle introduced the killed cholera vaccine.

5111.1   GOTSCHLICH, FELIX. 1874-
Über Cholera- und choleraähnliche Vibrionen unter den aus Mekka zurückkehrenden Pilgern. *Z. Hyg. InfektKr.*, 1906, **53**, 281-304.
Isolation of El Tor vibrio.

5111.2   MACPHERSON, JOHN. 1817-1890
Annals of cholera: from the earliest periods to the year 1817. London, *Ranken & Co.*, 1872.

5111.3   MACNAMARA, NOTTIDGE CHARLES. 1832-1918
A history of Asiatic cholera. London, *Macmillan*, 1876.

5111.4   POLLITZER, ROBERT.
Cholera. Geneva, *World Health Organization*, 1959.
Includes a section on the history of cholera. *WHO Monograph Series*, No. 43.

5112   STICKER, GEORG. 1860-1960
Abhandlungen aus der Seuchengeschichte und Seuchenlehre. II. Die Cholera. Giessen, *A. Töpelmann*, 1912.

5113 VALESCUS DE TARANTA. 1382-1417
Tractatus de epidemia et peste. [Basel, *Martin Flach*, c. 1474]
    One of the earliest works written on public health, and one of the
earliest printed medical books. It was first printed in Arnaldus de Villanova's
De arte cognoscendi venena (Padua, 1473; Mantua, 1473). Above is the
first separate edition.

5114 STEINHÖWEL, HEINRICH. 1420-1482
Buchlein der Ordnung der Pestilenz. Ulm, *Johann Zainer*, 1473.
    This was a famous book and was often reprinted. It is reproduced in
facsimile in A. C. Klebs: *Die ersten gedruckten Pestschriften*, 1936.

5115 JACME, JEAN [JOHANNES JACOBI]. *d.* 1384
Incipit perutilis tractatus de pestilencia. [Augsburg, *Johann Keller*, between 1478 and 1482.]
    The most widely disseminated of all plague tracts from the time of the
Black Death. A French rhymed version appeared in 1476, but this version
is very different from the prose, and from the pre-printing manuscripts that
are known. The plague tracts from the Black Death represent the first
productions of a large-scale public health effort in Europe. The English
version, *A litil boke the whiche traytied and reherced many gode thinges
necessaries for the ... pestilence*, [London, *Willelmus de Machlinia*, 1485?]
is the first medical book printed in England. Facsimile reprint from the copy
in the John Rylands Library, misattributing the work to Bengt Knutson (*d.*
1462), Manchester & London, 1910.

5117 DIEMERBROECK, YSBRAND VAN. 1609-1674
De peste libri quatuor, truculentissimi morbi historiam ratione et experientiâ
confirmatum exhibentes. Arenaci, *ex off. J. Jacobi*, 1646.
    Important early account of plague. English translation, 1722.

5118 KIRCHER, ATHANASIUS. 1602-1680
Scrutinium physico-medicum contagiosae luis, quae pestis dicitur. Romae,
typ. Mascardi, 1658.
    Kircher was probably the first to employ the microscope in investigating
the cause of disease. He mentioned that the blood of plague patients was
filled with a "countless brood of worms not perceptible to the naked eye,
but to be seen in all putrefying matter through the microscope" (Garrison).
He could not have seen the plague bacillus with his low-power microscope,
but he probably saw the larger micro-organisms. He was the first to state
explicitly the theory of contagion by animalculae as the cause of infectious
diseases.

5119 LONDON.
London's dreadful visitation, or, a collection of all the Bills of Mortality for
the present year: beginning the 27th of December 1664, and ending the
19th of December following...By the Company of Parish Clerks of London.
London, *E. Cotes*, 1665.
    This is a valuable statistical record of the great plague of 1665. (No. 6052
in the *Bibliotheca Osleriana*.)

5120   BOGHURST, WILLIAM. 1631-1685
        Loimographia. An account of the great plague of London in the year 1665.
        By William Boghurst. Now first printed from the British Museum Sloane
        Ms. 349, for the Epidemiological Society of London. Edited by J. F. PAYNE.
        London, *Shaw & Sons*, 1894.
        This work was written in 1666 and first published as above. Boghurst,
        an apothecary, did good work during the great plague; in his book he
        differentiated plague from typhus. Payne's introduction to the book
        contains some valuable historical data.

5121   HODGES, NATHANIEL. 1629-1688
        Λοιμόλόγια sive pestis nuperae apud populum Londinensem grassantis
        narratio historica. Londini, *J. Nevill*, 1672.
        Best medical record of the Great Plague of 1665. Hodges was physician
        to the City of London and the medical hero of the great epidemic. English
        translation by John Quincy, 1720.

5122   HASEIAH, LAURENTIUS [HASEIAC].
        De postrema Melitensi lue praxis historica. Panormi, 1677.
        This work, recording the epidemic of plague in Malta in 1675, is of
        interest as being the first medical work to be published by a Maltese.

5123   MEAD, RICHARD. 1673-1754
        A short discourse concerning pestilential contagion, and the methods to be
        used to prevent it. London, *S. Buckley*, 1720.
        Mead was asked for advice concerning the plague, and replied with the
        above tract. It was afterwards expanded into a book and is almost a
        prophecy of what was to develop as the English public health system.

5124   WESZPRÉMI, STEFAN. 1723-1799
        Tentamen de inoculandi peste. Londini, *J. Tuach*, 1755.
        Weszprémi proposed preventive inoculation against plague.

5125   YERSIN, ALEXANDRE EMILE JEAN. 1863-1943
        La peste bubonique à Hong-Kong. *Ann. Inst. Pasteur*, 1894, **8**, 662-67.
        Yersin discovered the plague bacillus *Pasteurella (Yersinia) pestis*,
        isolating it from excised buboes. He published the first account of this
        organism. Preliminary note in *C. R. Acad. Sci. (Paris)*, 1894, **119**, 356.

5126   RENNIE, ALEXANDER. 1859-1940
        The plague in the East. *Brit. Med. J.*, 1894, **2**, 615-16.
        Rennie appears to be the first seriously to support the theory of
        transmission of the plague bacillus by rats and to present evidence in
        support of that theory.

5127   YERSIN, ALEXANDRE EMILE JEAN. 1863-1943, *et al.*
        La peste bubonique. *Ann. Inst. Pasteur*, 1895, **9**, 589-92.
        Successful inoculation of animals with anti-plague vaccine. With L. C.
        A. Calmette and A. Borrel.

5128   OGATA, MASANORI. 1852-1919
        Ueber die Pestepidemie in Formosa. *Zbl. Bakt.*, 1897, Abt. I, **21**, 769-77.
        Ogata considered the flea (principally *Xenopsylla cheopis*) to be the
        principal, if not the sole, vector of bubonic plague infection.

5128.1   SIMOND, P. L.
La propagation de la peste. *Ann. Inst. Pasteur*, 1898, **12**, 625-87.
Simond provided substantial evidence to support Ogata that fleas transmitted plague from rat to man.

5129   HAFFKINE, WALDEMAR MORDECAI WOLFF. 1860-1930
Les inoculations antipesteuses. *Bull. Inst. Pasteur*, 1906, **4**, 825-40.
Haffkine developed an anti-bubonic plague vaccine (killed bouillon cultures), for use in man.

5129.1   BACOT, ARTHUR WILLIAM. 1866-1922, & MARTIN, *Sir* CHARLES JAMES. 1866-1955
Observations on the mechanism of the transmission of plague by fleas. *J. Hyg. (Camb.)*, 1914, Plague Suppl. 3, 423-39.
Bacot and Martin demonstrated the method by which the rat-flea transmitted the plague bacillus from rat to man.

5130   WU LIEN-TEH. 1879-1959
A treatise on pneumonic plague. Geneva, *League of Nations*, 1926.
Publication of the League of Nations, III. Health III, 13.

5131   POLLITZER, ROBERT.
Plague. Geneva, *World Health Organization*, 1954.
Includes a section on the history of plague. *WHO Monograph Series*, No. 22.

History of Plague

5132   PFEIFFER, LUDWIG. 1842-1921, & RULAND, C.
Pestilentia in nummis. Tübingen, *H. Laupp*, 1882.
A study of medals and tokens relating to epidemics of plague and other infectious diseases.

5135   HEITZ, PAUL.
Pestblätter des XV. Jahrhunderts. Hrsg. von P. Heitz, mit einleitendem Text von W. L. SCHEIBER. Strassburg, *Heitz u. Mündel*, 1901.

5136   STICKER, GEORG. 1860-1960
Abhandlungen aus der Seuchengeschichte und Seuchenlehre. I. Die Pest. Giessen, *A. Töpelmann*, 1908.
Exhaustive history of the subject by a prominent epidemiologist.

5137   GAFFAREL, PAUL. 1843- , & DURANTY, *Marquis de*.
La peste de 1720 à Marseille et en France d'après des documents inédits. Paris, *Perrin & Cie.*, 1911.

5138   CRAWFURD, *Sir* RAYMOND HENRY PAYNE. 1865-1938
Plague and pestilence in literature and art. Oxford, *Clarendon Press*, 1914.
Deals with the subject up to the end of the 18th century. Revised ed., 1951.

5140   KLEBS, ARNOLD CARL. 1870-1943, & DROZ, EUGÉNIE.
Remèdes contre la peste. Facsimilés, notes et liste bibliographique des incurables sur la peste. Paris, *Droz*, 1925.
     Includes facsimile reproduction of "La régime de l'epidémie et remède contre icelle" of Jean Jacme (Johannes Jacobi), [5115], together with the "Remède trèsutile contre fièvre pestilencieuse" by the same writer. *See* No. 5115.

5141   ———. & SUDHOFF, KARL FRIEDRICH JAKOB. 1853-1938
Die ersten gedruckten Pestschriften. München, *Verlag der Münchener Druck*, 1926.
     Includes description of 130 incunabula.

5142   WILSON, FREDERICK PERERA. 1876-1926
The plague in Shakespeare's London. Oxford, *Clarendon Press*, 1927.

5142.1   CAMPBELL, ANNA MONTGOMERY. 1888-
The black death and men of learning. New York, *Columbia University Press*, 1931.

5143   HIRST, LEONARD FABIAN. 1882-1964
Conquest of plague. A study of the evolution of epidemiology. Oxford, *Clarendon Press*, 1953.

5145   SHREWSBURY, JOHN FINDLAY DREW. 1898-1971
A history of bubonic plague in the British Isles. Cambridge, *University Press*, 1970.

5145.1   DOLS, MICHAEL W.
The black death in the Middle East. Princeton, *Princeton University Press*, [1977].

5145.2   ALEXANDER, JOHN T.
Bubonic plague in early modern Russia. Public health & urban disaster. Baltimore, *Johns Hopkins University Press*, [1980].

TETANUS

5146   ARETAEUS, *the Cappadocian*. A.D.81-?138
On tetanus. *In:* Extant works, ed. F. ADAMS, London, 1856, pp. 246-49, 400-04.
     Aretaeus left a full account of tetanus.

5147   CARLE, ANTONIO. 1854-1927, & RATTONE, GIORGIO.
Studio experimentale sull' eziologia del tetano. *G. r. Accad. Med. Torino*, 1884, 3 ser., **32**, 174-80.
     Demonstration of the transmissibility of tetanus by inoculation into rabbits of pus from a human case.

5148   NICOLAIER, ARTHUR. 1862-1942
Ueber infectiösen Tetanus. *Dtsch. med. Wschr.*, 1884, **10**, 842-44.
     The discovery of the tetanus bacillus is attributed to Nicolaier; he was, however, unable to isolate the organism in pure culture.

5149   KITASATO, Shibasaburo, *Baron*. 1852-1931
        Ueber den Tetanusbacillus. *Z. Hyg. InfektKr.*, 1889, **7**, 225-34.
        Kitasato obtained a pure culture of the tetanus bacillus, *Cl. tetani*.

5150   BEHRING, Emil Adolf von. 1854-1917, & KITASATO, Shibasaburo, *Baron*.
        1852-1931
        Ueber das Zustandekommen der Diphtherie-Immunität und der Tetanus-
        Immunität bei Thieren. *Dtsch. med. Wschr.*, 1890, **16**, 1113-14, 1145-48.
        Discovery of antitoxins and their immunizing powers (*see also* No. 5060).

5151   RAMON, Gaston Léon. 1886-1963, & ZOELLER, Christian. 1888-1934
        Sur la valeur et la durée de l'immunité conférée par l'anatoxine tétanique
        dans la vaccination de l'himme contre le tétanos. *C. R. Soc. Biol. (Paris)*,
        1933, **112**, 347-50.
        Tetanus toxoid first employed in the immunization of humans.

GLANDERS: MELIOIDOSIS

5152   CHABERT, Philibert. 1737-1814
        Mémoire sur la morve. *Hist. Soc. roy. Méd. (Paris)*, (1779), 1782, **3**, pt. 2,
        361-91.
        Chabert, the most celebrated veterinarian of his time, left a fine account
        of glanders.

5153   ELLIOTSON, John. 1791-1868
        On the glanders in the human subject. *Med.-chir. Trans.*, 1830, **16**, 171-218;
        1833, **18**, 201-07.
        Proof that glanders in the horse is communicable to man.

5154   RAYER, Pierre François Olive. 1793-1867
        De la morve et du farcin chez l'homme. *Mém. Acad. roy. Méd. (Paris)*,
        1837, **6**, 625-873.
        A classic contribution to the knowledge of glanders and farcy in man.
        Rayer showed that glanders is contagious but is not a form of tuberculosis.
        This work is a landmark in the history of bacteriology.

5156   LOEFFLER, Friedrich. 1852-1915
        Die Aetiologie der Rotzkrankheit. *Arb. k. GesundhAmte*, 1886, **1**, 141-98.
        Discovery of *Pfeifferella mallei*, causative organism of glanders. Pre-
        liminary notice in *Dtsch. med. Wschr.*, 1882, **8**, 707.

5157   STRAUS, Isidore. 1845-1896
        Sur un moyen de diagnostic rapide de la morve. *Arch. Méd. exp. Anat.
        path.*, 1889, **1**, 460-62.
        Straus reaction for the diagnosis of glanders.

5158   BABÉS, Victor. 1854-1926
        Observations sur la morve. *Arch. Méd. exp. Anat. path.*, 1891, **3**, 619-45.
        Mallein reaction for the diagnosis of glanders.

5159   WHITMORE, ALFRED. 1876-1946, & KRISHNASWAMI, C. S.
An account of the discovery of a hitherto undescribed infective disease occurring among the population of Rangoon. *Indian med. Gaz.*, 1912, **47**, 262-67.
First description of melioidosis. The organism isolated was subsequently named *Pfeifferella whitmori* by Stanton and Fletcher.

5159.1 STANTON, *Sir* AMBROSE THOMAS. 1875-1938
A form of pseudo-tuberculosis (melioidosis). *Studies Inst. Med. Res. Fed. Malay States*, No. 14, 1917.
Stanton identified the bacillus of melioidosis and reproduced the disease in animals by feeding and inoculation of cultures.

5159.2 ———. & FLETCHER, WILLIAM. ?-1938
Melioidosis. London, *John Bale*, 1932.
Studies from the Institute for Medical Research, F.M.S., No. 21. Stanton gave melioidosis its present name and, with Fletcher, wrote the authoritative work on the subject.

5160   HARTMAN, HARTMANNUS.
Thesis de carbunculo. Lugduni Batavorum, *ex off. F. Moyardi*, 1653.

5161   FRISCHMUTH, JOHANN.
Epistola...qua simul de anthrace, carbunculo, bubone et altauna, philologice disseritur. Jenae, *typ. vid. Krebsianae*, 1681.

5162   CHABERT, PHILIBERT. 1737-1814
Description et traitement du charbon dans les animaux. Paris, *Imp. Royale*, 1780.
First important clinical description of anthrax. For some time after the appearance of Chabert's little book, the condition was known as "Chabert's disease".

5163   RAYER, PIERRE FRANÇOIS OLIVE. 1793-1867
Inoculation du sang de rate. *C. R. Soc. Biol. (Paris)*, 1850, **2**, 141-44.
Rayer inoculated sheep with blood of other sheep dead of anthrax. Microscopically he saw the anthrax bacillus in the blood of the inoculated sheep. Rayer was associated with Davaine, who later, in *Bull. Acad. Méd.*, 1875, 2 sér., **4**, 581-84, said that he had written the above account and had sent it to Rayer for publication.

5164   POLLENDER, FRANZ ALOYS ANTOINE. 1800-1879
Mikroskopische und mikrochemische Untersuchung des Milzbrandblutes sowie über Wesen und Kur des Milzbrandes. *Vjschr. gerichtl. öff. Med.*, 1855, **8**, 103-14.
Pollender discovered the *B. anthracis* in 1849, but did not record this fact until 1855. He gave a more exact account of the organism than did Rayer (No. 5163).

5165 DAVAINE, CASIMIR JOSEPH. 1812-1882
Recherches sur les infusoires du sang dans la maladie connue sous le nom de sang de rate. *C. R. Acad. Sci. (Paris)*, 1863, **57**, 220-23, 351-53.

 Davaine showed that anthrax could be transmitted to sheep, horses, cattle, guinea-pigs, and mice, and that in such animals the bacilli did not appear in the blood until 4–5 hours before death.

5166 ——. Recherches sur la nature et la constitution anatomique de la pustule maligne. *C. R. Acad. Sci. (Paris)*, 1865, **60**, 1296-99.

 Davaine was the first conclusively to prove that a definite disease (anthrax) was due to a definite micro-organism (*B. anthracis*), and was thus one of the first to prove the germ theory of disease. He showed that the virulence of anthrax was in proportion to the number of bacteria present.

5167 KOCH, ROBERT. 1843-1910
Die Aetiologie der Milzbrand-Krankheit, begründet auf die Entwicklungsgeschichte des Bacillus anthracis. *Beitr. Biol Pflanzen*, 1876, **2**, 277-310.

 In 1876 Koch first obtained pure cultures of *B. anthracis* and described its complete life history. With Davaine (Nos. 5165–66) he did much to prove that infectious diseases are caused by living reproductive micro-organisms. The postulates suggested by Koch on this occasion had fundamental importance and have become the bases on which bacteriology largely rests. The paper also marks the beginning of exact knowledge of bacterial infectious diseases. It is reproduced with translation in *Med. Classics*, 1938, **2**, 745-820. *See also* Nos. 2331 and 2536.

5168 PASTEUR, LOUIS. 1822-1895, & JOUBERT, JULES FRANÇOIS.
Étude sur la maladie charbonneuse. *C. R. Soc. Biol. (Paris)*, 1877, **84**, 900-06.

 Pasteur confirmed Koch's results regarding anthrax; with Joubert he carried the bacillus through 100 generations and succeeded in producing anthrax from the last, thus disposing of the idea of a separate virus.

5169 – . & CHAMBERLAND, CHARLES. 1851-1908, & ROUX, PIERRE PAUL EMILE. 1853-1933
Sur l'étiologie du charbon. *C. R. Acad. Sci. (Paris)*, 1880, **91**, 86-94.

 First use of attenuated bacterial virus for therapeutic purposes. See also the same journal, 1881, **92**, 1378-83.

5170 SCLAVO, ACHILLE. 1861-1930
Sulla preparazione del siero anti-carbonchioso. *Riv. Ig. San. pubbl.*, 1895, **6**, 841-43.

 Specific anti-anthrax serum. German translation in *Zbl. Bakt.*, 1895, 1 Abt., **18**, 744-45.

5171 ASCOLI, ALBERTO. 1877-1957
La precipitina nella diagnosi del carbonchio ematico. *Clin. vet. (Milano)*, 1911, **34**, 2-20.

 Ascoli's thermoprecipitin reaction for the diagnosis of anthrax. German translation in *Zbl. Bakt.*, 1911, 1 Abt., **58**, Orig., 63-70. Preliminary note in *Pathologica*, 1910, **3**, 101.

5172   BECKER, GEORG.
Die bakteriologische Blutuntersuchung beim Milzbrand des Menschen.
Dtsch. Z. Chir., 1911, **112**, 265-83.
Salvarsan first used in the treatment of anthrax.

5172.1   STERNE, MAX. 1905-
The use of anthrax vaccines prepared from avirulent (uncapsulated)
variants of *Bacillus anthracis. Onderstepoort J. vet. Sci.*, 1939, **13**, 307-12.
Nonencapsulated spore vaccine.

TULARAEMIA

5173   McCOY, GEORGE WALTER. 1876-1952
A plague-like disease of rodents. *Publ. Hlth. Bull. (Wash.)*, 1911, **43**, 53-
71.
Tularaemia first recorded (in rodents).

5174   ——. & CHAPIN, CHARLES WILLARD. 1877-?
Further observations on a plague-like disease of rodents with a preliminary
note on the causative agent, Bacterium tularense. *J. infect. Dis.*, 1912, **10**,
61-72.
Isolation of *Pasteurella tularensis*, causal organism in tularaemia.

5175   WHERRY, WILLIAM BUCHANAN. 1875-1936. & LAMB, BENJAMIN HARRISON. 1889-
Infection of man with Bacterium tularense. *J. infect. Dis.*, 1914, **15**, 331-40.
Wherry and Lamb were first to isolate *P. tularensis* from lesions in man.

5176   FRANCIS, EDWARD. 1872-1957
Tularemia. *J. Amer. med. Assoc.*, 1925, **84**, 1243-50.
The important work of Francis on tularaemia, summarized in the above
paper, included his demonstration of its transmission to man from rodents
through insects, particularly the deerfly. He gave the disease its present
name; it is also called "Francis's disease" by some writers.

5177   OHARA, HACHIRO.
Ueber Identität von "Yato-Byo" (Ohara's disease) und "Tularämie", sowie
ihren Erreger. *Zbl. Bakt.*, 1930, Abt. 1, **117**, 440-50.
In Japan tularaemia is known as "Ohara's disease".

5178   FOSHAY, LEE. 1896-1960
Tularemia: accurate and earlier diagnosis by means of the intradermal
reaction. *J. infect. Dis.*, 1932, **51**, 286-91.
Skin test for the diagnosis of tularaemia.

5179   ——. Serum treatment of tularemia. *J. Amer. med. Assoc.*, 1932, **98**, 552;
1933, **101**, 1047-49.
Foshay devised a serum for the treatment of tularaemia.

5180   ——. & PASTERNACK, A. BERNARD. 1916-
Streptomycin treatment of tularemia. *J. Amer. med. Assoc.*, 1946, **130**, 393-
98.

See also 5089-5096, Bacillary Dysentery.

5180.1   ABREU, Alexo de. 1568-1630
Tratado de las siete enfermedades, *etc.* Lisboa, *P. Craesbeeck*, 1623.
An account of amoebiasis is given on fol. 1-42v., 61-72v., and 117v-150.
For full title of the book, *see* No. 2262.1.

5181   KNEUSSEL, Christophe Friedrich.
De ipecacuanha novo Gallorum antidysenterico. Gissae-Hassorum, *typ. Mülleri*, 1698.
There is evidence that amoebic dysentery was known to Hippocrates. The history of treatment begins with the use of ipecacuanha, first mentioned as a remedy in Purchas's *Pilgrimes*, 1625. Ipecacuanha was used as a secret remedy against dysentery in Paris about 1680, and was bought by the French Government for 20,000 francs in 1688.

5182   MAGENDIE, François. 1783-1855, & PELLETIER, Pierre Joseph. 1788-1842
Mémoire sur l'émétine, et sur les trois espèces d'ipecacuanha. *J. gén. Méd. Chir. Pharm.*, 1817, **59**, 223-31.
Isolation of emetine. It was not until a century later that Vedder demonstrated its value in the treatment of amoebiasis.

5182.1   BALLINGALL, *Sir* George. 1780-1855
Practical observations on fever, dysentery and liver complaints as they occur amongst European troops in India. Edinburgh, *D. Brown and A. Constable*, 1818.
Ballingall distinguished between amoebic and bacillary dysentery.

5183   BARDSLEY, *Sir* James Lomax. 1801-1876
Hospital facts and observations. London, *Burgess & Hill*, 1830.
First record (p. 149) of the use of emetine in the treatment of amoebiasis.

5183.1   GROS, G.
Fragments d'helminthologie et de physiologie microscopique. *Bull. Soc. imp. Nat. Moscou*, 1849, **22**, 549-73.
First observations of entozoic amoebae.

5183.2   JIMENEZ, Miguel F.
Clinica médica. Abcesos del higado. México, *M. Murguia*, 1856.
Jimenez gave a classic account of liver abscess in amoebiasis.

5184   LÖSCH, Friedrich. [Lesh, Fedor.] 1840-1903
Massenhafte Entwickelung von Amöben im Dickdarm. *Virchows Arch. path. Anat.*, 1875, **65**, 196-211.
Lösch discovered *Entamoeba histolytica* as the infective agent in amoebic dysentery. Before this time distinction between the different forms of dysentery had been made on purely clinical grounds. English translation in Kean (No. 2268.1).

5185   WOODWARD, Joseph Janvier. 1833-1884
Diarrhoea and dysentery. *In*: U.S. War Dept.: Medical and surgical history of the War of the Rebellion, 1879, pt. 2, **1**, 1-869.

Garrison considers this the greatest single monograph on dysentery. Woodward saw the Lösch amoeba, but without recognizing its significance; he was part author of the *Medical and surgical history of the War of the Rebellion. See* No. 2171.

5186   KARTULIS, STEPHANOS. 1852-1920
Zur Aetiologie der Dysenterie in Aegypten. *Virchows Arch. path. Anat.*, 1886, **105**, 521-31.
Kartulis discovered amoebae in liver abscess. It was principally through the work of Kartulis that amoebae came to be considered the cause of dysentery in man.

5186.1 HLAVA, JAROSLAV. 1855-1924
O úplavici. Předběžné sdělení. *Cas. Lék. čes.*, 1887, **26**, 70-74.
Hlava induced experimental amoebiasis in cats by intrarectal inoculation of stools. In an abstract of this paper Kartulis confused the author's name with that of the title, a mistake copied by writers for many years; see C. Dobell, *Parasitology*, 1938, **30**, 239-41.

5187   COUNCILMAN, WILLIAM THOMAS. 1854-1933, & LAFLEUR, HENRI AMADÉE. 1863-1939
Amoebic dysentery. *Johns Hopk. Hosp. Rep.*, 1890-91, **2**, 395-548.
These workers introduced the term "amoebic dysentery" in their important investigation of the condition.

5188   QUINCKE, HEINRICH IRENAEUS. 1842-1922, & ROOS, ERNST. 1866-
Ueber Amöben-Enteritis. *Berl. klin. Wschr.*, 1893, **30**, 1089-94.
Entamoeba histolytica distinguished from *Entamoeba coli*. English translation in Kean (No. 2268.1).

5189   VEDDER, EDWARD BRIGHT. 1878-1952
Experiments undertaken to test the efficacy of the ipecac treatment of dysentery. *Bull. Manila med. Soc.*, 1911, **3**, 48-53.
Vedder demonstrated the amoebicidal action of emetine; his work led to the general adoption of emetine in the treatment of amoebic dysentery.

5190   ROGERS, *Sir* LEONARD. 1868-1962
The rapid cure of amoebic dysentery and hepatitis by hypodermic injections of soluble salts of emetine. *Brit. med. J.*, 1912, **1**, 1424-25.
Following up the work of Vedder, Rogers showed that the soluble salts of emetine could be safely injected subcutaneously. The general use of emetine, introduced by Rogers, diminished the incidence of liver abscess – a grave sequel.

5191   WALKER, ERNEST LINWOOD. 1870-1952, & SELLARDS, ANDREW WATSON. 1884-1941
Experimental entamoebic dysentery. *Philipp. J. Sci.*, 1913, B, **8**, 253-331.
Walker and Sellards made important additions to our knowledge of amoebiasis, including the determination of the incubation period and the demonstration that *E. tetragena* and *E. minuta* are identical with *E. histolytica*.

5192   MÜHLENS, PETER. 1874-1943, & MENK, W.
Ueber Behandlungsversuche der chronischen Amoebenruhr mit Yatren.
Münch. med. Wschr., 1921, **68**, 802-03.
Introduction of Yatren.

5193   MARCHOUX, ÉMILE. 1862-1943
Le stovarsol guérit rapidement la dysenterie amibienne. *Bull. Soc. Path.
exot.*, 1923, **16**, 79-81.
Introduction of stovarsol (oxyaminophenylarsenic acid) in the treatment
of amoebiasis.

5194   BOECK, WILLIAM CHARLES. 1894- , & DRBOHLAV, JAROSLAV. 1893-1946
The cultivation of Endamoeba histolytica. *Amer. J. Hyg.*, 1925, **5**, 371-407.
Pure cultivation of *Entamoeba histolytica* was first accomplished by D.
W. Cutler (*J. Path. Bact.*, 1918, **22**, 22), but Boeck and Drbohlav evolved
the first media upon which amoebae could be cultivated for indefinite
periods.

5194.1   DOBELL, CLIFFORD. 1886-1949
Researches on the intestinal protozoa of monkeys and man. *Parasitology*,
1928, **20**, 357-412.
Classic account of the life-cycle of *E. histolytica*.

5194.2   REED, ALFRED CUMMINGS. 1884-1951, *et al.*
Carbarsone in the treatment of amebiasis. *J. Amer. med. Assoc.*, 1932, **98**,
189-94.
With H. H. Anderson, N. A. David, and C. D. Leake.

SEXUALLY TRANSMITTED DISEASES

See also 2362-2432.1, SYPHILIS; 4772-4806, NEUROSYPHILIS.

5195   ASTRUC, JEAN. 1684-1766
De morbis veneris libri sex. Lutetiae Parisiorum, *G. Cavelier*, 1736.
Considering the period in which it was written, this is an admirable and
comprehensive book on the subject. It includes a careful review of the
existing literature. Of syphilis, Astruc says that it made appearances in
Europe in 1493. The book was translated into English in 1737.

5196   BALFOUR, FRANCIS. ?-1812
De gonorrhoea virulenta. Edinburgh, *Balfour, Auld & Smellie*, 1767.
Balfour is said to have been the first to re-affirm the duality of gonor-
rhoea and syphilis.

5197   HUNTER, JOHN. 1728-1793
A treatise on the venereal disease. London, 1786.
In Hunter's day the venereal diseases were thought to be due to a single
pathogen. In order to test this theory Hunter inoculated matter from a
gonorrhoeal patient who, unknown to Hunter, also had syphilis. The
inoculee developed syphilis, supporting Hunter's view of a single pathogen.
Backed by the weight of Hunter's authority, this experiment held back for
many years the development of knowledge regarding gonorrhoea and
syphilis. The hard ("Hunterian") chancre eponymizes Hunter; his book

also contains the first suggestion of lymphogranuloma venereum as a separate disease. *See* No. 2377.

5198   NISBET, WILLIAM. 1759-1822
First lines of theory and practice in venereal diseases. Edinburgh, *C. Elliot,* 1787.
  First complete description of lymphatic chancre – "Nisbet's chancre".

5199   GIRTANNER, CHRISTOPH. 1760-1800
Abhandlung über die venerische Krankheit. 3 vols. Göttingen, *J. C. Dieterich,* 1788-89.
  Girtanner's important textbook on the venereal diseases contains some history.

5200   BELL, BENJAMIN. 1749-1806
A treatise on gonorrhoea virulenta, and lues venerea. 2 vols. Edinburgh, *J. Watson & G. Mudie,* 1793.
  Bell was the first to differentiate between gonorrhoea and syphilis.

5201   COLLES, ABRAHAM. 1773-1843
Practical observations on the venereal disease, and on the use of mercury. London, *Sherwood, Gilbert & Piper,* 1837.
  See No. 2380.

5202   RICORD, PHILIPPE. 1800-1889
Traité pratique des maladies vénériennes. Paris, *De Just Rouvier & E. Le Bouvier,* 1838.
  Repeating Hunter's experiment, Ricord proved that syphilis and gonorrhoea were separate diseases. After Hunter, he was the greatest authority on venereal disease. *See also* No. 2381. The first of several English translations appeared in 1842.

5203   BASSEREAU, LÉON. 1811-1888
Traité des affections de la peau symptomatiques de la syphilis. Paris, *J. B. Baillière,* 1852.
  Bassereau defined chancroid clearly for the first time.

5204   ROLLET, JOSEPH PIERRE. 1824-1894
Coincidence du chancre syphilitique primitif avec la gale, la blénorrhagie, le chancre simple et la vaccine. *Gaz. méd. Lyon,* 1866, **18**, 160-63.
  Rollet recognized the possibility of mixed infection of one sore with syphilis and chancroid, thus establishing the dualist theory of venereal infection. The mixed chancre is named "Rollet's disease".

5204.1   MACLEOD, KENNETH. 1840-1922
Precis of operations performed in the wards of the first surgeon, Medical College Hospital, during the year 1881. *Indian med. Gaz.,* 1882, **17**, 113-23.
  MacLeod was first to draw attention to granuloma inguinale.

5205   DUCREY, AUGUSTO. 1860-1940
Il virus dell' ulcera venerea. *Gazz. int. Sci. med.,* 1889, **11**, 44.
  Announcement of the discovery of *Haemophilus ducreyi* (Ducrey's bacillus), causal organism in chancroid.

5205.1 CONYERS, JAMES SALTERS. 1841-1896, & DANIELS, CHARLES WILBERFORCE. 1862-1927
The lupoid form of the so-called "groin ulceration" of this colony. *Brit. Guiana med. Annu.*, 1896, **8**, 13-29.
    Granuloma inguinale distinguished from other similar lesions in the genital region.

5206 JADASSOHN, JOSEF. 1863-1936
Handbuch der Haut- und Geschlechtskrankheiten. Hrsg...von J. JADASSOHN. 24 vols. [in 42]. Berlin, *J. Springer*, 1927-37.

Gonorrhoea and Trichomonas Infection

5207 DONNÉ, ALFRED. 1801-1878
Animalcules observés dans les matières purulentes et le produit des sécrétions des organes génitaux de l'homme et de la femme. *C. R. Acad. Sci. (Paris)*, 1836, **3**, 385-86.
    First description of *Trichomonas vaginalis*, which Donné at first believed to be the pernicious agent in gonorrhoea. He later admitted the organism to be a normal inhabitant of the female genital tract. Donné was, by this work, the first to describe living organisms in pathological conditions, as observed by modern methods. English translation in Kean (No. 2268.1).

5208 NEISSER, ALBERT LUDWIG SIEGMUND. 1855-1916
Ueber eine der Gonorrhoe eigentümliche Micrococcusform. *Zbl. med. Wiss.*, 1879, **17**, 497-500.
    Discovery of the gonococcus – causal organism in gonorrhoea.

5209 LEISTIKOW, LEO. 1847-1917
Ueber Bacterien bei den venerischen Krankheiten. *Charité-Ann.*, 1880, (1882), **7**, 750-72.
    Leistikow was first to report the cultivation of the gonococcus.

5210 BUMM, ERNST VON. 1858-1925
Der Mikro-Organismus der gonorrhöischen Schleimhaut-Erkrankungen, Gonococcus-Neisser. *Dtsch. med. Wschr.*, 1885, **11**, 508-09.
    Bumm cultured the gonococcus. By human inoculations he demonstrated its pathogenicity in pure culture.

5210.1 FRAENKEL, EUGEN. 1853-1925
Bericht über eine bei Kindern beobachtete Endemie infectiöser Colpitis. *Virchows Arch. path. Anat.*, 1885, **99**, 251-76.
    The gonococcus shown to be the cause of vulvovaginitis in children.

5211 FINGER, ERNST ANTON FRANZ. 1856-1939
Die Blenorrhöe der Sexualorgane und ihre Complicationen. Leipzig, Wien, *F. Deuticke*, 1888.

5212 THAYER, WILLIAM SYDNEY. 1864-1932, & BLUMER, GEORGE ALBERT. 1858-1940
Ulcerative endocarditis due to the gonococcus; gonorrheal septicemia. *Johns Hopk. Hosp. Bull.*, 1896, **7**, 57-63.

Thayer and Blumer found the gonococcus in cases of gonorrhoeal endocarditis.

5213   MÜLLER, RUDOLF. 1877- , & OPPENHEIM, MORITZ. 1876-1949
Ueber den Nachweis von Antikörpern im Serum eines an Arthritis gonorrhoica Erkrankten mittels Komplementablenkung. *Wien. klin. Wschr.*, 1906, **19**, 894-95.
"Müller–Oppenheim reaction" – a complement fixation test for the diagnosis of gonorrhoea.

5213.1 LEVADITI, CONSTANTIN. 1874-1953, & VAISMAN, A.
La toxi-infection gonococcique expérimentale et son traitement chimiothérapique. *Presse méd.*, 1937, **45**, 1371-73.
Levaditi and Vaisman showed that sulphanilamide protected mice against gonococcal infection.

5214   DEES, JOHN ESSARY. 1910- , & COLSTON, JOHN ARCHIBALD CAMPBELL. 1886-
The use of sulfanilamide in gonococcic infections. Preliminary report. *J. Amer. med. Assoc.*, 1937, **108**, 1855-58.

5214.1 HERRELL, WALLACE EDGAR. 1909- , *et al.*
Use of penicillin in sulfonamide resistant gonorrheal infections. *J. Amer. med. Assoc.*, 1943, **122**, 289-92.
With E. N. Cook and L. Thompson.

Lymphogranuloma Venereum

5215   WALLACE, WILLIAM. 1791-1837
A treatise on the venereal disease and its varieties. London, *Burgess & Hill*, 1833.
On p. 371 commences the first description of lymphogranuloma venereum, which Wallace called "indolent primary syphilitic bubo".

5216   HUGUIER, PIERRE CHARLES. 1804-1873
Mémoire sur l'esthiomène, ou dartre rongeante de la région vulvo-anale. *Mém. Acad. nat. Méd (Paris)*, 1849, **14**, 501-96.
Huguier gave the name esthiomène to the characteristic induration and discoloration of the affected parts in lymphogranuloma venereum.

5217   DURAND, JOSEPH. 1876- , NICOLAS, JOSEPH. 1868-1960, & FAVRE MAURICE. 1876-1955
Lymphogranulomatose inguinale subaiguë d'origine génitale probable, peut-être vénérienne. *Bull. Soc. méd. Hôp. Paris*, 1913, 3 sér., **35**, 274-88.
First important description. Sometimes called "Nicolas–Favre disease" and "Nicolas–Durand–Favre disease".

5218   FREI, WILHELM SIEGMUND. 1885-1943
Eine neue Hautreaktion bei "Lymphogranuloma inguinale". *Klin. Wschr.*, 1925, **4**, 2148-49.
The Frei skin test for the diagnosis of lymphogranuloma venereum.

5219   GAY PRIETO, José Antonio. 1905-
Contribución al estudio de la linfogranulomatosis inguinal subaguda o ulcera venérea adenógena de Nicolás y Favre. *Act. dermo-sifiliogr. (Madr.)*, 1927, **20**, 122-75.
      Gay Prieto was the first actually to see the infective agent of lymphogranuloma venereum.

5220   HELLERSTRÖM, Sven Curt Alfred. 1901- , & WASSÉN, Erik.
Meningo-enzephalitische Veränderungen bei Affen nach intra-cerebraler Impfung mit Lymphogranuloma inquinale. *VIII Congr. int. Derm. Syph.*, Copenhague, 1930, *C. R. Séances*, 1931, 1147-49.
      The authors transmitted lymphogranuloma venereum to animals and attributed it to a virus. See also *C. R. Soc. Biol. (Paris)*, 1931, **106**, 802-03.

5221   STANNUS, Hugh Stannus. 1877-1957
A sixth venereal disease. Climatic bubo, lymphogranuloma inguinale, esthiomène, chronic ulcer and elephantiasis of the genito-ano-rectal region, inflammatory stricture of the rectum. London, *Baillière, Tindall & Cox*, 1933.
      In this exhaustive review of the literature, Stannus considered all the conditions he discussed to be different manifestations of infection by the same organisms – the agent causing lymphogranuloma venereum. Includes historical summary and full bibliography.

5222   TAMURA, Joseph Takao. 1903-
Cultivation of the virus of lymphogranuloma inguinale and its use in therapeutic inoculation. Preliminary report. *J. Amer. Med. Assoc.*, 1934, **103**, 408-09.

5224   MCKEE, Clara M., *et al.*
Complement-fixation test in lymphogranuloma venereum. *Proc. Soc. exp. Biol. (N.Y.)*, 1940, **44**, 410-13.
      Diagnosis of lymphogranuloma venereum by complement-fixation test. With G. W. Rake and M. F. Shaffer.

5224.1   OTTOLINA, Carlos.
The vesicular test. Diagnostic method of infection by poradenic (lymphogranuloma inguinale) virus. *Amer. J. trop. Med.*, 1941, **21**, 597-602.
      Vesicular test for diagnosis of lymphogranuloma venereum.

5225   BEDSON, *Sir* Samuel Phillips. 1886-1969, *et al.*
The laboratory diagnosis of lymphogranuloma venereum. *J. clin. Path.*, 1949, **2**, 241-49.
      Skin-test antigen. With C. F. Barwell, E. J. King, and L. W. J. Bishop.

History of Sexually Transmitted Diseases

See also 2420-2432.1, History of Syphilis.

5226   PROKSCH, Johann Karl. 1840-1923
Die Litteratur über die venerischen Krankheiten von der ersten Schriften über Syphilis aus dem Ende des fünfzehnten Jahrhunderts bis zum Jahre 1889. (Supplement Band I. Enthält die Litteratur von 1889-99 und Nachträge aus früherer Zeit.) 5 vols. Bonn, *P. Hanstein*, 1889-1900.
      Reprinted Nieuwkoop, *De Graaf*, 1966.

5227 ————. Die Geschichte der venerischen Krankheiten. 2 vols. Bonn, *P. Hanstein*, 1895 (-1900).
   Vol. 1. Alterthum und Mittelalter. Vol. 2. Neuzeit.

5227.1 STICKER, Georg. 1860-1960
   Entwurf einer Geschichte der ansteckenden Geschlechtskrankheiten. In Jadassohn, J.: *Handbuch der Haut- und Geschlechtskrankheiten*, Berlin, 1931, **23**, 264-603, 606-16, 632-42.

5228 HIPPOCRATES, 460-375 B.C.
   Epidemics I and III. In [Works], with an English translation by W. H. S. Jones. London, *W. Heinemann*, 1923, **1**, 139-287.
   Hippocrates may be regarded as the first malariologist; he clearly and fully described the intermittent fevers; he was acquainted with seasonal and topographical variations in the distribution of malaria; and he recognized an association between marshes and fevers.

5229 SPIEGHEL, Adriaan van den [Spigelius]. 1578-1625
   De semitertiana libri quatuor. Francofurti, *apud haered. J. T. de Bry*, 1624.
   First extensive account of malaria.

5230.1 BADO, Sebastiano [Baldi]. *fl.* 1640-1676.
   Anastasis corticis Peruviae, seu chinae defensio. Genuae, typ. *P. I. Calenzani*, 1663.
   A defence of the virtues of Peruvian bark. Bado includes evidence to show that "fever bark" was introduced into Spain in 1632.

5231 TORTI, Francesco. 1658-1741
   Therapeutice specialis ad febres quasdam perniciosas, inopinato, ac repente lethales, una vera china china, peculiare methodo ministrata, sanabiles. Mutinae, *typ. B. Soliani*, 1712.
   Torti's work finally established the specific nature of cinchona bark. His demonstration of its effectiveness in periodic over continuous fevers finally overthrew the doctrine of the common origin of all fevers. He is also credited with the introduction of the term "malaria".

5232 LANCISI, Giovanni Maria. 1654-1720
   De noxiis paludum effluviis, eorumque remediis. Romae, *typ. J. M. Salvioni*, 1717.
   Lancisi suggested that since malaria disappears after drainage it was due to some sort of poison emanating from marshes and possibly transmitted by mosquitoes. He planned a drainage scheme for marshy regions.

5233 PELLETIER, Pierre Joseph. 1788-1842, & CAVENTOU, Joseph Bienaimé. 1795-1877
   Recherches chimique sur les quinquinas. *Ann. Chim. Phys. (Paris)*, 1820, **15**, 289-318, 337-65.
   Isolation of quinine.

5234 MITCHELL, JOHN KEARSLEY. 1793-1858
On the cryptogamous origin of malarious and epidemic fevers. Philadelphia, *Lea & Blanchard*, 1849.

Although Hensinger in 1844 had suggested a parasite as the cause of malaria, Mitchell was the first to approach this theory in a scientific spirit. He was Professor of Medicine at Jefferson College, and the father of S. Weir Mitchell.

5234.1 DRAKE, DANIEL. 1785-1852
A systematic treatise, historical, etiological, and practical, on the principal diseases of the interior valley of North America. Cincinnati, *W. B. Smith & Co.*, 1850. Second series, ed. S.H. SMITH and F.G. SMITH, Philadelphia, *Lippincott, Grambo*, 1854.

Includes the most important work on the natural history of malaria published up to that time.

5235 BERENGER-FÉRAUD, LAURENT JEAN BAPTISTE. 1832-1901
De la fièvre bilieuse mélanurique des pays chauds comparée avec la fièvre jaune. Paris, *A. Delahaye*, 1874.

An important description of blackwater fever. Berenger-Féraud had experience of the disease in French West Africa.

5236 LAVERAN, CHARLES LOUIS ALPHONSE. 1845-1922
Un nouveau parasite trouvé dans le sang plusieurs malades atteints de fièvre palustre. *Bull. Soc. méd. Hôp. Paris. (Mém.)*, 1881, 2 sér., **17**, 158-64.

Laveran first saw the malaria parasite on 20 October 1880; he at once grasped its significance. He named it *Oscillaria malariae*. English translation in Kean (No. 2268.1). Laveran also published a monograph on the discovery: Nature parasitaire des accidents de l'impaludisme. Description d'un nouveau parasite trouvé dans le sang...Paris, *Baillière*, 1881. He was awarded the Nobel Prize in 1907.

5237 KING, ALBERT FREEMAN AFRICANUS. 1841-1914
Insects and disease; mosquitoes and malaria. *Pop. Sci. Monthly, (N.Y.)*, 1883, **23**, 644-58.

The first reasoned argument in support of the belief of transmission of malaria by mosquitoes. Reproduced in part in Major, *Classic descriptions of disease*, 3rd ed., 1945, p. 104.

5238 MARCHIAFAVA, ETTORE. 1847-1935, & CELLI, ANGELO. 1857-1914
Weitere Untersuchungen über die Malariainfection. *Fortschr. Med.*, 1885, **3**, 787-806.

First accurate description of the malaria *Plasmodium*, discovered by Laveran in 1880. These writers were the first to adopt the name *P. malariae*.

5238.1 DANILEVSKI, VASILI IAKOVLEVICH. 1852-1934
Zur Parasitologie des Blutes. *Biol. Zbl.*, 1885, **5**, 529-37.

Discovery of malaria parasites in birds. See also *Ann. Inst. Pasteur*, 1890, **4**, 427-31.

5239 GOLGI, CAMILLO. 1844-1926
Sull' infezione malarica. *Arch. Sci. med. (Torino)*, 1886, **10**, 109-35.

Description of the development of the parasite of quartan malaria. Golgi differentiated the tertian and quartan parasites by the periods of their respective developments.

5240 ——. Sul ciclo evolutivo dei parassiti malarica nella febbre terzana. *Arch. Sci. med. (Torino)*, 1889, **13**, 173-96.

Golgi showed that the parasite of quartan differs from that of tertian malarial fever. English translation in Kean (No. 2268.1).

5240.1 CANALIS, PIETRO. 1856-1939
Études sur l'infection malarique. Sur la variété parasitaire des corps en croissant de Laveran et sur les fièvres palustres qui en dérivent. *Arch. ital. Biol.*, 1890, **13**, 262-86.

Canalis demonstrated and clearly differentiated *Plasmodium falciparum* from the species *vivax* and *malariae*.

5241 GRASSI, GIOVANNI BATTISTA. 1854-1925, & FELETTI, RAIMONDO. 1851-1928
Malariaparasiten in den Vögeln. *Zbl. Bakt.*, 1891, **9**, 403-09, 429-33, 461-67.

Confirmation of the work of Laveran.

5241.1 GUTTMANN, PAUL, & EHRLICH, PAUL. 1854-1915
Ueber die Wirkung des Methylenblau bei Malaria. *Berl. klin. Wschr.*, 1891, **28**, 953-56.

Guttmann and Ehrlich demonstrated methylene blue to be lethal *in vitro* for the malaria parasite – the beginning of Ehrlich's work on chemotherapy.

5242 ROMANOVSKY, DMITRIY LEONIDOVICH. 1861-1921
K voprosu o parazitologii i terapii bolotnoi likhoradki. [Parasitology and treatment of malarial fever.] St. Petersburg, *I. N. Skovokhodoff,* 1891.

Romanovsky made important studies of the malaria parasite and introduced a special stain for its demonstration. German version in *St. Petersburger med. Wschr.*, 1891, **8**, 297-302, 306-15. English translation in Kean (No. 2268.1).

5243 GOLGI, CAMILLO, 1844-1926
Azione della chinina sui parasite malarici e sui corrispondente accessi febbrili. *Gazz. med. Pavia*, 1892, **1**, 34, 79, 106.

French translation in *Arch. ital. Biol.*, 1892, **17**, 456-71.

5244 MARCHIAFAVA, ETTORE. 1847-1935, & BIGNAMI, AMICO. 1862-1929
Sulle febbre malariche estivo-autumnali. Roma, *E. Loescher,* 1892.

A summary of the Italian work on malaria. English translation, 1894.

5245 MANSON, *Sir* PATRICK. 1844-1922
On the nature and significance of the crescentic and flagellated bodies in malarial blood. *Brit. med. J.*, 1894, **2**, 1306-08.

Manson's mosquito–malaria hypothesis. See also his Gulstonian Lectures in *Lancet*, 1896, **1**, 695-98, 751-55, 831-33.

5246 MacCALLUM, WILLIAM GEORGE. 1874-1944
On the flagellated form of the malarial parasite. *Lancet*, 1897, **2**, 1240-41.

MacCallum reported at a meeting of the British Association his observation of the mode of fertilization of the malarial parasite of birds; two months later he announced that he had found the same to hold good for the human parasite.

5247   ROSS, *Sir* RONALD. 1857-1932
On some peculiar pigmented cells found in two mosquitoes fed on malarial blood. *Brit med. J.*, 1897, **2**, 1786-88.
Ross proved that the mosquito was responsible for the transmission of malaria. On 20 August 1897, he found Laveran's *Plasmodium* in the stomach of the *Anopheles* mosquito after it had fed on the blood of malaria patients. See also the earlier paper in the same journal, 1897, **1**, 251-55.

5248   LAVERAN, CHARLES LOUIS ALPHONSE. 1845-1922
Traité du paludisme. Paris, *Masson & Cie.*, 1898.

5249   OPIE, EUGENE LINDSAY. 1873-1971
On the haemocytozoa of birds. *J. exp. Med.*, 1898, **3**, 79-101.
Demonstration of sexual conjugation in the malaria parasite. *See also* No. 5250.

5250   MacCALLUM, WILLIAM GEORGE. 1874-1944
Notes on the pathological changes in the organs of birds infected with haemocytozoa. *J. exp. Med.*, 1898, **3**, 103-16, 117-36.
MacCallum and Opie discovered the sexual phase of malaria parasites.

5251   ROSS, *Sir* RONALD. 1857-1932
The rôle of the mosquito in the evolution of the malarial parasite. *Lancet*, 1898, **2**, 488-89.
Ross provided the last link in the chain demonstrating the complete life-cycle of the parasite of bird malaria. He found that mosquitoes which had fed on malaria-infected birds, and which had allowed the parasites to develop and lodge in their salivary glands, could then infect healthy birds, which in turn became malarious. Ross was awarded the Nobel Prize for Medicine in 1902.

5252   GRASSI, GIOVANNI BATTISTA. 1854-1925, & BIGNAMI, AMICO. 1862-1929
Ciclo evolutivo della semilune nell' Anopheles claviger. *Ann. Ig. sper.*, 1899, n.s. **9**, 258-64.
Grassi and Bignami showed that the *Plasmodium* undergoes its sexual phase only in the *Anopheles* mosquito.

5252.1 GRASSI, GIOVANNI BATTISTA. 1854-1925
Studi di uno zoologo sulla malaria. Roma, *V. Salviucci*, 1900.
Includes the best illustrations of the various stages of the malaria parasite published up to that time.

5252.2 MANSON, *Sir* PATRICK. 1844-1922
Experimental proof of the mosquito-malaria theory. *Brit. med. J.*, 1900, **2**, 949-51.
In a classic demonstration Manson allowed infected mosquitoes from Rome to bite a volunteer (his son) in London, who developed malaria 15 days later with tertian parasites in the blood, and who was cured by quinine.

5253   LEISHMAN, *Sir* WILLIAM BOOG. 1865-1926
        Note on a simple and rapid method of producing Romanowsky staining in
        malarial and other blood films. *Brit. med. J.*, 1901, **2**, 757-58.
        "Leishman's stain", a modification of that introduced by Romanovsky in
        1891.

5254   SCHAUDINN, FRITZ RICHARD. 1871-1906
        Studien über krankheitserregende Protozoen. II. Plasmodium vivax (Grassi
        & Feletti), der Erreger des Tertianfiebers beim Menschen. *Arb. k.
        GesundhAmte*, 1903, **19**, 169-250.
        Confirmation of the work of Ross and of Grassi.

5255   CRAIG, CHARLES FRANKLIN. 1872-1950
        Intracorpuscular conjugation in the malarial plasmodia and its significance.
        Amer. Med., 1905, **10**, 982-86, 1029-32.
        Demonstration of the existence of malarial carriers.

5255.1 BASS, CHARLES CASSEDY. 1875- , & JOHNS, FOSTER MATTHEW. 1889-
        The cultivation of malaria plasmodia *(Plasmodium vivax* and *Plasmodium
        falciparum)* in vitro. *J. exp. Med.*, 1912, **16**, 567-79.
        Cultivation of the malaria parasite.

5255.2 STEPHENS, JOHN WILLIAM WATSON. 1865-1946
        A new malaria parasite of man. *Ann. trop. Med. Parasit.*, 1922, **16**, 383-88.
        Plasmodium ovale described.

5256   ROEHL, WILHELM. *d.* 1929
        Die Wirkung des Plasmochins auf die Vogelmalaria. *Arch. Schiffs- u.
        Tropenhyg.*, 1926, **30**, Beihefte, 311-18; 1927, **31**, Beihefte, 48-58.
        Introduction of plasmoquine (pamaquin) in the treatment of malaria.

5256.1 SINTON, JOHN ALEXANDER. 1884-1956, & BIRD, WILLIAM.
        Studies in malaria, with special references to treatment. Part IX. Plasmoquine
        in the treatment of malaria. *Indian J. med. Res.*, 1928, **16**, 159-77.
        Clinical trials of pamaquin.

5257   KIKUTH, WALTER. 1896-1968
        Zur Weiterentwicklung synthetisch dargestellter Malariamittel. I. Ueber
        die chemotherapeutische Wirkung des Atebrin. *Dtsch. med. Wschr.*, 1932,
        58, 530-31.
        Introduction of atebrin (mepacrine, quinacrine).

5258   JAMES, SYDNEY PRICE. 1870-1946, & TAIT, P.
        Exo-erythrocytic schizogony in *Plasmodium gallinaceum* Brumpt, 1935.
        Parasitology, 1938, **30**, 128-39.
        The term "exo-erythrocytic stage" introduced to describe the
        unpigmented schizonts found in tissue cells.

5259   MUDROW, LILI. 1908-1957
        Klinische und parasitologische Befunde und chemotherapeutische
        Ergebnisse bei der Hühnermalaria. *Arch. Schiffs-u. Tropenhyg.*, 1940, **44**,
        257-75.
        Discovery of the developmental forms of *P. gallinaceum* in the incu-
        bation period.

5259.1   SHORTT, HENRY EDWARD. 1887-1987, *et al.*
The form of *Plasmodium gallinaceum* present in the incubation period of the infection. *Indian J. med. Res.*, 1940, **28**, 273-76.
    Independently of Mudrow, H. E. Shortt, K. P. Menon, and P. V. Seetharama Iyer found pre-erythrocytic forms of *P. gallinaceum* in the tissues.

5259.2   HUFF, CLAY G. 1900- , & COULSTON, FREDERICK. 1914-
The development of *Plasmodium gallinaceum* from sporozoite to erythrocytic trophozoite. *J. infect. Dis.*, 1944, **75**, 231-49.
    First detailed account of the full cycle of development of the avian malaria parasite *P. gallinaceum.*

5260   CURD, FRANCIS HENRY SWINTON. 1909-1948, *et al.*
Studies on synthetic antimalarial drugs. *Ann. trop. Med. Parasit.*, 1945, **39**, 139-64, 208-16.
    F. H. S. Curd, D. G. Davey, and F. L. Rose synthesized proguanil ("paludrine") and first tested it in avian malaria.

5261   ADAMS, ALFRED ROBERT DAVIES, *et al.*
Studies on synthetic antimalarial drugs. XIII. Results of a preliminary investigation of the therapeutic action of 4888 (paludrine) on acute attacks of benign tertian malaria. *Ann. trop. Med. Parasit.*, 1945, **39**, 225-31.
    First use of proguanil in human malaria. With B. G. Maegraith, J. D. King, R. H. Townsend, T. H. Davey, and R. E. Havard.

5261.1   MOST, HARRY. 1907- , *et al.*
Chloroquine for treatment of acute attacks of *vivax* malaria. *J. Amer. med. Assoc.*, 1946, **131**, 963-67.
    Clinical trials of chloroquine. With I. M. London, C. A. Kane, P. H. Lavietes, E. F. Schroeder, and J. M. Hayman. See also *J. Amer. med Assoc.*, 1946, **130**, 1069.

5261.2   ALVING, ALF SVEN. 1902- , *et al.*
Pentaquine (Sn-13,276), a therapeutic agent effective in reducing the relapse rate in *vivax* malaria. *J. clin. Invest.*, 1948, **27**, No. 3, pt. 2, 25-33.
    Clinical trials of pentaquine. With B. Craige, R. Jones, C. M. Whorton, T. N. Pullman, and L. Eichelberger.

5262   SHORTT, HENRY EDWARD. 1887-1987, *et al.*
The pre-erythrocytic stage of mammalian malaria. *Brit. med. J.*, 1948, **1**, 192-94.
    Demonstration of the pre-erythrocytic stage of *P. cynomolgi* in the monkey. With P. C. C. Garnham and B. Malamos. Preliminary communication in *Nature (Lond.)*, 1948, **161**, 126.

5262.1   ———. The pre-erythrocytic stage of human malaria, *Plasmodium vivax.* *Brit. med. J.*, 1948, **1**, 547 (only).
    With P. C. C. Garnham, G. Covell, and P. G. Shute.

5262.2   ———. The pre-erythrocytic stage of *Plasmodium falciparum*. A preliminary note. *Brit. med. J.*, 1949, **2**, 1006-08.
    With N. H. Fairley, G. Covell, P. G. Shute, and P. C. C. Garnham. See also *Trans. roy. Soc. trop. Med. Hyg.*, 1951, **44**, 405-19.

5262.3 EDGCOMB, JOHN HAROLD. 1924- , *et al.*
Primaquine, S.N. 13,272, a new curative agent in vivax malaria: a preliminary report. *J. nat. Malaria Soc.*, 1950, **9**, 285-92.
Introduction of primaquine.

5262.4 FALCO, E. A., *et al.*
2:4-Diaminopyrimidines – a new series of antimalarials. *Brit. J. Pharmacol.*, 1951, **6**, 185-200.
Preparation and laboratory tests of pyrimethamine. With L. G. Goodwin, G. H. Hutchings, I. M. Rollo, and P. B. Russell.

5262.5 ROLLO, IAN McINTOSH. 1926-
A 2:4-diamino pyrimidine in the treatment of proguanil-resistant laboratory malarial strains. *Nature (Lond.)*, 1951, **168**, 332-33.
Pyrimethamine (daraprim).

History of Malaria

5263 JONES, WILLIAM HENRY SAMUEL. 1876-1963
Malaria and Greek history. To which is added the history of Greek therapeutics and the malaria theory, by E. T. WITHINGTON. Manchester, *Univ. Press*, 1909.
The view is put forward by the writer that malarial infection was the cause of the decadence of the Greeks.

5264 CELLI, ANGELO. 1857-1914
The history of malaria in the Roman Campagna from ancient times. Edited and enlarged by ANNA CELLI-FRAENTZEL. London, *John Bale*, 1933.
Reprinted New York, 1977.

5264.1 STEPHENS, JOHN WILLIAM WATSON. 1865-1946
Blackwater fever, a historical survey and summary of observations made over a century. Liverpool, *University Press*, 1937.

5264.2 JARAMILLO-ARANGO, JAIME. 1897-1962
The conquest of malaria. London, *William Heinemann*, 1950.

5264.3 RUSSELL, PAUL FARR. 1894-
Man's mastery of malaria. London, *Oxford University Press*, 1955.
Heath Clark Lectures, 1953.

TRYPANOSOMIASIS

5265 ATKINS, JOHN. 1685-1757
The navy-surgeon: or, a practical system of surgery. London, *Caesar Ward*, 1734.
Includes (pp. 364-7) the first English description of African trypanosomiasis (sleeping sickness).

5266 WINTERBOTTOM, THOMAS MASTERMAN. 1765-1859
An account of the native Africans in the neighbourhood of Sierra Leone. Vol. 2. London, *J. Hatchard & J. Mawman*, 1803.

In his travels in Africa, Winterbottom saw sleeping sickness, which he described (pp. 29-31) as a species of lethargy. He also noticed that slave-dealers would not buy slaves whose neck glands showed signs of enlargement.

5267   CLARKE, ROBERT.
Observations on the disease lethargus: with cases and pathology. *Lond. med. Gaz.*, 1840, **26**, 970-76.
Clarke left a detailed account of African trypanosomiasis; he saw cases of the disease whilst a colonial surgeon at Sierra Leone and named it "narcoleptic dropsy".

5267.1 VALENTIN, GABRIEL GUSTAV. 1810-1883
Ueber ein Entozoon im Blute von Salmo fario. *Arch. Anat. Physiol. wiss. Med.*, 1841, 435-36.
Valentin was the first to discover a trypanosome; this was in a salmon. English translation in Kean (No. 2268.1).

5268   GRUBY, DAVID. 1810-1898
Recherches et observations sur une nouvelle espèce d'hématozoaire, Trypanosoma sanguinis. *C. R. Acad. Sci. (Paris)*, 1843, **17**, 1134-36.
Gruby discovered trypanosomes in the frog. He first suggested the name "trypanosome" to describe the parasite.

5269   LIVINGSTONE, DAVID. 1813-1873
Missionary travels and researches in South Africa. London, *John Murray*, 1857.
Livingstone gave an accurate account of the tsetse fly *Glossina morsitans* and of the disease in cattle following its bite (see pp. 80-83; picture of the tsetse fly on p. 571). In his time the bite of the fly was thought to be (and perhaps was) harmless to man.

5270   ——. Arsenic as a remedy for the tsetse bite. *Brit. med. J.*, 1858, 360-61.
Livingstone was probably the first to administer arsenic for the treatment of "nagana", a disease of horses caused by trypanosomes. This followed a suggestion by James Braid.

5270.1 LEWIS, TIMOTHY RICHARDS. 1841-1886
The microscopic organisms found in the blood of man and animals, and their relation to disease. *Ann. rep. sanit. Comm. India* (1877), 1878, **14**, Appendix B, 157-208.
First description of a trypanosome *(T. lewisi)* in a mammal.

5271   EVANS, GRIFFITH. 1835-1935
On a horse disease in India known as "surra", probably due to a haematozoon. *Vet. J.*, 1881, **13**, 1-10, 82-88, 180-200, 326-33.
While serving in India as a veterinary surgeon, Evans discovered parasites in the blood of horses suffering from surra; this was the first pathogenic trypanosome to be described.

5272   NEPVEU, GUSTAVE. 1841-1903
Étude sur les parasites du sang chez les paludiques. *C. R. Soc. Biol. (Paris)*, 1891, **43**, 39-50.
Nepveu, whilst in Algeria, was the first to see trypanosomes in human blood.

5273   BRUCE, *Sir* DAVID. 1855-1931
Preliminary report on the tsetse fly disease or nagana, in Zululand. Durban, *Bennett & Davis*, 1895.

In 1895 Bruce found that *nagana*, the tsetse fly disease of Zululand, was due to a trypanosome *(T. brucei).*

5274   FORDE, ROBERT MICHAEL. 1861-1948
Some clinical notes on a European patient in whose blood a trypanosoma was observed. *J. trop. Med. Hyg.*, 1902, **5**, 261-63.

In 1901 Forde saw (but did not at first recognize as such) trypanosomes in the blood of a patient in Gambia. (*See* No. 5275.)

5275   DUTTON, JOSEPH EVERETT. 1876-1905
Preliminary note upon a trypanosome occurring in the blood of man. *Thompson Yates Lab. Rep.*, 1902, **4**, 455-68.

Dutton was the first to recognize human trypanosomiasis. He saw Forde's patient (*see* No. 5274) and named the trypanosome *T. gambiense*. Sleeping sickness itself has been referred to as "Dutton's disease". The first announcement was in the form of a telegram to Ronald Ross, published in *Brit. med. J.*, 1902, **1**, 42.

5276   CASTELLANI, ALDO. 1877-1971
On the discovery of a species of trypanosoma in the cerebrospinal fluid of cases of sleeping sickness. *Proc. roy. Soc.*, 1903, **71**, 501-08.

Whilst in Uganda, Castellani discovered *T. gambiense* in human cerebrospinal fluid. A paper in *Notes Rec. roy. Soc.*, 1973, **23**, 93-110, discounts Castellani's claim that although he first discovered trypanosomes in the cerebrospinal fluid of sleeping sickness patients, he failed to appreciate the etiological significance of this until it was brought home to him by Sir David Bruce.

5277   ROYAL SOCIETY OF LONDON.
Reports of the Sleeping Sickness Commission of the Royal Society, 1903-1912. 17 pts. London, *H.M.S.O.*, 1903-19.

Bruce and D.N. Nabarro were sent to Africa by the Royal Society to study sleeping sickness, and in their report they showed that the tsetse fly was the vector of trypanosomiasis. They also found that Gambia fever and sleeping sickness were two stages of the same infection.

5278   LAVERAN, CHARLES LOUIS ALPHONSE. 1845-1922, & MESNIL, FÉLIX. 1868-1938
Trypanosomes et trypanosomiases. Paris, *Masson & Cie.*, 1904.

Laveran and Mesnil discovered that trypanosomes could be maintained indefinitely in rats and mice by serial passage.

5279   THOMAS, HAROLD WOLFERSTAN, & BREINL, ANTON.
Report on trypanosomes, trypanosomiasis, and sleeping sickness, being an experimental investigation into their pathology and treatment. London, *Williams & Norgate*, 1905.

Thomas and Breinl discovered that atoxyl, an organic derivative of arsenic acid, was more potent in the treatment of laboratory trypanosomiasis than arsenic in inorganic form. The above is Memoir XVI of the Liverpool School of Tropical Medicine.

5280 NICOLLE, Maurice. 1862-1932, & MESNIL, Félix. 1868-1938
Traitement des trypanosomiases par les "couleurs de benzidine". *Ann. Inst. Pasteur*, 1906, **20**, 417-48, 513-38.
Introduction of trypan-blue in the treatment of trypanosomiasis. Second paper by Mesnil and Nicolle.

5281 EHRLICH, Paul. 1854-1915
Chemotherapeutische Trypanosomen-Studien. *Berl. klin. Wschr.*, 1907, **44**, 233-36, 280-83, 310-14, 341-44.
Includes an account of "Trypanrot", by which Ehrlich succeeded in curing experimental trypanosomiasis. It was his work on this subject which led Ehrlich eventually to the production of salvarsan. He shared the Nobel Prize for Medicine with Metchnikoff in 1908.

5282 PLIMMER, Henry George. 1856-1918, & THOMSON, John D.
Further results of the experimental treatment of trypanosomiasis in rats. *Proc. roy. Soc. B.*, 1908, **80**, 1-12.
Trial of antimony in the treatment of trypanosomiasis.

5283 CHAGAS, Carlos Justiniano Ribeiro. 1879-1934
Nova tripanozomiaze humana. Estudos sobre a morfolojia e o ciclo evolutivo do *Schizotrypanum cruzi* n.gen., n.sp., ajente etiolojico de nova entidade morbida do homen. *Mem. Inst. Osw. Cruz*, 1909, **1**, 159-218.
Chagas discovered *T. cruzi*, causal organism in American trypanosomiasis ("Chagas's disease"). Partial English translation in Kean (No. 2268.1).

5283.1 KLEINE, Friedrich Karl. 1861-1950
Positive Infektionsversuche mit *Trypanosoma brucei* durch *Glossina palpalis*. *Dtsch. med. Wschr.*, 1909, **35**, 469-70.
Glossina was believed to transmit *Trypanosoma* mechanically to the new host until Kleine showed that the latter undergoes a developmental cycle in *Glossina*. English translation in Kean (No. 2268.1).

5284 LEVADITI, Constantin. 1874-1953
Le mécanisme d'action des dérivés arsenicaux dans les trypanosomiases. *Ann. Inst. Pasteur*, 1909, **23**, 604-43.
A study of the action of atoxyl and arsacétine.

5285 STEPHENS, John William Watson. 1865-1946, & FANTHAM, Harold Benjamin. 1875-1937
On the peculiar morphology of a trypanosome from a case of sleeping sickness and the possibility of its being a new species. *(T. rhodesiense)*. *Proc. roy. Soc. B.*, 1910, **83**, 28-33.
T. rhodesiense discovered.

5285.1 VIANNA, Gaspar Oliveira de. 1885-1914
Contribuiçao para o estudo da anatomia patolojica da "molestia de Carlos Chagas". *Mem. Inst. Osw. Cruz*, 1911, **3**, 276-94.
Demonstration of the mode of reproduction of *T. cruzi*. Text in Portuguese and German. See also the paper by Chagas in pp. 219-75 of the same journal.

5285.2 KINGHORN, ALLAN. 1880-1955, & YORKE, WARRINGTON. 1883-1943
On the transmission of human trypanosomes by *Glossina morsitans,* Westw.;
and on the occurrence of human trypanosomes in game. *Ann. trop. Med.
Parasit.,* 1912, **6**, 1-23.
Glossina morsitans shown to be the transmitting fly of *T. rhodesiense.*

5285.3 BRUMPT, ALEXANDRE JOSEPH EMILE. 1877-1951
Le trypanosoma cruzi évolue chez *Conorhinus megistus, Cimex lectularius,
Cimex Boueti* et *Ornithodorus moubata.* Cycle évolutif de ce parasite.
Bull. Soc. Path. exot., 1912, **5**, 360-64.
Life cycle of *T. cruzi* described. English translation in Kean (No. 2268.1).

5286 HAENDEL, LUDWIG. 1869-1939, & JOETTEN, KARL WILHELM. 1886-?
Ueber chemotherapeutische Versuche mit "205 Bayer", einen neuen
trypanoziden Mittel von besonderer Wirkung. *Berl. klin. Wschr.,* 1920, **57**,
821-23.
Introduction of "Bayer 205" (germanin, suramin, naphuride).

5287 PEARCE, LOUISE. 1886-1959
Studies on the treatment of human trypanosomiasis with tryparsamide (the
sodium salt of N-phenylglycineamide-*p*-arsonic acid). *J. exp. Med.,* 1921,
34, Suppl., 1-104.
Introduction of tryparsamide in the treatment of trypanosomiasis.

5288 FOURNEAU, ERNEST. 1872-1949
Chimiothérapie des trypanosomiasis. *Paris méd.,* 1923, **49**, 501-08.
Introduction of moranyl ("Fourneau 309").

5289 LEVADITI, CONSTANTIN. 1847-1953, *et. al.*
Essai de prophylaxie des trypanosomiases par des dérivés phénylarsiniques
administré *per os. Bull. Soc. Path. exot.,* 1926, **19**, 737-46.
First attempt to induce prophylaxis by chemical means in
trypanosomiasis. With S. Nicolau and I. Galloway.

5289.1 WIJERS, D. J. B.
Factors that may influence the infection rate of *Glossina palpalis* with
Trypanomosoma gambiense. 1. The age of the fly at the time of the infected
feed. *Ann. trop. Med. Parasit.,* 1958, **52**, 385-90.
Wijers showed that the tsetse fly is infected during its first or second
blood meal, but not afterwards, information of considerable importance in
determining the criteria for the transmission of trypanosomiasis.

5289.2 THIMM, C. A.
Bibliography of trypanosomiasis. London, *Sleeping Sickness Commission,
Royal Society,* 1909.
Subject index...with additional references and corrections, 1910.

5289.3 MILES, M. A., & ROUSE, JEAN E.
Chagas's disease (South American trypanosomiasis. A bibliography com-
piled from Sleeping Sickness Bureau Bulletin 1908-1912, and Tropical
Diseases Bulletin, 1912-1970. London, *Bureau of Hygiene and Tropical
diseases,* 1970.
Supplement to *Trop. Dis. Bull.,* vol. 67.

5289.4   OLIVIER, MARGARET C., *et al.*
A bibliography on Chagas's disease (1909-1969). By Margaret C. Olivier, Louis J. Olivier, Dorothy B. Segal. Washington, *U.S. Govt. Printing Office*, 1972.
Index-Catalogue of Medical and Veterinary Zoology, Special Publication No. 2.

LEISHMANIASIS

5290   RUSSELL, ALEXANDER. ?1715-1768
Natural history of Aleppo and parts adjacent. London, *A. Millar*, 1856 [1756].
Includes (Chap. iv) a good account of "Aleppo boil", which Russell found to be endemic in Aleppo.

5291   ALIBERT, JEAN LOUIS MARC, *le baron*. 1768-1837
Sur la pyrophlyctide endémique, ou pustule d'Aleppo. *Rev. méd. Franç., étrang.*, 1829, n.s. **3**, 62-71.
Important description of "Aleppo boil", furunculosis orientalis.

5292   BRISCOE, THOMAS BENJAMIN.
[Kala azar]. *Proc. Govt. Bengal in the Med. Dept.*, 1870, No. 52, pp. 31-33.
Kala azar is mentioned briefly in the *Proceedings* in 1869 (No. 34, p. 19) but the above is the first full description, given by Briscoe in a report dated 1 Dec 1869.

5293   CUNNINGHAM, DAVID DOUGLAS. 1843-1914
On the presence of peculiar parasitic organisms in the tissue of a specimen of Delhi boil. *Sci. Med. mem. Off. Army India*, [1884], 1885, **1**, 21-31.
Cunningham saw and described bodies in Delhi boil; these were almost certainly Leishman–Donovan bodies.

5293.1   BREDA, ACHILLE. 1850-1933
Beitrag zum klinischen und bacteriologischen Studium der brasilianischen Framboesie oder "Boubas". *Arch. Dermat. Syph. (Wien)*, 1895, **33**, 3-28.
"Breda's disease" – Brazilian yaws. English translation *New Sydenham Society*, 1897.

5294   BOROVSKII, PETR FOKICH. 1863-1932
[On sart sore.] *Voenno med. Zhur.*, 1898, **76**, 925-41.
First description of the protozoon later named *Leishmania tropica*. The paper is in Russian; for a translation, see C. A. Hoare, in *Trans. roy. Soc. trop. Med. Hyg.*, 1938, **32**, 78-90.

5295   LEISHMAN, *Sir* WILLIAM BOOG. 1865-1926
On the possibility of the occurrence of trypanosomiasis in India. *Brit. med. J.*, 1903, **1**, 1252-54; **2**, 1376-77.
An organism found by Leishman in 1900 was later described by him as possibly a trypanosome. C. Donovan found the same organism in blood in July 1903. The name *Leishmania donovani* (Leishman-Donovan bodies) was later attached to these organisms.

5296   DONOVAN, CHARLES. 1863-1951
On the possibility of the occurrence of trypanosomiasis in India. *Brit. med. J.*, 1903, **2**, 79.
See No. 5295, and *Med. Hist.*, 1983, **27**, 203-13..

5297   WRIGHT, JAMES HOMER. 1870-1928
Protozoa in a case of tropical ulcer (Delhi sore). *J. med. Res.*, 1903, 10, 472-82.
Wright found *Leishmania tropica* in Delhi sore. He was unaware of Borovskii's paper (No. 5294).

5298   LEISHMAN, *Sir* WILLIAM BOOG. 1865-1926
Note on the nature of the parasitic bodies found in tropical splenomegaly. *Brit. med. J.*, 1904, **1**, 303

5299   ROGERS, *Sir* LEONARD. 1868-1962
Note on the occurrence of Leishman–Donovan bodies in "cachexial fevers" including kala-azar. *Brit. med. J.*, 1904, 1, 1249-51.
Rogers demonstrated the Leishman–Donovan bodies in kala-azar. See also the same journal, 1904, **2**, 645-50. At about the same time Bentley reported similar findings in India.

5299.1   LINDENBERG, ADOLFO CARLOS. 1872-1944
L'ulcère de Bauru ou le bouton d'orient au Brésil. *Bull. Soc. Path. exot.*, 1909, **2**, 252-54.
Muco-cutaneous leishmaniasis of South America. English translation in Kean (No. 2268.1).

5300   NICOLLE, CHARLES JULES HENRI. 1866-1936
Le kala azar infantile. *Ann. Inst. Pasteur*, 1909, **23**, 361-401, 441-71.
Nicolle considered infantile kala-azar to be caused by a distinct species of *Leishmania*; to this he gave the name *L. infantum*.

5300.1   MIGONE, LUIS ENRIQUE.
Un cas de kala-azar à Asuncion (Paraguay). *Bull. Soc. Path. exot.*, 1913, **6**, 118-20.
Migone first noted the existence of visceral leishmaniasis in the Americas (Paraguay).

5301   VIANNA, GASPAR OLIVEIRA DE. 1885-1914
Sobre o tratemento de leishmaniose tegumentar. *Ann. paulist. Med. Cir.*, 1914, **2**, 167-69.
Vianna introduced tartar emetic in the treatment of S. American leishmaniasis. His preliminary announcement on this form of treatment was made to the Brazilian Dermatological Society and appears in *Arch. brasil. Med.*, 1912, **2**, 426-28. English translation of earlier paper in Kean (No. 2268.1).

5301.1   KNOWLES, ROBERT. 1883-1936, *et al.*
On a *Herpetomonas* found in the gut of the sandfly, *Phlebotomus argentipes*, fed on kala-azar patients. *Indian med. Gaz.*, 1924, **59**, 593-97.
Demonstration that *L. donovani* is capable of reproduction in *Phlebotomus*. With L. E. Napier and R. O. Smith.

5301.2   ADLER, SAUL. 1895-1956, & BER, MORDEHAI. *d*-1952
The transmission of *Leishmania tropica* by the bite of *Phlebotomus papatasii*. *Indian J. med. Res.*, 1941, **29**, 803-09.
Proof of the transmission of *L. tropica* by P. papatasii.

5302   SWAMINATH, C. S., *et al.*
Transmission of Indian kala-azar to man by the bites of *Phlebotomus argentipes*, Ann. and Brun. *Indian J. med. Res.*, 1942, **30**, 473-77.
Successful transmission of kala-azar to man by the bite of *Phlebotomus argentipes* reported, showing it to be the vector of *Leishmania*. With H. E. Shortt and L. A. P. Anderson.

TREPONEMATOSES

5303   PISO, WILLEM [LE POIS (GUILLAUME)]. 1611-1678
De lue Indica. In his *Historia naturalis Brasiliae*, (De medica Brasiliensi, p. 35), Lugduni Batavorum, *apud F. Hackium*; Amstelodami, *apud L. Elzevirum*, 1648.
Piso was the first to separate yaws from syphilis. *See* No. 2263.1.

5304   BANCROFT, EDWARD. 1774-1821
Essay on the natural history of Guiana, in South America. London, *T. Becket*, 1769.
Bancroft was an English physician who lived for many years in America. He noted the transmission of yaws by flies (p. 385 of his book).

5306   CASTELLANI, ALDO. 1877-1971
On the presence of spirochaetes in two cases of ulcerated parangi (yaws). *Brit med. J.*, 1905, **2**, 1280, 1330-31, 1430.
Castellani demonstrated in scrapings of yaws tissue a spirochaete, *T. pertenue*, later found to be the causal organism. He thus finally established it as a distinct organism from the syphilis spirochaete. Preliminary note in *J. Ceylon. Br. Brit. med. Ass.*, 1905, **2**, pt. 1, 54.

5307   WELLMANN, FREDERICK CREIGHTON. 1871-1960
On a spirochaete found in yaws papules. *J. trop. Med. Hyg.*, 1905, **8**, 345.
Independently of Castellani (No. 5306) Wellmann discovered *Treponema pertenue*.

5308   NICHOLS, HENRY JAMES. 1877-1927
Experimental yaws in the monkey and rabbit. *J. exp. Med.*, 1910, **12**, 616-22; 1911, **14**, 196-216.
A monkey was first infected and from it the infection was transmitted to a rabbit.

5308.1   SAENZ, BRAULIO, *et al.*
Demonstración de un treponema en el borde activo un caso de pinto de las manos y pies y en la linfa de ganglios superficiales (reporte preliminar). *Arch. Med. interna*, 1938, **4**, 112-17.
B. Saenz, J. Grau Triana, and J. Alfonso Armenteros indicated that pinta is caused by a treponeme, *T. carateum*.

5308.2 HACKETT, CECIL JOHN. 1905-
On the origin of the human treponematoses (pinta, yaws, endemic syphilis and venereal syphilis). *Bull. Wld. Hlth. Org.*, 1963, **29**, 7-41.
"Perhaps the most scholarly investigation of the origin of syphilis" (Wesley Spink).

5308.3 WORLD HEALTH ORGANIZATION.
Bibliography of yaws, 1905-62. Genève, *World Health Organization*, 1963.
Over 1,700 items.

5309 RUTTY, John. 1698-1775
A chronological history of the weather and seasons and of the prevailing diseases in Dublin. London, *Robinson & Roberts*, 1770.
Rutty kept continuous records of weather and diseases in Dublin from 1724-64. On page 75 of the above book is given the first clear description of relapsing fever.

5310 CORMACK, *Sir* JOHN ROSE. 1815-1882
Natural history, pathology and treatment of the epidemic fever at present prevailing in Edinburgh and other towns. London, *J. Churchill*, 1843.
The epidemic of relapsing fever in Edinburgh in 1843 was well described by Cormack. He was first editor of the *Association Medical Journal* which later became the *British Medical Journal.*

5311 CRAIGIE, DAVID. 1793-1866
Notice of a febrile disorder which has prevailed at Edinburgh during the summer of 1843. *Edinb. med. surg. J.*, 1843, **60**, 410-18.
Relapsing fever was given its name by Craigie, in his description of the Edinburgh epidemic.

5311.1 HENDERSON, WILLIAM. 1810-1872
On some of the characters which distinguish the fever at present epidemic from typhus fever. *Edinb. med. surg. J.*, 1844, **61**, 201-25.
Henderson, professor of pathology at Edinburgh, gave a good account of relapsing fever seen during the epidemic in 1843. He was one of the first to differentiate it from typhus.

5312 SILLIAU, PIERRE MARIE.
Fièvre à rechutes. Paris, *Thèse No.* 205, 1869.
Silliau gave a good account of the epidemic of relapsing fever at Réunion, 1865. He showed the contagious nature of the disease.

5313 PARRY, JOHN S. 1843-1876
Observations on relapsing fever, as it occurred in Philadelphia in the winter of 1869 and 1870. *Amer. J. med. Sci.*, 1870, n.s. **60**., 336-58.
Parry called attention to infection from articles of clothing worn by victims of the epidemic of relapsing fever in Philadelphia in 1869.

5314   OBERMEIER, OTTO HUGO FRANZ. 1843-1873
        Vorkommen feinster, eine Eigenbewegung zeigender Fäden im Blute von
        Recurrenskranken. *Zbl. med. Wiss.*, 1873, **11**, 145-47.
        Discovery (in 1868) of *Borrelia recurrentis*, causative agent in relapsing fever.

5315   MOCHUTKOVSKI, OSIP OSIPOVICH [MOSCHUTKOWSKY]. 1845-1903
        Materialien zur Pathologie und Therapie des Rückfallstyphus. *Dtsch. Arch.
        klin. Med.*, 1879, **24**, 80-97.
            By inoculating healthy subjects with blood of patients suffering from
        replasing fever, and producing the fever in the former, Mochutkovski
        demonstrated not only the communicability of the disease but also the
        specific pathogenic significance of the spirochaete.

5316   CARTER, HENRY VANDYKE. 1831-1897
        Spirillum fever. London, *J. & A. Churchill*, 1882.
            Asiatic relapsing fever; original work on this disease by Carter is
        remembered by the eponym "Carter's fever" and the name *Borrelia carteri*.
        He reproduced the disease in the monkey.

5317   ROSS, PHILIP HEDGELAND, 1876-1929, & MILNE, ARTHUR DAWSON. *d.*1932
        "Tick fever". *Brit. med. J.*, 1904, **2**, 1453-54.
            Ross and Milne discovered the causative agent in the African variety of
        relapsing (tick) fever.

5318   DUTTON, JOSEPH EVERETT. 1877-1905, & TODD, JOHN LANCELOT. 1876-1949
        The nature of tick fever in the eastern part of the Congo Free State. *Brit.
        med. J.*, 1905, **2**, 1259-60.
            Independently of Ross and Milne, Dutton and Todd demonstrated
        relapsing fever in monkeys conveyed by infected ticks, *Ornithodorus
        moubata.* The organism was named *Sp.* (now *Borrelia) duttoni.* Both Dutton
        and Todd contracted the disease, and the former died of it before the paper
        was published.

5319   NORRIS, CHARLES. 1867-1935, *et al.*
        Study of a spirochete obtained from a case of relapsing fever in man, with
        notes on morphology, animal reactions, and attempts at cultivation. *J. infect.
        Dis.*, 1906, **3**, 266-90.
            Spirochaete causing the American variety of relapsing fever first isolated.
        With A. W. Pappenheimer and T. Flournoy.

5320   NOVY, FREDERICK GEORGE. 1864-1957, & KNAPP, RICHARD EDWARD. 1884-
        Studies in *Spirillum obermeieri* and related organisms. *J. infect. Dis.*, 1906,
        3, 291-393.
            Novy and Knapp made important observations on the spirochaete
        isolated by Norris *et al.* from a case of (American) relapsing fever, proving
        it to be different from *Borrelia obermeieri,* sometimes referred to as "Novy's
        bacillus", *Borrelia novyi.* The above paper includes work on the immunol-
        ogy of the disease.

5321   MACKIE, FREDERICK PERCIVAL. 1875-1944
        The part played by Pediculus corporis in the transmission of relapsing
        fever. *Brit. med. J.*, 1907, **2**, 1706-09.
            Proof that relapsing fever is conveyed by the body louse, *Pediculus
        corporis.*

5322   WILCOX, Whitman.
        Violent symptoms from the bite of a rat. *Amer. J. med. Sci.*, 1840, **26**, 245-46.
        First report of rat-bite fever to appear in a medical journal.

5323   CARTER, Henry Vandyke. 1831-1897.
        Note on the occurrence of a minute blood-spirillum in an Indian rat. *Sci. Mem. med. Off. Army India*, (1887), 1888, **3**, 45-48.
        Demonstration of *Spirillum minus,* later shown to be a cause of rat-bite fever. (*See also* No. 5327).

5324   HATA, Sahachiro. 1873-1938
        Salvarsantherapie der Rattenbisskrankheit in Japan. *Münch. med. Wschr.*, 1912, **59**, 854-57.
        Salvarsan first used in the treatment of rat-bite fever.

5325   SCHOTTMÜLLER, Hugo. 1867-1936
        Zur Aetiologie und Klinik der Bisskrankheit. *Derm. Wschr.*, 1914, **58**, Suppl., 77-103.
        Isolation of *Streptothrix (Actinomyces) muris ratti* from human patients bitten by rats.

5326   FUTAKI, Kenzo. 1873-1966, *et al.*
        The cause of rat-bite fever. *J. exp. Med.*, 1916, **23**, 249-50; 1917, **25**, 33-44.
        K. Futaki, I. Takaki, T. Taniguchi, and S. Osumi found a spirillum (Sp. morsus muris) in the lymphatic glands and blood stream in cases of rat-bite fever (sodoku).

5327   ROBERTSON, Andrew.
        Observations on the causal organism of rat-bite fever in man. *Ann. trop. Med. Parasit.*, 1924, **16**, 157-75.
        Robertson proved one of the causal organisms of rat-bite fever to be *Sp. morsus muris*. He re-named it *Spirillum minus* Carter, 1887, identifying it as the first spiral micro-organism to be described from a rodent.

5328   PLACE, Edwin Hemphill. 1880-, *et al.*
        Erythema arthriticum epidemicum; preliminary report. *Boston med. surg. J.*, 1926, **194**, 285-87.
        "Haverhill fever" first reported. The writers isolated an organism, later found to be identical with *Streptothrix muris ratti* and *Streptobacillus moniliformis*. With L. E. Sutton and O. Willner.

5329   LEMIERRE, André. 1875- , *et al.*
        Sur une nouvelle fièvre par morsure de rat. *Bull. Acad. Méd. (Paris)*, 1937, 3 sér., **117**, 705-13.
        A. Lemierre, J. Reilly, A. Laporte, and M. Morin isolated *Streptobacillus moniliformis* from a case of rat-bite fever.

LEPTOSPIROSES

5330   MARSTON, JEFFERY ALLEN. 1831-1911
        Report on fever (Malta). *Army med. Dept. statist. sanit. Rep.* (1861), 1863,
        3, 486-521.
        Marston was apparently the first to describe "Weil's disease" (p. 513).

5331   LANDOUZY, LOUIS THÉOPHILE JOSEPH. 1845-1917
        Fièvre bilieuse ou hépatique. *Gaz. Hôp. (Paris)*, 1883, **56**, 809-10, 913-14.
        An early account of "Weil's disease", Leptospirosis icterohaemorrhagica.

5332   WEIL, ADOLF. 1848-1916
        Ueber eine eigenthümliche, mit Milztumor, Icterus und Nephritis
        einhergehende, acute Infectionskrankheit. *Dtsch. Arch. klin. Med.*, 1886,
        39, 209-32.
        In his classic description of Leptospirosis icterohaemorrhagica Weil
        differentiated the disease from other types of acute jaundice. It is better
        known as "Weil's disease".

5333   STIMSON, ARTHUR MARSTON. 1876-
        Note on an organism found in yellow-fever tissue. *Publ. Hlth. Rep. (Wash.)*,
        1907, **22**, 541.
        Stimson discovered a spirochaete in the organs of persons dying of (?)
        yellow fever. He called it *Sp. interrogans*, but it was almost certainly
        Leptospira icterohaemorrhagiae.

5334   INADA, RYUKICHI. 1874-1950, *et al.*
        The etiology, mode of infection, and specific therapy of Weil's disease
        (Spirochaetosis icterohaemorrhagica). *J. exp. Med.*, 1916, **23**, 377-402.
        Inada, Y. Ido, R. Hoki, R. Kaneko, and H. Ito proved that *Sp. (Leptospira)
        icterohaemorrhagiae* is the causal organism in Weil's disease. Preliminary
        report (in Japanese) in *Tokyo Ijishinshi*, 1915, No. 1908.

5334.1 IDO, YUTAKA, 1881-1919, *et al.*
        The rat as a carrier of Spirochaeta icterohaemorrhagiae, the causative agent
        in Weil's disease (spirochaetosis icterohaemorrhagica). *J. exp. Med.*, 1917,
        26, 341-53.
        Rats shown to be the carriers of *Leptospira*. With R. Hoki, H. Ito, and H.
        Wani.

5334.2 ———. Spirochaeta hebdomadis, the causative agent of seven-day fever
        (nanukayami). *J. exp. Med.*, 1918, **28**, 435-48.
        Discovery of *Leptospira hebdomadis*, carried by a mouse. With H. Ito
        and H. Wani.

5335   KLARENBEEK, ARIE. 1888-, & SCHÜFFNER, WILHELM AUGUST PAUL. 1867-
        1949
        Het voorkomen van een afwijkend Leptospira-ras in Nederland. *Ned. T.
        Geneesk.*, 1933, **77**, 4271-76.
        Leptospira canicola first isolated (1913) from the urine of a dog.

5335.1   WANI, HIDETSUNE.
Ueber die Prophylaxe der Spirochaetosis icterohaemorrhagica Inada (Weilschen Krankheit) durch Schutzimpfung. *Z. ImmunForsch.*, 1933, **79**, 1-26.
Prophylactic vaccination against leptospirosis.

5336   DHONT, C. M., *et al.*
De leptospiroses bij den hond, en de beteekenis der *Leptospira canicola. Ned. T. Geneesk.*, 1934, **78**, 5197-209.
First reported cases of human infection with *L. canicola.* With A. Klarenbeek, W. A. P. Schüffner, and J. Voet.

DISEASES DUE TO METAZOAN PARASITES

5336.1   WELSCH, GEORG HIERONYMUS. 1624-1677
Exercitatio de vena Medinensi. Augustae Vindelicorum. *T. Goebel*, 1674.
An exhaustive survey of dracontiasis.

5336.2   MONGIN.
Sur un ver trouvé sous la conjunctive, à Maribou, isle Saint-Domingue. *J. Méd Chir. Pharm.*, 1770, **32**, 338-39.
First description of the worm *Loa loa*. Mongin was a French surgeon working in the West Indies. English translation in Kean (No. 2268.1).

5336.3   CHISHOLM, COLIN. 1755-1825
An essay on the malignant pestilential fever introduced into the West Indian Islands from Boullam, on the coast of Guinea, as it appeared in 1793 and 1794. London, *C. Dilly*, 1795.
Chisholm was apparently the first to observe the mode of transmission of the Guinea worm, *Dracunculus medinensis.*

5336.4   TIEDEMANN, FRIEDRICH. 1781-1861
Notiz. a. d. Geb. d. Natur-u. Heilk., Weimar, 1821, **1**, col. 64.
Description of the calcified cysts of trichinosis in human muscle. No title.

5336.5   HILTON, JOHN. 1804-1878
Notes of a peculiar appearance observed in human muscle, probably depending upon the formation of very small cysticerci. *Lond. med. Gaz.*, 1833, **11**, 605.
Hilton described *Trichinella spiralis* and suggested its parasitic nature.

5337   OWEN, *Sir* RICHARD. 1804-1892
Description of a microscopic entozoon (Trichina spiralis) infesting the muscles of the human body. *Lond. med. Gaz.*, 1835, **16**, 125-127; *Trans. zool. Soc. Lond.*, 1835, **1**, 315-24.
While a first-year student at St. Bartholomew's Hospital, James Paget discovered trichina in muscle during dissection. Owen, his teacher, named it *Trichina spiralis* and published an account. It was renamed *Trichinella spiralis* in 1896. Paget communicated his discovery to the Abernethian Society at St. Bartholomew's on 6 Feb, 1835; an abstract of his paper is

published in the *Transactions* of the society, vol. 2. Paget recorded the chronology of the discovery in a letter to the *Lancet*, 1866, **1**, 269. This and his unpublished article intended for *Lond. med. Gaz.*, 1835, is reproduced by Kean (No. 2268.1), p. 458-62. The letter is also published in *Bull. Hist. Med.*, 1979, **53**, 547.

5338   LEIDY, JOSEPH. 1823-1891
[Entozoon in the superficial part of the extensor muscles of the thigh of the hog.], [Abstract]. *Proc. Acad. nat. Sci. Phila.*, 1846, **3**, 107-8.
    First description of trichinosis in the pig.

5338.1   HERBST, ERNST FRIEDRICH GUSTAV. 1803-1893
Beobachtungen über *Trichina spiralis* in Betriff der Uebertragung der Eingeweidewürmer. *Nachrichten Georg-August Univ. Königl. Wiss. Göttingen*, 1851, 260-64; 1852, 183-204.
    Herbst was the first to demonstrate that an animal eating trichinous flesh would thereby develop trichinae in its own muscles. English translation of part 1 in Kean (No. 2268.1).

5339   BILHARZ, THEODOR MAXIMILIAN. 1825-1862
Ein Beitrag zur Helminthographia humana aus brieflichen Mittheilungen des Dr. Bilharz in Cairo, nebst Bemerkungen von C. T. v. Siebold. *Z. wiss. Zool.*, 1852, **4**, 53-76.
    Discovery, in 1851, of *Schistosoma haematobium*, the parasite of bilharziasis. Bilharz was Professor of Zoology at Cairo. English translation in *Rev. infect. Dis.*, 1984, **4**, 727-32, and in Kean (No. 2268.1).

5340   SIEBOLD, CARL THEODOR ERNST VON. 1804-1885
Ueber die Band- und Blasenwürmer. Leipzig, *W. Engelmann*, 1854.
    Siebold succeeded in infecting dogs with *Taenia echinococcus*. Translation by T. H. Huxley *Sydenham Society* London, 1857.

5341   KÜCHENMEISTER, GOTTLOB FRIEDRICH HEINRICH. 1821-1890
Die in und an dem Körper des lebenden Menschen vorkommenden Parasiten. 2 vols. Leipzig, *B. G. Teubner*, 1855.
    English translation of 2nd ed. by Edwin Ray Lankester, 2 vols. London, *Sydenham Society*, 1857.

5342   ZENKER, FRIEDRICH ALBERT. 1825-1898
Ueber die Trichinen-Krankheit des Menschen. *Virchows Arch. path. Anat.*, 1860, **18**, 561-72.
    The intestinal and muscular forms of trichinosis were first noted by Zenker, who established their connection with the disease. English translation in Kean (No. 2268.1).

5343   LEUCKART, KARL GEORG FRIEDRICH RUDOLF. 1823-1898
Untersuchungen über Trichina spiralis. Leipzig, *C. F. Winter*, 1860.
    Leuckart provided an articulate and detailed description of *Trichinella spiralis*.

5344   ——. Die menschlichen Parasiten und die von ihnen herrührenden Krankheiten. 2 vols. Leipzig, *C. F. Winter*, 1863-76

Includes the first complete and accurate account of the life history and morphology of *Taenia echinococcus*. Leuckart proved the relationship between hydatid cysts and minute tape-worms in dogs.

5344.1   FRIEDREICH, NIKOLAUS. 1825-1882
Ein Beitrag zur Pathologie der Trichinenkrankheit beim Menschen. *Virchows Arch. path. Anat.*, 1862, **25**, 399-413.
First confirmed diagnosis of trichinosis in a living person.

5344.2   BASTIAN, HENRY CHARLTON. 1837-1915
On the structure and nature of the Dracunculus or Guinea worm. *Trans. Linn. Soc.*, 1863, **24**, 101-34.
First detailed description.

5344.3   DEMARQUAY, JEAN NICOLAS. 1811-1875
Note sur une tumeur des bourses contenant un liquide laiteux (galactocèle de Vidal) et renfermant de petits êtres vermiformes que l'on peut considérer comme les helminthes hématoïdes à l'état d'embryon. *Gaz. méd. Paris*, 1863, **33**, 665-67.
Description of the embryonic stage of *Wuchereria bancrofti* in hydrocele fluid.

5344.4   COBBOLD, THOMAS SPENCER. 1828-1886
Entozoa. London, *Groombridge & Sons*, 1864.
Cobbold suggested (p. 36) that a mollusc was the intermediate host in bilharziasis.

5344.5   HARLEY, JOHN. 1833-1921
On the endemic haematuria of the Cape of Good Hope. *Med.-chir. Trans.*, 1864, **47**, 55-74.
Like Cobbold, Harley expressed the view that a mollusc was the intermediate host in bilharziasis.

5344.6   WUCHERER, OTTO EDUARD HEINRICH. 1820-1873
Noticiar preliminar sobre vermes de uma especie ainda nao descripta, encontrados na urina de doentes de hematuria intertropical no Brazil. *Gaz. med. Bahia*, 1868, **3**, 97-99.
In 1866 Wucherer saw the embryo form of the filaria worm. Later the name *Wuchereria bancrofti* was applied to it. English translation in Kean (No. 2268.1).

5344.7   FEDCHENKO, ALEKSIEI PAVLOVICH. 1844-1873
[On the structure and reproduction of Filaria medinensis L.] Izvest. imp. Obsh. Liub. Estes. (Mosk.), 1869-70, 8, 71-82.
Fedchenko elucidated the life cycle of Dracunculus medinensis, the parasite of dracontiasis. English translation in *Amer. J. Med.*, 1971, **20**, 511-23, and in Kean (No. 2268.1) pp. 426-34.

5344.8   LEWIS, TIMOTHY RICHARDS. 1841-1886
On a haemotozoon inhabiting human blood. Its relation to chyluria and other diseases. *Ann. Rep. sanit. Comm. India* (1871), **8**, Appendix E 241-60.

Independently of Demarquay (No. 5344.3) and Wucherer (No. 5344.6), Lewis found microfilariae in the urine and blood in chyluria. He was first to use the term *Filaria sanguinis hominis* for the parasite.

5344.9   McCONNELL, JAMES FREDERICK PARRY. 1848-1896
Remarks on the anatomy and pathological relations of a new species of liver fluke. *Lancet*, 1875, **2**, 271-74.
First complete description of *Chlonorchis sinensis*.

5344.10   O'NEILL, JOHN.
On the presence of a Filaria in "craw-craw". *Lancet*, 1875, **1**, 265-66.
Onchocerca was described by O'Neill, an Irish naval surgeon, fifty years before the worm was linked with blindness (onchocerciasis).

5344.11   NORMOND, LOUIS ALEXIS. 1834-1885?
Sur la maladie dite diarrhée de Cochinchine. *C. R. Acad. Sci. (Paris)*, 1876, **83**, 316-18.
Normond found *Strongyloides stercoralis*, the causal parasite in strongyloidiasis. English translation in Kean (No. 2268.1).

5345   MANSON, *Sir* PATRICK. 1844-1922
Filaria sanguinis hominis. *Med. Rep. Imperial Maritime Customs, China*, 1877, 13th issue, 30-38.

5345.1   ——. Further observations on Filaria sanguinis hominis. *Med. Rep. Imperial Maritime Customs, China*, 1877 (1878), Special series No. 2, 14th issue, 1-26.
Manson showed that *Wuchereria bancrofti,* the cause of filarial elephantiasis in man, develops in, and is transmitted by, the *Culex* mosquito. This was the first proof that infective diseases are spread by animal vectors. See also his later paper in *J. Linnean Soc.*, 1878 (Zool.), *14*, 304-11.

5346   BANCROFT, JOSEPH. 1836-1894
Cases of filarious disease. *Trans. path. Soc. Lond.*, 1878, **29**, 406-19.
Discovery (1876) of *Wuchereria bancrofti*. Bancroft's first report on this was in the form of a letter to T. S. Cobbold, who published it in *Lancet*, 1877, **2**, 70-71.

5346.1   BAELZ, ERWIN OTTO EDUARD VON. 1849-1913
Ueber parasitäre Hämoptoë (Gregarinosis pulmonum). *Zbl. med. Wiss.*, 1880, **18**, 721-22.
Description of the ova of *Paragonimus* (which Baelz named *Gregarina pulmonalis)* and its relationship to endemic haemoptysis. Translation in Kean (No. 2268.1), p. 602.

5346.2   MANSON, *Sir* PATRICK. 1844-1922
Distoma ringeri. *Med. Rep. Imperial Maritime Customs, China*, 1880, Special series No. 2, 20th issue, pp. 10-12.
Manson made a fundamental contribution to knowledge on paragonimiasis with his description of its aetiology and of the parasite. He named it *Distoma ringeri* after Dr. Ringer, who recovered it from the lung at necropsy; it was later named *Paragonimus ringeri*. Reproduced in Kean (No. 2268.1), p. 603.

5346.3 ———. The metamorphosis of *Filaria sanguinis hominis* in the mosquito. *Trans. Linn. Soc. Lond., Zool.*, 1884, **2**, 367-88.

Manson reported that the changes he had observed in ingested filariae took place in the mosquito thorax, not in the stomach as previously thought.

5347 THOMAS, JOHN DAVIES. 1844-1893
Notes upon the experimental breeding of *Taenia echinococcus* in the dog from the echinococci of man. *Proc. roy. Soc. Lond.*, 1885, **38**, 449-57.

Thomas succeeded in transmitting *Taenia echinococcus* to the dog from human sources.

5347.1 ROBERTSON, DOUGLAS MORAY COOPER LAMB ARGYLL. 1837-1909
Case of *Filaria loa* in which the parasite was removed from under the conjunctiva. *Trans. ophthal. Soc. U.K.*, 1895, **15**, 137-67.

First detailed description of *Loa loa*. See also *Trans. ophthal. Soc. U.K.*, 1897, **17**, 227-32.

5348 BROWN, THOMAS RICHARDSON. 1872-1950
Studies on trichinosis, with especial reference to the increase of the eosinophilic cells in the blood and muscle, the origin of these cells and their diagnostic importance. *J. exp. Med.*, 1898, **3**, 315-47.

Brown pointed out the occurrence of eosinophilia in trichinosis. A preliminary communication upon the subject, by W. S. Thayer, was published in *C. R. XII Congr. int. Med.*, Moscou, 1897, 126-31.

5349 LOW, GEORGE CARMICHAEL. 1872-1952
A recent observation on *Filaria nocturna* in *Culex*: probable mode of infection of man. *Brit. med. J.*, 1900, **1**, 1456-57.

Demonstration of the complete chain of filarial infection from man-to-mosquito-to-man.

5349.1 KATSURADA, FUJIRO. 1867-1946
[The aetiology of a parasitic disease (in Japanese)]. *Ijo Shimbun*, 1904, No. 669, 1325-32.

First description of *Schistosoma japonicum*. Translation in Kean (No. 2368.1), p. 518.

5349.2 SYMMERS, WILLIAM ST CLAIR. 1863-1937
Note on a new form of liver cirrhosis due to the presence of the ova of Bilharzia haematobia. *J. Path. Bact.*, 1904, **9**, 237-39.

"Symmers's fibrosis", pipe stem fibrosis of the liver, occurring in cases of certain forms of schistosomiasis.

5350 FLEIG, CHARLES AUGUSTE. 1883-1912, & LISBONNE, MARCEL. 1883-
Recherches sur un séro-diagnostic du kyste hydatique par la méthode des précipitines. *C. R. Soc. Biol. (Paris)*, 1907, **62**, 1198-1201.

Precipitin reaction for the diagnosis of hydatid disease.

5350.1 FUJINAMI, AKIRA. 1870-1934, & NAKAMURA, HACHITARO.
Ueber den Wohnort von *Schistosomum japonicum*. [Japanese text.] *Kyoto Igaku Zassi*, 1907, **4**, No. 4.

Fujinami and Nakamura identified the intermediate host of *S. japonicum*. Abstract in *Arch. Schiffs- u. Tropenhyg.*, 1908, **12**, 471. Later (1909, **6**, 224-

52) they demonstrated that infection occurred by skin penetration. English translation of 1909 paper in Kean (No. 2268.1).

5350.2   MIYAIRI, KEINOSUKE. 1865-1946, & SUZUKI, MASATSUGU.
Der Zwischenwirt des *Schistosomum japonicum* Katsurada. *Mitt. med. Fak. Univ. Kyushu*, 1914, **1**, 187-97.
Miyairi and Suzuki confirmed that snails are the intermediate hosts of *S. japonicum*, and their paper completed the description of the life cycle from ova to snail intermediate host. Translation in Kean (No. 2268.1), p. 532.

5350.3   TURKHUD, DNYANESHVAR ATMARAN. 1868-1926
Report of the Bombay Bacteriological laboratory for the year 1913. Bombay, *Govt. Central Press*, 1914, pp. 14-16.
Experimental demonstration of the complete life cycle of Dracunculus medinensis.

5350.4   LEIPER, ROBERT THOMSON. 1881-1969
Reports of the results of the bilharzia mission in Egypt, 1915. *J. roy. Army med. Cps*, 1915, **25**, 1-55, 147-92, 253-67; 1916, **27**, 171-90; 1918, **30**, 235-60.
Leiper identified the snail responsible for the transmission of *Schistosoma mansoni* and *S. haematobium*.

5350.5   ——. & ATKINSON, EDWARD LEICESTER. 1882-1928
Observations on the spread of Asiatic schistosomiasis. *Brit. med. J.*, 1915, **1**, 201-03.
First paper in English giving a detailed account of the development of *S. japonicum* in the snail and its subsequent development in man. Atkinson, a surgeon in the Royal Navy, was a member of Scott's Antarctic expedition and led the search party which found the bodies of Scott and his companions.

5350.6   CHRISTOPHERSON, JOHN BRIAN. 1868-1955
The successful use of antimony in bilharziosis. *Lancet*, 1918, **2**, 325-27.
Introduction of tartar emetic (antimony) in the treatment of schistosomiasis.

5350.7   NAKAGAWA, KOAN. 1874-1959
On the life cycle of *Fasciolopsis buski* Lankester. *Kitasato Arch. exp. Med.*, 1921, **4**, 159-67.

5350.8   BLACKLOCK, DONALD BREADALBANE. 1879-1955
The insect transmission of *Onchocerca volvulus* (Leuckart, 1893), the cause of worm nodules in man in Africa. *Brit. med. J.*, 1927, **1**, 129-33.
The fly *Simulium damnosum* shown to be the vector of onchocerciasis.

5351   DEW, *Sir* HAROLD ROBERT. 1891-1962
Hydatid disease. Its pathology, diagnosis and treatment. Sydney, *Australasian Med. Publ. Co.*, 1928.
Dew's book remains the authoritative source. His many contributions to the knowledge of hydatid disease are summarized in it.

5351.1   AUGUSTINE, DONALD LESLIE. 1895- , & THEILER, HANS. 1894-
         Precipitin and skin tests as aids in diagnosing trichinosis. *Parasitology*, 1932,
         24, 60-86.
         Intradermal test for trichinosis.

5351.2   KIKUTH, WALTER. 1896-1968, *et al.*
         Miracil, ein neues Chemotherapeuticum gegen die Darmbilharziose.
         Naturwissenschaften, 1946, **33**, 253 (only).
         Lucanthone hydrochloride (Miracil D). With R. Gönnert and H. Mauss.

5351.3   HEWITT, REGINALD IRVING. 1911- , *et al.*
         Experimental chemotherapy of filariasis. III. Effect of 1-diethylcarbamyl-4-
         methyl-piperazine hydrochloride against naturally acquired filarial infec-
         tions in cotton rats and dogs. *J. Lab. clin. Med.*, 1947, **32**, 1314-29.
         Proof of antifilarial action of diethylcarbarmazine citrate (hetrazan).
         With S. Kushner, H. W. Stewart, E. White, W. S. Wallace, and Y. Subbarow.

5351.4   HOOF, L. VAN, *et al.*
         Sur la chimiothérapie de l'onchocercose. (Note préliminaire). *Ann. Soc.
         belge Méd. trop.*, 1947, **27**, 173-77.
         First effective chemotherapy (suramin). With C. Heurard, E. Peel, and
         M. Wanson.

5351.5   RASI, D., *et al.*
         A new, active metabolite of 'Miracil D'. *Nature (Lond.)*, 1965, **208**, 1005-
         06.
         Lucanthone. With five co-authors.

5351.6   LAMBERT, C. R.
         Chemotherapy of experimental *Schistosoma mansoni* infections with a
         nitro-thiazole derivative, CIBA 32,644-Ba. *Ann. trop. Med. Parasit.*, 1964,
         58, 292-303.
         Introduction of niridazole (Ambilhar).

5351.7   RICHARDS, HUGH COLIN, & FOSTER, RAYMOND.
         A new series of 2-aminomethyltetrahydroquinoline derivatives displaying
         schistosomicidal activity in rodents and primates. *Nature (Lond.)*, 1969, **222**,
         581-82.
         Oxamniquinine.

5352   KHALIL, MOHAMED.
         The bibliography of schistosomiasis (bilharziasis). Cairo, *Egyptian Uni-
         versity*, 1931.

5352.1   BOUILLON, ALBERT.
         Bibliographie des schistosome et des schistosomiases (bilharzioses)
         humaines et animales de 1931 à 1948. *Mémoires, Institut Royal Colonial
         Belge, Section des Sciences Naturelles et Médicales*, 1949, **18**, fasc. 5.
         Continues and supplements No. 5352.

5352.2   PAN AMERICAN SANITARY BUREAU.
         Bibliography of onchocerciasis. Washington, *Pan American Sanitary
         Bureau*, 1950.
         Publication No. 242.

5352.3   IYENGAR, MANDAYAM OSURI TIRUNARAYANA. 1895-
Annotated bibliography of filariasis and elephantiasis. 5 parts. Nouméa, *South Pacific Commission*, 1954-60.
South Pacific Commission Technical Papers, Nos. 65, 88, 109 (and Supplement), 124, and 160.

5352.4   WORLD HEALTH ORGANIZATION.
Bibliography of bilharziasis, 1949-1958. Genève, *World Health Organization*, 1960.
Continues and supplements Nos. 5352 and 5352.1

5352.5   WARREN, KENNETH S. 1929- , & NEWILL, VAUN ARCHIE. 1923-
Schistosomiasis. A bibliography of the world's literature from 1852 to 1962. 2 vols. Cleveland, *Western Reserve University Press*, 1967.

5352.6   WARREN, KENNETH S. 1929-
Schistosomiasis: the evolution of a medical literature. Selected abstracts and citations, 1852-1952. Cambridge, Mass., *M.I.T. Press*, 1973.
Includes 384 core references and bibliography (without abstracts) covering 1963-72.

Hookworm Disease

5353   DUBINI, ANGELO. 1813-1902
Nuovo verme intestinale umano (Agchylostoma duodenale), constituente un sesto genere dei nematoidei proprii dell' uomo. *Ann. univ. Med. (Milano)*, 1843, **106**, 5-51.
Dubini first found the hookworm of ankylostomiasis in 1838. His account of 1843, describing it, named it *Agchylostoma duodenale*, a name etymologically erroneous. Partial English translation in Kean (No. 2268.1).

5354   SIEBOLD, CARL THEODOR ERNST VON. 1804-1885
Bericht über die Leistungen im Gebiete der Helminthologie während des Jahres 1843 und 1844. *Arch. Naturgesch.*, 1845, **2**, 202-55.
Siebold classified the hookworm as belonging to the *Strongyloidae* (pp. 220-21).

5355   GRIESINGER, WILHELM. 1817-1868
Klinische und anatomische Beobachtungen über die Krankheiten von Aegypten. *Arch. physiol. Heilk.*, 1854, **13**, 528-75.
Griesinger connected the worm of ankylostomiasis with Egyptian chlorosis, a condition in which the worm had previously been noted without its being considered the causal agent (pp. 555-61). Apparently Bilharz in 1853 came to the same conclusion. The disease was for a time called "Griesinger's disease". Partial English translation in Kean (No. 2268.1).

5356   WUCHERER, OTTO EDUARD HEINRICH. 1820-1873
Sobre a molestia vulgarmente denominada oppilaçao ou cançaço. *Gaz. med. Bahia*, 1886, **1**, 27-29, 39-41, 52-54, 63-64.
Wucherer confirmed Griesinger's conclusion that the cause of tropical anaemia was hookworm infestation. See also the same journal, 1869, **3**, 170-72, 183-84, 198-200. English translation in Kean (No. 2268.1).

5357   GRASSI, GIOVANNI BATTISTA. 1854-1925, *et al.*
Intorno all' Anchilostoma duodenale (Dubini). *Gazz. med. ital. lomb.*, 1878,
7 ser., **5**, 193-96.
Faecal diagnosis of hookworm disease. Before this time hookworm had
been diagnosed only post mortem. With C. Parona and E. Parona. English
translation in Kean (No. 2268.1).

5358   BOZZOLO, CAMILLO. 1845-1920
L'anchilostomiasi e l'anemia che ne conseguita (anchilostomanemia). *G.
int. Sci. med.*, 1879, n.s. **1**, 1054-69, 1245-53.
Introduction of thymol as a hookworm vermifuge.

5359   LEIDY, JOSEPH. 1823-1891
Remarks on parasites and scorpions. *Trans. Coll. Phys. Philad.*, 1886, 3 ser.,
8, 441-43.
Leidy found the hookworm in the cat and suggested that it might also
be found in man as a cause of pernicious anaemia.

5360   BLICKHAHN, WALTER L.
A case of ankylostomiasis. *Med. News (Philad.)*, 1893, **63**, 662-63.
First recognition of ankylostomiasis in America. It had previously been
reported and described under various names.

5361   LOOSS, ARTHUR. 1861-1923
Notizen zur Helminthologie Aegyptens. Die Lebensgeschichte des
Anchylostomum duodenale(Dub.). *Zbl. Bakt.*, I Abt., 1896, **20**, 865-70; 1898,
24, 441-49, 483-88.
Looss elucidated the life cycle and mode of transmission of the
hookworm. *See also* No. 5365. English translation in Kean (No. 2268.1).

5362   ———. Ueber das Eindringen der Ankylostomalarven in die menschliche
Haut. *Zbl. Bakt.*, Abt.1, 1901, **29**, Orig., 733-39.
Looss discovered that hookworms can penetrate the skin; he himself
became infected when hookworm culture accidentally spilled on his
hands. English translation in Kean (No. 2268.1).

5362.1 BENTLEY, CHARLES ALBERT. 1873-1949
On the causal relationship between "ground itch", or "pani-ghao", and the
presence of the larvae of the *Ankylostoma duodenale* in the soil. *Brit. med.
J.*, 1902, **1**, 190-93.
While a medical officer in the tea plantations in Assam, Bentley
demonstrated the mode of entry of *Ankylostoma* into the body.

5363   STILES, CHARLES WARDELL. 1867-1941
A new species of hookworm (Uncinaria americana) parasitic in man.
Amer. Med., 1902, **3**, 777-78.
Discovery of the American species of hookworm, afterward re-named
Necator americanus. It was later believed to have originated in Africa,
being brought over by slaves.

5365   LOOSS, ARTHUR. 1861-1923
The anatomy and life history of Agchylostoma duodenale Dub. A.
monograph. 2 pts. Cairo, *National Printing Office*, 1905-11.

Vols. 3 and 4 of *Records of the School of Medicine, Cairo*. In 1898 Looss discovered that hookworm larvae can penetrate the skin. His monograph epitomized all knowledge of the condition to 1911.

5366   PERRONCITO, Edoardo. 1847-1936
La malattia dei minatori dal S. Gottardo al Sempione. Torino, *C. Pasta*, 1910.
Includes reprints of Perroncito's earlier papers. He insisted on the parasitic origin of the disease as it occurred among the St. Gotthard tunnellers in 1880, and he introduced *Felix mas* as a vermifuge against hookworm.

5367   SCHÜFFNER, Wilhelm. 1867-1949, & VERVOORT, Herman.
Das Oleum chenopodii anthelmintici gegen Ankylostomiasis im Vergleich zu anderen Wurmmitteln. *Trans. int. Congr. Hyg. Demogr.*, 1912, Washington, 1913, **1**, 734-39.
Schüffner and Vervoort introduced oil of chenopodium for the treatment of ankylostomiasis as early as 1900.

5368   HALL, Maurice Crowther. 1881-1938
The use of carbon tetrachloride for the removal of hookworms. *J. Amer. med. Assoc.*, 1921, **77**, 1641-43.
Introduction of the carbon tetrachloride treatment of ankylostomiasis.

5369   ROCKEFELLER FOUNDATION.
Bibliography of hookworm disease. New York, *Rockefeller Foundation*, 1922.
Contains 5,680 references to all aspects of hookworm disease, prefaced by a short history.

5369.1   WORLD HEALTH ORGANIZATION.
Bibliography of hookworm disease (ancylostomiasis) 1920-62. Genève, *World Health Organization*, 1965.

RICKETTSIAL INFECTIONS

5370   CARDANO, Girolamo [cardanus (hieronymus)]. 1501-1576
De malo recentiorum medicorum medendi usu libellus. Venetiis, *apud O. Scotum*, 1536.
Includes (cap. XXXVI) an early account of typhus, *morbus pulicaris*. English translation in Major, *Classic descriptions of disease*, 3rd ed., Springfield, 1945, p. 163.

5371   FRACASTORO, Girolamo [Fracastorius]. 1478-1553
De sympathia et antipathia rerum liber unus. De contagione et contagiosis morbis et curatione. Venetiis, *apud heredes L. Iuntae*, 1546.
This book, which contains one of the first accounts of typhus (pp. 43-44), marks an epoch in the history of medicine, since Fracastorius enunciated in it, perhaps for the first time, the modern doctrine of the specific characters and infectious nature of fevers. He is remembered for his poem on syphilis, but he was also eminent as a physicist, geologist, astronomer, and pathologist. *See* No. 2528.

5372   BRAVO, Francisco. *circa* 1530-1594
Tavardete. In his *Opera medicinalia*, Mexico, *P. Ocharte*, 1570, ff. 1-90.
Original description of tabardillo (Spanish or Mexican typhus). The *Opera* was the first medical book published in the New World; it includes references to native drugs and to parturition and its complications. It was reprinted, with bibliographical and biographical introduction by F. Guerra, 2 vols., London, *Dawson*, 1970.

5372.1   COYTTARUS, Joannes. *d.* 1590
De febre purpura epidemiali et contagiosa libri duo. Parisiis, *apud M. Juvenem*, 1578.
Coyttarus distinguished between petechial typhus and typhoid.

5373   COBER, Tobias. *d*1625
Observationum medicarum Castrensium Hungaricarum. Helmstadii, *F. Lüderwald*, 1685.
Pp. 49-51: Cober, a German physician, reported the relationship between typhus and pediculosis.

5374   PRINGLE, *Sir* John. 1707-1782
Observations on the nature and cure of hospital and jayl-fevers. London, *A. Millar & D. Wilson*, 1750.
Pringle was a strong advocate of better ventilation in prisons and hospitals as a means of preventing typhus, which he showed to be identical with "hospital fever".

5375   HILDENBRAND, Johann Valentin von. 1763-1818
Ueber den ansteckenden Typhus. Wien, 1810.
Hildenbrand gave a classic description of typhus. The French literature sometimes refers to the condition as "Hildenbrand's disease". English translation by S. D. Gross, 1829.

5376   VIRCHOW, Rudolf Ludwig Karl. 1821-1902
Ueber den Hungertyphus und einige verwandte Krankheitsformen. Berlin, *A. Hirschwald*, 1868.
Virchow was instrumental in introducing into Germany an epidemiology based on the study of multiple factors – sociological as well as bacteriological. In the above report on the reappearance of typhus in Berlin and East Prussia, he showed the connection between famine conditions and typhus outbreaks and strongly emphasized the social element in the generation of typhus. English translation, London, 1868.

5376.1   BAELZ, Erwin. 1849-1913, & KAWAKAMI.
Das japanische Fluss- oder Ueberschwemmings-fieber, eine acute Infectionskrankheit. *Virchows Arch. path. Anat.*, 1879, **78**, 373-420, 528-30.
Early scientific account of tsutsugamushi fever.

5377   MAXEY, Edward Ernest. 1867-1934
Some observations on the so-called spotted fever of Idaho. *Med. Sentinel (Portland, Ore.)*, 1899, **7**, 433-38.
Rocky Mountain spotted fever first described.

5378   RICKETTS, HOWARD TAYLOR. 1871-1910
The transmission of Rocky Mountain spotted fever by the bite of the wood-tick (*Dermacentor occidentalis*). *J. Amer. med. Assoc.*, 1906, **47**, 358.
     Ricketts (who himself died of typhus) demonstrated that the wood tick *Dermacentor andersoni* is a vector of Rocky Mountain spotted fever.

5379   ———. A micro-organism which apparently has a specific relationship to Rocky Mountain spotted fever. A preliminary report. *J. Amer. med. Assoc.*,1909, **52**, 379-80.
     Description of the causal organism, in blood smears.

5380   ———. & WILDER, RUSSELL MORSE. 1885-1952
The relation of typhus fever (tabardillo) to Rocky Mountain spotted fever. *Arch. intern. Med.*, 1910, **5**, 361-70.
     Ricketts and Wilder differentiated Rocky Mountain spotted fever and typhus.

5380.1   ———. The etiology of the typhus fever (tabardillo) of Mexico City. A further preliminary report. *J. Amer. med. Assoc.*, 1910, **54**, 1373-75.
     Demonstration of the causal organism of typhus.

5381   WILSON, WILLIAM JAMES. 1879-1954
On heterologous agglutinins more particularly those present in the blood serum of cerebro-spinal fever and typhus fever cases. *J. Hyg. (Camb.)*, 1909, **9**, 316-40.
     The reaction described by Wilson was later developed by Weil and Felix and named after them (*see* No. 5390). See also the paper by Wilson in *J. Hyg.*, 1920, **19**, 115-30.

5382   BRILL, NATHAN EDWIN. 1860-1925
An acute infectious disease of unknown origin. A clinical study based on 221 cases. *Amer. J. med. Sci.*, 1910, **139**, 484-502.
     "Brill's disease" – recrudescent typhus; first description.

5383   CONOR, ALFRED LEON JOSEPH. 1870-1914, & BRUCH, A.
Une fièvre éruptive observée en Tunisie. *Bull. Soc. Path. exot.*, 1910, **3**, 492-96.
     First description of fièvre boutonneuse, a form of tick-borne typhus found in Tunisia.

5384   NICOLLE, CHARLES JULES HENRI. 1866-1936
Recherches expérimentales sur le typhus exanthématique. *Ann. Inst. Pasteur*, 1910, **24**, 243-75; 1911, **25**, 97-144; 1912, **26**, 250-80, 332-50.
     Nicolle demonstrated the transmission of typhus by the body louse *Pediculus corporis*. He also produced the disease in monkeys and guinea-pigs by the injection of infected blood. He was awarded the Nobel Prize in 1928. Preliminary communication in *C. R. Acad. Sci. (Paris)*, 1909, **149**, 486-89.

5384.1   PROWAZEK, STANISLAUS JOSEPH MATTHIAS VON. 1875-1915
Ätiologische Untersuchungen über den Flecktyphus in Serbien 1913 und in Hamburg 1914. *Beitr. Klin. InfektKr.*, 1915, **4**, 5-31.
     Prowazek, like Ricketts and Wilder, demonstrated the specific causal agent in typhus. Like Ricketts he died of the disease.

5385   GRAHAM, JOHN HENRY PORTEUS. ?1869-1957
        A note on a relapsing febrile illness of unknown origin. *Lancet*, 1915, **2**, 703-04.
           First reported case of "trench fever".

5386   HUNT, GOERGE HERBERT. 1884-1926, & RANKIN, ALLAN COATS. 1877-1959
        Intermittent fever of obscure origin, occurring among British soldiers in France. The so-called "trench-fever". *Lancet*, 1915, **2**, 1133-36.
           In this paper trench fever is so named for the first time.

5387   HIS, WILHELM, *Jnr*. 1863-1934
        Ueber eine neue periodische Fiebererkrankung (Febris Wolhynica). *Berl. klin. Wschr.*, 1916, **53**, 322-23.
           His encountered a form of "trench fever" in Volhynia, Russia, and named it after that district.

5388   ROCHA-LIMA, HENRIQUE DA. 1879-1956
        Zur Aetiologie des Fleckfiebers. *Berl. klin. Wschr.*, 1916, **53**, 567-69.
           Rickettsia prowazeki, cause of typhus, was first isolated by da Rocha-Lima, who named it after Ricketts and Prowazek, both of whom died of the disease.

5389   TÖPFER, HANS WILLI. 1876-
        Zur Ursache und Uebertragung des Wolhynischen Fiebers. *Münch. med. Wschr.*, 1916, **63**, 1495-96.
           Isolation of *Rickettsia quintana* from lice found on patients suffering from trench fever.

5390   WEIL, EDMUND. 1880-1922, & FELIX, ARTHUR. 1887-1956
        Zur serologischen Diagnose des Fleckfiebers. *Wien. klin. Wschr.*, 1916, **29**, 33-35.
           Weil–Felix reaction for the diagnosis of typhus. See also the later paper in the same journal, 1916, **29**, 974-78.

5391   WOLBACH, SIMEON BURT. 1880-1954
        Studies on Rocky Mountain spotted fever. *J. med. Res.*, 1919, **41**, 1-197.
           In his important aetiological and pathological studies of Rocky Mountain spotted fever, Wolbach mentioned the causal agent *Dermacentroxenus rickettsi*.

5392   LOEWE, LEO. 1896- , *et al.*
        Cultivation of rickettsia-like bodies in typhus fever. *J. Amer. med. Assoc.*, 1921, **77**, 1967-69.
           Isolation of *Rickettsia prowazeki* from the blood. With S. A. Ritter and G. Baehr.

5393   WOLBACH, SIMEON BURT. 1880-1954, *et al.*
        The etiology and pathology of typhus. Cambridge, *Harvard Univ. Press*, 1922.
           The carefully controlled experiments of Wolbach, J. L. Todd, and F. W. Palfrey eliminated all doubt that *R. prowazeki* was the causal agent in typhus.

5394   FLETCHER, WILLIAM. *d*.1938, & LESSLAR, J. E.
Tropical typhus in the Federated Malay States, with a compilation on epidemic typhus. London, *John Bale*, 1925.
    Bull. Inst. med. Res., F. M. S., No. 2. Drew attention to scrub typhus in Malaya.

5395   ——. The Weil–Felix reaction in sporadic tropical typhus. London, *John Bale*, 1926.
Bull. Inst. Med. Res., F. M. S., 1926, No. 1.Demonstration that scrub-typhus patients developed agglutinins against the OX-K strain of *B. proteus* but not the OX-19 strain.

5396   MAXCY, KENNETH FULLER. 1889-1966
Clinical observations on endemic typhus (Brill's disease) in Southern United States. *Publ. Hlth. Rep. (Wash.)*, 1926, **41**, 1213-20, 2967-95.
    Maxcy described murine (flea-borne) typhus ("Maxcy's disease").

5396.1   MOOSER, HERMANN. 1891-1971
Experiments relating to the pathology and the etiology of Mexican typhus (tabardillo). *J. infect. Dis.*, 1928, **43**, 241-72.
    Mooser differentiated murine from epidemic typhus. The causative organism was later named *Rickettsia mooseri*.

5396.2   DYER, ROLLO EUGENE. 1886-, *et al.*
Typhus fever. A virus of the typhus type derived from fleas collected from wild rats. *Publ. Hlth. Rep. (Wash.)*, 1931, **46**, 334-38.
    Murine typhus shown to be caused by an organism later named *Rickettsia mooseri*, transmitted by fleas from rats to man. With A. Rumreich and L. F. Badger.

5396.3   OGATA, NORIO. 1883-
Aetiologie der *Tsutsugamushi*-Krankheit: *Rickettsia tsutsugamushi. Zbl. Bakt.*, I Abt., Orig., 1931, **122**, 249-53.
    Ogata isolated the causal agent of tsutsugamushi disease in 1927.

5396.4   ZINSSER, HANS. 1878-1940
Varieties of typhus virus and the epidemiology of the American form of European typhus fever (Brill's disease). *Amer. J. Hyg.*, 1934, **20**, 513-32.
    Zinsser advanced the theory that Brill's disease is a recrudescence of epidemic typhus in persons who have contracted the typhus some time previously. The condition has subsequently been renamed "Brill–Zinsser disease".

5397   DERRICK, EDWARD HOLBROOK. 1898-1976
"Q" fever, a new fever entity: clinical features and laboratory investigation. *Med. J. Aust.*, 1937, **2**, 281-99.
    First account of "Q" (query) fever. *See also* No. 5398.

5398   BURNET, *Sir* FRANK MACFARLANE. 1899-1985, & FREEMAN, MAVIS.
Experimental studies on the virus of "Q" fever. *Med. J. Aust.*, 1937, **2**, 299-305.
    Discovery of *Rickettsia burneti*, causal agent in Q fever.

5398.1   COX, HERALD REA. 1907- , & BELL, E. JOHN.
Epidemic and endemic typhus. Protective value for guinea pigs of vaccines prepared from infected tissues of the developing chick embryo. *Publ. Hlth. Rep. (Wash.)*, 1940, **55**, 110-15.
Typhus vaccine.

5398.2   LEWTHWAITE, RAYMOND. 1894-1972, & SAVOOR, S. R. 1900-1980
Rickettsia disease of Malaya. Identity of tsutsugamushi and rural typhus. *Lancet*, 1940, **1**, 255-59, 305-11.
Lewthwaite and Savoor showed scrub typhus to be identical to tsutsugamushi fever.

5398.3   YEOMANS, ANDREW. 1907- , *et al.*
The therapeutic effect of para-aminobenzic acid in louse-borne typhus fever. *J. Amer. med. Assoc.*, 1944, **126**, 349-56.
With J. C. Snyder, E. S. Murray, C. J. D. Zarafonetis, and R. S. Ecke.

5399   FULTON, FORREST. 1913- , & JOYNER, L.
Cultivation of *Rickettsia tsutsugamushi* in lungs of rodents. Preparation of a scrub-typhus vaccine. *Lancet*, 1945, **2**, 729-34.
Scrub-typhus vaccine.

5400   HUEBNER, ROBERT JOSEPH. 1914- , *et al.*
Rickettsialpox. A newly recognized rickettsial disease. IV. Isolation of a rickettsia apparently identical with the causative agent of rickettsialpox from *Allodermanyssus sanguineus*, a rodent mite. *Publ. Hlth. Rep. (Wash.)*, 1946, **61**, 1677-82.
Isolation of *Rickettsia akari*, aetiologic agent of rickettsialpox. With W. L. Jellison and C. Pomerantz.

5401   SUSSMAN, LEON NATHANIEL. 1907-
Kew Gardens spotted fever. *New York Med.*, 1946, **2**, No. 15, 27-28.
Rickettsialpox described.

5402   SMADEL, JOSEPH EDWIN. 1907-1963, & JACKSON, ELIZABETH B.
Chloromycetin, an antibiotic with chemotherapeutic activity in experimental rickettsial and viral infections. *Science*, 1947, **106**, 418-419.
Chloramphenicol used in treatment of typhus.

5402.1   STOKER, *Sir* MICHAEL GEORGE PARKE. 1918-
Serological evidence of Q fever in Great Britain. *Lancet*, 1949, **1**, 178-79.
Relationship of primary atypical pneumonia and Q fever.

5403   ZINSSER, HANS. 1878-1940
Rats, lice and history: being a study in biography, which, after 12 preliminary chapters indispensable for the preparation of the lay reader, deals with the life history of typhus fever. Boston, *Little, Brown & Co.*, 1935.

SMALLPOX (AND VACCINATION)

5404   RHAZES, [ABU BAKR MUHAMMAD IBN ZAKARIYA AL-RAZI]. *circa* 854-925 or 935
De variolis et morbillis commentarius. Londini, *G. Bowyer*, 1766.

The first medical description of smallpox was written by Rhazes, about the year 910. . The above work is the first edition of the Arabic text with a parallel Latin translation by the English pharmacist and scholar, John Channing, concerning whom see E. Savage-Smith, John Channing: Eighteen-century apothecary and arabist. *Pharmacy in history*, 1988, **30**, 63-80. For an English translation see *Med. Classics*, 1939, **4**, 22-84. A translation was also published by the Sydenham Society, 1848. See Nos. 2527 & 5441.

5405   VOLLGNAD, HEINRICH. 1634-1682
Globus vitulinus. *Misc. Curiosa sive Ephem. nat. cur.*, Jenae, 1671, **2**, 181-82.
First authentic report on variolation.

5406   THACHER, THOMAS. 1620-1678
A brief rule to guide the common-people of New-England how to order themselves and theirs in the small pocks, or measels. Boston, *J. Foster,* 1677 [i.e. 1678].
Broadside. The first medical publication of North America and the only one to appear in the 17th century. The sheet was reprinted, with a bibliographical and biographical study, in *Bibliotheca Medica Americana*, Vol. 1, Baltimore, 1937.

5407   SYDENHAM, THOMAS. 1624-1689
Observationes medicae circa morborum acutorum historiam et curationem. Ed. quarta. Londini, *G. Kettilby*, 1685.
Contains (Book 3, Cap. 2; Book 5, Cap. 4) an important account of smallpox, particularly the epidemics of 1667-69 and 1674-75. Sydenham attributed smallpox to a specific inflammation of the blood; he clearly distinguished it from measles. His treatment of fevers with fresh air and cooling drinks was an improvement on the sweating methods previously employed. English translation in his *Works*, ed. R. G. Latham, London, 1848, **1**, 123, 219.

5409   TIMONI, EMANUELE. *d.* 1718
An account, or history, of the procuring of the smallpox by incision or inoculation, as it has for some time been practised at Constantinople. *Phil. Trans.*, 1714-16, **29**, 72-82.
A letter dated December, 1713 from Timoni of Constantinople to John Woodward and read to the Royal Society in May, 1714 described the practice in that city of inoculation against smallpox. The letter aroused interest in inoculation in England. A fellow of the Royal Society since 1703, Timoni was the first to write on this subject for Western physicians, although Pylarini's researches had commenced in 1701.

5409.1   PILARINO, GIACOMO [PYLARINI]. 1659-1718
Nova et tuta variolas excitandi per transplantationem methodus; nuper inventa et in usum tracta. Venetiis, *apud J. G. Hertz*, 1715.
Inoculation was practised in ancient times. Pilarino in 1701 inoculated three children at Constantinople with smallpox virus. He is accredited with the "medical" discovery of variolation, and thus is the first immunologist. His book records his many researches on the subject.

5410   PILARINO, GIACOMO. 1659-1718
Nova & tuta variolas excitandi per transplantationem methodus, nuper inventa & in usum tracta. *Phil. Trans.*, 1714-16, **29**, 393-99.

This reprint of No. 5409.1 appeared in the same volume as Timoni's paper. Both were republished in Latin: *Tractatus bini de nova variolas per transplantationem excitandi methodo*, Leyden, 1721.

5410.1   BOYLSTON, ZABDIEL. 1680-1766.
Some account of what is said of inoculating or transplanting the small pox by the learned Dr. Emmanuel Timonius, and Jacobus Pylarinus. With some remarks theron...Boston, *S. Gerrish*, 1721.
    An abridgement of Nos. 5409 & 5410 together with Boylston's remarks. From internal evidence this would appear to be the first North American publication on inoculation. *See* No. 5415.

5411   COLMAN, BENJAMIN. 1673-1747
Some observations on the new method of receiving the smallpox by ingrafting or inoculating. Boston, *B. Green, for S. Gerrish*, 1721.
    This work offers general support for the practice of Zabdiel Boylston, detailing some of Boylston's cases, including accounts of occasions when patients died. Reprinted with additional material by Daniel Neal, as *A narrative of the method and success of inoculating the small-pox in New England, by Mr. Benj. Colman*...London, 1722.

5412   DOUGLASS, WILLIAM. 1691-1752
Inoculation of the smallpox as practised in Boston. Boston, *J. Franklin*, 1722.

5413   ——. The abuses and scandals of some late pamphlets in favour of inoculation of the small-pox. Boston, *J. Franklin*, 1722.
    Douglass at first opposed inoculation for smallpox, but by 1730 he had changed his views and had become an advocate of inoculation.

5414   MATHER, COTTON. 1663-1728
An account of the method and success of inoculating the small pox in Boston in New England. London, *Peele*, 1722.
    Mather republished reports of earlier writers on inoculation. He persuaded Boylston to adopt the practice in June 1721, and he supported Boylston during a period of great opposition to inoculation.

5414.1   MAITLAND, CHARLES. 1668-1748
Mr. Maitland's account of inoculating the small pox. London, *For the author by J. Downing*, 1722.
    Maitland inoculated the children of Lady Mary Wortley Montagu in 1721, and also inoculated six condemned prisoners as part of the so-called "Royal Experiment". Success with these trials lead to his inoculation of the children of the Prince of Wales, and to the popularization of inoculation in England.

5415   BOYLSTON, ZABDIEL. 1680-1766
An historical account of the small-pox inoculated in New England. London, *S. Chandler*, 1726.
    Boylston was the first in America to inoculate for smallpox, at Boston on 26 June 1721.

5416   KIRKPATRICK, JAMES [KILLPATRICK]. *d.* 1770
An essay on inoculation, occasioned by the small-pox being brought into South Carolina in the year 1738. London, *J. Huggonson*, 1743.

After its initial popularity, inoculation fell into disuse in England. Kirkpatrick, who became a prominent inoculator in England after experience in America, helped considerably in reviving its popularity. He attempted the attenuation of the virus by his arm-to-arm method of inoculation.

5417   MEAD, RICHARD. 1673-1754
De variolis et morbillis liber. Londini, *J. Brindley*, 1747.
Includes a Latin translation of Rhazes's commentary. Mead favoured inoculation, and his great authority and influence helped towards a more general acceptance of this measure. English translation entitled *A discourse on the small pox and measles*, London, 1748.

5418   THOMSON, ADAM. *d.*1767
A discourse on the preparation of the body for the small-pox; and the manner of receiving the infection. Philadelphia, *B. Franklin & D. Hall*, 1750.
Thomson was the originator of the American method of inoculation against smallpox.

5419   FRANKLIN, BENJAMIN. 1706-1790
Some account of the success of inoculation for the small-pox in England and America. Together with plain instructions, by which any person may be enabled to perform the operation. London, *W. Strahan*, 1759.
Franklin's statistical account of smallpox inoculation in Boston during the epidemic of 1753-54, showing the beneficial effects of the practice, was written for William Heberden, who contributed the "Plain instructions" mentioned on the title. Early in his life Franklin had actively opposed inoculation but he became one of its strongest advocates after the tragic death of his son from smallpox in 1736.

5420   DIMSDALE, THOMAS, *Baron Dimsdale*. 1712-1800
The present method of inoculating for the small-pox. London, *W. Owen*, 1767.
Dimsdale is notable as having inoculated Catherine of Russia and her son. For this he received a fee of £10,000 and a life pension. His reputation and the exalted rank of his patient helped in popularizing the measure in England. Dimsdale used material from the inoculated site of another patient.

5421   HUNTER, JOHN. 1728-1793
Account of a woman who had the smallpox during pregnancy, and who seemed to have communicated the same disease to the foetus. *Phil. Trans.*, 1780, **70**, 128-42.

5422   RUSH, BENJAMIN. 1745-1813
The new method in inoculating for the small pox. Philadelphia, *C. Cist*, 1781.

5423   JENNER, EDWARD. 1749-1823
An inquiry into the causes and effects of the variolae vaccinae. London, *S. Low*, 1798.
Jenner established the fact that a "vaccination" or inoculation with vaccinia (cowpox) lymph matter protects against smallpox. He performed his first vaccination on May 14, 1796. The above work, describing 23 successful vaccinations, announced to the world one of the greatest

triumphs in the history of medicine. Jennerian vaccination soon superseded the protective inoculation of material from human cases of smallpox, which had previously been in vogue. What is probably the first
mention of anaphylaxis appears on p. 13 of the pamphlet. See W.R. Lefanu,
A *Bio-bibliography of Edward Jenner*, 1749-1823, rev. 2nd. ed., Winchester, *St. Paul's Bibliographies*, 1985. Several facsimile editions have
been published. As a result of the success of Jenner's vaccine natural
smallpox was eradicated. The official declaration was made by the World
Health Organization on May 8, 1980. *See* No. 5434.2. *See also* No. 2529.1.

5424   WATERHOUSE, BENJAMIN. 1754-1846
A prospect of exterminating the small-pox. 2 pts. Boston, *W. Hilliard*,
(Cambridge [Mass.], *Univ. Press)*, 1800-02.
  Waterhouse introduced Jennerian vaccination into the U.S.A. He
inoculated his own child as his first case. See J. B. Blake, *Benjamin
Waterhouse and the introduction of vaccination. A reappraisal.* Phila-
delphia, 1957.

5425   COXE, JOHN REDMAN. 1773-1864
Practical observations on vaccination: or inoculation for the cow pock.
Philadelphia, *J. Humphreys*, 1802.
  Coxe did much to destroy ignorant prejudice against vaccination; he
was the first in Philadelphia to practise it. Like Waterhouse he inoculated
his own child as his first case.

5425.1 CHAUVEAU, JEAN BAPTISTE AUGUSTE. 1827-1917
Nature des virus vaccin. Détermination expérimentale des éléments qui
constituent le principe virulent dans le pus varioleux et le pus morveux. *C.
R. Acad. Sci. (Paris)*, 1868, **66**, 359-63.
  Chauveau first used the term "elementary bodies" to describe the
minute bodies inside the inclusions and which were the infective particles.

5426   WEIGERT, CARL. 1845-1904
Anatomische Beiträge zur Lehre von den Pocken. 2 pts. Breslau, *M. Cohn
u. Weigert*, 1874-75.
  In the course of his important studies on smallpox, Weigert carried out
the first successful staining of bacteria (*see* No. 2482). His fine description
of the destructive effects of the smallpox virus on the skin led to the coining
of the term "coagulation necrosis" as a name for the process causing the
development of the lesions.

5427   BUIST, JOHN BROWN. 1846-1915
The life-history of the micro-organisms associated with variola and vaccinia.
An abstract of results obtained from a study of smallpox and vaccination
in the surgical laboratory of the University of Edinburgh. *Proc. roy. Soc.
Edinb.*, 1886, **13**, 603-20.
  The "Paschen elementary bodies" (No. 5430) were first recognized and
demonstrated by Buist. Republished as an appendix to his *Vaccinia and
variola*, London, 1887.

5428   GUARNIERI, GUISEPPE. 1856-1918
Ricerche sulla patogenesi ed etiologia dell' infezione vaccinica e vaiolosa.
Arch. Sci. méd., 1893, **16**, 403-24.

Guarnieri described bodies found in the specific lesions of smallpox. *Cytorrhyctes variolae guarnieri*, which he believed to be the causative organism of the disease.

5429   COPEMAN, SYDNEY ARTHUR MONCKTON. 1862-1947
Vaccination, its natural history and pathology. London, *Macmillan & Co.*, 1899.
Milroy Lectures, Royal College of Physicians, 1898. Copeman's bacteriological studies permanently determined the validity of vaccination as a preventive of smallpox.

5429.1 MAGRATH, GEORGE BURGESS. 1870-1938, & BRINCKERHOFF, WALTER REMSEN. 1875-1911
On experimental variola in the monkey. *J. med. Res.*, 1904, **11**, 230-46.
Inoculation of smallpox into the monkey. An earlier report of successful inoculation by W. Zuelzer (*Zbl. med. Wiss.*, 1874, **12**, 82) is not generally accepted.

5430   PASCHEN, ENRIQUE. 1860-1936
Was wissen wir über den Vakzineerreger? *Münch. med. Wschr.*, 1906, **53**, 2391-93.
"Paschen elementary bodies"; *see also* No. 5427.

5430.1 NOGUCHI, HIDEYO. 1876-1928
Pure cultivation in vivo of vaccine virus free from bacteria. *J. exp. Med.*, 1915, **21**, 539-70.
Noguchi obtained a pure culture of vaccinia virus.

5431   PAUL, GUSTAV. 1859-1935
Zur Differentialdiagnose der Variola und der Varicellen. Die Erscheinungen an der variolierten Hornhaut des Kaninchens und ihre frühzeitige Erkennung. *Zbl. Bakt.*, I Abt., 1915, **75**, Orig., 518-24.
Paul's test for the diagnosis of smallpox.

5432   GORDON, MERVYN HENRY. 1872-1953
Studies of the viruses of vaccinia and variola. London, *H. M. Stationery Office*, 1925.
Medical Research Council Special Report No. 98; a summary of the more important additions to the knowledge of the subject.

5433   LEDINGHAM, *Sir* JOHN CHARLES GRANT. 1875-1944
Studies on variola, vaccinia, and avian molluscum. *J. State Med.*, 1926, **34**, 125-43.
Ledingham's diagnostic test.

5434   McKINNON, NEIL E. 1894- , & DEFRIES, ROBERT DAVIES. 1889-
The reaction of the skin of the normal rabbit following intradermal injection of material from smallpox lesions: the specificity of this reaction and its application as a diagnostic test. *Amer. J. Hyg.*, 1928, **8**, 93-106.
McKinnon's diagnostic test.

5434.1 MAITLAND, HUGH BETHUNE. 1895-1972, & MAITLAND, MARY COWAN. *d.* 1972
Cultivation of vaccinia virus without tissue culture. *Lancet,* 1928, **2**, 596-97.
Introduction of "Maitland's medium".

5434.2 WORLD HEALTH ORGANIZATION
The global eradication of smallpox. Final report of the Global Commission for the Certification of Smallpox Eradication, Geneva, *World Health Organization*, 1980.

On 8 May 1980, the World Health Organization officially announced that "smallpox eradication has been achieved throughout the world". The upper cover of this report reproduces an electron micrograph of a specimen of variola virus taken from the last case of endemic smallpox in the world, 26 October 1977. This was the successful conclusion of worldwide vaccination efforts initiated by Jenner in 1798. *See* No. 5423.

History of Smallpox and Vaccination

5435 CROOKSHANK, EDGAR MARCH. 1858-1928
History and pathology of vaccination. 2 vols. London, *H. K. Lewis*, 1889.

This very full history of the subject caused a good deal of controversy; see the review of it in *Lancet*, 1890, **1**, 470-72. Crookshank was an opponent of vaccination.

5435.1 EDWARDES, EDWARD JOSHUA.
A concise history of small-pox and vaccination in Europe. London, *H. K. Lewis*, 1902.

A comprehensive summary, in tabular form.

5436 KLEBS, ARNOLD CARL. 1870-1943
The historic evolution of variolation. *Johns Hopk. Hosp. Bull.*, 1913, **24**, 69-83.

5436.1 MILLER, GENEVIEVE. 1914-
The adoption of inoculation for smallpox in England and France. Philadelphia, *University of Pennsylvania Press*, 1957.

The appendices contain the early histories of inoculation and a list of German doctoral dissertations on inoculation, 1720-52. There is also an excellent bibliography.

5436.2 HOPKINS, DONALD R.
Princes and peasants: Smallpox in history. Chicago, *University of Chicago Press*, 1983.

CHICKENPOX

5437 INGRASSIA, GIOVANNI FILIPPO. 1510-1580
De tumoribus praeter naturam. Neapoli, 1553.

Ingrassia was first to differentiate varicella from scarlet fever (pp. 194-95).

5438 HEBERDEN, WILLIAM, *Snr.* 1710-1801
On the chickenpox. *Med. Trans. Coll. Phys. Lond.*, 1768, **1**, 427-36.

In a paper read before the (Royal) College of Physicians on 11 August 1767, Heberden first definitely differentiated chickenpox from smallpox.

5439   HUTCHINSON, *Sir* JONATHAN. 1828-1913
On gangrenous eruptions in connection with vaccination and chickenpox.
Med.-chir. Trans., 1882, **65**, 1-12.
Original description of varicella gangrenosa.

5439.1   BOKAY, JANOS. 1858-1937
Das Auftreten von Varizellen unter eigentümlichen Verhältnissen. *Magy.
orv. Arch.*, 1892, (Nov. 3).
Bokay was the first to suggest an aetiological relationship between
varicella and herpes zoster. See also his paper in *Wien. klin. Wschr.*, 1909,
22, 1323-26.

5440   TYZZER, ERNEST EDWARD. 1875-1965
The histology of the skin lesions in varicella. *J. med. Res.*, 1905-06, **14**, 361-
92.
Tyzzer was first to recognize inclusion bodies in varicella.

5440.1   WELLER, THOMAS HUCKLE. 1915-
Serial propagation *in vitro* of agents producing inclusion bodies derived
from varicella and herpes zoster. *Proc. Soc. exp. Biol. (N.Y.)*, 1953, **83**, 340-
46.
Isolation of the varicella-herpes virus.

5440.2   BRUNELL, PHILIP ALFRED. 1931- , *et al.*
Prevention of varicella by zoster immune globulin. *New Engl. J. Med.*, 1969,
280, 1191-94.
With A. Ross, L. H. Miller, and B. Kuo.

MEASLES

5441   RHAZES [ABU BAKR MUHAMMAD IBN ZAKARIYA AL-RAZI]. ?850-?923
A treatise on the smallpox and measles. Translated from Arabic by William
Alexander Greenhill. London, *Sydenham Society*, 1848.
Rhazes differentiated measles from smallpox. Reprinted in *Med. Clas-
sics*, 1939, **4**, 22-84. For original publication *see* No. 5404. The first English
translation appeared in No. 5417.

5441.1   SYDENHAM, THOMAS. 1624-1689
Observationes medicae circa morborum acutorum historiam et curationem.
Londini, *G. Kettilby*, 1676.
Includes (pp. 272-80) the most minute and careful description of
measles that had so far appeared; this is reprinted in *Med. Classics*, 1939,
4, 313-19.

5442   HOME, FRANCIS. 1719-1813
Medical facts and experiments. London, *A. Millar*, 1759.
Experimental human transmission of measles (pp. 266-88).

5443   PANUM, PETER LUDVIG. 1820-1885
Iagttagelser, anstillede under Maeslinge-Epidemien paa Faerøerne i Aaret
1846. *Bibl. Laeger*, 1847, 3 R., **1**, 270-344.
When only 26 years of age, Panum was sent by the Danish Government
to investigate the epidemic of measles then raging in the Faroes. His report

on the subject was a valuable contribution to medical literature. A translation of his papers is in *Med. Classics*, 1939, **3**, 829-86. It was also published in translation by the Delta Omega Society, New York, 1940.

5444   KOPLIK, HENRY. 1858-1927
The diagnosis of the invasion of measles from a study of the exanthema as it appears on the buccal mucous membrane. *Arch. Pediat.*, 1896, **13**, 918-22.
Koplik, American paediatrician, was the first to note and report on "Koplik's spots", the buccal spots which are an important early diagnostic sign in measles.

5445   JOSIAS, ALBERT HENRI LOUIS. 1852-1906
Recherches expérimentales sur la transmissibilité de la rougeole animaux. *Méd. mod.* (Paris), 1898, **9**, 153.
Measles transmitted to animals.

5446   HEKTOEN, LUDVIG. 1863-1951
Experimental measles. *J. infect. Dis.*, 1905, **2**, 238-55.
Experimental human transmission of measles.

5447   CENCI, FRANCESCO.
Alcune esperienze di sieroimmunizzazione e sieroterapia nel morbillo. *Riv. Clin. pediat.*, 1907, **5**, 1017-25.
First use of convalescent serum in prophylaxis against measles.

5448   ANDERSON, JOHN F. 1873-1958, & GOLDBERGER, JOSEPH. 1874-1929
Experimental measles in the monkey. *Publ. Hlth. Rep. (Wash.)*, 1911, **26**, 847-48, 887-95.
Measles transmitted to monkeys.

5449   PLOTZ, HARRY, 1890-1947
Culture "in vitro" du virus de la rougeole. *Bull. Acad. Méd. (Paris)*, 1938, **119**, 598-601.
Successful cultivation of measles virus.

5449.1   ORDMAN, CHARLES WILLIAM. 1914- , *et al.*
Chemical, clinical, and immunological studies on the products of human plasma fractionation. XII. The use of concentrated normal human serum gamma globulin (human immune serum globulin) in the prevention and attenuation of measles. *J. clin. Invest.*, 1944, **23**, 541-49.
Gamma globulin used for passive immunization against measles. With C. G. Jennings and C. A. Janeway.

5449.2   ENDERS, JOHN FRANKLIN. 1897-1985, & PEEBLES, THOMAS C. 1921-
Propagation in tissue cultures of cytopathogenic agents from patients with measles. *Proc. Soc. exp. Biol. (N.Y.)*, 1954, **86**, 277-86.
Isolation of measles virus.

5449.3   KATZ, SAMUEL LAWRENCE. 1927- , *et al.*
Propagation of measles virus in cultures of chick embryo cells. *Proc. Soc. exp. Biol. (N.Y.)*, 1958, **97**, 23-29.
With M. V. Milovanovič and J. F. Enders.

5449.4   ENDERS, JOHN FRANKLIN. 1897-1985, *et al.*
Studies on an attenuated measles-virus vaccine. I. Development and preparation of the vaccine: technics for assay of effects of vaccination. *New Engl. J. Med.*, 1960, **263**, 153-59.
Live virus vaccine. With S. L. Katz, M. V. Milovanovič, and A. Holloway.

YELLOW FEVER

5449.5   ABREU, ALEXO DE. 1568-1630
Tratado de las siete enfermedades, *etc.* Lisboa, *P. Craesbeeck,* 1623.
Contains (fol. 193v-199v) an account of yellow fever. For full title of the book, *see* No. 2262.1

5450   DU TERTRE, JEAN BAPTISTE.
Histoire générale des Antilles habités par les Français. Tom. 1. Paris, 1667.
Du Tertre, a priest, described (pp. 81, 99, 423) the outbreaks of yellow fever at Guadeloupe in 1635, 1640, and 1648.

5451   CAREY, MATHEW. 1760-1839
A short account of the malignant fever, lately prevalent in Philadelphia. Philadelphia, *The Author,* 1793.
In this little book, which passed through four editions in a few months, Carey left a graphic description of the great yellow fever epidemic of Philadelphia in 1793. He gave a good clinical description of the disease, mentioning the efficacy and the failure of many forms of treatment.

5452   CURRIE, WILLIAM. 1754-1828
A description of the malignant, infectious fever prevailing at present in Philadelphia. Philadelphia, *T Dobson,* 1793.

5453   RUSH, BENJAMIN. 1745-1813
An account of the bilious remitting yellow fever, as it appeared in the city of Philadelphia in the year 1793. Philadelphia, *T. Dobson,* 1794.
Benjamin Rush was the most eminent figure in Philadelphia medicine in his day. His description of the yellow fever epidemic of 1793 is classic. He did magnificent work in treating the sick during the epidemic and in proposing measures to prevent a recurrence.

5453.1   J[ONES], A[BSOLOM]. 1746-1818, & A[LLEN], R[ICHARD]. 1760-1831
A narrative of the proceedings of the black people during the late awful calamity in Philadelphia, in the year 1793: and a refutation of some censures thrown upon them in some late publications. Philadelphia, *W. W. Woodward,* 1794.
A refutation of slights by Carey in the 2nd and 3rd editions of his *Account* (No. 5451) to the important contributions of black people who played a major role in relief efforts during the epidemic. One of the earliest of Afro-American medical publications.

5454   NOTT, JOSIAH CLARK. 1804-1873
Yellow fever contrasted with bilious fever – reasons for believing it a disease sui generis – its mode of propagation – remote cause – probable insect or animalcular origin. *New Orleans med. surg. J.*, 1848, **4**, 563-601.

Nott advanced the theory that yellow fever was caused by minute animalcula. Reproduced in part in R. H. Major, *Classic descriptions of disease*, 3rd ed., 1945, p. 122.

5454.1   BEAUPERTHUY, Louis Daniel. 1807-1871
Fiebre amarilla. *Gaceta Oficial de Cumaná*, Año 4, No. 57, Mayo 23, 1854.
    Beauperthuy was the first protagonist of the mosquito theory of the transmission of yellow fever. Reprinted in Beauperthuy's *La Obra*, Caracas, 1963, pp. 260-70; French translation in *Travaux scientifiques de Louis-Daniel Beauperthuy*, Bordeaux, 1891, pp. 131-42.

5454.2   LA ROCHE, René. 1795-1872
Yellow fever...2 vols. Philadelphia, *Blanchard & Lea*, 1855.
    The most important 19th century American monograph on yellow fever. La Roche's work sketched the disease in its appearances from 1699 to 1854 at Philadelphia, which saw some of the worst yellow fever epidemics, and provided a splendid bibliography along with discussion of the pathology, aetiology and therapeutics of the disease.

5455   FINLAY, Carlos Juan. 1833-1915
El mosquito hipoteticamente considerado como agente de transmisión de la fiebre amarilla. *Ann. r. Acad. Cienc. méd. Habana*, 1881-82, **18**, 147-69.
    Finlay was the first to suggest that the mosquito carried yellow fever infection from man to man. The paper is reprinted, with translation, in *Med. Classics*, 1938, **2**, 569-612.

5456   CARTER, Henry Rose. 1852-1925
A note on the interval between infecting and secondary cases of yellow fever from the records of yellow fever at Orwood and Taylor, Mississippi, in 1898, *New Orleans med. surg. J.*, 1900, **52**, 617-36.
    Carter did important work on yellow fever. His determination of its incubation period decided the direction of Reed's later researches, which in turn ended in the discovery of the mode of transmission of the yellow fever virus.

5457   REED, Walter. 1851-1902, CARROLL, James. 1854-1907, AGRAMONTE Y SIMONI, Aristide. 1868-1931, & LAZEAR, Jesse William. 1866-1900
The etiology of yellow fever. *Philad. med. J.*, 1900, **6**, 790-96.
    First definite proof that the organism causing yellow fever is transmitted to man by the mosquito *Aëdes aegypti*. During the period spent by these workers in the investigation of the disease, Lazear died from yellow fever after having been accidentally bitten by a mosquito. Reproduced in part in Major, *Classic descriptions of disease*, 3rd ed., 1945, p. 131. Further account in *J. Hyg. (Camb.)*, 1902, **2**, 101-19.

5459   MARCHOUX, Emile. 1862-1943, *et al.*
La fièvre jaune. *Ann. Inst. Pasteur*, 1903, **17**, 665-731.
    Yellow fever convalescent serum employed. With A. T. Salimbeni and P. L. Simond.

5460   GORGAS, William Crawford. 1854-1920
Sanitation of the tropics with special reference to malaria and yellow fever. *J. Amer. med. Assoc.*, 1909, **52**, 1075-77.

In 1901 Gorgas was sent to Havana to undertake a special campaign against the yellow fever mosquito *Aëdes aegypti*. His methods of sanitation were so successful that in three months yellow fever was practically eradicated from Havana. Gorgas outlined the main principles of his methods in the above paper.

5460.1 FRANCO, R., *et al.*
Fiebre amarilla y fiebre espiroquetal; endemias y epidemias en Muzo, de 1907 a 1910. *Acad. nac. Med. Ses. Cient. Centen., Bogotá*, 1911, **1**, 169-228.
Franco, J. Martínez-Santamaria, and G. Toro-Villa described epidemics of yellow fever spread by mosquitoes other than *Ae. aegypti*. Later F. L. Soper, *et al., Amer. J. Hyg.*, 1933, **18**, 555-87, substantiated this.

5461 HINDLE, EDWARD. 1886-1973
A yellow fever vaccine. *Brit. med. J.*, 1928, **1**, 976-77.
First vaccine for immunization against yellow fever. Hindle devised a method for the transportation of frozen infected material from West Africa to London, making it possible to carry on experimental work in Britain.

5462 STOKES, ADRIAN. 1887-1927, *et al.*
Experimental transmission of yellow-fever to laboratory animals. *Amer. J. trop. Med.*, 1928, **8**, 103-64.
Experimental infection of the monkey, *Macacus rhesus*, with the yellow fever virus. Stokes succumbed to yellow fever while investigating the disease. With J. H. Bauer and N. P. Hudson.

5463 THEILER, MAX. 1899-1972
Studies on the action of yellow fever virus in mice. *Ann. trop. Med. Parasit.*, 1930, **24**, 249-72.
The intracerebral protection test in mice, a test for the diagnosis of yellow fever and for the determination of its past existence in a community, was made possible by Theiler's discovery that white mice are susceptible to the intracerebral inoculation of the virus. He was awarded the Nobel Prize in 1951.

5464 SAWYER, WILBUR AUGUSTUS. 1879-1951, & LLOYD, WRAY DEVERE MARR. 1902-1936
The use of mice in tests of immunity against yellow fever. *J. exp. Med.*, 1931, **54**, 533-35.
Intraperitoneal protection test.

5465 ———. *et al.*
Vaccination against yellow fever with immune serum and virus fixed for mice. *J. exp. Med.*, 1932, **55**, 945-69.
These workers devised an immune serum for prophylactic inoculation against yellow fever. With S. F. Kitchen and W. D. M. Lloyd.

5465.1 HAAGEN, EUGEN, & THEILER, MAX. 1899-1972
Untersuchungen über das Verhalten des Gelbfiebervirus in der Gewebekultur. Mit besonderer Berücksichtigung seiner Kultivierbarkeit. *Zbl. Bakt.*, I Abt., Orig., 1932, **125**, 145-58.
Yellow fever virus grown in tissue culture.

5466   THEILER, Max. 1899-1972
A yellow fever protection test in mice by intracerebral injection. *Ann. trop. Med. Hyg.*, 1933, **27**, 57-77.
Intracerebral protection test.

5467   ——. & SMITH, Hugh Hollingsworth. 1902-
The use of yellow fever virus modified by *in vitro* cultivation for human immunization. *J. exp. Med.*, 1937, **65**, 787-800.
Immunization without the use of immune serum.

5467.1   SHANNON, Raymond Corbett. 1894- , *et al.*
Yellow fever virus in jungle mosquitoes. *Science*, 1938, **88**, 110-11.
Haemagogus sp. shown to be vectors of yellow fever. With L. Whitman and M. Frania.

5468   CARTER, Henry Rose. 1852-1925
Yellow fever: an epidemiological and historical study of its place of origin. Edited by Laura Armistead Carter and Wade Hampton Frost. Baltimore, *Williams & Wilkins*, 1931.

DENGUE

5469   BYLON, David.
Korte aantekening wegens eene algemeene ziekte, doorgaans genaamd knokkel-koorts. *Verh. Batav. Genootsch. Kunst en Wet.*, Batavia, 1780, **2**, 17-30.
Bylon described an epidemic of dengue which appeared in the Dutch East Indies in 1779, the first definite description of the disease. O. H. P. Pepper has published a photographic reproduction of the article in *Ann. med. Hist.*, 1941, 3rd ser., **3**, 363-68.

5470   RUSH, Benjamin. 1745-1813
An account of the bilious remitting fever. In his *Medical inquiries and observations*, Philadelphia, 1789, **1**, 104-21.
One of the first important accounts of dengue ("breakbone fever"). Rush described the Philadelphia outbreak of 1780.

5471   DICKSON, Samuel Henry. 1798-1872
On dengue; its history, pathology, and treatment. Philadelphia, *Haswell, Barrington & Haswell*, 1839.

5472   BANCROFT, Thomas Lane. 1860-1933
On the etiology of dengue fever. *Aust. med. Gaz.*, 1906, **25**, 17-18.
Bancroft was the first to produce evidence that *Aëdes aegypti* is a vector of dengue.

5473   ASHBURN, Percy Moreau. 1872-1940, & CRAIG, Charles Franklin. 1872-1950
Experimental investigations regarding the aetiology of dengue fever, with a general consideration regarding the disease. *Philipp. J. Sci. B.*, 1907, **2**, 93-152.
Proof that the causal organism of dengue is a filterable virus. Published also in *J. infect. Dis.*, 1907, **4**, 440-75.

5474　　CLELAND, *Sir* JOHN BURTON. 1878-1971, *et al.*
On the transmission of Australian dengue by the mosquito Stegomyia fasciata. *Med. J. Aust.*, 1916, **2**, 179-84, 200-05.
These workers proved that *Aëdes aegypti (Stegomyia fasciata)* is capable of transmitting dengue fever. See also *J. Hyg. (Camb.)*, 1918, **16**, 317-418. With C. H. Bradley and W. McDonald.

5475　　SIMMONS, JAMES STEVENS. 1890-1954, *et al.*
Experimental studies of dengue. *Philipp. J. Sci.*, 1931, **44**, 1-251.
Proof that *Aëdes albopictus* is a vector of dengue. See also the earlier paper in the same journal, 1930, **41**, 215-29. With J. H. St. John and F. H. K. Reynolds.

5475.1　　SABIN, ALBERT BRUCE. 1906- , & SCHLESINGER, ROBERT WALTER. 1913-
Production of immunity to dengue with virus modified by propagation in mice. *Science*, 1945, **101**, 604-42.
Successful propagation of dengue in mice and production of a vaccine.

5475.2　　KUNO, G. & FLORES, B.
Bibliography of dengue fever and dengue-like illnesses, 1780-1981. Noumea, New Caledonia, *South Pacific Commission*, 1982.

PHLEBOTOMUS (PAPPATACI) FEVER

5476　　PICK, ALOIS. 1859-1945
Zur Pathologie und Therapie einer eigenthümlichen endemischen Krankheitsform. *Wien. med. Wschr.*, 1886, **36**, 1141-45, 1168-71.
This is generally regarded as the first description of pappataci fever.

5477　　DOERR, ROBERT. 1871-1952
Ueber ein neues invisibles Virus. *Berl. klin. Wschr.*, 1908, **45**, 1847-49.
Doerr showed the relation of phlebotomus fever to the sandfly, *Phlebotomus.*

5478　　———. & RUSS, VIKTOR KARL. 1879-
Weitere Untersuchungen über das Pappatacifieber. *Arch. Schiffs- u. Tropenhyg.*, 1909, **13**, 693-706.
Doerr and Russ suggested that the virus of phlebotomus fever may be transmitted from one generation of infected *Phlebotomus papatasii* to another.

5479　　DOERR, ROBERT. 1871-1952, *et al.*
Das Pappatacifieber. Leipzig, Wien, *F. Deuticke*, 1909.
An Austrian military commission consisting of R. Doerr, K. Franz, and S. Taussig proved that the causal organism of pappataci fever was a virus and that *Phlebotomus papatasii* was the vector.

5480　　SHORTT, HENRY EDWARD. 1887-1987, *et al.*
Cultivation of the viruses of sandfly fever and dengue fever on the chorio-allantoic membrane of the chick-embryo. *Indian J. Med. Research*, Calcutta, 1936, **23**, 865-70.
Cultivation of the virus of phlebotomus fever. With R. S. Rao and C. S. Swaminath.

5481   ZINKE, Georg Gottfried.
Neue Ansichten der Hundswuth, ihrer Ursachen und Folgen, nebst einer sichern Behandlungsart der von tollen Thieren gebissenen Menschen. Jena, *C. E. Gabler*, 1804.
Zinke transmitted rabies from a rabid dog to a normal one, and to a rabbit and a hen, by injection of saliva and proved the disease to be infectious.

5481.1   KRÜGELSTEIN, Franz Christian Karl. 1779-1864
Die Geschichte der Hundswuth und der Wasserscheu und deren Behandlung. Gotha, *In der Hennings'schen Buchhandlung*, 1826.
A full account of rabies, summarizing current knowledge, with a bibliography of about 300 items.

5481.2   GALTIER, Victor. 1846-1908
Études sur la rage. *Ann. Méd. vét.*, 1879, **28**, 627-39.
Galtier demonstrated the transmissibility of rabies from dog to rabbit to rabbit in a series, a matter of considerable interest to Pasteur.

5481.3   ——. Les injections de virus rabique dans le torrent circulatoire ne provoquent pas l'éclosion de la rage et semblant conférer l'immunité. La rage peut être transmise par l'ingestion de la matière rabique. *C. R. Acad. Sci. (Paris)*, 1881, **93**, 284-85.
Galtier immunized sheep by inoculating rabid saliva in the veins; this did not produce the disease and protected the animals from a further inoculation. His work aroused the interest of Pasteur.

5481.4   PASTEUR, Louis. 1822-1895, *et al.*
Sur la rage. *C. R. Acad. Sci. (Paris)*, 1881, **92**, 1259-60.
This paper marks the beginning of Pasteur's studies on rabies. With C. Chamberland, P. P. E. Roux, and T. Thuillier. English translation in R. Suzor, *Hydrophobia: An account of M. Pasteur's system...*London, 1887.

5482   ——. Nouvelle communication sur la rage. *C. R. Acad. Sci. (Paris)*, 1884, **98**, 457-63, 1229-31.
Demonstration in the blood of the rabies virus. With C. Chamberland and P.P.E. Roux. English translation in R. Suzor, *Hydrophobia: An account of M. Pasteur's system...*London, 1887.

5483   ——. Méthode pour prévenir la rage après morsure. *C. R. Acad. Sci. (Paris)*, 1885, **101**, 765-74; 1886, **102**, 459-69, 835-38; **103**, 777-85.
Pasteur's papers describing his rabies vaccine, and the results he attained with it gave further proof of the value of attenuated virus as a protective inoculum against infective diseases in man and animals. This is considered Pasteur's greatest triumph. A grateful public subscribed two and a half million francs and made possible the erection of the Institut Pasteur, Paris. English translation of first part in Bibel, *Milestones in immunology* (1988). *See* No. 2541.

5484   NEGRI, ADELCHI. 1876-1912
Contributo allo studio dell' eziologia della rabia. *Boll. Soc. med.-chir. Pavia,*
1903, 88, 229; 1904, 22; 1905, 321.
        Discovery of the "Negri bodies" in rabies, making possible prompt
microscopic diagnosis. German translation in *Z. Hyg. InfektKr.,* 1903, **43**,
507-28.

5484.1   FERMI, CLAUDIO. 1862-
Über die Immunisierung gegen Wutkrankheit. *Z. Hyg. InfektKr.,* 1908, **58**,
233-76.
        Fermi was the first to use chemical treatment of tissue suspensions of
fixed rabies virus for the preparation of vaccine (Fermi vaccine). He
introduced the use of carbolic acid for this purpose.

5484.2   WEBSTER, LESLIE TILLOTSON. 1894-1943, & CLOW, ANNA D.
Propagation of rabies virus in tissue culture and the successful use of
culture virus as antirabic vaccine. *Science,* 1936, **84**, 487-88.
        Webster and Clow succeeded in growing rabies virus in tissue culture.

5484.3   DAWSON, JAMES ROBERTSON. 1908-
Infection of chicks and chick embryos with rabies. *Science,* 1939, **89**,
300-01.
        Cultivation of rabies virus in the chick embryo. Soon afterwards I. J.
Kligler and H. Bernkopf, *Nature,* 1939, **143**, 899, made a similar report.

5484.4   WIKTOR, TADEUSZ J., *et al.*
Human cell culture rabies vaccine. Antibody response in man. *J. Amer. med.
Assoc.,* 1973, **224**, 1170-71.
        Human diploid cell vaccine. With S. A. Plotkin and D. W. Grella. See also
Develop. biol. Standard., 1978, **40**, 3-9.

INFECTIOUS MONONUCLEOSIS

5485   FILATOV, NIL FEODOROVICH. 1847-1902
Lektsii ob ostrikh infektsionnîkh bolierznyakh u dietei. [Lectures on acute
infectious diseases of children.] 2 vols. Moskva, *A. Lang,* 1885-87.
        Glandular fever (infectious mononucleosis) was first described by
Filatov under the name of idiopathic adenitis ("Filatov's disease"). A
German translation of his book appeared in 1895-97.

5486   PFEIFFER, EMIL. 1846-1921
Drüsenfieber. *Jb. Kinderheilk.,* 1889, **29**, 257-64.
        "Pfeiffer's disease". He is by some accredited with the original descrip-
tion of infectious mononucleosis, ascribed to Filatov. Pfeiffer's paper is a
most comprehensive discussion of the clinical aspects of the disease.

5486.1   SPRUNT, THOMAS PECK. 1884-, & EVANS, FRANK ALEXANDER. 1889-
Mononucleosis leukocytosis in reaction to acute infections ("infectious
mononucleosis"). *Bull. Johns Hopk. Hosp.,* 1920, **31**, 410-17.
        Classic account, with first use of the term "infectious mononucleosis".

5487　PAUL, John Rodman. 1893-1971, & BUNNELL, Walls Willard. 1902-
The presence of heterophile antibodies in infectious mononucleosis.
Amer. J. med. Sci., 1932, **183**, 90-104.
The Paul–Bunnell test for the diagnosis of infectious mononucleosis.

5487.1　HENLE, Gertrude, *et al.*
Relation of Burkitt's tumor-associated herpes-type virus to infectious
mononucleosis. *Proc. nat. Acad. Sci. (Wash.)*, 1968, **59**, 94-101.
Epstein–Barr virus shown to be the aetiological agent in infectious
mononucleosis. With W. Henle and V. Diehl.

5488　SAILLANT, Charles Jacques. 1747-1804
Tableau historique et raisonné des épidémies catharrales vulgairement
dites la grippe; depuis 1510 jusques et y compris celle de 1780. Paris, *Didot*,
1780.

5489　THOMPSON, Theophilus. 1807-1860
Annals of influenza or epidemic catarrhal fever in Great Britain from 1510-
1837. London, *Sydenham Society*, 1852.

5490　PFEIFFER, Richard Friedrich Johannes. 1858-1945
Vorläufige Mittheilungen über die Erreger der Influenza. *Dtsch. med. Wschr.*,
1892, **18**, 28.
Pfeiffer discovered a bacillus, *Haemophilus influenzae*, "Pfeiffer's bacillus", which he believed to be the causal organism of influenza.

5491　LEICHTENSTERN, Otto. 1845-1900
Influenza und Dengue. Wien, *A. Hölder*, 1896.
Forms Bd. IV, Teil 1 of Nothnagel's *Specielle Pathologie und Therapie*.

5492　GREAT BRITAIN. *Ministry of health.*
Report on the pandemic of influenza 1918-19. London, *H. M. Stationery
Office*, 1920.
Reports on Public Health and Medical Subjects, No. 4. The most
widespread and serious pandemic of influenza occurred in 1918-19. It
spread throughout Europe, Russia, Canada, S. America, New Zealand,
Australia, Africa, India, China, and Japan. About 21,000,000 people died
from the disease (2,000,000 in Europe alone).

5493　SHOPE, Richard Edwin. 1901-1966
Swine influenza. III. Filtration experiments and etiology. *J. exp. Med.*, 1931,
54, 373-85.
Shope's important work on the aetiology of influenza included the
isolation of the Shope virus.

5494　SMITH, Wilson. 1897-1965, *et al.*
A virus obtained from influenza patients. *Lancet*, 1933, **2**, 66-68.
W. Smith, C. H. Andrewes, and P. P. Laidlaw successfully infected
ferrets with filtered throat-washings from influenzal patients by intranasal
instillation (influenza A virus).

5495   THOMSON, DAVID. 1884-1969, & THOMSON, ROBERT. 1888-
Influenza. 2 vols. London, *Baillière, Tindall & Cox*, 1933-34.
Annals of the Pickett Thomson Research Lab., Monograph 16.

5496   BURNET, *Sir* FRANK MACFARLANE. 1899-1985
Propagation of the virus of epidemic influenza on the developing egg.
Med. J. Aust., 1935, **2**, 687-89.
Cultivation of the influenza virus.

5497   SMITH, WILSON. 1897-1965, & STUART-HARRIS, *Sir* CHARLES HERBERT. 1909-
Influenza infection of man from the ferret. *Lancet*, 1936, **2**, 121-23.
First record of successful passage of influenza from animal to man. The
ferret had previously been infected with a virus from a case of influenza.

5498   FRANCIS, THOMAS. 1900-1969
A new type of virus from epidemic influenza. *Science*, 1940, **92**, 405-08.
Recovery of influenza B virus.

5499   MAGILL, THOMAS PLEINES. 1903-
A virus from cases of influenza-like upper-respiratory infection. *Proc. Soc.
exp. Biol. (N.Y.)*, 1940, **45**, 162-64.
Recovery of influenza B virus.

5500   TAYLOR, RICHARD MORELAND. 1887-
Studies on survival of influenza-virus between epidemics and antigenic
variants of the virus. *Amer. J. publ. Hlth.*, 1949, **39**, 171-78.
Recovery of influenza C virus.

5500.1   SCHÄFER, WERNER. 1912-
Vergleichende sero-immunologische Untersuchungen über die Viren der
Influenza und klassischen Geflügelpest. *Z. Naturf.*, 1955, **10b**, 81-91.
Schäfer showed the close serological relationship between human
influenza viruses and their avian counterparts and suggested that members
of this group might change their host specificity.

5500.2   BEVERIDGE, WILLIAM IAN BEARDMORE.
Influenza: the last great plague. London, *Heinemann*, 1977.

RUBELLA AND ALLIED CONDITIONS

5501   WAGNER.
Die Rötheln, als für sich bestehende Krankheit. *Litt. Ann. ges. Heilk.*, 1829,
13, 420-28.
Wagner separated rubella from measles and scarlet fever.

5502   VEALE, HENRY RICHARD LOBB. 1832-1908
History of an epidemic of rötheln, with observations on its pathology.
Edinb. med. J., 1866, **12**, 404-14.
Veale introduced the term "rubella" to describe German measles.

5503   FILATOV, NIL FEODOROVICH. 1847-1902
Lektsii ob ostrikh infektsionnîkh bolieznyakh u dietei. [Lectures on acute
infectious diseases of children.] Vol. 2, Moskva, *A. Lang*, 1887.

On p. 113 is Filatov's account of a form of rubella with a scarlatiniform rash. To this he gave the name "rubeola scarlatinosa". (*See also* No. 5505.)

5504 TSCHAMER, ANTON.
Ueber örtliche Rötheln. *Jb. Kinderheilk.*, 1889, n.F., **29**, 372-79.
First description of acute infectious erythema, "fifth disease", called also "Sticker's disease" after the latter's description of it in *Z. prakt. Aerzte*, 1899, **8**, 353.

5505 DUKES, CLEMENT. 1845-1925
On the confusion of two different diseases under the name of rubella (rose-rash). *Lancet*, 1900, **2**, 89-94.
Dukes described a condition similar to that noted earlier by Filatov (No. 5503). Dukes called it the "fourth disease", distinguishing it from scarlet fever, measles, and rubella on the ground that an attack of any of these diseases gives no immunity. The autonomy of this disease ("Filatov–Dukes disease") is not universally accepted.

5506 ZAHORSKY, JOHN. 1871-
Roseola infantilis. *Pediatrics (N.Y.)*, 1910, **22**, 60-64.
Roseola (exanthema) subitum first described as a distinct entity.

5506.1 HESS, ALFRED FABIAN. 1875-1933
German measles (rubella): an experimental study. *Arch. intern. Med.*, 1914, **13**, 913-16.
Experimental proof that rubella is caused by a virus.

5506.2 HIRO, Y., & TASAKA, S.
Die Röteln sind eine Viruskrankheit. *Mschr. Kinderheilk.*, 1938, **76**, 328-32.
Successful transfer of rubella to children by means of filtered nasal washings.

5507 GREGG, *Sir* NORMAN MCALISTER. 1892-1966
Congenital cataract following German measles in the mother. *Trans. ophthal. Soc. Aust.*, 1941, **3**, 35-46.
Gregg drew attention to congenital defects in infants following rubella in the mother during the early part of pregnancy.

5508 HABEL, KARL. 1908-
Transmission of rubella to *Macacus mulatta* monkeys. *Publ. Hlth. Rep. (Wash.)*, 1942, **57**, 1126-39.
Successful transmission of rubella.

5509 SWAN, CHARLES SPENCER, *et al.*
Congenital defects in infants following infectious diseases during pregnancy. *Med. J. Aust.*, 1943, **2**, 201-10.
Figures demonstrating that rubella in the first or second month of pregnancy always results in an abnormal infant. With A. L. Tostevin, B. Moore, H. Mayo, and G. H. B. Black.

5509.1 WELLER, THOMAS HUCKLE. 1915- , & NEVA, FRANKLIN ALLEN. 1922-
Propagation in tissue culture of cytopathic agents from patients with rubella-like illness. *Proc. Soc. exp. Biol. (N.Y.)*, 1962, **111**, 215-25.
Isolation of rubella virus. It was simultaneously isolated by P. D. Parkman, *et al.* (No. 5509.2.)

5509.2 PARKMAN, PAUL DOUGLAS. 1932- , *et al.*
Recovery of rubella virus from army recruits. *Proc. Soc. exp. Biol. (N.Y.),* 1962, **111**, 225-30.
With E. L. Buescher and M. S. Artenstein.

5509.3 MEYER, HARRY MARTIN. 1928- , *et al.*
Attenuated rubella virus. II. Production of an experimental live-virus vaccine and clinical trial. *New Engl. J. Med.,* 1966, **275**, 575-80.
With P. D. Parkman and T. C. Panos.

5509.4 STEWART, GEORGE LOUIS. 1936- , *et al.*
Rubella-virus hemagglutination-inhibition test. *New Engl. J. Med.,* 1967, **276**, 554-57.
With five co-authors.

ACTINOMYCOSIS: NOCARDIOSIS

5510 BOLLINGER, OTTO. 1843-1909
Ueber eine neue Pilzkrankheit beim Rinde. *Zbl. med. Wiss.,* 1877, **15**, 481-85.
First effective description of *Actinomyces bovis.*

5511 ISRAEL, JAMES. 1848-1926
Neue Beobachtungen auf dem Gebiete der Mykosen des Menschen. *Virchows Arch. path. Anat.,* 1878, **74**, 15-53.
Israel contributed an important early paper on the ray fungus *Actinomyces.* He included some drawings made by Langenbeck in 1845 and was the first to describe a human case of actinomycosis.

5512 PONFICK, EMIL. 1844-1913
Ueber Actinomykose. *Berl. klin. Wschr.,* 1880, **17**, 660-61.
Ponfick recognized the causative role of *Actinomyces* in human actinomycosis; he established the identity of the human and animal forms of the disease. He published a book on the subject in 1882.

5512.1 NOCARD, EDMOND ISIDORE ETIENNE. 1850-1903
Note sur la maladie des boeufs de la Guadeloupe, connue sous le nom de farcin. *Ann. Inst. Pasteur,* 1888, **2**, 293-302.
The first pathogenic aerobic actinomycete to be described. It was later named *Nocardia farcinica* and is probably identical with *N. asteroides.*

5513 BOSTROEM, EUGEN. 1850-1928
Untersuchungen über die Aktinomykose des Menschen. *Beitr. path. Anat.,* 1890, **9**, 1-240.
Isolation of *Actinomyces graminis* from human actinomycosis, and staining method for *Actinomyces.*

5513.1 EPPINGER, HANS. 1846-1916
Ueber eine neue, pathogene Cladothrix und eine durch sie hervorgerufene Pseudotuberculosis (cladothrichica). *Beitr. path. Anat.,* 1891, **9**, 287-328.
Eppinger isolated *Cladothrix (Nocardia) asteroides* in a patient suffering from pseudotuberculosis with brain abscesses and meningitis.

5514   WOLFF, Max. 1844-1923, & ISRAEL, James. 1848-1926
Ueber Reincultur des Actinomyces und seine Uebertragbarkeit auf Thiere.
Virchows Arch. path. Anat., 1891, **126**, 11-59.
Isolation of *Actinomyces bovis*.

5515   CUTTINO, John Tindal. 1912- , & McCABE, Anne M.
Pure granulomatous nocardiosis: a new fungus disease distinguished by
intracellular parasitism. A description of a new disease in man due to a
hitherto undescribed organism, *Nocardia intracellularis*, n.sp., including
a study of the biological and pathogenic properties. *Amer. J. Path.*, 1949,
25, 1-48.
Nocardiosis described.

CANDIDIASIS

5516   UNDERWOOD, Michael. 1737-1820
Aphthae of thrush. In his *Treatise on the diseases of children*, London, *J.
Mathews*, 1784, pp. 43-52.

5517   LANGENBECK, Bernhard Rudolph Conrad von. 1810-1887
Auffindung von Pilzen auf der Schleimhaut der Speiseröhre einer Typhus-
Leiche. *Neue Notiz. Geb. Natur -u. Heilk.* (Froriep), 1839, **12**, cols. 145-47.
Discovery of *Candida albicans*, which Berg (No. 5518) showed to be
the causal organism in thrush.

5518   BERG, Fredrik Theodor. 1806-1887
Torsk i mikroskopiskt anatomiskt hänseende. *Hygiea (Stockh.)*, 1841, **3**, 541-
50.
Discovery of *Candida albicans* in thrush.

5519   GRUBY, David. 1810-1898
Recherches anatomiques sur une plante cryptogame qui constitue le vrai
muguet des enfants. *C. R. Acad. Sci. (Paris)*, 1842, **14**, 634-36.
Independently of Berg, Gruby found *Candida albicans* in thrush. He
demonstrated its fungal nature.

OTHER COMMUNICABLE DISEASES

5520   CORDUS, Euricius. 1486-1535
Ein Regiment: wie man sich vor der newen Plage der Englische Schwaisz
genannt, bewaren, unnd so mann damit ergryffen wirt, darinn halten soll.
Marpurg, 1529.
Euricius Cordus, father of Valerius, wrote an important account of
sweating sickness. Another edition was published at Nuremberg, also in
1529. Reproduced in Gruner's *Scriptores*, 1847 (No. 5524).

5521   SCHYLLER, Joachim [Schiller]. *fl.* 1529
De peste Brittanica commentariolus vere aureus. Basileae, *H. Petrus*, 1531.
Schyller's book on sweating sickness deals with the German epidemic
of 1528-30.

5522   CAIUS, JOHN [KAYE]. 1510-1573
        A boke, or conseill against the disease commonly called the sweate, or
        sweatyng sicknesse. London, *Richard Grafton*, 1552.
        First English book on sweating sickness, and the first devoted to a single
        disease to be published in England. Caius's work appeared a year after the
        last epidemic visit of the disease. From it we learn that the disease was
        febrile, the sweating merely a manifestation of the fever, and that it was
        accompanied by pain in the limbs, nausea, vomiting, and delirium. A
        facsimile edition of the book was published in New York, 1937; it also
        appears in Gruner (No. 5524) and in the 1844, 1846, and 1859 editions of
        No. 1678.

5523   HAMILTON, ROBERT. 1721-1793
        An account of a distemper, by the common people in England vulgarly
        called the mumps. *Trans. roy. Soc. Edinb.*, 1790, **2**, 59-72.
        First modern account of the occurrence of parotitis and orchitis com-
        plicating it. Hamilton's paper, read in 1773, by its fullness and clarity made
        the disease more generally known, so that within a few years many text
        books included descriptions of it.

5524   GRUNER, CHRISTIAN GOTTFRIED. 1744-1815
        Scriptores de sudore anglico superstites. Colliget C. G. Gruner. Post
        mortem auctoris adornavit et edidit H. HAESER. Jenae, *F. Mauk*, 1847.
        A collection of all the important earlier writings on sweating sickness.

5525   SALAZAR, TOMAS. 1830-1917
        Historia de la verrugas. *Gac. méd. Lima*, 1858, **2**, 161-64, 175-78.
        Verruga peruana.

5526   BOLLINGER, OTTO. 1843-1909
        Mycosis der Lunge beim Pferde. *Virchows Arch. path. Anat.*, 1870, **49**, 583-
        86.
        Botriomycosis first described.

5527   RITTER, JACOB.
        Beitrag zur Frage des Pneumotyphus. (Eine Hausepidemie in Uster [Schweiz]
        betreffend.) *Dtsch. Arch. klin. Med.*, 1879, **25**, 53-96.
        First description of psittacosis in a human.

5528   PALTAUF, ARNOLD. 1860-1893
        Mycosis mucorina. *Virchows Arch. path. Anat.*, 1885, **102**, 543-64.
        First authentic case reported in man.

5528.1 POSADAS, ALEJANDRO. 1870-1902
        Un nuovo caso de micosis fungoides con psorospermias. *An Circ. med.
        argent.*, 1892, **15**, 585-97.
        See No. 5528.2.

5528.2 WERNICKE, ROBERT JOHANN. 1873-
        Pentastomas. *Rev. Asoc. med. argent.*, 1892, **1**, 186-89.
        Posadas (No. 5528.1) and Wernicke were the first to report cases of
        coccidioidomycosis. German translation of Wernicke's paper in *Zbl. Bakt.*,
        1892, **12**, 859-61.

5529   SMITH, THEOBALD. 1859-1934, & KILBORNE, FREDERICK LUCIUS. 1858-1936
Investigations into the nature, causation and prevention of Texas or
Southern cattle fever. Washington, *Govt. Printing Office*, 1893.
U.S. Bureau of Animal Industry, Bulletin No. 1. Discovery of the parasite
of Texas cattle fever, *Pyrosoma bigeminum,* and proof that its transmission
is due to the cattle tick, *Boöphilus bovis.* This was the first demonstration
of arthropod transmission of disease. *Pyrosoma bigeminum* is now known
as *Babesia bigemina,* and *Boöphilus bovis* as *B. annulatus.*

5529.1 BUSSE, OTTO. 1867-1922
Ueber parasitäre Zelleinschlüsse und ihre Züchtung. *Dtsch. med. Wschr.,*
1895, **21**, Vereins-Beilage, 14.
"Busse–Buschke disease" – blastomycosis of the skin due to *Cryptococcus
neoformans.* See also No. 5529.2. Busse first described it in *Zbl. Bakt.,* 1894,
16, 175-80.

5529.2 BUSCHKE, ABRAHAM. 1868-1943
Ueber eine durch Coccidien hervorgerufene Krankheit des Menschen.
Dtsch. med. Wschr., 1895, **21**, Vereine-Beilage, 14.
See No. 5529.1.

5530   ODRIOZOLA, ERNESTO. 1862-1921
La erupción en la enfermedad de Carrión (verruga peruana). *Monitor méd.,*
1895, **10**, 309-11.
"Carrion's disease" (Oroya fever) was so named by Odriozola, after
Daniel Carrión (1859-85), a student. In order to prove or disprove the
connection between Oroya fever and verruga peruana Carrión had himself
inoculated with blood from a patient suffering from verruga peruana and
later died of the disease.

5530.1 GILCHRIST, THOMAS CASPAR. 1862-1927
A case of blastomycetic dermatitis in man. *Johns Hopk. Hosp. Rep.,* 1896,
1, 269-83.
Gilchrist's description of blastomycosis ("Gilchrist's disease", "Busse-
Buschke disease", Nos. 5529.1 and 5529.2), is an important contribution to
the knowledge of the infectious granulomata involving the skin.

5530.2 LAVERAN, CHARLES LOUIS ALPHONSE. 1845-1922
Au sujet de l'hématozoaire endoglobulaire de *Padda oryzivora. C. R. Soc.
Biol. (Paris),* 1900, **52**, 19-20.
Toxoplasma described.

5530.3 OPHÜLS, WILLIAM. 1871-1933, & MOFFITT, HERBERT C.
A new pathogenic mould (formerly described as a protozoon: Coccidioides
immitis pyogenes). Preliminary report. *Philad. med. J.,* 1900, **5**, 1471-72.
Recognition that the protozoan was the pathogenic phase of a mycelial
fungus.

5531   LIGNIE"RES. JOSEPH LÉON MARCEL. 1868-1933, & SPITZ, J.
Actinobacilosis. *Semana méd.,* 1902, **9**, 207-15.
Discovery of the actinobacillus.

5531.1   STRONG, RICHARD PEARSON. 1872-1948
           A study of some tropical ulcerations of skin with particular reference to
           their etiology. *Philipp. J. Sci.*, 1906, **1**, 91-116.
           Strong described organisms consistent with *Histoplasma capsulatum*
           before Darling, although his work was overshadowed by the latter.

5532   DARLING, SAMUEL TAYLOR. 1872-1925
           A protozoon general infection producing pseudotubercles in the lungs and
           focal necroses in the liver, spleen and lymphnodes. *J. Amer. med. Assoc.*,
           1906, **46**, 1283-85.
           Histoplasmosis (*Histoplasma capsulatum*), "Darling's disease".

5532.1   LUTZ, ADOLFO. 1855-1940
           Uma mycose pseudococcidica localisada na bocca e observada no Brazil.
           Contribuiçao ao conhecimento das hyphoblastomycoses americanas.
           Brazil-méd., 1908, **22**, 121-24, 141-44.
           South American blastomycosis.

5533   BARTON, A. L.
           Descripción de elementos endo-globulares hallados en las enfermos de
           fiebre verrucosa. *Crón. méd. (Lima)*, 1909, **26**, 7-10.
           The causal organism of Oroya fever and verruga peruana was named
           Bartonella bacilliformis after Barton, who was one of the first to observe
           it.

5534   NICOLLE, CHARLES JULES HENRI. 1866-1936, & MANCEAUX, LOUIS HERBERT.
           1865-1943
           Sur une infection à corps de Leishman (ou organismes voisins) du gondi.
           C. R. Acad. Sci. (Paris), 1908, **147**, 763-66.
           Toxoplasma described. English translation in Kean (No. 2268.1).

5534.1   SPLENDORE, ALFONSO. 1871-1953
           Un nuovo protozoa parassito de' conigli incontrato nelle lesioni anatomiche
           d'una malattia che ricorda in molti punti il kala azar dell'uomo. *Rev. Soc.
           Sci. S. Paulo*, 1908, **3**, 109-12. English translation in Kean (No. 2268.1).
           Splendore discovered *Toxoplasma* in a rabbit; it was named *T. cuniculi.*

5535   GOUGEROT, HENRI. 1881-1955, & CARAVEN, PIERRE JEAN BAPTISTE. 1879-
           1958
           Mycose nouvelle: l'hémisporose. Ostéite humaine primitive du tibia due à
           l'*Hemispora Stellata. C. R. Soc. Biol. (Paris)*, 1909, **66**, 474-76.
           Hemisporosis described.

5535.1   CASTELLANI, ALDO. 1877-1971
           Note on certain protozoa-like bodies in a case of protracted fever with
           splenomegaly. *J. trop. Med.*, 1914, **17**, 113-14.
           Castellani was first to suspect that toxoplasmosis could affect humans.

5536   MAGROU, JOSEPH EMILE. 1883-
           Les grains botryomycotiques. Leur signification en pathologie et en biologie
           générales. Laval, *L. Barnéoud*, 1914.
           Thèse de Paris, No. 267, 1914. Magrou showed botriomycosis (granuloma
           pyogenicum) to be due to a staphylococcus.

5537   STODDARD, JAMES LEAVITT. 1889-, & CUTLER, ELLIOTT CARR. 1888-1947
        Torula infection in man. *Monograph 6, Rockefeller Inst. med. Res.*, 1916.
        Description of *Torula histolytica* infection in man, later shown to be
        identical with *Cryptococcus neoformans*.

5538   ZAHORSKY, JOHN. 1871-
        Herpetic sore throat. *Sth. med. J. (Nashville)*, 1920, **13**, 871-72.
        First description of herpangina, an acute infection associated with
        Coxsackie viruses.

5538.1 ASHWORTH, JAMES HARTLEY. 1874-1936
        On *Rhinosporidium seeberi* (Wernicke, 1903), with special reference to its
        sporulation and affinities. *Trans. roy. Soc. Edinb.*, 1923, **53**, 301-42.
        Ashworth was the first to show that *Rhinosporidium* was a fungus.

5538.2 NOGUCHI, HIDEYO. 1876-1928, *et al.*
        Etiology of Oroya fever. XIV. The insect vectors of Carrión's disease. *J. exp.
        Med.*, 1929, **49**, 993-1008.
        Phlebotomus shown to be the vector of Oroya fever. With R. C.
        Shannon, E. B. Tilden, and J. B. Tyler.

5538.3 BECKER, FREDERICK EDWARD. 1888-
        Tick-borne infections in Colorado. I. The diagnosis and management of
        infections transmitted by the wood tick. *Colorado Med.*, 1930, **27**, 36-44.
        Becker first clearly described Colorado tick fever as a separate entity
        and suggested that the causal organism was transmitted by the tick,
        Dermacentor andersoni.

5539   LEVINTHAL, CLAUDE WALTER. 1886-1963
        Die Ätiologie der Psittakosis. *Klin. Wschr.*, 1930, **9**, 654.
        Discovery of the causal agent of psittacosis, *Chlamydia psittaci*. Si-
        multaneously A. C. Coles (*Lancet*, 1930, **1**, 1011-12) and R. D. Lillie (*Publ.
        Hlth. Rep., Wash.*, 1930, **45**, 773-78) made the same discovery, and the
        elementary bodies of psittacosis are known as the Levinthal–Coles–Lillie
        (LCL) bodies.

5540   SYLVEST, EJNAR OLUF SORENSON. 1880-1931
        En Bornholmsk epidemi-myositis epidemica. *Ugeskr. Laeg.*, 1930, **92**, 798-
        801.
        First full description of epidemic myositis, "Bornholm disease". See also
        Sylvest's monograph on the subject, London, 1934.

5541   DAUBNEY, ROBERT. 1891- , & HUDSON, JOHN RICHARD.
        Enzootic hepatitis or Rift Valley fever. An undescribed virus disease of
        sheep, cattle and man from East Africa. *J. Path. Bact.*, 1931, **34**, 545-79.
        First description.

5541.1 BEDSON, *Sir* SAMUEL PHILLIPS. 1886-1969, & BLAND, J. O. W.
        A morphological study of psittacosis virus, with the description of a
        developmental cycle. *Brit. J. exp. Path.*, 1932, **13**, 461-66.
        Conclusive proof of the causal relationship of the psittacosis agent to
        the infection.

5541.2   HANSMANN, GEORGE HENRY. 1890- , & SCHENKEN, JOHN RUDOLPH. 1905-
A unique infection in man caused by a new yeast-like organism, a
pathogenic member of the genus Sepedonium. *Amer. J. Path.*, 1934, **10**, 731-
38.
  Cultivation of *Histoplasma capsulatum* before DeMonbreun (No.
5542); preliminary announcement in *Science*, 1933, **77**, Suppl. 2002, p. 8.
DeMonbreun and Hansmann & Schenken independently and almost
simultaneously demonstrated the fungal nature of the pathogen.

5542   DeMONBREUN, WILLIAM ANDREW. 1899-
The cultivation and cultural characteristics of Darling's Histoplasma
capsulatum. *Amer. J. trop. Med.*, 1934, **14**, 93-125.
  Demonstration of the fungal nature of the pathogen.

5543   JOHNSON, CLAUD D., & GOODPASTURE, ERNEST WILLIAM. 1886-1960
An investigation of the etiology of mumps. *J. exp. Med.*, 1934, **59**, 1-19.
  Isolation of mumps virus.

5544   RIVERS, THOMAS MILTON. 1888-1962, & BERRY, GEORGE PACKER. 1898-
Diagnosis of psittacosis in man by means of injections of sputum into white
mice. *J. exp. Med.*, 1935, **61**, 205-12.

5544.1   WOLF, ABNER. 1902- , & COWEN, DAVID. 1907-
Granulomatous encephalomyelitis due to an encephalitozoon
(encephalitozoic encephalomyelitis), a new protozoon disease of man.
Bull. neurol. Inst. N.Y., 1937, **6**, 306-71.
  Definite recognition of human toxoplasmosis. See also their later paper
in the same journal, 1938, **7**, 266-83.

5544.2   STOKES, JOSEPH. 1896-1972, *et al.*
Immunity in mumps. VI. Experiments on the vaccination of human beings
with formolized mumps virus. *J. exp. Med.*, 1946, **84**, 407-28.
  With J. F. Enders, E. P. Maris, and L. W. Kane.

5545   DALLDORF, GILBERT JULIUS. 1900- , & SICKLES, GRACE MARY. 1898-1959
An unidentified, filterable agent isolated from the feces of children with
paralysis. *Science*, 1948, **108**, 61-62.
  Isolation of the Coxsackie virus.

5546   CURNEN, EDWARD CHARLES. 1909- , *et al.*
Disease resembling nonparalytic poliomyelitis associated with a virus
pathogenic for infant mice. *J. Amer. med. Assoc.*, 1949, **141**, 894-901.
  Isolation of the Coxsackie virus from patients with poliomyelitis. With
E. W. Shaw and J. L. Melnick.

5546.1   FLORIO, LLOYD JOSEPH. 1910- , *et al.*
Colorado tick fever. Isolation of the virus from *Dermacentor andersoni* in
nature and a laboratory study of the transmission of the virus in the tick. *J.
Immunol.*, 1950, **64**, 257-63.
  Isolation of the virus of Colorado tick fever. With M. S. Miller and E. R.
Mugrage.

862

5546.2   GREER, WILLIAM EDWARD R. 1918- , & KEEFER, CHESTER SCOTT. 1897-1972
          Cat-scratch fever. A disease entity. *New Engl. J. Med.*, 1951, **244**, 545-48.
          First description.

5546.3   HENLE, GERTRUDE. 1912- , & DEINHARDT, FRIEDRICH.
          Propagation and primary isolation of mumps virus in tissue culture. *Proc. Soc. exp. Biol. (N.Y.)*, 1955, **89**, 556-60.

5546.4   FRAME, JOHN D., *et al.*
          Lassa fever, a new virus disease of man from West Africa. I. Clinical description and pathological findings. *Amer. J. trop. Med. Hyg.*, 1970, **19**, 670-76.
          An arenovirus infection first noted in Lassa, N. E. Nigeria, in 1969. With J. M. Baldwin, D. J. Gocke, and J. M. Troup.

5546.5   BUCKLEY, SONJA MARGARET. 1918- , & CASALS, JORDI. 1911-
          Lassa fever, a new virus disease of man from West Africa. III. Isolation and characterization of the virus. *Amer. J. trop. Med. Hyg.*, 1970, **19**, 680-91.
          Preliminary note in *Nature (Lond.)*, 1970, 227, 174.

History of Communicable Diseases

5546.6   BLOOMFIELD, ARTHUR LEONARD. 1888-
          A bibliography of internal medicine. Communicable diseases. Chicago, *University of Chicago Press*, 1958.
          An extensive bibliography, and substantial excerpts from practically every important reference made to each of 30 communicable diseases, from 1800 onwards.

5546.7   COCKBURN, AIDAN.
          The evolution and eradication of infectious diseases. Baltimore, *Johns Hopkins Press*, 1963.

5546.8   HOOGSTRAAL, HARRY. 1917-
          Bibliography of ticks and tickborne diseases from Homer (about 600 B.C.) to 31 December, 1969. Vol. 1- . Cairo, *U. S. Medical Research Unit No. 3*, 1970- .

5546.9   SPINK, WESLEY WILLIAM. 1904-1988
          Infectious diseases. Prevention and treatment in the nineteenth and twentieth centuries. Minneapolis, *University of Minnesota Press*, 1978.

5546.10   AINSWORTH, GEOFFREY CLOUGH. 1905-
          Introduction to the history of medical and veterinary mycology. Cambridge, *Cambridge University Press*, [1986].
          Authoritative and well-illustrated history with excellent chronological bibliography.

SURGERY

See also 3021-3047.25, Cardiovascular Surgery; 4850-4914.7, Neurological surgery; and under organs and regions.

5547   EDWIN SMITH PAPYRUS.
The Edwin Smith Surgical Papyrus. Published in facsimile and hieroglyphic transliteration with translation and commentary by James Henry Breasted. 2 vols. Chicago, *Univ. Press,* 1930.

Edwin Smith, pioneer Egyptologist, purchased at Luxor in 1862 the papyrus which bears his name. It is now in the possession of the New York Academy of Medicine. The original text was written about 3000 B.C., and the present manuscript is a copy dating about 1600 B.C. It is the oldest known surgical treatise and consists entirely of case reports; it describes 47 different cases of injuries and affections of the head, nose, and mouth, together with methods of bandaging.

5548   HIPPOCRATES, 460-375 B.C.
Chirurgie d'Hippocrate. 2 vols. Paris, *Imprimérie nationale,* 1877-78.

A Greek–French edition with extensive notes and commentaries by J. E. Pétrequin, surgeon-in-chief of the Hôtel-Dieu of Lyon. Hippocrates performed trephining and paracentesis; his most important successes were in the reduction of fractures and dislocations.

5548.1   CELSUS, Aulus Aurelius Cornelius. 25 B.C.-A.D. 50
De medicina. Florentiae, *Nicolaus [Laurentius],* 1478.

The surgical chapters of *De medicina* contain the first accounts of the use of ligature, excellent descriptions of lateral lithotomy and herniotomy. and the earliest discussion of the surgical remedies for mutilations – what we now call plastic surgery. First edition in English, London, 1756. *See* Nos. 20, 3666.81, & 5733.50.

5549   PAUL *of Aegina.* A.D. 625-690
The seven books of Paulus Aegineta. Translated from the Greek...by Francis Adams. 3 vols. London, *Sydenham Society,* 1844-47.

Book VI is entirely devoted to operative surgery. Adams himself says that it "contains the most complete system of operative surgery which has come down to us from ancient times". Book IV contains much information on surgical diseases. (*See also* No. 36.)

5550   ABUL QASIM [Albucasis]. 936-1013
De chirurgia. Arabice et Latine cura Johannis Channing. 3 vols. Oxonii, *e typ. Clarendoniano,* 1778.

The surgical section of Albucasis's *Altasrif,* the first rational, complete and illustrated treatise on surgery and surgical instruments. During the Middle Ages it was the leading textbook on surgery until superseded by Saliceto. This is the first edition in Arabic, and the first modern edition of the text. A Latin translation by Gerard of Cremona was printed in Venice in 1497. The standard edition is *Albucasis on surgery and instruments. A definitive edition of the Arabic text, with English translation and commentary by M. S. Spink and G. L. Lewis,* London, *Wellcome Institute for the*

History of Medicine, 1973. A superbly illustrated 14th century MS of Albucasis was reproduced in full colour facsimile as Codex Vindobonensis Series Nova 2641, Graz, *Akademische Druck*, 1979. *See* No. 3666.82.

5551 ROGER OF SALERNO [RUGGERIO FRUGARDI]. *fl.* late 12th century
Glossulae quatuor magistrorum super chirurgiam Rogerii et Rolandi. Ed. C. DAREMBERG. Neapoli et Parisiis, *J. B. Baillière*, 1854.

In Roger of Palermo's *Practica chirurgiae*, which appeared about 1180, end-to-end suture is described, as is the value of mercurial inunction in chronic skin diseases; in his recommendation of seaweed for the treatment of goitre Roger anticipated Coindet (No. 3812). Roland of Parma [Rolando Capelluti or Capezutti] (*fl.* early 13th century) was a pupil of Roger, and edited his master's books about A.D. 1230. The work was one of the most important emanating from the School of Salerno. A colour facsimile with Italian translation of an illuminated medieval manuscript of Roland's version of Roger's work in the Bibliotheca Casanatense Roma was published in Rome, 1927.

5551.1 THEODORIC, *Bishop of Cervia*. 1210-1298
The surgery of Theodoric ca. 1267. Translated from the Latin by ELDRIDGE CAMPBELL and JAMES COLTON. 2 vols. New York, *Appleton-Century-Crofts*, 1955-60.

Theodoric, a Dominican friar, was a pupil of Hugh of Lucca (*circa* 1160-1257), whose teachings are reflected in his writings. Allbutt considered Theodoric to be one of the most original surgeons of all time.

5552 SALICETO, GULIELMO DA [WILLIAM OF SALICET]. 1210-1280
La ciroxia vulgarmente fata. [Venice, *F. de Pietro*, 1474.]

Saliceto was Professor of Surgery at Bologna about 1268. He was a skilful surgeon and his book on surgery was the most important on the subject during the 13th century. It was written about 1275. This Italian translation is the first medical book printed in Italian and probably the first work on surgery ever printed; the original Latin text was printed two years after the above Italian edition. Book IV contains the first known treatise on surgical anatomy. A French translation by P. Pifteau was published in Toulouse in 1898.

5553 LANFRANCHO, *of Milan* [LANFRANC]. *fl.* 1290-1296
La chirurgie d'Alanfranc traduit du latin par GUILLAUME YVOIRE. Lyon, *Jean de la Fontaine*, 1490.

Lanfranc, the founder of French surgery, was a pupil of William of Salicet. He enjoyed a great reputation for his lecturing and bedside teaching. His *Chirurgia magna* was completed in 1296. According to Hirsch and others it was first published in Venice in 1490, but no copy of this edition has been traced. Above is a French translation; an English version appeared in 1565 and the Early English Text Society published an Old English version, *Science of cirurgie*, 1894. Lanfranc was the first surgeon to describe cerebral concussion and to distinguish between simple hypertrophy and cancer of the breast. He wrote a *Chirurgia parva* about 1295.

5554 MONDEVILLE, HENRI DE. ?1260-1320
Die Chirurgie des Heinrich de Mondeville. Hrsg. VON JULIUS LEOPOLD PAGEL. Berlin, *A. Hirschwald*, 1892.

Henri de Mondeville was the teacher of Guy de Chauliac; he belonged to the School of Montpellier. His work was first printed as above; French translations by E. Nicaise, 1893, and A. Bos, 1897; the latter was reprinted in 1965.

5555   YPERMAN, JAN. 1295-1351
La chirurgie de maître Jean Yperman...Mise au jour et annotée par J. M. F. CAROLUS. Gand, *F. & E. Gyselynck*, 1854.

Jan Yperman, a pupil of Lanfranc, became the first authority on surgery in the Low Countries during the 14th century. His work was first printed in *Ann. Soc. Méd. Gand*, 1854, **32**, and re-issued as above. Another edition was published in Paris, 1936.

5556   GUY DE CHAULIAC. ?1298-1368
La pratique en chirurgie du maistre Guidon de Chauliac. Lyon, *Barthelemy Buyer*, 1478.

Guy de Chauliac was the most eminent surgeon of his time; his authority remained for some 200 years. He distinguished the various kinds of hernia from varicocele, hydrocele, and sarcocele, and described an operation for the radical cure of hernia. The book, which was originally written about 1363, includes Guy's views on fractures, and gives an excellent summary of the dentistry of that period. It is the greatest surgical text of the time. The first edition is the first important medical book printed in French. The standard edition in French is that of Edouard Nicaise (1838-96) published in Paris, 1890. It includes a very extensive bibliography of both manuscript and printed versions. English translation of sections on wounds and fractures, Chicago, 1923. See No. 3666.83.

5557   JOHN *of Arderne*. 1307-?1380
De arte phisicale et de cirurgia. Translated by D'ARCY POWER from a transcript made by Eric Millar from the replica of the Stockholm manuscript in the Wellcome Historical Medical Museum. London, *John Bale*, 1922.

John of Arderne was the first English surgeon of note. The Stockholm manuscript, an illustrated scroll nearly 18 feet long and 15 inches wide, written in England c. 1420, was reproduced in black & white facsimile in an edition limited to 100 copies, Stockholm, *Generalstabens Litografiska Anstalt*, 1929. *See* No. 3416.

5558   PFOLSPEUNDT, HEINRICH VON. *fl.* 1460
Buch der Bündth-Ertznei. Hrsg. von H. HAESER und A. MIDDELDORPF. Berlin, *G. Reimer*, 1868.

Although not printed until 1868, this work was written about 1460, and is the first work of the early German surgeons. Pfolspeundt was a Bavarian army surgeon; his book includes the first allusion to the extraction of bullets, and gives an account of rhinoplasty. Some authorities have used the name "Pfolsprundt"; for an explanation of this mistake, see Muffat, in *S. B. k. bayer. Akad. Wiss. München*, 1869, **1**, 564. *See* No. 5733.51

5559   BRUNSCHWIG, HIERONYMUS [BRAUNSCHWEIG]. *circa* 1450-*circa* 1512
Dis ist das buch der Cirurgia Hantwirckung der wundartzny von Hyeronimo brunschwig. Strassburg. [*J. Grüninger]*, 1497.

First important printed surgical treatise in German. It combines a compilation of the ancient and medieval authorities with Brunschwig's own extensive experience. It contains the first detailed account of gunshot wounds in medical literature and is notable for its wood-cuts, some of the earliest specimens of medical illustration. It was reproduced in facsimile in 1911 (Munich), 1923 (Milan), and 1967 (Gertenbach). English translation, Southwark (London), 1525.

5559.1 VIGO, GIOVANNI DE. 1460?-1525?
Practica in arte chirurgica copiosa...continens novem libros. [Rome, *per S. Guillireti et H. Bononiensem*], 1514.
The first complete system of surgery after that of Guy de Chauliac. It contains an account of gunshot wounds and a section on syphilis. It was "a book which especially suited a practitioner who knew nothing of anatomy and feared or disliked to make use of the knife" (J. S. Billings). The book went through 40 editions; an English translation by B. Traheron was published in London, 1543. Facsimile reproduction of 1543 edition, Amsterdam, 1968.

5560 GERSDORFF, HANS VON. *fl.* 1500
Feldtbuch der wundartzney. Strassburg. *J. Schott*, [1517].
Gersdorff performed nearly 200 amputations. He opposed Paré's abandonment of boiling oil for the cauterization of wounds. The book contains some instructive pictures of early surgical procedures and includes the first printed picture of an amputation. Reprinted, Darmstadt, 1967.

5561 PARACELSUS [BOMBASTUS VON HOHENHEIM, THEOPHRASTUS PHILIPPUS AUREOLUS]. 1493-1541
Grosse Wund Artzney von allen Wunden, Stich, Schüssz, Bränd, Bissz, Beynbrüch, und alles was die Wundartzney begreifft. Ulm, *Hans Varnier*, [1536].
Paracelsus was a doctor, chemist, lecturer, and reformer. His novel doctrines gained him many followers. He disbelieved in the use of boiling oil for the purification of gunshot wounds. His *Chirurgia magna* attained many editions and translations.

5562 GESNER, CONRAD. 1516-1565
De chirurgia scriptores optimi quique veteres et recentiores, plerique in Germania antehac non editi. Tiguri, *apud A. et J. Gesnerum*, 1555.
A collection made by Gesner of various surgical works by M. A. Blondus, A. Bolognini, G. Dondi, A. Ferri, Galen, C. Gesner, J. Langius, B. Maggi, Marianus Sanctus, Oribasius, and J. Tagault. The list of surgical writers and their works which Gesner appended to this book is one of the earliest bibliographies of surgery.

5563 WÜRTZ, FELIX [WIRTZ]. 1518-1574
Practica der Wundartzney. Basel, 1563.
Würtz, famous surgeon in the 16th century, studied at Nuremberg. He was a friend of Gesner and an admirer of Paracelsus; his book went through many editions and was translated into English, French, and Dutch. It describes the treatment of gunshot wounds, fractures, and dislocations, but does not include operative surgery. *See* No. 6357.50.

5564 PARÉ, AMBROISE. 1510-1590
Dix livres de la chirurgie avec le magasin des instruments necessaires à icelle. Paris, *imp. Jean Le Royer*, 1564.

Paré's first surgical work; it includes his first description of the use of the ligature in amputations. *See* No. 5565. English translation, Athens, Ga., 1969. *See also* No. 3668.1.

5565 ———. Les oeuvres de M. Ambroise Paré. Paris, *G. Buon*, 1575.

Paré was the greatest of the army surgeons before Larrey. Born in poor circumstances, he became the most famous surgeon in France. He is particularly remembered for his abandonment of boiling oil and the cautery (No. 2139), for his revival of podalic version (No. 6140), his re-introduction of the ligature and his invention of many new surgical instruments. He was the first to suggest that syphilis is a cause of aneurysm. He popularized the truss, introduced artificial limbs, and (in dentistry) re-implantation of the teeth. *See also* No. 59. The fifth and most complete edition, containing the first printing of Paré's final revisions, was published in Paris, 1598. English translation by Thomas Johnson, London, 1634 (from the 1582 Latin translation of the second [1579] edition). *See* No. 3668.1.

5566 FABRY VON HILDEN, WILHELM [FABRICIUS HILDANUS]. 1560-1634
De gangraena et sphacelo. Cölln, *P. Keschedt*, 1593.

Fabricius, the "Father of German Surgery", was the first to advocate the amputation above the gangrenous or injured part. He is accredited with the first amputation of the thigh. In his work he makes no reference to Paré's methods; he believed in the efficacy of the "weapon-salve". *See also* No. 5570.

5666.1 GUILLEMEAU, JACQUES. 1550-1613
La chirurgie françoise recueillie des antiens medecins et chirurgiens. Paris, *N. Gilles*, 1594.

Guillemeau was Paré's son-in-law. His splendidly illustrated work is of special importance for dentistry and for surgery for cleft lip. English translation, Dordrecht, 1597. *See* No. 3669.

5567 LOWE, PETER. 1560-1610
A discourse on the whole art of chyrurgerie. London, *T. Purfoot*, 1596.

The first systematic work on the whole subject of surgery written in England. Lowe was the founder of the Faculty of Physicians and Surgeons of Glasgow. This was the first medical organization in Great Britain to include physicians and surgeons together. Lowe trained in Paris but settled in Glasgow after practising on the Continent and in London.

5568 UFFENBACH, PETER. 1566-1635
Thesaurus chirurgiae. Francofurti, *Typ N. Hoffmanni, imp. J. Fischeri*, 1610.

An anthology of 16th century writers; a good summary of the surgical knowledge of that period.

5569 BRADWELL, STEPHEN. 1594-1636
Helps for suddain accidents endangering life. London, *T. Purfoot*, 1633.

First book on first-aid.

5570 FABRY VON HILDEN, WILHELM [FABRICIUS HILDANUS]. 1560-1634
Observationum et curationum chirurgicarum centuriae. 6 vols. Basle, Frankfort, & Lyons, 1606-1641.

Fabricius's most important work; it was the best collection of case-records available for many years. Among other things, Fabricius used a magnet to extract an iron splinter from the eye – an idea suggested to him by his wife – and he described the first field-chest of drugs for army use. He was first to remove a gallstone from a living patient (1618).

5571   SCHULTES, JOHANN [SCULTETUS]. 1595-1645
Χειροπλοθήκη seu armamentarium chirurgicum. Ulmae Suevorum, *imp. B. Kühnen*, 1655.
Scultetus is famous for his illustrations of surgical procedures and instruments. The first edition was the only edition published in folio format. This was the most popular surgical text of the 17th century. It underwent numerous editions and translations. That with the most expanded text and illustrations was published in Amsterdam, 1672. English translation from a less expanded Dutch edition, London, 1674.

5572   MARCHETTI, PIETRO DE. *circa* 1589-1673
Observationum medico-chirurgicarum rariorum sylloge. Patavii, *Typis Matthaei de Cadorinis*, 1664.
Pietro de Marchetti was Professor of Surgery at Padua. His book contains many valuable observations in surgery.

5573   WISEMAN, RICHARD. 1622-1676
Severall chirurgicall treatises. London, *R. Royston*, 1676.
Wiseman ranks in surgery as high as does Sydenham in medicine. He made many valuable contributions to the subject; he was the first to describe tuberculosis of the joints ("tumor albus") and he gave a good account of gunshot wounds. Wiseman became surgeon to Charles II in 1672. Books V, VI, and VII reprinted, Bath, *Kingsmead*, 1977.

5574   LE CLERC, CHARLES GABRIEL. 1644-1700?
La chirurgie complète. Paris, *E. Michallet*, 1695.
This "quiz-compend" passed through eighteen editions. Among other things it mentions the use of vitriol buttons for checking haemorrhage and the mode of manual compression used at the Hôtel-Dieu. English translation, London, 1696.

5575   DIONIS, PIERRE. *d.*1718
Cours d'opérations de chirurgie, de demonstrées au Jardin Royal. Paris, *L. d'Houry*, 1707.
Dionis taught operative surgery at the Jardin-du-Roi, Paris, a famous training ground for surgeons. English translation, London, 1710.

5576   HEISTER, LORENZ. 1683-1758
Chirurgie in welcher alles was zur Wund-Artzney gehöret, nach der neuesten und besten Art. Nürnberg, *J. Hoffmann*, 1718.
Heister is the founder of scientific surgery in Germany. His book contains many interesting illustrations and includes an account of tourniquets used in his time; Heister introduced a spinal brace. This was the most popular surgical text of the 18th century; it underwent numerous editions and translations. First English translation, London, 1743.

5578   BELL, BENJAMIN. 1749-1806
A treatise on the theory and management of ulcers. Edinburgh, *C. Elliot*, 1778.
Important classification of ulcers.

5579 ———. A system of surgery. 6 vols. Edinburgh, *C. Elliot*, 1782-87.

Bell studied under the Monros at Edinburgh. He was surgeon to the Royal Infirmary, Edinburgh, for 29 years. He improved the methods of amputation, introducing the "triple incision of Bell". Above is his best work.

5580 DESAULT, PIERRE JOSEPH. 1744-1795

Œuvres chirurgicales. 3 vols. Paris, *C. Ve. Desault*, an VI [1798]-1803.

Desault was a great French surgeon, one of the first professors at the Ecole Pratique de Chirurgie, Paris. He made many suggestions regarding the treatment of fractures and dislocations and is one of the founders of modern vascular surgery. He was Xavier Bichat's teacher, and Bichat edited vols. 1 & 2. Vol. 3, edited by P.J. Roux, concerns urological diseases. *See* No. 4165.02. Vol. 1 was translated into English as *A treatise on fractures, luxations and other affections of the bones*, Philadelphia, 1805. The translation of vols. 2 & 3 was entitled *The surgical works*, 2 vols., Philadelphia, 1814. *See also* No. 2927. Desault edited the first journal specifically on surgery, *Journal de chirurgie*, 4 vols., 1791-92. *See* No. 3250.

5581 BELL, JOHN. 1763-1820

The principles of surgery. 3 vols. [in 4]. Edinburgh, London, *T. Cadell & W. Davis*, 1801-08.

John Bell, the Scottish anatomist and brother of Charles Bell, is regarded as a founder of surgical anatomy. He was first to ligate the gluteal artery and tied the common carotid and internal iliac. His illustrations were his own work, and were of a high standard.

5582 HEY, WILLIAM. 1736-1819

Practical observations in surgery. London, *T. Cadell, jun., & W. Davies*, 1803.

Hey is remembered for "Hey's saw" and "Hey's internal derangement of the knee". He was an outstanding surgeon in his day; he founded and was senior surgeon of the General Infirmary, Leeds. He devised a type of amputation of the foot ("Hey's amputation"). His book includes the description of the falciform ligament of the saphenous opening, "Hey's ligament". *See* No. 4308.1.

5583 BELL, *Sir* CHARLES. 1774-1842

A system of operative surgery. 2 vols. London, *Longman*, 1807-09.

Famous as anatomist, physiologist, and neurologist, Charles Bell was also, like his brother John, an eminent surgeon. His artistic talent was even greater than that of his brother. (*See* No. 5588.)

5584 ABERNETHY, JOHN. 1764-1831

Surgical observations on the constitutional origin and treatment of local diseases. London, *Longman*, 1809.

A pupil of John Hunter, Abernethy became a leading surgeon in London. He was most industrious, and it is said that not even on his wedding day did he fail to give his usual daily lecture at St. Bartholomew's Hospital. His book was, in the view of D'Arcy Power, epoch-making; on pp. 234-92 is recorded the first successful ligation of the external iliac artery for aneurysm, an operation carried out by Abernethy in 1796. *See* No. 2928.

5585   COOPER, Samuel. 1780-1848
        A dictionary of practical surgery. London, *J. Murray*, 1809.
            Cooper was surgeon on the field at Waterloo, and was later appointed
        to the chair of surgery at University College, London. His great dictionary
        went through seven editions during his lifetime and was translated into
        French, German and Italian.

5585.1 DORSEY, John Syng. 1783-1818
        Elements of surgery; for the use of students. 2 vols. Philadelphia, *E.
        Parker...*1813.
            The first systematic treatise on surgery written by an American. The
        work is notable for containing not only Dorsey's original contributions, but
        for its publication of the work of Dorsey's uncle and teacher, the pioneer
        American surgeon, Philip Syng Physick (1768-1837). Physick, who never
        learned to become a competent writer, asked his nephew to organize his
        teachings into a surgical handbook.

5586   PHYSICK, Philip Syng. 1768-1837
        [Buck-skin and kid ligatures]. *Eclect. Repert.*, 1816, **6**, 389-90.
            Physick, the "Father of American surgery", graduated at Edinburgh,
        having been a pupil of John Hunter. He introduced several new procedures
        in surgery, one of which was the use of absorbable kid and buckskin
        ligatures to replace silk or flax sutures then in use.

5587   COOPER, *Sir* Astley Paston, *Bart.* 1768-1841, & TRAVERS, Benjamin. 1783-
        1858
        Surgical essays. 2 vols. London, *Cox & Son*, 1818-19.
            Cooper, the pupil and great interpreter of Hunter, was the most popular
        surgeon in London during the Regency. In 1802 he gained the Copley
        Medal of the Royal Society. Travers was surgeon to St. Thomas's Hospital,
        and particularly distinguished himself in vascular surgery and ophthal-
        mology. The book includes a description of "Cooper's tumour".

5588   BELL, *Sir* Charles. 1774-1842
        Illustrations of the great operations of surgery, trepan, hernia, amputation,
        aneurism, and lithotomy. London, *Longman*, 18[20]-21.
            One of the most dramatically and beautifully illustrated works in the
        entire literature of surgery. Hand-coloured copies show more blood than
        is usual for surgical treatises of this period. From publication in fascicules,
        1820-21. A second, undated issue appeared *circa* 1830.

5589   JAMESON, Horatio Gates. 1778-1855
        Observations upon traumatic haemorrhage, illustrated by experiments
        upon living animals. *Amer. med. Recorder*, 1827, **11**, 3-70.
            Jameson was for twenty years surgeon to Baltimore Hospital. This essay
        described some of the earliest multiple animal experiments used in
        American medical research.

5589.1 LARREY, Dominique Jean, *le baron*. 1766-1842
        Clinique chirurgicale, exercée particulièrement dans les camps et les
        hôpitaux militaires depuis 1792 jusqu'en 1829. 5 vols. plus atlas to vols. 1-
        3, and atlas to vol. 5. Paris, *Gabon* [vols. 1-3]; Paris, *J.-B. Baillière* [vols. 4-
        5], 1829-36.

Larrey's most comprehensive surgical treatise, and the only one of his works that is extensively illustrated. Many of the plates concern surgical pathology.

5590 DUPUYTREN, GUILLAUME, *le baron*. 1777-1835
Leçons orales de clinique chirurgicale. 4 vols. Paris, *Germer-Baillière*, 1832-34.
    Dupuytren was born in poverty and died a millionaire. He became the best surgeon of his time in France. He was a "shrewd diagnostician, an operator of unrivaled aplomb, a wonderful clinical teacher, and a good experimental physiologist and pathologist" (Garrison); his greatest contributions were in the field of surgical pathology. *See* No. 4322.

5591 MALGAIGNE, JOSEPH FRANÇOIS. 1806-1865
Manuel de médecine opératoire. Paris, *Germer-Ballière*, 1834.
    Malgaigne was a brilliant lecturer, notable also as a historian of medieval surgery. His *Manuel* was an important work on operative surgery, and was translated into English, German, Italian, and Arabic.

5592 VELPEAU, ALFRED ARMAND LOUIS MARIE. 1795-1867
Nouveaux éléments de médecine opératoire. 3 vols. and atlas, Paris, *Ballière*, 1832.
    In its time this was the most comprehensive work on operative surgery in France; it contains some useful historical information. The first English translation appeared in New York, 1835. The atlas for that edition was never published. The best edition was the English translation annotated and significantly expanded by Valentine Mott (1785-1865), 3 vols. and atlas, New York, 1845-47.

5593 LISTON, ROBERT. 1794-1847
Practical surgery. London, *J. Churchill*, 1837.
    In his day Liston was the most dexterous and resourceful surgeon in the British Isles. He was the first in the country to remove the scapula and the first – on 21 Dec. 1846 – to perform a major operation with the aid of an anaesthetic. His method of laryngoscopy is described on p. 350 of the above work.

5594 MALGAIGNE, JOSEPH FRANÇOIS. 1806-1865
Traité d'anatomie chirurgicale et de chirurgie expérimentale. 2 vols. Paris, *J. B. Baillière*, 1838.

5595 AMMON, FRIEDRICH AUGUST VON. 1799-1861
Die angeborenen chirurgischen Krankheiten des Menschen in Abbildungen dargestellt. 2 vols. Berlin, *F.A. Herbig*, 1842.

5596 FERGUSSON, *Sir* WILLIAM. 1808-1877
A system of practical surgery. London, *J. Churchill*, 1842.
    Fergusson was the founder of conservative surgery. He was surgeon of the Royal Infirmary, Edinburgh, before being appointed to the chair of surgery at King's College Hospital, London, a position to which he was succeeded by Lister.

5597   NÉLATON, AUGUSTE. 1807-1873
        Elémens de pathologie chirurgicale. 5 vols. Paris, *Germer-Baillière*, 1844-59.
        Nélaton was a great teacher and operator at the Hôpital St. Louis. He invented several surgical instruments. In vol. 2, p. 46 of the above work is to be found the description of "Nélaton's tumour" of bone, and on p. 441, "Nélaton's line".

5598   PANCOAST, JOSEPH. 1805-1882
        A treatise on operative surgery. Philadelphia, *Carey & Hart*, 1844.
        Pancoast was Professor of Anatomy and Surgery at Jefferson Medical College. He was a fine operator and devised a number of new surgical operations and instruments. This was work contains 80 fine lithographed plates, and among its important contributions was the first extensive section on plastic surgery in an American surgical textbook. See No. 5746.2.

5598.1 DIEFFENBACH, JOHANN FRIEDRICH. 1794-1847
        Die operative Chirurgie. 2 vols., Leipzig, *F.A. Brockhaus*, 1845-48.
        Dieffenbach's most comprehensive work, covering in addition to reconstructive procedures, virtually all other types of procedures including amputations, paracentesis, laparotomy, hysterectomy, dental extractions, etc. See No. 5746.3.

5599   SYME, JAMES. 1799-1870
        Contributions to the pathology and practice of surgery. Edinburgh, *Sutherland & Knox*, 1848.
        Syme, one-time colleague of Liston, succeeded to the latter's extensive practice in Scotland. He came to London for a short time as Professor of Surgery at University College, but soon returned to Scotland. He was a popular teacher and a fine, conservative surgeon, one of the first to adopt ether anaesthesia and to welcome the antiseptic principles laid down by his son-in-law, Lister.

5600   NÉLATON, AUGUSTE. 1807-1873
        De l'influence de la position dans les maladies chirurgicales. Paris, *Germer-Baillière*, 1851.

5601   PIROGOV, NIKOLAI IVANOVICH. 1810-1881
        Klinische Chirurgie. 3 pts. Leipzig, *Breitkopf u. Härtel*, 1851-54.
        Pirogov is considered the greatest Russian surgeon and one of the greatest military surgeons of all time. He was among the first in Europe to employ ether anaesthesia. He served in the Crimean campaign and was responsible for the introduction there of female nursing of the wounded. This edition in German predates the first edition in Russian.

5602   ERICHSEN, *Sir* JOHN ERIC. 1818-1896
        The science and art of surgery. London, *Walton & Maberly*, 1853.
        The most popular textbook on the subject for many years. Erichsen was surgeon to University College Hospital, London, and Lister served as his house surgeon.

5603   PRAVAZ, CHARLES GABRIEL. 1791-1853
        Sur un nouveau moyen d'opérer la coagulation du sang dans les artères,
        applicable à la guérison des anévrismes. *C. R. Acad. Sci. (Paris)*, 1853, **36**,
        88-90.
        Pravaz invented the modern galvanocautery.

5604   MIDDELDORPF, ALBRECHT THEODOR. 1824-1868
        Die Galvanokaustik. Breslau, *J. Max u. Co.*, 1854.
        Middeldorpf improved the galvano-cautery and introduced it in major
        surgery.

5605   SIMS, JAMES MARION. 1813-1883
        Silver sutures in surgery. New York, *S. S. & S. W. Wood*, 1858.
        Sims, famous American gynaecologist, introduced a silver wire suture,
        in order to avoid sepsis. *See* No. 6037.

5606   CHASSAIGNAC, EDOUARD PIERRE MARIE. 1804-1879
        Traité pratique de la suppuration et du drainage chirurgical. 2 vols. Paris,
        V. Masson, 1859.
        Chassaignac, who introduced india-rubber tubes to drain abscesses,
        put the whole subject of surgical drainage on a scientific and methodical
        footing.

5607   GROSS, SAMUEL DAVID. 1805-1884
        A system of surgery; pathological, diagnostic, therapeutic, and operative.
        2 vols. Philadelphia, *Blanchard & Lea*, 1859.
        A profound intellect in 19th-century American surgery, Gross was both
        a surgical innovator and an outstanding author of numerous works which
        have become classics. This massive treatise containing nearly 2500 pages
        was intended to be "the most elaborate, if not the most complete treatise
        in the English language". It remains his greatest work.

5608   BILLROTH, CHRISTIAN ALBERT THEODOR. 1829-1894
        Die allgemeine chirurgische Pathologie und Therapie. Berlin, *G. Reimer*,
        1863.
        Billroth, professor of surgery at Zürich and Vienna, was the founder of
        the Vienna School of Surgery. He has also been called the founder of
        modern abdominal surgery, and he was one of the first to introduce
        antisepsis into the Continental operating room. The above work, which
        placed him in the front rank, was translated into ten languages. English
        translation from the 4th edition as General surgical pathology and therapy,
        N.Y., 1871, and from the 8th German edition, 2 vols., London, *New Sydenham
        Society*, 1877-78. Biography by K. B. Absolon, 3 vols., Lawrence, Kansas,
        1979-1987.

5609   HILTON, JOHN. 1804-1878
        On the influence of mechanical and physiological rest in the treatment of
        accidents and surgical diseases, and the diagnostic value of pain. London,
        G. Bell, 1863.
        Hilton, surgeon to Guy's Hospital, suggested that symptoms are dis-
        ordered reflexes. He advocated complete rest in the treatment of surgical
        disorders of all parts of the body. His book is a surgical classic, still in
        demand among students (sixth edition 1950). Second and later editions are
        entitled *On rest and pain*.

5610   RIZZOLI, FRANCESCO. 1809-1880
        Collezione della memorie chirurgiche ed ostetriche. 2 vols. Bologna,
        Regia Tipog., 1869.
        Rizzoli was Professor of Surgery at Bologna and an outstanding operative
        surgeon. He introduced a compressor for aneurysms, a tracheotome,
        cystotome, lithotrite, enterotome, osteoclast, and performed acupressure
        as early as 1854.

5611   ESMARCH, JOHANN FRIEDRICH AUGUST VON. 1823-1908
        Ueber künstliche Blutleere bei Operationen. *Samml. klin. Vortr.*, 1873, Nr.
        58 (Chir., Nr. 19), 373-84.
        Esmarch bandage for surgical haemostasis. English translation *New
        Sydenham Society*, 1876.

5612   VERNEUIL, ARISTIDE AUGUSTE STANISLAS. 1823-1895
        De la forcipressure. *Bull mém. Soc. méd. chir. Paris*, 1875, n.s., **1**, 17, 108,
        273, 522, 646.
        Introduction of forcipressure in the control of haemorrhage. Repub-
        lished in book form, 1875.

5613   ———. Mémoires de chirurgie. 5 vols. Paris, *G. Masson*, 1877-88.
        Verneuil, Paris surgeon, introduced forcipressure in haemorrhage (see
        No. 5612), dry bandaging, and iodoform in the treatment of abscesses. All
        his works are included in his *Mémoires*.

5614   PAQUELIN, CLAUDE ANDRÉ. 1836-1905
        Du cautère Paquelin. *Bull. gén. Thérap.*, 1877, **93**, 145-58.
        Paquelin introduced a thermocautery ("Paquelin's cautery").

5615   WELLS, *Sir* THOMAS SPENCER. 1818-1897
        Remarks on forcipressure and the use of pressure-forceps in surgery. *Brit.
        med. J.*, 1879, **1**, 926-28; **2**, 3-4.
        Spencer Wells forceps.

5616   LISTER, JOSEPH, 1*st Baron Lister.* 1827-1912
        [An address on the catgut ligature]. *Trans. clin. Soc. Lond.*, 1881, **14**, pp.
        xliii-lxiii.

5617   VOLKMANN, RICHARD VON. 1830-1889
        Die ischaemischen Muskellähmungen und Kontrakturen. *Zbl. Chir.*, 1881,
        8, 801-03.
        "Volkmann's ischaemic contracture" first described. English translation
        in Bick, *Classics of orthopaedics.*

5618   MOSETIG-MOORHOF, ALBERT VON. 1838-1907
        Der Jodoform-Verband. *Samml. klin. Vortr.*, Leipzig, 1882, Nr. 211, (Chir.,
        Nr. 68), 1811-64.
        Introduction of iodoform dressing in surgery.

5619   ROSENBACH, ANTON JULIUS FRIEDRICH. 1842-1923
        Mikro-Organismen bei den Wund-Infections-Krankheiten des Menschen.
        Wiesbaden, *J. F. Bergmann*, 1884.
        Rosenbach proved that streptococci and staphylococci are distinct and
        differentiated two strains of staphylococci ("aureus" and "albus"). He

cultured cocci from a considerable range of septic conditions, thus more accurately defining their pathological signficance for humans, and confirmed Pasteur's prediction that acute osteomyelitis was a "furuncle of the bone marrow" (Foster).

5619.1   KOCHER, EMIL THEODOR. 1841-1917
Eine einfache Methode zur Erzielung sicherer Asepsis. *CorrespBl. schweiz. Aerzte*, 1888, **18**, 3-20.
Kocher introduced silk sutures.

5620   SENN, NICHOLAS. 1844-1908
Experimental surgery. Chicago, *W. T. Keener,* 1889.
Senn was one of the leading surgeons in North America. He made important experimental studies on air embolism, introduced a method of diagnosing intestinal perforation by means of insufflation of hydrogen (*see* No. 3494), and used Roentgen rays in the treatment of leukaemia. He was professor of surgery at Rush Medical College.

5620.1   TIEMANN, GEORGE CHRISTOPH. 1793-1868
The American armamentarium chirurgicum. Chicago, *George Tiemann & Co.,* 1889.
The most comprehensive trade catalogue of medical and surgical instruments and equipment published in America during the 19th century. Reprinted with introduction by James M. Edmondson and F. Terry Hambrecht, San Francisco, *Norman Publishing*, and Boston, *The Printers' Devil,* 1989.

5621   WELCH, WILLIAM HENRY. 1850-1934
Conditions underlying the infection of wounds. *Trans. Congr. Amer. Phys. Surg.,* 1892, **2**, 1-28.
Discovery of *Staph. epidermidis albus* and its relation to the infection of wounds.

5622   CRILE, GEORGE WASHINGTON. 1864-1943
An experimental research into surgical shock. Philadelphia, *J. B. Lippincott,* [1899].
Crile saw and recorded elevations in systemic and portal venous pressures under experimental shock.

5622.1   TRUAX, CHARLES. 1852-1918
The mechanics of surgery. Chicago, *Charles Truax & Co.,* 1899.
Truax described, illustrated, and analysed the entire range of instrumentation employed in medicine and surgery. No one else has ever undertaken this extremely ambitious task. Reprinted with introduction by James M. Edmonson, San Francisco, *Norman Publishing,* 1988.

5623   FOWLER, GEORGE RYERSON. 1848-1906
Diffuse septic peritonitis, with special reference to a new method of treatment, namely, the elevated head and trunk posture, to facilitate drainage into the pelvis, with a report of nine consecutive cases of recovery. *Med. Rec. (N.Y.),* 1900, **57**, 617-23, 1029-31.
First description of the "Fowler position". Reprinted in *Med. Classics,* 1940, **4**, 551-80. Fowler was preceded in this innovation by Charles White. *See* No.6270.

5624   CRILE, GEORGE WASHINGTON. 1864-1943
An experimental and clinical research into certain problems relating to surgical operations. Philadelphia, *J. B. Lippincott Co.*, 1901.
     Crile made important contributions to the knowledge regarding shock. He originated the theory that it is due to exhaustion of the vasomotor centre. (*See also* No. 5629.)

5625   OCHSNER, ALBERT JOHN. 1858-1925
The cause of diffuse peritonitis complicating appendicitis and its prevention. *J.Amer. med. Ass.*, 1901, **36**, 1747-54.
     Ochsner was professor of clinical surgery at the University of Illinois. The above is reprinted in *Med. Classics*, 1940, **4**, 600-26.

5626   BIER, AUGUST KARL GUSTAV. 1861-1949
Hyperaemie als Heilmittel. Leipzig, *F. C. W. Vogel*, 1903.
     Bier introduced hyperaemia, active and passive, as an adjuvant in surgical therapy. English translation, New York, *Rebman*, 1909.

5627   CRILE, GEORGE WASHINGTON. 1864-1943
Blood-pressure in surgery. Philadelphia, *J. B. Lippincott Co.*, 1903.

5628   ——. Hemorrhage and transfusion. New York, *D. Appleton & Co.*, 1909.

5629   ——. The kinetic theory of shock and its prevention through anoci-association (shockless operation). *Lancet*, 1913, **2**, 7-16.
     Crile advanced the anoci-association concept in which local and general anaesthesia are combined in a sequence to eliminate pre-operative fear and tension.

5630   DALE, *Sir* HENRY HALLETT. 1875-1968, & LAIDLAW, *Sir* PATRICK PLAYFAIR. 1881-1940
Histamine shock. *J. Physiol. (Lond.),* 1919, **52**, 355-90.
     Experimental shock produced by histamine and shown to be similar to traumatic and surgical shock.

5630.1   DUNHILL, *Sir* THOMAS PEEL. 1876-1957
Removal of intrathoracic tumours by the trans-sternal route. *Brit J. Surg.*, 1922, **10**, 4-14.
     Dunhill's operation for the removal of intrathoracic tumours.

5630.2   BLALOCK, ALFRED. 1899-1964
Mechanism and treatment of experimental shock. I. Shock following hemorrhage. *Arch. Surg. (Chicago)*, 1927, **15**, 762-98.
     First of a series of papers in the *Archives. See also* No. 5630.3.

5630.3   ——. Experimental shock. The cause of the low blood pressure produced by muscle injury. *Arch. Surg. (Chicago)*,1930, **20**, 959-96.
     Blalock "demonstrated that surgical shock is not due to the elaboration of toxins nor to reflex neurologic mechanisms, but ... to decrease in circulating the blood volume" (M.M. Ravitch). He wrote many papers on the subject, principally experimental studies; Ravitch considers the above the most important (see *Johns Hopk. med. J.*, 1977, **140**, 57-67, for bibliography).

5631   BURGER, KARL. 1893-
Künstliche Scheidenbildung mittels Eihäuten. *Zbl. Gynak.*, 1937, **61**, 2437-40.
Introduction of amnioplastin.

5632   TRUETA, JOSEP. 1897-1977
El tratamiento de la fractura de guerra. Barcelona, *Biblioteca Médica de Cataluña*, 1938.
    Trueta's method of treatment of wounds – application of closed plaster after packing the excised wound with sterile vaselined gauze. English translation, London, 1939. *See* No. 4435.1.

ANTISEPSIS: ASEPSIS

5633   LABARRAQUE, ANTOINE GERMAIN. 1777-1850
De l'emploi des chlorures d'oxide de sodium et de chaux. Paris, *Mme Hazard*, 1825.
    First chlorine solution for disinfecting purposes. English translation,1826.

5634   LISTER, JOSEPH, 1*st Baron Lister.* 1827-1912
On a new method of treating compound fracture, abscess, etc., with observations on the conditions of suppuration. *Lancet.*, 1867, **1**, 326-29, 357-59, 387-89, 507-09; **2**, 95-96.
    Lister's work on the antiseptic principle in surgery. He believed that bacteria could enter wounds and cause suppuration and putrefaction and that it was necessary to kill the bacteria already in wounds and to apply dressings impregnated with some bactericidal substance. He finally hit on carbolic acid for this purpose. When this work was done it had not yet been proved that bacteria were the cause of disease. The above work is reprinted in *Med. Classics*, 1937, **2**, 28-71. *See* No. 4423.1.

5635   ——. On the antiseptic principle in the practice of surgery. *Lancet*, 1867, **2**, 353-56, 668-69.
    Having realized the significance of Pasteur's work on fermentation, Lister evolved the idea of the antiseptic prevention of wound infection. This and the preceding entry represent two of the most epoch-making contributions to surgery. The paper in reprinted in *Med. Classics*, 1937, **2**, 72-83.

5636   LUCAS-CHAMPIONNIÈRE, JUST MARIE MARCELLIN. 1843-1913
Chirurgie antiseptique. Paris, *J. B. Baillière*, 1876.
    Lucas-Championnière, eminent French surgeon, was one of the first to adopt the principles of Listerism. He wrote the first authoritative work on antiseptic surgery and introduced antisepsis into France.

5636.1   KOCH, ROBERT. 1843-1910
Ueber Desinfection. *Mitt. k. Gesundheitsamte,* 1881, **1**, 234-82.
    Koch showed that mercuric chloride was superior to carbolic acid, and that live steam surpassed hot air in sterilizing power.

5637   NEUBER, GUSTAV ADOLF. 1850-1932
Die aseptische Wundbehandlung in meinen chirurgischen Privat-Hospitälern, Kiel, *Lipsius u. Tischer*, 1886.
    The first attempts at asepsis were made by Neuber.

5638 BERGMANN, ERNST VON. 1836-1907
Zur Sublimatfrage. *Therap. Mb.*, 1887, **1**, 41-44.
   Bergmann was a pioneer in the evolution of asepsis. His corrosive sublimate method of antisepsis was gradually merged into steam sterilization and the present-day elaborate ritual of asepsis.

5639 TARNIER, STÉPHANE. 1828-1897
De l'asepsie et antisepsie en obstétrique. Paris, *G. Steinheil*, 1894.
   Tarnier was the first to adopt Listerism in obstetrics. In the discussion following a paper in *Trans. int. med. Congr.*, London, 1881, **4**, 390-391, he showed that he was the first to employ carbolic acid solution in obstetrics.

5640 HALSTED, WILLIAM STEWART. 1852-1922
The results of operations for the cure of cancer of the breast performed at the Johns Hopkins Hospital from June, 1889, to January, 1894. *Johns Hopk. Hosp. Rep.*, 1894-95, **4**, 297-350, plate XII.
   Depicts the use of rubber gloves during an operation by Halsted. In a later paper (*J. Amer. med. Ass.*, 1913, **60**, 1123-24) he gives some account of this, from which it appears that he was responsible for this innovation. In *Johns Hopk. Hosp. Rep.*, 1891, **2**, 308-10, he advised the assistant to use rubber gloves while treating wounds. Halsted originally developed rubber gloves to protect the hands of his operating room nurse, who was allergic to the antisepsis chemicals. That nurse later became Mrs. Halsted. Also published in *Ann. Surg.*, 1894, **20**, 497-555. *See also* No. 5777.

5641 BERGER, PAUL. 1845-1908
De l'emploi du masque dans les opérations. *Bull Soc. Chirurgiens Paris*, 1899, n.s., **25**, 187-96.
   Introduction of the gauze face mask, October 1897.

5642 CARREL, ALEXIS. 1873-1944, *et al.*
Traitement abortif de l'infection des plaies. *Bull Acad. Méd. (Paris)*, 1915, 3 sér., **74**, 361-68.
   Carrel–Dakin treatment of wounds. With Dakin, Daufresne, Dehelly, and Dumas.

5643 DAKIN, HENRY DRYSDALE. 1880-1952
On the use of certain antiseptic substances in the treatment of infected wounds. *Brit med. J.*, 1915, **2**, 318-20.
   "Dakin's solution" was employed by Carrel (No. 5642) in the Carrel–Dakin method of irrigation of wounds.

5644 MORISON, JAMES RUTHERFORD. 1853-1939
The treatment of infected suppurating war wounds. *Lancet*, 1916, **2**, 268-72.
   Introduction of "Bipp" in the treatment of wounds.

5645 JENSEN, NATHAN KENNETH. 1910- , *et al.*
The local implantation of sulfanilamide in compound fractures. *Surgery*, 1939, **6**, 1-12.
   Sulphonamide dressing of wounds. With L. W. Johnsrud and M. C. Nelson.

5645.90   BARTHOLIN, THOMAS. 1616-1680
De nivis usu medico observationes variae...Hafniae, *Petri Haubold,* 1661.
The first work after Avicenna to discuss the use of snow as an anaesthetic.

5645.91   MOORE, JAMES CARRICK. 1763-1834
A method of preventing or diminishing pain in several operations of
surgery. London, *T. Cadell,* 1784.
Moore revived the ancient concept of nerve compression, developing
a special clamp for its use. John Hunter used Moore's clamp in a leg
amputation in 1784 in which analgaesia was successfully obtained.

5646   DAVY, *Sir* HUMPHRY. 1778-1829
Researches, chemical and philosophical, chiefly concerning nitrous oxide.
London, *J. Johnson,* 1800.
Davy discovered the anaesthetic properties of nitrous oxide and sug-
gested its use during surgical operations, a suggestion which was not
turned to useful account until 1844. Reprinted, London, *Butterworths,* 1972.

5647   HICKMAN, HENRY HILL. 1800-1830
A letter on suspended animation, containing experiments showing that it
may be safely employed during operations on animals, with a view of
ascertaining its probable utility in surgical operations on the human
subject. Ironbridge, *W. Smith,* 1824.
Hickman was the first to prove that the pain of surgical operations could
be abolished by the inhalation of a gas. He rendered animals unconscious,
first through partial asphyxiation by the exclusion of air, then by inhalation
of carbon dioxide. He amputated limbs without pain and with good
surgical results. His work, the first in the field of surgical anaesthesia, was
received with apathy, and no use was made of it. His "Letter" is republished in the *Hickman centenary volume,* published by the Wellcome
Historical Medical Museum, London, 1930.

5648   GUTHRIE, SAMUEL. 1782-1848
New mode of preparing a spirituous solution of chloric ether. *Amer. J. Sci.
Arts.,* 1832, **21**, 64-65; **22**, 105-06.
Guthrie, Liebig, and Soubeiran discovered chloroform independently
of one another. Guthrie discovered the modern method of making
chloroform by distilling alcohol with chlorinated lime. The second paper
has the title: On pure chloric ether.

5649   SOUBEIRAN, EUGÈNE. 1793-1858
Recherches sur quelques combinaisons du chlore. *Ann Chim. (Paris),* 1831,
48, 113-57.
Soubeiran, like Liebig and Guthrie, discovered chloroform; it is difficult
to determine priority as each may have allowed an interval of time to elapse
between discovery and publication.

5650   LIEBIG, JUSTUS VON. 1803-1873
Ueber die Verbindungen, welche durch die Einwirkung des Chlors auf
Alkohol, Aether, ölbildenes Gas und Essiggeist entstehen. *Ann. Pharm.
(Lemgo),* 1832, **1**, 182-230.
Discovery, in 1831, of chloroform and chloral.

5650.1   TOPHAM, *Sir* WILLIAM. 1810-1895, & WARD, W. SQUIRE.
          Account of a case of sccessful amputation of the thigh during the mesmeric
          state. London, *Baillière*, 1842.
          The original account of the first major operation performed in England
          using hypnosis as a form of anaesthesia. The amputation was performed
          by Ward. Topham, a lawyer interested in mesmerism, performed the
          hypnosis. The controversy caused by this operation led to Elliotson's book
          (No. 5650.2).

5650.2   ELLIOTSON, JOHN. 1791-1868
          Numerous cases of surgical operation without pain in the mesmeric state.
          London, *H. Baillière*, 1843.
          Elliotson was one of the first in England to perform surgical operations
          with the aid of hypnotism. He was a great friend of Dickens and Thackeray,
          but his views on hypnotism were bitterly opposed by Thomas Wakley,
          editor of the *Lancet*, whose onslaughts eventually led to his downfall.

5650.3   ESDAILE, JAMES. 1808-1859
          Mesmerism in India, and its practical application in surgery and medicine.
          London, *Longman, etc.*, 1846.
          Esdaile performed a variety of surgical operations on Hindus, upon
          many of whom he appears successfully to have induced hypnotic anaes-
          thesia. However, his similar attempts with Europeans were not so successful.

5651   BIGELOW, HENRY JACOB. 1818-1890
          Insensibility during surgical operations produced by inhalation. *Boston
          med. surg. J.*, 1846, **35**, 309-17, 379-82.
          For an operation performed by John Collins Warren (1778-1856) at
          Massachusetts General Hospital on 16 October 1846, William Morton used
          ether as an anaesthetic for the first time. Warren removed a benign angioma
          under the jaw of his patient. It was immediately recognized that complete
          anaesthesia could be produced by the inhalation of ether vapour. Bigelow,
          a surgeon who witnessed the operation, left an excellent account in the
          above paper, which was read before the Boston Society of Medical Im-
          provement on 9 November 1846, an abstract having been previously read
          before the American Academy of Arts and Sciences on 3 November.

5652   MORTON, WILLIAM THOMAS GREEN. 1819-1868
          Circular. Morton's Letheon. Boston, *Dutton & Wentworth*, [1846].
          Unaware of Long's results with ether, Morton discovered independ-
          ently its anaesthetic effects. At first he tried to patent his discovery and
          published the above circular, in which he called his anaesthetic by the
          name of "Letheon". Fortunately Bigelow had detected the nature of
          Morton's discovery; his paper (No. 5651) soon spread the news throughout
          the world. *See* Nos. 5653 & 5660.

5653   MORTON, WILLIAM THOMAS GREEN. 1819-1868
          Remarks on the proper mode of administering sulphuric ether by inhalation.
          Boston, *Dutton & Wentworth*, 1847.
          Morton announced that his method of producing anaesthesia was
          obtained by the inhalation of sulphuric ether. He subsequently gave up a
          lucrative practice in order to devote himself to the study of surgical
          anaesthesia and the dissemination of information concerning it. He spent
          more than £20,000 in furthering the use of ether, and in so doing reduced

himself to poverty. His sacrifice was recognized when a national subscription was organized in the U. S. A. in order to pay his debts and to assure him of comfort during the last years of his life. *See* No. 5660.

5654   FLOURENS, MARIE JEAN PIERRE. 1794-1867
Note touchant l'action de l'ether sur les centres nerveux. *C. R. Acad. Sci. (Paris)*, 1847, **24**, 340-44.
On 8 March 1847, Flourens announced that chloroform had an anaesthetic effect analogous to that of ether. Little notice seems to have been taken of his paper, but later in the year Simpson independently demonstrated the value of chloroform.

5655   PIROGOV, NIKOLAI IVANOVICH. 1810-1881
Nouveau procédé pour produire, au moyen de la vapeur d'éther, l'insensibilité chez les individus soumis à des opérations chirurgicales. *C. R. Acad. Sci. (Paris)*, 1847, **24**, 789.
Pirogov was the first to practise rectal etherization, suggested by Roux earlier in 1847.

5656   ——. Recherches pratiques et physiologiques sur l'éthérisation. St. Pétersbourg, *Imprimérie Française*, 1847.
Pirogov, the great military surgeon, was with Syme the first in Europe to adopt ether anaesthesia, and he left an interesting account of his experiences with it.

5657   SIMPSON, *Sir* JAMES YOUNG. 1811-1870
Discovery of a new anaesthetic agent, more efficient than sulphuric ether. *Lond. med. Gaz.*, 1847, n.s., **5**, 934-37; *Lancet*, 1847, **2**, 549.
In an attempt to find an anaesthetic less irritating than ether, Simpson discovered the advantages of chloroform. He had previously used ether with great benefit in midwifery, but now substituted chloroform, being the first to do so. Preliminary announcements in *Lond. med. Gaz.*, 1847, n.s. **5**, 906.

5657.1 ROBINSON, JAMES. 1813-1861
A treatise on the inhalation of the vapour of ether for the prevention of pain in surgical operations. London, *Webster & Co.* 1847.
The first textbook of ether anaesthesia, published in March, 1847. Robinson, a British dentist, was the first to use anaesthesia in England, after receiving information from Henry Jacob Bigelow and Francis Boott. Facsimile edition, Park Ridge, Illinois, 1983.

5658   SNOW, JOHN. 1813-1858
On the inhalation of the vapour of ether in surgical operations. London, *J. Churchill*, 1847.
Includes an account of Snow's regulating inhaler, the first to control the amount of ether vapour by the patient. Snow forecast this apparatus in *Lond. med. Gaz.*, 1847, n.s. **4**, 156. This pamphlet was the second treatise on ether anaesthesia, appearing in October, 1847. Facsimile edition, Philadelphia, 1959.

5659   SYME, JAMES. 1799-1870
On the use of ether in the performance of surgical operations. *(Lond. Edinb.) Month. J. med. Sci.*, 1847-48, **8**, 73-76.

Syme was, with Pirogov, the first in Europe to adopt ether anaesthesia in surgical operations.

5659.1   DIEFFENBACH, JOHANN FRIEDRICH. 1792-1847
Die Aether gegen den Schmerz. Berlin, *Hirschwald*, 1847.
First application of ether anaesthesia for plastic operations. Dieffenbach made his first use of the anaesthetic in reconstructing a nose. He modified Morton's inhaler. Dieffenbach's work helped bring about the early acceptance of anaesthesia in Germany.

5660   WELLS, HORACE. 1815-1848
A history of the discovery of the application of nitrous oxide gas, ether, and other vapours, to surgical operations. Hartford, *J. G. Wells*, 1847.
In 1844 Wells, a Hartford dentist, successfully used nitrous oxide as a dental anaesthetic. To publicize his discovery, he arranged a demonstration at Harvard Medical School in January 1845, but this proved a fiasco. He discussed his discovery with a former pupil, W.T.G. Morton (Nos. 5652-53). Morton got the idea of using ether instead of nitrous oxide from Charles T. Jackson (1805-80). Jackson suffered from mental illness and later tried to claim that he had discovered surgical anaesthesia, as well as guncotton, and that he had described to Samuel F.B. Morse the essential features of the telegraph. Wells, who was not in very good mental health himself, eventually committed suicide by opening a vein in his arm and at the same time inhaling ether vapour.

5661   CHANNING, WALTER. 1786-1876
A treatise on etherization in childbirth. Boston, *W. D. Ticknor & Co.*, 1848.
Channing was an early advocate of anaesthesia in obstetrics. In his book, and in several earlier papers, he brought the importance of this branch of anaesthetics into the foreground.

5662   HEYFELDER, JOHANN FERDINAND MARTIN. 1798-1869
Die Versuche mit dem Schwefeläther, Salzäther und Chloroform. Erlangen, *C. Heyder*, 1848.
Introduction of ethyl chloride in anaesthesia.

5663   SNOW, JOHN. 1813-1858
On the inhalation of chloroform and ether. With description of an apparatus. *Lancet*, 1848, **1**, 177-80.
Snow's chloroform inhaler.

5664   LONG, CRAWFORD WILLIAMSON. 1815-1878
An account of the first use of sulphuric ether by inhalation as an anaesthetic in surgical operations. *South med. surg. J.*, 1849, **5**, 705-713.
There is no doubt that Long was the first successfully to use ether vapour as an anaesthetic. This was on 30 March 1842, at Jefferson, Georgia. Unfortunately he did not publish his results until others, notably Morton, had independently introduced it. See also the biography of Long by Frances Long Taylor, New York, 1928.

5665   SNOW, JOHN. 1813-1858
On narcotism by the inhalation of vapours. *Lond. med. Gaz.*, 1850. n.s., **11**, 749-54; 1851, n.s., **12**, 622-27.
Snow attempted carbon dioxide absorption.

5666   ———. On chloroform and other anaesthetics: their action and administration. London, *J. Churchill*, 1858.

Snow, the first specialist in anaesthesiology, delivered Queen Victoria with the aid of chloroform in 1853 and 1857. This work put the administration of chloroform and ether on a scientific basis. Snow also investigated amylene, which he was the first to administer. Reproduced in facsimile, 1950.

5667   FISCHER, E.
Ueber die Einwirkung von Wasserstoff auf Einfach-Chlorkohlenstoff. *Jena. Z. Naturw.*, 1864, **1**, 123-24.

Discovery of trichlorethylene.

5668   JUNKER, FERDINAND ETHELBERT. 1828-?1901
Description of a new apparatus for administering narcotic vapors. *Med. Times Gaz.*, 1867, **2**, 590; 1868, **1**, 171-73.

Junker's chloroform inhaler.

5669   ANDREWS, EDMUND. 1824-1904
The oxygen mixture; a new anesthetic combination. *Med Examiner*, 1868, **9**, 665-61.

Andrews advocated the use of an oxygen-nitrous mixture.

5669.1   TRENDELENBURG, FRIEDRICH. 1844-1924
Beiträge zu den Operationen an den Luftwegen. *Arch. klin. Chir.*, 1871, **12**, 112-33.

Endotracheal anaesthesia by means of a tracheostomy.

5670   LABBE:, LÉON. 1832-1916, & GUYON, E.
Sur l'action combinée de la morphine et du chloroforme. *C. R. Acad. Sci. (Paris)*, 1872, **74**, 627-29.

Labbé and Guyon developed pre-anaesthetic medication.

5671   CLOVER, JOSEPH THOMAS. 1825-1882
Description of a new double current inhaler for administering ether. *Brit. med. J.*, 1873, **1**, 282-83.

Clover's gas-ether inhaler.

5672   ORÉ, PIERRE CYPRIEN. 1828-1889
De l'anesthésie produite chez l'homme par les injections de chloral dans des veines. *C. R. Acad. Sci. (Paris)*, 1874, **78**, 515-17, 651-54.

First successful human intravenous anaesthesia. Oré, professor of physiology at Bordeaux, reported the successful use of this method in animals in *Bull. Soc. Chir. Paris,* 1972, 3 sér., **1,** 400-12. See also his monograph on the subject, Paris, 1875.

5673   BERNARD, CLAUDE. 1813-1878
Leçons sur les anesthésiques et sur l'asphyxie. Paris, *J. B. Baillière,* 1875.

As early as 1864 Bernard discovered that chloroform anaesthesia could be prolonged and intensified by the injection of morphine. J. N. von Nussbaum also observed this. English translation by B.Fink, Park Ridge, 1989.

5674   CLOVER, JOSEPH THOMAS. 1825-1882
On an apparatus for administering nitrous oxide gas and ether, singly or combined. *Brit med. J.*, 1876, **2**, 74-75.

    Clover's ether inhaler. See also the same journal, 1877, **1**, 69. He invented an inhaler in 1862; this was described, but not by Clover, in *Med. Times Gaz.*, 1862, **2**, 149.

5675   ANREP, VASILI KONSTANTINOVICH. 1852-
Ueber die physiologische Wirkung des Cocain. *Pflügers Arch. ges. Physiol.*, 1880, **21**, 38-77.

    Anrep studied the action of cocaine and, likely Moréno y Maiz, suggested its use as a local anaesthetic.

5676   MACEWEN, *Sir* WILLIAM. 1848-1924
Clinical observations on the introduction of tracheal tubes by the mouth instead of performing tracheotomy or laryngotomy. *Brit. med. J.*, 1880, **2**, 122-24, 163-65.

    First administration of an anaesthetic (chloroform) through a metal tracheal tube introduced by the mouth (endotracheal anaesthesia).

5677   FREUND, AUGUST VON. 1835-1892
Über Trimethylene. *Mh. Chem.*, 1882, **3**, 625-35.

    Cyclopropane (trimethylene) first prepared.

5678   KOLLER, CARL. 1857-1944
Vorläufige Mitteilung über locale Anästhesirung am Auge. *Klin. Mbl. Augenheilk.*, 1884, **22**, Beilageheft, 60-63.

    Introduction of cocaine as a local anaesthetic; this was the first local anaesthetic employed (16 September 1884). Freud (No. 1880.1) is accredited by some with this innovation, but in this connection see the letter by Koller in *J. Amer. med. Ass.*, 1941, **117**, 1284. English translation by H. Knapp in *Arch. Ophthal. (Chicago)*, December, 1884. This was reprinted in book form with extensive supplementary material as H. Knapp, *Cocaine and its use in ophthalmic and general surgery*, New York, *G.P. Putnam's Sons*, 1885.

5679   HALSTED, WILLIAM STEWART. 1852-1922
Practical comments on the use and abuse of cocaine; suggested by its invariably successful employment in more than a thousand minor surgical operations. *N.Y. med. J.*, 1885, **42**, 294-95.

    The first experiments on local infiltration anaesthesia were made by Halsted, who even produced anaesthesia by the intradermal injection of water. Through the process of self-experimentation Halsted became addicted to cocaine for the remainder of his life. This fact was kept a secret from all but his closest associates until after his death.

5680   CORNING, JAMES LEONARD. 1855-1923
Spinal anaesthesia and local medication of the cord. *N.Y. med. J.*, 1885, **42**, 483-85.

    Spinal anaesthesia introduced. Corning showed experimentally that cocaine exerts a prolonged anaesthetic effect while arresting the circulation in the anaesthetized area. He first described injection of cocaine between the spinous processes of the lower dorsal vertebrae in a dog (see his earlier paper in the same journal, 1885, **42**, 317-19) and then in a human being.

5680.1 ——.Local anesthesia in general medicine and surgery. New York, *D. Appleton*, 1886.

The first textbook on local anaesthesia.

5681 PERNICE, LUDWIG.

Ueber Cocainanasthesie. *Dtsch. med. Wschr.*, 1890, **16**, 287-89.

Max Oberst's method of conduction anaesthesia was first reported by Pernice, his pupil.

5682 HEWITT, *Sir* FREDERIC WILLIAM. 1857-1916

Anaesthetics and their administration. London, *C. Griffin & Co.*, 1893.

Hewitt, anaesthetist to Edward VII, did much to develop the use of ether, and advanced our knowledge of the pharmacology of anaesthetics. In 1892 he introduced the first practical gas and oxygen apparatus.

5682.1 ——. Further observations on the use of oxygen with nitrous oxide. *J. Brit. dent. Ass.*, 1894, **15**, 380-87.

Includes description of Hewitt's nitrous oxide/oxygen stopcock.

5683 SCHLEICH, CARL LUDWIG. 1859-1922

Infiltrationsanästhesie (locale Anästhesie) und ihr Verhältniss zur allgemeinen Narcose (Inhalationsanästhesie). *Verh. Dtsch. Ges. Chir.*, 1892, **21**, 121-7.

Infiltration anaesthesia was developed by Schleich after pioneer work by Halsted (No. 5679). Schleich published a paper in English on the subject in *Int. Clin.*, 1895, 5 ser., **2**, 177-92.

5684 BIER, AUGUST KARL GUSTAV. 1861-1949

Versuche über Cocainisirung des Rückenmarkes. *Dtsch. Z. Chir.*, 1899, **51**, 361-69.

Bier introduced the use of cocaine as a spinal anaesthetic.

5685 EINHORN, ALFRED. 1856-1917

Ueber die Chemie der localen Anaesthetica. *Münch. med. Wschr.*, 1899, **46**, 1218-20, 1254-56.

Synthesis of procaine (novocaine).

5685.1 MEYER, HANS HORST. 1853-1939

Zur Theorie der Alkoholnarkose. Erste Mitteilung. *Arch. exp. Path. Pharmak.*, 1899, **42**, 109-18.

Meyer's theory of narcosis.

5686 CATHELIN, FERNAND. 1873-

Une nouvelle voie d'injection rachidienne. Méthode des injections épidurales par le procédé du canal sacré.

Applications à l'homme. *C. R. Soc. Biol. (Paris)*, 1901, **53**, 452-53.

Caudal anaesthesia.

5687 CRILE, GEORGE WASHINGTON. 1864-1943

On the physiologic action of cocain and eucain when injected into tissues. *In*: Experimental and clinical research into certain problems relating to surgical operations. Philadelphia, 1901, 88-163.

Anaesthetic blocking of nerve trunks.

5688   OVERTON, CHARLES ERNEST. 1865-1933
Studien über die Narkose. Jena, *G. Fischer*, 1901.
Overton developed the lipid theory of narcosis.

5689   CUSHING, HARVEY WILLIAMS. 1869-1939
On the avoidance of shock in major amputations by cocainization of large nerve-trunks preliminary to their division. *Ann. Surg.*, 1902, **36**, 321-45.
W. S. Halsted was first to use infiltration anaesthesia (*see* No. 5679) and it was later developed by Cushing.

5690   FOURNEAU, ERNEST. 1872-1949
Stovaine, anesthésique locale. *Bull Soc. Pharmacol. (Paris)*, 1904, **10**, 141-48.
Introduction of stovaine, 1903.

5691   BRAUN, HEINRICH FRIEDRICH WILHELM. 1862-1934
Die Lokalanästhesie, ihre wissenschaftliche Grundlagen und praktische Anwendung. Leipzig, *J. A. Barth*, 1905.
Braun's important book on local anaesthesia greatly stimulated the development of that subject. English translation, Philadelphia, 1914.

5692   ———. Ueber einige neue örtliche Anaesthetica (Stovain, Alypin, Novocain). *Dtsch. med. Wschr.*, 1905, **31**, 1667-71.
Procaine (novocaine), synthesized by Einhorn, was first used clinically by Braun.

5693   KUHN, FRANZ. 1866-1929
Perorale Tubagen mit und ohne Druck. *Dtsch. Z. Chir.*, 1905, **76**, 148-207.
Kuhn introduced the intratracheal insufflation method of anaesthetization about 1900; he used a flexible metal tube and a curved introducer. He also experimented with positive and negative pressure insufflation.

5693.1   OMBRÉDANNE, LOUIS. 1871-1956
Un appareil pour l'anesthésie par l'éther. *Gaz., Hôp. (Paris)*, 1908, **81**, 1095-1100.
Ombrédanne ether inhaler.

5694   MELTZER, SAMUEL JAMES. 1851-1920, & AUER, JOHN. 1875-1948
Continuous respiration without respiratory movements. *J. exp. Med.*, 1909, **11**, 622-25.
Meltzer and Auer experimented further with the intratracheal insufflation method introduced by Kuhn (No. 5693).

5695   ELSBERG, CHARLES ALBERT. 1871-1948
Zur Narkose beim Menschen mittelst der kontinuierlichen intratrachealen Insufflation von Meltzer. *Berl. klin. Wschr.*, 1910, **47**, 957-58.
The clinical introduction of Meltzer and Auer's method of intratracheal insufflation marks the beginning of modern endotracheal anaesthesia. Also reported in *Ann. Surg.*, 1910, **52**, 23-29.

5696   LEHMANN, KARL BERNHARD. 1858-1940
Experimentelle Studien über den Einfluss technisch und hygienisch
wichtiger Gase und Dämpfe auf den Organismus. Die gechlorten
Kohlenwasserstoffe der Fettreihe. *Arch. Hyg. (Berl.)*, 1911, **74**, 1-60.
Introduction of trichlorethylene ("trilene").

5697   McKESSON, ELMER ISAAC. 1881-1935
Nitrous oxide-oxygen anaesthesia. With a description of a new apparatus.
Surg. Gynec. Obstet., 1911, **13**, 456-62.
Intermittent gas-oxygen machine.

5698   COTTON, FREDERIC JAY. 1869-1938, & BOOTHBY, WALTER MEREDITH. 1880-
1953
Nitrous oxide-oxygen-ether anesthesia: notes on administration; a perfected
apparatus. *Surg. Gynec. Obstet.*, 1912, **15**, 281-89.
Boothby and Cotton's flowmeter.

5699   GWATHMEY, JAMES TAYLOE. 1865-1944
Oil-ether anaesthesia. *N. Y. med. J.*, 1913, **98**, 1101-04.
Gwathmey produced anaesthesia by injection into the rectum of liquid
ether with olive oil dissolved in it (synergistic anaesthesia). Faulconer &
Keys report that by 1930 Gwathmey was able to report 20,000 successful
cases of the use of rectal ether in midwifery.

5699.1   ——. Anesthesia. New York, *Appleton*, 1914.
Gwathmey was one of the first physicians in the United States to
specialize exclusively in anaesthesiology. This work includes (p. 334) a
description of his nitrous oxide-oxygen-ether apparatus.

5699.2   KELLY, *Sir* ROBERT ERNEST. 1879-1944
Intratracheal anaesthesia. *Brit. J. Surg.*, 1913, **1**, 90-95.
Kelly's intratracheal ether apparatus.

5699.3   SHIPWAY, *Sir* FRANCIS EDWARD. 1875-1968
The advantages of warm anaesthetic vapours, and an apparatus for their
administration. *Lancet*, 1916, **1**, 70-74.
Shipway apparatus.

5700   BOYLE, HENRY EDMUND GASKIN. 1875-1941
Nitrous oxide-oxygen-ether outfit. *Proc. roy. Soc. Med.*, 1917-18, **11**, Sect.
Anaesth., 30.
Boyle's continous-flow anaesthetic machine.

5701   KAPPIS, MAX. 1881-1938
Zur Technik der Splanchnicusanästhesie. *Zbl. Chir.*, 1920, **47**, 98.
Splanchnic anaesthesia. See also *Dtsch. med. Wschr.*, 1920, **46**, 535.

5702   PAGÉS MIRAVÉ, FIDEL. *d*.1924.
Anestesia metamérica. *Rev. Sanid. milit. (Madr)*, 1921, **11**, 351-65, 389-96.
Introduction of peridural anaesthesia.

5703   ROWBOTHAM, EDGAR STANLEY. 1890-1979, & MAGILL, *Sir* IVAN WHITESIDE. 1888-1986
Anaesthetics in the plastic surgery of the face and jaws. *Proc. roy. Soc. Med.*, 1921, **14**, Sect. Anaesth., 17-27.
    Intratracheal insufflation method of anaesthetization. See also Magill, I. W., *Lancet*, 1921, **1**, 918; 1923, **2**, 229.

5704   LABAT, GASTON LOUIS. 1877-1934
Regional anesthesia: its technic and clinical application. Philadelphia, *W. B. Saunders*, 1922.

5705   LUCKHARDT, ARNO BENEDICT. 1885-1957, & CARTER, JAY BAILEY. 1898-
Physiologic effects of ethylene; a new gas anesthetic. *J. Amer. med. Ass.*, 1923, **80**, 765-70.
    Introduction of ethylene.

5706   PAGE, IRVINE HEINLY. 1901-
Isoamyl ethyl barbituric acid - an anesthetic without influence on blood sugar regulation. *J. Lab. clin. Med.*, 1923, **9**, 194-96.
    Sodium amytal described.

5707   HENDERSON, YANDELL. 1873-1944
A lecture on respiration in anaesthesia: control by carbon dioxide. *Brit. med. J.*, 1925, **2**, 1170-75.
    Henderson's important investigations on the physiology of respiration included his demonstration of the relation of acapnia to anaesthesia and the recommendation that carbon dioxide inhalation be used to overcome collapse due to anaesthesia.

5707.1   McKESSON, ELMER ISAAC. 1881-1935
Some physical factors in the administration of gaseous ether. *Brit med. J.*, 1926, **2**, 1113-17.
    McKesson introduced the intermittent flow method.

5708   EICHHOLTZ, FRITZ. 1889-
Ueber rektale Narkose mit Avertin (E 107). *Dtsch. med. Wschr.*, 1927, **53**, 710-12.
    Experimental use of "avertin" (tribromethanol).

5709   BUTZENGEIGER, O.
Klinische Erfahrungen mit Avertin (E 107). *Dtsch. med. Wschr.*, 1927, **53**, 710-12.
    First clinical use of "avertin".

5709.1   BROWNE, *Sir* DENIS. 1892-1942
Anaesthesia for tonsillectomy and removal of adenoids. *Brit. med. J.*, 1928, **2**, 632 (only).
    Denis Browne ether inhaler.

5710   KIRSCHNER, MARTIN. 1879-1942
Eine psycheschonende und steuerbare Form der Allgemeinbetäubung. *Chirurg.*, 1929, **1**, 673-82.
    Intravenous use of "avertin".

5711   LUCAS, George Herbert William. 1894- , & HENDERSON, Velyien Ewart. 1877-1945
A new anaesthetic gas: cyclopropane. A preliminary report. *Canad. med. Ass. J.*, 1929, **21**, 173-75.

5712   ZERFAS, Leon Grotius. 1897- , *et al.*
Induction of anesthesia in man by intravenous injection of sodium iso-amyl-ethyl barbiturate. *Proc. Soc. exp. Biol. (N.Y.)*, 1929, **26**, 399-403.
     Sodium amytal. With J. T. C. McCallum, H. A. Shonle, E. E. Swanson, J. B. Scott, and G. H. A. Clowes.

5712.1   FITCH, Richard Homer. 1903- , *et al.*
The intravenous use of the barbituric acid hypnotics in surgery. *Amer. J. Surg.*, 1930, **9**, 110-14.
     Intravenous use of pentobarbitone sodium. With R. M. Waters and A. L. Tatum.

5713   LEAKE, Chauncey Depew. 1896-1978, & CHEN, Mei-Yu.
The anesthetic properties of certain unsaturated ethers. *Proc. Soc. exp. Biol. (N.Y.)*, 1930, **28**, 151-54.
     Demonstration of the anaesthetic properties of divinyl ether.

5714   WEESE, Hellmut. 1897-1954, & SCHARPFF, Walther.
Evipan, ein neuartiges Einschlafmittel. *Dtsch. med. Wschr.*, 1932, **58**, 1205-07.
     Introduction of evipan (hexobarbitone).

5715   GELFAN, Samuel. 1903- , & BELL, I.R.
The anesthetic action of divinyl oxide on humans. *J. Pharmacol.*, 1933, **47**, 1-3.
     Clinical application of divinyl ether.

5716   JACKSON, Dennis Emerson. 1878-
A study of anesthesia and analgesia, with special reference to such substances as trichlorethylene and vinesthene (divinyl ether), together with apparatus for their administration. *Curr. Res. Anesth.*, 1934, **13**, 198-203.
     Experimental use of trichlorethylene as anaesthetic.

5717   STILES, John Alden. 1905- , *et al.*
Cyclopropane as an anesthetic agent: a preliminary clinical report. *Curr. Res. Anesth.*, 1934, **13**, 56-60.
     First clinical use of cyclopropane. With W. B. Neff, E. A. Rovenstine, and R. M. Waters.

5718   WATERS, Ralph Milton. 1883- , & SCHMIDT, Erwin Rudolph. 1890-
Cyclopropane anesthesia. *J. Amer. med. Ass.*, 1934, **103**, 975-83.
     Closed circuit method.

5719   KING, Harold. 1887-1956
Curare. *Nature (Lond.)*, 1935, **135**, 469-70.
     Isolation from curare of *d*-tubocurarine chloride.

5720   LUNDY, JOHN SILAS. 1894-
Intravenous anesthesia: preliminary report of the use of two new thiobarbiturates. *Proc. Mayo Clin.*, 1935, **10**, 536-43.
Introduction of thiopentone sodium.

5721   STRIKER, CECIL. 1897- , *et al.*
Clinical experiences with the use of trichlorethylene in the production of over 300 analgesias and anesthesias. *Curr. Res. Anesth.*, 1935, **14**, 68-71.
Human anaesthetization with trichlorethylene. With S. Goldblatt, I. S. Warm, and D. E. Jackson.

5721.1   FLAGG, PALUEL JOSEPH. 1886-1970
The art of anesthesia. 6th ed. Philadelphia, *J. B. Lippincott*, 1939.
Flagg had an important influence on American anaesthesia. The Flagg can is described on p. 148 of his book.

5722   LEMMON, WILLIAM THOMAS. 1896-
A method of continous spinal anesthesia. A preliminary note. *Ann. Surg.*, 1940, **111**, 141-44.
Continous spinal analgesia introduced.

5723   EPSTEIN, HANS GEORG, *et al.*
The Oxford vaporiser No. 1. *Lancet*, 1941, **2**, 62-64.
With R. R. Macintosh and K. Mendelssohn. The Oxford vaporiser No. 2 is described in the same journal, pp. 64-66 by S. L. Cowan, R. D. Scott, and S. F. Suffolk.

5724   GRIFFITH, HAROLD RANDALL. 1894- , & JOHNSON, G. ENID.
The use of curare in general anesthesia. *Anesthesiology*, 1942, **3**, 418-20.
Introduction of curare in anaesthesia.

5725   BOVET, DANIEL. 1907- , *et al.*
Propriétés curarisantes du di-iodoéthylate de *bis*-[quinoléyloxy-8'] 1.5-pentane. *C. R. Acad. Sci. (Paris)*, 1946, **223**, 597-98.
Introduction of gallamine triethiodide ("flaxedil"). With S. Courvoisier, R. Ducrot, And R. Horclois. See also the same journal, 1947, **225**, 74.

5726   PATON, *Sir* WILLIAM DRUMMOND MACDONALD. 1917- , & ZAIMIS, ELEANOR. 1915-1982
Curare-like action of polymethylene *bis*-quaternary ammonium salts. *Nature (Lond.)*, 1948, **161**, 718-19.
Methonium compounds. See also the same journal, 1948, **162**, 810.

5727   ———. The pharmacological actions of polymethylene bistrimethyl-ammonium salts. *Brit. J. Pharmacol.*, 1949, **4**, 381-400.
Introduction of hexamethonium bromide.

5728   BOVET, DANIEL. 1907- , *et al.*
Proprietà farmacodinamiche di alcuni derivati della succinilcolina dotati di azione curarica. Esteri di trialchiletanolammonio di acidi bicarbossilici alifatici. *R. C. Ist. sup. Sanità*, 1949, **12**, 106-37.
Introduction of succinylcholine chloride. With F. Bovet-Nitti, S. Guarino, V. G. Longo, and M. Marotta.

5729   BRÜCKE, H. *et al.*
Bis-Cholinester von Dicarbonsäuren als Muskelrelaxantien in der Narkose.
Wien. klin. Wschr., 1951, **63**, 464-66.
    Clinical use of succinylcholine chloride. With K. H. Ginzel, H. Klupp,
F. Pfaffenschlager, and G. Werner.

5729.1   KRANTZ, JOHN CHRISTIAN. 1899- *et al.*
Anesthesia: XL. The anesthetic action of trifluoroethyl vinyl ether. *J.
Pharmacol.*, 1953, **108**, 488-95.
    Fluroxene, first fluorine-containing anaesthetic. With C. J. Carr, Go Lu
and F. K. Bell.

5729.2   JOHNSTONE, MICHAEL WILLIAM.
The human cardiovascular response to fluothane. *Brit J. Anaesth*, 1956,
28, 392-410.
    Clinical introduction of halothane ("fluothane").

5729.3   RAVENTÓS, J.
The action of fluothane – a new volatile anaesthetic. *Brit J. Pharmacol.*, 1956,
11, 394-410.
    Halothane ("fluothane") a non-inflammable and non-irritant anaesthetic,
was synthesized by C. W. Suckling at the I. C. I. Laboratories in Manchester.

History of Anaesthesia

5730   BIGELOW, HENRY JACOB. 1818-1890
Ether and chloroform: a compendium of their history, surgical use,
dangers and discovery. Boston, *D. Clapp*, 1848.
    Bigelow's speedy publication of Morton's discovery (No. 5651), and his
subsequent advocacy of ether assured its adoption throughout the civilized
world. The above work deals with the priority claims in general and with
a defence of Morton's claim in particular.

5732   KEYS, THOMAS EDWARD. 1908-
The history of surgical anesthesia. New York, *Schuman's*, 1945.
    Reprinted with corrections and additions, 1963. Reprint, 1978.

5732.1   FULTON, JOHN FARQUHAR. 1899-1960, & STANTON, MADELINE.
The centennial of surgical anesthesia. An annotated catalogue of books
and pamphlets bearing on the early history of surgical anesthesia exibited
at the Yale Medical Library. New York, *Henry Schuman*, 1946.

5733   DUNCUM, BARBARA MARY.
The development of inhalation anaesthesia, with special reference to the
years 1846-1900. London, *Oxford Univ. Press*, 1947.
    Publications of the Wellcome Historical Medical Museum, New series,
No. 2.

5733.1   COLE, FRANK. 1909-
Milestones in anesthesia. Readings in the development of surgical
anesthesia, 1665-1940. Lincoln, *University of Nebraska Press*, 1965.
    First-hand accounts of discoveries and advances in anaesthesia.

5733.2 FAULCONER, Albert. 1911- , & KEYS, Thomas Edward. 1908-
Foundations of anesthesiology. 2 vols. Springfield, Ill., *C. C. Thomas*, 1965.
An anthology of 150 papers on anaesthesia and related topics, from the 16th century to 1961.

5733.3 THOMAS, Kenneth Bryn. 1916-1978
The development of anaesthetic apparatus. A history based on the Charles King Collection of the Association of Anaesthetists of Great Britain and Ireland. Oxford, *Blackwell*, 1975.

5733.4 SMITH, William Denis Ashley.
Under the influence. A history of nitrous oxide and oxygen anaesthesia. London, *Macmillan*, 1982.
The most comprehensive work on the subject. Articles reprinted primarily from *Brit. J. Anaesth.*, with new introduction and index.

5733.41 ATKINSON, Richard Stuart, & BOULTON, Thomas Babington.
The history of anesthesia. London, *Royal Society of Medicine and Parthenon Publishing*, 1989.
Proceedings of the 1987 Second International Symposium on the History of Anaesthesia at the Royal College of Surgeons of England. Over 100 contributors. International Congress and Symposium Series 134.

PLASTIC AND RECONSTRUCTIVE SURGERY

5733.50 CELSUS, Aulus Aurelius Cornelius. 25 b.c.-a.d. 50
De medicina. Florentiae, *Nicolaus [Laurentius]*, 1478.
Celsus provides the earliest account in Western literature of surgical remedies for mutilations, including plastic operations for restoration of the nose, lips, eyelids, ears, etc. First edition in English, London, 1756. *See* Nos. 20, 3666.81, & 5548.1.

5733.51 PFOLSPEUNDT, Heinrich von. *fl.* 1460
Buch der Bündth-Ertznei. Hrsg. von H. Haeser und A. Middeldorpf. Berlin, *G. Reimer*, 1868.
Although not printed until 1868, this treatise was written about 1460, and is the first work of the early German surgeons. It includes the earliest western account of rhinoplasty after Celsus, probably learned from one of the Brancas, itinerant Sicilian surgeons of the early 15th century. Pfolspeundt also described harelip and its treatment. *See* No. 5558.

5733.52 MERCURIALE, Girolamo. 1530-1606
De decoratione liber...Additi nunc primum duo tractatus, alter, de varicibus, alter de reficiendo naso. Francofurdi, *Apud Joannem Wechelum*, 1587.
This work on cosmetics contains Tagliacozzi's first publication on rhinoplasty – *De reficiendo naso* – a letter written to Mercuriale in response to inaccurate statements about his methods made by Mercuriale in *De decoratione* (1585).

5734 TAGLIACOZZI, Gaspare. 1545-1599
De curtorum chirurgia per insitionem. Venetiis, *apud G. Bindonum, jun.*, 1597.

Tagliacozzi of Bologna became famous for his work on rhinoplasty, but Paré and Fallopius both abused him and his work, and the Church (which regarded such operations as meddling with the work of God) exhumed his body and reburied it in unconsecrated ground.   English translation of Book II in Read, *Chirurgorum comes: or the whole practice of chirurgery*, London, 1687. The definitive biography of Tagliacozzi by Martha T. Gnudi, and J. P. Webster, New York, 1950 reprints this translation and reproduces the woodcuts from Tagliacozzi's book. It also contains a history of plastic surgery after Tagliacozzi. A pirated edition published by R. Meietti, Venice, 1597, was reprinted, Mexico, 1974.

5735   MEEKEREN, Job Janszoon van. 1611-1666
Heel- en geneeskonstige aanmerkkingen. Amsterdam, *C. Commelijn*, 1668.
    Van Meekeren was first to record a bone graft. He states (Chap. 1) that he read a report of it in a letter received by the Rev. Engebert Sloot of Slooterdijk from John Kraanwinkel, a missionary in Russia, where the operation had been performed. It consisted of the transplantation of a piece of bone from a dog's skull into a cranial defect in a soldier. Although healing was perfect, the Church ordered the removal of the graft. German translation of the book, 1675; Latin translation, 1682. The original was reprinted Alphen a.d. Rijn, *Stafleu*, 1979.

5735.1   B. L.
Article on Indian rhinoplasty. *Gentleman's Magazine*, 1794, **64**, pt.2, 891-92.
    The first report published in Europe on the so-called Indian or Hindu method of rhinoplasty using a forehead flap, accompanied by an engraving of the patient, Cowasjee, with a restored nose and showing the stages of the operation.

5736   BARONIO, Giuseppe. 1759-1811
Degli innesti animali. Milano, *stemp. e. fond. del Genio*, 1804.
    Baronio was among the first to attempt transplantation and experimental surgery in animals. He successfully carried out full-thickness skin grafts after detachment from the body, and the first purely scientific research in the history of plastic surgery.   English translation and definitive edition, Boston, *Countway Library of Medicine*, 1985.

5737   CARPUE, Joseph Constantine. 1764-1846
An account of two successful operations for restoring a lost nose from the integuments of the forehead. London, *Longman, Hurst, etc.*, 1816.
    Carpue revived the Hindu method of rhinoplasty (*see* No. 5735.1), and reported two successful cases. Facsimile edition, with biography of Carpue by Frank C. McDowell and bibliography of his writings, Birmingham, *Classics of Medicine Library*, 1981. German translation by C.F. von Graefe, Berlin, *Realschulbuchhandlung*, 1817.

5738   GRAEFE, Carl Ferdinand von. 1787-1840
Rhinoplastik, oder die Kunst den Verlust der Nase organisch zu ersetzen. Berlin, *Reimer*, 1818.
    Von Graefe revived rhinoplasty in Germany with this survey what of he called the three methods: the Italian, the Indian, and the "German" method, his own variation on the Italian method. On p. 13 he described the first truly

successful case of blepharoplasty, performed in 1809. Latin translation by J. Hecker, 1818.

5739   ——. Die Gaumennath, ein neuentdecktes Mittel gegen angeborene Fehler der Sprache. *J. Chir. Augenheilk.*, 1820, **1**, 1-54.

Graefe devised an operation for the treatment of congenital cleft palate. He reported his first closure of a cleft in the soft palate to the Med.-Chir. Gesellschaft, Berlin, on 27 December 1816 (see *J. pract Heilk.*, 1817, **44**, 1 St., p. 116). Abridged English translation in No. 5768.2.

5739.1   ROUX, PHILIBERT JOSEPH. 1780-1854

Observation sur une division congénitale du voile du palais et de la luette guérie au moyen d'une opération analogue à celle de bec-de-lièvre. *J. univ. Sci. med.*, 1819, **16**, 356.

Report of Roux's operation on Stephenson (No. 5740). English translation in No. 5768.2. Roux recorded it more fully in his *Quarante années de pratique chirurgicale*, vol. 1. Paris, *Masson*, 1854. *See* No. 5741.2.

5740   STEPHENSON, JOHN. 1797-1842

Dissertatio chirurgo-medica inauguralis de velosynthesi. Edinburgi, *J. Moir*, 1820.

Stephenson, a medical student from Montreal, was the first to be operated upon by Roux (No. 5739.1) for the repair of cleft of the soft palate. He described the operation in his graduation thesis. Stephenson later founded the Montreal Medical Institution, from which the Medical Faculty at McGill University developed. For translations see *J. Hist. Med.*, 1963, **18**, 209-19, and *Brit J. plast. Surg.*, 1966, **19**, 1-14.

5740.1   BÜNGER, CHRISTIAN HEINRICH. 1782-1842

Gelungener Versuch einer Nasenbildung aus einem völlig getrennten Hautstück aus dem Beine. *J. Chir. Augen-Heilk.*, 1822, **4**, 569-582.

First well-documented full-thickness skin graft, used for a rhinoplasty on a patient whose nose and forehead had been destroyed by uncontrolled lupus. English translation in No. 5768.2.

5741   DIEFFENBACH, JOHANN FRIEDRICH. 1792-1847

Nonnula de regeneratione et transplantatione. Herbipoli, *typ. Richterianis*, 1822.

Dieffenbach's thesis for the degree of M.D., Würzburg.

5741.1   DELPECH, JACQUES MATLHIEU. 1777-1832

Chirurgie clinique de Montpellier. 2 vols. Paris, *Gabon*, 1823-28.

The first account of rhinoplasty in France. On 4 June 1823, Delpech performed the first of six cases of rhinoplasty by the Indian forehead flap method, and one (unsuccessful) with a flap from the arm following von Graefe (No. 5738). Delpech also was the first to restore the lower lip by means of a skin graft from the throat.

5741.2   ROUX, PHILIBERT JOSEPH. 1780-1854

Mémoire sur la staphyloraphie, ou la suture du voile du palais. *Arch. gén. Méd.*, 1825, **7**, 516-38.

Roux's first detailed paper on his operation for cleft of the soft palate in which he first proposed the name, "staphylorrhaphy". The greatly expanded edition in book form, Paris, *Chaudé*, 1825, was translated into German by Dieffenbach, Berlin, *Enslin*, 1826.

5742   WARREN, JOHN COLLINS. 1778-1856
On an operation for the cure of natural fissure of the soft palate. *Amer. J. med. Sci.*, 1828, **3** , 1-3.
Operation in May 1824 – the first staphylorraphy in America – performed without direct knowledge of Roux's operations. Nathan Smith (1762-1829) published an earlier paper on staphylorrhaphy in America: *Am. med. Rev.*, 1826, **3**, 396.

5742.1   FRICKE, JOHANN KARL GEORG. 1790-1841
Die Bildung neuer Augenlider (Blepharoplastik) nach Zerstörungen und dadurch hervorgebrachten Auswärtsweundungen derselben. Hamburg, *Perthes & Besser*, 1829.
First extensive treatise on the use of pedicle grafts from the temple and cheek for supplying necessary skin for the reconstruction of deformed eyelids.

5743   DIEFFENBACH, JOHANN FRIEDRICH. 1792-1856
Chirurgische Erfahrungen besonders über die Wiederherstellung zerstörter Theile des menschlichen Körpers nach neuen Methoden. 3 vols. [in 4] and atlas. Berlin, *T. C. F. Enslin*, 1829-34.
Dieffenbach was Professor of Surgery in Berlin. He was a pioneer in the field of plastic and orthopaedic surgery, performing tenotomy and skingrafting successfully. English translation of the section on rhinoplasty, with additional cases and notes by the translator, J.S. Bushnan, London, 1833.

5743.1   BLANDIN, PHILIPPE-FRÉDÉRIC. 1798-1849
Autoplastie, ou restauration des parties du corps, qui ont été détruites, à la faveur d'un emprunt fait à d'autres parties plus ou mains éloigneés. Paris, *Urtubie*, 1836.
The first treatise on plastic surgery in general, criticised by Zeis (No. 5743.4) for its bias against the achievements of German surgeons. This is the first commerical edition. The work was published slightly earlier as a thesis with title, *De l'autoplastie. Thèse présentée et soutenue...pour une chaire de clinique chirurgicale*, Paris, *Urtubie*, 1836.

5743.2   MUTTER, THOMAS DENT. 1811-1859
Case of deformity of the mouth, from a burn, successfully treated by Dieffenbach's method. *Am. J. med. Sci.*, 1837, **20**, 341-46.
Mutter was probably the first in America to perform plastic operations to correct deformities.

5743.3   WARREN, JONATHAN MASON. 1811-1867
Rhinoplastic operation. *Bost. med. surg. J.*, 1837, **16**, 69-79.
First rhinoplasty reported in the United States. For this Warren used the Hindu method. He reported his first use of the Italian or Tagliacotian method in *Bost. med. surg. J.*, 1840, **22**, 261-69. Jonathan Mason Warren was the son of John Collins Warren.

5743.4   ZEIS, EDUARD. 1807-1868
Handbuch der plastischen Chirurgie. Nebst einer Vorrede von J.F. Dieffenbach. Berlin, *G. Reimer*, 1838.

In this work Zeis introduced the term "plastic surgery". The first half of the work covers the general principles of plastic surgery, and the first history of the subject. The second half describes the special operative techniques required for the individual parts of the body. Annotated English translation by T.J.S. Patterson, Oxford, *Oxford University Press*, 1988. *See* No. 5767.

5744   AMMON, FRIEDRICH AUGUST VON. 1799-1861
Die plastische Chirurgie. Berlin, *G. Reimer*, 1842.

5745   WARREN, JONATHAN MASON. 1811-1867
Operations for fissure of the hard and soft palate (palatoplastie). *New Engl. quart. J. Med. Surg.*, 1842-43, **1**, 538-47.
        Warren devised the first operation for closure of complete clefts of the palate.

5746   MALGAIGNE, JOSEPH FRANÇOIS. 1806-1865
Nouvelle méthode pour l'opération du bec-de-lièvre. *J. Chir. (Malgaigne)*, 1844, **2**, 1-6.
        Malgaigne's two-flap method for repair of cleft lip. English translation by R. Ivy in No. 5768.2.

5746.1 MIRAULT, GERMANICUS. 1796-1879
Lettre (Deuxième lettre) sur l'opération du bec-de-lièvre, considérée dans ses divers états de simplicité et de complication. *J. Chir. (Malgaigne)*, 1844, **2**, 257-65; 1845, **3**, 5-20.
        Mirault modified Malgaigne's technique for cleft lip repair by discarding the medial flap and bringing the lateral flap of mucosa across. Abridged English translation by R. Ivy in No. 5768.2.

5746.2 PANCOAST, JOSEPH. 1805-1882
A treatise on operative surgery. Philadelphia, *Carey & Hart*, 1844.
        This splendidly illustrated work contains the first extensive section on plastic surgery in an American surgical textbook. *See* No. 5598.

5746.3 DIEFFENBACH, JOHANN FRIEDRICH. 1794-1847
Die operative Chirurgie. 2 vols., Leipzig, *F.A. Brockhaus*, 1845-48.
        This is Dieffenbach's most comprehensive work. It also contains his most detailed exposition of his methods of performing plastic operations. *See* No. 5598.1.

5746.4 FRITZE, HERMANN EDUARD. 1811-66, & REICH, O.F.G.
Die plastische Chirurgie. Berlin, *Hirschwald*, 1845.
        Fritze and Reich studied under Dieffenbach. This is the first extensively illustrated general treatise on plastic surgery published in Europe.

5747   HAMILTON, FRANK HASTINGS. 1813-1886
Elkoplasty, or anaplasty applied to the treatment of old ulcers. New York, *Holman, Gray & Co.*, 1854.
        Hamilton was among the first to treat ulcers by skin-grafting. He made the flap smaller than the space which it was intended to fill, "trusting to growth and expansion of the graft to complete the cure". Also published in *N.Y.J. Med.*, 1854, **13**, 163-73. See his earlier theoretical paper in *Buffalo med. J.*, 1847, **2**, 501-509.

5748   LANGENBECK, Bernhard Rudolph Conrad von. 1810-1887
Die Uranoplastik mittelst Ablösung es mucös-periostalen
Gaumenüberzuges. *Arch. klin. Chir.*, 1862, **2**, 205-87.
Langenbeck has several operations named after him, one of the most
important being that for cleft palate. Abridged English translation in No.
5768.2.

5749   SIMON, Gustav. 1824-1876
Mittheilungen aus der chirurgischen Klinik des Rostocker Krankhauses...II.
Abtheilung. Beiträge zur plastischen Chirurgie. Prag. Vierteljschr. prakt.
Heilk. (1866-67). Prag, *C. Reichendecker*, 1868.
Simon was the first to report a procedure capable of preserving the
cupid's bow in repair of the lip – a critical procedure for the development
of cheiloplasty. A separate edition in book form was also published. *See*
No. 5766.1.

5750   REVERDIN, Jacques Louis. 1842-1929
Greffe épidermique. Expérience faite dans le service de M. le docteur
Guyon à l'hôpital Necker. *Bull. Soc. imp. Chir. Paris,* (1869), 1870, 2 sér.,
10, 511-15.
Reverdin's work on the transplantation of free skin, as contrasted with
the previous method of pedunculated flaps, attracted much attention.
English translation in No. 5768.2.

5751   LAWSON, George. 1831-1903
On the transplantation of portions of skin for the closure of large granulating
surfaces. *Trans. clin. Soc. Lond.*, 1871, **4**, 49-53.
Lawson, surgeon to the Middlesex Hospital, London, was the first
successfully to transplant sizeable areas of skin, as compared with the small
grafts of Reverdin, and of whole thickness skin as well. Reprinted in No.
5768.2.

5752   OLLIER, Louis Xavier Edouard Léopold. 1830-1900
Greffes cutanées ou autoplastiques. *Bull Acad. Méd. (Paris)*, 1872, 2 sér.,
1, 243-50.
First description of intermediate thickness skin grafts. Ollier used large
grafts and carried out complete excision of scar tissue and its replacement
with skin.

5753   THIERSCH, Carl. 1822-1895
Ueber die feineren anatomischen Veränderungen bei Aufheilung von
Haut auf Granulationen. *Verh. dtsch. Ges. Chir.*, 1874, **3**, 69-75.
Thiersch's first paper on transplantation of skin. Simultaneous publication
in *Arch. klin. Chir.*, 1874, **17**, 318-24. English translation in No. 5768.2.

5754   WOLFE, John Reissberg. 1824-1904
A new method of performing plastic operations. *Brit. med. J.*, 1875, **2**, 360-
61.
Wolfe insisted that in free skin grafts the subcutaneous tissue at the site
of the graft must be removed, and that the graft should consist of skin only.
His name is perpetuated in the "Wolfe–Krause graft rest".

5754.1   BUCK, GURDON. 1807-1877
           Contributions to reparative surgery; showing its application to the treatment
           of deformities produced by destructive disease or injury; congenital
           defects from arrest or excess of development; and cicatrical contractions
           from burns. New York, *D. Appleton*, 1876.
           First American work exclusively on reconstructive surgery.

5754.2   ELY, EDWARD TALBOT. 1850-1885
           An operation for prominence of the auricles. *Arch. Otol. (N.Y.)*, 1881, **10**,
           97-99.
                 Otoplasty first described. Ely died very young from tuberculosis.

5754.3   HAGEDORN, WERNER. 1831-1894
           Über eine Modifikation der Hasenschartenoperation. *Zbl. Chir.*, 1884, **11**,
           756-8.
                 Hagedorn's operation is important as forming the basis of most modern
           methods of unilateral cleft lip repair.

5754.4   ROE, JOHN ORLANDO. 1848-1915
           The deformity termed "pug nose" and its correction, by a simple operation.
           Med. Rec., 1887, **31**, 621-23.
                 Roe invented the intranasal approach for corrective rhinoplasty.

5754.5   ——.The correction of angular deformities of the nose by a subcutaneous
           operation, *Med. Rec.*, 1891, **40**, 57-59.
                 The first reduction rhinoplasty to enhance the appearance of a patient.
           See No. 5755.3.

5754.6   WEIR, ROBERT FULTON. 1838-1927
           On restoring sunken noses without scarring the face. *N. Y. med. J.*, 1892,
           56, 449-54.
                 Reduction rhinoplasty by the endonasal approach. "The beginnings of
           the logical step-by-step rhinoplasty in use today" (McDowell).

5755   KRAUSE, FEDOR. 1856-1937
           Ueber die Transplantation grosser ungestielter Hautlappen. *Verh. dtsch.
           Ges. Chir.*, 1893, **22**, pt. 2, 46-51.
                 Krause popularized the use of whole thickness skin grafts. English
           translation in No. 5768.2.

5755.1   ISRAEL, JAMES. 1848-1926
           Zwei neue Methoden der Rhinoplastik. *Arch. klin. Chir.*, 1896, **53**, 255-
           265.
                 First free bone graft to the nose. Abridged English translation in No.
           5768.2.

5755.2   ABBE, ROBERT. 1851-1928
           A new plastic operation for the relief of deformity due to double harelip.
           Med. Rec. (N.Y), 1898, **53**, 477-8.
                 Abbe's lip-switch flap, transferring a full-thickness flap from one lip of
           the oral cavity to fill a defect in the other lip. This is also known eponymically
           as the Abbe–Estlander operation, crediting Jakob Estlander (1831-1881).
           See No. 5768.2.

5755.3 JOSEPH, JACQUES. 1865-1934
Über die operative Verkleinerung eine Nase (Rhinomiosis). *Berl. klin. Wschr.*, 1898, **35**, 882-5.
  Joseph rhinoplasty, developed independently of Roe (Nos. 5754.4-5) and Weir (No. 5754.6). Translation in *Plast. reconstr. Surg.*, 1970, **46**, 178-81.

5755.4 MONKS, GEORGE HOWARD. 1853-1933
Correction, by operation, of some nasal deformities and disfigurements. BOST. MED. SURG. J., 1898, 139, 262-69.
  Monks developed the modern surgical treatment of rhinophyma.

5756 MORESTIN, HIPPOLYTE. 1869-1919
De l'ablation esthétique des tumeurs bénignes du sein. *Presse méd.*, 1902, **10**, 975-77.
  Morestin's method of mammaplasty. He was also responsible for several of the techniques employed in maxillo-facial surgery. Reprinted, Pittsburgh, 1959.

5756.1 MILLER, CHARLES CONRAD. 1880-1950
The correction of featural imperfections. Chicago, *Published by the Author*, [1907].
  The first book on cosmetic surgery. Miller "was both a quack and surgical visionary, years ahead of his more academic colleagues" (Rogers).

5756.2 BLAIR, VILRAY PAPIN. 1871-1955
Underdeveloped lower jaw, with limited excursion. Report of two cases with operation. *J. Amer. Med. Assoc.*, 1909, **53**, 178-183.
  Closed ramisection of the mandible for micrognathia or prognathism.

5756.3 DAVIS, JOHN STAIGE. 1872-1946
A method of splinting skin grafts. *Ann Surg.*, 1909, **49**, 416-18.
  The Davis graft was devised by Halsted but Davis popularized its use.

5756.4 LUCKETT, WILLIAM HENRY. 1872-1929
A new operation for prominent ears based on the anatomy of the deformity. *Surg. Gynec. Obst.*, 1910, **10**, 635-7.
  Luckett developed the modern operation for the correction of protruding ears.

5756.5 KOLLE, FREDERICK STRANGE. 1872-1929
Plastic and cosmetic surgery. New York, *D. Appleton*, 1911.
  First comprehensive work on cosmetic surgery.

5756.6 GUTHRIE, CHARLES CLAUDE. 1880-1963
Blood-vessel surgery and its applications. London, *E. Arnold*, 1912.
  This book describes Guthrie's pioneer work in tissue and organ transplantation.

5756.7 BLAIR, VILRAY PAPIN. 1871-1955
Surgery and diseases of the mouth and jaws. St. Louis, *C. V. Mosby Co.*, 1912.
  First comprehensive work on maxillofacial surgery. After World War I Blair established the first separate Plastic Surgery Service in the United States at Barnes Hospital and Washington University in St. Louis.

5756.8   HOLLÄNDER, Eugen. 1867-1932
Die kosmetische Chirurgie. *In:* Joseph, M. (ed.) Handbuch der Kosmetik, Leipzig, *Verlag von Veit*, 1912.
Briefly describes (p. 688) the first facelift operation. Holländer later stated that the operation was performed in 1901. A pupil of James Israel (No. 5755.1), Holländer is better known today for his series of books on medicine in art. See Rogers, The development of aesthetic plastic surgery: a history, *Aesth. Plast. Surg.*, 1976, **1**, 3-24.

5757   ALBEE, Fred Houdlett. 1876-1945
Bone-graft surgery. Philadelphia, *W. B. Saunders Co.*, 1915.
Albee was the first to employ living bone grafts as internal splints. He used cutting machines and saws to make inlaid, perfectly-fitting grafts. See especially his "Transplantation of a portion of the tibia into the spine for Pott's disease. A preliminary report", *J. Amer. med. Ass.*, 1911, **57**, 885-86. *See* No. 4384.1.

5757.1   FILATOV, Vladimir Petrovich. 1875-1956
Plastika na kruglom stebl. [Plastic procedure using a round pedicle]. *Vestn. Oftal.*, 1917, **34**, No. 4-5, 149-58.
Filatov used a tubed pedicle flap in September 1916. English translation in *Surg. Clin. N. Amer.*, 1959, **39**, 277-87.

5757.2   GANZER, Hugo.
Weichteilplastik des Gesichts bei Kieferschuss-Verletzungen. *Dtsch. Z. Zahnheilk.*, 1917, **35**, 348-54.
Independantly of Filatov, Ganzer devised a tubed flap for repairs about the mouth and jaw.

5757.3   ROBERTS, John Bingham. 1852-1924
Congenital clefts of the face. *Ann. Surg.*, 1918, **67**, 110-114.
Roberts introduced the push-back procedure - backward displacement of the velum to ensure adequate speech.

5757.4   DAVIS, John Staige. 1872-1946
Plastic surgery: Its principles and practice. Philadelphia, *Blakiston*, [1919].
Davis was the first surgeon to limit his work exclusively to plastic surgery. This was the first comprehensive textbook on the subject.

5758   GILLIES, *Sir* Harold Delf. 1882-1960
Plastic surgery of the face. London, *H. Frowde*, 1920.
Gillies introduced a tubed pedical flap in 1917.

5759   ——, & FRY, *Sir* William Kelsey. 1889-1963
A new principle in the surgical treatment of "congenital cleft palate", and its mechanical counterpart. *Brit. med. J.*, 1921, **1**, 335-38.
Gillies's operation for cleft palate.

5760   KRASKE, Hans.
Die Operation der atrophischen und hypertrophischen Hängebrust. *Munch. med. Wschr.*, 1923, **70**, 672.
Plastic operation for enlarged breasts.

5761   WARDILL, WILLIAM EDWARD MANDALL. 1894-1960
        Cleft palate. *Brit J. Surg.*, 1928, **16**, 127-48.
            Wardill's operation for cleft palate.

5761.1 BLAIR, VILRAY PAPIN. 1871-1955, & BROWN, JAMES BARRETT. 1899-1971
        The use and uses of large split skin grafts of intermediate thickness. *Surg. Gynec. Obstet.*, 1929, **49**, 82-97.
            Split-skin grafts for covering large areas of granulating surfaces introduced.

5762   ——, ——. Mirault operation for single harelip. *Surg. Gynec. Obstet.*, 1930, **51**, 81-98.
            Modern refinement of Mirault's precedure for repair of cleft lip.

5763   VEAU, VICTOR. 1871-1949
        Division palatine. Paris, *Masson*, 1931.
            Includes Veau's operation for cleft palate.

5763.01 JOSEPH, JACQUES. 1865-1934
        Nasenplastik und sonitige Gesichtsplastik nebst einem Anhang über Mammaplastik. Leipzig, *C. Kabitsch*, 1931,
            A masterpiece of 20th century plastic surgery, and Joseph's most comprehensive work. English translation by S. Milstein, following original text and illustrations page for page, Phoenix, *Columnella Press*, 1987.

5763.1 PADGETT, EARL CALVIN. 1893-1946
        Calibrated intermediate skin-grafts. *Surg. Gynec. Obstet.*, 1939, **69**, 779-93.
            Padgett dermatome.

5764   INCLAN, ALBERTO FRANCIS. 1916-
        The use of preserved bone grafts in orthopaedic surgery. *J. Bone Jt. Surg.*, 1942, **24**, 81-96.
            These studies form the basis of the modern use of bone preserved by refrigeration.

5765   SANO, MACHTELD ELISABETH. 1903-
        Skin grafting. A new method based on the principles of tissue culture. *Amer. J. Surg.*, 1943, **61**, 105-06.
            First use of fibrin glue for skin grafting. See also *Surg. Gynec. Obstet.*, 1943, **77**, 510-13.

5766   THOREK, MAX. 1880-1960
        Plastic surgery of the breast and abdominal wall. Springfield, *C. C. Thomas*, 1942.

5766.1 LeMESURIER, ARTHUR BAKER. 1889-
        A method of cutting and suturing the lip in the treatment of complete unilateral clefts. *Plast. reconstr. Surg.*, 1949, **4**, 1-12.
            LeMesurier's cheiloplasty procedure was based on Hagedorn's method. He was first to attempt construction of the cupid's bow of the vermilion.

5766.2 ORTICOCHEA, MIGUEL.
        A new method of total reconstruction of the penis. *Brit. J. Plast. Surg.*, 1972, **25**, 347-66.

The first description of the use of a musculocutaneous flap in reconstructive surgery. The resulting penis was fully-functional.

5766.3   DANIEL, ROLLIN K. and TAYLOR, G. IAN.
Distant transfer of an island flap by microvascular anastomoses. A clinical technique. *Plast. reconstr. Surg.*, 1973, **52**, 111-17.
Successful direct flap transfer by vascular anastomosis. See also *Austr. N. Z. J. Surg.*, 1973, **43**, 1-3.

5766.4   TAYLOR, G. IAN. *et al.*
The free vascularized bone graft. A clinical extension of microvascular techniques. *Plast. reconstr. Surg.*, 1975, 55, 533-54.
First clinically successful free bone graft with microvascular anastomosis in which a fibular segment was transferred to the contralateral leg to reconstruct a large tibial defect. With G.D.H. Miller and F. J.Ham.

5766.5   MILLARD, DAVID RALPH. 1919-
Cleft craft: the evolution of its surgery. 3 vols. Boston, *Little, Brown & Co.*, 1976-80.
An encyclopaedic monograph on cleft palate surgery, exceptionally well written, illustrated, and produced, incorporating an historical approach.

5766.6   HARTRAMPF, CARL R., SCHEFLAN, MICHAEL, & BLACK, PAUL W.
Breast reconstruction with a transverse abdominal island flap. *Plast. reconstr. Surg.*, 1982, **69**, 216-24.
Breast reconstruction without the use of an artificial implant.

5766.7   RADOVAN, CHADOMIR.
Tissue expansion in soft-tissue reconstruction. *Plast. reconstr. Surg.*, 1984, **74**, 482-90.

History of Plastic and Reconstructive Surgery

5767   ZEIS, EDUARD. 1807-1868
Die Literatur and Geschichte der plastichen Chirurgie. Leipzig, *W. Engelmann*, 1863.
A history of plastic surgery and an annotated bibliography of its literature prior to 1860. Nachträge, 1864. Reprint, including Nachträge, Bologna, 1963. The main bibliography has 2008 references, the supplement 275 more. Both parts were collated and translated, with additions and revisions by T.J.S. Patterson, as *The Zeis index and history of plastic surgery*, and published as volume 1 of No. 5768.2. *See also* No. 5743.4.

5768   DORRANCE, GEORGE MORRIS. 1877-1948
The operative story of cleft palate. Philadelphia, *W.B. Saunders*, 1933.

5768.1   HUGHES, WENDELL L.
Reconstructive surgery of the eyelids. St. Louis, *C.V. Mosby Co.*, 1943.
Most of this work is a very carefully documented history of the subject. Bibliography of 451 references.

5768.2 McDOWELL, Frank. 1911-1981
McDowell series of plastic surgical indexes. Edited by Frank McDowell. 5 vols. Baltimore, *Williams & Wilkins*, 1977-81.
Vol. I: 900 B.C. TO A.D. 1863 (Zeis [*see* No. 5767] translated, with additions and revisions); Vol. II: 1864-1920; Vol. III: 1921-1946; [Vol. IV]: 25-year index of *Plastic and Reconstructive Surgery*, 1946-71; Vol. V: 1971-76. Titles of nearly all foreign citations have been translated into English. Only Vol. I. is annotated.

5768.3 ——. The source book of plastic surgery. Compiled and edited by Frank McDowell. Baltimore, *Williams & Wilkins*, 1977.
Reprints, translated into English where necessary, of classic papers on plastic surgery, with commentary.

5768.4 KLASEN, Henk J.
History of free skin grafting. Berlin & New York, *Springer-Verlag*, [1981].
Comprehensive work, with hundreds of bibliographical references. No index.

5768.5 WALLACE, Antony F.
The progress of plastic surgery: An introductory history. Oxford, *Meeuws*, 1982.

5768.6 GABKA, Joachim, & VAUBEL, Ekkehard.
Plastic surgery past and present. Origin and history of modern lines of incision. Basel, *S. Karger*, [1983].
Well-documented history of current plastic operations using both recent surgical photographs and illustrations from classics in the historical literature. Includes brief biographies of the most important pioneers.

5768.7 GONZALEZ-ULLOA, Mario, (ed.)
The creation of aesthetic plastic surgery. New York, *Springer-Verlag*, [1985].
Reprints useful papers from *Aesthetic plast. Surg.*, 1976-85. No index.

5768.8 BOSNIAK, Stephen L. (Ed.)
History and tradition [of ophthalmic plastic surgery]. *Advances in Ophthalmic Plastic and Reconstructive Surgery*, 1986, 5.
A collection of articles by various authors, including partial reprint of No. 5768.1.

DISEASES OF THE BREAST

5769 COOPER, *Sir* Astley Paston, *Bart*. 1768-1841
Illustrations of the diseases of the breast. London, *Longman, Rees & Co.*, 1829.
Includes one of the earliest descriptions of hyperplastic cystic disease of the breast, which Cooper referred to as "hydatid disease".

5769.1 ——. On the anatomy of the breast. 2 vols. London, *Longman...*1840.
Anatomical sequel to No. 5769, with outstanding illustrations.

5770 BRODIE, *Sir* Benjamin Collins, *Bart*, 1783-1862
Lecture on sero-cystic tumors of the breast. *Lond. med. Gaz.*, 1840, **25**, 808-14.
"Brodie's tumour". Reprinted inn *Med. Classics*, 1938, **2**, 941-54.

5771   VELPEAU, ALFRED ARMAND LOUIS MARIE. 1795-1867
Traité des maladies du sein et de la région mammaire. Paris, *V. Masson*, 1854.
Velpeau was the leading French surgeon of the first half of the 19th century. His great treatise on tumours of the breast, his best work, was the most important of its time on the subject. It includes a good account of hyperplastic disease of the breast. English translation, 1856.

5772   PAGET, *Sir* JAMES *Bart.* 1814-1899
On disease of the mammary areola preceding cancer of the mammary gland. *St. Barth. Hosp. Rep.*, 1874, **10**, 87-89.
First description of "Paget's disease of the nipple" – eczema of the nipple with cancer. The paper is reprinted in *Med. Classics*, 1936, **1**, 75-78. Paget was Serjeant Surgeon to Queen Victoria, and a great surgical pathologist. He was associated with St. Bartholomew's Hospital during most of his life.

5773   BILLROTH, CHRISTIAN ALBERT THEODOR. 1829-1894
Die Krankheiten der Brustdrüsen. Stuttgart, *F. Enke*, 1880.

5774   RECLUS, PAUL. 1847-1914
La maladie kystique des mamelles. *Bull Soc. Anat. Paris*, 1883, **58**, 428-33.
"Reclus's disease". Reclus was professor of surgery in Paris; he left a classic description of chronic cystic mastitis.

5775   SCHIMMELBUSCH, CURT. 1860-1895
Das Cystadenom der Mamma. *Arch. klin. Chir.*, 1892, **44**, 117-34.
"Schimmelbusch's disease".

5776   HALSTED, WILLIAM STEWART. 1852-1922
The treatment of wounds with especial reference to the value of the blood clot in the management of dead spaces. *Johns Hopk. Hosp. Rep.*, 1890-91, **2**, 255-314.
Halsted showed that optimum wound healing was most easily obtained by avoiding haematoma formation. Contains description of Halsted's method of radical mastectomy – one of the greatest contributions ever made to the treatment of mammary cancer. This paper also contains the first mention of the use of rubber gloves (a Halsted invention) in an operating room. This paper and No. 5777 contain the first illustrations published by Max Brödel after he moved to Johns Hopkins Hospital.

5777   ——. The results of operations for the cure of cancer of the breast performed at the Johns Hopkins Hospital from June, 1889 to January, 1894. *Johns Hopk. Hosp. Rep.*, 1894-95, **4**, 297-350.
Halsted's operation invariably excised the pectoralis major muscle in radical mastectomy. His operation, modified by the retention of the pectoral muscles, remains the cornerstone of surgical treatment of carcinoma of the breast. Plate 12 shows the first use of rubber gloves during an operation. *See* No. 5640. Reprinted in *Med. Classics*, 1938, **3**, 441-509.

5778   ——. A clinical and histological study of certain adenocarcinomata of the breast, and a brief consideration of the supraclavicular operations for cancer of the breast from 1889 to 1898 at Johns Hopkins Hospital. *Trans. Amer. surg. Ass.*, 1898, **16**, 144-81.

5778.1   BEATSON, *Sir* GEORGE THOMAS. 1848-1933
On the treatment of inoperable cases of carcinoma of the mamma: suggestions for a new method of treatment, with illustrative cases. *Lancet*, 1896, **2**, 104-07, 162-65.
Öophorectomy in the treatment of breast cancer.

5779   ———. The treatment of cancer of the breast by öophorectomy and thyroid extract. *Brit med. J.*, 1901, **2**, 1145-48.

5780   BLOODGOOD, JOSEPH COLT. 1867-1935
Senile parenchymatous hypertrophy of female breast. *Surg. Gynec. Obstet.*, 1906, **3**, 721-30.
Bloodgood's theory of the causation of chronic mastitis.

5781   CORNIL, ANDRÉ VICTOR. 1837-1908
Les tumeurs du sein. Paris, *F. Alcan*, 1908.

5782   HANDLEY, WILLIAM SAMPSON. 1872-1962
Cancer of the breast and its treatment. 2nd ed. London, *J. Murray*, 1922.
Sampson Handley advanced the theory that in mammary cancer metastasis is due to extension along lymphatic vessels – "lymphatic permeation" – and not to dissemination by way of the blood stream. The book was first published in 1906.

5782.1   LANE-CLAYPON, JANET ELIZABETH. 1877-1967
A further report on cancer of the breast, with special reference to its associated antecedent conditions. *Rep. Minist. Hlth, London, No. 32.* London, H. M. S. O., 1926.
First modern case-control study.

5783   DARTIGUES, LOUIS. 1869-1940
Mammectomie totale et autogreffe libre aréolomamelonnaire; mammectomie bilatérale esthétique. *Bull. Soc. Chirurgiens Paris*, 1928, **20**, 739-44.
The modern operation of total bilateral mammectomy, with transplantation of the nipple and areola, was especially developed by Dartigues.

5784   CHEATLE, *Sir* GEORGE LENTHAL. 1865-1951, & CUTLER, MAX. 1899-1984
Tumours of the breast. Their pathology, symptoms, diagnosis, and treatment. London, *E. Arnold & Co.*, 1931.

5785   CUTLER, MAX. 1899-1984
The cause of "painful breasts" and treatment by means of ovarian residue. *J. Amer. med. Ass.*, 1931, **96**, 1201-05.
Cutler was the first to employ ovarian hormone systematically in the treatment of chronic mastitis.

5786   KEYNES, *Sir* GEOFFREY LANGDON. 1887-1982
The radium treatment of carcinoma of the breast. *Brit J. Surg.*, 1932, **19**, 415-80.
Keynes's successes with radium in breast cancer established this method of conservative treatment. His first paper on the subject, with the same title, was published in *St. Barth. Hosp. Rep.*, 1927, **60**, 91-95.

5787 LACASSAGNE, Antoine Marcellin. 1884-1971
Apparition de cancers de la mamelle chez la souris mâle, soumise à des injections de folliculine. *C. R. Acad. Sci. (Paris)*, 1932, **195**, 630-632.
Demonstration of the carcinogenic effect of ovarian hormone.

5788 ADAIR, Frank Earl. 1887-
Plasma cell mastitis – a lesion simulating mammary carcinoma. *Arch. Surg. (Chicago)*, 1933, **26**, 735-49.
First description of plasma-cell mastitis.

History of Surgery

5788.9 PORTAL, Antoine. 1742-1832
Histoire de l'anatomie et de la chirurgie. 6 vols. [in 7]. Paris, *P.F. Didot le jeune*, 1770-73.
A biobibliographical survey to 1755.

5789 HALLER, Albrecht von. 1708-1777
Bibliotheca chirurgica. 2 vols. Bernae & Basileae, *Haller & Schweighauser*, 1774-75.
Reprinted, Hildesheim, *G. Olms*, 1971.

5790 MALGAIGNE, Joseph François. 1806-1865
Histoire de la chirurgie en Occident depuis de VIe jusqu'au XVIe siècle, et histoire de la vie et des travaux d'Ambroise Paré. Paris, *J. B. Baillière*, [1840].
Billings considered Malgaigne "the greatest surgical historian and critic the world has ever seen"; Leonardo (No. 5812) says that his greatest contribution to surgery was his unique manner of evaluating surgical techniques and innovations by which the then new methods of statistical computation were conjoined with actual surgical experiments. This work was also published in vol. 1 of No. 59. English translation by W. Hamby, Norman, Oklahoma, 1965.

5791 GRÜNDER, Johann Wilhelm Ludwig. 1819-1866
Geschichte der Chirurgie von den Urzeiten bis zu Anfang des achtzehnten Jahrhunderts. Breslau, *Trewendt & Granier*, 1859.

5792 TRENDELENBURG, Friedrich. 1844-1924
De veterum Indorum chirurgia. Berolini, *G. Schade*, [1866].
Trendelenburg's graduation thesis.

5793 FERGUSSON, Sir William. 1808-1877
Lectures on the progress of anatomy and surgery during the present century. London, *J. Churchill & Sons*, 1867.

5794 FISCHER, Georg. 1836-1921
Chirurgie vor 100 Jahren; historische Studie. Leipzig, *F. C. W. Vogel*, 1876.
Reprinted Berlin, *Springer*, 1978.

5795 GROSS, Samuel David. 1805-1884
A century of American surgery. *Amer. J. med. Sci.*, 1876, n.s., **71**, 431-84.
The first serious history of American surgery to 1876. Also published in No. 6586.

5796 ROHLFS, Heinrich. 1827-1898
Die chirurgischen Classiker Deutschlands. 2 vols. Leipzig, *C. L. Hirschfeld*, 1883-85.

5797 SOUTH, John Flint. 1797-1882
Memorials of the craft of surgery in England ... Edited by D'Arcy Power. London, *Cassell & Co.*, 1886.
South, trained in Germany, became surgeon to St. Thomas's Hospital. Through his efforts John Hunter's body was reburied in Westminster Abbey and South himself wrote the inscription on the tablet there.

5798 YOUNG, Sidney.
The annals of the Barber-Surgeons of London, compiled from their records and other sources. London, *Blades, East & Blades*, 1890.

5799 BILLINGS, John Shaw. 1838-1913
The history and literature of surgery. *In*: F. S. Dennis: Systems of surgery, New York, 1895, **1**, 17-144.
Reprinted, New York, *Argosy*, 1970.

5800 GURLT, Ernst Julius. 1825-1899
Geschichte der Chirurgie und ihrer Ausübung. 3 vols. Berlin, *A. Hirschwald*, 1898.
A history of surgery to the end of the 16th century. Includes translations from the literature and illustrations of instruments. Reprinted, Hildesheim, *G. Olms*, 1964.

5801 TILLMANS, Robert Hermann. 1844-1927
Hundert Jahre Chirurgie. *Verh. Ges. dtsch. Naturf. Aerzte*, 1898, **70**, 1 Heft, 38-60.
History of 18th-century German surgery.

5802 BUSCHAN, Georg Hermann Theodor. 1863-1942
Chirurgisches aus der Völkerkunde. Leipzig, *B. Konegen*, 1902.

5803 ALLBUTT, *Sir* Thomas Clifford. 1836-1925
The historical relations of medicine and surgery to the end of the sixteenth century. London, *Macmillan & Co.*, 1905.

5804 HELFREICH, Friedrich. 1842-1927
Geschichte der Chirurgie. *In*: T. Puschmann's Handbuch der Geschichte der Medizin, Jena, 1905, **3**, 1-306.

5805 SMITH, Stephen. 1823-1922
The evolution of American surgery. In *American practice of surgery*, edited by J. D. Bryant and A. H. Buck, New York, 1906, **2**, 1-67.

5806 MILNE, John Stewart. *d.*1913
Surgical instruments in Greek and Roman times. Aberdeen, & London, *Clarendon Press*, 1907.
Reprinted, N.Y., 1970.

5807 FOURMESTRAUX, Jacques de. 1879-
Histoire de la chirurgie française (1790-1920). Paris, *Masson*, 1934.

5808   BLANCHARD, Charles Elton. 1868-
        The romance of proctology, which is the story of the history and devel-
        opment of this much neglected branch of surgery. Youngstown, *Medical
        Success Press*, 1938.

5811   THOMPSON, Charles John Samuel. 1862-1943
        The history and evolution of surgical instruments. New York, *Schuman*,
        1942.

5812   LEONARDO, Richard Anthony. 1895-
        History of surgery. New York, *Froben Press*, 1943.

5813   KILLIAN, Hans. 1892- , & KRÄMER, G.
        Meister der Chirurgie und die Chirurgenschulen im Deutschen Raum.
        Stuttgart, *G. Thieme*, 1951.

5813.1 HURWITZ, Alfred. 1909- & DEGENSHEIN, George A. 1918-
        Milestones in modern surgery. New York, *Hoeber-Harper*, 1958.
            Each chapter contains prefatory comments, a short biography of each
        main builder of the particular milestone (with portrait), and his surgical
        contribution reprinted or translated in full.

5813.2 RANDERS-PEHRSON, Justine. 1910-
        The surgeon's glove. Springfield, *C. C. Thomas*, 1960.
            Contains an extensive bibliography.

5813.3 ZIMMERMAN, Leo M. 1898-1980, & VEITH, Ilza. 1915-
        Great ideas in the history of surgery. Baltimore, *Williams & Wilkins*, 1961.

5813.4 WHIPPLE, Allen Oldfather. 1881-1963
        The story of wound healing and wound repair. Springfield, *C. C. Thomas*
        [1963].
            See No. 3659.1.

5813.5 ELLIOTT, Isabelle Mary Zena.
        A short history of surgical dressings. London, *Pharmaceutical Press*, 1964.
            Based on material collected by James Rawling Elliott (1905-1958).

5813.6 COPE, *Sir* Vincent Zachary. 1881-1974
        A history of the acute abdomen. London, *Oxford University Press*, 1965.

5813.7 HUARD, Pierre Alphonse. 1901-1983, & GRMEK, Mirko Dražen.
        Mille ans de chirurgie en occident: Ve-XVe siècles. Paris, *Roger Dacosta*,
        [1966].

5813.8 ———. La chirurgie moderne. Ses debuts en Occident: XVIe-XVIIe-XVIIIe
        siècles. Paris, *Editions Dacosta*, 1968.

5813.9 CARTWRIGHT, Frederick Fox.
        The development of modern surgery. London, *Arthur Barker*, 1967.

5813.10 MAJNO, Guido.
        The healing hand: Man and wound in the ancient world. Cambridge, Mass.,
        Harvard University Press, [1975].

Emphasizing surgery, this is an exceptionally imaginative and exquisitely designed and illustrated history of medicine in ancient Egypt,
Greece, Rome, and China.

5813.11 WANGENSTEEN, Owen Harding. 1898-1981, & WANGENSTEEN, Sarah D.
The rise of surgery from empiric craft to scientific discipline. Minneapolis,
University of Minnesota Press, 1978.
Not a systematic history but an assessment of those technical factors that
contributed to or retarded the advance of surgery.

5813.12 BENNION, Elisabeth.
Antique medical instruments. Berkeley, *University of California Press*, 1979.
Well-illustrated work coving the history of medical and surgical instruments from the Middle Ages to 1870, with emphasis on pre-19th century
material. Includes useful information on instrument makers.

5813.13 EARLE, A. Scott.
Surgery in America. From the colonial era to the twentieth century. Second
edition. New York, *Praeger*, [1983].
Well-chosen readings from original published sources, with informa-
tive commentary.

5813.14 RUTKOW, Ira Michael. 1948-
The history of surgery in the United States 1775-1900. Volume 1- . San
Francisco, *Norman Publishing*, 1988.
Volume one is an annotated bibliography of all textbooks, mono-
graphs, and treatises written by American surgeons and published in the
United States before 1900. Its chapters include separate bibliographies for
general surgery, ophthalmology, oto-rhino-laryngology, orthopaedic sur-
gery, gynaecology, urology, colon–rectal surgery, and neurological surgery.

5813.15 ORGAN, Claude H. Jr, and KOSIBA, Margaret M.
A century of black surgeons. The U.S.A. experience. 2 vols., Norman,
Oklahoma, *Transcript Press*, [1987].

OPHTHALMOLOGY

5814 AETIUS *of Amida*. a.d. 502-575
Βιβλιων ιατρικῶν τόμος A Librorum medicinalium tomus primus, primi
scilicet libri octo nunc primum in lucem editi. [Venetiis, *in aedibus haeredum
Aldi Manutii et Andreae Asulani*], 1534.
Aetius left an exhaustive treatise on diseases of the eye. Although he did
not describe cataract, he was familiar with 61 different affections of the eye.
Most of his work consists of compilations of earlier writers, but he recorded
his own observations on ophthalmic therapeutics. Julius Hirschberg
translated the section of Aetius's text on ophthalmology into German,
Berlin, 1899. *See* No. 33.

5814.1 HUNAYN IBN ISHAQ AL-IBADI, ABU ZAYD [Johannitius]. 808-873
The book of the ten treatises on the eye. The Arabic text from the only two
known manuscripts, with an English translation and glossary by Max
Meyerhof. Cairo, *Government Press*, 1928.

The earliest extant systematic textbook of ophthalmology. The Arabs were the first to make a specialty of ophthalmology.

5815   'ALI IBN-'ISA [JESU HALY]. *circa* 940-1010
Memorandum book of a tenth-century oculist for the use of modern ophthalmologists. A translation of the Tadhkirat. First edition in English by CASEY A. WOOD. Chicago, *Northwestern University*, 1936.
The *Tadhkirat al-Kahhalin* was one of the oldest and best of the medieval Arabic works on ophthalmology. It carefully described 130 diseases of the eye and became the standard work on the subject in the Middle East. German translation, 1904.

5815.1   AL-GHAFIQI, MOHAMMAD IBN QASSOUM IBN ASLAM. *d.* 1165
Le guide d'oculistique...Traduction des parties ophtalmologiques d'après le manuscrit conservé á la bibliothèque l'Escurial par MAX MEYERHOF. Barcelona, *Laboratoires du Nord de l'Espagne*, 1933.

5816   GRASSI, BENVENUTO [GRAPHEUS]. *fl.* 12th cent.
De oculis eorumque egritudinibus et curis. [Ferrara, *Severinus de Ferrara*, 1474].
The earliest printed book on ophthalmology. Grassi was the most celebrated ophthalmic surgeon of the Middle Ages. English translation by Casey A. Wood, 1929.

5816.1   STROMAYR, CASPAR. *fl.* 16th cent.
Die Handschrift des Schnitt-und Augenartztes...in der Lindauer Handschift...vom 4. Juli 1559...Einführung...von Dr. med. Walter von Brunn.... Berlin, *Idra*, [1925].
Like Bartisch (No. 5817) Stromayr specialized in hernia repair and eye surgery. His unique manuscript with 186 large coloured paintings of surgical instruments and procedures was first published in the above edition. The portrait-like illustrations of eye diseases at the end of this work bear a striking resemblance to the woodcuts in Bartisch. *See* No. 3573.1.

5817   BARTISCH, GEORG. 1535-1606
Ὀφθαλμοδούλεια das ist, Augendienst. Dresden, *M. Stöckel*, 1583.
In this treatise on ophthalmic surgery Bartisch, who limited his practice to ophthalmology and hernia repair, left the first extensively illustrated account of any surgical specialty.Bartisch was a skilful operator and the first to practise the extirpation of the bulbus in cancer of the eye. The illustrations in his book form a comprehensive pictorial record of Renaissance eye-surgery; some of the woodcuts show the parts of the eye in various layers as they are viewed in dissection by means of movable anatomical flaps. This is one of the earliest uses of movable flaps to illustrate a medical book. Facsimile reprints, Folkstone,1966, and Hannover, 1983.

5818   GUILLEMEAU, JACQUES. 1550-1612
Traité des maladies de l'oeil. Paris, *chez Charles Massé*, 1585.
The first French work on ophthalmology. Guillemeau was a pupil and son-in-law of Ambroise Paré; his book was an epitome of the existing knowledge on the subject, chiefly from Greek and Arabian sources. English translation, London, [1587?]. *See also* No. 5820.

5819　BAYLEY, WALTER [BAILEY; BALEY]. 1529-1592
A briefe treatise touching the preseruation of the eie sight. [London, *R. Waldegrave]*, 1586.
This is the first separate work on ophthalmology printed in England.

5820　BANISTER, RICHARD. *fl.* 1620
A treatise of one hundred and thirteene diseases of the eyes. London, *F. Kynaston for T. Man*, 1622.
Although much of this is a translation of Guillemeau (No.5818), the first 112 pages are Banister's own work, "Banister's Breviary". He was an itinerant but honest oculist; he was the first to point out that hardness of the eyeball is an essential diagnostic sign of glaucoma.

5821　DAZA DE VALDES, BENITO. *fl.* 17th cent.
Uso del los antojos para todo genero de vistas, en que se enseña a conocer los grados que a cada uno le faltan de su vista, y los que tienen qualesquier antojos.. Sevilla, *Diego Perez*, 1623.
The earliest scientific work dealing with spectacles. It includes sight-testing tables and points out the value of convex lenses after cataract operations.

5821.1　ROLFINCK, GUERNER [WERNER]. 1599-1673
Dissertationes anatomicae methodo synthetica exaratae...Nuremberg, *Endter*, 1656.
Rolfinck was the first to demonstrate the location of cataract in the lens.

5822　BRIGGS, WILLIAM. 1642-1704
Two remarkable cases relating to vision. *Phil Trans.*, 1684, **14**, 561-65.
Includes the first known description of nyctalopia.

5823　STAHL, GEORG ERNST. 1660-1734
Propempticon inaugurale, De fistula lacrimali. *Published as addendum to:* LANGE, ERNST CHRISTIAN. Disputatio inauguralis medica de affectibus oculorum in genere...sub praesidio...Stahl. Halle, *Henckel*, 1702.
Stahl was the first to treat lacrimal fistula on the basis of correct anatomical understanding. He described his treatment in an addendum to the thesis on eye disease of his student, Lange.

5824　MAÎTRE-JAN, ANTOINE [MAÎTRE-JEAN] 1650-1730
Traité des maladies de l'oeil. Troyes, *J. le Febure*, 1707.
Called "the Father of French ophthalmology", Maître-Jan energetically supported Brisseau's doctrine, ensuring its acceptance. As far back as 1692, Maître-Jan had proved that the opaque lens is cataract, but before Brisseau's work appeared it had been regarded as a sort of skin or pellicle immediately inside the capsule of the lens.

5825　BRISSEAU, MICHEL. 1676-1743
Traité de la cataracte et du glaucoma. Paris, *L. d'Houry*, 1709.
Brisseau was the first to demonstrate the true nature and location of cataract. His book was reprinted in facsimile, 1921.

5826   ANEL, DOMINIQUE. 1679-1730

Observation singulière sur la fistule lacrimale, dans la quelle l'on verra, que la matière des fistules lacrimales s'evacuë très souvent par les points lacrimaux; en même tems l'on aprendra la méthode de les guérir radicalement, *etc.* Turin, *P. J. Zappatte*, 1713.

Lacrimal duct catheterized for the first time. *See* No. 5823.

5827   SAINT-YVES, CHARLES DE. 1667-1733

Nouveau traité des maladies des yeux. Paris, *P. A. Le mercier*, 1722.

Records the removal of a cataract "en masse" from a living subject. English edition, 1741.

5828   CHESELDEN, WILLIAM. 1688-1752

An account of some observations made by a young gentleman who was born blind, or lost his sight so early, that he had no remembrance of ever having seen, and was couch'd between 13 and 14 yrs. of age. *Phil Trans.*, (1727-28), 1729, **35**, 447-52.

The versatile Cheselden made an artificial pupil in an eye in which the products of inflammation had closed or obscured the natural pupil. This iridotomy operation was, next to Daviel's cataract operation, the most important contribution to ophthalmology during the 18th century.

5829   DAVIEL, JACQUES. 1693-1762

Sur une nouvelle méthode de guérir la cataracte par l'extraction du cristalin. *Mém. Acad. roy. Chir. (Paris)*, 1753, **2**, 337-54.

Daviel originated the modern method of treating cataract by extraction of the lens. By the time he made this official scientific report to the Academy of Surgery, Daviel had already tested his method on 206 cases, with success in 182. See D.B. Weiner, An 18th century battle for priority: Jacques Daviel (1693-1762) and the extraction of cataracts. *J. Hist. Med. All. Sci.*, 1986, **41**, 129-55.

5831   HEBERDEN, WILLIAM *Sr.* 1710-1801

Of the night-blindness or nyctalopia. *Med. Trans. Coll. Phys. Lond.*, 1768, **1**, 60-63.

A classic description of nyctalopia. Report of a single case.

5832   HUDDART, JOSEPH. 1741-1816

An account of persons who could not distinguish colours. *Phil Trans.*, 1777, **667**, 260-65.

First reliable record of colour blindness. Written in the form of a letter to Joseph Priestley, who communicated it to the Royal Society.

5833   HAÜY, VALENTIN. 1745-1822

Essai sur l'education des aveugles. Paris, *Imp. d. Enf. Aveugles*, 1786.

Haüy founded the first school for the blind. To him belongs the honour of being the first to emboss paper as a means of reading for the blind. His *Essai* originated modern methods of teaching and caring for blind persons. English translation by the celebrated blind poet, Thomas Blacklock (1721-91), who lost his sight at the age of 6 months, in *Poems by the late Reverend Dr. Thomas Blacklock*, Edinburgh, 1793.

5833.1   PELLIER DE QUENGSY, GUILLAUME. 1750 or 1751-1835
Précis ou cours d'opérations sur la chirurgie des yeux. 2 vols., Paris, *Didot*, 1789-90.
The first separate book on ophthalmic surgery.

5833.2   BEER, GEORG JOSEPH. 1763-1821
Praktische Beobachtungen über verschiedene, vorzüglich aber über jene Augenkrankheiten, welche aus allgemeinen Krankheiten des Körpers entspringen. Vienna, *F.J. Kaiserer*, 1791.
"This is the first monograph ever published dealing with ocular signs of systemic disease. It deals with lacrimal fistulas, trichiasis, adhesions of the lids, lid ulcers, ephiphora, and ocular inflammations.   He illustrates through anecdotal cases the ocular changes caused by smallpox, measles, venereal afflictions, gouty and rheumatic diseases, scrofula, and dietary deficiencies" (D.M. Albert).

5834   DALTON, JOHN. 1766-1844
Extraordinary facts relating to the vision of colours. *Mem. lit. phil. Soc. Manch.*, 1798, **5** pt. 1, 28-45.
Firt scientific description of colour-blindness, or "Daltonism". Dalton himself suffered from red–green blindness. His paper was read to the Society in 1794.

5834.1   HIMLY, KARL GUSTAV. 1772-1837
Ophthalmologische Beobachtungen und Untersuchungen oder Beyträge zur richtigen Kenntniss und Behandlung der Augen im gesunden und kranken Zustande. Erstes Stück. Bremen, *F. Wilmans*, 1801.
Himly used hyoscyamine to dilate the pupil to facilitate removal of the lens. (p. 97).

5835   SCARPA, ANTONIO. 1752-1832
Saggio di osservazioni e d'esperienze sulle principali malattie degli occhi. Pavia, *B. Comino*, 1801.
This beautifully illustrated work was the first textbook on the subject to be published in the Italian language. Its author has been called "the father of Italian ophthalmology". English translation, London, 1806.

5836   SCHMIDT, JOHANN ADAM. 1759-1809
Ueber Nachstaar und Iritis nach Staaroperationen. *Abhandl. k. k. med.-chir. Josephs-Acad. Wien*, 1801, **2**, 209-92.
Inflammation of the iris was named iritis by Schmidt. In 1801, with Himly, he founded the first journal devoted to ophthalmology, the *Ophthalmologische Bibliothek*.

5837   LARREY, DOMINIQUE JEAN, *le baron*. 1766-1842
Mémoire sur l'ophtalmie régnante en Egypte. Kaire, *Imprimerie Nationale*, an IX [1800-01].
The great military surgeon Larrey served during the Napoleonic campaign in Egypt, where he was the first to observe the contagiousness of trachoma shortly after the successful invasion in 1798. The disease spread to Europe thereafter under the name of "military ophthalmia" or "Egyptian ophthalmia". Reprinted in Larrey's, *Relation historique et chirurgicale de l'expedition de l'Armée d'Orient*, Paris, 1803.

5838   SCHMIDT, JOHANN ADAM. 1759-1809
Ueber die Krankheiten des Thränenorgans. Wien, *J. Geissinger*, 1803.
Schmidt was Professor of Ophthalmology at Vienna.

5839   VETCH, JOHN. 1783-1835
An account of the ophthalmia which has appeared in England since the
return of the British Army from Egypt. London, *Longman*, 1807.
Vetch described trachoma.

5840   WARDROP, JAMES. 1782-1869
Essays on the morbid anatomy of the human eye. 2 vols. Edinburgh, *G.
Ramsay & Co.*, 1808-18.
Wardrop was the first to classify the various inflammations of the eye
according to the structures attacked. He was also the first to use the term
"keratitis".

5841   LANGENBECK, CONRAD JOHANN MARTIN. 1776-1851
Prüfung der Keratonyxis, einer neuen Methode den grauen Staar durch die
Hornhaut zu recliniren oder zu zerstückeln. Göttingen, *J. F. Danckwerts*,
1811.
Langenbeck's operation of iridencleisis for construction of artificial
pupil. He was Professor of Anatomy and Surgery at Göttingen.

5842   BEER, GEORG JOSEPH. 1763-1821
Lehre von den Augenkrankheiten. 2 vols. Wien, *Camesina; Heubner &
Volke*, 1813-17.
Beer is remembered for his textbook; the doctrines in it dominated
practice for many years. He described the symptoms of glaucoma and
noted the luminosity of the fundus in aniridia. He also presented for the
first time the general principles of treating post-traumatic inflammations,
including penetrating and perforating injuries as well as injuries to the
orbit. He describes the first use of the loupe for the examination of the
living eye. The plates in this work were both hand-coloured and signed by
Beer. He was a distinguished iridectomist. Many of his pupils bacame
famous ophthalmic surgeons. Beer opened the first known eye hospital,
in 1786, in Vienna. He was the first Jew to graduate in Austria. English
translation, Glasgow, 1821.

5842.1   DEMOURS, ANTOINE P. 1762-1836
Traité des maladies des yeux. 3 vols. and atlas. Paris, *l'Auteur et Crochard*,
1818.
Includes the first description of glaucoma in which heightened intraocular
pressure is recognized, credit for which goes to the author's father, Pierre
Demours (1702-95), whose portrait appears in the atlas in recognition of
this. The atlas also contains the first French translation of Soemmerring
(No. 1489) with additional plates.

5843   TRAVERS, BENJAMIN. 1783-1858
A synopsis of the diseases of the eye. London, *Longman*, 1820.
The earliest systematic treatise in English on diseases of the eye. The
book became the authority in Europe and America. Travers, a pupil of Sir
Astley Cooper, became surgeon to St. Thomas's Hospital.

5844   FRICK, GEORGE. 1793-1870
A treatise on the diseases of the eye. Baltimore, *F. Lucas jnr.*, 1823.
First American textbook of ophthalmology by the first American who is believed to have restricted his practice to diseases of the eye. Frick studied under Georg Beer in Vienna.

5845   GUTHRIE, GEORGE JAMES. 1785-1856
Lectures on the operative surgery of the eye. London, *Burgess & Hill*, 1823.
Guthrie founded the Royal Westminster Ophthalmic Hospital, London, in 1816. He was the earliest teacher of the subject in the British Isles. The above includes important work on the artificial pupil.

5847   AIRY, *Sir* GEORGE BIDDELL. 1801-1892
On a peculiar defect in the eye, and a mode of correcting it. *Trans. Cambr. phil Soc.* (1825), 1827, **2**, 267-73.
Airy drew attention to astigmatism from which he himself suffered, and he fitted cylindrical lenses for its correction.

5848   MACKENZIE, WILLIAM. 1791-1868
A practical treatise on diseases of the eye. London, *Longman*, 1830.
In this book Mackenzie, one of the foremost ophthalmologists of his time, included a classic description of the symptomatology of glaucoma, and was probably the first to draw attention to the increase of intra-ocular pressure as a characteristic of the condition. He introduced the term "asthenopia", and was the first to describe sympathetic ophthalmia as a distinct disease.

5849   LAWRENCE, *Sir* WILLIAM. 1783-1867
A treatise on the diseases of the eye. London, *J. Churchill*, 1833.
This comprehensive work marks an epoch in ophthalmic surgery. It is based on lectures delivered by Lawrence at the London Ophthalmic Infirmary. He was a surgeon to St. Bartholomew's Hospital; he succeeded Abernethy as lecturer on surgery and did much to advance the surgery of the eye.

5850   JULLIARD, ETIENNE FRANÇOIS.
De l'emploi de l'excision et de la cautérisation à l'aide du nitrate d'argent fondu dans l'ophtalmie blenorrhagique. Paris, *Thèse* No. 26, 1835.
Silver nitrate for treatment of gonococcal ophthalmia.

5850.1   BIGGER, SAMUEL L. L.
An inquiry into the possibility of transplanting the cornea, with the view of relieving blindness...*Dublin J. med. Sci.*, 1837, **11**, 408-17.
Bigger, a Dublin surgeon, successfully grafted a cornea of one gazelle onto that of another. According to this paper, he first performed this operation in 1835 while he was "a prisoner with a Nomadic tribe of Arabs, about twelve or fourteen days' journey from Grand Cairo". By the time this account of his work was published by a "Mr. Swift", Bigger had not attempted the operation on a human subject.

5851   BRAILLE, LOUIS. 1809-1852
Procéde pour écrire au moyen des points. Paris, 1837.
Braille, himself blind, modified the system of elevated points first suggested by Charles Barbier in 1820 for enabling the blind to read. His types are today used throughout the world.

5852   AMMON, FRIEDRICH AUGUST VON. 1799-1861
Klinische Darstellungen der Krankheiten und Bildungsfehler des menschlichen Auges, der Augenlider und der Thränenwerkzeuge nach eigenen Beobachtungen und Untersuchungen. 4 pts. Berlin, *G. Reimer*, 1838-47.
This great colour-plate atlas is probably the best summary of the knowledge of diseases of the eye prior to the introduction of the ophthalmoscope.

5853   CARRON DU VILLARDS, CHARLES JOSEPH FRÉDÉRIC. 1801-1860
Guide pratique pour l'étude et le traitement des maladies des yeux. 2 vols. Paris, *Soc. encycl.*, 1838.
Carron du Villards taught ophthalmology in Paris; his book is one of the best of the period.

5854   FERRALL, JOSEPH MICHAEL [*afterwards* O'FERRALL]. 1790-1860
On the anatomy and pathology of certain structures in the orbit not previously described. *Dublin J. med. Sci.*, 1841, **19**, 329-56.
Ferrall's operation for enucleation of the eyeball (p. 354).

5855   BOLTON, JAMES. 1812-1869
A treatise on strabismus, with a description of new instruments designed to improve the operation for its cure. Richmond, Va., *P. D. Bernard*, 1842.

5856   DIEFFENBACH, JOHANN FRIEDRICH. 1792-1847
Ueber das Schielen und die Heilung desselben durch eine Operation. Berlin, *A. Förstner*, 1842.
The first successful attempt at treating strabismus by myotomy. The operation was later abandoned owing to the frequently disastrous final effects. A preliminary paper appeared in *Med. Ztg.*, 1839, **8**, 227.

5857   HIMLY, KARL GUSTAV. 1772-1837
Die Krankheiten und Missbildungen des menschlichen Auges und deren Heilung. 2 vols. Berlin, *A. Hirschwald*, 1843.
Himly was professor of ophthalmology at Jena and later at Göttingen. He introduced clinical teaching in ophthalmology.

5858   KÜCHLER, HEINRICH. 1811-1873
Schriftnummerprobe für Gesichtsleidende. Darmstadt, *J. P. Diehl*, 1843.
Küchler introduced test readings of print at a distance, for examination of patients.

5859   BRÜCKE, ERNST WILHELM VON, *Ritter.* 1819-1892
Anatomische Untersuchungen über die sogenannten leuchtenden Augen bei den Wirbelthieren. *Arch. Anat. Physiol. wiss. Med.*, 1845, 387-406.
Von Brücke studied the luminosity of the eye in animals, and by passing a tube through a candle flame, was able to see the fundus. See also the same journal, 1847, 225-27.

5860   WALTHER, PHILIPP FRANZ VON. 1782-1849
Ueber die Hornhautflecken. *J. Chir Augenheilk.*, 1845, **34**, 1-90.
First description of corneal opacity.

5861 CUMMING, WILLIAM. 1812-1886
On a luminous appearance of the human eye, and its application to the
detection of disease of the retina and posterior part of the eye. *Med.-chir.*
Trans., 1846, **29**, 283-96.
　　While a student at the London Hospital, Cumming, by shading the eye
of a fellow student from the light, was able to look directly into it and obtain
both the retinal reflex and the white light from the entrance of the optic
nerve. He made the first suggestion for the construction of a device for
examining the fundus.

5862 JONES, THOMAS WHARTON. 1808-1891
A manual of the principles and practice of ophthalmic medicine and
surgery. London, *J. Churchill*, 1847.
　　The last important English work on opthalmology published before the
invention of the ophthalmoscope. Jones did not appreciate the prototype
ophthalmoscope devised by Charles Babbage, and shown to him in 1847.
After the success of Helmholtz's invention (No. 5866) Jones wrote about
Babbage's invention and his role in discouraging it. *See* No. 5874.

5863 DESMARRES, LOUIS AUGUSTE. 1810-1882
Traité théorique et pratique des maladies des yeux. Paris, *Germer-Baillère*,
1847.

5864 ———. Opérations qui se pratiquent sur les yeux. Paris, [1850].

5865 ARLT, CARL FERDINAND VON. 1812-1887
Die Krankheiten des Auges. 3 vols. Prag. *F. A. Credner & Kleinbub*, 1851-56.
　　Arlt described granular conjunctivitis ("Arlt's trachoma") and an opera-
tion for transplantation of the ciliary bulbs in the treatment of distichiasis.

5866 HELMHOLTZ, HERMANN LUDWIG FERDINAND VON. 1821-1894
Beschreibung eines Augen-Spiegels zur Untersuchung der Netzhaut im
lebenden Auge. Berlin, *A. Förstner*, 1851.
　　Invention of the ophthalmoscope, one of the greatest events in the
history of ophthalmology. English translation by T. H. Shastid, Chicago,
Cleveland Press, 1916.

5866.1 RUETE, CHRISTIAN G.T. 1810-1867
Der Augenspiegel und des Optometer für practische Aerzte. Göttingen,
Dieterich, 1852.
　　Ruete introduced a practical lens system for examining the inverted
image, and improved the illumination, producing the first practical oph-
thalmoscope.

5867 BOWMAN, *Sir* WILLIAM. 1816-1892
Observations on artificial pupil, with a description of a new method of
operating in certain cases. *Med. Times Gaz.*, 1852, n.s., **4**, 11-14, 33-35.
　　Bowman devised an operation for the formation of an artificial pupil.

5868 SICHEL, JULES. 1802-1868
Iconographie ophtalmologique. 1 vol. and atlas. Paris, *J. B. Baillière*, 1852-59.
　　This work and that of Ammon (No. 5852) remain the greatest pre-
ophthalmoscopic atlases of ophthalmology.

5869   STELLWAG VON CARION, CARL. 1823-1904
        Die Ophthalmologie vom naturwissenschaftlichen Standpunkte aus
        bearbeitet. 2 vols. [in 3]. Freiburg, Erlangen, *Herder, F. Enke*, 1853-58.
        English translation, 1868.

5869.1 TRIGT, ADRIAN CHRISTOPHER VAN. 1825-1864
        Dissertatio ophthalmologica inauguralis de speculo oculi. Trajecti ad
        Rhenum, *P.W. van de Weijer*, 1853.
        Contains the first printed illustrations of the fundus of the eye.

5870   TÜRCK, LUDWIG. 1810-1868
        Ein Fall von Hämorrhagie der Netzhaut beider Augen. *Z. k. k. Ges. Aerzte
        Wien*, 1853, **9**, 1 Abt., 214-18.
        Türck was the first to note the correlation of retinal haemorrhage with
        tumours of the brain.

5871   GRAEFE, FRIEDRICH WILHELM ERNST ALBRECHT VON. 1828-1870
        Notiz über die Behandlung der Mydriasis. *v. Graefes Arch. Ophthal.*, 1854-
        55, **1**, 1 Abt., 351-19.

5872   ———. Vorlaüfige Notiz über das Wesen des Glaucoms. *v. Graefes Arch.
        Ophthal.*, 1854-55, **1**, 1 Abt., 371-82.

5873   ———. Ueber die Coremorphosis als Mittel gegen chronische Iritis und
        Iridochorioiditis. *v. Graefes Arch. Ophthal.*, 1855-56, **2**, 2 Abt., 202-57.
        Graefe introduced iridectomy in the treatment of iritis and
        iridochoroiditis.

5874   JONES, THOMAS WHARTON. 1808-1891
        Report on the ophthalmoscope. *Brit. for. med.-chir. Rev.*, 1854, **14**, 549-
        57.
        Jones reported that Charles Babbage (1792-1871), the computer pio-
        neer, had produced a simple ophthalmoscope in 1847. After the success of
        Helmholtz's instrument in 1851 (No. 5866) Jones wrote about Babbage's
        instrument and of his role in discouraging it. *See* No. 5862.

5875   MECKEL VON HEMSBACH, HEINRICH. 1821-1856
        Die pyämische Ophthalmie in Beziehung zur feinsten Organisation des
        Entzündungs-Produkts und zu der eigenthümlichen Struktur des
        Glaskörpers. *Ann. Charité-Krankenh.*, 1854, **5**, 2 Heft, 276-89.
        First account of metastatic ophthalmia.

5876   BENDZ, JACOB CHRISTIAN. 1802-1858
        Quelques considérations sur la nature de l'ophthalmie dite militaire, par
        rapport à son apparition dans l'armée danoise depuis 1851. *Ann Oculist.
        (Brux.)*, 1855, **33**, 164-76.
        Description of trachoma.

5877   LIEBREICH, RICHARD. 1830-1917
        Ophthalmoskopische Notizen 4. Seitliche Beleuchtung und mikroskopische
        Untersuchung am lebenden Auge. *v. Graefes Arch Ophthal.*, 1855, **1**, 2 Abt.,
        351-56.
        Liebreich introduced lateral illumination in microscopic investigation
        of the living eye.

5878   WILLIAMS, HENRY WILLARD. 1821-1895
Iritis – non-mercurial treatment. *Boston med. surg. J.*, 1856, **55**, 49-55, 69-74, 92-99.
The second and third papers are entitled "On the treatment of iritis without mercury".

5879   BOWMAN, *Sir* WILLIAM. 1816-1892
On the treatment of lacrymal obstructions. *Ophthal. Hosp. Rep.*, 1857-59, **1**, 10-20, 88.

5880   GRAEFE, FRIEDRICH WILHELM ERNST ALBRECHT VON. 1828-1870
Beiträge zur Lehre vom Schielen und von der Schiel-Operation. *v. Graefes Arch Ophthal.*, 1857, **3**, 1 Abt., 177-286.
Graefe's operation for strabismus.

5881   ———. Ueber die Iridectomie bei Glaucom und über den glaucomatösen Process. *v. Graefes Arch. Ophthal.*, 1857, **3**, 2 Abt., 456-560; 1858, **4**, 2 Abt., 127-61; 1862, **8**, 2 Abt., 242-313.
Iridectomy for the treatment of glaucoma was introduced by Graefe.

5882   ———. Ueber Embolie der Arteria centralis retinae als Ursache plötzlicher Erblindung. *v. Graefes Arch. Opthal.*, 1859, **5**, 1 Abt., 136-57.
Discovery of embolism of the retinal artery as a cause of sudden blindness.

5883   GRAEFE, ALFRED CARL. 1830-1899
Klinische Analyse der Motilitätsstörungen des Auges. Berlin, *H. Peters*, 1858.
Alfred Carl Graefe, cousin of Albrecht, made a careful clinical analysis of disordered movements of the eye. He also invented a special "localization ophthalmoscope", and, with Saemisch, edited the great *Handbuch der gesamten Augenheilkunde* (*see* No. 5944).

5884   KNAPP, HERMANN JAKOB. 1831-1911
Die Krümmung der Hornhaut des menschlichen Auges. Heidelberg, *J. C. B. Mohr*, 1859.
Knapp wrote valuable monographs on curvature of the cornea (above) and on intraocular tumours (*see* No. 5902). He became one of the leading ophthalmologists in America.

5885   DEMARQUAY, JEAN NICHOLAS. 1811-1875
Ueber Complication von Sehnervenentzündung mit Gehirnkrankheiten. *v. Graefes Arch. Ophthal.*, 1860, **7**, 2 Abt., 58-71.
Graefe showed that most cases of blindness and impaired vision connected with cerebral disorders are a result of optic neuritis rather than of paralysis of the optic nerve.

5887   JAEGER, EDUARD, *Ritter von Jaxtthal*. 1818-1884
Schriftskalen. 3te. Aufl. Wien, *L. W. Seidel*, 1860.
Jaeger first introduced his test types in 1854; Emil Fuchs improved them in 1895.

5888   MITCHELL, SILAS WEIR. 1829-1914
On the production of cataract in frogs by the administration of sugar. *Amer J. med. Sci.*, 1860, n.s., **39**, 106-10.

5889   DONDERS, FRANS CORNELIS. 1818-1889
Astigmatisme en cilindrische glazen. Utrecht, *Post*, 1862.
    Includes statement of "Donders's law" – the rotation of the eye around the line of sight is not voluntary. French and German translations, 1862.

5890   SNELLEN, HERMANN. 1834-1908
Probebuchstaben zur Bestimmung der Sehschärfe. Utrecht, *P. W. van de Weijer*, 1862.
    Snellen's test-types ("Optotypi") which soon gained acceptance in all civilized countries.

5891   JACOBSON, JULIUS. 1828-1889
Ein neues und gefahrloses Operations-Verfahren zur Heilung des grauen Staares. Berlin, *Peters*, 1863.
    Jacobson used a peripheral incision in his operation for cataract.

5892   LIEBREICH, RICHARD. 1830-1917
Atlas der Ophthalmoscopie. Darstellung des Augengrundes im gesunden und krankhaften Zustande enthalten. Berlin, *A. Hirschwald*, 1863.
    First atlas of the fundus. The author was an assistant to Helmholtz at the time of the invention of the ophthalmoscope. The work is illustrated with reproductions of his own paintings. Text in French and German. English translation by M. R. Swanzy, 1870 and 1884. Leibreich became ophthalmic surgeon to St. Thomas's Hospital, London.

5893   DONDERS, FRANS CORNELIS. 1818-1889
On the anomalies of accommodation and refraction of the eye ... Translated from the author's manuscript by W. D. MOORE, London, *New Sydenham Soc.*, 1864.
    Donders's greatest work, the basis for all succeeding studies of the subject, and a classic of physiological optics. It contains Donders's explanation of astigmatism, his definition of aphakia and hypermetropia, his sharp distinctions between myopia and hypermetropia, etc. This English translation from the Dutch is the first published edition.

5894   AGNEW, CORNELIUS REA. 1830-1888
A method of operating for divergent squint. *Trans. Amer ophthal. Soc.*, 1865-72, **1**, 3rd Ann. Mtg, 31-34.
    Agnew devised an operation for the treatment of divergent squint.

5895   WILLIAMS, HENRY WILLARD. 1821-1895
Suture of the flap, after extraction of cataract. *Trans. Amer. ophthal Soc.*, 1865-72, **1**, 3rd Ann. Mtg, 45-46.
    A method of suturing the flap after cataract extraction was introduced by Williams.

5896   PAGENSTECHER, ALEXANDER. 1828-1879
Ueber die Extraktion des grauen Staares bei uneröffneter Kapsel durch den Scleralschnitt. In *Klinische Beobachtungen aus der Augenheilanstalt zu Wiesbaden,* hrsg. von E. H. PAGENSTECHER U. T. SAEMISCH. Heft 3, 10-46. Wiesbaden, *J. Niedner*, 1866.
    Extraction of the lens in the closed capsule through a scleral incision, for the treatment of cataract.

5897   GRAEFE, FRIEDRICH WILHELM ERNST ALBRECHT VON. 1828-1870
Ueber mordificirte Linearextraction. *v. Graefes Arch. Ophthal.*, 1865, **11**,
3 Abt., 1-106; 1866, **12**, 1 Abt., 150-223; 1868, **14**, 3 Abt., 106-48.
    Graefe's improvement of the operation for cataract by the modified
linear extraction reduced the incidence of eye loss from 10 to 2.3 per cent.

5898   ——. Zur Lehre der sympathischen Ophthalmie, *v. Graefes Arch. Ophthal.*,
1866, **12**, 2 Abt., 149-74.
    A classic contribution to the literature of sympathetic ophthalmia.

5899   ——. Symptomenlehre der Augenmuskellähmungen. Berlin, *H. Peters*,
1867.
    The first thorough account of paralysis of the eye muscles, and the basis
for their surgical treatment. The first section describes conditions resulting
from injuries to the eye muscles. The second part outlines physiologic laws
governing eye movements and the effects of impaired function in each of
the ocular muscles.

5900   ——. Ueber Ceratoconus. *Berl. klin. Wschr.*, 1868, **5**, 241-44, 249-254.
    Classic description of conical cornea (keratoconus).

5901   JAVAL, LOUIS EMILE. 1839-1907
Sur un nouvel instrument pour la détermination de l'astigmatisme. *Ann.
Oculist. (Brux.)*, 1867, **57**, 39-43.
    Javal invented the astigmometer, and described it in the above paper.

5902   KNAPP, HERMANN JAKOB. 1831-1911
Die intraocularen Geschwülste nach eigenen klinischen Beobachtungen
und anatomischen Untersuchungen. Carlsruhe, *C. F. Müller*, 1868.
    English translation, New York, 1869.

5903   HORNER, JOHANN FRIEDRICH. 1831-1886
Ueber eine Form von Ptosis. *Klin Mbl. Augenheilk.*, 1869, **7**, 193-98.
    "Horner's syndrome" – due to lesion of the cervical sympathetic. The
same syndrome was evoked in animals by du Petit in 1727 (*see* No. 1313).
It was also described by Claude Bernard, *Leçons sur la physiologie et la
pathologie du système nerveux*, 1858, **2**, 473-74, and, less impressively, by
E. S. Hare, *Lond. med. Gaz.*, 1838-39, **1**, 16-18.

5904   JAEGER, EDUARD, *Ritter von Jaxtthal*. 1818-1884
Opthalmoskopischer Hand-Atlas. Wien, 1869.
    A fine atlas which was for many years unsurpassed. The illustrations
were reproduced from Jaeger's own paintings, each of which required
from 20 to 50 sittings of from two to three hours each. English translation,
London & New York, 1890. Jaeger's original paintings were reproduced in
colour with new descriptions, and revisions, by Daniel M. Albert as *Atlas
of diseases of the ocular fundus*, Philadelphia, *Saunders*, 1972.

5905   SAEMISCH, EDWIN THEODOR. 1833-1909
Das Ulcus corneae serpens und seine Therapie. Bonn, *M. Cohen u. Sohn*,
1870.
    First description of serpiginous ulcer of the cornea and its treatment.
Called also "Saemisch's ulcer".

5906 LEBER, THEODOR. 1840-1917
Ueber hereditäre und congenital-angelegte Sehnervenleiden. *v. Graefes Arch. Ophthal.*, 1871, **17**, 2 Abt., 249-91.
First description of hereditary optic atrophy, "Leber's optic atrophy".

5907 BERLIN, RUDOLF. 1833-1897
Zur sogenannten Commotio retinae. *Klin. Mbl. Augenheilk.*, 1873, **11**, 42-78.
Berlin, professor of ophthalmology at Rostock, described the traumatic oedema of the retina which is sometimes referred to as "Berlin's oedema".

5908 CUIGNET, FERDINAND LOUIS JOSEPH. 1823-
Kératoscopie. *Rec. Ophtal.*, 1873-74, **1**, 14-23.
Introduction of the shadow test (retinoscopy), sometimes called "Cuignet's method".

5909 MOON, WILLIAM. 1818-1894
Light for the blind: a history of the origin and success of Moon's system of reading ... for the blind. London, 1873.
Moon became totally blind at the age of 22. He taught other blind people and devised a simplified form of roman letters, embossed on paper, for use by blind readers. This was in 1845, and two years later he published his first book in Moon type.

5910 PAGENSTECHER, ERNST HERMANN. 1844-1932, & GENTH, CARL PHILIPP. 1844-1904
Atlas der pathologischen Anatomie des Augapfels. Weisbaden, *C. W. Kreidel*, 1873-75.
Text in German and English; Sir W. R. Gowers was responsible for the English translation.

5911 HOLMGREN, ALARIK FRITHIOF. 1831-1897
Om den medfödda, färgblindhetens diagnostik och teori. *Nord. med. Ark.*, 1874, **6**, Nr. 24, 1-21; Nr. 28, 1-35.
Holmgren introduced the wool-skein test for the diagnosis of colour-blindness.

5912 ARLT, CARL FERDINAND VON. 1812-1887
Ueber die Verletzungen des Auges mit besonderer Rücksicht auf deren gerichtsärztliche Würdigung. Wien, *W. Braumuller*, 1875.
An important work dealing with the medico-legal aspects of eye injuries. English translation by C. S. Turnbull, 1878.

5913 LAQUEUR, LUDWIG. 1839-1909
Ueber eine neue therapeutische Verwendung des Physostigmin. *Zbl. med. Wiss.*, 1876, **14**, 421-22.
Introduction of physostigmine in the treatment of glaucoma.

5914 SAEMISCH, EDWIN THEODOR. 1833-1909
Der Frühjahrskatarrh. *In*: GRAEFE and SAEMISCH, Handbuch der gesammten Augenheilkunde, Leipzig, 1876, **4**, Theil 2, 25-29.
First description of vernal conjunctivitis.

5915   FÖRSTER, CARL FRIEDRICH RICHARD. 1825-1902
Beziehungen der Allgemein-Leiden und Organ-Erkrankungen zu
Veränderungen und Krankheiten des Sehorgans. *In*: GRAEFE and SAEMISCH,
Handbuch der gesammten Augenheilkunde, Leipzig, 1877, **7**, Theil 5, 59-
234.
Förster was among the first to study the relationship between eye
disease and general and organic disease of the body.

5916   HOLMGREN, ALARIK FRITHIOF. 1831-1897
Om färgblindheten i dess förhallande till jernvägstrafiken och sjöväsendet.
Upsala Läkaref. Förh., 1876-77, **12**, 171-251, 267-358.
A serious railway accident in Sweden in 1875 was believed by Holmgren
to be due to colour-blindness, and resulted in the above important paper
dealing with the condition and its relation to railway and maritime traffic.
Translation in *Rep. Smithsonian Inst.*, 1877. Washington, 1878, 131-200.

5916.1 SELLERBECK, HEINRICH. 1842-
Ueber Keratoplastik. *Graefe's Arch. Ophthal.*, 1878, **24**, 4 Abt., 1-46, 321-24.
Sellerbeck was first to use human donor corneas for transplants. He was
not very successful, probably because the antiseptics employed were too
strong.

5917   THOMSON, WILLIAM. 1833-1907
On astigmatism as a cause for persistent headache and other nervous
symptoms. *Med. News (Philad.)*, 1879, **27**, 81-88.
Thomson was a pioneer in the study of refraction. He was much
interested in colour-blindness and modified Holmgren's wool-skein test.
Himself affected with hypermetropia, he made important investigations on
this condition, and (above) on astigmatism as a cause of headache.

5918   TAY, WAREN. 1843-1927
Symmetrical changes in the region of the yellow spot in each eye of an
infant. *Trans. ophthal. Soc. U. K.*, 1880-81, **1**, 55-57.
Tay was the first to describe amaurotic familial idiocy, his paper dealing
mainly with the ocular manifestations. The condition later became known
as "Tay–Sachs's disease" (*see also* No. 4705).

5919   WECKER, LOUIS DE. 1832-1909, & LANDOLT, EDMOND. 1846-1926
Traité complet de l'ophtalmologie. 4 vols. Paris, *Vve. A. Delahaye et Cie.*,
1880-89.

5920   JAVAL, LOUIS EMILE. 1839-1907, & SCHIÖTZ, HJALMAR. 1850-1927
Un ophtalmomètre pratique. *Ann Oculist. (Brux.)*, 1881, **86**, 5-21.
Javal and Schiötz here describe an ophthalmometer invented by them.

5921   DEUTSCHMANN, RICHARD. 1852-1935
Ein experimenteller Beitrag zur Pathogenese der sympathischen Augen-
Entzündung. *v. Graefes Arch. ophthal.*, 1882, **28**, 2 Abt., 291-300.
Deutschmann was the chief protagonist of the infective theory of
sympathetic ophthalmia.

5922   PLACIDO DA COSTA, ANTONIO. 1849-1916
Neue Instrumente. *Zbl. prakt. Augenheilk.*, 1882, **6**, 30-31.
Introduction of the keratoscope.

5923   KOCH, ROBERT. 1843-1910
Bericht über die Thätigkeit der deutschen Cholerakommission in Aegypten
und Ostindien. *Wien. med. Wschr.*, 1883, **33**, 1548-51.
Koch–Weeks bacillus. Koch discovered the bacilli of two varieties of
Egyptian conjunctivitis. *See also* No. 5930.

5924   CREDÉ, CARL SIGMUND FRANZ. 1819-1892
Die Verhütung der Augenentzündung der Neugeborenen. Berlin, *A.
Hirschwald*, 1884.
Credé introduced the practice of instilling silver nitrate into the eyes of
newborn infants as a preventive measure against ophthalmia neonatorum.

5925   KOLLER, CARL. 1857-1944
Vorläufige Mittheilung über locale Anästhesirung am Auge. *Klin. Mbl.
Augenheilk.*, 1884, **22**, Beilageheft, 60-63.
Koller was first to demonstrate the practical value of cocaine as a local
anaesthetic in ophthalmology. *See* No. 5678.

5926   FUCHS, ERNST. 1851-1930
Die periphere Atrophie des Sehnerven. *v. Graefes Arch. Ophthal.*, 1885,
31, 1 Abt., 177-200.
Peripheral atrophy of the optic nerve was described by Fuchs and called
"Fuchs's optic atrophy".

5927   HIRSCHBERG, JULIUS. 1843-1925
Der Electromagnet in der Augenheilkunde. Leipzig, *Veit & Co.*, 1885.
The introduction of the electromagnet into ophthalmology. A pupil of
Helmholtz, Hirschberg was one of the most voluminous writers in the field
of ophthalmology. Besides his dictionary (*see* No. 5932) he wrote a classic
history of the subject (*see* No. 5996) which today remains the authoritative
history of ophthalmology. He founded the *Centralblatt für praktische
Augenheilkunde* in 1877.

5928   MULES, PHILIP HENRY. 1843-1905
On the surgical, physiological, and aesthetic advantages of the artificial
vitreous body. *Brit. med. J.*, 1885, **2**, 1153-55.
"Mules's operation", evisceration of the eyeball with insertion of artificial vitreous.

5929   PANAS, PHOTINOS. 1832-1903
D'un nouveau procédé opératoire applicable au ptosis congénital et au
ptosis paralytique. *Arch. Ophtal.*, 1886, **6**, 1-14.
An operation for congenital and paralytic ptosis was introduced by
Panas.

5930   WEEKS, JOHN ELMER. 1853-1949
The bacillus of acute conjunctival catarrh or "pink eye". *Arch. Ophthal.
(N.Y.)*, 1886, **15**, 441-51.
In 1883 Koch discovered the bacilli of two different forms of infectious
conjunctivitis (Egyptian ophthalmia); in 1886 Weeks discovered the same
organism to be the cause of "pink-eye". The organism has become known
as the Koch–Weeks bacillus (*see also* No. 5923).

5931 COHN, HERMANN LUDWIG. 1828-1906
Die ärztliche Ueberwachung der Schulen zur Verhütung der Verbreitung der Kurzsichtigkeit. *Arb VII. int Congr. Hyg. Demogr.*, Wien, 1887-88, **1**, Heft 12, 9-28.
Cohn was a pioneer in his advocacy of the routine examination of the eyes of schoolchildren.

5932 HIRSCHBERG, JULIUS. 1843-1925
Wörterbuch der Augenheilkunde. Leipzig, *Veit & Co.*, 1887.

5933 HIPPEL, ARTHUR VON. 1841-1917
Eine neue Methode der Hornhauttransplantation. *v. Graefes Arch. Ophthal.*, 1888, **34**, 1 Abt., 108-30.
Modern keratoplasty is based on the technique introduced by von Hippel.

5934 FUCHS, ERNST. 1851-1930
Keratitis punctata superficialis. *Wien. klin. Wschr.*, 1889, **2**, 837-41.
Epidemic keratoconjunctivitis first described.

5935 ——. Lehrbuch der Augenheilkunde. Leipzig u. Wien, *F. Deuticke*, 1889.
Fuchs's textbook was an outstanding contribution to the literature, and was translated into many languages. The last English edition appeared in 1933.

5936 PARINAUD, HENRI. 1844-1905, & GALEZOWSKI, XAVIER. 1832-1907
Conjonctivite infectieuse transmise par les animaux. *Ann. Oculist. (Brux.)*, 1889, **101**, 252.
Parinaud described an infectious tuberculous conjunctivitis transmissible from animals to man. In 1924 Gifford suggested the name "Parinaud's oculo-glandular syndrome" as a more suitable description. See also *Rec. Ophtalmologie*, 1889, 3 sér., **11**, 176-80.

5937 EDRIDGE-GREEN, FREDERICK WILLIAM. 1863-1953
Colour-blindness and colour-perception. London, *Kegan Paul, Trench, Trübner & Co.*, 1891.
Includes (p. 262 *et seq.*) description of Edridge-Green's lantern test for colour-blindness. This was officially adopted in Great Britain in 1915 in place of the Holmgren test.

5938 AXENFELD, KARL THEODOR PAUL POLYKARPOS. 1867-1930
Ueber die eitrige metastatische Ophthalmie, besonders ihre Aetiologie und prognostische Bedeutung. *v. Graefes Arch. Ophthal.*, 1894, **40**, Abt. 3, 1-129.
Classic account of metastatic ophthalmia.

5939 PARINAUD, HENRI. 1844-1905
Conjonctivite lacrymale à pneumocoques des nouveau-nés. *Ann. Oculist. (Paris)*, 1894, **112**, 369-73.

5940 HIPPEL, EUGEN VON. 1867-1939
Vorstellung eines Patientin mit einem sehr ungewöhnlichen Netzhautbeziehungsweise Aderhautleiden. *Ber. ophthal. Ges. Heidelb.*, 1895, **24**, 269.
First description of angiomatosis of the retina – "Hippel's disease".

5941 AXENFELD, KARL THEODOR PAUL POLYKARPOS. 1867-1930
Beiträge zur Aetiologie der Bindehautenzündungen. Ueber chronische
Diplobacillenconjunctivitis. *Ber. ophthal. Ges. Heidelb.*, (1896), 1897, **25**,
140-55.
Description of the diplobacillary form of chronic conjunctivitis.

5942 MORAX, VICTOR. 1866-1935
Note sur un diplobacille pathogène pour la conjunctiva humaine. *Ann.
Inst. Pasteur.*, 1896, **10**, 337-45.
Morax and Axenfeld (No. 5941) independently isolated a diplobacillus
which causes a chronic conjunctivitis – the Morax–Axenfeld haemophilus.

5943 SCHMIDT-RIMPLER, HERMANN. 1838-1915
Die Erkrankungen des Auges im Zusammenhang mit anderen Krankheiten.
Wien, *A. Hölder*, 1898.
Like Förster (No. 5915), Schmidt-Rimpler was interested in the relationship between eye diseases and general organic diseases; like Cohn (No.
5931), he was an advocate of the routine examination of the eyes of
schoolchildren.

5944 GRAEFE, ALFRED CARL. 1830-1899, & SAEMISCH, EDWIN THEODOR. 1833-1909
Handbuch der gesamten Augenheilkunde. 2te. Aufl. 15 vols. [in 41].
Leipzig, *W. Engelmann*, 1899-1918.
The first edition of this great collective work, of which Graefe and
Saemisch were the editors, appeared between 1874 and 1880.

5945 GULLSTRAND, ALLVAR. 1862-1930
Allgemeine Theorie der monochromatischen Aberrationen und ihre
nächsten Ergebnisse für die Ophthalmologie. Uppsala, *E. Berling*, 1900.
Gullstrand was professor of ophthalmology at Uppsala. He was
awarded the Nobel Prize in 1911. The above work is the exposition of his
general theory of monochromatic aberrations. This is an offprint from
Nova Acta Reg. Soc. Sci. Ups., 1900-01, ser. 3, **20**.

5946 SMITH, HENRY. 1862-1948
Extractions of cataract in the capsule. *Indian med. Gaz.*, 1900, **35**, 241-46;
1901, **36**, 220-25; 1905, **40**, 327-30.
Smith, an officer in the Indian Medical Service, had remarkable success
with his method of extraction of cataract within the capsule, one of the
most important contributions of recent times. He modified his operation
in 1926 (*Arch. Ophthal. N.Y., ***55**, 213-24).

5947 PARSONS, *Sir* JOHN HERBERT. 1868-1957
The pathology of the eye. 4 vols. London, *Hodder & Stoughton, Henry
Frowde*, 1904-08.

5948 TOTI, ADDEO. 1861-
Nuovo metodo conservatore di cura radicale delle suppurazioni croniche
del sacco lacrimale (dacriocistorinostomia). *Clin. mod. (Pisa)*, 1904, **10**,
385-87.
Toti's account of dacryocystorhinostomy, a procedure he himself
introduced.

5949   HEINE, LEOPOLD. 1870-
Die Cyklodialyse, eine neue Glaukomoperation. *Dtsch. med. Wschr.*, 1905, **31**, 824-26.
Introduction of cyclodialysis in glaucoma.

5950   MARKUS, CHARLES.
Notes on a peculiar pupil phenomenon in cases of partial iridoplegia. *Trans. ophthal. Soc. U. K.*, 1906, **26**, 50-56.
Markus was among the first to describe the condition known as "Adie's syndrome" (No. 4611).

5950.1   ZIRM, EDUARD KONRAD. 1863-1944
Eine erfolgreiche totale Keratoplastik. *v. Graefes Arch. Ophthal.*, 1906, **64**, 580-93.
First successful corneal transplantation (keratoplasty).

5951   HALBERSTAEDTER, LUDWIG. 1876- , & PROWAZEK, STANISLAUS JOSEPH MATTHIAS VON. 1875-1915
Über Zelleinschlüsse parasitärer Natur beim Trachom. *Arb. k. Gesundh-Amte*, 1907, **26**, 44-47.
Halberstaedter and Prowazek first described the cytoplasmic inclusion bodies of trachoma, *Chlamydia trachomatis.*

5952   HOLTH, SÖREN. 1863-1937
Iridencleisis antiglaucomatosa. *Ann Oculist. (Paris)*, 1907, **137**, 345-75.
Introduction of iridencleisis for glaucoma.

5953   LAGRANGE, PIERRE FÉLIX. 1857-1928
Nouveau traitement du glaucome chronique; iridectomie et sclérectomie combinée. *Gaz. hebd. Sci. méd Bordeaux,* 1907, **28**, 2-4.
Sclerectomy for the treatment of glaucoma.

5954   COATS, GEORGE. 1876-1915
Forms of retinal disease with massive exudation. *Ophthal. Hosp. Rep.*, 1908, **17**, 440-525.
"Coats's disease" (retinitis circinata).

5955   ELLIOT, ROBERT HENRY. 1864-1936
A preliminary note on a new operative procedure for the establishment of a filtering cicatrix in the treatment of glaucoma. *Ophthalmoscope*, 1909, **7**, 804-06.
The operation of sclero-corneal trephining for glaucoma was introduced by Elliot in 1909.

5956   STARGARDT, KARL BRUNO. 1875-1927
Über Epithelzellveränderungen beim Trachom und andern Conjunctivalerkrankungen. *v. Graefes Arch. Ophthal.*, 1909, **69**, 525-42.
Demonstration of the inclusion bodies in ophthalmia neonatorum.

5957   ELSCHNIG, ANTON. 1863-1939
Studien zur sympathischen Ophthalmie. 1. Wirkung von Antigenen vom Augeninnern aus. *v. Graefes Arch. Ophthal.*, 1910, **75**, 459-73.
Elschnig suggested the anaphylactic theory of the pathogenesis of sympathetic ophthalmia.

5958   HERBERT, HERBERT. 1865-1942
The small flap incision for glaucoma. *Trans. ophthal. Soc. U. K.*, 1910, **30**, 199-215.
Herbert's small flap sclerotomy.

5959   HULEN, VARD HOUGHTON. 1865-1939
Vacuum fixation of the lens and flap suture in the extraction of a cataract in its capsule. *J. Amer. med. Ass.*, 1911, **57**, 188-89.
Hulen devised a vacuum method of cataract extraction.

5960   BOTTERI, ALBERT. 1879-1955
Klinische, experimentelle und mikroskopische Studien über Trachom, Einschlussblenorrhöe und Frühjahrskatarrh. *Klin. Mbl. Augenheilk.*, 1912, **50**, i, 653-90.
Filtration of the virus of inclusion conjunctivitis.

5961   NICOLLE, CHARLES JULES HENRI. 1866-1936, *et al.*
Le magot animal réactif du trachôme. Filtrabilité du virus. Pouvoir infectant des larmes. *C. R. Acad. Sci (Paris)*, 1912, **155**, 241-43.
Filtration of the trachoma agent, *Chlamydia trachomatis*. With L. Blaisot and A. Cuénod.

5962   PURTSCHER, OTTMAR. 1852-1927
Angiopathia retinae traumatica. Lymphorrhagien des Augengrundes. *v. Graefes Arch. Ophthal.*, 1912, **82**, 347-71.
"Purtscher's disease", traumatic angiopathy of the retina, first described.

5963   STANCULEANU, GHEORGHE. 1874-
Intrakapsuläre Staroperationen. *Klin. Mbl. Augenheilk.*, 1912, **50**, 527-37.
Stanculeanu's technique for cataract extraction.

5964   KNAPP, ARNOLD HERMANN. 1869-1956
Report of one hundred successive extractions of cataract in the capsule after subluxation with the capsule forceps. *Arch. Ophthal.*, (N.Y.), 1915, **44**, 1-9.
Knapp's method of extraction of cataract with forceps. See also his later paper in the same journal, 1921, **50**, 426-30.

5965   BARRAQUER, IGNACIO. 1884-1965, & ANDUYNED.
Un procédé d'extrême douceur pour l'extraction "in toto" de la cataracte. *Clin Ophthal.*, 1917, **22**, 328-33.
Attempts to extract cataract by suction and aspiration date from ancient times. Barraquer employed a special machine of his own invention.

5966   ISHIHARA, SHINOBU. 1879-1963
Tests for colour-blindness. Tokyo, *Kanehira Shuppan*, & London, *H.K. Lewis*, 1917.
Ishihara's colour tests. 15th ed., 1960.

5967   TSCHERNING, MARIUS HANS ERIK. 1854-1939
L'adaption compensatrice de l'oeil. *Ann. Oculist. (Brux.)*, 1922, **159**, 625-37.
Introduction of the photometric spectacle lens.

5968   URIBE TRONCOSO, MANUEL. 1867-
Gonioscopy and its clinical applications. *Amer. J. Ophthal.*, 1925, **8**, 433-49.
Troncoso's gonioscope.

5969   WOODS, ALAN CHURCHILL. 1889-1963
Diseases of the uvea. I. Sympathetic ophthalmia: the use of uveal pigment
in diagnosis and treatment. *Trans. ophthal. Soc. U. K.*, 1925, **45**, 208-51.
Intradermal pigment test in sympathetic ophthalmitis.

5970   HAMBURGER, CARL. 1870-1944
Glaukosantropfen, Glaukom und Akkommodation. *Klin. Mbl. Augenheilk.*,
1926, 76, 400-03.
Introduction of glaucosan.

5971   LINDAU, ARVID VILHELM. 1892-
Studien über Kleinhirncysten. Bau, Pathogenese und Beziehungen zur
Angiomatosis retinae. *Acta path. microbiol. scand.*, 1926, Suppl. **1**.
Lindau's important histological study of haemangiomatosis retinae
("Lindau's disease").

5972   GONIN, JULES. 1870-1935
Nouveaux cas de guérison opératoire de décollements rétiniens. *Ann.
Oculist. (Paris)*, 1927, **164**, 817-26.
Gonin's operation of ignipuncture for treatment of detachment of the
retina.

5973   NOGUCHI, HIDEYO. 1876-1928
Experimental production of a trachoma-like condition in monkeys by
means of a micro-organism isolated from American Indian trachoma. *J.
Amer. med. Ass.*, 1927, **89**, 739-42.
Isolation of *Bact. granulosis*, believed by Noguchi to be the causal
organism in trachoma. See also his monograph in *J. exp. Med.*, 1928, **48**,
Suppl. 2.

5974   VERHOEFF, FREDERICK HERMAN. 1874-
A new operation for removing cataracts with their capsules. *Trans. Amer.
ophthal. Soc.*, 1927, **25**, 54-64.
Verhoeff's buttonhole iridectomy.

5975   ELSCHNIG, ANTON. 1863-1939
Keratoplasty. *Arch. Ophthal. (N.Y.)*, 1930, **4**, 165-73.
Elschnig developed the method of corneal grafting introduced by von
Hippel (No. 5933) and produced good results on the human eye.

5976   HEINE, LEOPOLD. 1870-
Ueber den Ausgleich sämtlicher Brechungsfehler des Auges durch
geschliffene Haftgläser (unter den Lidern getragene Schalen). *Münch. med.
Wschr.*, 1930, **77**, 6-7, 271-72.
The manufacture of modern contact glasses has been made possible by
the work of Heine. See also his paper in *Lancet*, 1931, **1**, 631-32. For a brief
history of this subject, see *Schweiz. med. Wschr.*, 1946, **76**, 719.

5977   LARSSON, SVEN.
Operative Behandlung von Netzhautabhebung mit Elektroendothermie und Trepanation; vorläufige Mitteilung. *Acta ophthal., (Kbh.)*, 1930, **8**, 172-83.
    Superficial diathermy treatment of retinal detachment. See also *Arch Ophthal. (N.Y.)*, 1932, **7**, 661-80.

5978   MOORE, ROBERT FOSTER. 1878-1963
Choroidal sarcoma treated by the intra-ocular insertion of radon needles. *Brit. J. Ophthal.*, 1930, **14**, 145-52.
    Foster Moore's technique for the radiation treatment of choroidal neoplasms.

5979   THOMAS, *Sir* JAMES WILLIAM TUDOR. 1893-1976
Transplantation of cornea: a preliminary report on a series of experiments on rabbits. *Trans. ophthal. Soc. U. K.*, 1930, **50**, 127-41.
    See also his paper in *Brit. J. Ophthal.*, 1934, **18**, 129-42.

5980   GUIST, GUSTAV.
Eine neue Ablatiooperation. *Z. Augenheilk.*, 1931, **74**, 232-42.
    Guist's operation for detachment of the retina (multiple trephining and chemical cauterization of the choroid).

5981   CASTROVIEJO, RAMON. 1904-1987
Keratoplasty. A historical and experimental study, including a new method. *Amer. J. Ophthal.*, 1932, **15**, 825-38, 905-16.
    Castroviejo's method of keratoplasty.

5983   LOPEZ LACARRERE, JULIO.
Nuestro método original de extracción total de la catarata senil: la electrodiafaquia. Primeros ensayos. *Arch. Oftal. hisp.-amer.*, 1932, **32**, 293-303.
    Intracapsular extraction of cataract by diathermy with the electro-diaphake. Preliminary report in *Klin. Mbl. Augenheilk.*, 1932, **88**, 778-83.

5984   SAFR, KARL.
Behandlung der Netzhautabhebung mit Elektroden für multiple diathermische Stichelung. *Klin. Mbl. Augenheilk.*, 1932, **88**, 814.
    Safr's method of treatment of retinal detachment.

5985   DALLOS, JOSEF. 1905-1979
Ueber Haftgläser und Kontaktschalen. *Klin, Mbl. Augenheilk.*, 1933, **91**, 640-59.
    Contact lenses introduced. *See also* No. 5976.

5986   FILATOV, VLADIMIR PETROVICH. 1875-1956
Transplantation of the cornea. *Arch. Ophthal. (N.Y.)*, 1935, **13**, 321-47.
    Earlier papers recording the important work of Filatov on corneal transplantation appeared in Russian journals.

5987   MANN, IDA CAROLINE. 1893-
Developmental abnormalities of the eye. Cambridge, *Univ. Press*, 1937.

5988   VOGT, ALFRED. 1879-1943
Ergebnisse der Diathermiestichelung des Corpus ciliare (Zyklodiathermiestichelung) gegen Glaukom. *Klin. Mbl. Augenheilk.*, 1937, **99**, 9-15.
Vogt's operation of cyclodiathermy for glaucoma.

5988.1   MARZIO, QUIRINO DI. 1883-1954
Fundus oculi: diagnostica oftalmoscopica...[Torino, *Rosenberg & Sellier*, 1937].
The first atlas of ophthalmoscopy published in Italy, considered by many to be the most beautiful ever published. German translation, Torino, *Rosenberg und Sellier*, [1941]. Some copies of that edition contain an English translation of the text by G. Bonaccolto enclosed in a pocket of the binding.

5989   TERRY, THEODORE LASATER. 1899-1946
Extreme prematurity and fibroblastic overgrowth of persistent vascular sheath behind each crystalline lens. I. Preliminary report. *Amer. J. Ophthal.*, 1942, **25**, 203-04.
Retrolental fibroplasia first described. See also the same volume, pp. 1409-23, and *Trans. Sect. Ophthal. Amer. med. Ass.*, 1942, 213-29, for later papers.

5990   SANDERS, MURRAY JONATHAN. 1910-1987, & ALEXANDER, R. C.
Epidemic keratoconjunctivitis. I. Isolation and identification of a filterable virus. *J. exp. Med.*, 1943, **77**, 71-96.

5990.1   BARRAQUER MONER, JOSÉ IGNACIO.
Actual técnica de elección en queratoplastia penetrante. *Arch. Soc. oftal. hispano-amer.*, 1949, **9**, 152-9.
Barraquer's method of corneal graft fixation by minute direct interrupted stitches.

5991   RIDLEY, NICHOLAS HAROLD LLOYD. 1906-
Intra-ocular acrylic lenses. *Trans. ophthal. Soc. U.K.*, 1951, **71**, 617-21.
Ridley implanted the first intra-ocular lens on 19 November 1949. At the time of this first report the lens had remained in place for 17 months.

5991.1   T'ANG, FEI FAN, *et al.*
Studies on the etiology of trachoma with special reference to isolation of the virus in chick embryo. *Chinese med. J.*, 1957, **75**, 429-47.
Isolation of trachoma agent, *Chlamydia trachomatis*. With H. L. Chang, Y. T. Huang, and K. C. Wang.

History of Ophthalmology

5991.9   MANNI, DOMENICO MARIA. 1690-1788
Degli occhiali da naso inventati da Salvino Armati...Firenze, *Albizzini*, 1738.
The first book on the history of spectacles. Manni gave credit for the invention to the Florentine Armati (*fl.* 1300).

5992   JUGLER, JOHANN HEINRICH. 1758-1812
Bibliothecae ophthalmicae specimen primum eruditorum examini subjicit. Hamburg, *J. P. C. Reuse*, 1783.
The earliest bibliography and history of ophthalmology.

5993   MAGNUS, Hugo Friedrich. 1842-1907
        Geschichte des grauen Staares. Leipzig, *Veit & Co.*, 1876.
            An early history of cataract.

5994   HIRSCH, August. 1817-1894
        Geschichte der Ophthalmologie. *In*: Graefe and Saemisch, Handbuch der
        gesammten Augenheilkunde, Leipzig, 1877, **7**, Theil 5, 235-554.
            The first systematic history of the subject.

5996   HIRSCHBERG, Julius. 1843-1925
        Geschichte der Augenheilkunde. 10 pts. Leipzig, *W. Engelmann*, 1899-1918.
            This monumental work remains the authoritative encyclopaedic his-
        tory of ophthalmology, up to the first decade of the 20th century. Its
        thoroughness and critical judgement mark it as one of the greatest of all
        histories of scientific subjects. Forms Bde. 12-15 of Graefe–Saemisch
        Handbuch der gesamten Augenheilkunde, 2te Aufl. Reprinted Hildesheim,
        G. Olms, 1977. Extensively illustrated English translation by F.C. Blodi, 11
        vols. plus supplements, (In progress). Bonn, *J.P. Wayenborgh*, 1982-   .

5997   MAGNUS, Hugo Friedrich. 1842-1907
        Die Augenheilkunde der Alten. Breslau, *J.V. Kern*, 1901.
            A history of ancient ophthalmology in which the writer has attempted
        to reconstruct the anatomical concepts of the ancient Greeks.

5998   PANSIER, Pierre. 1864-1939
        Histoire des lunettes. Paris, *A. Maloine*, 1901.

5999   ——. Histoire de l'ophtalmologie. In P.F. Lagrange and E. Valude:
        Encyclopédie française d'ophtalmologie, Paris, 1903, **1**, 1-86.

6000   BOCK, Emil. 1857-1916
        Die Brille und ihre Geschichte. Wien, *J. Safar*, 1903.

6001   HORSTMANN, Carl. 1847-1912
        Geschichte der Augenheilkunde. *In*: Puschmann, T., Handbuch der
        Geschichte de Medizin, Jena, 1905, **3**, 489-572.

6002   HUBBELL, Alvin Allace. 1846-1911
        The development of ophthalmology in America, 1800 to 1870. Chicago,
        Amer. Med. Assoc. Press, 1908.
            Of limited value, but the only available history of early American
        ophthalmology.

6003   GREEFF, Carl Richard. 1862-1938
        Die Erfindung der Augengläser. Berlin, *Optische Bücherei*, 1921.

6004   JAMES, Robert Rutson. 1881-1959
        Studies in the history of ophthalmology in England prior to the year 1800.
        Cambridge, *University Press*, 1933.

6005   HUGHES, Wendell L.
        Reconstructive surgery of the eyelids. St. Louis, *C.V. Mosby Co.*, 1943.
            Most of this work is a very carefully documented history of the subject.
        Bibliography of 451 references.

6006 SORSBY, ARNOLD.1900-1980
A short history of ophthalmology. 2nd ed. London, *Staples Press*, 1948.

6007 DRAEGER, JÖRG
Geschichte der Tonometrie. Basel, *S. Karger*, 1961.
Revised and enlarged English translation with deceptive title: *Tonometry: physical fundamentals, development of methods and clinical application*, New York, *Hafner*, 1966.

6007.1 RUCKER, C. WILBUR.
A history of the ophthalmoscope. Rochester, *Privately printed*, [1971].

6007.2 HAUGWITZ, THILO VON
Ophthalmologisch-optische Untersuchungsgeräte. Stuttgart, *Ferdinand Enke*, 1981.
English translation by F.C. Blodi, Bonn, *J.P. Wayenborgh*, 1986.

6007.3 BOSNIAK, STEPHEN L. (Ed.)
History and tradition [of ophthalmic plastic surgery]. *Advances in Ophthalmic Plastic and Reconstructive Surgery*, 1986, 5.
A collection of articles by various authors, including partial reprint of No.6005.

GYNAECOLOGY

6008 SORANUS *of Ephesus*. A.D. 98-138
De arte obstetricia morbisque mulierum quae supersunt. Ex apographo F. R. DIETZ. Regimontii Prus., *Graefe et Unzer*, 1838.
Greek *editio princeps* of Soranus, based on manuscripts Dietz discovered in Paris and Rome. Soranus is the leading authority on the gynaecology and obstetrics of antiquity. He recognized atresia of the vagina as being congenital or acquired from inflammation. He packed the uterus for haemorrhage and performed hysterectomy for prolapse. He described podalic version. English translation by O. Temkin, Baltimore, 1956.

6009 ———. Gynaeciorum libri iv...ed. I. Ilberg. Corpus Medicorum Graecorum IV. Lipsiae et Berolini, *B.G. Teubner*, 1927.
Standard Greek edition of the works of Soranus.

6009.1 TROTULA [*also* TROTTA, TROCTA]. *fl.* 11th century A.D.
Experimentarius medicinae. Continens Trotulae curandarum aegriudinum muliebrium ante, in & post partium lib. unicum, nusquam antea editum...Argent[orati], *Apud Joannem Schottum*, 1544.
The gynaecological writings attributed to the woman physician, Trotula, who is said to have taught at Salerno during the 11th century. Trotula is the earliest woman physician to write a significant medical treatise. English translation by E. Mason-Hohl, Los Angeles, 1940.

6010 BERENGARIO DA CARPI, GIACOMO.*circa* 1460-1530?
Commentaria cum amplissimis additionibus super anatomia Mundini. (Bononiae, *per H. de Benedictis*, 1521.)
On fol. ccxxv Berengario gives the first authentic report of vaginal hysterectomy for prolapse. He describes two cases, one performed by himself in 1507 and the other by his father. *See* No. 367.

6011   WOLFF, Caspar [Wolf]. 1525-1601
Volumen gynaeciorum, hoc est, de mulierum tum aliis, tum gravidarum, parientium et puerperarum affectibus et morbis. Basileae, *per T. Guarinum*, 1566.
The first encyclopaedia of gynaecology and obstetrics, originally conceived by Conrad Gesner, who collected material for the purpose. Wolff, Gesner's literary executor, added material and published the collection one year after Gesner's death. This contains the first edition of Moschion (No. 6136).

6012   BAUHIN, Caspar [Bauhinus]. 1560-1624
Gynaeciorum sive de mulierum affectibus commentarii. 4 vols. Basileae, *per T. Guarinum*, 1586-88.
An enlarged version of No. 6011, now edited by Bauhin.

6013   SPACH, Israel. 1560-1610
Gynaeciorum sive de mulierum tum communibus, tum gravidarum, parientum, et puerperarum affectibus et morbis, libri. Argentinae, *sumpt. L. Zetzneri*, 1597.
Spach was the editor of this collection of gynaecological writings. It is in effect the third edition of the collection previously issued by Wolff (No. 6011) and Bauhin (No. 6012).

6013.1 GUINTERIUS, Johannes, *Andernacus*. 1505-1574
Gynaeciorum commentarius, de gravidarum parturientium, puerperarum & infantium, cura...Accessit elenchus auctorum in re medica cluentium, qui gynaecia scriptis clararunt & illustrarunt. Opera e studio Joan. Georgii Schenkii...Argentorati, *Impensis Lazari Zetzneri*, 1606.
The first bibliography of gynaecology, covering physicians who wrote on the subject from the earliest times to the beginning of the 17th century, was written by Johann Georg Schenck (*d.* 1620) and appended to his posthumous first edition of Guinter's treatise on gynaecology.

6014   BAILLOU, Guillaume de [Ballonius]. 1538-1616
De virginum et mulierum morbis liber. Parisiis, *J. Quisnel*, 1643.

6015   ROONHUYZE, Hendrik van. 1622-1672
Heel-konstige aanmerkkingen betreffende de gebreeken der vrouwen. Amsterdam, *weduwe van T. Jacobsz*, 1663.
Roonhuyze's book is regarded as the first work on operative gynaecology in the modern sense. He successfully performed caesarean section several times, and he used retractors for the repair of vesico-vaginal fistulae. English translation, London, 1676.

6016   STAHL, Georg Ernst. 1660-1734
Ausführliche Abhandlung von den Zufällen und Kranckheiten des Frauenzimmers. Leipzig, *J. C. Eyssel*, 1724.

6017   HOUSTOUN, Robert [Houston]. 1678-1734
An account of a dropsy of the left ovary of a woman, aged 58, cured by a large incision made in the side of the abdomen. *Phil. Trans.*, (1724-25), 1726, **33**, 8-15.
Houstoun was the first to treat ovarian dropsy by tapping the cyst, 1701. For biographical note, see *J. Obst. Gynaec. Brit. Comw.*, 1973, **80**, 193-200.

6018   EISENMANN, GEORGE HEINRICH. 1693-1768
Tabulae anatomicae quatuor uteri duplicis. Argentorati, *ex. off. A. Königii*, 1752.
      Atlas of bipartite and double uterus.

6019   ASTRUC, JEAN. 1684-1766
Traité des maladies des femmes. 6 vols. Paris, *P. G. Cavelier*, 1761-1765.
      Mettler considers this "the most pretentious gynecologic work of the [eighteenth] century...chiefly useful for its historical orientation". English translation, 3 vols., London, 1762-67.

6020   HUNTER, WILLIAM. 1718-1783.
[Appendix to Lynn's The history of a fatal inversion of the uterus]. *Med. Obs. Inqu.*, 1771, **4**, 400-09; 1776, **5**, 388-93.
      First accurate description of retroversion of the uterus.

6021   BAILLIE, MATTHEW. 1761-1823
An account of a particular change of structure in the human ovarium. *Phil Trans.*, 1789, **79**, 71-78.
      Matthew Baillie's notable anatomico-pathological studies on dermoid cysts of the ovary. Also published in *Lond. med. J.*, 1789, **10**, 322-32.

6022   SOEMMERRING, SAMUEL THOMAS. 1755-1830
Ueber die Wirkungen der Schnürbrüste. Berlin, *Voss*, 1793.
      Soemmerring enumerated the bad effects of tight corsets on the internal organs of women. His paper created much interest and resulted in a great decline in the fad of tight lacing and hoop skirts. The first edition was published at Leipzig, 1788, but is less important as it had no illustrations.

6023   McDOWELL, EPHRAIM. 1771-1830
Three cases of extirpation of diseased ovaria. *Eclect. Repert. Analyt. Rev.*, 1817, **7**, 242-44.
      McDowell was a pioneer ovariotomist. Although not the first to perform this operation, he deserves credit for putting it upon a permanent basis. The above records his first ovariotomy, performed in 1809, together with two later cases. Reprinted in *Med. Classics*, 1938, **2**, 651-53.

6024   SMITH, NATHAN. 1762-1829
Case of ovarian dropsy, successfully removed by a surgical operation. *Amer. Med. Recorder*, 1822, **5**, 124-26.
      Smith was the first in the U.S.A. after McDowell to perform ovariotomy, for ovarian dropsy. Smith was apparently without knowledge of the previous operations of McDowell.

6025   SIEBOLD, ADAM ELIAS VON. 1775-1826
Ueber den Gebärmutterkrebs, dessen Entstehung und Verhütung. Berlin, *F. Dummler*, 1824.
      Classic account of cancer of the uterus.

6026   LIZARS, JOHN. 1794-1860
Observations on extraction of diseased ovaria. Edinburgh, *D. Lizars*, 1825.
      Lizars performed the first (unsuccessful) ovariotomy in Britain. His book made generally known the practical possibility of this operation.

6026.1 DEWEES, WILLIAM POTTS. 1768-1841
A treatise on the diseases of females. Philadelphia, *Carey & Lea*, 1826.
First American textbook on gynaecology.

6027 STRACHAN, JOHN B.
Case of successful excision of the cervis uteri in a scirrhous state. *Amer. J. med. Sci.*, 1829, **5**, 307-09.
First successful excision of the cervix in America. Reported by T. F. Gillan.

6028 BOIVIN, MARIE ANNE VICTOIRE, *née Gillain*. 1773-1841, & DUGÈS, ANTOINE. 1798-1838
Traité pratique des maladies de l'utérus et de ses annexes. 2 vols. and atlas. Paris, *J. B. Baillière*, 1833.
Boivin and Dugès practised amputation of the cervix for chronic ulceration. On page 648 of vol. 2 is the first recorded case of cancer of the female urethra. English translation, 1834.

6028.1 GOSSET, MONTAGUE. 1792-1854
Calculus in the bladder. Incontinence of urine. Vesico-vaginal fistula. Advantages of the gilt-wire suture. *Lancet*, 1834-5, **1**, 345-6.
Gosset repaired a vesicovaginal fistula of eleven years' duration, using silver gilt-wire, removed after 9, 12 and 21 days respectively.

6029 ROUX, PHILIBERT JOSEPH. 1780-1854
Mémoire sur la restauration du périnée chez la femme dans les cas de division ou de rupture complète de cette partie. *Gaz. méd. Paris*, 1834, 2 sér., **2**, 17-22.
Roux was the first to suture the ruptured female perineum.

6030 HAYWARD, GEORGE. 1791-1863
Case of vesico-vaginal fistula, successfully treated by an operation. *Amer. J. med. Sci.*, 1839, **24**, 283-88.
Hayward's successful treatment of vesico-vaginal fistula was performed after Mettauer's, although reported earlier.

6031 METTAUER, JOHN PETER. 1787-1875
Vesico-vaginal fistula. *Boston med. surg. J.*, 1840, **22**, 154-55.
The first successful operation for vesico-vaginal fistula is believed to be that performed in August 1838, by Mettauer, a Virginian gynaecologist. He introduced metallic sutures and a retention catheter.

6031.1 WILTON, WILLIAM. 1809-1899
Hydatids, terminating fatally, by haemorrhage. *Lancet,* 1840, **1**, 691-693.
First report of a chorionic tumour.

6032 CLAY, CHARLES. 1801-1893
Cases of peritoneal section, for the extirpation of diseased ovaria, by the large incision from sternum to pubes, successfully treated. *Med. Times,* 1842, **7**, 43, 59, 67, 83, 99, 139, 153, 270.
Clay, pioneer ovariotomist in Great Britain, introduced the word "ovariotomy". (*See also* his later paper, No. 6054.)

6033   RÉCAMIER, Joseph Claude Anthelme. 1774-1852
Invention du spéculum plein et brisé. *Bull. Acad. Méd. (Paris)*, 1842-1843, **8**, 661-68.
Description of the speculum invented by Récamier.

6034   ATLEE, John Light. 1799-1885
Case of ovarian tumors – both the right and the left being removed at the same operation. *N. Y. J. Med.*, 1843, **1**, 168-70.
First successful double oöphorectomy. Communicated in a letter to the editor by J. M. Foltz.

6035   SIMPSON, *Sir* James Young. 1811-1870
Contributions to the pathology and treatment of disease of the uterus. *Lond. Edinb. month. J. med. Sci.*, 1843, **3**, 547-56, 701-15, 1009-27; 1844, **4**, 208-17.
Simpson introduced many important procedures into gynaecology and obstetrics; among them may be mentioned his use of the uterine sound for diagnosing retro-positions of the uterus

6036   BENNET, James Henry. 1816-1891
A practical treatise on inflammation, ulceration, and induration of the neck of the uterus. London, *J. Churchill*, 1845.
Bennet was the first to differentiate between benign and malignant uterine tumours.

6037   SIMS, James Marion. 1813-1883
On the treatment of vesico-vaginal fistula. *Amer. J. med. Sci.*, 1852, n.s., **23**, 59-82.
Original description of Sims's operation for the treatment of vesico-vaginal fistula; also describes "Sims's position, the knee–chest position. Reprinted in *Med. Classics*, 1938, **2**, 677-712.

6038   ATLEE, Washington Lemuel. 1808-1878
A table of all the known operations of ovariotomy. From 1701-1851. *Trans. Amer. med. Ass.*, 1851, **4**, 286-314.
Atlee is said to have performed ovariotomy 387 times; with his brother John he firmly established the operation in the U.S.A.

6039   ——. The surgical treatment of certain fibrous tumours of the uterus. Philadelphia, *T. K. & P. G. Collins*, 1853.
Atlee was among the first to study the surgical removal of uterine fibroids.

6040   BURNHAM, Walter. 1808-1883
Extirpation of the uterus and ovaries for sarcomatous disease. *Nelson's Amer. Lancet*, 1854, **8**, 147.
First successful abdominal hysterectomy, 25 May, 1853. An account of Burnham's work is given by J. C. Irish in *Trans. Amer. med. Ass.* 1878, **29**, 447-61.

6041   SIMON, Gustav. 1824-1876
Ueber die Heilung der Blasen-Scheidenfisteln. Gissen, *E. Heinemann*, 1854.
Simon is perhaps best remembered as being the first in Europe to excise the kidney; he also wrote a fine monograph on vesico-vaginal fistula.

6042   KIMBALL, GILMAN. 1804-1892
Successful case of extirpation of the uterus. *Boston med. surg. J.* 1855, **52**, 249-55.
First successful abdominal hysteromyomectomy (for fibromyoma), 1 September 1853.

6043   FERGUSSON, *Sir* WILLIAM. 1808-1877
System of practical surgery. 4th ed. London, *J. Churchill,* 1857.
On p. 724 is described Fergusson's vaginal speculum.

6043.1   HODGE, HUGH LENNOX. 1796-1873
On diseases peculiar to women, including displacements of the uterus. Philadelphia, *Blanchard & Lea,* 1860.
Chapter 5 includes a lengthy description of the "Hodge pessary". *See* No. 6185.

6044   NOEGGERATH, EMIL. 1827-1895
On epicystotomy. *N. Y. J. Med.,* 1858, 3 ser., **4**, 9-24.
Noeggerath, who devised the operation of epicystotomy, spent many years in America, where he became a leading gynaecologist and obstetrician.

6045   WAGNER, ERNST LEBERECHT. 1829-1888
Der Gebärmutterkrebs. Leipzig, *B. G. Teubner,* 1858.
In this work Wagner presented the first important contribution to the knowledge of the gross pathology of uterine cancer.

6046   AYRES, DANIEL. 1822-1892
Congenital exstrophy of the urinary bladder, complicated with prolapsus uteri following pregnancy; successfully treated by a new plastic operation. *Amer. med. Gaz.,* 1859, **10**, 81-89.
First successful plastic operation for exstrophy of the female bladder.

6047   ATLEE, WASHINGTON LEMUEL. 1808-1878
Case of successful operation for vesico-vaginal fistula. *Amer J. med. Sci.,* 1860, n.s., **39**, 67-82.
Atlee's operation for vesico-vaginal fistula.

6048   BERNUTZ, GUSTAVE LOUIS RICHARD. 1819-1887, & GOUPIL, JEAN ERNEST. 1829-1864
Clinique médicale sur les maladies des femmes. 2 vols. Paris, *F. Chamerot,* 1860-62.
One of the most important texts on the subject during the mid nineteenth century. English translation, *New Sydenham Society,* 1867.

6049   SIMS, JAMES MARION. 1813-1883
Amputation of the cervix uteri. *Trans N.Y. med. Soc.,* 1861. 367-71.
Sims's method for amputating the cervix.

6050   ——. On vaginismus. *Trans. obstet. Soc. Lond.,* (1861), 1862, **3**, 356-67.

6051   KOEBERLÉ, EUGÈNE. 1828-1915
De l'ovariotomie. *Mém. Acad. imp. Méd (Paris),* 1863, **26**, 321-472.
The introduction of ovariotomy into France was in part due to Koeberlé. He made great advances in gynaecological operative technique.

6052 ———. Exstirpation de l'utérus et des ovaires. *Gaz. méd. Strasbourg,* 1863, **23**, 101.

First successful excision of uterus and ovaries for tumour.

6053 ———. Documents pour servir à l'histoire de l'extirpation des tumeurs fibreuses de la matrice par la méthode suspubienne. *Mém. Soc. de Méd. de Strasbourg,* (1863-64), 1865, **4**, 84-158.

6054 CLAY, CHARLES. 1801-1893

Observations on ovariotomy, statistical and practical. Also, a successful case of entire removal of the uterus and its appendages. *Trans. obstet. Soc. Lond.,* (1863), 1864, **5**, 58-74.

For many years Clay was the most eminent ovariotomist in Great Britain. In all, he performed 395 ovariotomies, with a mortality of 25 per cent.

6055 EMMET, THOMAS ADDIS. 1828-1919

On the treatment of dysmenorrhoea and sterility, resulting from anteflexion of the uterus. *N.Y. med. J.,* 1865, **1**, 205-19.

Emmet was an outstanding American gynaecological surgeon, a disciple of Sims.

6056 WELLS, *Sir* THOMAS SPENCER. 1818-1897

Diseases of the ovaries. London, *J. Churchill,* 1865.

Wells was perhaps the greatest of the pioneer ovariotomists; he performed his first ovariotomy in 1858. The title page to this work states that a second volume would be published. By the time Wells issued the intended Volume two he considered it an entirely separate work and not a continuation of his 1865 treatise. The second work, published in 1872, has frequently been miscatalogued as Volume two because it bears the same title and was issued by the same publisher. However, it is not called Volume two on its title page.

6057 SIMS, JAMES MARION. 1813-1883

Clinical notes on uterine surgery, with reference to the management of the sterile condition. London, *R. Hardwicke,* 1866.

A revolutionary and controversial work, written in Paris while Sims was in voluntary exile because of the U.S. Civil War, and first serialized in *Lancet,* 1864-65. Includes, pp. 16-18, the description of Sims's duck-billed speculum. Also includes important and pioneering work on the treatment of infertility, including analysis of the conditions essential to conception, and record of a successful artificial insemination. American edition, N.Y., 1866.

6058 EMMET, THOMAS ADDIS. 1828-1919

Vesico-vaginal fistula from parturition and other causes: with cases of recto-vaginal fistula. New York, *William Wood,* 1868.

A comprehensive and valuable account of the management of vesico-vaginal fistula based on Sims's technique.

6059 ———. Surgery of the cervix in connection with the treatment of certain uterine diseases. *Amer J. Obstet. Dis. Wom.,* 1869, **1**, 339-62.

Surgical repair of lacerations of the cervix.

6060   THOMAS, THEODORE GAILLARD. 1831-1903
        A practical treatise on diseases of women. Philadelphia, *H. C. Lea,* 1868.
        The most complete and systematic treatise on the subject in its day.

6061   ——. Vaginal ovariotomy. *Amer. J. med. Sci.,* 1870, **59**, 387-90.
        First vaginal ovariotomy.

6062   BATTEY, ROBERT. 1828-1895
        Normal ovariotomy. *Atlanta med. surg. J.,* 1872, **10**, 321-39: also in *Trans. med. Ass. Georgia,* 1873, **24**, 36-69.
        Battey's ovariotomy operation for the treatment of non-ovarian conditions. This operation later acquired a greater significance in connection with more modern work on endocrinology. Preliminary communication in *J. gynaec. Soc. Boston,* 1872, **7**, 331-35.

6063   EMMET, THOMAS ADDIS. 1828-1919
        Chronic cystitis in the female, and mode of treatment. *Amer. Practit.,* 1872, **5**, 65-92.
        Vaginal cystotomy for chronic cystitis.

6064   NOEGGERATH, EMIL. 1827-1895
        Die latente Gonorrhoe im weiblichen Geschlecht. Bonn, *M. Cohen & Sohn,* 1872
        Noeggerath was the first to point out the late effects of gonorrhoea in women, particularly its role in the production of sterility.

6065   PRIESTLEY, *Sir* WILLIAM OVEREND. 1829-1901
        Cases of intermenstrual or intermediate dysmenorrhoea. *Brit. med. J.,* 1872, **2**, 431-32.
        First report of cases of Mittelschmerz.

6066   MARTIN, AUGUST EDUARD. 1847-1933
        Zur Enucleation der intraparietalen Myome des Corpus uteri. *Z. Geburtsh. Frauenkr.,* 1876, **1**, 143-67

6066.1 CHIARI, HANS. 1851-1916
        Uber drei Fälle von primärem Carcinom im Fundus und Corpus des Uterus. *Med. Jb.,* 1877, 364-68.
        Choriocarcinoma first reported.

6067   HEGAR, ALFRED. 1830-1914
        Ueber die Exstirpation normaler und nicht zu umfänglichen Tumoren degenerirter Eierstöcke. *Zbl Gynäk.,* 1877, **1**, 297-307; 1878, **2**, 25-39.
        Hegar developed Battey's operation (No. 6062) and employed it for the treatment of various ovarian conditions.

6068   LE FORT, LÉON CLÉMENT. 1829-1893
        Noveau procédé pour la guérison du prolapsus utérin. *Bull. gén. Thérap.,* 1877, **92**, 337-44.
        Le Fort's operation for prolapse.

6069   RUGE, CARL ARNOLD. 1846-1926, & VEIT, JOHANN. 1852-1917
        Anatomische Bedeutung der Erosionen am Scheidentheil. *Zbl. Gynäk.,* 1877, **1**, 17-19.

6070   FREUND, WILHELM ALEXANDER. 1833-1918
Eine neue Methode der Exstirpation des ganzen Uterus. *Berl. klin. Wschr.*,
1878, **15**, 417-18.
Freund performed the first successful abdominal hysterectomy for
cancer. Although removal of the uterus by the abdominal route had been
carried out earlier, to Freund belongs the credit for the invention of the
operation, in which he utilized Lister's antiseptic method.

6071   TAIT, ROBERT LAWSON. 1845-1899
Removal of normal ovaries. *Brit. med. J.*, 1879, **1**, 813-14.
Lawson Tait reported that he had performed Battey's operation on
1 August 1872, 16 days before Battey. *See* No. 6062.

6072   CZERNY, VINCENZ. 1842-1916
Ueber die Ausrottung des Gebärmutterkrebses. *Wien. med. Wschr.*, 1879,
29, 1171-74.
First total hysterectomy by the vaginal route.

6073   ———. Ueber die Enukleation subperitonealer Fibrome der Gebärmutter
durch das Scheidengewölbe; vaginale Myoniotomie. *Wien. med. Wschr.*,
1881, **31**, col. 501-05, 525-29.
The operation of enucleation of subperitoneal uterine fibroids by the
vaginal route was introduced by Czerny. In the second paper the words
"Fibromyome" and "Myomotomie" replace "Fibrome" and "Myoniotomie"
in the title.

6074   SCHRÖDER, KARL LUDWIG ERNST. 1838-1887
Ueber die theilweise und vollständige Ausschneidung der carcinomatösen
Gebärmutter. *Z. Geburtsh. Gynäk.*, 1881, **6**, 213-30.

6075   TAIT, ROBERT LAWSON. 1845-1899
A case of removal of the uterine appendages. *Brit. med. J.*, 1881, **1**, 766-67.
Oöphorectomy, February 1881.

6076   ADAMS, JAMES ALEXANDER. 1857-1930
A new operation for uterine displacements. *Glasg. med. J.*, 1882, **17**, 437-
46.
Adams devised an operation for retroversion of the uterus, similar to
that performed by Alexander (No. 6077).

6077   ALEXANDER, WILLIAM. 1844-1919
A new method of treating inveterate and troublesome displacements of the
uterus. *Med. Times Gaz.*, 1882, **1**, 327-28.
Alexander's suspension operation for retroversion of the uterus, first
performed by him in 1881.

6078   EMMET, THOMAS ADDIS. 1828-1919
A study of the etiology of perineal laceration, with a new method for its
proper repair. *Trans. Amer. gynec. Soc.*, (1883), 1884, **8**, 198-216.
First description of Emmet's technique for perineorrhaphy.

6079   APOSTOLI, GEORGES. 1847-1900
Sur la faradisation utérine double ou bipolaire. *Union méd.*, 1884, 3 sér.,
38, 709-13, 733-36.

Apostoli was the first to employ the double faradic current in the electrotherapy of uterine diseases.

6080   SCHRÖDER, KARL LUDWIG ERNST. 1838-1887
Ueber die Enucleation interstitieller Myome. *Z. Geburtsh. Gynäk.*, 1884, **10**, 156-62.

6081   TAIT, ROBERT LAWSON. 1845-1889
General summary of conclusions from one thousand cases of abdominal section. Birmingham, *R. Birbeck,* 1884.
        Tait was probably the greatest of the ovariotomists. He abandoned Listerian principles of antisepsis, relying on "scrupulous attention to cleanliness of every kind and in all directions".

6082   BREISKY, AUGUST. 1832-1889
Ueber Kraurosis vulvae, eine wenig beachtete Form von Hautatrophie am pudendum muliebre. *Z. Heilk.,* 1885, **6**, 69-80.
        Although not the first to describe kraurosis vulvae, Breisky left an important account, and the condition became known as "Breisky's disease".

6083   OLSHAUSEN, ROBERT VON. 1835-1915
Ueber ventrale Operation bei Prolapsus und Retroversio uteri. *Zbl. Gynäk.,* 1886, **10**, 698-701.
        First account of Olshausen's operation for retroversion of the uterus.

6084   PÉAN, JULES ÉMILE. 1830-1898
Ablation des tumeurs fibreuses ou myomes du corps de l'utérus par la voie vaginale. *Gaz. Hôp. (Paris),* 1886, **59**, 445-47.
        Péan's method of morcellement of the uterus for the removal of tumours.

6085   BOZEMAN, NATHAN. 1825-1905
The gradual preparatory treatment of the complications of urinary and faecal fistulae in women. *Trans. int. med. Congr.,* Washington, 1887, **2**, 514-58.
        Pyelitis complicating vesical and faecal fistulae in women was successfully treated by Bozeman.

6086   KELLY, HOWARD ATWOOD. 1858-1943
Hysterorrhaphy. New York, *W. Wood & Co.,* 1887.

6087   TAIT, ROBERT LAWSON. 1845-1899
On the method of flap-splitting in certain plastic operations. *Brit. gynaec. J.,* 1887-88, **3**, 367-76; 1891-92, **7**, 195-214.
        Tait devised a flap-splitting operation for retocele which, with some modifications, is in use today.

6088   SÄNGER, MAX. 1853-1903
Die Tripperansteckung beim weiblichen Geschlechte. Leipzig, *O. Wigand,* 1889.

6089   PFANNENSTIEL, HERMANN JOHANN. 1862-1909
Ueber die Pseudomucine der cystischen Ovariengeschwülste. Leipzig, *A. T. Engelhardt,* 1890.

6090 PRICE, JOSEPH. 1853-1911
Pus in the pelvis and how to deal with it. *Trans sth. surg. gynec. Ass.,* (1889), 1890, **2**, 102-12.

6091 TRENDELENBURG, FRIEDRICH. 1844-1924
Ueber Blasenscheidenfisteloperationen und über Beckenhochlagerung bei Operationen in der Bauchhöhle. *Samml. klin. Vortr.,* 1890, Nr. 355 (Chir., Nr. 109), 3372-92.
 Includes description of the "Trendelenburg position". Reprinted with translation, in *Med. Classics,* 1940, **4**, 936-88. The first description of Trendelenburg's elevated pelvic position was given by one of his students, W. Meyer, in *Arch. klin. Chir.,* 1885, **31**, 494-525.

6092 WILLIAMS, JOHN WHITRIDGE. 1866-1931
Contributions to the histogenesis of the papillary cystoma of the ovary. *Johns Hopk. Hosp. Bull.,* 1891, **2**, 149-57.

6093 BAER, BENJAMIN FRANKLIN. 1846-1920
Supravaginal hysterectomy without ligature of the cervix, in operation for uterine fibroids; a new method. *Amer J. Obstet. Dis. Wom.,* 1892, **26**, 489-504.
 Baer's operation.

6093.1 TAIT, ROBERT LAWSON. 1845-1899
On the occurrence of pleural effusion in association with disease of the abdomen. *Med.-chir. Trans.,* 1892, **75**, 109-18.
 Lawson Tait was apparently the first to describe what is now known as Meigs's syndrome (ovarian fibroma combined with pleural effusion).

6094 SANGER, MAX. 1853-1903
Ueber Sarcoma uteri deciduo-cellulare und andere deciduale Geschwülste. *Arch. Gynäk.,* 1893, **44**, 89-148
 A detailed classification of "deciduomata", chorionic neoplasms, and a review of the literature.

6095 HENROTIN, FERNAND. 1847-1906
Vaginal hysterectomy in bilateral peri-uterine suppuration. *Amer. J. Obstet. Dis. Wom.,* 1892, **26**, 448-60.
 Henrotin's method of removing the uterus.

6096 ——, Conservative surgical treatment of para- and peri-uterine septic diseases. *Amer. gynaec. obstet. J.,* 1895, **6**, 769-83.

6097 KAHLDEN, CLEMENS VON. 1859-1903
Ueber eine eigenthümliche Form des Ovarialcarcinoms. *Zbl. allg. Path.,* 1895, **6**, 257-64.
 Granulosa cell tumour first described.

6097.1 MARCHAND, FELIX JACOB. 1846-1928
Über die sogenannten "decidualen" Geschwülste im Anschluss an normale Geburt, Abort, Blasenmole und Extrauterinschwangerschaft. *Mschr. Geburtsh.,* 1895, **1**, 419-38, 513-62.

Marchand's theory of the histogenesis of choriocarcinoma (chorionepithelioma). He considered that such tumours derived from trophoblast and not from decidua.

6098   OLSHAUSEN, Robert von. 1835-1915
Über Exstirpation der Vagina. *Zbl. Gynäk.*, 1895, **19**, 1-6.
The operation of excision of the vagina was introduced by Olshausen.

6099   WERTHEIM, Ernst. 1864-1920
Ueber Uterus-Gonorrhöe. *Verh. dtsch. Ges. Gynäk.*, 1895, **6**, 199-223.
Wertheim emphasized the importance of latent uterine gonorrhoea.

6100   WILLIAMS, John Whitridge. 1866-1931
Deciduoma malignum. *Johns Hopk. Hosp. Rep.*, 1895, **4**, 461-504.
First case of choriocarcinoma reported in N. America.

6101   KRUKENBERG, Friedrich Ernst. 1870-1946
Ueber das Fibrosarcoma ovarii mucocellulare (carcinomatodes). *Arch. Gynäk.*, 1896, **50**, 287-321.
Original description of "Krukenberg's tumour".

6102   MACKENRODT, Alwin Karl. 1859-1925
Ueber den künstlichen Ersatz der Scheide. *Zbl. Gynäk.*, 1896, **20**, 546-50.
Mackenrodt's operation for the plastic reconstruction of the vagina.

6103   WERTHEIM, Ernst. 1864-1920
Über Blasen-Gonorrhöe. *Z. Geburtsh. Gynäk.*, 1896, **35**, 1-10.
Wertheim demonstrated the gonococcus in acute cystitis.

6105   FAURE, Jean Louis. 1863-1944
Sur un nouveau procédé d'hystérectomie abdominale totale; la section médiane de l'utérus. *Presse méd.*, 1897, **5**, **ii**, 237-38.

6106   MENGE, Karl. 1864-1945, & KRÖNIG, Claus Ludwig Theodor Bernhard. 1863-1918
Bakteriologie des weiblichen Genital-Kanales. 2 vols. Leipzig, *A. Georgi*, 1897.

6107   ALEXANDER, William. 1844-1919
Enucleation of uterine fibroids. *Brit. gynaec. J.*, 1898, **14**, 47-61.
An outstanding account of myomectomy.

6108   KELLY, Howard Atwood. 1858-1943
Operative gynecology. 2 vols. New York, *D. Appleton & Co.*, 1899.
Kelly, professor of gynaecology at Pennsylvania and Johns Hopkins University, was a leading gynaecologist in America.

6109   ———. The removal of pelvic inflammatory masses by the abdomen after bisection of the uterus. *Amer. J. Obstet. Dis Wom.*, 1900, **42**, 818-39.

6109.1   ORTHMANN, Ernst Gottlob. 1858-1922
Zur Casuistik einiger seltenerer Ovarial- und Tuben-Tumoren. *Mschr. Geburtsh. Gynäk.*, 1899, **9**, 771-82.
"Brenner tumour" first described; *see also* No. 6118.

6110   CULLEN, THOMAS STEPHEN. 1868-1953
        Cancer of the uterus. New York, *Appleton & Co.*, 1900.
        Includes first clinical and pathological study of hyperplasia of the
        endometrium. Cullen is remembered eponymically for "Cullen's sign", a
        discoloration of the skin about the umbilicous, regarded as a sign of
        ruptured ectopic gestation. *See* Nos. 6220 & 6124.1.

6111   GILLIAM, DAVID TOD. 1844-1923
        Round-ligament ventrosuspension of the uterus: a new method. *Amer. J.
        Obstet. Dis. Wom.*, 1900, **41**, 299-303.
        Gilliam's operation for prolapse.

6112   NOBLE, GEORGE HENRY. 1860-
        A flap operation for atresia of the vagina. *Trans. sth. surg. gynec. Ass.*, 1900,
        13, 78-83.
        Noble introduced a flap operation for atresia of the vagina.

6113   PFANNENSTIEL, HERMANN JOHANN. 1862-1909
        Ueber die Vortheile der suprasymphysären Fascienquerschnitts für die
        gynäkologischen Koeliotomieen. *Samml. klin. Vortr.*, Leipzig, 1900, n.F.,
        Nr.268 (Gynäk. Nr. 97), 1735-56.
        "Pfannenstiel's incision".

6114   WERTHEIM, ERNST. 1864-1920
        Zur Frage der Radicaloperation beim Uteruskrebs. *Arch. Gynäk.*, 1900, **61**,
        627-68; 1902, **65**, 1-39.
        Wertheim's radical operation for cancer of the uterus.

6115   EDEBOHLS, GEORGE MICHAEL. 1853-1908
        Panhysterokolpectomy; a new prolapsus operation. *Med Rec. (N.Y.)*, 1901,
        60, 561-64.

6116   WEBSTER, JOHN CLARENCE. 1863-1950
        A satisfactory operation for certain cases of retroversion of the uterus. *J.
        Amer. med. Ass.*, 1901, **37**, 913.
        "Baldy–Webster operation". Webster's method of treating retrodis-
        placement of the uterus was later modified by J. M. Baldy, *Amer. J. Obstet.
        Dis. Wom.*, 1902, **45**, 650-54, and *N.Y. med. J.*, 1903, **78**, 167-69.

6117   BALDWIN, JAMES FAIRCHILD. 1850-1936
        The formation of an artificial vagina by intestinal transplantation. *Ann. Surg.*,
        1904, **40**, 398-403.
        Baldwin's operation.

6118   BRENNER, FRITZ. 1877-
        Das Oophoroma folliculare. *Frankf. Z. Path.*, 1907, **1**, 150-71.
        "Brenner tumour", earlier described by Orthmann (No. 6109.1). See the
        historical note in *Cancer*, 1956, **9**, 217.

6119   DONALD, ARCHIBALD. 1860-1937
        Operation in cases of complete prolapse. *J. Obstet. Gynaec. Brit. Emp.*,
        1908, **13**, 195-96.
        Donald's operation for prolapse.

6120   SCHAUTA, FRIEDRICH. 1849-1919
        Die erweiterte vaginale Totalexstirpation des Uterus bei Kollumkarzinom.
        Wien, Leipzig, *J. Safar*, 1908.
        Radical vaginal hysterectomy for carcinoma of the cervix.

6121   BELL, WILLIAM BLAIR. 1871-1936
        The principles of gynaecology. London, *Longmans, Green & Co.*, 1910.
        Blair Bell was an outstanding figure in British gynaecology and one of
        the founders of the Royal College of Obstetricians and Gynaecologists.

6122   CARY, WILLIAM HOLLENBACK. 1883-
        Note on determination of patency of Fallopian tubes by the use of collargol
        and x-ray shadow. *Amer. J. Obstet. Dis. Wom.*, 1914, **69**, 462-64.
        Cary was the first to perform salpingography.

6123   RUBIN, ISADOR CLINTON. 1883-1958
        X-ray diagnosis in gynecology with the aid of intra-uterine collargol
        injection. *Surg. Gynec. Obstet.*, 1915, **20**, 435-43.
        Independently of Cary (No. 6122) Rubin performed salpingography.
        Preliminary communication in *Zbl Gynäk.*, 1914, **38**, 658-60.

6124   FOTHERGILL, WILLIAM EDWARD. 1865-1926
        Anterior colporrhaphy and its combination with amputation of the cervix
        as a single operation. *J. Obstet Gynaec. Brit. Emp.*, 1915, **27**, 146-47.
        Fothergill's modification of Donald's operation for prolapse.

6124.1 CULLEN, THOMAS STEPHEN. 1868-1953
        Embryology, anatomy, and diseases of the umbilicus together with diseases
        of the urachus. Philadelphia, *Saunders*, 1916.
        Contains the first reference to what would become known as "Cullen's
        sign", discoloration of the skin about the umbilicus, as a sign of ruptured
        ectopic gestation. This work contains extraordinary illustrations by Max
        Brödel, including a series of truly remarkable variations in belly buttons.

6125   FORSSELL, CARL GUSTAF [GÖSTA] ABRAHAMSSON. 1876-1950
        Översikt över resultaten av kräftbehandling vid Radiumhemmet i Stock-
        holm 1910-1915. *Hospitalstidende*, 1917, 8R., **10**, 273-83.
        The Stockholm method of radium treatment of cancer of the uterus, as
        carried out at the Radiumhemmet, Stockholm, follows the technique
        devised by Forssell.

6126   SCHROEDER, ROBERT. 1884-1959
        Die pathogenese der Meno- und besonders der Metrorrhagien. *Arch.
        Gynäk.*, 1919, **110**, 633-58.
        First description of metropathia haemorrhagica.

6127   RUBIN, ISADOR CLINTON. 1883-1958
        Nonoperative determination of patency of Fallopian tubes in sterility.
        Intra-uterine inflation with oxygen, and production of an artificial
        pneumoperitoneum. *J. Amer. med. Ass.*, 1920, **74**, 1017; **75**, 661-67.
        Tubal insufflation method for the diagnosis and treatment of sterility
        due to occlusion of the Fallopian tubes.

6128   SAMPSON, JOHN ALBERTSON. 1873-1946
Perforating hemorrhagic (chocolate) cysts of the ovary. *Arch. Surg. (Chicago)*, 1921, **3**, 245-323.
The true nature of ovarian endometriomata was elucidated by Sampson.

6129   HALBAN, JOSEF VON. 1870-1937, & SEITZ, LUDWIG. 1872-
Biologie und Pathologie des Weibes. Hrsg. von J. HALBAN und L. SEITZ. 8 vols. [in 15]. Berlin, *Urban & Schwarzenberg*. 1924-29.
Second edition, 10 vols. & index, 1941-55.

6130   KAUFMANN, CARL.
Die Behandlung der Amenorrhöe mit hohen Dosen der Ovarialhormone. *Klin. Wschr.*, 1933, **12**, 1557-62.
First use of oestrogenic hormone for the treatment of amenorrhoea.

6131   REGAUD, CLAUDE. 1870-1940
Considérations sur la radiothérapie des cancers cervico-uterins, d'après l'experience et les résultats acquis à l'Institut du Radium de Paris. *Radiophysiol. et Radiothérap.*, 1933-39. **3**, 155-70.
The Paris method of radium treatment of cancer of the uterus was devised by Regaud.

6132   SCHILLER, WALTER. 1887-1960
Early diagnosis of carcinoma of the cervix. *Surg. Gynec. Obstet.*, 1933, **56**, 210-22.
Schiller's test for carcinoma of the cervix.

6132.01   MEIGS, JOE VINCENT. 1892-
Tumors of the female pelvic organs. New York, *Macmillan*, 1934.
"Meigs's syndrome" – fibroma of the ovary with pleural effusion – is described on pp. 262-63.

6132.1   STEIN, IRVING FREILER. 1887- & LEVENTHAL, MICHAEL LEO. 1901-
Amenorrhea associated with bilateral polycystic ovaries. *Amer. J. Obstet. Gynec.*, 1935, **29**, 181-91.
Stein–Leventhal syndrome.

6133   McINDOE, *Sir* ARCHIBALD HECTOR. 1900-1960, & BANISTER, JOHN BRIGHT. 1880-1938
An operation for the cure of congenital absence of the vagina. *J. Obstet. Gynaec. Brit. Emp.*, 1938, **45**, 490-94.
McIndoe's operation for the construction of an artificial vagina.

6135   PAPANICOLAOU, GEORGE NICHOLAS. 1883-1962, & TRAUT, HERBERT FREDERICK. 1894-
The diagnostic value of vaginal smears in carcinoma of the uterus. *Amer. J. Obstet. Gynec.*, 1941, **42**, 193-206.
Smear diagnosis of carcinoma of the cervix. Papanicolaou first reported in 1928 that he could recognize cancer cells (*Proc. Third Race Betterment Conf.*, p. 528) but the importance of his findings was not generally accepted and he abandoned the work for some years.

For history of gynaecology, see Nos. 6287, 6295-7, 6300-03, 6305-6, 6309-10, 6311.1-6311.7

OBSTETRICS

6136   MOSCHION [Muscio or Mustio]. *fl. circa* A.D. 500
Moschionos Peri gynaikeion pathon, id est...De morbis muliebribus liber
unus; cum Conardi Gesneri...scholiis & emendationibus nun primum editus
opera ac studio Caspari Wolphii. Basileae, *Per Thomam Guarinum*, 1566.
     The earliest text specifically for midwives, based on the teachings of
Soranus, the greatest obstetrical writer of antiquity. Muscio was a pupil of
Soranus. His book is arranged in catechism form; it was first published as
above and in Caspar Wolff's *Gynaeciorum*, 1566 (No. 6011). A Greek–
Latin bilingual text was edited by F. O Dewez, Vienna, 1793. Until the 19th
century Moschion was lauded as the greatest obstetrical writer of antiquity
while Soranus's works remained hidden. See V. Rose, *Sorani Gynaeciorum
vetus translatio latina*, Leipzig, 1882.

6137   AETIUS *of Amida* A.D. 502-575
Aetii Amideni quem alii antiochenum vocant...libri XVI. in tres tomos
divisi, quorum primus & ultimus Joan. Baptista Montano... secundus Jano
Cornario....Basileae, *In Officina Frobeniana*, 1533-35.
     Aetius epitomized all previous knowledge regarding obstetrics. The
first half of his writings were published in Greek by the Aldine Press in
1534. However that did not include the section on obstetrics. This is the first
Latin edition of the complete work. An annotated translation of Aetius's
obstetrical writings from the improved Latin edition of Basel, 1542, was
published by J. V. Ricci, Philadelphia, 1950. *See* No. 33.

6137.1   ORTOLFF VON BAYRLANT. *circa* 1400.
Büchlein der schwangeren Frauen. [Augsburg, *Anonymous printer*, about
1495].
     The first obstetrical book printed in the vernacular. Facsimile edition,
Munich, 1910. Ortoloff also wrote the first German pharmacopoeia. *See*
No. 1794.

6138   RÖSSLIN, Eucharius [Rhodion; Röslin]. *d*.1526
Der swangern frawen und hebammen roszgarten. [Hagenau, *H. Gran,*] 1513.
     Earliest printed textbook for midwives. It survived 40 editions, being
used as late as 1730. An English translation by Richard Jonas was published
in 1540, printed by Thomas Raynalde. This translation, entitled "The Byrth
of Mankynde" was the first book on the subject to be printed in English.
There were three variant editions in 1513, for which no clear priority has
been established. All were printed from different type by different printers.
One is dated and the other two are not. One was reproduced in facsimile
in 1910 at Munich and at Zürich, *J. Stocker*, 1977. For a bibliographical study
of the work, see Sir D'Arcy Power's article in The Library, 1927, 4 ser. 8, 1-
37, subsequently reprinted in book form. See also A.M. Hellman, *A collection of early obstetrical books...including 25 editions of Roesslin's
Rosengarten*, New Haven, Privately printed, 1952.

6139   ———. The byrth of mankynde by Thomas Raynalde. London, *T.R.*, 1540.
     English translation of No. 6138. The first edition contained copperplate
illustrations by Thomas Geminus (*See* No. 376.1). and is the first book printed
in England with illustrations of this type. In the numerous later editions
these illustrations were replaced by woodcuts.

6140   PARÉ, AMBROISE. 1510-1590
Briefve collection de ladministration anatomique: avec la maniere de
conjoindre les os: et d'extraire les enfans tant mors que vivans du ventre
de la mere, lors que nature de soy ne peult venir a son effect. Paris, *G.
Cavellat*, 1549.

     Paré's revival of podalic version repopularized the procedure, which
had been described by Soranus of Ephesus (No. 6008). English translation
in *The Workes of Ambroise Parey* [sic], London, 1634.

6141   RUEFF, JACOB [RÜFF; RUOFF]. 1500-1558
Ein schön lustig Trostbüchle von den Empfengknussen und Geburten der
Menschen...Tiguri, *Apud Frosch[overu*m], 1554.

     An improved version of Rösslin's *Swangern frawen*. This contains the
first true anatomical pictures in an obstetrics book. Rueff described
smooth-edged forceps for delivery of a live baby, preceding Chamberlen,
and a toothed forceps for extraction of the dead foetus. He developed a
method of celphic version combining internal and external manipulation.
A Latin translation of his book, *De conceptu et generatione hominis*, was
published by Froschouer in the same year. English translation, London,
1637.

6142   RATISBON.
Ordnung eines erbarn Raths der Statt Regenspurg, die Hebammen
betreffende. (Regenspurg, *H. Kohl*, 1555.]

     Earliest public document in the vernacular containing legislation gov-
erning midwives.

6143   LONITZER, ADAM [LONICERUS]. 1528-1586
Reformation oder Ordnung für die Hebammen. Franckfurt a. M., *getruckt
bey C. Egenolffs Erben*, 1573.

     Legislation governing the practice of midwifery was introduced in the
city of Frankfurt in 1573,

6144   MERCURIO, GERONIMO SCIPIONE. 1550-1616
La commare o riccoglitrice. Venitia, *G. B. Ciotti*, 1596.

     First Italian book on obstetrics. It is a work of importance for the study
of the history of Caesarean section; in it Mercurio advocated the Caesarean
operation in cases of contracted pelvis.

6144.1   BONAVENTURA, FEDERICO. 1555-1602
De natura partus octomestris adversus vulgatam opinionem. Urbini, *Apud
Bartholomaeum, & Simonem Ragusios*, 1600.

     An encyclopaedic work on ancient and contemporary medical, scientific
and juridical opinion on premature birth and the period of gestation.

6145   BOURGEOIS, LOUISE [dite *Boursier*]. 1563-1636
Observations diverses sur la sterilite, perte de fruict, foecondite,
accouchements, et maladies des femmes, et enfants nouveaux naiz. Paris,
A. Saugrain, 1609.

     The first book on obstetrics published by a midwife. Louise Bourgeois
was accoucheuse to the French court. She was one of the pioneers of
scientific midwifery; her *Observations* was the vade mecum of contemporary midwives. She induced premature labour in patients with contracted
pelvis, an idea probably derived from Paré.

6145.1   GUILLEMEAU, JACQUES. 1550-1613
De l'heureux accouchement des femmes. Paris, *Nicolas Buon*, 1609.

Actual origin of the so-called "Mauriceau" manoeuvre, usually credited to Mauriceau (No. 6147). Guillemeau was not only responsible for this technique for delivery of the aftercoming head so important before the forceps and Caesarian section, but he was also the first to employ podalic version in placenta praevia. English translation, London, 1612.

6146   HARVEY, WILLIAM. 1578-1657
Exercitationes de generatione animalium. Londini, *O. Pulleyn*, 1651.

The chapter on labour ("De partu") in this book represents the first original work on obstetrics to be published by an English author. English translation, 1653.

6146.1   LA COURVEÉ, JEAN CLAUDE DE. 1615-1664
De nutritione foetus in utero paradoxa. Dantisci, *G. Förster*, 1655.

Page 245 contains a report of successful symphysiotomy.

6147   MAURICEAU, FRANÇOIS. 1637-1709
Des maladies des femmes grosses et accouchées. Paris, *chez l'Auteur*, 1668.

The outstanding textbook of the time. Mauriceau, leading obstetrician of his day, introduced the practice of delivering his patients in bed instead of in the obstetrical chair. It was to Mauriceau that Hugh Chamberlen attempted to sell the secret of his forceps; Chamberlen translated the *Traité* into English in 1672. This book established obstetrics as a science.

6148   PORTAL, PAUL. 1630-1703
La pratique des accouchemens soutenue d'un grand nombre d'observations. Paris, *G. Martin*, 1685.

Portal's important treatise included his demonstration that version could be done with one foot. He also taught that face presentation usually ran a normal course. English translation, 1705.

6149   SIEGEMUNDIN, JUSTINE [DITTRICHIN]. 1650-1705
Die Chur-Brandenburgische Hoff-Wehe-Mutter. Cölln an der Spree, *U. Liebperten*, 1690.

With Mauriceau, Justine Siegemundin was responsible for introducing the practice of puncturing the amniotic sac to arrest haemorrhage in placenta praevia. She was midwife to the Court of the Elector of Brandenburg, and the most celebrated of the German midwives of the 17th century.

6150   MAUQUEST DE LA MOTTE, GUILLAUME. 1665-1737
Traité complet des accouchemens. Paris, *L. d'Houry*, 1721.

This was an important treatise in its time; it shows that Mauquest de la Motte applied podalic version to head presentations. English translation, prepared at the suggestion of William Smellie, 1746.

6151   OULD, *Sir* FIELDING. 1710-1789
A treatise of midwifry. Dublin, *O. Nelson & C. Conner*, 1742.

The teaching of Ould did much towards the advancement of midwifery in the British Isles. His *Treatise* is the first text-book of obstetrics of any importance in English.

6152   LEVRET, ANDRÉ. 1703-1780
        Observations sur les causes et les accidens de plusieurs accouchemens
        laborieux. Paris, *C. Osmont*, 1747.
           Levret, who improved the obstetric forceps, was a famous teacher in Paris.

6153   ——. L'art des accouchemens. Paris, *Delaguette*, 1753.
           Besides introducing a curved forceps (*see* No. 6152) Levret invented
        several other obstetric instruments and made fundamental observations
        on pelvic anomalies. His book covered the whole field of obstetrics and
        remained a standard work for many years.

6154   SMELLIE, WILLIAM. 1697-1763
        A treatise on the theory and practice of midwifery. London, *D. Wilson*, 1752.
           Smellie contributed more to the fundamentals of obstetrics than virtually
        any individual. In his *Treatise* he described more accurately than any pre-
        vious writer the mechanism of parturition, stressing the importance of exact
        measurement of the pelvis. He was the first to lay down safe rules regarding
        the use of forceps, and personally introduced the steel-lock, the curved, and
        the double forceps. He invented the "Smellie manoeuvre" to deliver breech
        cases. His book was followed by two volumes of case reports, 1754 and 1764;
        it was re-published by the New Sydenham Society, 3 vols., 1876-78. It
        includes the first illustration of a rachitic pelvis. Facsimile reproduction of
        the original edition, London, 1974. The first American edition, *An abridge-
        ment of the practice of midwifery: and a set of anatomical tables*, Boston,
        J. Norman, [1786] is the first illustrated medical book published in North
        America, and also the first book on obstetrics published in the United States.
        Biography by R.W. Johnstone, Edinburgh, 1952.

6154.1 ——. A sett [sic] of anatomical tables, with explanations, and an abridg-
        ment, of the practice of midwifery...London, *Printed in the year* 1754.
           The celebrated atlas for No. 6154, which is a complete work in itself. The
        39 superb engravings include 26 after drawings by Jan van Rymsdyk,
        which are preserved in the Hunterian Collection at the University of
        Glasgow Library. The remainder were by Smellie, "assisted by a pupil
        called [Pieter] Camper". Camper's drawings are preserved in the Royal
        College of Physicians, Edinburgh, and Leiden University. Camper's illus-
        trated MS of his studies with Smellie and his third visit to England in 1785
        is preserved in Amsterdam University. It was translated into English with
        notes, and published as *Opuscula selecta Neerlandicorum de arte medica*,
        1939, **15**. See J.L. Thornton, *Jan van Rymsdyk: Medical artist of the
        eighteenth century*, Cambridge, *Oleander Press*, 1982.

6155   BARD, JOHN. 1716-1799
        A case of extra-uterine foetus. *Med. Obs. Soc. Physicians Lond.*, 1764, **2**,
        369-72.
           This description of an abdominal pregnancy, successfully operated on by
        Bard was "the first scientific paper on a surgical subject to come from the
        North American Colonies" (Earle). John Bard was the father of Samuel Bard.

6156   HARVIE, JOHN.
        Practical directions, shewing a method of preserving the perinaeum in
        birth, and delivering the placenta without violence. London, *D. Wilson &
        G. Nicol*, 1767.

Harvie, Smellie's successor, advocated external expression of the placenta instead of traction on the cord, anticipating Credé in this connection by almost a century (*see* No. 6183). Reprinted in H. Thoms: *Classic contributions to obstetrics and gynecology*, 1935, pp.131-38.

6156.1   SHARP, JANE. *fl.* 1650
The midwives book. London, *Miller*, 1671.
The first book written by an English midwife. Sharp was the most accomplished midwife of 17th-century England.

6156.2   CHAPMAN, EDMUND. 1680?-1756
An essay on the improvement of midwifery. London, *A. Bettsworth*, 1733.
Gives the first published account of the forceps, kept secret by the Chamberlen family for generations. Chapman was the second person in England to teach midwifery publicly. The first edition of his book was not illustrated. In the second edition of 1735 he included an illustration of the forceps.

6156.3   GIFFARD, WILLIAM. *d.* 1731
Cases in midwifry. Revised by EDWARD HODY. London, *B. Motte*, 1734.
Contains, under case 14, the earliest published record of the use of the hitherto secret Chamberlen forceps, in 1726, together with illustrations of two variant types. Giffard is considered the first English obstetrician to publish substantial contributions to clinical midwifery.

6156.4   JENTY, CHARLES NICHOLAS. *fl.* 1720-1770
The demonstrations of a pregnant uterus of a woman at her full term. London, *Printed for...the author*, 1757.
Atlas of six superb life-size mezzotint plates after paintings by Jan van Rymsdyk. A separate 16-page text was published in octavo.

6157   HUNTER, WILLIAM. 1718-1783
Anatomia uteri humani gravidi tabulis illustrata. The anatomy of the human gravid uterus exhibited in figures. Birmingham, *John Baskerville*, 1774.
Hunter originally trained as Smellie's assistant. Once he achieved brilliant professional and financial success he became a great collector of rare books, coins, and paintings. Reflecting Hunter's interests in anatomical art and fine printing, this work contains 34 copper plates depicting the gravid uterus, life-size. It is William Hunter's best work and one of the finest anatomical atlases ever to be produced, "anatomically exact and artistically perfect" (Choulant). Except for J. Dalby's little book, *Virtues of cinnabar and musk against the bite of a mad dog*, 1762, it is the only medical publication to come from the famous Baskerville Press. The letterpress is in both Latin and English. The plates are engraved by several artists from drawings by Jan van Rymsdyk. The Sydenham Society published a reprint of the atlas in 1851. See J. L. Thornton's *Jan van Rymsdyk, medical artist of the eighteenth century*, Cambridge, *Oleander Press*, 1982. Van Rymsdyk's original drawings for the above work are preserved in the Hunterian Collection at the University of Glasgow Library.

6157.1   ——. An anatomical description of the human gravid uterus and its contents. London, *J. Johnson; and G. Nicol*, 1794.
Hunter's text for No. 6157, posthumously edited by Matthew Baillie.

6158 RIGBY, EDWARD. 1747-1821
An essay on the uterine haemorrhage, which precedes the delivery of the full grown foetus: illustrated with cases. London, *J. Johnson,* 1775.
  Rigby differentiated between premature separation of the normal placenta (accidental haemorrhage) and placenta praevia (unavoidable haemorrhage).

6160 BÖER, LUCAS JOHANN [BOOGERS]. 1751-1835
Abhandlungen und Versuche geburtshilflichen Inhalts. 2 vols. Vienna, *C.F. Wappler*, 1791-1806.
  Böer, a pioneer of "natural childbirth", was the founder of the Viennese school of obstetrics.

6161 MOHRENHEIM, JOSEPH JACOB VON, *Freiherr. d.* 1789
Abhandlung über die Entbindungskunst. St. Petersburg, *K. Akad. D. Wiss, 1791.*
  This work was edited by order of Catherine II of Russia, to whom von Mohrenheim was accoucheur. The importance of this work lies mainly in its splendid engravings, some of which were taken from Smellie (*see* No. 6154.1). It includes a brief literary history of obstetrics.

6162 HOME, *Sir* EVERARD. 1763-1832
Account of the dissection of an hermaphrodite dog. *Phil. Trans.*, 1799, **18**, 157-78.
  Home records (p. 162) that John Hunter suggested artificial insemination. The actual insemination was performed by the patient's husband with a syringe.

6163 SCHMITT, WILHELM JOSEPH. 1760-1827
Drey Wahrnehmungen von Schwangerschaften ausserhalb der Gebähr-mutter. *Beobacht. k. k. med-chir. Josephs Acad. Wien*, 1801, **1**, 59-96.
  Interstitial pregnancy first reported.

6163.1 BARD, SAMUEL. 1742-1821
A compendium of the theory and practice of midwifery. New York, *Collins & Perkins*, 1807.
  First significant textbook on obstetrics written by an American. Bard gave an excellent description of the mechanism of labour, and of pre-eclampsia.

6164 STEARNS, JOHN. 1770-1848
Accounts of the pulvis parturiens, a remedy for quickening childbirth. *Med. Reposit.*, 1808, 2 Hex., **5**, 308-09.
  First use of ergot in the induction of labour in America. Reprinted in H. Thoms: *Classic contributions to obstetrics and gynecology*, 1935, pp. 21-23.

6165 BOIVIN, MARIE ANNE VICTOIRE, *née Gillain.* 1773-1841
Mémorial de l'art des accouchements. Paris, *Méquignon père*, 1812.
  Mme Boivin was one of the most famous of the Paris midwives. She improved the speculum and wrote intelligently on hydatidiform mole.

6166 KING, JOHN.
Case of an extra-uterine foetus, produced alive through an incision made into the vagina of the mother, who recovered after delivery, without any alarming symptoms. *Med. Reposit.*, 1817, n.s., **3**, 388-94.
  First successful operation for abdominal pregnancy.

6167 ——. An analysis of the subject of extrauterine foetation and of the retroversion of the gravid uterus. Norwich, *G. Wright*, 1818.

  Expansion of No. 6166. First book on the subject.

6168 WENZEL, CARL. 1769-1827

Allgemeine geburtshülfliche Betrachtungen und über die künstliche Frühgeburt. Mainz, *F. Kupferberg*, 1818.

  Artificial induction of premature labour.

6169 NAEGELE, FRANZ CARL. 1778-1851

Ueber den Mechanismus der Geburt. *Dtsch. Arch. Physiol.*, 1819, **5**, 483-531.

  Best work of its time on the mechanism of labour. English translation, London, 1829.

6170 LA CHAPELLE, MARIE LOUISE, *Mme*. [DUGÈS]. 1769-1821

Pratique des accouchemens... Publiés par ANTOINE DUGÈS. 3 vols. Paris, *J.B.Baillère*, 1821-25.

  Mme La Chapelle was a famous midwife and a colleague of Baudelocque. She supervised 5,000 deliveries and her vast experience enabled her to write her book. She reduced the 94 theoretical presentations suggested by Baudelocque to 22. The above, posthumously edited by her nephew, represents her life work.

6171 LEJUMEAU, JEAN ALEXANDRE, *Vicomte de Kergaradec*. 1787-1877

Mémoire sur l'auscultation appliquée à l'étude de la grossesse. Paris, *Méquignon-Marvis*, 1822.

  Although not the first to record the auscultation of the fetal heart sound, Lejumeau, a pupil of Laennec, brought the importance of this diagnostic procedure to the notice of the medical profession. Laennec reprinted Lujumeau's paper in the later editions of *De l'auscultation médiate* (No. 2673).

6172 BOIVIN, MARIE ANNE VICTOIRE, *née Gillian*. 1773-1841

Nouvelles recherches sur l'origine, la nature et le traitement de la mole vésiculaire ou grossesse hydatique. Paris, *Méquignon l'âiné pére*, 1827.

  Classic description of hydatidiform mole.

6173 MONTGOMERY, WILLIAM FETHERSTON. 1797-1859

An exposition of the signs and symptoms of pregnancy. London, *Sherwood, Gilbert & Piper*, 1837.

  "Montgomery's glands", the sebaceous glands of the areola, were previously described by Morgagni. They are described, with his "tubercles" (the secondary areola seen in pregnancy) in the above work.

6174 JACQUEMIER, JEAN MARIE. 1806-1879

Recherches d'anatomie et de physiologie sur le système vasculaire sanguin de l'utérus humain pendant la gestation, et plus spécialement sur les vaisseaux utéro-placentaires. *Arch gén. Méd.*, 1838, 3 sér., **3**, 165-94.

  Jacquemier's sign, diagnostic of pregnancy.

6175 NAEGELE, HERMANN FRANZ JOSEPH. 1810-1858
Die geburtshülfiche Auscultation Mainz, *v. von Zabern*, 1838.
 Pioneering work on obstetric auscultation, including the sounds of the foetal heart. English translation by C. West, London, 1839.

6176 LEVER, JOHN CHARLES WEAVER. 1811-1858
Cases of puerperal convulsions, with remarks. *Guy's Hosp. Rep.*, 1843, 2 ser., **1**, 495-517.
 Lever, of Guy's Hospital, was the first to report the finding of albuminous urine in connection with puerperal convulsions.

6177 MEIGS, CHARLES DELUCENA. 1792-1869
The heart-clot. *Med. Exam.*, 1849, **5**, 141-52.
 Meigs drew attention to embolism as a cause of sudden death in childbed. Previously such deaths had been attributed to syncope.

6178 NÉLATON, AUGUSTE. 1807-1873
Leçons sur l'hématocèle rétro-utérine. *Gaz. Hôp. (Paris)*, 1851, 3sér., **3**, 573, 578-79, 581; 1852, 3 sér., **4**, 45-46, 66-67.
 Classic description of pelvic haematocele.

6179 DU BOIS, PAUL. 1795-1871
Considérations sur l'avortement provoqué dans les cas de vomissements. *Bull. Acad. Méd. (Paris)*, 1852, **17**, 557-83.
 Classic description of hyperemesis gravidarum.

6180 TALIAFERRO, VALENTINE H. 1831-1888
Rigidity of the soft parts – delivery effected by incision in the perineum. *Stethoscope & Virginia med. Gaz.*, 1852, **2**, 382.
 First episiotomy in America, 2 December 1851.

6181 DUNCAN, JAMES MATTHEWS. 1826-1890
On the displacements of the uterus. *Edinb. med. surg. J.*, 1854, **81**, 321-48.
 "Duncan's folds", the peritoneal folds of the uterus. Republished in book form, Edinburgh, 1854. Duncan, a leading Edinburgh obstetrician, became lecturer on the subject at St. Bartholomew's Hospital.

6182 WRIGHT, MARMADUKE BURR. 1803-1879
Difficult labors and their treatment. Cincinnati, *Jackson, White & Co.*, 1854.
 Wright was responsible for the introduction of combined cephalic version.

6183 CREDÉ, CARL SIEGMUND FRANZ. 1819-1892
De optima in partu naturali placentum amovendi ratione. Lipsiae, *A. Edelmannum*, [1860].
 Credé's method of removing the placenta by external manual expression. It is first mentioned in his *Klinische Vorträge über Geburtshilfe*, Berlin, 1854, 599-603.

6184 BRAUN, GUSTAV AUGUST. 1829-1911
Ueber das technische Verfahren bei vernachlässigten Querlagen und über Decapitationsinstrumente. *Wien. med. Wschr.*, 1861, **11**, 713-16.
 Braun's decapitation hook.

6185　HODGE, HUGH LENOX. 1796-1873
The principles and practice of obstetrics. Philadelphia, *Blanchard & Lea*, 1864.

Hodge, nearly blind, dictated this superb textbook from memory to his son. It includes his concept of "parallel planes" at the various levels of the pelvic canal, and his placental forceps for the completion of abortion. The book is very well illustrated. Hodge invented the "Hodge pessary". *See* No. 6043.1.

6186　HICKS, JOHN BRAXTON. 1823-1897
On combined external and internal version. *Trans. obstet. Soc. Lond.* (1863), 1864, **5**, 219-67,
Introduction of combined podalic version.

6187　——. On the condition of the uterus in obstructed labour. *Trans. obstet. Soc. Lond.*, (1867), 1868, **9**, 207-39.

6188　BRAUNE, CHRISTIAN WILHELM. 1831-1892
Die Lage des Uterus und Foetus am Ende der Schwangerschaft nach Durchschnitten an gefrornen Cadavern. Leipzig, *Veit u. Co.*, 1872.

A classic atlas of frozen sections of the uterus and foetus. Published as a supplement to No. 424.

6189　HICKS, JOHN BRAXTON. 1823-1897
On the contradictions of the uterus throughout pregnancy: their physiological effects and their value in the diagnosis of pregnancy. *Trans. obstet. Soc. Lond.*, (1871), 1872, **13**, 216-31.
"Braxton Hicks's sign".

6190　BANDL, LUDWIG. 1842-1892
Ueber das Verhalten des Uterus und Cervix in der Schwangerschaft und während der Geburt. Stuttgart, *F. Enke*, 1876.
"Bandl's ring". Bandl was professor of obstetrics and gynaecology at Vienna and Prague.

6191　PARRY, JOHN S. 1843-1876
Extra-uterine pregnancy. Philadelphia, *H. C. Lea*, 1876.
Lawson Tait regarded this as the first authoritative work on the subject. Parry showed the necessity for operation in such cases and it was this book, more than anything else, which determined Tait (No. 6196) to do so.

6192　TARNIER, ETIENNE STÉPHANE. 1828-1897
Description de deux nouveaux forceps. Paris, *Lauwereyns*, 1877.
Tarnier invented the axis-traction forceps. See also *Ann. Gynéc.*, 1877, **7**, 241-64

6193　PINARD, ADOLPHE. 1844-1934
Traité du palper abdominal au point de vue obstétrical. Paris, *H. Lauwereyns*, 1878.
Pinard, professor of obstetrics in Paris, showed the importance of abdominal palpation as an aid to obstetrical diagnosis. English translation, 1885.

6194   DUNCAN, JAMES MATTHEWS. 1826-1890
Clinical lecture on hepatic disease in gynaecology and obstetrics. *Med. Times Gaz.*, 1879, **1**, 57-59.
Matthews Duncan pointed out that pernicious vomiting in pregnancy may be associated with hepatic lesions.

6195   CREDÉ, CARL SIEGMUND FRANZ. 1819-1890
Die Verhütung der Augenentzüngung der Neugeborenen. Arch. Gynäk., 1881, 17, 50-53.
Credé introduced the practice of instillation of silver nitrate into the eyes of all newborn children as a preventive measure against ophthalmia neonatorum. Separate expanded edition, Berlin, 1884.

6196   TAIT, ROBERT LAWSON. 1845-1899
Five cases of extra-uterine pregnancy operated upon at the time of rupture. *Brit med. J.*, 1884, **1**, 1250-51.
The first successful operation for ruptured ectopic pregnancy was performed by Lawson Tait on 1 March 1883.

6197   WERTH, RICHARD. 1850-1918
Beiträge zur Anatomie und zur operativen Behandlung der Extrauterinschwangerschaft. Stuttgart, *F. Enke*, 1887.

6198   CHAMPETIER DE RIBES, CAMILLE LOUIS ANTOINE. 1848-1935
De l'accouchement provoqué; dilatation du canal génital (col de l'utérus, vagin et vulve) à l'aide de ballons introduits dans la cavité utérine pendant la grossesse. *Ann. Gynéc. Obstet.*, 1888, **30**, 401-38.
The "Champetier de Ribes bag".

6199   TAIT, ROBERT LAWSON. 1845-1899
Lectures on ectopic pregnancy and pelvic haematocele. Birmingham, *Journal Printing Works*, 1888.

6200   WALCHER, GUSTAV ADOLF. 1856-1935
Die Conjugata eines engen Beckens ist keine konstante Grosse, sondern lässt sich durch die Körperhaltung der Trägerin verändern. *Zbl. Gynäk.*, 1889, **13**, 892-93.
Description of the "Walcher position".

6201   BOSSI, LUIGI MARIA. 1859-1919
Sulla provocazione artificiale del parto e sul parto forzato col mezzo della dilatazione meccanica del collo uterino. *Ann. Ostet. Ginec.*, 1892, **14**, 881-928.
Bossi originated the method of induction of premature labour by means of forced dilatation of the cervix.

6202   BREUS, CARL. 1852-1914
Das tuberöse subchoriale Hämatom der Decidua. Eine typische Form der Molenschwangerschaft. Leipzig, Wien, *F. Deuticke*, 1892.
Tuberous ("Breus") mole first described.

6203   WEBSTER, JOHN CLARENCE. 1863-1950
Tubo peritoneal ectopic gestation. Edinburgh, *Y. J. Pentland*, 1892.

6204 GIGLI, LEONARDO. 1863-1908
Taglio lateralizzato del pube, suoi vantaggi, sua technica. *Ann. Obstet.
Ginec.*, 1894, **16**, 649-67.
 Gigli's saw, first used for pubiotomy. German translation, *Zbl. Chir.*, 1894,
21, 409-11.

6205 HEGAR, ALFRED. 1830-1914
Diagnose der frühesten Schwangerschaftsperiode. *Dtsch. med. Wschr.*,
1895, **21**, 565-67.
 Hegar's sign – softening of the lower segment of the uterus, an early
diagnostic sign of pregnancy. It was first described by his assistant, C.
Reinl, in *Prag. med. Wschr.*, 1884, **9**, 253-54.

6206 KOUWER, BENJAMIN JAN. 1861-1933
Een geval van ovariaalzwangerschap (zwangerschap in een Graafschen
follikel). *Ned. T. Verlosk. Gynaec.*, 1897, **8**, 157-68.
 First description of ovarian pregnancy.

6207 STROGANOFF, VASILI VASILIEVICH. 1857-1938
[On the treatment of eclampsia]. *Vrach*, St. Petersburg, 1900, **21**, 1137-40.
 The first of Stroganoff's important papers on the pathogenesis and
treatment of eclampsia.

6208 BALLANTYNE, JOHN WILLIAM. 1861-1923
Manual of antenatal pathology and hygiene. 2 vols. Edinburgh, *William
Green & Sons*, 1902-04.
 Ballantyne was a pioneer advocate of antenatal care.

6209 GIGLI, LEONARDO. 1863-1908
Sinfisiotomia classica e taglio lateralizzato del pube. *Clin. mod.*, 1902, **8**,
302-08.
 "Gigli's operation". Gigli substituted pubiotomy for symphysiotomy.

6210 STEINBÜCHEL, RICHARD VON.
Vorläufige Mittheilung über die Anwendung von Skopolamin-Morphium-
Injecktionen in der Geburtshilfe. *Zbl. Gynäk.*, 1902, **26**, 1304-06.
 "Twilight sleep".

6210.1 WILLIAMS, JOHN WHITRIDGE. 1866-1931
Obstetrics. New York, *D. Appleton*, 1903.
 The most famous American textbook of obstetrics, still in print under
modern editorship.

6212 GAUSS, CARL JOSEPH. 1875-1957
Geburten in künstlichem Dämmerschlaf. *Arch. Gynäk.*, 1906, **78**, 579-631.
 "Twilight sleep". Gauss developed the method introduced by
Steinbüchel (No. 6210).

6213 SELLHEIM, HUGO. 1871-1936
Die Mechanik der Geburt. *Samml. klin. Vortr.*, 1906, n.F., Nr. 421, (Gynäk.,
Nr. 156), 659-82.

6214   MOMBURG, FRITZ AUGUST. 1870-1939
Die künstliche Blutleere der unteren Körperhälfte. *Zbl. Chir.*, 1908, **35**, 697-99.
Abdominal ligature in prevention of post-partum haemorrhage.

6215   BELL, WILLIAM BLAIR. 1871-1936
The pituitary body and the therapeutic value of the infundibular extract in shock, uterine atony, and intestinal paresis. *Brit. med. J.*, 1909, **2**, 1609-13.

6216   EDLING, LARS. 1878-
Ueber die Anwendung des Roentgenverfahrens bei der Diagnose der Schwangerschaft. *Fortschr. Röntgenstr.*, 1911, **17**, 345-55.
First use of *x* rays for the diagnosis of pregnancy.

6218   LYNCH, FRANK WORTHINGTON. 1871-1945
Eutocia by means of nitrous oxide gas analgesia; a safe substitute for the Freiburg method. *J. Amer. med. Ass.*, 1915, **64**, 1187-89.

6219   KIELLAND, CHRISTIAN. 1871-1941.
Ueber die Anlegung der Zange am nicht rotierten Kopf mit Beschreibung eines neuen Zangenmodelles und einer neuen Anlegungsmethode. *Mschr. Geburtsh. Gynäk.*, 1916, **43**, 48-78.
Kielland forceps. English translation and historical background in E.P. Jones, *Kielland's forceps*, London, 1952.

6220   CULLEN, THOMAS STEPHEN. 1868-1953
Bluish discoloration of the umbilicus as a diagnostic sign where ruptured uterine pregnancy exists. *In*: Contributions to medical and biological research dedicated to Sir William Osler, 1919, **1**, 420-21.
"Cullen's sign".

6221   POTTER, IRVING WHITE. 1868-1956
Version. *Amer J. Obstet. Gynec.*, 1921, **1**, 560-73.
Potter's operation of podalic version.

6221.1   SPALDING, ALFRED BAKER. 1874-1942
A pathognomonic sign of intra-uterine death. *Surg. Gynec. Obstet.*, 1922, **34**, 754-57.
"Spalding's sign".

6222   ASCHHEIM, SELMAR. 1878-1965, & ZONDEK, BERNHARD. 1891-1966
Schwangerschaftsdiagnose aus dem Harn (durch Hormonnachweis). *Klin. Wschr.*, 1928, **7**, 8-9, 1404-11, 1453-57.
The Aschheim–Zondek test for the diagnosis of pregnancy.

6223   MENEES, THOMAS ORVILLE. 1890-1937, *et al.*
Amniography; preliminary report. *Amer. J. Roentgenol.*, 1930, **24**, 363-66.
Introduction of amniography. With J. D. Miller and L. E. Holly.

6224   FRIEDMAN, MAURICE HAROLD. 1903- , & LAPHAM, MAXWELL EDWARD. 1899-1983
A simple, rapid procedure for the laboratory diagnosis of early pregnancies. *Amer. J. Obstet. Gynec.*, 1931, **21**, 405-10.
Friedman test for the diagnosis of pregnancy.

6225   READ, GRANTLY DICK. 1890-1959
Natural childbirth. London, *W. Heinemann*, 1933
    Read advocated natural childbirth for many years; he demonstrated that prenatal education in methods of relaxation in many cases makes labour almost painless.

6226   BELLERBY, CHARLES WILLIAM.
A rapid test for the diagnosis of pregnancy. *Nature, (Lond)*, 1934, **133**, 494-95.
    The *Xenopus* toad test for the diagnosis of pregnancy; this preliminary note followed Hogben's demonstration that *Xenopus* responds by ovulation to the gonadotrophic hormone (*Trans. roy. Soc. S. Africa*, 1930, Ser. A, **5**, 19). For detailed history of the development of this test, see *Brit. med. J.*, 1946, **2**, 554.

6227   KAPELLER-ADLER, REGINE.
Über eine neue chemische Schwangerschaftsreaktion. *Klin. Wschr.*, 1934, **13**, 21-22.
    Kapeller-Adler test for diagnosis of pregnancy.

6228   MINNITT, ROBERT JAMES. 1889-1974
A new technique for the self-administration of gas-air analgesia in labour. *Lancet*, 1934, **1**, 1278-79.
    Introduction of the "Minnitt apparatus".

6229   SNOW, WILLIAM. 1898- , & POWELL, CLILIAN BETHANY. 1894-
Roentgen visualization of the placenta. *Amer. J. Roentgenol.*, 1934, **31**, 37-40.
    Direct radiography of the placenta.

6230   DUDLEY, HAROLD WARD. 1887-1935, & MOIR, JOHN CHASSAR. 1900-1977
The substance responsible for the traditional clinical effect of ergot. *Brit. med. J.*, 1935, **1**, 520-23.
    Isolation and introduction of ergometrine.

6231   WHITE, PRISCILLA. 1900- , *et al.*
Prediction and prevention of late pregnancy accidents in diabetes. *Amer. J. med. Sci.*, 1939, **198**, 482-92.
    First report of hormone treatment. Written with R.S. Titus, E.P. Joslin, and H. Hunt.

6232   STEINER, PAUL EBY. 1902- , & LUSHBAUGH, CLARENCE CHANCELUM. 1916-
Maternal pulmonary embolism by amniotic fluid as a cause of obstetric shock and unexpected deaths in obstetrics. *J. Amer. med. Ass.*, 1941, **117**, 1245-54, 1340-45.
    Amniotic fluid embolism described.

6232.1   HINGSON, ROBERT ANDREW. 1913- , & EDWARDS, WALDO BERRY. 1905-
Continuous caudal anesthesia during labor and delivery. *Curr. Res. Anesth. Analg.*, 1942, **21**, 301-11.

6233   O'SULLIVAN, JAMES VINCENT.
Acute inversion of the uterus. *Brit. med. J.*, 1945, **2**, 282-83.
    O'Sullivan's method of replacement by intravaginal hydraulic pressure.

6234　GALLI MAININI, CARLOS. 1914-1961
Reacción diagnóstica del embarazo en la que se usa el sapo macho como animal reactivo. *Sem. méd. (B. Aires),* 1947, **1**, 337-40.
　　Male toad test. An English account is in *J. clin. Endocr.,* 1947, **7**, 653-58.

6235　RAPP, GUSTAV WILLIAM. 1917- , & RICHARDSON, GARWOOD COLVIN. 1897-
A salive test for prenatal sex determination. *Science,* 1952, **115**, 265.

6235.1　DONALD, IAN. 1910-1987, & BROWN, T.G.
Demonstration of tissue interfaces within the body by ultrasonic echo sounding. *Brit. J. Radiol.,* 1961, **34**, 539-46.
　　Biparietal foetal cephalometry by ultrasound.

6235.2　JACOBSON, CECIL BRYANT. 1936- , & BARTER, ROBERT HENRY. 1913-
Intrauterine diagnosis and management of genetic defects. *Amer. J. Obstet. Gynec.,* 1967, **99**, 796-807.
　　Amniocentesis used to diagnose genetic disorders *in utero.* First detailed report. See also Fuchs, F., Genetic information from amniotic fluid contents. *Lancet,* 1960, **2**, 180.

CAESAREAN SECTION

6236　ROUSSET, FRANÇOIS [ROUSSETUS; ROSSETUS]. 1535-1590?
Traitte nouveau de l'hysterotomotokie, ou enfantement caesarien. Paris, *Denys du Val,* 1581.
　　Rousset records 15 successful Caesarean sections carried out by various persons during the preceding 80 years.

6236.1　BARLOW, JAMES. 1767-1839
A case of the caesarean operation performed, and the life of the woman preserved. *Medical Records and Researches Selected from the Papers of a Private Medical Association,* London, *T. Cox,* 1789, pp. 154-62.
　　This is apparently the first Caesarean section in England from which the mother recovered. It was performed on 27 November 1793. Barlow's account is reproduced by Young (No. 6307), pp. 54-58. A note on Barlow is in *Practitioner,* 1965, **195**, 103-08.

6237　OSIANDER, FRIEDRICH BENJAMIN. 1759-1822
Handbuch der Entbindungskunst. 4 vols. Tübingen, *C. F. Osiander,* 1818-25.
　　Includes (Bd. 2, Abt II, p. 302) description of Osiander's lower-segment Caesarean operation.

6238　RITGEN, FERDINAND AUGUST MARIE FRANZ. 1787-1867
Geschichte eines mit ungünstigem Erfolge verrichteten Bauchscheidenschnitts und Folgerung daraus. *Heidelb. klin. Ann.,* 1825, **1**, 263-77.
　　Ritgen first performed extraperitoneal Caesarean section in 1821.

6239　THOMAS, THEODORE GAILLARD. 1831-1903
Gastro-elytrotomy; a substitute for the Caesarean section. *Amer. J. Obstet. Dis. Wom.,* 1870, **3**, 125-39.
　　Thomas revived and modified Ritgen's operation.

6240 PORRO, EDOARDO. 1842-1902
Della amputazione utero-ovarica come complemento di taglio cesareo.
Ann. univ. Med. Chir., 1876, **237**, 289-350.
Caesarean section with excision of the uterus and adnexa ("Porro's operation").

6241 KEHRER, FERDINAND ADOLF. 1837-1914
Ueber ein modificirtes Verfahren beim Kaiserschnitte. *Arch. Gynäk.*, 1882, **19**, 177-209.
Kehrer improved the technique of the Caesarean operation.

6242 SÄNGER, MAX. 1853-1903
Der Kaiserschnitt bei Uterusfibromen nebst vergleichender Methodik der Sectio Caesarea und der Porro-Operation. Leipzig, *W. Engelmann*, 1882.
"Sänger's operation" – the so-called "classic Caesarean section". A preliminary note is in *Arch. Gynäk.*, 1882, **19**, 370.

6243 CHAMPNEYS, *Sir* FRANCIS HENRY. 1848-1930
A case of Caesarean section for contracted pelvis. *Trans. obstet. Soc. Lond.*, 1889, **31**, 136-60.
Champney's advocacy for the Sänger operation was a powerful factor in its adoption in Britain.

6244 HALBERTSMA, TJALLING. 1841-1898
Eclampsia gravidarum: eene nieuwe indicatie voor sectie caesarea. *Ned. T. Geneesk.*, 1889, 2D., **25**, 485-91.
Halbertsma first performed Caesarean section in puerperal convulsions.

6245 TAIT, ROBERT LAWSON. 1845-1899
An address on the surgical aspect of impacted labour. *Brit. med. J.*, 1890, **1**, 657-61.
The Tait–Porro operation, by which Tait performed Caesarean section in cases of placenta praevia.

6246 DÜHRSSEN, ALFRED. 1862-1933
Über vaginalen Kaiserschnitt. *Samml. klin. Vortr.*, 1898, n.F., Nr. 232 (Gynäkol., Nr. 84), 1365-88.
The vaginal Caesarean operation was introduced by Dührssen in April, 1895.

6247 FRANK, FRITZ. 1856-1923
Die suprasymphysäre Entbindung und ihr Verhältniss zu den anderen Operationen bei engen Becken. *Arch. Gynäk.*, 1907, **81**, 46-94.
Suprasymphyseal transperitoneal Caesarean section.

6248 SELLHEIM, HUGO. 1871-1936
Die extraperitoneale Uterusschnitt. *Zbl. Gynäk.*, 1908, **32**, 133-42.
Sellheim's operation. For his three subsequent modifications, see the same journal, 319-31, 641-51, and *Mschr. Geburtsh. Gynäk.*, 1911, **34**, 34-45.

6249 LATZKO, WILHELM. 1863-1945
Der extraperitoneale Kaiserschnitt. Seine Geschichte, seine Technik und seine Indikationen. *Wien. klin. Wschr.*, 1909, **22**, 477-82.

Latzko's extraperitoneal lower-segment Caesarean operation. Preliminary report in the same journal, 1908, **21**, 737.

6250 DÖDERLEIN, ALBERT SIEGMUND GUSTAV. 1860-1941, & KRÖNIG, BERNARD. 1863-1917
Operative Gynäkologie. 3rd ed. Leipzig, *Georg Thieme*, 1912.
Includes (p. 879) first description of Krönig's operation of transperitoneal lower-segment Caesarean section.

6251 DELEE, JOSEPH BOLIVAR. 1869-1942
The newer methods of cesarean section. Report of 40 cases. *J. Amer. med. Ass.*, 1919, **73**, 91-95.
DeLee's low cervical operation (laparotrachelotomy).

6252 PORTES, LOUIS. 1891-1950
Césarienne suivie d'extériorisation temporaire de l'utérus et de réintégration secondaire dans le bassin. *Bull. Soc. Obstét. Gynéc. Paris*, 1924, **13**, 171-76.
Portes operation – the classic Caesarean section followed by temporary exteriorization of the uterus. More fully described in *Gynéc. et Obstét.*, 1924, **10**, 225-50.

For history, see No. 6307

PELVIS: PELVIC ANOMALIES

6253 DEVENTER, HENDRIK VAN. 1651-1724
Manuale operatien, I. deel zijnde een neiuw ligt voor vroed-meesters en vroed-vrouen. The Hague, *The author*, 1701.
This work gives the first accurate description of the female pelvis and its deformities, and the effect of the latter in complicating labour. The first edition contains a relatively unattractive frontispiece portrait of the author, engraved by himself. Latin translation, Leiden, 1701. English translation, London, 1724.

6254 HUNTER, WILLIAM. 1718-1783
A singular case of the separation of the ossa pubis. *Med. Obs. Inqu.*, 1762, **2**, 321-33, 415-18.
A case of osteomalacic pelvis was reported to Hunter by a country practitioner.

6255 BAUDELOCQUE, JEAN LOUIS. 1746-1810
L'art des accouchemens. 2 vols. Paris, *Méquignon*, 1781.
Baudelocque invented a pelvimeter and advanced the knowledge of pelvimetry and of the mechanism of labour. The external conjugate diameter is known as "Baudelocque's diameter". English translation, London, 1790.

6256 NAEGELE, FRANZ CARL. 1778-1851
Das weibliche Becken. Carlsruhe, *C.F. Muller*, 1825.

6257 ———. Das schräg verengte Becken nebst einem Anhange über die wichtigsten Fehler des weiblichen Beckens überhaupt. Mainz, *V. von Zabern*, 1839.

First description of the obliquely contracted pelvis, or "Naegele pelvis". Because of its rarity and the difficulty of recognizing it clinically in living subjects, the obliquely contracted pelvis, with its most often fatal consequences at delivery, was unknown until Naegele's study of 37 cases. He suggested diagnostic aids for its recognition. English translation, Manchester, 1848. Centennial English translation by Pynson Printers, 1939.

6258   ROKITANSKY, CARL, *Freiherr von*. 1804-1878
Beyträge zur Kenntniss der Rückgrathskrümmungen, und der mit demselben zusammentreffenden Abweichungen des Brustkorbes und Beckens. *Med Jb. österr. Staates*, 1839, **19**, 41, 195.
Original description of spondylolisthesis.

6259   MICHAELIS, GUSTAV ADOLF. 1798-1848
Das enge Becken: nach eigenen Beobachtungen und Untersuchungen. Leipzig, *G. Wigand*, 1851.
First important work dealing with pelvic deformities since the time of van Deventer. It is a pioneer work in the literature dealing with pelvic architecture; Michaelis was one of the first to differentiate between the non-rachitic flat pelvis and the rachitic pelvis. This book was completed and published by C.C.T. Litzmann (No. 6260) three years after Michaelis's death.

6260   LITZMANN, CARL CONRAD THEODOR. 1815-1890
Das schräg-ovale Becken. Kiel, *Akad. Buchhandlung*, 1853.
Litzmann (*see also* No. 6263) described in this work the coxalgic, scoliotic and kyphoscoliotic forms of pelvis.

6261   KILIAN, HERMANN FRIEDRICH. 1800-1863
Schilderungen neuer Beckenformen und ihres Verhaltens im Leben. Mannheim, *Bassermann & Malthey*, 1854.
First description of pelvis spinosa.

6262   ——. De spondylolisthesi gravissimae pelvangustiae causa nuper detecta. Bonnae, *C. Georg*, [1854].
An important study of the spondylolisthetic pelvis, which Kilian called "pelvis obtecta".

6263   LITZMANN, CARL CONRAD THEODOR. 1815-1890
Die Formen des Beckens, insbesondere des engen weiblichen Beckens. Berlin, *G. Reimer*, 1861.
Litzmann devised a clinical classification of pelves which was for many years generally used, and he described various deformities of the female pelvis.

6263.1   ——. Ueber die hintere Scheitelbeinstellung, eine nicht selten Art von fehlerhafter Einstellung des Kopfes unter der Geburt. Arch. Gynäk., 1871, 2, 433-40.
"Litzmann's obliquity" or posterior parietal presentation.

6264   NEUGEBAUER, FRANZ LUDWIG. 1856-1914
Neuer Beitrag zur Aetiologie und Casuistik der Spondyl-olisthesis. *Arch. Gynäk.*, 1885, **25**, 182-252.

6265 BREUS, CARL. 1852-1914, & KOLISKO, ALEXANDER. 1847-1918
Die pathologischen Beckenformen. Leipzig, *F. Deuticke*, 1900-04.
Classic description and classification of pelvic deformities.

6266 CALDWELL, WILLIAM EDGAR. 1880-1943, & MOLOY, HOWARD CARMAN. 1903-1953
Anatomical variations in the female pelvis and their effect in labour, with a suggested classification. *Amer. J. Obstet Gynec.*, 1933, **26**, 479-505.
The modern classification of the female pelvis is based on the work of Caldwell and Moloy.

PUERPERAL FEVER

6267 HIPPOCRATES. 460-375 B.C.
Epidemics 1, case 4. *In*: [Works] with an English translation by W.H. JONES. London, *W. Heinemann*, 1923, **1**, 193-95.
The earliest known description of puerperal fever.

6268 BURTON, JOHN. 1697-1771
An essay towards a complete new system of midwifery, theoretical and practical. London, *J. Hodges*, 1751.
Burton was the first to suggest that puerperal fever is contagious, and the first to give a detailed discussion of Caesarean section. Sterne satirized him as "Dr. Slop" in *Tristram Shandy*.

6269 LEAKE, JOHN. 1729-1792.
Practical observations on the child-bed fever. London, *J. Walter*, [1772].
Leake insisted on the contagious nature of puerperal fever. Reprinted, London, *Sydenham Society*, 1949.

6270 WHITE, CHARLES. 1728-1813
A treatise on the management of pregnant and lying-in women. London, *E. & C. Dilly*, 1773.
White was the first to state clearly in a text on midwifery the necessity of absolute cleanliness in the lying-in chamber, the isolation of infected patients, and adequate ventilation. He instituted the principle of uterine drainage, placing his patients in a sitting position shortly after delivery using a special bed and chair. In this he preceded Fowler (No. 5623). White was also the first after Hippocrates to make any substantial contributions towards the solution of the aetiology and management of puerperal fever.

6271 ——. An inquiry into the nature and cause of that swelling, in one or both of the lower extremeties, which sometimes happens to lying-in-women. Warrington, *printed by W. Eyres, for C. Dilly in the Poultry London*, 1784.
First clinical description of phlegmasia alba dolens. White ascribed it to destruction of the lymphatics due to pressure of the foetal head.

6272 GORDON, ALEXANDER. 1752-1799
A treatise on the epidemic puerperal fever of Aberdeen. London, *G.G. & J. Robinson*, 1795.
Gordon was the first to advance as a definite hypothesis the contagious nature of puerperal fever, thus preceding Holmes and Semmelweis by half a century. He also advocated the disinfection of the clothes of the doctor and midwife.

6273　　DAVIS, David Daniel. 1777-1841
An essay on the proximate cause of the disease called phlegmasia dolens.
Med.-chir. Trans., 1823, **12**, 419-60.

Davis was the first to state that phlegmasia alba dolens was due to
inflammation of the veins. He was physician-accoucheur at the birth of
Queen Victoria.

6274　　HOLMES, Oliver Wendell. 1809-1894
The contagiousness of puerperal fever. *N. Engl. quart. J. Med. Surg.*, 1842-
43, **1**, 503-30.

Oliver Wendell Holmes was the first to establish the contagious nature
of puerperal fever. His essay on the subject took a strong line against the
opinions then prevailing, stirring up violent opposition among the obstetricians of Philadelphia. Reprinted in *Med. Classics*, 1936, **1**, 211-43.

6275　　SEMMELWEIS, Ignaz Philipp. 1818-1865
Höchst wichtige Erfahrungen über die Aetiologie der in Gebäranstalten
epidemischen Puerperalfieber. *Z.k.k. Ges. Aerzte Wien*, 1847-48, **4**, pt. 2,
242-44; 1849, **5**, 64-65.

Semmelweis, pioneer of antisepsis in obstetrics, was the first to recognize that puerperal fever is a septicaemia. He concluded that the doctors
and students of Vienna's First Obstetrical Clinic carried the infection on
their hands from the autopsy room to the maternity wards, and instituted
a programme of hand-washing in chlorinated lime between autopsy work
and examination of patients. One month later the First Clinic's mortality
rate had dropped by 10 per cent. Despite this spectacular success
Semmelweis refused to communicate his results officially. The above
papers were written for Semmelweis by his friend, Ferdinand von Hebra,
editor of the *Zeitschrift*. (*See also* No. 6277).

6276　　HOLMES, Oliver Wendell. 1809-1894
Puerperal fever, as a private pestilence. Boston, *Ticknor & Fields*, 1855.

Because his first paper (No. 6274) had been published in a short-lived
journal with very small circulation, Holmes enlarged his famous essay on
the contagiousness of puerperal fever, and in this reiteration mentioned
the steps already being taken by Semmelweis. Reprinted in *Med. Classics*,
1936, **1**, 245-68.

6277　　SEMMELWEIS, Ignaz Philipp. 1818-1865
Die Aetiologie, der Begriff und die Prophylaxis des Kindbettfiebers. Pest,
Wien & Leipzig, *C.A. Hartleben*, 1861.

One of the epoch-making books in medical literature. Semmelweis,
who earlier had shown puerperal fever to be a septicaemia, strove to
improve conditions in the lying-in wards of Vienna and Budapest. Mis-
understood and maligned by many, he eventually published this book in
support of his views on the aetiology of puerperal sepsis. He had no
literary style and his book is difficult reading; it had an overwhelming mass
of badly-presented statistics. Sir W. J. Sinclair, his biographer, said of him
that "if he could have written like Oliver Wendell Holmes, his 'Aetiology'
would have conquered Europe in 12 months". Semmelweis died in an
asylum on 13 August 1865. An English translation of the book, by F. P.
Murphy, is in *Med. Classics*, 1941, **5**, 350-773. This translation was reprinted
with translations of Semmelweis's other works by Ferenc Gyorgyey,
Birmingham, *Classics of Medicine Library*, 1980. Original edition re-

printed, Budapest, 1970. New English translation, somewhat abridged, Madison, Wisc., 1983.

6278   PASTEUR, LOUIS. 1822-1895
Septicémie puerpérale. *Bull. Acad. Méd. (Paris)*, 1879, 2 sér., **8**, 505-508.
Description of the streptococcus of puerperal sepsis.

6279   DÖDERLEIN, ALBERT SIEGMUND GUSTAV. 1860-1941
Das Scheidensekret und seine Bedeutung für das Puerperalfieber. Leipzig, *O. Durr*, 1892.
A classic study of the vaginal secretion in relation to puerperal fever. Includes the first description of "Döderlein's bacillus".

6280   HALBAN, JOSEF VON. 1870-1937, & KÖHLER, ROBERT. 1884-
Die patholigische Anatomie des Puerperalprozesses. Wien, Leipzig, *W. Braumüller*, 1919.

6280.1 ANSELM, EUGEN.
Unsere Erfahrungen mit Prontosil bei Puerperalfieber. *Dtsch. med. Wschr.*, 1935, **61**, 264 (only).
First report of the use of an antimicrobial agent in the treatment of obstetric infections.

6281   COLEBROOK, LEONARD. 1883-1967, & KENNY, MÉAVE.
Treatment of human puerperal infections, and of experimental infections in mice, with prontosil. *Lancet*, 1936, **1**, 1279-86.
Chemotherapeutic treatment of puerperal sepsis.

History of Gynaecology and Obstetrics

6282   AVELING, JAMES HOBSON. 1828-1892
English midwives. London, *J.& A. Churchill*, 1872.
Reprinted with biographical sketch by J. L. Thornton, London, 1967.

6283   —. The Chamberlens and the midwifery forceps. London, *J.&A. Churchill*, 1882.

6284   ENGELMANN, GEORGE JULIUS. 1847-1903
Labor among primitive peoples. St.Louis, *J. H. Chambers & Co.*, 1882.
Third edition, revised, 1884.

6285   WITKOWSKI, GUSTAVE JULES A. 1843-?
Les accouchements à la cour. Paris, *G. Steinheil*, 1887.

6286   ——. Histoire des accouchements chez tous les peuples. 1 vol. and Appendix. Paris, *G.Steinheil*, [1887].

6287   McKAY, WILLIAM JOHN STEWART. 1866-1948
The history of ancient gynaecology. London, *Baillière, Tindall & Cox*, 1901.

6288   SIEBOLD, EDUARD CASPAR JACOB VON. 1801-1861
Versuch einer Geschichte der Geburtshilfe. 2te. Aufl. 2 vols. Tübingen, *F. Pietzcker*, 1901-02.

First edition, 1839-45. Continuation by R. Dohrn, for the period 1840-80, forming Bd. 3 (see No. 6289).

6289   DOHRN, RUDOLF. 1836-1915
Geschichte der Geburtshülfe der Neuzeit. 2 pts. Tübingen, *F. Pietzcker,* 1903-04.
A supplement to No. 6288.

6290   MÜLLERHEIM, ROBERT NATHAN. 1862-
Die Wochenstube in der Kunst. Stuttgart, *F. Enke,* 1904.

6291   FASBENDER, HEINRICH. 1843-1914
Geschichte der Geburtshülfe. Jena, *G. Fischer,* 1906.
Probably the most valuable history of the subject. Reprinted, Hildesheim. *TIG. Olms,* 1964.

6293   WEINDLER, FRITZ.
Geschichte der gynäkologische-anatomischen Abbildungen. Dresden, *Zahn u. Jaensch,* 1908.

6295   LA TORRE, FELICE. 1846-1923
L'utero attraverso i secoli da Erofilo al giorni nostri; storia, iconografia, struttura, fisiologia. Città di Castello, *Unione Arti Grafiche,* 1917.
Contains an important collection of illustrations.

6296   FISCHER, ISIDOR. 1868-1943
Geschichte der Gynäkologie. *In:* J. VON HALBAN and L. SEITZ: Biologie und Pathologie des Weibes, Berlin, 1924, **1**, 1-202.

6297   FEHLER, HERMANN JOHANN KARL. 1847-1925
Entwicklund der Gerurtshilfe und Gynäkologie im 19. Jahrhundert. Berlin, *J. Springer,* 1925.

6298   SONDEREGGER, ALBERT.
Missgeburten und Wundergestalten in Einblattdrucken und Handzeichnungen des 16. Jahrhunderts. Zürich, *O. Füssli,* 1927.

6299   SPENCER, HERBERT RITCHIE. 1860-1941
History of British midwifery from 1650-1800. London, *John Bale,* 1927.

6299.1   DAS, KEDARNATH.
Obstetric forceps, its history and evolution. St. Louis, *C.V. Mosby,* 1929.

6300   VIANA, ODORICO. 1877-1942, & VOZZA, FRANCESCO.
L'ostretricia e la ginecologia in Italia. Milano, *A. Cordani,* 1933.

6301   THOMS, HERBERT. 1885-1972
Classical contributions to obstetrics and gynecology. Springfield, *C.C. Thomas,* 1935.

6303   DIEPGEN, PAUL. 1878-1966
Geschichte der Frauenheilkunde. 1 Teil. Die Frauenheilkunde der alten Welt. München, *J.F. Bergmann,* 1937.

Forms Bd. 12, Teil 1, of *Handbuch der Gynäkologie*, hrsg. J. Veit u. Stoeckel. *See also* No. 6311.4

6304   CLAYE, *Sir* ANDREW MOYNIHAN. 1896-1977
        The evolution of obstetric analgesia. London, *Oxford University Press*, 1939.

6305   RICCI, JAMES VINCENT. 1890-
        The genealogy of gynaecology. History of the development of gynaecology throughout the ages 2000 B.C.-A.D. 1800. Philadelphia, *Blakiston* (1943).
        Second edition, 1950.

6306   LEONARDO, RICHARD ANTHONY. 1895-
        History of gynecology. New York, *Froben Press*, 1944.

6307   YOUNG, JOHN HARLEY.
        Caesarean section. The history and development of the operation from earliest times. London, *H. K. Lewis*, 1944.

6309   RICCI, JAMES VINCENT. 1890-
        One hundred years of gynaecology, 1800-1900. Philadelphia, *Blakiston*, (1945).

6310   ——. The development of gynaecological surgery and instruments ... from the Hippocratic age to the Antiseptic period. Philadelphia, *Blakiston*, 1949.
        Reprint, San Francisco, *Norman Publishing*, 1990.

6311   RADCLIFFE, WALTER.
        The secret instrument. The birth of the midwifery forceps. London, *W. Heinemann*, 1947.
        Reprinted with No. 6311.5, San Francisco, *Norman Publishing*, 1989.

6311.1 KERR, JOHN MARTIN MUNRO. 1868-1960, *et al.*
        Historical review of British obstetrics and gynaecology, 1800-1950. Edinburgh, *E. & S. Livingstone*, 1954.
        Edited by J. M. Munro Kerr, R. W. Johnstone, and M.H. Phillips. Supplements No. 6299.

6311.2 SPEERT, HAROLD. 1915-
        Obstetric and gynecologic milestones: essays in eponymy. New York, *Macmillan*, 1958.
        79 essays with historical accounts, excerpts from sources. etc.

6311.4 DIEPGEN, PAUL. 1878-1966
        Frau und Frauenheilkunde in der Kultur des Mittelalters. Stuttgart, *G. Thieme*, 1963.
        A continuation of No. 6303.

6311.5 RADCLIFFE, WALTER.
        Milestones in midwifery. Bristol, *John Wright*, 1967.
        Reprinted with No. 6311, San Francisco, *Norman Publishing*, 1989.

6311.6 SPEERT, HAROLD. 1915-
        Iconographia gyniatrica: a pictorial history of gynecology and obstetrics. Philadelphia, *F. W. Davis*, 1973.
        French translation, 1976.

6311.7 ———. Obstetrics and gynecology in America: a history. Chicago, *American College of Obstetricians and Gynecologists*, 1980.

PAEDIATRICS

6312 SORANUS, *of Ephesus*. A.D. 98-138
Gynaecology. Translated with an introduction by OSWEI TEMKIN. Baltimore, *Johns Hopkins Press*, 1956.
Soranus included full instructions on the care and management of infants.

6313 RHAZES [ABU BAKR MUHAMMAD IBN ZAKARIYA AL-RAZI]. *c*. 850-923
De curis puerorum in prima aetate. *In his* Opuscula. Mediolani, *per L. Pachel et V. Scincenzeller*, 1481.
Rhazes was the first to devote an entire treatise to diseases of children. Although he lived so many years before the advent of printing, he was still regarded as an authority in the 15th century and his works were amongst the earliest medical books to be printed. Sudhoff includes the above work in his *Erstlinge der pädiatrischen Literatur*, München, 1925.

6314 LOUFFENBERG, HEINRICH VON. *d*. 1458
Versehung des Leibs. Augsburg, [*Erhard Ratdolt*], 1491.
Includes the first poem on paediatrics. It is written in old Swabian; its author was a monk. For details of this rare work, see J. Ruhräh, *Pediatrics of the past*, New York, 1925, pp. 465-86.

6315 BAGELLARDO, PAOLO. *d*. 1494
De infantium aegritudinibus et remediis. [Padua, *B. de Valdezoccho & Matinus de Septum Arboribus*, 1472].
First printed book dealing exclusively with paediatrics; this is also the first medical treatise to make its original appearance in printed form, rather than having prior circulation in manuscript. The book is based mainly on the writings of Avicenna and Rhazes. It appears in facsimile in Sudhoff's *Erstlinge* (*see* No. 6355), and there is a translation by H.F. Wright in J. F. Ruhräh's *Pediatrics of the past,* 1925 (No.6354).

6316 METLINGER, BARTHOLOMAEUS. *d*. 1492
Regiment der jungen Kinder. [Augsburg, *G. Zainer*, 1473].
This work has very little originality, being mainly derived from the Arabic physicians of 500 years before, but is noteworthy as being the first book on paediatrics printed in German. It includes what is probably the first reference in medical literature to microcephaly. It was reprinted several times before 1500. Facsimile in Sudhoff's *Erstlinge* (*see* No. 6355). The edition of 1497 is the first printed work on paediatrics to contain an illustration. Facsimile reproduction with commentary, Zürich, *J. Stocker*, 1976. English translation in Ruhräh (No. 6354).

6316.1 ROELANS, CORNELIUS. 1450-1525
De aegritudinibus infantium. Louvain, *Jan Veldener*, [not before 16 February 1486].
A work on disorders of pregnant women as well as on paediatrics. Facsimile reprint in Sudhoff (No. 6355). Curiously all recorded copies lack

the first 77 leaves. which apparently were not issued. Recently six of the missing leaves have been discovered as endpapers. See D.E. Rhodes, *A volume from the monastery library of Hayles. Trans. Camb. Bibl. Soc.*, 1985, **8**, 598-603. English translation in Rührah, No. 6354.

6317 PHAER, THOMAS [PHAYER; PHAYR]. 1510-1560
The regiment of life, whereunto is added a treatise of the pestilence, with the boke of children. London, 1545.
The "boke of children" is the first work on diseases of children to be written by an Englishman. Phaer enabled Englishmen to read and think of paediatrics in their own language. Reprint of 1553 edition, edited by A.V. Neale and H.R.E. Wallis, Edinburgh, 1955. Also reprinted in Rühräh (No. 6354).

6318 VALLAMBERT, SIMON DE [VALLEMBERT]. *fl.* 1537-1565
Cinq livres, de la maniere de nourrir et gouverner les enfans des leur naissance. Poictiers, *de Marnesz, & Bouchetz*, 1565.
The first French work on paediatrics. Vallambert considered a wider range of diseases than any previous writer, including the first reference to syphilis in children, and gave the best commentary up to his time on infant feeding, including the first mention of baby-feeding apparatus.

6320 PEMELL, ROBERT. *d.* 1653
De morbis puerorum, or, a treatise of the diseases of children. London, *J. Legatt for P. Stevens*, 1653.
More than 100 years after the publication of Phaer's book appeared this, the second work in English on paediatrics. Pemell was a general practitioner living at Cranbrook in Kent; he was buried only five days after the publication of his book. Reprint, Tuckahoe, 1971.

6321 HARRIS, WALTER. 1647-1732
De morbis acutis infantum. Londini, *Samuel Smith*, 1689.
Harris was physician to William and Mary. His book served for nearly a century as a standard work on paediatrics. He anticipated the modern treatment of tetany by using calcium salts in infantile convulsions. For a study of the book, see *Ann. med. Hist.*, 1919, **2**, 228-40. English translation 1693, 1742.

6322 CADOGAN, WILLIAM. 1711-1797
An essay upon nursing, and the management of children, from their birth to three years of age. London, *J. Roberts*, 1748.
Cadogan's famous essay laid down rules on the nursing, feeding, and clothing of infants, and filled a great need at a time when infant welfare was much neglected through the ignorance of those concerned. As a result of this work, Cadogan was elected a physician of the Foundling Hospital in 1754. He became a friend of Garrick, and was present at that great actor's deathbed. 10th ed., 1772.

6323 ROSÉN VON ROSENSTEIN, NILS. 1706-1773
Underrättelser om barn-sjukdomar och deras botemedel. Stockholm, *Kongl. Wet. Acad.*, 1764.
Sir Frederic Still considered this work "the most progressive which had yet been written"; it gave an impetus to research which influenced the future course of paediatrics. Rosén was particularly interested in infant

feeding. The *Underrättelser* were originally published in the calenders of the Academy and were later collected and issued in book form in 1764. English and German translations in 1776. For a biography, bibliography, and essays on this book, see *Nils Rosen von Rosenstein and his textbook on paediatrics*, ed. B. Vahlquist and A. Wallgren. *Acta paediat.*, 1964. Suppl. 156.

6324   AMRSTRONG, GEORGE. 1719-1789
An essay on the diseases most fatal to infants. London, *T. Cadell*, 1767.
One of the best paediatric works of the period. Armstrong is noteworthy as the founder of the first children's dispensary in Europe, the Dispensary for Sick Children, London, in 1769.

6325   ——. An account of the diseases most incident to children, from their birth till the age of puberty. London, *T. Cadell*, 1777.
An enlarged and more important (third) edition of No. 6324. *See also* No. 3425.

6326   UNDERWOOD, MICHAEL. 1737-1820
A treatise on the diseases of children. London, *J. Mathews*, 1784.
Underwood laid the foundation of modern paediatrics. His work was superior to anything that had previously appeared and remained the most important book on the subject for sixty years, passing through many editions. Includes (p.76) the first description of sclerema neonatorum ("Underwood's disease"); the second edition (1789) contains a description of congenital heart disease in children, being the first paediatric treatise to do so.

6327   HEBERDEN, WILLIAM *Jr.* 1767-1845
Morborum puerilium epitome. London, *T. Payne*, 1804.
English translation, Uttoxeter, 1805. Like his father, Heberden junior was a great clinician. It is probable that the above was compiled from notes left by Heberden senior.

6328   CLARKE, JOHN. 1761-1815
Commentaries on some of the most important diseases of children. Part the first. London, *Longman, etc.*, 1815.
Clarke died before this work was published. In it he gave a clear description of tetany and of laryngismus stridulus.

6329   GOELIS, LEOPOLD ANTON. 1765-1827
Praktische Abhandlungen über die vorzüglicheren Krankheiten des kindlichen Alters. 2 vols. Wien, *C. Gerold*, 1815-18.

6330   DAVIS, JOHN BUNNELL. 1780-1824
A cursory inquiry into some of the principal causes of mortality among children. London, *T. & G. Underwood*, 1817.
Davis called attention to the high infant mortality rate, especially in London. His suggestion that poor mothers should be instructed in the care of their infants resulted in a system of health-visiting by benevolent ladies. He founded a dispensary for sick and indigent children at St. Andrew's Hill, London, in 1816; this was later removed to the Waterloo Road and eventually became the Royal Waterloo Hospital for Children and Women.

6331   DEWEES, WILLIAM POTTS. 1768-1841
Treatise on the physical and medical treatment of children. Philadelphia,
H.C. Carey & I. Lea, 1825.
First American textbook on paediatrics.

6332   BILLARD, CHARLES MICHEL. 1800-1832
Traité des maladies des enfans nouveau-nés et à la mamelle. 1 vol. and
atlas. Paris, *J. B. Bailliére*, 1828.
Billard performed several hundred autopsies on infants and children
and correlated the data obtained with clinical observations he had made.
This pioneer work on the pathological anatomy of infants includes interesting observations on cerebral congestion, intestinal disturbances, the
pulse, teething, etc. It includes the first classification of infantile diseases
of any importance (Abt/Garrison). English translation of the third edition,
1839, does not include the atlas of coloured plates. *See* No. 2285.1.

6333   RILLIET, FRÉDÉRIC. 1814-1861, & BARTHIEZ, ANTOINE CHARLES ERNEST. 1811-
1891
Traité clinique et pratique des maladies des enfants. 3 vols. Paris, *G. Balliére*,
1843.

6334   WEST, CHARLES. 1816-1898
Lectures on the diseases of infancy and childhood. London, *Longman*, 1848.
In its day this was the best English work on the subject, and was
translated into several languages. West was one of the founders of the
Hospital for Sick Children, Gt. Ormond Street, London.

6335   BEDNAŘ, ALOIS. 1816-1888
Die Krankheiten der Neugebornen und Säuglinge. 4 vols. Wien, *C. Gerold*,
1850-53.
Bednař was a famous Viennese paediatrician. His description of
aphthae of the palate in the newborn ("Bednař's aphthae") is in vol. 1, p.
104 of his book.

6336   HENOCH, EDUARD. 1820-1910
Beiträge zur Kinderheilkunde. Berlin, *A. Hirschwald*, 1861.

6337   GERHARDT, CARL ADOLPH CHRISTIAN JACOB. 1833-1902
Handbuch der Kinderkrankheiten. Hrsg. von C. GERHARDT. 9 vols. [in16].
Tübingen, *H. Laupp*, 1877-93.
Gerhardt edited this great work, which was written by the foremost
paediatricians of the time and which gives a close-up view of paediatric
knowledge at the end of the 19th century.

6338   WINCKEL, FRANZ CARL LUDWIG VON. 1837-1911
Ueber eine bisher nicht beschriebene endemisch aufgetretene Erkrankung
Neugeborener. *Dtsch. med. Wschr.*, 1879, **5**, 303-07, 415-18, 431-36, 447-
50.
First description of "Winckel's disease" of the newborn, characterized
by icterus, haemorrhage, haemoglobinuria, and cyanosis.

6339   HENOCH, EDUARD. 1820-1910
Vorlesungen über Kinderkrankheiten. Berlin, *A. Hirschwald*, 1881.

Henoch, whose name is remembered for his description of purpura, initiated the modern concept of paediatrics. English translation, New York, 1882.

6340   ESCHERICH, THEODOR. 1857-1911
Die Darmbakterien des Säuglings und ihre Beziehungen zur Physiologie der Verdauung. Stuttgart, *F. Enke*, 1886.
    Escherich described *Bact. coli* infection. The genus *Escherichia* is named after him.

6341   SOXHLET, FRANZ VON. 1848-1926
Ueber Kindermilch und Säuglings-Ernährung. *Münch. med. Wschr.*, 1886, **33**, 253, 276.
    Soxhlet wrote on the nature of milk droplets, estimated the specific gravity of milk with his lactodensimeter, described an apparatus for the sterilization of milk, and devised a test for the estimation of fats in milk.

6342   JACOBI, ABRAHAM. 1830-1919
The intestinal diseases of infancy and childhood. Detroit, *G.S. Davis*, 1887.
    Jacobi was the first in the United States to specialize in the teaching of paediatrics, and in 1862 founded the first paediatric clinic there (in New York). He wrote extensively on paediatrics; the above is probably his best work.

6342.1   HOLT, LUTHER EMMETT. 1855-1924
The care and feeding of children. New York, *D. Appleton*, 1894.
    A commonsense work written for parents and caretakers of children rather than for physicians. This brief book achieved a popular success unrivalled by any previous American medical publication. It was the forerunner of "Dr. Spock" and related works.

6342.2   ———. The diseases of infancy and childhood. New York, *D. Appleton*, 1897.
    The first really complete and authoritative American text on the subject.

6343   HEUBNER, JOHANN OTTO LEONARD. 1843-1926
Lehrbuch der Kinderheilkunde. 2 vols. Leipzig, *J.A. Barth*, 1903-1906.
    Heubner was professor of paediatrics at Berlin. With Rubner he determined the caloric requirement of infants and did other important work on infant feeding.

6344   SELTER, PAUL. 1866-
Ueber Trophodermatoneurose. *Verh. Ges. Kinderheilk.*, 1903, **20**, 45-50.
    First clear description of infantile acrodynia ("pink disease").

6344.1   BUDIN, PIERRE-CONSTANT. 1846-1907
Le nourisson. Alimentation et hygiène. Paris, *O. Doin*, 1900.
    Pioneer treatise on the care and feeding of premature and newborn infants. Budin sponsored the idea that an infant should be given milk equal in amount to one-tenth of its body weight. English translation, London, 1907.

6347   PFAUNDLER, MEINHARD VON. 1872-1947, & SCHLOSSMANN, ARTHUR. 1867-1932
        Handbuch der Kinderheilkunde. 2te. Aufl. 6 vols. Leipzig, *F.C.W. Vogel*, 1910-12.
        English translation, 1912-24.

6348   SWIFT, HARRY. 1858-1937
        Erythroedema. *Trans. 10th Australasian med. Congr.*, 1914, 547-52.
        Acrodynia ("pink disease", "Swift's disease"); first full description.

6348.1 HESS, JULIUS H. 1876-1955
        Premature and congenitally diseased infants. Philadelphia, *Lea & Febiger*, 1922.
        "The first book ever written dealing solely with premature and congenitally diseased infants" (Cone). Hess founded the first premature infant centre in the United States at Michael Reese Hospital in Chicago.

6349   FEER, EMIL. 1864-1955
        Eine eigenartige Neurose des vegetativen Systems beim Kleinkinde. *Ergeb. inn. Med. Kinderheilk.*, 1923, **24**, 100-22.
        Feer described a vegetative neurosis ("Feer's disease") affecting infants and characterized by cyanosis of the extremities, recurrent sweating, tremor, motor weakness, rapid pulse, and insomnia. It was first described by Selter (No. 6344) and later by Swift, with whose names it is sometimes associated; it is also termed infantile acrodynia and pink disease.

6350   MARRIOTT, WILLIAMS McKIM. 1885-1936
        The food requirements of malnourished infants with a note on the use of insulin. *J. Amer. med. Ass.*, 1924, **83**, 600-03.
        Marriott introduced the insulin-fattening method of treatment of malnutrition in infants.

History of Paediatrics

6351   MEISSNER, FRIEDRICH LUDWIG. 1796-1860
        Grundlage der Literatur der Pädiatrik.   Leipzig, *Fest'sche Verlagsbuchhandlung*, 1850.
        An extensive bibliography of paediatric literature, containing about 7,000 references.

6352   BÓKAY, JÁNOS. 1858-1937
        Die Geschichte der Kinderheilkunde. Berlin, *J. Springer*, 1922.

6353   GARRISON, FIELDING HUDSON. 1870-1935
        History of pediatrics. In I. Abt, *System of pediatrics*, Philadelphia, 1923, **1**, 1-170.
        Re-issued separately with an appendix on the history of paediatrics in recent times by A. F. Abt, Philadelphia, *W. B. Saunders*, 1965.

6354   RUHRÄH, JOHN. 1872-1935
        Pediatrics of the past: an anthology. New York, *P.B. Hoeber*, 1925.
        Contains sketches of the lives of the more important paediatricians of the past, with a comprehensive selection of their works, translated where necessary into English. Ruhräh has thrown much light on the important

contributions of long-forgotten writers, and he has carefully traced the progress of paediatrics from ancient times to the 19th century. The book includes a valuable bibliography.

6355   SUDHOFF, KARL FRIEDRICH JAKOB. 1853-1938
Erstlinge der pädiatrischen Literatur. München, *Münchener Drucke*, 1925.
     Facsimile reproductions of the three earliest printed works on paediatrics: Bagellardo, Metlinger, and Roelans, together with a valuable prefatory essay on their importance.

6356   STILL, *Sir* GEORGE FREDERIC. 1868-1941
The history of paediatrics. The progress of the study of diseases of children up to the end of the XVIIIth century. London, *Oxford Univ. Press*, 1931.
     This work covers the whole field of paediatrics to the end of the 18th century. It is a very readable, interesting and accurate history of the subject. Reprinted Folkstone, 1965. *See* No. 4503.

6357   LEVINSON, ABRAHAM. 1888-1955
Pioneers of pediatrics. 2nd ed. New York, *Froben Press*, 1943.

6357.01   HENKLE, HERMANN HENRY. 1900-
Catalogue of the Clifford G. Grulee collection on pediatrics. Chicago, *John Crerar Library*, [1959].
     4404 entries. The rare books formerly in the John Crerar Library are now in the Regenstein Library at the University of Chicago.

6357.1   PEIPER, ALBRECHT. 1889-1968
Chronik der Kinderheilkunde. 4te. Aufl. Leipzig, *G., Theime*, 1966.

6357.2   CONE, THOMAS E., JR. 1915-
History of American pediatrics. Boston, *Little, Brown*, [1979].

6357.3   TANNER, JAMES MOURILYAN.
A history of the study of human growth. Cambridge, *Cambridge University Press*, [1981].

PAEDIATRIC SURGERY

6357.50   WÜRTZ, FELIX [Wirtz]. *circa* 1510- *circa* 1590
Ein schönes und nützliches Kinderbuchlein. In his *Practica der Wundartzney*, Basel, *S. Henricpetri*, 1616, pp. 725-84.
     This has been traditionally considered the first work on paediatric surgery. However Würtz did not describe any operations – only splinting and bandaging of deformed limbs. English translation, London, 1656, which is reprinted in J. Ruhräh's *Pediatrics of the past*, 1925. *See* No. 5563.

6357.51   FATIO, JOHANNES. 1649-1691
Helvetisch-Vernünftige Wehe-Mutter. Basel, *Johann Rudolph Imhof*, 1752.
     Fatio was probably the first surgeon to study systematically and treat surgical conditions of children. In the last section of this handbook of obstetrics written primarily for midwives, Fatio includes the earliest section on paediatric surgery in a medical book. He describes operations for hypospadias, hydrocolpos, imperforate anus and many more. Because of

revolutionary political activity in the city of Basel, Fatio was imprisoned, tortured, and executed in 1691. All of his manuscripts except the text of above work were burned by the authorities. See Rickham, *The dawn of paediatric surgery: Johannes Fatio (1649-1691)- His life, his work and his horrible end*, in No. 6357.90.

6357.52   BODENHAMER, WILLIAM. 1808-1905
A practical treatise on the etiology, pathology, and treatment of the congenital malformations of the rectum and anus. New York, *Samuel & William Wood*, 1860.
The first comprehensive work ever published on the subject. *See* No. 3459.1.

6357.53   HILLIER, THOMAS. 1831-1868
Hydronephrosis in a boy four years old, repeatedly tapped; recovery. *Proc. roy. med. chir. Soc.*, 1865, **5**, 59-60.
Hillier performed the first therapeutic percutaneous nephrostomy for giant hydronephrosis with ureteropelvic junction obstruction in a four-year old boy.

6357.54   HUTCHINSON, *Sir* JONATHAN. 1828-1913
A successful case of abdominal section for intussusception. *Med.-chir. Trans.*, 1874, **57**, 31-75.
In 1871 Hutchinson was the first successfully to operate on a case of intussusception in a two year-old infant. Preliminary account in *Med. chir. Trans.*, 1876, **41** (2nd ser.), 99-102.

6357.55   HIRSCHSPRUNG, HARALD. 1830-1916
Et Tilfaelde af Subakut Tarminvagination. *Hosp. Tid.*, 1876, **3**, 321-27.
Discouraged by the high mortality of intussusception, Hirschsprung instituted a plan of controlled hydrostatic pressure reduction. By 1905 he was able to present a 35 per cent mortality based on 107 personal cases in a disease that was usually fatal in over 80 per cent of cases.

6357.56   RAMMSTEDT, WILHELM CONRAD. 1867-1963
Zur Operation der angeborenen Pylorusstenose. *Med. Klin.*, 1912, **8**, 1702-05.
"Rammstedt's operation" for congenital pyloric stenosis. In 1920 Rammstedt discovered that the family name had originally been spelt Ramstedt; he therefore reverted to the original spelling for the rest of his life (see *Lancet*, 1963, **1**, 674).

6357.57   LADD, WILLIAM E. 1880-1967, & GROSS, ROBERT EDWARD. 1905-1988
Abdominal surgery of infancy and childhood. Philadelphia, *W.B. Saunders*, 1941.
Ladd pioneered the development of paediatric surgery in the United States. Robert E. Gross, his chief resident, succeeded to his position at Boston Children's Hospital.

6357.58   HAIGHT, CAMERON. 1901-1970 & TOWSLEY, HARRY A.
Congenital atresia of the esophagus with tracheo-esophageal fistula. Extrapleural ligation of fistula and end-to-end anastomosis of esophageal segments. *Surg. Gynecol. Obstet.*, 1943, **76**, 672-88.
Ablation of the tracheo-oesophageal fistula and primary end-to-end oesophageal anastomosis, first achieved in 1941.

6357.59 GROSS, ROBERT EDWARD. 1905-1988
The surgery of infancy and childhood. Philadelphia, *W.B. Saunders*, 1953.
 Gross developed the specialty of paediatric surgery, inventing numerous operations. This was the first modern comprehensive textbook on the subject.

History of Paediatric Surgery

6357.90 RICKHAM, P.P. (ed.)
Historical aspects of pediatric surgery. *Prog. pediat. Surg.*, **20**. Berlin & New York, *Springer-Verlag*, [1986].
 Well-documented illustrated series of historical articles by various authors.

CONDITIONS AND SYNDROMES NOT CLASSIFIED ELSEWHERE

6358 DANZ, FERDINAND GEORG. 1761-1793
Von Menschen ohne Haare und Zähne. *Arch. Geburtsh. (Jena)*, 1792, **4**, 684.
 Hereditary ectodermal dysplasia first described.

6358.1 AXMANN, EDMUND.
Merkwürdige Fragilität der Knochen ohne dyskrasische Ursache als krankhafte Eigenthümlichkeit dreier Geschwister. *Ann ges. Heilk (Karlsruhe)*, 1831, **4**, 58-68.
 Axmann of Wertheim described osteogenesis imperfecta occurring in himself and his two brothers. He referred to the occurrence of articular dislocations and blue sclerotics. *See also* No. 6367.

6359 SMITH, *Sir* THOMAS. 1833-1909
Skull-cap showing congenital deficiencies of bone. *Trans. path. Soc. Lond.*, 1865, **16**, 224-25.

6360 ——. Haemorrhagic periostitis of the shafts of several of the long bones, with separation of the epiphyses. *Trans. path. Soc. Lond.*, 1876, **27**, 219-22
 Craniohypophyseal xanthomatosis was first reported by Sir Thomas Smith (*see also* No. 6359). Hand in 1893 (No. 6361), Schüller in 1915 (No. 6362), and Christian in 1919 (No. 6363) also reported cases, and the condition became known as the "Hand–Schüller–Christian syndrome".

6361 HAND, ALFRED. 1868-1949
Polyuria and tuberculosis. *Proc. path. Soc. Philad.*, 1893, **16**, 282-84; *Arch. Pediat.*, 1893, **10**, 673-75.
 "Hand–Schüller–Christian syndrome", which Hand called polyuria and tuberculosis.

6362 SCHÜLLER, ARTUR. 1874-1958
Ueber eigenartige Schädeldefekte im Jugendalter. *Fortschr. Röntgenstr.*, 1915-16, **23**, 12-18.
 Schüller described two more cases of the condition to which his name, with those of Hand and Christian, has been attached.

6363   CHRISTIAN, HENRY ASBURY. 1876-1951
        Defects in membranous bones, exophthalmos, and diabetes insipidus;
        an unusual syndrome of dyspituitarism; a clinical study. In *Contributions
        to medical and biological research, dedicated to Sir William Osler.* New
        York, *P.B. Hoeber,* 1919, **1**, 390-401.
        "Hand–Schüller–Christian syndrome".

6365   RENDU, ROBERT. 1886-
        Sur un syndrome caractérisé par l'inflammation simultanée de toutes les
        muqueuses externes (conjunctivale, nasale, linguale, buccopharyngée,
        anale et balano-préputiale) coexistant avec une éruption varicelliforme
        puis purpurique des quatres membres. *J. Prat. (Paris)*, 1916, **30**, 351.
        First description of the "Stevens–Johnson syndrome" (*see* No. 4150).

6366   ROWLAND, RUSSELL STURGIS., 1874-
        Xanthomatosis and the reticulo-endothelial system. *Arch intern. Med.*, 1928,
        42, 611-74.
        "Rowland collected 14 cases of the Hand–Schüller–Christian syndrome,
        and made the important generalization that it was due to xanthomatosis"
        (Rolleston).

6367   EDDOWES, ALFRED. 1850-1946
        Dark sclerotics and fragilitas ossium. *Brit. med. J.*, 1900, **2**, 222.
        "Eddowes's syndrome" – blue sclerotics and fragility of the bones,
        occurring as a familial syndrome; osteogenesis imperfecta. *See also* No.
        6358.1.

6368   LAURENCE, JOHN ZACHARIAH. 1830-1874, & MOON, ROBERT CHARLES. 1844-
        1914.
        Four cases of "retinitis pigmentosa", occurring in the same family, and
        accompanied by general imperfections of development. *Ophthal. Rev.*,
        1866, **2**, 32-41.
        Laurence–Moon (–Biedl) syndrome first described. *See also* No. 6369.

6369   BIEDL, ARTUR. 1869-1933
        Geschwisterpaar mit adiposo-genitaler Dystrophie. *Dtsch. med. Wschr.*,
        1922, **48**, 1630.
        Laurence–Moon–Biedl syndrome (*see also* No. 6368). Biedl's cases
        were more fully described by W. Raab, in *Wien. Arch. inn. Med.*, 1924, **7**,
        443-530.

6370   FIESSINGER, NOEL. 1881-1946, & LEROY, EDGAR.
        Contribution à l'étude d'une épidémie de dysenterie dans la Somme
        (juillet–octobre 1916). *Bull Soc. méd. Hôp. Paris*, 1916, **40**, 2030-69.
        Includes several references to the condition later known as "Reiter's
        syndrome" (No. 6371).

6371   REITER, HANS CONRAD JULIUS. 1881-1969
        Ueber eine bisher unerkannte Spirochäteninfektion (Spirochaetosis
        arthritica). *Dtsch, med. Wschr.*, 1916, **42**, 1535-36.
        "Reiter's syndrome", a disease of males characterized by initial diar-
        rhoea, urethritis, conjunctivitis, and arthritis. *See also* No. 6370.

6371.1   HUNTER, CHARLES. 1872-1955
          A rare disease in two brothers. *Proc. roy. Soc. Med.*, 1917, **10**, Sect. Dis.
          Child., 104-16.
             First definite description of the Hurler syndrome (No. 6371.2). Hunter
          became Professor of Medicine in the University of Manitoba.

6371.2   HURLER, GERTRUD.
          Ueber einen Typ multipler Abartungen, vorwiegend am Sklettsystem.
          Z. Kinderheilk., 1919, **24**, 220-34.
             Hurler syndrome (lipochondrodystrophy, gargoylism), earlier described
          by Hunter (No. 6371.1).

6372   LETTERER, ERICH. 1895-1982
          Aleukämische Reticulose. (Ein Beitrag zu den proliferativen Erkrankungen
          des Retikuloendothelialapparates.) *Frankf. Z. Path.*, 1924, **30**, 377-94.
             "Letterer–Siwe disease"; *see also* No. 6373.

6372.1   WEVE, HENRICUS JACOBUS MARIE. 1888-1962
          Ueber Arachnodaktylie (Dystrophia mesodermalis congenita, Typus
          Marfan). *Arch Augenheilk.*, 1931, **104**, 1-46.
             Weve of Utrecht first clearly demonstrated the heritable nature of the
          Marfan syndrome (*see* No. 4365.1).

6373   SIWE, STURE AUGUST. 1897-
          Die Reticuloendotheliose - eine neues Krankheitsbild unter den
          Hepatosplenomegalien. *Z. Kinderheilk.*, 1933, **55**, 212-47.
             See No. 6372.

6374   BEHÇET, HULÜSI. 1889-1948
          Über rezidivierende, aphthöse, durch ein Virus verursachte Geschwüre
          am Mund, am Auge und an den Genitalien. *Derm. Wschr.*, 1937, **105**, 1152-
          57.
             "Behçet's syndrome", previously described by H. Planner and F.
          Remenovsky, *Arch. Derm. Syph. (Berlin),* 1922, **140**, 162-88.

ALTERNATIVE MEDICINE

ACUPUNCTURE (WESTERN REFERENCES)

6374.10   TEN RHIJNE, WILLEM. 1647-1700
          Dissertatio de arthritide: mantissa schematica: de acupunctura: et orationes
          tres...London, *R. Chiswell*, 1683.
             This work by the resident physician at Deshima, the Dutch East India
          Company's trading station in Nagasaki Bay, Japan, contains the first
          detailed description of acupuncture, and the first illustration of acu-points
          published in the West. Ten Rhijne correctly described fourteen acu-tracts
          but confused them with blood-vessels, a misidentification that persisted in
          later Western studies of acupuncture.

6374.11   KAEMPFER, ENGELBERT. 1651-1716
          Amoentitatum exoticarum politico-physico-medicarum fasciculi V. Lemgo,
          Meyer, 1712.

Kaempfer's illustrated accounts of Japanese acupuncture and moxibustion are among the best of the 17th century. They appear for the first time in the above work and are translated into English in his *The History of Japan*, 2 vols., London, 1727.

6374.12   DUJARDIN, FRANÇOIS. 1738-1775
Histoire de la chirurgie depuis son origine jusqu'a nos jours. 2 vols.,Paris, *l'Imprimérie Royale*, 1774-1780.
    Dujardin seems to be the first European to discuss acupuncture within its historical context as an ancient remedy still found to be of practical value. His section on Chinese and Japanese medicine appears on pp. 75-104 of Vol. 1, and includes reproductions of Ten Rhijne's plates. Volume 2 was edited by Bernard Peyrilhe (1735-1804).

6374.13   BERLIOZ, L.V.J.
Mémoires sur les maladies chroniques, les évacuations sanguines et l'acupuncture. 2 vols., Paris, *Croullebois*, 1816.
    Berlioz, father of the composer, published the first French monograph on acupuncture. He had his best success with muscle and joint stiffness after falls, and rheumatic and arthritic states.

6374.14   CHURCHILL, JAMES MORSS. *d.* 1863
A treatise on acupuncturation....London, *Simpkin & Marshall*, [1821].
    The first English monograph on acupuncture. Churchill had most success with rheumatic conditions, sciatica, back-pain, etc.

6374.15   MORAND, J.
Memoir on acupuncturation, embracing a series of cases drawn up under the inspection of M. Julius Cloquet. Paris, 1825. Translated from the French by FRANKLIN BACHE. Philadelphia, *Robert Desilver*, 1825.
    The first American book on acupuncture, translated by the grandson of Benjamin Franklin. Little is known about Morand. He does, however, refer to his association with JULES CLOQUET (1790-1883) throughout the text.

6374.16   SARLANDIÈRE, JEAN-BAPTISTE. 1787-1838
Mémoires sur l'électro-puncture, considerée comme moyen nouveau de traiter efficacement la goutte, les rheumatisme et les affections nerveuses...Paris, *Chez l'Auteur*, 1825.
    The first treatise on electro-puncture – the only significant Western contribution to acupuncture, and one of the most widely used methods of acupuncture today.

History of Acupuncture

6374.90   LU, GWEI-DJEN, and NEEDHAM, JOSEPH. 1900-
Celestial lancets: a history and rationale of acupuncture and moxa. Cambridge, *Cambridge University Press*, [1980].
    A section of Needham's *Science and civilisation in China* series, separately published. Includes the best bibliography of early Western treatises on acupuncture.

HISTORY OF MEDICINE

GENERAL

6375   CELSUS, Aulus Aurelius Cornelius. 25 b.c.-a.d. 50
De medicina. Florentiae, *Nicolaus [Laurentius]*, 1478.
The *De Medicina* is the oldest medical document after the Hippocratic
writings. Written about a.d. 30, it remains the greatest medical treatise from
ancient Rome, and the first Western history of medicine. Celsus's superb
literary style won him the title of *Cicero medicorum*. First English translation by J. Grieve, London, 1756. *See* Nos. 20, 3666.81, 5548.1, and 5733.50.

6376   CHAMPIER, Symphorien. 1472-1539
De medicine claris scriptoribus in quinque partitus tractatus. *In his* Libelli
duo [Lyon, *J. de Campis*, 1506?].
The first history of medicine of any importance. Champier's biographical
study of famous medical writers also includes the earliest attempt at a
medical bibliography. A bibliographical study of Champier by P.A. Allut
appeared from Lyons in 1859; a check-list of his writings was published by
J.F. Ballard and M. Pijoan in *Bull. med. Libr. Ass.*, 1940, **28**, 182-88.

6377   DONATI, Marcello. 1538-1602
De medica historia mirabili libri sex. Mantuae, *per Fr. Osanam*, 1586.
See Nos. 3417 & 4011.2.

6378   FREIND, John. 1675-1728
The history of physick; from the time of Galen to the beginning of the
sixteenth century. 2 vols. London, *J. Walthoe*, 1725-26.
Freind was the first English historian of medicine; his book is the best
English work on the period of which it treats. Freind dabbled in politics and
planned the above work while committed to the Tower of London on a
charge of high treason, a charge of which he was innocent. Sir Robert
Walpole, Prime Minister at the time, suffered much from renal calculi and
called in Mead, a great friend of Freind. Mead refused to treat Walpole until
Freind was released, and this was speedily arranged!

6379   LE CLERC, Daniel. 1652-1728
Histoire de la médecine. A La Haye, *I. van der Kloot*, 1729.
The first large history of medicine. It is still consulted today. Le Clerc is
sometimes called the "Father of the History of Medicine". The first edition of
this work appeared in 1696, but later editions are more useful. English
translation, 1699. Reprint of 1729 edition, Amsterdam, *B. M. Israel*, 1967.

6380   MIDDLETON, Peter. *d.* 1781
A medical discourse, or an historical inquiry into the ancient and present
state of medicine. New York, *Hugh Gaine*, 1769.
First American publication on medical history.

6381   LETTSOM, John Coakley. 1744-1815
History of the origin of medicine. London, *J. Phillips for E. & C. Dilly*, 1778.

6382   SPRENGEL, Kurt Polykarp Joachim. 1766-1833
Versuch einer pragmatischen Geschichte der Arzneikunde. 5 vols. Halle,
J. J. Gebauer, 1792-1803.

A monumental work, full of important information which has been of great assistance to later historians. Includes a useful chronology. Third edition, 1821-28; fourth edition of vol. 1, 1846.

6383   HECKER, JUSTUS FRIEDRICH KARL. 1795-1850
Geschichte der Heilkunde. 2 vols. Berlin, *Enslin*, 1822-29.
An important early German work on the history of medicine.

6384   HAESER, HEINRICH. 1811-1884
Lehrbuch der Geschichte der Medicin und der Volkskrankheiten. Jena, *F. Mauke*, 1845.
An important German work on the history of medicine and one of the most outstanding contributions. Haeser was eclipsed only by his fellow-countryman Sudhoff. A third edition, in three volumes, appeared in 1875-82 and was reprinted, Hildesheim, *G.Olms*, 1971.

6385   PUCCINOTTI, FRANCESCO. 1794-1872
Storia della medicina. 3 vols. [in 4]. Livorno, *M. Wagner,* 1850-66.

6386   WUNDERLICH, CARL REINHOLD AUGUST. 1815-1877
Geschichte der Medicin. Stuttgart, *Ebner & Seubert*, 1859.

6387   DAREMBERG, CHARLES VICTOR. 1817-1872
Histoire des sciences médicales. 2 vols. Paris, *J.B. Baillère*, 1870.

6388   LITTRÉ, MAXIMILIEN PAUL EMILE. 1801-1881
Médecine et médecins. Paris, *Didier & Cie.*, 1872.

6389   BAAS, JOHANN HERMANN. 1838-1909
Grundriss der Geschichte der Medicin. Stuttgart, *F. Enke*, 1876.
Until superseded by Garrison, Baas's book was the most important one-volume text on the history of medicine. For an expert evaluation of it, see Garrison's *History*, 4th ed., p. 884. An English translation, by H.E. Handerson was published in New York in 1889, and reprinted, New York, *Krieger,* 1971.

6390   HOLMES, OLIVER WENDELL. 1809-1894
Medical essays: 1842-1882. Boston, *Houghton Mifflin & Co.*, 1883.
"The most important American book dealing with the history of medicine up to its day" (Garrison).

6391   PUSCHMANN, THEODOR. 1844-1899
Geschichte des medizinischen Unterrichtes von den ältesten Zeiten bis zur Gegenwart. Leipzig, *Veit & Co.*, 1889.
English translation, 1891, reprinted, New York, 1966. German edition reprinted Amsterdam, 1961.

6392   PETERSON, JAKOB JULIUS. 1840-1912
Hauptmomente in der älteren Geschichte der medicinischen Klinik. Kopenhagen, *A.F. Host*, 1890.
Reprinted Hildesheim, *G. Olms*, 1966.

6393   BOUCHUT, EUGENE. 1818-1891
Histoire de la médecine et des doctrines médicales. 2 vols. Paris, *Germer-Ballière*, 1873.

6395   WITHINGTON, Edward Theodore. 1860-1947
Medical history from the earliest times. London, *Scientific Press*, 1894.
A classic brief history up to the early 19th century. Reprinted 1964.

6396   PAGEL, Julius Leopold. 1851-1912
Geschichte der Medicin. 2 vols. Berlin, *S. Karger*, 1898.
A collection of lectures. The bibliography of the revised edition of 1922, for which Sudhoff was responsible, is a great improvement upon the first edition.

6397   VIRCHOW, Rudolf Ludwig Karl. 1821-1902
Die neueren Fortschritte in der Wissenschaft und ihr Einfluss auf Medicin und Chirurgie. Berlin, *A. Hirschwald*, 1898.
English translation in *Disease, life and man. Selected essays by Rudolf Virchow*. Selected, translated, annotated, and introduced by L. J. Rather, Stanford, 1958.

6398   PUSCHMANN, Theodor. 1844-1899
Handbuch der Geschichte der Medizin. Begründet von Theodor Puschmann. 3 vols. Jena, *G. Fischer*, 1902-05.
Puschmann died before the completion of this work, and it was then edited by Pagel and Neuburger. It is one of the most important books on the subject, ranking with the work of Haeser; many authorities collaborated in the writing of the histories of the various subjects treated. Reprinted, Hildesheim, *G. Olms*, 1971.

6399   SUDHOFF, Karl Friedrich Jakob. 1853-1938
Iatromathematiker vornehmlich im 15. und 16. Jahrundert. Breslau, *J. U. Kern*, 1902.

6400   ALLBUTT, *Sir* Thomas Clifford. 1836-1925
The historical relations of medicine and surgery to the end of the sixteenth century. London, *Macmillan*, 1905.

6401   NEUBURGER, Max. 1868-1955
Geschichte der Medizin. Vol. 1-2, pt. 1. Stuttgart, *F. Enke*, 1906-1911.
An English translation was published in London, 2 vols., 1910-25.

6403   PAGEL, Julius Leopold. 1851-1912
Zeittafeln zur Geschichte der Medizin. Berlin, *A. Hirschwald*, 1908.

6404   FOSSEL, Viktor. 1846-1913
Studien zur Geschichte der Medizin. Stuttgart, *F. Enke*, 1909.

6406   VIERORDT, Karl Hermann. 1853-1944
Medizinisches aus der Geschichte. 3te. Aufl. Tübingen, *H. Laupp*, 1910.

6408   GARRISON, Fielding Hudson. 1870-1935
An introduction to the history of medicine. Philadelphia, London, *W.B. Saunders*, 1913.
Still one of the best single-volume histories of medicine. A rather compressed work with much detail, this is really more of a reference work than something to read from cover to cover. Garrison had a special gift for distilling the complex lifetime achievements of great physicians into a few

paragraphs. In his time he was the leading American authority on the subject and wrote many papers on various aspects of medical history. Those published in *Bull. N.Y. Acad. Med.*, 1925-35 were collected under the title of *Contributions to the history of medicine*, New York, *Hafner*, 1966. Garrison saw his so-called *Introduction* through four editions, the last of which appeared in 1929. That edition has been frequently reprinted. See the biography by S.R. Kagan, Boston, 1948. See also Fielding H. Garrison: the man and his book, by G. H. Brieger, *Trans. Stud. Coll. Phycns. Philad., Med. Sci.*, 1981, **3**, 1-21.

6409 VIERORDT, KARL HERMANN. 1853-1944
Medizin-geschichtliches Hilfsbuch mit besonderer Berücksichtigung der Entdeckungsgeschichte und der Biographie. Tübingen, *H. Laupp*, 1916.

6411 SINGER, CHARLES JOSEPH. 1876-1960
Studies in the history and method of science. Edited by CHARLES SINGER. 2 vols. Oxford, *Clarendon Press*, 1917-21.
A collection of essays by several authorities.

6413 MEYER-STEINEG, THEODOR. 1873-1936, & SUDHOFF, KARL FRIEDRICH JAKOB. 1853-1938
Geschichte der Medizin im Überblick. Jena, *G. Fischer*, 1921.
5th edition, 1965, under the title *Illustrierte Geschichte der Medizin*.

6414 OSLER, *Sir* WILLIAM, *Bart.* 1849-1919
The evolution of modern medicine. New Haven, *Yale Univ. Press*, 1921.
This book is based on the Silliman Lectures delivered at Yale in 1913. It remained unfinished at Osler's death, and Osler requested in his will that it and his other unfinished works not be published. In spite of this, work was prepared for the press by Harvey Cushing, Archibald Malloch and others. It is one of the most interesting short histories of medicine, written in Osler's usual charming style, and is still one of the best books with which to commence the study of medical history. Reprinted, New York, 1963 and 1972.

6415 CUMSTON, CHARLES GREENE. 1868-1927
An introduction to the history of medicine from the time of the Pharaohs to the end of the XVIIIth century ... With an essay on the relation of history and philosophy to medicine, by F.G. CROOKSHANK. London, *Kegan Paul*, 1926.

6417 NEUBURGER, MAX. 1868-1955
Die Lehre von der heilkraft der Natur im Wandel der Zeiten. Stuttgart, *F. Enke*, 1926.
The standard work on the history of the doctrine of "the healing power of Nature". English translation, New York, 1932.

6418 CASTIGLIONI, ARTURO. 1874-1953
Storia della medicina. Milano, *Soc. Ed. Unitas*, 1927.
This work is similar in plan and scope to that of Garrison (No. 6408). Much attention is devoted to palaeopathology, while the accounts of the School of Salerno, and mediaeval and Renaissance Italian medicine are especially valuable. The bibliographies are excellent. This is one of the most accurate and comprehensive textbooks on the subject. An English

translation by E.B. Krumbhaar was published in 1941 and revised in 1947; new Italian editions, 1936 and 1938.

6419   SARTON, GEORGE ALFRED LÉON. 1884-1956
        Introduction to the history of science. Vol. 1-3 [in5]. Baltimore, *Williams & Wilkins*, 1927-48.
        An invaluable annotated bibliographical survey to the end of the 14th century of the progress of science throughout the world. Reprinted, Huntington, N.Y., *Krieger*, 1975.

6421   SINGER, CHARLES JOSEPH. 1876-1960
        A short history of medicine. Oxford, *Clarendon Press*, 1928.
        A highly readable outline history of the subject. It is especially valuable for non-medical readers and for those who have time to deal only with the principal events of medical history. A second edition revised by E.A. Underwood was published in 1962.

6422   THORNDIKE, LYNN. 1882-1965
        A history of magic and experimental science. 8 vols. New York, *Columbia University Press*, 1923-58.
        Vols. 1-2 deal with the first 13 centuries of the Christian era; vols. 3-4 with the 14th and 15th centuries, vols. 5-6 with the 16th century, and vols. 7-8 with the 17th century.

6423   CAMAC, CHARLES NICOLL BANCKER. 1868-1940
        Imhotep to Harvey: backgrounds of medical history. Foreword by HENRY FAIRFIELD OSBORN. New York, *Hoeber*, 1931.

6424   SIGERIST, HENRY ERNEST. 1891-1957
        Einführing in die Medizin. Leipzig, *G. Thieme*, 1931.
        Traces the evolution of medicine from the stage of superstition and magic to the present time, and shows how our knowledge of the subject has developed through the study of anatomy and physiology. English translation, *Man and Medicine*, was published in New York, 1932.

6425   GARCIA DEL REAL, EDUARDO. 1870-1947
        Historia contemporánea de la medicina. Madrid, *Espasa-Calpe*, 1934.

6429   FÜLÖP-MILLER, RENÉ. 1891-
        Kulturgeschichte der Heilkunde. München, *Bruckmann*, 1935-37.

6430   LAIGNEL-LAVASTINE, MAXIME PAUL MARIE. 1875-1953
        Histoire générale de la médicine, de la pharmacie, de l'art dentaire et de l'art vétérinaire. 3 vols. Paris, *Michel*, 1936-49.
        This splendidly produced work, beautifully illustrated, was written by experts in each branch of the subject, with Laignel-Lavastine as general editor.

6431   LLOYD, WYNDHAM EDWARD BUCKLEY.
        A hundred years of medicine. London, *Duckworth*, [1936].
        New edition 1968.

6432   MAJOR, RALPH HERMON. 1884-1970
        Disease and destiny. New York, *Appleton-Century*, 1936.

6433   SHRYOCK, RICHARD HARRISON. 1893-1972
The development of modern medicine, an interpretation of the social and
scientific factors involved. Philadelphia, *University of Pennsylvania Press,*
1936.
Revised edition, 1947, reprinted, Madison, 1980.

6435   GALDSTON, IAGO. 1895-
Progress in medicine: a critical review of the last hundred years. New
York, *Knopf,* 1940.

6436   CLENDENING, LOGAN, 1884-1945
Source book of medical history. New York, *Hoeber,* 1942.
Reprinted, *Dover Publications,* 1960.

6437   NEUBURGER, MAX. 1868-1955
British medicine and the Vienna School: contacts and parallels. London,
Heinemann, 1943.

6439   GUTHRIE, DOUGLAS JAMES. 1885-1975
A history of medicine. London, *Nelson,* (1945).

6440   METTLER, CECILIA CHARLOTTE. 1909-1943
History of medicine. A correlative text arranged according to subjects.
Edited by FRED A. METTLER. Philadelphia, *Blakiston Co.,* 1947.

6441   PAZZINI, ADALBERTO. 1898-1975
Storia della medicina. 2 vols. Milano, *Soc. Editrice Libraria,* 1947

6443   CREUTZ, RUDOLPH, & STEUDEL, JOHANNES. 1901-1973
Einführung in die Geschichte der Medizin in Einzeldarstellungen Iserlohn,
Silva Verlag, 1948.

6444   ARTELT, WALTER. 1906-1976
Einführung in die Medizinhistorik. Ihr Wesen, ihre Arbeitsweise und ihre
Hilfsmittel. Stuttgart, *F. Enke,* 1949.

6445   DIEPGEN, PAUL. 1878-1966
Geschichte der Medizin. Die historische Entwicklung der Heilkunde und
des ärztlichen Lebens. 2 vols. [in 3]. Berlin, *W. de Gruyter,* 1949-55.

6447   GOTFREDSEN, EDVARD. 1899-1963
Medicinens historie. Kjobenhavn, *Busck, 1950.*
2nd edition, 1964.

6448   SIGERIST, HENRY ERNEST. 1891-1957
A history of medicine. Vol. 1-2 New York, *Oxford University Press,* 1951-61.
1. Primitive and archaic medicine. 2. Early Greek, Hindu and Persian
medicine.

6449   SARTON, GEORGE ALFRED LÉON. 1884-1956
Horus. A guide to the history of science. A first guide for the study of the
history of science. With introductory essays on science and tradition.
Waltham, Mass., *Chronica Botanica Co.,* 1952.
Contains extensive bibliographies.

6450 ————. A history of science. Vol. 1-2. Cambridge, Mass., *Harvard Univ. Press*, 1953-59.
1. Ancient science through the Golden age of Greece. 2. Hellenistic science and culture in the last three centuries B.C.

6451 ARTELT, W. & STEUDEL, J.
Index zur Geschichte der Medizin. Vol. 1-2. München, *Urban & Schwarzenberg*, 1953-66.
Vol. 1 contains over 10,000 and vol. 2 over 7,000 references to books and papers. Vol. 1 edited by W. Artelt, vol.2 edited by J. Steudel. Covers the years 1945-48 and 1949-52.

6451.1 WELLCOME INSTITUTE FOR THE HISTORY OF MEDICINE
Current work in the history of medicine. An international bibliography. No. 1- . London, *Wellcome Institute for the History of Medicine*, 1954-
A quarterly subject index to periodical literature on the history of medicine. Also lists new books alphabetically by author. *See* No. 6451.11.

6451.2 MAJOR, RALPH HERMON. 1884-1970
A history of medicine. 1 vol. [in 2]. Springfield, *C.C. Thomas*, 1954.

6451.4 BARIÉTY, MAURICE JACQUES CLÉMENT. 1897-1971 & COURY, CHARLES RENÉ. 1916-1973
Histoire de la médecine. Paris, *Fayard,*, 1963.

6451.5 NATIONAL LIBRARY OF MEDICINE
Bibliography of the history of medicine. No. 1-. Bethesda, Md., 1965-
Annual. Quinquennial cumulations 1964-69, 1970-74, 1975-79 *et seq.* Published by the National Library of Medicine.

6451.6 METTE, ALEXANDER & WINTER, IRENE
Geschichte der Medizin. Einführung in ihre Grundzüge. Berlin, *Volk und Gesundheit*, 1968.
A general history of medicine from a Marxist perspective.

6451.7 LAI:N ENTRALGO, PEDRO. 1908-
Historia universal de la medicina. 7 vols. Barcelona, *Salvat*, 1972-75.

6451.8 SMIT, PIETER. 1925-
History of the life sciences. An annotated bibliography. Amsterdam, *A. Asher*, 1974.
Over 4,000 annotated citations of works dealing with all aspects of the history of medicine and biology, including a section on individual and collected biographies.

6451.9 LICHTENTHAELER, CHARLES. 1915-
Geschichte der Medizin. 2 vols. Köln, *Deutsche Ärzte-Verlag*, 1975.
French translation, 1978.

6451.10 LYONS, ALBERT S. 1912- , & PETRUCELLI, R. JOSEPH. 1943-
Medicine, an illustrated history. New York, *Harry N. Abrams*, 1978.
Includes over 1,000 illustrations, many in colour.

6451.11 WELLCOME INSTITUTE FOR THE HISTORY OF MEDICINE
Subject catalogue of the history of medicine and related sciences. 18 vols.
Munich, *Kraus International*, 1980.
Subject section: 9 vols.; Biographical section: 5 vols.; Topographical
section: 4 vols. Reproduces the card subject catalogue of the library and
includes a cumulation of *Current Work in the History of Medicine* (No.
6451.1). Includes material published to 1977.

PREHISTORIC, PRIMITIVE, AND FOLK MEDICINE

6451.90 RUSH, Benjamin. 1745-1813
An oration...containing an enquiry into the natural history of medicine
among the Indians in North-America; and a comparative view of their
diseases and remedies, with those of civilized nations. Philadelphia, *Joseph
Cruikshank*, [1774].
Rush was the first American physician to publish a detailed study of
American Indian medicine.

6452 BLACK, William George. 1857-1932
Folk-medicine; a chapter in the history of culture. London, *E. Stock*, 1883.
Folk-Lore Society Publication No. 12. The authoritative English work
on medical folk-lore.

6452.1 BOURKE, John Gregory. 1846-1896
The medicine-men of the Apache. *Ann. Rep. Bur. Amer. Ethnol.*, 1892, **9**,
451-603.
Bourke, a U.S. Army officer with experience on the American Indian
frontier, was a pioneer student of American Indian medicine and anthropology.

6453 BARTELS, Maximillian Carl August. 1843-1904
Die Medicin der Naturvölker. Leipzig, *T. Grieben*, 1893.

6455 HOVORKA, Oscar von. 1866-1930, & KRONFELD, Adolf. 1861-09
Vergleichende Volksmedizin. 2 vols. Stuttgart, *Strecker & Schröder*, 1908-09.
Most authoritative work so far available on the subject.

6455.1 HRDLICKA, Ales. 1869-1943
Physiological and medical observations among the Indians of Southwestern
United States and Northern Mexico. *Bur. Amer. Ethnol. Bull.* No. 34.
Washington, D.C., *Government Printing Office*, 1908.

6456 MADDOX, John Lee. 1878-
The medicine man; a sociological study of the character and evolution of
shamanism...New York, *Macmillan*, 1923.

6458 JAYNE, Walter Addison. 1853-
The healing gods of ancient civilizations. New Haven, *Yale Univ., Press*,
1925.

6459 McKENZIE, Dan. 1870-1935
The infancy of medicine. An enquiry into the influence of folk-lore upon
the evolution of scientific medicine. London, *Macmillan*, 1927.

6460   STONE, ERIC PERCY. 1892-
Medicine among the American Indians. New York, *P.B. Hoeber*, 1932.
Reprinted, New York, *Hafner*, 1962.

6461   CORLETT, WILLIAM THOMAS. 1854-1948
The medicine-man of the American Indian and his cultural background.
Springfield, *Thomas*, 1935.

6462   KEMP, PHYLIS.
Healing ritual: studies of the technique and tradition of the southern Slavs.
London, *Faber*, 1935.

6463   CHAUVET, STEPHEN. 1885-1950
La médecine chez les peuples primitifs. Paris, *A. Maloine*, 1936.

6464   PARDAL, RAMÓN. 1896-1955
Medicina aborigen americana. Buenos Aires, *Anesi*, [1937].

6465   WECK, WOLFGANG. 1881-
Heilkunde und Volkstum auf Bali. Stuttgart, *Enke*, 1937.

6465.1   MIGUELITO. *circa* 1865-1936
Navajo medicine man. Sandpaintings and legends of Miguelito by GLADYS
A. REICHARD. New York, *Augustin*, [1939].
      Navajo sandpaintings are traditionally made only for the healing cer-
emony in which they are used, and then destroyed. This book contains
superb reproductions on sand-coloured paper of watercolour versions of
the sandpaintings painted by the medicine man, himself. The paintings are
accompanied by an essay on this ancient form of medicine, in which the
patient sat in the centre of the painting and the healer chanted, and a cure
was effected through the identification of the patient with divine powers
portrayed in the painting and chant.

6466   HARLEY, GEORGE WAY. 1894-
Native African medicine. Cambridge, *Harvard University Press*, 1941.

6467   PAZZINI, ADALBERTO. 1898-1975
La medicina primitiva. Milano, *"Arte e Storia"*, 1941.

6467.1   VOGEL, VIRGIL J.
American Indian medicine. Norman, *University of Oklahoma Press*, [1970].
      The best available work on the subject. Volume 95 of *The Civililization
of the American Indian Series*.

6467.2   ACKERKNECHT, ERWIN HEINZ. 1906-
Medicine and ethnology. Selected essays, edited by H.H. WALSER & H.M.
KOELBING. Baltimore, *Johns Hopkins Press*, [1971].
See also No. 6448

6467.9   EBERS PAPYRUS.
Papyros Ebers. Das älteste Buch über Heilkunde. Aus dem Aegyptischen zum erstenmal vollständig übersetzt von H. Joachim. Berlin, *G. Reimer,* 1890.
    The Ebers Papyrus dates from about 1552 B.C. The original, now at Leipzig, was discovered about 1862 and was purchased by Georg Ebers in 1873. The papyrus measures 20.23 m. in length and 30 cm. in height. It is the most important medical papyrus yet recovered; it is written in hieratic script and contains the most complete record of Egyptian medicine known. Ebers published a facsimile of the papyrus, with a partial translation, in 1875.

6467.91   ——. The papyrus Ebers. The greatest Egyptian medical document. Translated by B. Ebbell. Copenhagen, *Levin & Munksgaard,* 1937.
    Best English translation so far published.

6467.92   WRESZINSKI, Walter. 1880-
Der grosse medizinische Papyrus des Berliner Museums (Pap. Berl. 3038) in Facsimile und Umschrift mit Uebersetzung, Kommentar und Glossar. Herausg. von W. Wreszinski. Leipzig, *J. C. Hinrichs,* 1909.
    The Greater German Papyrus (Brugsch Papyrus) dates from about 1300 B.C. The above facsimile reproduction and translation forms vol. 1 of the *Medizin der alten Aegypter* series.

6467.93   CHESTER BEATTY PAPYRUS.
Le papyrus médical Chester Beatty. Par le Dr. Frans Jonckheere. Bruxelles, *Fondation Egyptologique Reine Elisabeth,* 1947. *La Médicine Egyptienne,* No. 2.
    A hieratic papyrus of the 13th-12th century B.C. It is a fragment of a monograph on diseases of the anus. It was reproduced with hieroglyphic transcription by A. H. Gardiner in 1935.

6468   ALPINI, Prospero. 1553-1617
De medicina Aegyptiorum, libri quatuor. Venetiis, *apud Fr. de Franciscis,* 1591.
    First important work on the history of Egyptian medicine. Alpini became professor of botany at Padua after having spent three years in Egypt. French translation by R. de Fenoyl, 2 vols, Cairo, *Inst. Française d'Archéologie Orientale,* 1979.

6469   SCHWIMMER, Ernst. 1837-1898
Die ersten Anfänge der Heilkunde und die Medizin im alten Aegypten. Eine kulturgeschichteliche Skizze. Berlin, *Habel,* 1876.
    Sammlung gemeinverständlicher wissenschaftlicher Vorträge, No. 255.

6470   HURRY, Jamieson Boyd. 1857-1930
Imhotep: the vizier and physician of Kind Zoser, and afterwards the Egyptian god of medicine. Oxford, *Univ. Press,* 1926.

6471   DAWSON, Warren Royal. 1888-1968
The beginnings. Egypt and Assyria. New York, *Hoeber,* 1930.
    Clio Medica series.

6471.1   LEAKE, Chauncey Depew. 1896-1978
          The old Egyptian medical papyri. Kansas, *University of Kansas Press*, 1952.
          A guide to the chief medical papyri, with particular attention to
          therapeutics.

6471.2   AKADEMIE-VERLAG
          Grundriss der Medizin der alten Ägypter. Vol. 1-9. Berlin, *Akademie-Verlag*,
          1954-73.
          Critical studies, texts, translations. Includes the best translations of Nos.
          2-5.

6471.9   HAMMURABI, *King of Babylon. fl.* 1792-1750 B.C.
          The code of Hammurabi, King of Babylon about 2000 B.C. Autographed text,
          transliteration, translation...by ROBERT FRANCIS HARPER. Chicago, *Callaghan &
          Co.,* 1904.
          The Code of Hammurabi was found among the clay tablets of the library
          of Ashurbanipal. It is now in the Louvre. It was first published in Scheil:
          Mémoires de la Délégation en Perse, Paris, 1902, **4,** 4-162. The Code
          mentions the fees payable to a physician following successful treatment;
          these varied according to the station of the patient. Similarly, the punishment
          for the failure of an operation is set out. At least this shows that in Babylon
          4,000 years ago the medical profession had advanced far enough in public
          esteem to warrant the payment of adequate fees. *See* No. 1.

6471.91   KÜCHLER, Friedrich.
          Beiträge zur Kenntnis der assyrisch-babylonischen Medizin. Texte mit
          Umschrift, Uebersetzung und Kommentar. Leipzig, *J. C. Hinrich,* 1904.
          Medical texts from the library of Ashurbanipal, together with German
          translations. A valuable paper on this subject is M. Jastrow's The medicine
          of the Babylonians and Assyrians, *Proc. roy. Soc. Med.* 1913-14, **7,** Sect. Hist.
          Med., 109-76.

6471.92   THOMPSON, Reginald Campbell. 1876-1941
          Assyrian medical texts. From the originals in the British Museum. London,
          Oxford Univ. Press, 1923.
          Facsimiles of the texts of 660 cuneiform medical tablets, many of which
          were hitherto unpublished, from the library of Ashurbanipal. The tablets date
          back to the seventh century B.C. No translations are included, but Thompson
          has interpreted and systematized many of the texts in a later work (*Proc. roy.
          Soc. Med.,* 1924, **17,** Sect. Hist. Med., 1-34; 1926, **19,** Sect. Hist. Med., 29-78).

6472   OEFELE, Felix, *Freiherr* von. 1861-
          Keilschriftmedicin. Breslau, *J.N. Kern,* 1902.
          Cuneiform medicine.

6473   CONTENAU, Georges.
          La médecine en Assyrie et en Babylonie. Paris, *Maloine,* 1938.

6473.1   KÖCHER, Franz.
          Die babylonisch-assyrische Medizin in Texten und Untersuchungen. Vol
          1-6. Berlin, *Walter de Gruyter,* 1963-80.

6474   DAREMBERG, CHARLES VICTOR. 1817-1872
        La médecine dans Homère. Paris, *Didier et Cie.*, 1865.

6475   ——. Etat de la médecine entre Homère et Hippocrate. Paris, *Didier et Cie.*, 1869.

6476   EDELSTEIN, EMMA J. & EDELSTEIN, LUDWIG. 1902-1965
        Asclepius. A collection and interpretation of the testimonies. 2 vols., Baltimore, *Johns Hopkins Press*, 1945.

6478   SUDHOFF, KARL FRIEDRICH JAKOB. 1853-1938
        Aerztliches aus griechischen Papyrus-Urkunden. Leipzig, *J.A. Barth*, 1907.

6479   ALLBUTT, *Sir* THOMAS CLIFFORD. 1836-1925
        Greek medicine in Rome. London, *Macmillan & Co.*, 1921.
        FitzPatrick Lectures, 1909-10. Allbutt was Regius Professor of Physic at Cambridge and a great literary stylist. Underwood described him as the most learned and distinguished physician of the last hundred years.

6482   SUDHOFF, KARL FRIEDRICH JAKOB. 1853-1938
        Kos und Knidos. München, *Münchner Drucke*, 1927.

6483   HEIDEL, WILLIAM ARTHUR.
        Hippocratic medicine. Its spirit and method. New York, *Columbia University Press*, 1941.

6484   BOURGEY, LOUIS. 1901-1979
        Observation et expérience chez les médecins de la Collection Hippocratique. Paris, *J. Vrin*, 1953.

6485   COHN-HAFT, LOUIS.
        The public physicians of ancient Greece. Northampton, Mass., *Smith College*, 1956.

6485.1 SCHUMACHER, JOSEPH. 1902-
        Antike Medizin. Die naturphilosophischen Grundlagen der Medizin in der griechischen Antike. 2nd ed. Berlin, *W. de Gruyter*, 1963.

6485.2 KUDLIEN, FRIDOLF. 1928-
        Der Beginn des medizinischen Denkens bei den Griechen von Homer bis Hippokrates. Zürich, *Artemis*, 1967.

6485.3 EDELSTEIN, LUDWIG. 1902-1965
        Ancient medicine: selected papers. Edited by O. TEMKIN and C. L. TEMKIN. Baltimore, *Johns Hopkins Press*, 1967.

6485.4 LAÍN ENTRALGO, PEDRO. 1908-
        La medicina Hipocratica. Madrid, *Revista de Occidente*, 1970.

6485.5 FLASHAR, Hellmut (ed.).
Antike Medizin. Wege der Forschung ccxxi. Darmstadt, *Wissenschaftliche Buchgesellschaft*, 1971.

6485.6 MAJNO, Guido.
The healing hand: Man and wound in the ancient world. Cambridge, Mass., *Harvard University Press*, [1975].
Emphasizing surgery, this is an exceptionally imaginative and exquisitely designed and illustrated history of medicine in ancient Egypt, Greece, Rome, and China.

6485.61 LONIE, Ian Malcolm. 1932-1988
The Hippocratic treatises "On generation" "On the nature of the child" "Diseases IV". A commentary. Berlin, *W. de Gruyter*, 1981.

6485.62 GRMEK, Mirko Drazen.
Les maladies à l'aube de la civilization occidentale. Paris, *Payot*, 1983.
English translation entitled, *Diseases in the ancient Greek world*, Baltimore, *Johns Hopkins Univ. Press*, 1989.

6485.63 KÜNZEL, Ernst.
Medizinische Instrumente aus Sepulkralfunden der römischen Kaiserzeit. Köln, *Rheinland Verlag*, 1983.

6485.64 NUTTON, Vivian.
From Democedes to Harvey: Studies in the history of medicine. London, *Variorum Reprints*, 1988.

6485.9 AYURVEDA
The Ayurvedic system of medicine. By Nagendra Nath Sen Gupta. 3 vols. Calcutta, *K. R. Chatterjee,* 1901-07.
Ayurveda is the most ancient system of Hindu medicine; only fragments of the original remain. The early Hindus believed it to be of divine origin and ascribed it to Brahma. It dates from *circa* 1400-1200 b.c. Reprinted Delhi, *Indian Book Centre*, 1984.

6485.91 CHARAKA SAMHITA.
[Charaka Samhita. Edited by Jibananda Vidyasagara.] Calcutta, *Sarasvati Press,* 1877.
Sanskrit text. Authorities vary as to the date of Charaka. He is said to have lived at times varying between 800 b.c. and a.d. 78. The Samhita, or Sanhita, is one of the most ancient and complete systems of Hindu medicine to have survived. It is arranged in the form of dialogues between master and pupil and is divided into eight books. Charaka's writing is superior to that of Susruta in the accuracy of his descriptions. What Susruta is to surgery, Charaka is to medicine.

6485.92 ——. The Charaka Samhita. Edited and published with translations in Hindi, Gujerati and English, *Shree Gulabkunverba Ayurvedic Society.* 6 vols. Jamnagar, 1949.

6485.93 SUŚRUTA SAMHITA.
[Suśruta Samhita. The system of Hindu medicine taught by Dhanwantari. Compiled by Suśruta. Edited and published by PANDIT-KULAPATI JIBANANDA VIDYASAGARA.] 5th ed. Calcutta, 1909.

Sanskrit text. The Suśruta Samhita required a good educational foundation of a student of medicine. Suśruta is said to have lived in the 6th or 5th centuries, B.C. The writings of Suśruta and Charaka formed the groundwork of all the Hindu medical and surgical systems which followed. The Suśruta Samhita is divided into six books and contains a fairly accurate description of the human body, besides some surgery. This work was first published in the West in the Latin translation of Franz Hessler (1799-1890), 5 vols., Erlangen, 1844-55.

6485.94 ———. An English translation of the Suśruta Samhita...translated and edited by K. K. BHISHAGRATNA. 2nd ed. Varanasi, *Chowkhamba Sanskrit Series Office,* 1963.

6486 BHAGVAT SIN HJEE, *Maharajah of Gondal.* 1865-1944
A short history of Aryan medical science. London, *Macmillan & Co.*, 1890. 2nd ed., Gondal, 1927, reprinted 1977.

6486.1 JOLLY, JULIUS.
Medicin. Grundriss der Indoarabischen Philologie und Altertumskunde. III. Band, 10. Heft. Strassburg, *K.J. Trübner,* 1901.

6487 HOERNLE, AUGUST FRIEDRICH RUDOLPH. 1841-1918
Studies in the medicine of ancient India. Part 1. Osteology or the bones of the human body. Oxford, *Clarendon Press,* 1907.
All published.

6488 MUKHOPADHYAYA, GIRANDRANATH. 1872-1935
The surgical instruments of the Hindus, with a comparative study of the surgical instruments of the Greek, Roman, Arab and the modern Eouropean [sic] surgeons. 2 vols. Calcutta, *University Press,* 1913-1914.
Vol. 2 consists of plates.

6488.1 ———. History of Indian medicine. 3 vols. Calcutta, *Univ. of Calcutta,* 1923-29. Reprinted New Delhi, 1974.

6489 BURMA. *Public Health Department.*
Report of the Committee of Enquiry into the Indigenous System of Medicine. Rangoon, *Supdt. Govt. Printing,* 1931.

6490 MARIADASSOU, PARAMANANDA.
Médecine traditionelle de l'Inde. Conférences faites à l'Ecole de Médecine de Pondichéry ... Préface de M. GEORGES BOURRET. 3 vols. [in 1]. Pondichéry, *Imp. Ste. Anne,* 1934-35.

6491 ZIMMER, HENRY ROBERT. 1890-1943
Hindu medicine. Edited with a foreword and preface by LUDWIG EDELSTEIN. Baltimore, *Johns Hopkins Press,* 1948.

6491.1 KUTUMBIAH, P.
Ancient Indian Medicine. Bombay, *Orient Longmans,* 1962.
Revised edition, Bombay, 1969.

6491.2   SANYAL, Promode Kumar.
A story of medicine and pharmacy in India. Pharmacy 2000 years ago and after. Calcutta, *Sanyal*, 1965.
A short history of the four systems of medicine practised in India today.

6491.9   ANONYMOUS
Les secrets de la Medicine des chinois, consistant en la parfaite connoissance du pouls. Envoyez de la Chine par un françois, homme de grand merite...Grenoble, *Philippes Charuys*, 1671.
The first Western book on Chinese medicine, with a few brief comments on Japanese methods. This anonymous collection of translations of early Chinese texts on pulse medicine has been variously attributed to different Jesuits working in China at the time.

6492   CLEYER, Andreas. *fl.* 1650
Specimen medicinae Sinicae. Francofurti, *J. P. Zubrodt*, 1682.
One of the earliest studies of Chinese medicine published in the West. (*See also* Nos.6472.10 *et seq.*). Cleyer edited these translations of Chinese medical texts, reproducing a series of 30 plates dealing with Chinese pulse-lore. Acu-tracts are illustrated but no acu-points. The book concerns Chinese doctrines of the pulse rather than acupuncture. Abridged English translation in No. 2670.

6492.1   BOYM, Michal Piotr [Dziurdzi-Boïm]. 1612-1659
Clavis medica ad Chinarum doctrinam de pulsibus...in lucem Europaeam produxit...Andreas Cleyerus...[Nuremberg], 1686.
Translations of Chinese treatises on pulse medicine with illustrations of hands and wrists to illustrate pulse-taking. The texts published here are different from those published by Cleyer in No. 6492. Previously published in *Misc. cur. Acad. Nat. Cur.* (Nürnberg), Dec. II, 4, 1686, 1-144.

6492.2   DABRY DE THIERSANT, Pierre.
La médicine chez les chinois. Corrigé et précédé d'une préface par M.J. Léon Soubeiran. Paris, *Henri Plon*, 1863.
The best account of Chinese medicine published in Europe during the 19th century, including translations from original Chinese medical texts. Dabry was French consul at Hang-Keou. Soubeiran, a physician, edited his work for publication.

6493   WONG, K. Chimin. 1889-1972, & WU LIEN-TEH. 1879-1959
History of Chinese medicine. Tientsin, *Tientsin Press*, [1932].
The writers spent 15 years in the compilation of this work, the first important contribution to the history of Chinese medicine for Western readers. Beginning with demonology, plant lore and folk medicine, the writers deal with the subject from the earliest times to the present. They tell of the high standards attained by the Chinese in the 8th century B.C., of the effect of Confucianism upon the development of surgery, of the "doctrine of the pulse", of Chinese pharmacy and acupuncture, and of the establishment of Western medicine in present day China. Second edition, Shanghai, *National Quarantine Service*, 1936, reprinted, New York, *AMS Press*, 1973.

6494   MORSE, WILLIAM REGINALD. 1874-1939
Chinese medicine. New York, *P.B. Hoeber*, 1934.

6495   HUME, EDWARD HICKS. 1876-1957
The Chinese way in medicine. Baltimore, *Johns Hopkins Press*, 1940.

6495.1   HUARD, PIERRE ALPHONSE. 1901-1983, & WONG, MING. 1926-
La médecine chinoise au cours des siècles. Paris, *Roger Dacosta* [1959].
English translation by B. Fielding, London, 1968.

6495.2   PORKERT, MANFRED.
The theoretical foundations of Chinese medicine. Systems of correspondence. Cambridge, Mass., *Massachusetts Institute of Technology Press*,
[1974].

6495.3   LU, GWEI-DJEN, and NEEDHAM, JOSEPH. 1900-
Celestial lancets: a history and rationale of acupuncture and moxa. Cam-
bridge, *Cambridge University Press*, [1980].
A section of Needham's *Science and civilisation in China* series,
separately published. Includes the best bibliography and analysis of early
Western treatises on Chinese medicine.

6495.4   UNSCHULD, PAUL ULRICH. 1943-
Medicine in China: a history of ideas. Berkeley, *University of California
Press*, [1985].
The first comprehensive and analytical history of therapeutic concepts
and practices in China, encompassing all aspects of Chinese medicine over
3500 years. Approximately one third of the work consists of primary texts
in translation.

TIBET

6495.5   KORVIN-KRASINSKI, P. CYRILL VON.
Die tibetische Medizinphilosophie. Der Mensch als Mikrokosmos. Zürich,
Origo, 1953.
2nd edition, 1965.

6495.6   RECHUNG, JAMPAL KUNZANG, *Rinpoche*.
Tibetan medicine, illustrated in original texts. London, *Wellcome Institute
for the History of Medicine*, 1973.

JEWISH: BIBLICAL

6495.7   MAIMON, MOSHE BEN [MAIMONIDES]. 1135/38-1204
[Incipit] Incipiunt aphorismi excellentissimi Raby Moyses secundum
doctrinam Galieni medicorum principis. [Venice, *Franciscus de Benedictis
for Benedictus Hector*, 1489].
The most popular and influential medical work of the most famous of
early Jewish physician/philosophers. This is a collection of aphorisms
derived from Galen, and divided into 24 topics. In the 25th and final
chapter Maimonides discusses Galen's teleological ideas from the Biblical
standpoint. *See also* No. 53.

6495.8   ———.The medical writings of Moses Maimonides, edited by Suessman
Muntner. Philadelphia, *J.B. Lippincott*, [1963-]
The following volumes have been published: *Treatise on asthma*
(1963), *Treatise on poisons and their antidotes* (1966), *Treatise on
hemorrhoids* with *Medical answers (responsa)* (1969).

6496   BARTHOLIN, THOMAS. 1616-1680
De morbis biblicis miscellanea medica. 2nd ed. Francofurti, *D. Paulli*, 1672.
A study of the diseases mentioned in the Bible.

6496.1   COHN, TOBIAS BEN MOSES [COHEN]. 1652-1729
Ma'aseh Tuviyyah [Works of Tobias]...Hebrew text. [Venice, *Stamperia
Bragadina*, [1708].
The only significantly illustrated early book on medicine in Hebrew.
This is an encyclopaedia, of which approximately half concerns medicine.
One of the first Jews from the Eastern ghetto to obtain a medical education
at a German university, Cohn completed his degree at Padua, and served
as court physician to the Turkish Sultan.

6496.2   LANDAU, RICHARD. 1864-1903
Geschichte der jüdischen Ärzte. Ein Beitrag zur Geschichte der Medicin.
Berlin, *S. Karger*, 1895.

6497   EBSTEIN, WILHELM. 1836-1912
Die Medizin im Alten Testamente. Stuttgart, *Enke*, 1901.

6498   PREUSS, JULIUS. 1861-1913
Biblisch-talmudische Medizin. Berlin, *S. Karger*, 1911.
3rd edition, 1923. Translated as *Biblical and Talmudic medicine.
Translated by Fred Rosner.* New York, *Sanhedrin Press*, 1978, with enlarged index and expanded references.

6499   BRIM, CHARLES JACOB. 1891-
Medicine in the Bible. The Pentateuch, Torah. New York, *Froben Press*,
1936.
References to medicine in the Old Testament, with notes and definitions,
and references to the Talmud.

6500   KAGEN, SOLOMON ROBERT. 1881-1955
Jewish medicine. Boston, *Medico-Historical Press*, 1952.

6501   SHORT, ARTHUR RENDLE. 1880-1953
The Bible and modern medicine: a survey of health and healing in the Old
and New Testaments. London, *Paternoster Press*, 1953.

6501.1   FRIEDENWALD, HARRY. 1864-1950
The Jews and medicine. Jewish luminaries in medical history. 3 vols. New
York, *Ktav Publishing House*, 1967.
First published 1944-46. Vol. 1 includes a classified bibliography of
ancient Hebrew medicine.

6501.2   FRAZIER, CLAUD ALBEE. 1920-
Through the Bible with a physician. Springfield, *C.C. Thomas* , 1971.

6501.3 ROSNER, FRED.
Medicine in the *Mishneh Torah* of Maimonides. New York, *Ktav Publishing*, [1984].

6502 WÜSTENFELD, HEINRICH FERDINAND. 1808-1899
Geschichte der arabischen Aerzte und Naturforscher. Göttingen, *Vandenhoeck & Ruprecht*, 1840.
Reprinted 1963.

6503 BERTHERAND, EMILE LOUIS.
Médecine et hygiène des Arabes. Etudes sur l'exercise de la médecine et de la chirurgie chez les Musulmans de l'Algérie ... Précédées de considérations sur l'état général de la médecine chez les principales nations Mahométanes. Paris, *Baillère*, 1855.

6504 DJELAL ED-DIN, ABOU SOLEIMAN DAOUD.
La médecine du Prophète. Traduit par N. PERRON, Paris, *Baillère*, 1860.
First appeared in *Gaz. méd. d'Algerie*, 1859, **4**.

6505 LECLERC, LUCIEN. 1816-1893
Histoire de la médecine arabe. Exposé complet des traductions du grec. Les sciences en Orient, leur transmission à l'Occident par les traductions latines. 2 vols. Paris, *E. Leroux*, 1876.
An exhaustive history of Arabian medical translations from East to West and *vice versa*. Reprint, New York, 1963.

6506 OPITZ, ADOLF HERMANN KARL. 1877-
Die Medizin im Koran. Stuttgart, *F. Enke*, 1906.

6507 BROWNE, EDWARD GRANVILLE. 1862-1926
Arabian medicine. Cambridge, *Univ. Press*, 1921.
FitzPatrick Lectures, 1919-20. Browne, an eminent authority on oriental languages, became professor of Arabic in the University of Cambridge. Reprint 1962.

6508 HILTON-SIMPSON, MELVILLE WILLIAM. 1881-1938
Arab medicine and surgery. A study of the healing art in Algeria. London, *Oxford Univ. Press*, 1922.
An interesting account of medicine, surgery and pharmacology as practised among the nomadic Arabs in Algeria at the present time.

6509 CAMPBELL, DONALD. -1949
Arabian medicine and its influence on the Middle Ages. 2 vols. London, *Kegan Paul*, 1926.
A survey of the Arabian medical writings of the Eastern and Western Caliphates. The second volume includes a list of translators into Latin of Arabic works and a reconstruction of the Galenic library.

6510 KHAIRALLAH, AMIN ASAD.
Outline of Arabic contributions to medicine and the allied sciences. Beirut, *American Press*, 1946.

6510.01   ULLMANN, MANFRED.
Die Medizin im Islam. Leiden, *E.J. Brill*, 1970.
See also Ullman, *Islamic medicine*, Edinburgh,1978.

6510.1   EBIED, RIFAAT Y.
Bibliography of medieval Arabic and Jewish medicine and allied sciences.
London, *Wellcome Institute for the History of Medicine*, 1971.

6510.2   SEZGIN, F.
Geschichte des arabischen Schriftums. Band 3. Medizin-Pharmazie,
Zoologie-Tierheilkunde. Leiden, *E.J. Brill*, 1971.

6510.3   HADDAD, SAMI I. 1890-1957
History of Arab medicine. Beirut, [*Privately printed,*] 1975.

6510.4   BRANDENBURG, DIETRICH.
Islamic miniature painting in medical manuscripts. Basel, *Editiones "Roche"*,
[1982].

PERSIA

6511   FONAHN, ADOLF. 1873-1940
Zur Quellenkunde der persischen Medizin. Leipzig, *J.A. Barth*, 1910.

6512   FICHTNER, HORST. 1893-
Die Medizin im Avesta. Leipzig, *Pfeiffer*, 1924.

6513   NAFICY, ABBAS. 1905-
La médecine en Perse des origines à nos jours. Ses fondements théoriques
d'après l'Encyclopédie médicale de Gorgani. Paris, *Editions Vega*, 1933.

6514   ELGOOD, CYRIL LLOYD. 1892-1970
Medicine in Persia. New York, *P.B. Hoeber*, 1934.

6515   ——. A medical history of Persia and the Eastern Caliphate from the
earliest times until the year A.D. 1932. Cambridge, *University Press*, 1951.
A continous history of the art and practice of medicine in Persia and
bordering countries from the earliest times. Reprinted, with additions and
corrections from the author's copy: edited by G. van Heusden. Amsterdam, *APA-Philo Press*, 1979.

MEDIEVAL

6516   HECKER, JUSTUS FRIEDRICH KARL. 1795-1850
Die Tanzwuth, eine Volkskrankheit im Mittelalter. Berlin, *T.C.F. Enslin*,
1832.
A study of the dancing mania of the Middle Ages. An English translation
(*see* No. 1678) appeared in 1835.

6517   ——. Kinderfahrten, eine historisch-pathologische Skizze. Berlin, *A.W.
Schade*, 1845.

6518   RENZI, Salvator de. 1801-1871
         Storia documentata della scuola medica di Salerno. 2nd. ed. Napoli,
         Nobile, 1857.
             Reprinted, Milan, *Ferro*, 1967. An account of the School is provided by
         P.O. Kristeller in *Bull. Hist. Med.*, 1945, **17**, 138-94.

6519   HENSLOW, George. 1835-1925
         Medical works of the fourteenth century; together with a list of plants
         recorded in contemporary writings, with their identification. London,
         Chapman & Hall, 1899.

6519.1   CLAY, Rotha Mary.
         The mediaeval hospitals of England. London, *Metheun* [1909].
             Reprinted London 1966.

6520   WALSH, James Joseph. 1865-1942
         Old time makers of medicine. The story of the students and teachers of the
         sciences related to medicine during the Middle Ages. New York, *Fordham
         Univ. Press*, 1911.

6521   ——. Medieval medicine. London, *A. & C. Black*, 1920.

6522   LARSEN, Henning.
         An old Icelandic medical miscellany. MS. Royal Irish Academy 23 D 43,
         with supplement from MS. Trinity College (Dublin) L.2.27. Oslo, *Dybwad*,
         1931.

6523   RIESMAN, David. 1867-1940
         The story of medicine in the Middle Ages. New York, *P.B Hoeber*, 1935.

6524   MacKINNEY, Loren Cary. 1891-1963
         Early medieval medicine with special reference to France and Chartres.
         The Hideyo Noguchi Lectures. Baltimore, *Johns Hopkins Press*, 1937.

6524.2   MacKINNEY, Loren Cary. 1891-1963
         Medical illustrations in medieval manuscripts. London, *Wellcome His-
         torical Medical Library*, 1965.

6524.3   GRAPE-ALBERS, Heide.
         Spätantike Bilder aus der Welt des Arztes. Medizinische Bilderhand-
         schriften der Spätantike und ihre mittelalterliche Überlieferung. Wiesbaden,
         Guido Pressler, 1977.

6524.4   SIRAISI, Nancy G.
         Taddeo Alderotti and his pupils. Two generations of Italian medical
         learning. Princeton, *Princeton University Press*, 1981.

6524.5   JONES, Peter Murray.
         Medieval medical miniatures. Austin, *University of Texas Press*, [1985].

AUSTRIA

6525   HIRSCHEL, Bernhard. 1815-1874
Compendium der Geschichte der Medicin von den Urzeiten bis auf die
Gegenwart, mit besonderer Berücksichtigung der Neuzeit und der Wiener
Schule. 2te Aufl. Wien, *Braumüller*, 1862.

6526   PUSCHMANN, Theodor. 1844-1899
Die Medicin in Wien während der letzten 100 Jahre. Wien, *M. Perles*, 1884.

6527   NEUBURGER, Max. 1868-1955
Die Entwicklung der Medizin in Oesterreich. Wien, *C. Fromme*, 1918.

6528   ———. Das alte medizinische Wien in zeitgenössischen Schilderungen.
Wien, *M. Perles*, 1921.

6529   SCHOENBAUER, Leopold. 1888-1963
Das medizinische Wien: Geschichte, Werden, Würdigung. 2nd ed. Wien,
Urban & Schwarzenberg, 1947.

6529.1 BREITNER, Burghard. 1884-
Geschichte der Medizin in Österreich. Wien, *Rohrer*, 1951.
        Forms Bd. 226 Heft 5, of *Österr. Akad. Wiss., Sitzungsber. Phil.-hist. Kl.*

6529.2 LESKY, Erna. 1911-1986
Die Wiener medizinische Schule im 19. Jahrhundert. Graz, *Verlag
Böhlaus*, 1965.
        English translation, Baltimore, 1976.

BELGIUM: FLANDERS: NETHERLANDS

6530   BROECKX, Corneille. 1807-1869
Essai sur l'histoire de la médecine belge avant le XIXe siècle. Grand, *L.
Hebbelynck*, 1837.

6531   ———. Coup d'oeil sur les institutions médicales belges, depuis les dernières
années du dix-huitième siècle jusqu'à nos jours, suivie de la Bibliographie
de cette époque. Bruxelles, *Soc. Encyclographique des Sciences Médicales*,
1841.

6532   FAIDHERBE, Alexandre Joseph. 1867-
Les médecins et les chirurgiens de Flandre avant 1789. Lille, *Danel*, 1892.

6533   BAUMANN, Evert D.
Uit drie eeuwen Nederlands geneeskunde. Amsterdam, *Meulenhoff*, 1951.

6533.1 LINDEBOOM, Gerrit Arie. 1905-1986
A classified bibliography of the history of Dutch medicine 1900-1974. The
Hague, *Martinus Nijhoff*, 1975.

6533.2 SONDERVORST, François André. 1909-
Histoire de la médecine belge. Zaventem, *Elsevier Librico*, 1981.

6534   COCKAYNE, THOMAS OSWALD. 1807-1873
Leechdoms, wortcunning, and starcraft of early England. 3 vols. London, *Longman*, 1864-66.
     One of the most important pieces of medical scholarship that has so far appeared from the pen of an English writer. Written by a clergyman, it contains a vast amount of material on Western barbarian medicine and on the Anglo-Saxon language. It contains the Herbal of Apuleius, in Anglo-Saxon English, the Leech Book of Bald, etc. Reprinted, 1961.

6535   PAYNE, JOSEPH FRANK. 1840-1910
English medicine in the Anglo-Saxon times. Oxford, *Clarendon Press*, 1904.
     FitzPatrick Lectures, 1903.

6536   MOORE, *Sir* NORMAN. 1847-1922
The history of the study of medicine in the British Isles. Oxford, *Clarendon Press*, 1908.
     FitzPatrick Lectures, 1905-06.

6537   ——. The physician in English history. Cambridge, *Univ. Press*, 1913.
     Linacre Lecture, 1913.

6537.1   CAMERON, *Sir* CHARLES ALEXANDER. 1857-1921
A history of the Royal College of Surgeons in Ireland and of the Irish schools of medicine, including a medical bibliography and a medical biography. 2nd ed. Dublin, *Fannin & Co.*, 1916.

6538   CHAPLIN, THOMAS HANCOCK ARNOLD. 1864-1944
Medicine in England during the reign of George III. London, *The Author*, 1919.
     FitzPatrick Lectures, 1917-18.

6539   SINGER, CHARLES JOSEPH. 1876-1960
Early English magic and medicine. London, *H. Milford*, [1920].
     Reprinted from *Proc. Brit. Acad.*, 1919-20, **9**, 341-74.

6540   POWER, *Sir* D'ARCY. 1855-1941
Medicine in the British Isles. New York, *P.B. Hoeber*, 1930.
     Clio Medica series.

6541   COMRIE, JOHN DIXON. 1875-1939
History of Scottish medicine. 2nd. ed. 2 vols. London, *Baillère, Tindall & Cox*, 1932.
     Traces fully and accurately the history of medicine in Scotland from the earliest times.

6544   COLLIS, WILLIAM ROBERT FITZGERALD. 1900-
The state of medicine in Ireland. Carmichael prize essay. Dublin, *Parkside Press*, 1943.

6545   FLEETWOOD, JOHN.
History of medicine in Ireland. Dublin, *Browne & Nolan Ltd.*, 1951.
     Second edition, Dublin, *Skellig Press*, 1983.

6546   GRATTAN, JOHN HENRY GRAFTON. 1878-1951, & SINGER, CHARLES JOSEPH. 1876-1960
Anglo-Saxon magic and medicine. London, *Oxford University Press*, 1952.

6548   DAVIDSON, MAURICE. 1883-1967
The Royal Society of Medicine: The realization of an ideal (1805-1955). London, *Royal Society of Medicine*, 1955.

6548.1   COPE, *Sir* VINCENT ZACHARY. 1881-1974
The Royal College of Surgeons of England: A history. London, *Blond*, 1959.

6548.2   COPEMAN, WILLIAM SYDNEY CHARLES. 1900-1970
Doctors and disease in Tudor times. London, *W. Dawson*, 1960.

6549   BONSER, WILFRID. 1887-1971
The medical background of Anglo-Saxon England; a study in history, psychology, and folklore. London, *Wellcome Historical Medical Library*, 1963.

6550   WALL, CECIL. 1869-1947, *et al.*
A history of the Worshipful Society of Apothecaries of London. Abstracted and arranged from the MS notes of Cecil Wall by H. Charles Cameron; revised, annotated and edited by E. ASHWORTH UNDERWOOD. Vol. 1: 1617-1815. London, *Wellcome Historical Medical Museum*, 1963.

6550.1   CLARK, *Sir* GEORGE NORMAN. 1890-1978
A history of the Royal College of Physicians of London. 3 vols. Oxford, *Clarendon Press*, 1964-72.
    Vol. 3 is by A.N. Cooke.

6550.2   POYNTER, FREDERICK NOEL LAWRENCE. 1908-1979
The evolution of hospitals in Britain. Edited by F. N. L. Poynter. London, *Pitman*, 1964.
    14 papers delivered at the 3rd British Congress on the History of Medicine and Pharmacy, 1962, and a classified bibliography of British hospital history by E. Gaskell (pp. 225-79).

6550.3   TALBOT, CHARLES HOLWELL.
Medicine in medieval England. London, *Oldbourne Press*, 1967.

6550.4   GIBSON, WILLIAM CARLETON. 1913-
British contributions to medical science. The Woodward–Wellcome symposium, University of British Columbia, 1970.
London, *Wellcome Institute of the History of Medicine*, 1971.

6550.5   THOMSON, *Sir* ARTHUR LANDSBOROUGH. 1890-
Half a century of medical research. 2 vols. London, *H. M. Stationery Office*, 1973-75.
    The origins, policy and programme of the (British) Medical Research Council.

6550.6   CULE, JOHN.
Wales and medicine. An historical survey from papers given at the Ninth British Congress on the History of Medicine. Edited by J. CULE. Llandysul, Dyfed, *Gomer Press*, 1975.

6550.7   WEBSTER, CHARLES.
         The great instauration. Science, medicine and reform, 1626-1660. New
         York, *Holmes & Meier*, [1976].

6551   CRAIG, WILLIAM STUART McRAE. 1903-1975
         History of the Royal College of Physicians of Edinburgh. Oxford, *Blackwell*,
         1976.

6551.1   CULE, JOHN
         Wales and medicine. A source-list for printed books showing the history
         of medicine in relation to Wales and Welshmen. Aberystwyth, *National
         Library of Wales*, 1980.

6551.2   HAMILTON, DAVID NINIAN HAY.
         The healers: a history of medicine in Scotland. Edinburgh, *Canongate*, 1981.

6551.3   O'BRIEN, EOIN, & CROOKSHANK, ANNE.
         A portrait of Irish medicine. An illustrated history of medicine in Ireland.
         Dublin, *Ward River Press*, [1984].
             Published for the bicentenary of the Royal College of Surgeons in
         Ireland. With Sir Gordon Wolstenholme.

6551.4   GOTTFRIED, ROBERT S.
         Doctors and medicine in medieval England 1340-1530. Princeton, *Princeton
         University Press*, [1986].
             A social, cultural, and intellectual history of medicine and medical
         practitioners between the Black Death and the foundation of the Royal
         College of Physicians.

                            CZECHOSLOVAKIA

6552   VINAR, JOSEF.
         Obrazy z minulosti českého lěkarstvi. Praha, *Státni Zdravotnické
         Nakladatelstvi*, 1959.

6553   VOJTOVA, MARIE, *et al*
         Dějiny československeho lekařstvi. Svazek 1. Do r. 1740. Praha, *Avicenum*,
         1970.

                                FRANCE

6554   WICKERSHEIMER, CHARLES ADOLPHE ERNEST. 1880-1965
         La médecine et les médecins en France à l'époque de la Renaissance. Paris,
         Maloine, 1906.
             Wickersheimer, librarian of University of Strasbourg, contributed sev-
         eral scholarly works on the history of medicine.

6555   LAIGNEL-LAVASTINE, MAXIME. 1875-1953, & MOLINÉRY, RAYMOND. 1876-
         1946
         French Medicine. Translated by E.B. KRUMBHAAR. New York, *P.B. Hoeber*,
         1934.
             Clio Medica series.

6555.1   DELAUNAY, Paul. 1878-1958
La vie médicale aux XVIe, XVIIe et XVIIIe siècles. Paris, *Editions Hippocrate*, 1935.

6556   GUIART, Jules. 1870-1945
Histoire de la médecine française: son passé, son présent, son avenir. Paris, *Editions Nagel*. 1947.

6556.1   PECKER, André.
La médecine à Paris du XIIIe au XXe siecle. [Paris,] *Editions Hervas*, [1984].
A collective work, edited by Pecker, superbly illustrated.

GERMANY

6558   HIRSCH, August. 1817-1894
Geschichte der medicinischen Wissenschaften in Deutschland. München, *Oldenbourg*, 1893.
Reprinted, Hildesheim, 1966.

6559   STICKER, Georg. 1860-1960
Die Entwickelung der ärztlichen Kunst in Deutschland. München, *Münchner Drucke*, 1927.

6560   HABERLING, Wilhelm Gustav Moritz. 1871-1940
German medicine. Translated by Jules Freund. New York, *P.B. Hoeber*, 1934.
Clio Medica series.

HUNGARY

6560.1   GORTVAY, György
Az újabbkori magyar orvosi müvelödés és egészégügy története. I Kötet. Budapest, *Akadémiai Kiadó*, 1953.

ITALY

6561   RENZI, Salvatore de. 1801-1971
Storia della medicina italiana. 5 vols. Napoil, tipog. del. *Filiatre-Sebezio*, 1845-48.
Reprinted Bologna, 1966.

6562   PITRÈ, Giuseppe. 1842-1916
Medicina popolare siciliana. Torino, *Clausen*, 1896.
English translation, Lawrence, Kansas, *Coronado Press*, 1971.

6563   CASTIGLIONI, Arturo. 1874-1953
Italian medicine. Translated by E. B. Krumbhaar. New York, *P.B. Hoeber*, 1932.
Clio Medica series.

6564   ——. The renaissance of medicine in Italy ... The Hideyo Noguchi Lectures. Baltimore, *Johns Hopkins Press*, 1934.

6565   PAZZINI, ADALBERTO. 1898-1975
Bibliografia di storia della medicine italiana. Roma, *Tosi*, 1939.
    Classified list of 7451 books and papers, some annotated, on Italian medical history and biography. Reprinted 1946.

6565.01   PERUTA, FRANCO DELLA.
Storia d'Italia. Vol. 7: Malattia e medicina. Torino, *Giulio Einaudi*, [1984].
    A collective work, edited by della Peruta.

6565.02   SIRAISI, NANCY G.
Avicenna in Renaissance Italy. The *Canon* and medical teaching in Italian Universities after 1500. Princeton, *Princeton University Press*, 1987.

MALTA

6565.1   CASSAR, PAUL.
Medical history of Malta. London, *Wellcome Historical Medical Library*, 1964.

RUSSIA: U.S.S.R.

6566   RICHTER, WILHELM MICHAEL VON. 1767-1822
Geschichte der Medicin in Russland. 3 vols. Moskwa, *N.S. Wsewolojsky*, 1813-17.

6567   GANTT, WILLIAM ANDREW HORSLEY. 1892-1980
Russian medicine. New York, *P. B. Hoeber*, 1937.

6569   SIGERIST, HENRY ERNEST. 1891-1957
Medicine and health in the Soviet Union. New York, *Citadel Press*, 1947.

6569.1   ORGANESIAN, LEON A.
Istoriia meditsiny v Armenii s drevneishikh vremen do nashikh dnei. 5 vols. Erevan, *Akademiia nauk Armanskoi SSSR*, 1946-47.
    Supplement, *Illustratskii k istorii meditsiny v Armenii*, Erevan, 1958

6569.2   ROSSIISKII, DMITRI M.
Istoriia vseobshchei i otechestvennoi meditsiny i zdravookhraneniia: Bibliografica (996-1954gg). Moskva, *Medgiz*, 1956.

6569.3   VASIL'EV, KONSTANTIN GEORGIEVICH. *et al.*
Materialy po istorii meditsiny i zdravookhraneniia Latvii. Riga, *Latviiskoe Gosud. Izd.-vo.*, 1959.
    With F.F. Grigorash and A. A. Krauss. Revised abridged version by Vasil'ev and Grigorash, Moscow, 1964.

SCANDINAVIA

6570   INGERSLEV, JOHAN VILHELM CHRISTIAN. 1835-1918
Danmarks Laeger og Laegevaesen fra de aeldste Tider indtil Aar 1800. 2 vols. Kjobenhavn, *E. Jespersen*, 1873.

6571   CARØE, Kristian Frederik. 1851-1921
Den Danske Laegestand, 1749-1900. 5 vols. Kobenhavn, *Gyldendal*, 1905-22
   Biographies of Danish physicians and surgeons. Supplements about
every ten years.

6572   LENNMALM, Frithiof. 1858-1924
Svenska Läkaresällskapets historia 1808-1908. Stockholm, *I. Marcus*, 1908.
   Continued (1908-38) by Gunnar Nilson, Stockholm, *General-Statens
litograf. Anstalt*, 1947.

6573   LAACHE, Soren Bloch. 1854-1941
Norsk medicin i hundrede aar. Kristiania, *Steenske Bogtrykkeri*, 1911.

6574   QVIGSTAD, Just knud. 1853-
Lappische Heilkunde. Oslo, *H. Aschehoug*, 1932.

6574.1   REICHBORN-KJENNERUD, Ingjald. 1865-1949, *et al.*
Medisinens historie i Norge. Oslo, *Grondal*, 1936.

6574.2   BONSDORFF, Bertel von. 1904-
The history of medicine in Finland 1828-1918. Helsinki, *Societas Scientarium
Fennica* , 1975.

6575   CHINCHILLA Y PIQUERAS, Anastasio. 1801-1867
Anales históricos de la medicina en general, y biografico-bibliográficos de
la española en particular. 8 vols. Valencia, *Lopez, Cervera*, 1841-46.
   Includes No. 6576, together with *Historia particular de las operaciones
quirúrgicas*, 1841; *Historia general de la medicina*, 2 vols. 1841-43; and
Vade mecum histórico y bibliográfico, etc., 1844. Facsimile reproduction,
1964.

6576   ——. Historia de la medicina española. 4 vols. Valencia, *Lopez, Cervera*,
1841-46.
   Forms Vols. 3-6 of No. 6575.

6576.1   HERNÁNDEZ MOREJØN, Antonio. 1773-1836
Historia bibliográfica de la medicina española. 7 vols. Madrid, 1842-52.
   Reprinted, New York, 1967.

6577   LEMOS, Maximiano Augusto d'Oliveira. 1860-1923
História da medicina em Portugal. 2 vols. Lisboa, *M. Gomes*, 1899.

6578   COMMENGE Y FERRER, Luis. 1854-1916
La medicina en Cataluña (bosquejo histórico). Barcelona, *Henrich*, 1908.

6579   GARCIA DEL REAL, Eduardo. 1870-1947
Historia de la medicina en España. Madrid, *Editorial Reus*, 1921.

6579.1   FERREIRA DE MIRA, Matias Boleto. 1875-
História da medicina portuguesa. Lisboa, *Empresa Nacional de Publicidade*,
1947.

6579.2   GRANJEL, Luis S.
Bibliográfia história de la medicina española. 2 vols. Salamanca, *Univ. Salamanca*, 1965-66.
A bibliography covering Spain and the former South American colonies.

6579.3   ———. Historia general de la medicina española. Vol. 1-4. Salamanca, *Ed. Universidad de Salamanca*, 1987-81.
Vol. 1: Ancient and medieval; Vol. 2: Renaissance; Vol. 3: 17th century; Vol.. 4: 18th century.

SWITZERLAND

6580   GAUTIER, Léon. 1853-1916
La médecine à Genève jusqu'à la fin du dix-huitième siècle. Genève, *Jullien*, 1906.

6581   BRUNNER, Conrad. 1859-1927
Über Medizin und Krankenpflege im Mittelalter in Schweizerischen Landen. Zürich, *Füssli*, 1922.

6581.1   BUESS, Heinrich.
Schweizer Aerzte als Forscher, Entdecker und Erfinder. Basel, *Ciba Aktiengesellschaft*, 1945.

YUGOSLAVIA

6581.2   GRMEK, Mirko Dražen.
Bibliographia medica Croatica. Hrvatska medicinska bibliografija. 2 vols. Zagreb, *Jugoslovenske Akad. Znanosti i Umjelnosti u Zagrebu*, 1955-70.
Croatian medical, pharmaceutical and veterinary bibliography; Dio 1, Sr. I, 1470-1875; Sr. II, 1875-1918.

CANADA

6582   CANNIFF, William. 1830-1910
The medical profession in Upper Canada, 1783-1850. Toronto, *W. Briggs*, 1894.
Rescues from oblivion many historical facts and discusses the pioneer medical men of Canada. Biographies of many famous physicians of Canada are included. Reprinted Toronto, 1980.

6583   HEAGERTY, John Joseph. 1879-
Four centuries of medical history in Canada. 2 vols. London, *Simpkin Marshall*, 1928.
The authoritative work on the history of medicine in Canada.

6584   HOWELL, William Boyman. 1873-
Medicine in Canada. New York, *P.B. Hoeber*, 1933.

6584.1   ROLAND, Charles G. 1933-
Secondary sources in the history of Canadian medicine. A bibliography. Waterloo, Ontario, *Wilfred Laurier University Press*, 1984.

This work is complemented by C.G. Roland and P. Potter, *An annotated bibliography of Canadian medical periodicals, 1826-1975*, Toronto, *Hannah Institute*, 1979.

6584.2   ROLAND, CHARLES G. 1933- (Ed.)
Health, disease and medicine. Essays in Canadian history. Toronto, *Hannah Institute*, 1984.

6584.9   THACHER, JAMES. 1574-1844
A military journal during the American Revolutionary War, from 1775-1783...Boston, *Richardson & Lord*, 1823.
The first American medical historian, Thacher gave the best contemporary account of medicine during the Revolutionary War, as well as an important history of the war in general. *See* No. 6710.

6585   TONER, JOSEPH MEREDITH. 1825-1896
Contributions to the annals of medical progress and medical education in the United States before and during the War of Independence. Washington, *Govt. Printing Office*, 1874.

6586   CLARKE, EDWARD HAMMOND, *et al.* 1820-1877
A century of American medicine 1776-1876. By EDWARD H. CLARKE, H.J. BIGELOW, S.D.GROSS, T. GAILLARD THOMAS and J.S BILLINGS. Philadelphia, *H.C.Lea*, 1876.

6588   BLANTON, WYNDHAM BOLLING. 1890-1960
Medicine in Virginia in the seventeenth (eighteenth, nineteenth) century. 3 vols. Richmond, *W. Byrd Press; Garrett & Massie*, 1930-33.

6590   PACKARD, FRANCIS RANDOLPH. 1870-1950
History of medicine in the United States. 2nd. ed. 2 vols. New York, *P. B. Hoeber*, 1931.
An authoritative source-book of the history of medicine in the United States. The first edition appeared in 1901. Dr. Packard edited the *Annals of Medical History* from its commencement in 1917 until its decease in 1942. Reprinted, New York, *Hafner*, 1963.

6592   SIGERIST, HENRY ERNEST. 1891-1957
Amerika und die Medizin. Leipzig, *G. Thieme*, 1933.
This is not a systematic history of American medicine, but an account of the most important landmarks in the development of medical science and teaching in the United States. An English translation, *American Medicine*, was published in New York in 1934.

6594   COBB, W. MONTAGUE.
The first Negro medical society. A history of the Medico-Chirurgical Society of the District of Columbia. Washington, D.C. *The Associated Publishers*, 1939.
A detailed history of the "first American Negro medical society formed in America and probably in the world". Also probably the first history concerning black physicians. Cobb is the first black American medical historian of note.

6595   SHRYOCK, RICHARD HARRISON. 1893-1972
       American medical research, past and present. New York, *Commonwealth Fund,* 1947.

6596   GORDON, MAURICE BEAR. 1916-
       Aesculapius comes to the Colonies. The story of the early days of medicine in the thirteen original colonies. Ventnor, N.J., *Ventnor Publishers,* 1949.

6596.1 POSTELL, WILLIAM DOSITE. 1908-1982
        The health of slaves on southern plantations. Baton Rouge, *Louisiana State Press,* 1951.
        Chiefly from contemporary MS records.

6596.2 SHRYOCK, RICHARD HARRISON. 1893-1972
        Medicine in America: historical essays. Baltimore, *Johns Hopkins Press,* 1966.

6596.3 BORDLEY, JAMES. 1900- , & HARVEY, ABNER MCGEHEE, 1911-
        Two centuries of American medicine 1776-1976. Philadelphia, *W.B. Saunders,* 1976.
        A valuable supplement to Packard (No. 6590), besides covering the main events in American medicine.

6596.4 CASH, PHILIP *et al.*
        Medicine in colonial Massachusetts, 1620-1820. [Edited by PHILIP CASH, ERIC H. CHRISTIANSON and J. WORTH ESTES.] Boston, *Colonial Society of Massachusetts,* [1980].
        A well-illustrated collection of essays covering medicine in Massachusetts but also applicable in some cases to the history of medicine and surgery throughout the American colonies.

6596.5 HALLER, JOHN H., JR.
        American medicine in transition, 1840-1910. Urbana, Ill., *University of Illinois Press,* [1981].

6596.6 STARR, PAUL.
        The social transformation of American medicine. New York, *Basic Books,* 1982.

6596.61 ROSENBERG, CHARLES E.
         The care of strangers: The rise of America's hospital system. New York, *Basic Books,* 1987.

6596.62 RUTKOW, IRA MICHAEL. 1948-
         The history of surgery in the United States. Vol. 1: Textbooks, monographs and treatises. San Francisco, *Norman Publishing,* 1988.

CARIBBEAN

6596.9 PARSONS, ROBERT P.
        History of Haitian medicine. New York, *Paul Hoeber,* 1930.

6597   FLORES, Francisco A.
Historia de la medicina en México desde la epoca de los Indios hasta la presente. 3 vols. México, 1886-88.

6598   SCHIAFFINO, Rafael. 1881-
Historia de la medicina en el Uruguay. 3 vols. Montevidoe, *Imprenta Nacional, "Rosgal"*, 1927-52.

6599   RIBEIRO, Leonidio.
Brazilian medical contributions. Rio de Janeiro, *Livraria José Olympio*, 1939.

6600   MOLL, Aristides Alcibiades. 1882-
Aesculapius in Latin America. Philadelphia, *Saunders*, 1944.

6601   SANTOS, Lycurgo de Castro.
Historia da medicina no Brasil. (Do século XVI ao século XIX). 2 vols. São Paulo, *Edit. Brasiliense*, 1947.

6601.1   REINA VALENZUELA, José.
Bosquejo histórico de la farmacia y la medicina en Honduras. Tegucigalpa, *Ariston*, 1947.

6602   LASTRES Y QUINONES, Juan B. 1902-1960
Historia de la medicina peruna. 3 vols. *Lima, Imprenta Santa Maria*, 1951.

6602.1   PERERA, Ambrosio.
Historia de la medicina en Venezuela. Caracas, *Imprenta Nacional*, 1951.
      Comprehensive account to end of ninteenth century.

6603   GUERRA, Francisco. 1916-
Historiografia de la medicina colonial hispanoamericana. México, *Abastecedora de Impresos*, 1953.

6603.1   BALCÁZAR, Juan Manuel. 1894-
Historia de la medicina en Bolivia. La Paz, *Ediciones Juventud*, 1956.

6603.2   SOMOLINOS D'ARDOIS, Germán. 1911-
Historia y medicina; figuras y hechos de la historiografia médica mexicana. México, *Imprenta Universitaria*, 1957.

6603.3   ARCHILA, Ricardo. 1909-
Historia de la medicina en Venezuela. Epoca colonial. Caracas, *Tip. Vargas*, 1961.

6603.4   PAREDES BORJA, Virgilio.
Historia de la medicina en el Ecuador. 2 vols. Quito, *Casa de la Cultura Ecuatoriana*, 1963.

6603.5   MARTINEZ DURAN, Carlos. 1906-1974
Las ciencias médicas en Guatemala: origen y evolución. 3rd ed. Guatemala, *Editorial Universitaria*, 1964.

6603.6   ROIG DE LEUCHSENRING, EMILIO. 1889-
Médicos y medicina en Cuba. Historia, biografia, costumbrismo. La
Habana, *Acad. Ciencias de Cuba*, 1965.

6603.7   CORTÉS, FERNANDO MARTÍNEZ
Historia general de medicina en México. Tomo I- México, Universidad
Nacional Autónoma de México, 1984- .
     A collective work under the general editorship of Cortés.

JAPAN

6604   WHITNEY, WILLIS NORTON.
Notes on the history of medical progress in Japan. Yokohama, *Meiklejohn*,
1885.
     From *Trans. Asiatic Soc. Japan*, 1885, **12**, 245-469.

6604.1   FUJIKAWA, YU. 1865-1940
Geschichte der Medizin in Japan. Tokyo, 1911.
     History of Japanese medicine from the earliest times to 1911.Expanded
English translation, New York, 1934.

6604.2   BOWERS, JOHN Z. 1913-
Western medical pioneers in feudal Japan. Baltimore, *Johns Hopkins Press*,
[1970].
     Covers the influence of Western medicine on Japan from the seventeenth
century through 1870.

6604.3   HUARD, PIERRE. 1901-1983, *et al.*
La médecine japonaise des origines à nos jours. Paris, *Roger Dacosta*, 1974.
     With Z. Ohya and Ming Wong.

6604.31   BOWERS, JOHN Z. 1913-
When the twain meet. The rise of western medicine in Japan. Baltimore,
Johns Hopkins Press, [1980].
     Suppl. to *Bull. Hist. Med.*, new ser., 5.

PHILIPPINES

6604.39   BANTUG, JOSÉ POLICARPIO. 1884-
A short history of medicine in the Philippines during the Spanish regime.
1565-1898. Manila, *Colegio Médico-Famacéutico de Filipinas*, 1953.

INDONESIA

6604.4   SCHOUTE, DIRK. 1873-
Occidental therapeutics in the Netherlands East Indies during three centuries of Netherlands settlement. 1600-1900. Batavia, *Netherlands Indies
Public Health Service*, 1937.
     An English summary of two earlier Dutch works by D. Schoute, 1929-
1936.

6604.5   LAIDLER, Percy Ward & GELFAND, Michael. 1912/13-1985
           South Africa; its medical history 1652-1898. Cape Town, *C. Struik*, 1971.

6604.6   GANDEVIA, Bryan. 1925-
           An annotated bibliography of the history of medicine in Australia. Glebe,
           N.S.W., *Australasian Medical Publishing Co.*, 1955.
               Revised and enlarged as *An annotated bibliography of the history of
           medicine and health in Australia.* Sydney, *Royal Australian College of
           Physicians*, 1984. With A. Holster and S. Simpson.

6604.7   FORD, *Sir* Edward. 1902-
           Bibliography of Australian medicine 1790-1900. Sydney, *University Press*,
           1976.
               2567 annotated entries providing a complete record for all printed
           works on the subject, including topics such as nursing, dentistry, etc.

6604.8   GANDEVIA, Brian. 1925-
           Tears often shed. Child health and welfare in Australia from 1788. Rushcutters
           Bay NSW, *Pergamon Press*, [1978].

6604.81   PEARN, John Hemsley & O'CARRIGAN, Catharine.
           Australia's quest for colonial health. Some influences on early health and
           medicine in Australia. Brisbane, Dept. of Child Health, *Royal Children's
           Hospital*, [1983].
               A collective work edited by Pearn and O'Carrigan.

6604.82   PEARN, John Hemsley.
           Pioneer medicine in Australia. Brisbane, *Amphion Press, [University of
           Queensland]*, [1988].
               Twenty illustrated essays by various authors, edited by Pearn.

See also ANATOMY and ANTHROPOLOGY

6604.90   MOEHSEN, Johann Karl Wilhelm. 1722-1795
           Verzeichnis einer Samlung von Bildnissen, gröstentheils berühmter Aerzte.
           Berlin, *Himburg*, 1771.
               "Very valuable reports on artistic anatomy and the history of anatomic
           illustration" (Choulant).

6604.91   CAMPER, Pieter. 1722-1789
           Redevoeringen over die wijze om de verscheidene hartstogten op onze
           wezens te verbeelden...Utrecht, *bij Wild en Altheer*, 1792.
               Lectures on the methods of representing the passions in the human
           face, and on other aspects of medicine and the arts. German translation,
           Berlin, 1793. *See* No. 158.

6604.92   BELL, *Sir* Charles. 1774-1842
Essays on the anatomy of expression in painting. London, *Longman*, 1806.
     Bell's artistic and literary skills combined with his knowledge of anatomy and physiology to make this work a *tour de force* of art history and the anatomical and physiological basis of facial expression.

6604.93   LORDAT, Jacques. 1773-1870
Essai sur l'iconologie médicale, ou sur les rapports d'utilité qui existent entre l'art du dessin et l'étude de la médecine. Montpellier, *Veuve Picot*, 1833.
     Pioneering study of art and medicine based on collections at Montpellier.

6604.94   FABRE, François. 1797-1853
Némésis médicale illustrée. 2 vols., Paris, *Bureau de la Gazette des Hôpitaux*, 1840.
     The only medical book illustrated by Honoré Daumier (1808-79), and a great satire in verse on the medical profession.

6605   CHARCOT, Jean Martin. 1825-1893, & RICHER, Paul Marie Louis Pierre. 1849-1933
Les démoniaques dans l'art. Paris, *A. Delahaye & E. Lecrosnier*, 1887.
     Charcot was a talented artist; he collaborated with Richer, artist at La Salpêtrière, in the production of interesting books on disease and deformity as portrayed by artists, books which have put the study of medicine in relation to art upon a sound footing. Reprinted, Amsterdam, *B.M. Israël*, 1972.

6606   ———. Les difformes et les malades dans l'art. Paris, *Lecrosnier & Babé*, 1889. Reprinted Amsterdam, *B.M. Israël*, 1972

6607   RICHER, Paul Marie Louis Pierre. 1849-1933
L'art et la médecine. Paris, *Gaultier & Cie.*, 1902.

6608   HOLLÄNDER, Eugen. 1867-1932
Die Medizin in der klassischen Malerei. Stuttgart, *F. Enke*, 1903.
     4th edition, 1950 (a re-impression of 3rd edition, 1923).

6608.1   FREUD, Sigmund. 1856-1939
Eine Kindheitserinnerung des Leonardo da Vinci. Leipzig, *F. Deuticke*, 1910.
     The first psychoanalytic investigation in art.

6609   HOLLÄNDER, Eugen. 1867-1932
Plastik und Medizin. Stuttgart, *F. Enke*, 1912.

6609.1   ———. Wunder, Wundgeburt und Wundergestalt in Einblattdrucken des 15.:-18. Jahrhunderts. Stuttgart, *Ferdinand Enke*, 1922.
     History of teratology in art from 15th to 18th centuries.

6610   VETH, Cornelis. 1880-
De arts in de caricatuur. Amsterdam, *Van Munster*, [c. 1925].
     German edition, Berlin, 1927.

6610.1   CABANÈS, Augustin. 1862-1928
Esculape chez les artistes. Paris, *Le François*, 1928.

Chapters and illustrations on deformities, infirmities, medicine, surgery, etc.

6610.2   HECKSCHER, William S.
Rembrandt's Anatomy of Dr. Nicholas Tulp. An iconological study. Washington Square, *New York University Press*, 1958.
    An important supplement to and revision of this work is W. Schupbach, The paradox of Rembrandt's 'Anatomy of Dr. Tulp'. *Med. Hist.* Suppl. 2, 1982.

6610.3   WOLSTENHOLME, *Sir* Gordon. 1913-
The Royal College of Physicians of London: portraits. London, *J. & A. Churchill,* 1964.
    Descriptions of the portraits by D. Piper. Wolstenholme and J.F. Kerslake edited Vol. 2 of the study, with essays by R. Ekkart and D. Piper, Oxford, *Elsevier,* 1977.

6610.4   HERRLINGER, Robert. 1914-1968
Geschichte der medizinische Abbildung. 2nd ed. 2 vols. München, *Moos,* 1967-72.
    A history of medical illustration, with the emphasis on anatomy. Vol.2 edited by Marielene Putscher, covers the subject from 1600 to the present. English translation of Vol. 1 (to 1600), London, *Pitman,* 1970.

6610.5   SCHOUTEN, Jan.
The rod and serpent of Asklepios: Symbol of medicine. Amsterdam, *Elzevier,* 1967.

6610.6   WOLF-HEIDEGGER, Gerhard and CETTO, Anna Maria.
Die anatomische Sektion in bildlicher Darstellung. Basel, *S. Karger,* 1967.
    Full descriptions and illustrations of 355 of the most important paintings, prints, sculpture, and book illustrations concerning anatomy in its widest sense.

6610.7   ROUSSELOT, Jean.
Medicine in art: a cultural history. Jean Rousselot, general editor. New York, *McGraw-Hill*, [1967].

6610.8   VOGT, Helmut.
Das Bild des Kranken. Die Darstellung äusserer Veränderungen Durch innere Leiden und ihrer Heilmassnahmen von der Renaissance bis in unsere Zeit. München, *J.F. Lehmanns Verlag*, [1969].

6610.9   BAUER, Veit Harold.
Das Antonius-Feuer in Kunst und Medizin. Berlin, *Springer-Verlag*, 1973.
    Superbly designed and illustrated with colour plates. *Sitzungsberichte der Heidelberger Akademie der Wissenschaften, Mathematisch-naturwissenschaftliche Klasse,* Supplement zum Jahrgang 1973.

6610.10   BURGESS, Renate.
Portraits of doctors & scientists in the Wellcome Institute of the History of Medicine. A catalogue. London, *Wellcome Institute of the History of Medicine,* 1973.

6610.11   DOHERTY, TERENCE.
The anatomical works of George Stubbs. Boston, *David R. Godine*, [1975].
Reproduces all of the known anatomical drawings of the painter,
George Stubbs (1724-1806), together with his midwifery illustrations and
the text and plates for his work on anatomy of the horse. (No. 308.1).

6610.12   BUCCI, MARIO.
Anatomia come arte. 2nd ed. Firenze, *Edizioni d'Arte il Fiorino*, [1976].
Includes spectacular colour plates of 19th-century wax models and
earlier sculptures concerning anatomy.

6610.13   THEOPOLD, WILHELM.
Votivmalerie und Medizin. Kulturgeschichte und Heilkunst im Spiegel der
Votivmalerei. München, *Verlag Karl Thiemig*, [1978].

6610.14   HELFAND, WILLIAM H.
Medicine and pharmacy in American political prints (1765-1870). Madison,
American Institute of the History of Pharmacy, 1978.

6610.15   GERDTS, WILLIAM H.
The art of healing. Medicine and science in American art. Birmingham,
Alabama, *Birmingham Museum of Art*, 1981.

6610.16   DUMAITRE, PAULE.
La curieuse destinée des planches anatomiques de Gerard de Lairese,
peintre en Hollande – Lairesse, Bidloo, Cowper. Amsterdam, *Rodopi*, 1982.

6610.17   SCHMIDT-VOIGT, JÖRGEN.
Russiche Ikonenmalerie und Medizin. Zugleich eine Einführung in die
Konographie. 2., Überarbeitete Auflage. München, *Karl Thiemeg AG*, [1983].

6610.18   KARP, DIANE R. 1948-
Ars medica: art, medicine, and the human condition. Philadelphia,
Philadelphia Museum of Art, [1985].
Fully annotated and illustrated catalogue of an exhibition of paintings,
prints, drawings, book illustrations, and photographs.

COSTUME IN MEDICINE

6611   CABANÈS, AUGUSTIN. 1862-1928
Le costume du médecin en France des origines au XVIIe siècle. Paris,
Longuet, [1921].

6612   ———. Le costume du médecin à l'étranger. Paris, *Longuet*, [c. 1925].

LITERATURE AND MEDICINE

6612.90   BROWNE, *Sir* THOMAS. 1605-1682
Religio medici. [London,] Andrew Crooke, 1642.
The most famous work of English literature written by a physician.
Browne did not intend to have it published, but manuscripts of the work

circulated privately. Two unauthorized and inaccurate editions were issued surreptitiously by the same publisher in the same year.

6613   BARTHOLIN, THOMAS. 1616-1680
De medicis poetis dissertatio. Hafniae, *apud D. Paulli*, 1669.

6614   MENIÈRE, PROSPER. 1799-1862
Etudes médicales sur les poètes latins. Paris, *Baillière*, 1858.

6615   BUCKNILL, *Sir* JOHN CHARLES. 1817-1897
The medical knowledge of Shakespeare. London, *Longman*, 1860.

6615.1   CONOLLY, JOHN. 1794-1866
A study of Hamlet. London, *E. Moxon*, 1863.
      The first psychiatric study of Hamlet.

6616   CHÉREAU, ACHILLE. 1817-1885
Le Parnasse médicale français. Paris, *A. Delahaye*, 1874.
      Dictionary of French medical poets.

6617   FLETCHER, ROBERT. 1823-1912
Medical lore in the older English dramatists and poets exclusive of Shakespeare. *Johns Hopk. Hosp. Bull.*, 1895, **6**, 73-84.
      Fletcher, who was born in Bristol, England, assisted J.S. Billings in the creation of the *Index-Catalogue* (No. 6763).

6618   MOYES, JOHN. 1848-1895
Medicine and kindred arts in the plays of Shakespeare. Glasgow, *J. MacLehose*, 1896.

6619   HOLLÄNDER, EUGEN. 1867-1932
Die Karikatur und Satire in der Medizin. Stuttgart, *F. Enke*, 1905.
      An encyclopaedic collection of medical wit and caricature of all ages. Second edition, 1921.

6620   BLANCHARD, RAPHAEL ANATOLE ÉMILE. 1857-1919
Épigraphie médicale. 2 vols. Paris, 1909-15.

6621   PIA, PASCAL.
Bouquet poëtique des médecins, chirurgiens, dentistes et apothicaires. Paris, *Coll de l'Ecritoire*, 1933.

6622   YEARSLEY, PERCIVAL MACLEOD, 1867-1951
Doctors in Elizabethan drama. London, *John Bale*, 1933.

6622.1   KEATS, JOHN. 1795-1821.
John Keats's anatomical and physiological note book...edited by MAURICE BUXTON FORMAN. [London,] *Oxford University Press*, 1934.
      Keats was a pupil and dresser at Guy's Hospital from 1815-16, and was licensed to practise upon completion of his studies. While struggling to launch his poetic career he was often tempted to practise medicine, but never did so.

6623 McDONOUGH, Mary Lou McCarthy.
Poet physicians: an anthology of medical poetry written by physicians. Springfield, *C.C. Thomas*, 1945.

6623.01 THOMAS, Dylan. 1914-1953
The doctor and the devils. London, *Dent*, 1953.
The great lyric poet's screenplay based on the notorious career of Robert Knox, the anatomist who purchased bodies for dissection from the resurrectionists/murderers, Burke and Hare. This was the first screenplay to be published before the film was produced.

6623.1 SIMPSON, Robert Ritchie.
Shakespeare and medicine. Edinburgh, *E.& S. Livingstone*, 1959.

6623.2 PENFIELD, Wilder Graves. 1891-1976
The torch. Boston, *Little, Brown*, 1960.
A romantic and inspirational historical novel about Hippocrates by the great Canadian neurological surgeon.

6623.3 DEWHURST, Kenneth. 1919-1985, and REEVES, Nigel.
Friedrich Schiller: Medicine, psychology and literature. With the first English edition of his complete medical and psychological writings. Berkeley, *University of California Press*, 1978.
The medical writings of Johann Christoph Friedrich von Schiller (1759-1805) and their influence on his poetry and plays.

6623.4 TRAUTMANN, Joanne, & POLLARD, Carol.
Literature and medicine. An annotated bibliography. Revised edition. Pittsburgh, *University of Pittsburgh Press*, [1982].
Annotated bibliography of medical references in Western literature from the ancient world to time of writing. Emphasis is on summaries of the medical content. Editions cited are usually modern and always in English.

6623.50 RODIN, Alvin E. and KEY, Jack D.
Medical case book of Doctor Arthur Conan Doyle. Melbourne, Fl., *Krieger*, 1983.
The first complete book on the medical aspects of the Sherlock Holmes stories as well as the non-fiction writings of Conan Doyle.

6623.51 KAIL, Aubrey C.
The medical mind of Shakespeare. Melbourne, *Williams & Wilkins-Adis*, [1986].

6623.52 RODIN, Alvin E., & KEY, Jack D.
Medicine, literature, and eponyms: Encyclopaedia of medical eponyms derived from literary characters. Malabar, Fl., *Krieger*, 1989.

MAGIC AND SUPERSTITION

6624 MAGNUS, Hugo Friedrich. 1842-1907
Der Aberglauben in der Medicin. Breslau, *M. Müller*, 1903.
English translation, 1905.

6625 MERCIER, CHARLES ARTHUR. 1852-1919
Astrology in medicine. London, *Macmillan*, 1914.

6626 SELIGMANN, SIEGFRIED. 1870-1926
Die magischen Heil- und Schutzmittel aus der unbelebten Natur. Stuttgart, *Strecker & Schröder*, 1927.

6627 VILLIERS, ELIZABETH.
Amulette und Talismane und andere geheime Dingen. München, *Drei Masken Verlag*, 1927.

6627.1 BUDGE, *Sir* ERNEST ALFRED THOMPSON WALLIS. 1857-1934
Amulets and superstitions: the original texts with translations and descriptions. London, *Oxford University Press*, 1930.
  Reprinted, 1961.

6628 MOON, ROBERT OSWALD. 1865-1953
Medicine and mysticism. London, *Longmans, Green & Co.*, 1934.

6629 THOMPSON, CHARLES JOHN SAMUEL. 1862-1943
Magic and healing. London, *Rider*, [1947].

MUSIC AND MEDICINE

6631.01 ROGER, JOSEPH-LOUIS. *d.* 1761.
Tentamen de vi soni et musices in corpus humanorum. Avenione, *Apud Jacobum Garrigan*, 1758.
  The first significant work on music and medicine. The best edition is the French translation by E. Sainte-Marie, augmented with 96pp. of notes: *Traité des effets de la musique sur le corps humain*. Paris, *Brunot*, An XI (1803).

6631.02 MARMELSZADT, WILLARD. 1919-
Musical sons of Aesculapius. New York, *Froeben Press*, 1946.

6631.1 SCHULLIAN, Dorothy May. 1906-1989, & SCHOEN, Max. 1888-
Music and medicine. Edited by DOROTHY M. SCHULLIAN and MAX SCHOEN. New York, *Schuman*, 1948.

MEDICAL NUMISMATICS

6631.90 KLUYSKENS, HIPPOLYTE.
Des hommes célèbres dans les sciences et les arts, et des médailles qui consacrent leur souvenir. 2 vols., Gand, *Leonaard Hebbelynck*, 1859.

6632 GARRISON, FIELDING HUDSON. 1870-1935
Medical numismatics. *Ann. med. Hist.*, 1926, **8**, 128-35.
  An excellent short paper on the subject, with references to the more important previous work.

6633 STORER, HORATIO ROBINSON. 1830-1922
Medicina in nummis. A descriptive list of the coins, medals, jetons relating to medicine, surgery and the allied sciences. Boston, *Wright & Potter Print Co.*, 1931.
This consists mainly of a catalogue of 6,000 medals collected by Storer, an eminent Boston gynaecologist. The collection is now in the Countway Medical Library, and the book, edited by M. Storer, includes some excellent reproductions, a select bibliography, and a short résumé of the subject.

6633.1 HOLZMAIR, EDUARD.
Katalog der Sammlung Dr. Josef Brettauer Medicina in Nummis. Wien, *J. Weimar*, 1937.
5557 items; references to works on numismatics and medical history.

6633.2 NEWMAN, SARAH ELIZABETH.
Medals relating to medicine and allied sciences in the numismatic collection of The Johns Hopkins University. Baltimore, *The Evergreen House Foundation*, 1964.
Full descriptions of 922 items; some illustrated.

NURSING

6634 HAESER, HEINRICH. 1811-1884
Geschichte christlicher Krankenpflege und Pflegerschaften. Berlin, *W. Hertz*, 1857.
Reprinted, Bad Reichenhall, *Kleinert*, 1966.

6635 NUTTING, MARY ADELAIDE. 1858-1948. & DOCK, LAVINIA LLOYD. 1858-1956
A history of nursing. 4 vols. New York, *G.P Putnam*, 1907-12.
Vols. 3-4 by L.L Dock only.

6636 JENSEN, DEBORAH MacLURG. 1900-
History of nursing. St Louis, *C. V. Mosby Co.*, 1943.
Second edition, *History and trends of professional nursing*, 1950.

6637 PAVEY, AGNES ELIZABETH. 1889-
The story of the growth of nursing as an art, a vocation, and a profession. Fifth edition. London, *Faber & Faber*, 1959.

6638 SHRYOCK, RICHARD HARRISON. 1893-1972
The history of nursing; an interpretation of the social and medical factors involved. Philadelphia, *W.B. Saunders*, 1959.

6639 ABEL-SMITH, BRIAN. 1926-
A history of the nursing profession. London, *Heinemann*, 1960.
Covers England and Wales only.

6639.1 THOMPSON, ALICE MARY CHARLOTTE. 1907-1981
A bibliography of nursing literature, 1859-1960. London, *Library Association for Royal College of Nursing*, 1968.
Includes sections on history and biography. Supplement 1961-70, 1974.

6639.11 DONAHUE, M. PATRICIA.
Nursing: the finest art. An illustrated history. St. Louis, *C.V. Mosby Co.*, 1985.
The most elaborately illustrated history available.

6639.12 BULLOUGH, VERN L.
American nursing: A biographical dictionary. New York, *Garland Publishing*, 1988.
Edited with O.M. Church and A.P. Stein.

6639.13 KAUFMAN, MARTIN
Dictionary of American nursing biography. Westport, Conn., *Greenwood Press*, 1988.
Edited with J.W. Hawkins, L.P. Higgins, and A.H. Friedman.

PHILATELY

6639.2 BISHOP, WILLIAM JOHN. 1903-1961, & MATHESON, NORMAN MURDOCH. 1897-1977
Medicine and science in postage stamps. London, *Harvey & Blythe*, 1948.

QUACKERY

6640 MAGNUS, HUGO FRIEDRICH. 1842-1907
Das Kurpfuscherthum. Breslau. *M. Müller*, 1905
History of quackery in medicine.

6641 ———. Die Kurierfreiheit und das Recht auf den eigenen Körper. Ein geschichtlicher Beitrag zum Kampf gegen das Kurpfuschertum. Breslau. *M. Müller*, 1905.

6643 THOMPSON, CHARLES JOHN SAMUEL. 1862-1943
The quacks of old London. London, *Brentano's* (1928).

6643.1 JAMESON, ERIC.
The natural history of quackery. London, *Michael Joseph*, 1961.

6643.2 YOUNG, JAMES HARVEY.
The medical messiahs. A social history of health quackery in twentieth-century America. Princeton, *Princeton University Press*, 1967.

RELIGION AND PHILOSOPHY IN RELATION TO MEDICINE

6643.9 GLOVER [EDDY], MARY BAKER. 1821-1910
Science and health. Boston, *Christian Science Publishing Company*, 1875.
Includes an exposition of the system of faith healing that holds a significant place in Christian Science.

6644 ALLBUTT, *Sir* THOMAS CLIFFORD. 1836-1953
Science and mediaeval thought. London, *C.J. Clay & Sons*, 1901.

6645 MOON, ROBERT OSWALD. 1865-1953
The relation of medicine to philosophy. London, *Longmans, Green*, 1909.

6646   CRAWFURD, *Sir* RAYMOND HENRY PAYNE. 1865-1938
The king's evil. Oxford, *Clarendon Press*, 1911.
    FitzPatrick Lectures, 1911. A classic account of the history of touching for the "king's evil", scrofula, a practice of kings from ancient times until the 18th century.

6647   MOON, ROBERT OSWALD. 1865-1953
Hippocrates and his successors in relation to the philosophy of their time. London, *Longmans, Green & Co.*, 1923.

6648   PAZZINI, ADALBERTO. 1899-1975
I santi nella storia della medicina. Roma, *Casa Ed. "Mediterranea"*, 1937.

6649   MAJOR, RALPH HERMON. 1884-1970
Faiths that healed. New York, *Appleton*, 1940.

WOMEN IN MEDICINE

6649.90   BLACKWELL, ELIZABETH. 1821-1910
Medicine as a profession for women. New York, *Trustees of the New York Infirmary for Women*, 1860.

6649.91   JEX-BLAKE, SOPHIA LOUISA. 1840-1912
Medical Women: Two essays. I. Medicine as a profession for women. II. Medical education for women, Edinburgh, *Oliphant*, 1872.
    From the time of her admission to medical school Jex-Blake became virtually the leader of the movement in Great Britain to open the medical profession to women. Greatly expanded second edition, Edinburgh, 1886.

6649.92   BLACKWELL, ELIZABETH. 1820-1910
Pioneer work in opening the medical profession to women; autobiographical sketches. London and New York, *Longmans, Green & Co.*, 1895.
    Blackwell led the movement in America to open the medical profession to women.

6649.93   LIPINSKA, MÉLANIE.
Histoire des femmes médecins depuis l'antiquité jusqu'à nos jours. Paris, *G. Jacques*, 1900.

6650   HURD-MEAD, KATE CAMPBELL. 1867-1941
A history of women in medicine from the earliest times to the beginning of the nineteenth century. Haddam, Conn., *Haddam Press*, 1938.
    Most complete and authentic work so far available upon the subject.

6650.1   SCHÖNFELD, WALTHER. 1888-1977
Frauen in der abendländischen Heilkunde, vom klassischen Altertum bis zum Ausgang des 19. Jahrhunderts. Stuttgart, *F. Enke*, 1947.

6650.2   LOVEJOY, ESTHER POHL. 1869-1967
Women doctors of the world. New York, *Macmillan*, 1957.

6650.3 CHAFF, Sandra L., *et al.*
Women in medicine: a bibliography of the literature on women physicians. Metuchen, N.J., *Scarecrow Press*, 1977.
Lists over 4,000 items published between 1750 and 1975. With R. Haimbach, C. Fenichel and N. B. Woodside.

SELECT LIST OF PERIODICALS
SPECIALIZING IN THE HISTORY OF MEDICINE

A comprehensive list of current periodicals specializing in the history of medicine and science was published in *Current Work in the History of Medicine,* No. 15, pp. 239-42, 1957, with supplementary lists in later issues.

6651 ACTA HISTORICA SCIENTIARUM NATURALIUM ET MEDICINALIUM.
1-, Kobenhavn, Odense, 1942-
Monographic series.

6652 ANNALS OF MEDICAL HISTORY.
1-10; New series, 1-10; 3rd series, 1-4, New York, 1917-42. Index (1917-42), 1946.

6653 ARCHIWUM HISTORII MEDYCYNY.
1- , Poznan, Warszawa, 1924-
Original title, *Archiwum Historii i Filozofii Medycyny;* title shortened 1957.

6654 BULLETIN OF THE HISTORY OF MEDICINE.
7- , Baltimore, 1939-.
Vol. 1-6, 1933-38 entitled *Bulletin of the Institute of the History of Medicine.*

6655 CENTAURUS.
International Magazine of the History of Science and Medicine. 1- , Copenhagen, 1950- .

6656 CLIO MEDICA.
Acta Academiae Internationalis Historiae Medicinae. 1- , Oxford, Amsterdam, 1965-

6657 GESNERUS.
Vierteljahrsschrift für Geschichte der Medizin und der Naturwissenschaften. 1- , Aarau, 1943-

6658 HISTOIRE DE LA MEDICINE.
1- , Paris, 1951- .

6659 ISIS.
1- , Wondelgem-lez-Gand, Bruges, Washington, 1913- .
Official publication of the History of Science Society.

6660   JANUS.
        Archives Internationales pour l'Histoire de la Médecine, 1- , Amsterdam,
        etc., 1896-
            Subtitle changed to Revue Internationale de l'Histoire des Sciences, de
        la Médicine, de la Pharmacie, et dela Technique.

6661   JOURNAL OF THE HISTORY OF BIOLOGY.
        1- , Cambridge, Mass., 1968-

6662   JOURNAL OF THE HISTORY OF MEDICINE AND ALLIED SCIENCES.
        1- , New Haven, 1946-

6662.1 MEDICAL CLASSICS.
        Compiled by Emerson C. Kelly. 1-5. Baltimore, 1936-41.
            Reprints of classic texts, with English translations where necessary.
        Includes biographical notes and full bibliographies.

6663   MEDICAL HISTORY.
        1- , London, 1957-

6664   MEDICINA NEI SECOLI.
        1- , Perugia, Roma, 1964-.

6665   NEUE MÜNCHENER BEITRÄGE ZUR GESCHICHTE DER MEDIZIN UND
        NATURWISSENSCHAFTEN; MEDIZINHISTORISCHE REIHE.
        1- , Munchen, 1970- .
            Monographic series. Continuation of *Münchener Beiträge*, etc., 1-17,
        1926-29.

6666   SUDHOFFS ARCHIV
        Zeitschrift für Wissenschaftsgeschichte. 53- , Wiesbaden, 1969- .
            Formerly *Archiv für Geschichte der Medizin*, 1-20, 1907-28; *Sudhoffs
        Archiv für Geschichte der Medizin (und der Naturwissenschaften)*, 21-52,
        1929-68.

6667   TRANSACTIONS AND STUDIES OF THE COLLEGE OF PHYSICIANS OF
        PHILADELPHIA. MEDICINE AND HISTORY.
        Series V, 1- , Philadelphia. 1979-

6668   CANADIAN BULLETIN OF MEDICAL HISTORY.
        1- , Waterloo, Ontario, 1984-

MEDICAL BIOGRAPHY

6703   MANDOSIO, Prospero. *circa* 1648-1709
        Theatron in quo maximorum Christiani orbis pontifcum
        archiatros...spectandos exhibet. Romae, *Typis Francisco de Lazaris*, 1696.
            The first book on the lives of papal physicians.

6704   ELOY, Nicolas François Joseph. 1714-1788
        Dictionnaire historique de la médecine ancienne et moderne, ou mémoires
        disposés en ordre alphabétique pour servir à l'histoire de cette science, et
        à celle des médecins, anatomistes, botanistes, chirurgiens et chymistes de
        toutes nations. 4 vols. Mons, *H. Hoyois*, 1778.

Earliest exhaustive collection of medical biographies. The first edition of this work appeared in 1775; the above edition is the most useful. Reprinted, Bruxelles, *Culture et Civilisation*, 1973.

6705   AIKIN, JOHN. 1747-1822
Biographical memoirs of medicine in Great Britain from the revival of literature to the time of Harvey. London, *J. Johnson*, 1780.
The first collection of British medical biographies.

6706   MARINI, G.
Degli archiatri pontifici. 2 vols. Roma, 1784.
Biographies of papal physicians.

6707   HUTCHINSON, BENJAMIN.
Biographia medica; or, historical and critical memoirs of the lives and writings of the most eminent medical characters that have existed from the earliest account of time to the present period; with a catalogue of their literary productions. 2 vols. London, *J. Johnson*, 1799.
British and foreign medical biographies.

6708   DICTIONNAIRE DES SCIENCES MÉDICALES.
Biographie médicale. 7 vols. Paris, *C.L.F.Panckoucke*, 1820-25.
Preface signed by A. J. L. Jourdan [1788-1848], to whom the work is by some attributed. Reprinted Amsterdam, *B.M. Israël*, 1967.

6709   MACMICHAEL, WILLIAM. 1784-1839
The gold-headed cane. London, *J. Murray*, 1827.
This charming "autobiography" tells of the adventures of the famous gold-headed cane, successively in the posession of Radcliffe, Mead, Askew, William and David Pitcairn, and Baillie, and then retired to a glass case in the library of the Royal College of Physicians of London. Besides good biographies of the several owners of the cane, the book gives interesting information on the condition of medicine in England in the 18th century. Several good reprints of the book are available; in particular may be mentioned that of 1915 which has an introduction by Osler and a preface by F. R. Packard, and one edited by H.S. Robinson, 1932; facsimile of author's own copy of the 1827 edition published by the Royal College of Physicians of London, 1968.

6709.1   DEZEIMERIS, JEAN EUGENE. 1799-1852, *et al.*
Dictionnaire historique de la médecine ancienne et moderne. 4 vols. Paris, *Bechet Jeune*, 1828-39.
Includes bibliographies of authors cited. With C.P. Ollivier and J. Raige-Delorme.

6710   THACHER, JAMES. 1754-1844
American medical biography. 2 vols. Boston, *Richardson, etc.*, 1828.
Thacher was the first American medical historian.   The above biography is a valuable source of information on the early medical history of the United States. Reprinted, New York, *Da Capo Press*, 1967.

6711   PETTIGREW, THOMAS JOSEPH. 1791-1865
Medical portrait gallery. Biographical memoirs of the most celebrated physicians, surgeons, etc. etc. who have contributed to the advancement of medical science. 4 vols. London, *Fisher, Son & Co., Whittaker & Co.*, [1838]-40.

6711.1   WILLIAMS, STEPHEN WEST. 1790-1855
American medical biography...Greenfield, Mass., *L. Merriam & Co.*, 1845.
   Biographies of American physicians who died after publication of Thacher (No. 6710). Reprint, New York, *Milford House*, 1967.

6712   BAYLE, ANTOINE LAURENT JESSÉ. 1799-1858, & THILLAYE, AUGUST JEAN.
Biographie médicale par ordre chronologique. 2 vols. Paris, *A. Delahaye*, 1855.
   Reprinted, Amsterdam, *B. M. Israël*, 1967.

6715   MUNK, WILLIAM. 1816-1898
The roll of the Royal College of Physicians of London; comprising biographical sketches. Second edition. 3 vols. London, *The College*, 1878.
   "Munk's Roll". Covers the period 1518-1825. Vol.4 (1826-1925), 1955; Vol.5 (1926-65), 1968; Vol. 6 (1966-75), 1982; Vol. 7 (1976-83), 1984; Vol. 8 (1984-88), 1989.

6715.1   ATKINSON, WILLIAM B.
The physicians and surgeons of the United States. Philadelphia, *Charles Robson*, 1878.
   The second edition was entitled, A biographical dictionary of contemporary American physicians and surgeons. Philadelphia, *D.G. Brinton*, 1880.

6716   HIRSCH, AUGUST. 1817-1894
Biographisches Lexikon der hervorragenden Ärzte aller Zeiten und Völker. 6 vols. Wien, Leipzig, *Urban & Schwarzenberg*, 1884-88.
   This is one of the best sources of medical biography up to 1880, with useful bibliographical notes. A revised edition, incorporating a revision of No. 6720, was completed in 1935 and reprinted, Munich, 1962. *See also* No. 6732.

6717   BETTANY, GEORGE THOMAS. 1850-1891
Eminent doctors; their lives and their work. Second edition. 2 vols. London, *J. Hogg*, 1885.
   Deals with British doctors only.

6719   WATSON, IRVING ALLISON. 1849-1918
Physicians and surgeons of America. Concord, *Rep. Press Assoc.*, 1896.

6719.1   BRADFORD, THOMAS L.
The pioneers of homeopathy. Philadelphia, *Boericke & Tafel*, 1897.
   Brief biographies of about 500 homeopathic physicians from all countries who were practitioners prior to 1835.

6720   PAGEL, JULIUS LEOPOLD. 1851-1912
Biographisches Lexikon hervorragender Aerzte des neunzehnten Jahrhunderts. Berlin, Wien, *Urban & Schwarzenberg*, 1901.

Second, revised edition, containing entries from 1880 to 1930, 2 vols., München & Berlin, *Urban & Schwarzenberg*, 1962.

6721   RICHARDSON, *Sir* BENJAMIN WARD. 1828-1896
Disciples of Aesculapius 2. vols. London, *Hutchinson & Co.* 1900.
   Biography of Richardson by Sir Arthur MacNalty, 1950.

6722   OSLER, *Sir* WILLIAM, *Bart*. 1849-1919
An Alabama student, and other biographical essays. London, *Oxford, Univ. Press,* 1908.

6723   JOHNSTON, WILLIAM. 1843-1914
Roll of commissioned officers in the medical service of the British Army. Aberdeen, *University Press,* 1917.
   Covers the period from the accession of George II in 1727 to the formation of the Royal Army Medical Corps, 1898. Reprinted 1968, together with the complementary *List of commissioned medical officers of the Army, Charles II to accession of George II, 1660 to 1727*, by Alfred Peterkin, Aberdeen, University Press, 1925, as vol. 1 of *Commissioned officers in the medical services of the British Army 1660-1960*, ed. by Sir Robert Drew. London, *Wellcome Historical Medical Library,* 1968. Vol. 2 covers the period 1898-1960.

6724   GROTE, LOUIS RUYTER RADCLIFFE. 1886-
Die Medizin der Gegenwart in Selbstdarstellungen. Hrsg. VON L.R. GROTE. Vol. 1-8. Leipzig, *F. Meiner,* 1923-29.

6725   CAPPARONI, PIETRO. 1868-1947
Profili bio-bibliografici di medici naturalisti celebri Italiani dal sec. XVo al sec. XVIIIo. 2 vols. Roma, *Ist. Naz. Med. Farm.*, 1925-28.

6727   GARRISON, FIELDING HUDSON. 1870-1935
Available sources and future prospects of medical biography. *Bull N.Y. Acad. Med.*, 1928, 2 ser., **4**, 586-607.
   Includes a valuable bibliography of sources of medical biography.

6728   KELLY, HOWARD ATWOOD. 1858-1943, & BURRAGE, WALTER LINCOLN. 1860-1935
Dictionary of American medical biography. Lives of eminent physicians of the United States and Canada, from the earliest times. New York, *D. Appleton & Co.*, 1928.
   Reprinted, New York, *Milford House,* 1971.

6729   CRAWFORD, DIROM GREY. 1857-1942
Roll of the Indian Medical Service 1615-1930. London, *W. Thacker & Co.*, 1930.
   Appendix and Errata, 1933.

6730   PLARR, VICTOR GUSTAVE. 1863-1929
Plarr's lives of the Fellows of the Royal College of Surgeons of England. Revised by Sir D'ARCY POWER, with the assistance of W. G. SPENCER and G. E. GASK. 2 vols. Bristol, *John Wright & Sons,* 1930.
   Supplement, 1930-51, by Sir D'Arcy Power and W. R. LeFanu, 1953. Second supplement, 1952-64, by R.H.O.B. Robinson and W. R. LeFanu,

1970. Third supplement. 1965-73 by Sir J. Paterson Ross and W. R. LeFanu, 1981. Fourth supplement, 1974-82 by E.H. Cornelius and S.F. Taylor, 1988.

6731   SACKLEN, JOHAN FREDRIC. 1763-1851, *et al.*
Sveriges läkare-historia ifran Konung Gustaf den I:s till närvarande tid. 1-4 series. Stockholm, *P.A Norstedt & Soner*, 1822-1935.

6732   FISCHER, ISIDOR. 1868-1943
Biographisches Lexikon der hervorragenden Ärzte der letzen fünfzig Jahre. 1 vol. [in 2]. Berlin & Wien, *Urban & Schwarzenberg*, 1932-33.
    A supplement to the *Biographisches Lexikon* compiled by A. Hirsch (No. 6716). Reprinted Munich, 1962. Covers the period 1880-1930.

6733   OLPP, GOTTLIEB. 1872-
    Hervorragende Tropenärzte in Wort und Bild. München, *Otto Gmelin*, 1932.

6734   ROYAL SOCIETY, LONDON.
Obituary notices of Fellows of the Royal Society. Vol. 1-9. London, 1932-54.
    Continued as *Biographical Memoirs of Fellows of the Royal Society*, vol. 1- 1955-

6735   SIGERIST, HENRY ERNEST. 1891-1957
Grosse Aerzte. Leipzig, *J. F. Lehmann*, 1932.
    A series of biographies of the great men in medical history. English translation, New York, 1933, reprinted 1972; second (German) edition, 1954.

6736   WICKERSHEIMER, CHARLES ADOLPHE ERNEST. 1880-1965
Dictionnaire biographique des médecins en France au moyen âge. 2 vols. Paris, *E. Droz*, 1936.
    Supplement by D. Jacquart, Geneva, *Droz*, 1979, containing 600 names.

6737   BAILEY, HAMILTON. 1894-1961, & BISHOP, WILLIAM JOHN. 1903-1961
Notable names in medicine and surgery. London, *H.K. Lewis*, 1944.
    Biographical notes and portraits of men and women whose names are perpetuated in well-known medical eponyms. 3rd. edition 1959.

6739   DOOLIN, WILLIAM. 1887-1962
Wayfarers in medicine. London, *W. Heinemann*, 1947.

6740   LEONARDO, RICHARD ANTHONY. 1895-
Lives of master surgeons. New York, *Froeben Press*, 1948-49.
    One volume and supplement.

6742   MONRO, THOMAS KIRKPATRICK. 1865-1958
The physician as man of letters, science and action. 2nd ed. Edinburgh, *E. & S. Livingstone*, 1951.

6742.1   GILBERT, JUDSON BENNETT. 1895-1950
Disease and destiny. A bibliography of medical references to the famous. London, *Dawsons*, 1962.

6742.2 NOBEL FOUNDATION.
Nobel lectures. Physiology or medicine. 4 vols. Amsterdam, *Elsevier*, 1964-72.
Prize lectures 1901-70, with biographies of prize-winners.

6742.3 TALBOT, CHARLES HOLWELL, & HAMMOND, E. A.
The medical practitioners in medieval England. A biographical register.
London, *Wellcome Historical Library*, 1965.
Precedes Munk's *Roll* (No. 6715) as a biographical record.

6742.4 GRANJEL, LUIS S.
Médicos españoles. Salamanca, *Seminario de História de la medicina
Española, Univ, de Salamanca*, 1967.

6742.5 SOURKES, THEODORE LIONEL. 1919-
Nobel prize winners in medicine and physiology, 1910-1965. London,
New York, *Abelard-Schuman*, 1967.
Gives for each laureate a biographical sketch, description of work and
its consequences, theoretical and practical.

6742.6 DICTIONARY OF SCIENTIFIC BIOGRAPHY.
CHARLES COULSTON GILLISPIE, editor in chief. 16 vols. New York, *Charles
Scribner's Sons*, 1970-80.
Over 5,000 biographies, each with detailed bibliographies of primary and
secondary sources. Medical biographies tend to be of physiologists and
other researchers rather than clinicians. Includes an exhaustive index and
some topical essays. The *Concise dictionary of scientific biography* (New
York, *Scribner's*, [1981]) contains in 1 vol. very useful abridged versions of
all biographies found in the 16 vol. work without the bibliographies.

6742.8 PEEL, *Sir* JOHN HAROLD. 1904-
The lives of the Fellows of the Royal College of Obstetricians and Gy-
naecologists 1929-1969. London, *W. Heinemann Medical Books*, 1976.

6742.9 HOLLOWAY, LISABETH M.
Medical obituaries. American physicians' biographical notices in selected
medical journals before 1907. New York, *Garland Publishing*, 1981.
With E.N. Feind and G.N. Holloway.

6742.10 KAUFMAN, MARTIN.
Dictionary of American medical biography. 2 vols., Westport, Conn.,
Greenwood Press, 1984.
Edited with S. Galishoff and T.L. Savitt.

6742.11 LINDEBOOM, GERRIT ARIE. 1905-1986
Dutch medical biography. A biographical dictionary of Dutch physicians
and surgeons 1475-1975. Amsterdam, *Rodopi*, 1984.

6742.12 MORTON, LESLIE THOMAS. 1907- , & MOORE, ROBERT JOHN. 1939-
A bibliography of medical and biomedical biography. Aldershot, *Scolar
Press, Gower Publishing Co. Ltd.*, 1989.
Collective and individual biographies. Confined to books in English
published in the 19th-20th centuries. Revised and enlarged version of J.L.
Thornton, *A select bibliography of medical biography*. 2nd ed., London, 1970.

1031

MEDICAL BIBLIOGRAPHY

6742.99   CHAMPIER, Symphorien. 1472-1539
De medicine claris scriptoribus in quinque partitus tractatus. *In his* Libelli
duo [Lyon, *J. de Campis*, 1506?].
　　First bibliography of medical literature, and an important early history
of medicine. *See* No. 6376.

6743   GESNER, Conrad. 1516-1565
Bibliotheca universalis, sive catalogus omnium scriptorum locupletissimus,
in tribus linguis. Latina, Graeca, and Hebraica. 3 vols. and appendix.
Tiguri, *apud C. Froschouerum*, 1545-55.
　　This was one of the first attempts at a universal bibliography. Unfor-
tunately the section on medicine (liber xxi) was never published. Osler
used the *Bibliotheca universalis* as one of the models for his own *Bibliotheca
Osleriana*. He placed Gesner in the most important section ("Bibliotheca
prima"), and once remarked: "I am not sure that this fellow should go into
'Prima', but I love him so much that I must put him there. Besides, he is the
Father of Bibliography".

6743.1   LECOQ, Pascal. 1567-1632
Bibliotheca medica. Sive catalogus illorum, qui ex professo artem medicam
in hunc usque annum scriptis illustrarunt. Basileae, *C. Waldkirch*, 1590.
　　The first systematic medical bibliography. Includes an annotated list of
1,224 authors writing in Latin, lists of French, German, and Italian writers,
and other material.

6743.2   SPACH, Israel. 1560-1610
Nomenclator scriptorum medicorum. Hoc est: elenchus eorum qui artem
medicam suis scriptis illustrarunt, secundum locos communes ipsius
medicinae. Francofurti, *impensis Nicolai Bassaei*, 1591.
　　The first attempt at a medical subject bibliography, arranged under very
broad subject headings with indexes of authors and subjects.

6744   LINDEN, Johannes Antonides van der. 1609-1664
De scriptis medicis, libri duo. Amstelredami, *J. Blaeu*, 1637.
　　Van der Linden's book was at the time of its appearance the most
complete medical bibliography yet produced. He issued corrected editions
in 1651 and 1662, and G.A. Mercklin published a considerably expanded
version as *Lindenius renovatus* in 1686.

6744.1   LIPEN, Martin. 1630-1692
Bibliotheca realis medica, omnium materiarum, rerum, et titulorum, in
universa medicina occurrentium. Francofurti ad Moenum, *Johannis
Friderici*, 1679.
　　The first large, well-printed bibliography of medicine, including twice
as many authors as van der Linden (No. 6744). An elaborate subject
anaylsis, with entries arranged alphabetically by subjects, with numerous
cross-references and an author index. This formed part of a six-volume
work covering various sectors of learning from the beginning of printing.

6745   DOUGLAS, James. 1675-1742
Bibliographiae anatomicae specimen, sive catalogus omnium penè
auctorum qui ab Hippocrate ad Harveum re anatomicam ex professo, vel
obiter, scriptis illustrârunt. Londini, *G. Sayes*, 1715.
　　First attempt at a systematic medical bibliography.

6746 BOERHAAVE, HERMAN. 1668-1738
Methodus discendi medicinam. London, 1726.
An introduction to medical literature. The edition of 1751, containing the additions of Haller, is the best.

6746.1 STOLLE, GOTTLIEB. 1673-1744 and KESTNER, CHRISTIAN WILHELM. 1694-1747
Anleitung zur Historie der medicinischen Gelahrheit. Jena, *Meyer*, 1731.
A pioneer history of medical writing, for which the historian, Stolle, collaborated with the medical historian/biographer/bibliographer Kestner.

6747 HALLER, ALBRECHT VON. 1708-1777
Bibliotheca medicinae practicae. 4 vols. Basle, *J. Schweighauser*, Berne, *E. Haller*, 1776-88.
Haller compiled four great bibliographies dealing respectively with botany, anatomy, surgery, and medicine. They formed the most complete reference work of the time, consisting of a classified analysis of over 52,000 publications of all countries. Additions and corrections to Haller's *Bibliothecae* were published by C.G. Murr, *Adnotationes ad bibliothecas Hallerianas*, Erlangen, 1805. A catalogue of Haller's library of 15,000 volumes, preserved in Milan, has been published as M.T. Monti, *Catalogo del fondo Haller della Bibliotheca Nazionale Braidense di Milano*, 9 vols., Milano, 1983-87.

6748 BLUMENBACH, JOHANN FRIEDRICH. 1752-1840
Medicinische Bibliothek. 3 vols. Göttingen, *J. C. Dieterich*, 1783-95.
Includes detailed abstracts of periodical literature.

6749 ———. Introductio in historiam medicinae litterarium. Gottingae, *J. C. Dieterich*, 1786.
An annotated subject biliography, arranged chronologically from antiquity to Blumenbach's time.

6750 PLOUCQUET, WILHELM GOTTFRIED. 1744-1814
Initia bibliothecae medico-practicae et chirurgicae realis sive repertorii medicinae practicae et chirurgiae. 8 vols. Tubingae, *J.G. Cotta*, 1793-97.
The first important classified bibliography of medical literature covering both monographic material and current periodicals.

6750.1 ———. Bibliotheca medico-practica et chirurgica realis recentior sive continuatio et supplementa initiorum bibliothecae medico-practicae et chirurgicae. 4 vols. Tubingae, *J. G. Cotta*, 1799-1803.
Continuation of No. 6750.

6750.2 ———. Literatura medica digesta sive repertorium medicinae practicae, chirurgiae atque rei obstetriciae. 4 vols. Tubingae, *J. G. Cotta*, 1808-9.
A revised edition, with 40,000 additional citations, of Nos. 6750 and 6750.1. A supplement (1 vol.) was published in 1813.

6750.3 REUSS, JEREMIAS DAVID.
Repertorium commentationum a societatibus litterariis editarum. 16 vols. Göttingen, *Dieterich*, 1801-21

A classified subject index to the contents of learned society journals to the end of the 18th century. Vols. 10-16 deal with medicine and surgery. Reprinted, New York, *Franklin*, 1961.

6751   YOUNG, Thomas. 1773-1829
An introduction to medical literature, including a system of practical nosology. Intended as a guide to students, and an assistant to practitioners. London, *B.R.Howlett*, 1813.
The remarkable Thomas Young compiled this bibliography which he considered necessary to a complete medical library. Second edition, 1823.

6752   HAIN, Ludwig Friedrich Theodor. 1781-1836
Repertorium bibliographicum. 2 vols. [in 4]. Stuttgartiae et Tubingae, *J. G. Cotta*, 1826-38.
Alphabetical author-index of 16,299 incunabula. Originally based on the contents of the Munich Hofbibliothek, it was made more useful when W. Copinger published a 3-volume supplement, 1895-1902, which added 6,619 items and corrected 7,000 of the original entries. In 1914, D. Reichling completed a further supplement containing 1,921 items.

6753   CHOULANT, Johann Ludwig. 1791-1861
Handbuch der Bücherkunde für die aeltere Medicin zur Kenntniss der griechischen, lateinischen und arabischen Schriften im ärztlichen Fache und zur bibliographischen Unterscheidung ihrer verschiedenen Ausgaben, Vebersetzungen und Erläuterungen. Leipzig, *L. Voss*, 1828.
This is one of the best check lists of the printed works of the older medical writers. It achieved a second edition in 1841, which was reprinted in 1911, 1926 and 1956.

6754   CALLISEN, Adolph Carl Peter. 1787-1866
Medicinisches Schriftsteller-Lexicon der jetzt lebenden Aerzte, Wundärzte, Geburtschelfer, Apotheker, und Naturforscher aller gebildeten Völker. 33 vols. Copenhagen & Altona, 1830-45.
In 25 vols. and and 8-vol. supplement, Callisen's great medical bibliography gives a complete view of the literature of the period from about 1780 to about 1830, describing over 99,000 items. It is, as Garrison points out, one of the greatest bibliographical achievements of a single man. Reprinted, Nieuwkoop *De Graaf*, 1962-64.

6754.1   ATKINSON, James. 1759-1839
Medical bibliography, A and B. York, *Printed at the Gazette-Office*, 1833.
Although of limited scientific value, this extensively annotated work is the most humorous bibliography of medical literature ever published. Atkinson, surgeon to the Duke of York and senior surgeon to York County Hospital, published this work when he was 74 years old. There is nothing in it to indicate that he ever intended to continue the work beyond the letter B. Most copies were issued with a cancel title, London, *John Churchill*, 1834.

6755   FORBES, *Sir* John. 1788-1861
A manual of select medical bibliography. London, *Sherwood, Gilbert, and Piper*, 1835.
"First serious attempt by anyone in the English-speaking world to give a subject classification for medical literature" (Fulton). This was first

published in volume 4 of *Cyclopaedia of practical medicine*, edited by Forbes, A. Tweedie, and J. Conolly, 4 vols., London, *Sherwood*, 1833-34.

6756   CHOULANT, JOHANN LUDWIG. 1791-1861
Bibliotheca medico-historica: sive, catalogus librorum historicorum de re medica et scientia naturali systematicus. Lipsiae, *W. Engelmann*, 1842.
    Additamenta, by Julius Rosenbaum, 2 parts, 1842-47. Reprinted (without *Additamenta*), 1960.

6757   ——. Graphische Incunabeln für Naturgeschichte und Medicin. Enthaltend Geschichte und Bibliographie des ersten naturhistorischen und medicinischen Drucke des XV. und XVI. Jahrhunderts, welche mit illustrirenden Abbildungen versehen sind. Leipzig, *R. Weigel*, 1858.
    Reprint, Munich, 1924, Hildesheim, 1963.

6759   POGGENDORFF, JOHANN CHRISTIAN. 1796-1877
Biographisch-litterarisches Handwörterbuch zur Geschichte der exacten Wissenschaften. Vol. 1- , Leipzig, *J.A Barth*, 1863-
    Brief biographies, fuller bibliographies. Facsimile reprint (10 vols.), Ann Arbor, 1945. Vol. 3-4 also reprinted Leipzig, 1972. Vol. 7b, Lief 2-5 appeared in 1980 (Berlin, *Akademie Verlag*).

6760   ROYAL SOCIETY OF LONDON.
Catalogue of scientific papers, compiled and published by the Royal Society of London. 19 vols. London, Cambridge, 1867-1925.
    An author catalogue of all important scientific papers published during the 19th century. Vol. 1-7: London, *Eyre & Spottiswoode*; vol. 8; London, *J. Murray*; Trübner; vol. 9-12; London, *CJ Clay*; vol. 13-19: Cambridge. *University Press*. Reprinted, *Johnson Reprint Corp.* and *Kraus Reprint Corp.*, New York, 1965

6760.1   PAULY, ALPHONSE. 1830-1909
Bibliographie des sciences Médicales. Paris, *Librairie Tross*, 1874.
    Cites books and articles. Author index. Begun by C. Daremberg (1817-1882) and completed by Pauly. Reprint, London, 1954.

6761   GROSS, SAMUEL DAVID. 1805-1884
History of American medical literature from 1776 to the present time. Philadelphia, *Collins*, 1876.

6761.1   WÜSTENFELD, HEINRICH FERDINAND. 1808-1899
Die Uebersetzungen arabischer Werke in das Lateinische seit dem XI. Jahrhundert. Göttingen, *J. F. Dieterich*, 1877.

6762   INDEX MEDICUS.
A monthly classified record of the current medical literature of the world. Compiled under the supervision of John S. Billings and Robert Fletcher. Vol. 1-21. New York, 1879-99.
    A second series, edited by Fletcher and F. H. Garrison, vols. 1-6, 1921-27. In 1927 the *Quarterly Cumulative Index to Current Medical Literature* (12 vols., 1916-26) was amalgamated with the *Index Medicus* to form *Quarterly Cumulative Index Medicus* (1927-56) which, with No. 6777, was superseded in 1960 by a new monthly *Index Medicus* with an annual *Cumulated Index Medicus*. The gap 1900-02 was partly filled by

Bibliographia Medica, 3 vols., Paris, 1900-1903, and by *Index Medicus Novus*, Vienna, No. 1-12, 1899; No. 1-3, 1900. The first three series of *Index Medicus* were reprinted New York, *Johnson Reprint*, 1967. *Bibliographia Medica* was reprinted New York, *Johnson Reprint*, 1972.

6763   UNITED STATES. War Dept. Surgeon General's Office.
        Index-catalogue of the library of the Surgeon General's Office. Vol. 1-16; 2nd ser., vol. 1-21; 3rd ser., vol. 1-10; 4th ser., vol. 1-11 (A-Mn); 5th ser., vol. 1-3. Washington, *Govt. Printing Office*, 1880-1961.
        In 1836 Surgeon General Lovell established a small collection of medical books for the use of his staff. From it grew the " Surgeon General's Library", one of the greatest medical libraries in the world. J.S. Billings did much to develop the library; he planned and started the *Index Catalogue*, one of the finest achievements of medical bibliography. Series 1-4 index about 3,000,000 books, journal articles, and pamphlets. In the 5th series only monographs and theses are included. For continuation *see* Nos. 6784, 6786.9. The name of the library was changed to Armed Forces Medical Library in 1952; it became the National Library of Medicine in 1956.

6764.1 BRADFORD, THOMAS L.
        Homeopathic bibliography of the United States, from the year 1825 to the year 1891. Philadelphia, *Boericke & Tafel*, 1892.

6765   STEINSCHNEIDER, MORITZ. 1816-1907
        Die hebräischen Uebersetzungen des Mittelalters. 2 vols. Berlin, 1893. Reprinted, 1956.

6766   GYÖRY, TIBOR. 1869-1938
        Bibliographia medica Hungariae, 1472-1899, Budapestini, *sumpt. Athenaei*, 1900.

6767   DIELS, HERMANN. 1848-1922
        Die Handschriften der antiken Aerzte. *Abhanl. k. preuss. Akad. Wiss. (Berl.)*, Phil.- hist. Cl., 1905, 1-158; 1906. 1-115; 1907, 1-72.
        A catalogue of manuscripts of texts and translations of classical Greek physicians. Republished in book form, 1905-08.

6768   SUDHOFF, KARL FRIEDRICH JAKOB. 1853-1938
        Deutsch medizinische Inkunabeln. Leipzig, *J. A. Brath*, 1908.

6768.1 YOUNG, JOHN.
        A catalogue of the manuscripts in the library of the Hunterian Museum. Planned and begun by John Young, contined and completed by P. Henderson Aitken. Glasgow, *James Maclehose*, 1908.
        Catalogue of the manuscripts collected and donated to the University of Glasgow by William Hunter (1718-83), now in the Hunterian Collection, University of Glasgow Library. The catalogue provides full descriptions of approximately 600 manuscripts dating mostly from the Middle Ages and Renaissance, covering a wide range of subjects in addition to medicine.

6769   OSLER, *Sir* WILLIAM, *Bart.* 1849-1919
        Incunabula medica. A study of the earliest printed medical books, 1467-1480. Oxford, *Univ. Press*, 1923.

Bibliographical Society Publication. Based on Osler's presidential address to the Bibliographical Society in 1914, the work opens with an essay showing the influence of printing upon the development of modern medicine. Next follows a descriptive list of 217 medical books printed to 1480. This list was edited by V. Scholderer.

6771   POLLARD, ALFRED WILLIAM. 1859-1944. & REDGRAVE, GILBERT R.
A short-title catalogue of books printed in England, Scotland, and Ireland and of English books printed abroad, 1475-1640. London, *Bibliographical Society,* 1926.

This has been completely superseded by the second edition, revised and enlarged. Begun by W. A. Jackson and F. S. Ferguson; completed by K. F. Pantzer. Vol. 1. A-H.; Vol. 2. I-Z. London, *Bibliographical Society,* 1972-86. In addition to countless works of medical interest, this includes in brief form many bibliographies of individual medical authors whose works appeared during the dates covered.

6772   OSLER, *Sir* WILLIAM, *Bart.* 1849-1919
Bibliotheca Osleriana. A catalogue of books illustrating the history of medicine and science, collected, arranged, and annotated by Sir WILLIAM OSLER, Bt. and bequeathed to McGill University. Oxford, *Clarendon Press,* 1929.

This bibliography of over 7,500 titles is the catalogue of Osler's magnificent library. It is one of the best well-annotated bibliographies in the history of medicine and stands as a monument to its author. Reprinted 1969 and 1988 with addenda and corrigenda, Montreal, *McGill-Queen's University Press.* See also *The Osler Library,* Montreal, *McGill University,* 1979.

6772.1   FERGUSON, MUNGO.
The printed books in the library of the Hunterian Museum...Glasgow, *Jackson, Wylie,* 1930.

Catalogue of the printed books in the celebrated library formed by William Hunter (1718-83), now called the Hunterian Collection, at the University of Glasgow Library. The catalogue was actually printed in 1916 but not issued until 1930 because of the First World War. *See* No. 6768.1.

6773   GARRISON, FIELDING HUDSON. 1870-1935
Revised students' check-list of texts illustrating the history of medicine, with references for collateral reading. *Bull. Inst. Hist. Med.,* 1933, **1**, 333-434.

An expansion of the list which appeared in the *Index-Catalogue of the Library of the Surgeon General's Office, Washington,* 1912, 2 ser. **17**, 89-178, also compiled by Garrison. The 1933 check-list formed the starting point for L.T. Morton's first edition of this bibliography, published in 1943.

6774   ———. The medical and scientific periodicals of the 17th and 18th centuries, with revised catalogue and check-list. *Bull. Inst. His. Med.,* 1934, **2**, 285-343.

Addenda and corrigenda by D.A. Kronick, *Bull. Hist. Med.* 1958, **32**, 456-74.

6775   LeFANU, WILLIAM RICHARD. 1904-
British periodicals of medicine. A chronological list. *Bull Inst. Hist. Med.,* 1937, **5**, 735-61, 827-55; 1938, **6**, 614-48.

Covers British periodicals published in the British Empire. Published in book form, Baltimore, 1938. Supplement, 1938-61, by A. M Shadrake, *Bull.*

med. Libr. Ass., 1963, **51**, 181-96, covers Gt Britain and Ireland, but excludes reports of societies and hospitals.

6776   KLEBS, ARNOLD CARL. 1870-1943
Incunabula scientifica et medica. Short title list. Bruges, *St. Catherine Press*, 1938.
     3,000 editions of 1,000 incunabula. Reprinted, Hildesheim, 1963.

6777   CURRENT LIST OF MEDICAL LITERATURE.
Vol. 1-36. Washington, 1941-59.
     Published weekly until June, 1950, then monthly, with author and subject indexes. Cumulated indexes semi-annually. Superseded in 1960 by *Index Medicus.*

6779   CUSHING, HARVEY WILLIAMS. 1869-1939
The Harvey Cushing collection of books and manuscripts. New York, *Schuman's*, 1943.
     Catalogue, without annotations, of the books and manuscripts bequeathed by Cushing to the Historical Library in the Cushing/Whitney Medical Library at Yale University School of Medicine.

6780   WING, DONALD GODDARD. 1904-1972
Short-title catalogue of books printed in England, Scotland, Ireland, Wales, and British America and of English books printed in other countries, 1641-1700. 3 vols. New York, *Columbia University Press*, 1945-51.
     Supplements the *Short title catalogue* (No. 6771). This has been superseded by the second edition, revised and enlarged, 3 vols., New York, *Modern Language Association of America*, 1972-88. In addition to countless works of medical interest, this bibliography includes in brief form many author bibliographies of individual physicians whose works appeared during 1640-1700.

6781   RUSSELL, KENNETH FITZPATRICK. 1911-1987
A check-list of medical books published in English before 1600. *Bull Hist. Med.*, 1947, **21**, 922-58.

6782   KELLY, EMERSON CROSBY. 1899-1977
Encyclopedia of medical sources. Baltimore, *Williams & Wilkins*, 1948.
     A valuable list of medical eponyms and original sources, arranged alphabetically by authors' names.

6783   SCHULLIAN, DOROTHY MAY, 1906-1989, & SOMMER, FRANCIS ERICH. 1890-
A catalogue of incunabula and manuscripts in the Army Medical Library. New York, *Henry Schuman*, 1950.
     For supplement *see* No. 6786.18.

6784   UNITED STATES. National Library of Medicine Catalogue.
18 vols. Washington, New York, *Ann Arbor*, 1950-66.
     Two quinquennial and one sexennial cumulations of annual volumes. 6 vols., 1950-54; 6 vols., 1955-59; 6 vols., 1960-65. Author and subject indexes. First series under title "U.S. Armed Forces Medical Library". *See also* No. 6763; continued by No. 6786.9.

6785   FULTON, JOHN FARQUHAR. 1899-1960
The great medical bibliographers. A study in humanism. Philadelphia, *University of Pennsylvania Press*, 1951.
Gives details of the life and work of all the outstanding contributors to medical bibliography.

6785.1   BRODMAN, ESTELLE. 1914-
The development of medical bibliography. Baltimore, *Medical Library Association*, 1954.
A historical study; includes a list of 255 medical bibliographies published since 1500. Reprinted 1981.

6786   POYNTER, FREDERICK NOEL LAWRENCE. 1908-1979
A catalogue of incunabula in the Wellcome Historical Medical Library, compiled by F. N. L. POYNTER. London, *Oxford Univ. Press*, 1954.
Gives full bibliographical description of 632 incunabula.

6786.1   SALLANDER, HANS.
Bibliotheca Walleriana. The books illustrating the history of medicine and science collected by Dr. [Axel] Erik Waller [1875-1955] and bequeathed to the library of the Royal University of Uppsala. A catalogue compiled by HANS SALLANDER. 2 vols. Stockholm, *Almqvist & Wiksell*, 1955.
Contains 23,000 printed items, including 150 incunabula. The catalogue does not include Waller's vast collection of autographs and manuscripts also preserved in Uppsala.

6786.2   PRIME, L. MARGUERIETE.
A catalogue of the H. Winnett Orr historical collection and other rare books in the library of the American College of Surgeons. Chicago, *American College of Surgeons*, 1960.
Describes 2289 rare books primarily concerning surgery, military medicine, and orthopaedics, donated by H. Winnett Orr (1877-1956).

6786.3   AUSTIN, ROBERT B.
Early American medical imprints. A guide to works printed in the United States 1668-1820. Washington, *U.S. Dept of Health, Education and Welfare*, 1961.
Describes 2105 items with paginations. Reprinted 1977.

6786.4   GUERRA, FRANCISCO. 1916-
American medical bibliography 1639-1783. New York, *Lathrop C. Harper*, 1962.
Lists and describes 719 books, pamphlets, and broadsides, 506 almanacs, 25 magazines, and 224 newspapers published in the area now forming the U.S.A.

6786.5   WELLCOME HISTORICAL MEDICAL LIBRARY.
A catalogue of printed books in the Wellcome Historical Medical Library Vol 1- . London, *Wellcome Historical Medical Library*, 1962- .
Vol. 1: Books printed before 1641; Vol. 2-3: Books printed from 1641-1850, A-E, F-L.

6786.6   MOORAT, Samuel Arthur Joseph. 1892-1974
A catalogue of western manuscripts on medicine and science in the
Wellcome Historical Medical Library. 3 vols. London, *Wellcome Institute*,
1962-72.
    I: MSS written before AD 1650. II-III: MSS written after AD 1650. Addenda
in *1. Anzeiger dtsch. Altertum dtsch. Lit.*, 1970, **81**, 49-55.

6786.7   HAHN, André. 1900-1975, & DUMAITRE, Paule.
Histoire de la médecine et du livre médical à la lumière des collections de
la Bibliothèque de la Faculté de Médecine de Paris. Paris, *Olivier Perrin*,
[1962].

6786.8   EMMERSON, Joan Stuart.
Translations of medical classics. A list. Newcastle upon Tyne, 1965.
    University Library Publication No. 3. Lists translations of medical works
of classical interest and importance published before 1900.

6786.9   UNITED STATES. National Library of Medicine Current catalog. Washington, 1966- .
    Published quarterly, with annual and quinquennial (one sexennial-
1965-70) cumulations.

6786.10   WICKERSHEIMER, Charles Adolphe Ernest. 1880-1965
Les manuscrits latins de médecine du haut moyen age dans les bibliothèques
de France. Paris, *Centre National de la Recherche Scientifique*, 1966.

6786.11   BLAKE, John Ballard. 1922- , & ROOS, Charles.
Medical reference works 1679-1966; a selected bibliography. Chicago,
Medical Library Association, 1967.
    Contains over 2,700 items with annotations. Probably the most authorita-
tive list of medical reference books available. Supplements: I(1967-68),
1970; compiled by M.V. Clark. II (1969-72), 1973; compiled by J. S.
Richmond. III (1973-74), 1975; compiled by J. S. Richmond. Further
supplements are being compiled from National Library of Medicine
databases.

6786.12   DURLING, Richard Jasper. 1932-
A catalogue of sixteenth century printed books in the National Library of
Medicine. Compiled by Richard J. Durling. Bethesda, Md, *U.S. Dept. of
Health, Education, and Welfare*, 1967.
    Describes with pagination and some collations, approximately 4,800
items printed between 1501 and 1600. There are geographical and alphabetical indices of printers and publishers. For supplement, *see* No.
6786.18.

6786.13   ISKANDAR, Albert Z.
A catalogue of Arabic manuscripts on medicine and science in the Wellcome
Historical Medical Library. London, *Wellcome Historical Medical Library*,
1967.

6786.14   THOMAS, Martha Lou.
Rare books and collections of the Reynolds Historical Library. A bibliography. Birmingham, Alabama, *University of Alabama Press*, [1968].

Describes 5119 rare books, manuscripts, and medieval anatomical mannequins donated by Lawrence Reynolds (1889-1961). Includes some fine colour plates.

6786.15   EALES, NELLIE B.
The Cole Library of early medicine and zoology. Catalogue of books and pamphlets. 2 parts. Reading, *Alden Press for the Library, University of Reading*, 1969-75.
The library of F.J. Cole (*see* No. 356). Part 1: 1472-1800 to the present day and Supplement to Part 1.

6786.16   STILLWELL, MARGARET BINGHAM.
The awakening interest in science during the first century of printing 1450-1550. An annotated checklist of first editions viewed from the angle of their subject content. Astronomy. Mathematics. Medicine. Natural science. Physics. Technology. New York, *Bibliographical Society of America*, 1970.

6786.17   BESTERMAN, THEODORE DEODATUS NATHANIEL. 1904-1977
Medicine; a bibliography of bibliographies. Totowa, N.J., *Rowman and Littlefield*, 1971.
Extracted from *A world bibliography of bibliographies* (4th ed., 1965-66).

6786.18   KRIVATSY, PETER. 1922-
A catalogue of incunabula and sixteenth century printed books in the National Library of Medicine. First supplement, compiled by PETER KRIVATSY. Bethesda, Md., *U.S. Dept of Health, Education & Welfare*, 1971.
Supplements Nos. 6783 and 6786.12. Records 27 15th century imprints and 272 16th century imprints acquired by the library since publication of these two catalogues.

6786.19   PARKINSON, ETHEL M.
Catalogue of medical books in Manchester University Library 1480-1700. Manchester, *Manchester University Press*, [1972].
Describes 2685 items with full title transcriptions, paginations, and some annotations.

6786.20   KRONICK, DAVID A.
A history of scientific and technical periodicals. The origins and development of the scientific and technical press, 1665-1790. 2nd ed. Metuchen, N.J., 1976.
"Includes much of medical interest and contains several tables indicating comparative numbers of periodicals on various subjects at different dates" (L.T. Morton).

6786.21   BLAKE, JOHN BALLARD. 1922-
A short title catalogue of eighteenth century printed books in the National Library of Medicine. Compiled by JOHN B. BLAKE. Bethesda, Md., *U.S. Dept. of Health, Education, and Welfare*, 1979.
Lists approximately 25,000 works (except dissertations) printed between 1701 and 1800.

6786.22   RUSSELL, KENNETH FITZPATRICK. 1911-1987
Catalogue of the historical books in the library of the Royal Australasian College of Surgeons. Melbourne, *Queensberry Hill Press*, 1979.

6786.23   ADAMS, Scott. 1909-1982
Medical bibliography in an age of discontinuity. Chicago, *Medical Library Association*, 1981.
A history of medical bibliography since World War II, focusing on the information requirements of biomedical research; supplements No. 6785.1

6786.24   EMMERSON, Joan Stuart.
Catalogue of the Pybus Collection of medical books, letters and engravings, 15th-20th centuries. Newcastle upon Tyne, *Manchester University Press for The University Library*, [1981].
Describes the collection of 2305 classics in the history of medicine formed by Frederick C. Pybus (1883-1975), giving pagination and plate counts. Also included are annotated descriptions of 158 autograph letters by physicians, and descriptions of about 1000 medical portraits and other prints. Completely indexed.

6786.25   IMBAULT-HUART, Marie-José.
La médecine médiévale à travers les manuscrits de la Bibliothèque Nationale. Paris, *Bibliothèque Nationale*, 1982.
Annotated exhibition catalogue, with introductory essays, describing 99 exceptionally important medieval medical manuscripts as well as a few very early medallions.

6786.26   BIRD, D. T.
A catalogue of sixteenth-century medical books in Edinburgh libraries. Edinburgh, *Royal College of Physicians of Edinburgh*, 1982.
Describes 2509 books with paginations and collations. Reproduces 89 illustrations.

6786.27   PRICE, Robin.
An annotated catalogue of medical Americana in the library of the Wellcome Institute for the History of Medicine. London, *Wellcome Institute for the History of Medicine*, 1983.
Books and printed documents 1557-1821 from Latin America and the Caribbean Islands. and manuscripts from the Americas 1575-1927. 540 items, usually with detailed notes.

6786.28   CORDASCO, Francesco. 1920-
American medical imprints, 1820-1910. 2 vols., Totowa, N.J., *Rowman & Littlefield*, 1985.
A work in progress for over 40 years, this catalogue describes over 36,000 books, pamphlets, and broadsides, arranged by decade, from 1820-1910, with a comprehensive index. Included is an essay: *19th century American medical literature: A gallery of Lea titles,* and an appendix: *Wood's Library of Standard Medical Authors: A checklist and biographical guide.*

6786.29   MEYNELL, Geoffrey Guy.
The two Sydenham Societies. A history and bibliography of the medical classics published by the Sydenham Society and the New Sydenham Society (1844-1911). Acrise, Kent, *Winterdown Books*, 1985.

6786.30   KESHAVARZ, Fateme.
A descriptive and analytical catalogue of Persian manuscripts in the Library of the Wellcome Institute for the History of Medicine. London, *The Wellcome Institute for the History of Medicine*, 1986.

6786.31   WYGANT, Larry J.
The Truman G. Blocker, Jr. history of medicine collections: books and manuscripts. Galveston, *The University of Texas Medical Branch*, 1986.
Describes approximately 13,000 books chiefly acquired for the Moody Medical Library by Truman G. Blocker, Jr. (1909-84).

6786.32   DAVIS, Aubrey B., & DREYFUSS, Mark S.
The finest instruments ever made. A bibliography of medical, dental, optical and pharmaceutical company trade literature; 1700-1939. Arlington, Mass., *Medical History Publishing Assoc. I*, [1986].

6786.33   KRIVATSY, Peter. 1922-
A catalogue of seventeenth century printed books in the National Library of Medicine. Bethesda, Md., *U.S. Depart. of Health and Human Services*, 1989.
Describes, with paginations, approximately 13,300 monographs, dissertations, broadsides, pamphlets and serials printed between 1601 and 1700.

6786.34   BESSON, Alain.
Thornton's medical books, libraries and collectors. A study of bibliography and the book trade in relation to the medical sciences. Third, revised edition, edited by Alain Besson. Aldershot, *Gower*, 1990.
A highly useful work, originally published by John L. Thornton (b. 1913) in 1949. This new edition includes the following fully-documented historical essays: P. Jones, *Medical books before the invention of printing*; D.E. Rhodes, *Medical incunabula*; Y. Hibbott, *Medical books of the sixteenth century*; C.R. English, *Seventeenth century medical books*; P.C. Want, *Medical books from 1701-1800*; G. Davenport, *Medical books of the nineteenth century*; L.T. Morton, *The growth of medical periodical literature*; J. Symonds, *Medical bibliographies and bibliographers*; A. Besson, *Private medical libraries*; R.B. Tabor, *Medical libraries of today*.

6786.35   EIMAS, Richard.
Heirs of Hippocrates. The development of medicine in a catalogue of historic books in the Hardin Library for the Health Sciences, The University of Iowa. *Iowa City, University of Iowa Press*, 1991.
Describes with detailed historical notes over 2300 books in the John Martin Rare Book Room, and chiefly donated to the library by John Martin. The books are arranged chronologically by date of the author's birth. Numerous illustrations, including some in colour.

6786.36   HOOK, Diana Hainault. 1955-   & NORMAN, Jeremy Michael. 1945-
The Haskell F. Norman library of science and medicine. 2 vols. San Francisco, *Jeremy Norman & Co., Inc.*, 1991.
Fully annotated descriptions, mostly with complete collations, paginations, and plate counts, of 2600 classics covering the spectrum of the sciences, emphasizing medicine, from *circa* 1470 to 1950, in the library of Haskell F. Norman. 1915- . Numerous illustrations, some in colour.

MEDICAL LEXICOGRAPHY

6787   ISIDORE, *Bishop of Seville* [ISIDORUS HISPALENSIS]. A.D.570-636
Etymologiarum libri xx. Augsburg, *G. Zainer*, 1472.
    The principal work of Isidore of Seville, one of the greatest education-
ists of the Middle Ages. The *Etymologiae*, an encyclopaedic work, presents
the sum of contemporary knowledge on all branches of science. Book IV
affords a survey of the entire range of medicine. An English translation of
the medical and anatomical sections of the *Etymologiae* is in *Trans. Amer.
philos. Soc.*, 1964, **54**, pt.2.

6788   CORDO, SIMONE [SIMON *Januensis* or *Genuensis*]. 1270-1303
Synonyma medicinae, seu clavis sanationis. Mediolani, *Antonio Zarothus*,
1473.
    First printed medical dictionary. It was originally published at Ferrara,
1471-2?, of which the only recorded copy is a fragment of 21 leaves in the
Bodleian Library.

6789   DONDI, GIACOMO DE [JACOBUS DE DONDIS]. 1298-1359
Aggregator, sive de medicinis simplicibus. Strassburg, *Adolph Rusch*,
[*circa* 1470].
    An encyclopaedic dictionary of medicine, containing a large number of
medical recipes based upon Greek and Arabic sources.

6790   FRIES, LORENZ [FRISIUS; PHRYESEN]. *d.*1532
Synonima und gerecht Uszlegung der Wörter so man dan in der Artzny,
allen Krütern, Wurtzlen, Blumen, Somen, *J. Grieninger*, 1519.]

6791   ESTIENNE, HENRI [STEPHANUS]. 1531-1598
Dictionarium medicum. [Genevae], *Henricus Stephanus*, 1564.
    This valuable Greek–Latin dictionary for the ancient medical writers
defined and fixed a large number of anatomical terms, and exercised
considerable influence on modern anatomical terminology. It was an
important aid to the full understanding of the ancient texts.

6792   GORRIS, JEAN DE [GORRAEUS]. 1505-1577
Definitionum medicarum libri xxiii. Lutetiae Parisiorum, *apud A. Wechelum*,
1564.
    This dictionary arranges in order of the Greek alphabet all Greek
medical terms and carefully explains them in Latin. It was widely used and
exerted much influence on modern medical terminology.

6793   FOES, ANUCE [FOESIUS]. 1528-1595
Oeconomia Hippocratis, aphabeti serie distincta. In qua dictionum apud
Hippocratem omnium, praesertim obscuriorum, usus explicatur, etc.
Francofurdi, *apud A. Wecheli heredes*, 1588.
    A Greek alphabetical dictionary of the vocabulary of the Hippocratic
writings, based on an exhaustive investigation of all ancient medical texts.

6794   CASTELLI, BARTOLOMMEO. *d.*1607
Lexicon medicum Graeco-Latinum ... ex Hippocrate et Galeno desumptum.
Messanae, *typ. P. Brae*, 1598.

The earlier lexicon of Gorraeus formed the basis of this work, which was reprinted in several editions, the last in 1792.

6795   NAUDÉ, GABRIEL. 1600-1653
Quaestio iatrophilologica. Romae, *G. Facciotte,* 1632.
    Learned bibliophile and at one period librarian of the Vatican, Gabriel Naudé eventually became Mazarin's librarian and built up for his master a famous collection of books. He wrote an important medical dictionary. Four further parts of the above, with varying titles and places of publication appeared, 1634-47.

6796   BAILLOU, GUILLAUME DE [BALLONIUS]. 1538-1616
Definitionum medicinarum liber. Parisiis, *J. Quesnel,* 1639.
    A glossary of Hippocratic terms.

6797   BLANKAART, STEVEN [BLANCARD]. 1650-1702
A physical dictionary; in which all the terms relating either to anatomy, chirurgery, pharmacy, or chemistry, are very accurately explain'd. London, *J.D. Crouch,* 1684.
    The English translation of Blankaart's dictionary was the first medical dictionary to be printed in the British Isles. The original Greek-Latin text was published in Amsterdam, 1679.

6798   CALLARD DE LA DUCQUERIE, JEAN BAPTISTE. 1630-1718
Lexicon medicum etymologicum. Cadomi, *J. Briard,* 1691.

6799   JAMES, ROBERT. 1705-1776
A medicinal dictionary. 3 vols. London, *T. Osborne,* 1743-45.
    The largest, most exhaustive and most learned medical dictionary written in English prior to the early 19th century. Samuel Johnson wrote the dedication and some of the articles. This was Johnson's first venture into lexicography, and when he was done, a syndicate of booksellers asked him to write his famous dictionary. Denis Diderot collaborated on the French translation, 6 vols., Paris, 1746-48. That experience gave him the idea to produce the famous Diderot et d'Alembert *Encyclopédie.*

6800   COPLAND, JAMES. 1791-1870
A dictionary of practical medicine. 3 vols. London, *Longman, etc.,* [1832]-58.

6801   DICTIONNAIRE ENCYCLOPÉDIQUE DES SCIENCES MÉDICALES.
100 Vols. Paris, *Asselin et Masson,* 1864-89.
    Includes a great number of articles written by the best-known French medical men of the period. A. Dechambre directed it until 1885 when he was succeeded by L. Lereboullet.

6803   POWER, HENRY. 1829-1911, & SEDGWICK, LEONARD W.
New Sydenham Society's lexicon of terms used in medicine and the allied sciences. Edited by HENRY POWER and LEONARD W. SEDGWICK. 5 vols. London, *New Sydenham Soc.,* 1881-99.

6804   FISCHER, ISIDOR. 1868-1943
Die Eigennamen in der Krankheitsterminologie. Wien, Leipzig, *M. Perles,* 1931.

This dictionary of medical eponyms gives references to the original publications involved and records wherever possible the first use of the eponym.

6805   LEIBER, BERNFRIED. 1919- , & OLBRICH, GERTRUDE.
Wörtenbuch der klinischen Syndrome. 3te. Auflage. München, *Urban & Schwarzenberg*, 1963.
    5th ed., 1972.

6806   LIEBER, BERNFRIED. 1919- , & OLBERT, THEODOR.
Die klinische Eponyme. München, *Urban & Schwarzenberg*, 1968.

6807   STRAUSS, MAURICE BENJAMIN. 1904-
Familiar medical quotations. Boston, *Little Brown*, 1968.
    Over 7,000 quotations, arranged under broad subject headings; author and subject indexes.

6808   JABLONSKI, STANLEY.
Illustrated dictionary of eponymic syndromes and diseases and their synonyms. Philadelphia, *W.B. Saunders*, 1969.
    Second edition as *Jablonski's Dictionary of syndromes and eponymic diseases*, Malabar, Fl., *Krieger*, 1989.

6809   MAGALINI, SERGIO. 1927-
Dictionary of medical syndromes. Philadelphia, *J.B. Lippincott*, 1971.
    Second edition with E. Scrasia, 1981.

6810   WALTON, *Sir* JOHN NICHOLAS. 1922- , BEESON, PAUL BRUCE. 1908- , & SCOTT, *Sir* RONALD BODLEY. 1906-1982
The Oxford companion to medicine. 2 vols., Oxford, *Oxford University Press*, 1986.
    A dictionary, biographical dictionary, and encyclopaedia covering selected aspects of the theory, practice and profession of medicine, including history, by the editors and 150 notable contributors. Produced in the style of previous volumes in the *Oxford Companion* series.

INDEX OF PERSONAL NAMES

References are to entry numbers; page numbers are not used in this index. References to original works are given in roman type; other references are given in *italic* type.

Dotter, C.T., 2924.4
Double, F.J., 2672.2
Douglas, C.G., 955, 957, *958*, *2137.7*
Douglas, G., *1314*
Douglas, J., 1217, 2162.1, 4281, 6745
Douglas, S.R., 2558
Douglass, W., 5076, 5412–3
Doumer, E., *3871*
Dowling, G.B., 4011
Down, J.L.H., 4936
Downes, *Sir* A.H., 1997
Downing, J., *5414.1*
Doyen, E.L., 3028.1
Doyle, *Sir* A.C., *2127.1*
Doyon, *4096.1*
Drabkin, D.L., *1415.1*
Drabkin, I.E., *1959.1*
Draeger, J., 6007
Dragendorff, G.J.N., 1746–7, 2039
Dragstedt, L.R., 1086.1, 3557
Drake, D., 1777, 5234.1
Drbohlav, J., 5194
Dresbach, M., 3132.1
Dreschfeld, J., 3772
Dreschsel, E., 716
Dreser, H., 1891
Dressler, L.A., 4169.2
Drew, *Sir* R., *6723*
Drey, R.E.A., 2068.19
Dreyfuss, M.S., 6786.32
Drier, J., 4005
Driesch, H.A.E., 129, 509
Drinker, P., 1978
Dripps, R.D., 3161.41
Droz, E., 5140
Drummond, *Sir* J.C., 1053, 1092.51
Dry, T.J., 3160
Dryander, J., 370–1, *461.3*
Du Bois, P., 6179
Du Bois-Reymond, E., 609–10, *621*
Du Laurens, A., 3806
Du Tertre, J.B., 5450
Du Verney, G.J., *295, 585, 1494*, 1545, 3351
Du Vigneaud, V., 1085, 1175.3–4
Düben, G.W.J., 2761.1
Dubilier, W., *4256.2*
Dubini, A., 4637, 5353
Dubois de Chemant, N., 3677
Dubois, E., 210
DuBois, E.F., 1036
Dubois, R.J., 1933.1
Dubost, C., 2993.1
Duchâteau, A., *3677*
Duchenne de Boulogne, G.B.A., 614, 624, 1995, *1996.3, 4548*, 4732, 4734, 4736, *4738*, 4739, 4774, 4973, *4975*
Duckworth, W.L.H., 347
Duclaux, E., *83*
Ducrey, A., 5205
Ducrot, R., *1931.1, 5725*

Ducuing, J., 3018
Duddell, B., 1482
Dudley, B.W., 4851.1
Dudley, H.W., 1345, *1916*, 6230
Duel, A.B., 4899
Dugès, A., 6028
Duhring, L.A., 4083
Dührssen, A., 6246
Dujardin, F., 2470, 6374.12
Duke-Elder, *Sir* W.S., 1530–1
Dukes, C., 5505
Dulbecco, R., 2526.1, 2660.13, *2660.20*, *2660.22*, 2660.27
Dumaître, P., *385, 401.1*, 6610.16, 6786.8
Dumas, J.B.A., 474.1, 478, 2016, *5642*
Duméril, C., *311*
Dumont, G., *4727*
Dumont, J., 3013
Dunant, J.H., 2166
Dunbar, W.P., 2592
Duncan, J., 3120
Duncan, J.M., 6181, 6194
Duncum, B.M., 5733
Dundas, D., 2739
Dungan, C.E., *4615*
Dungern, E. von, 898
Dunglison, R., 4691
Dunhill, *Sir* T.P., 3849.1, 5630.1
Dunn, L.C., 258.4
Dunstan, *Sir* W.R., 1886
Dupertuis, S.M., *3038*
Duplay, S., 4339.2
Duprat-Duverger, L., *313*
Dupuy, P.E., 1569.1
Dupuytren, G., *Baron, 2123.1*, 2163, 2247, 2943, 2947, 2976, 3437–8, 3788, 4290.1, 4317, 4322, 4411, 4413, 4444, 5590
Durand, J., 5217
Durand, P., 4661
Duranty, *Marquis de*, 5137
Dürer, A., 149
Duret, P., 3429
Durham, *2514, 2550*
Durham, H.E., 2513, 2549, 5036
Durlacher, L., 4325
Durling, R.J., 6786.12
Duroziez, P.L., 2762, 2780
Dusser de Barenne, J.G., 1442
Dutrochet, R.J.H., 108, 110, 670
Dutton, J.E., 5275, 5318
Duval, M.M., 446, 553
Duve, C. de, 566.4
Duvernoy, G.L., *311*
Duvillard, E.E., 1695
Dyer, R.E., 5396.2
Dyke, C.G., 4611.3
Dykshorn, S.W., *1171*
Daza de Valdes, B., 5821
Dziurdzi-Boim, M.P *See* Boym, M.P

Florey, H.W., *1933–4, 1934.1*
Florio, L.J., 5546.1
Florkin, M., *113*, 1588.10
Flosdorf, E.W., 2022
Flourens, M.J.P., *1256, 1388*, 1391, 1493, 1557, *1574*, 5654
Flournoy, T., *5319*
Floyer, *Sir* J., 1595, 2029, 2670, 3166
Flückiger, F.A., 2032
Flynn, E.H. *1946*
Fockens, P., 3536
Fodere, F.E., 1605, 1734
Fodéré, F.E., 3810
Foedisch, F., 3114
Foerster, H.R., *2416*
Foerster, O., 1377.1, 1450, 4604, 4613, 4880
Foerster, O.H., 2416
Foes, A., *13*, 6793
Foesius, A. *See* Foes, A.
Fogarty, T.J., 3020.2
Foix, C., 4721
Foley, F.E.B., 4250.1
Folff, W.J., 4257.1
Folin, O.K.O., 741.1, 3922
Folius, C. *See* Folli, C.
Folkers, K., *1088, 1091*
Folli, C., 1542
Folling, I.A., 3924
Fonahn, A., *365*, 6511
Fontaine, R., *3038*, 4902
Fontana, F., 1485, 2103, 3047.24
Fontius, B., *20*
Fonzi, G., 3679.2
Forbes, *Sir* J., *2673*, 6755
Forbes, S.A., 145.62
Forbes, T.R., 1757.2
Ford, *Sir* E., 6604.7
Ford, W.W., 2084, 2581
Forde, R.M., 5274, *5275*
Fordyce, J.A., 4123, 4137
Forel, A.H., 1368.2, 1411, 1635, 4952, 4996
Forestier, J., 2693, 3199, 4506.1, 4605
Forget, A., 3371
Forlanini, C., 3225
Forlivio, de, *363.1*
Forman, M.B., *6622.1*
Forssell, C.G.A., 6125
Forssmann, W.T.O., 2858, *2871*
Forst, J.J., 4563
Förster, A., 534.63
Förster, C.F.R., 5915
Forster, J.C., 3457
Fort, G.F., 1648
Forta, G.B.D., 150
Foshay, L., 5178–80
Fossel, V., 6404
Föster, *5943*
Foster, G.E., *1926*
Foster, M., *500, 600*
Foster, R., 5351.7

Foster, *Sir* M., 631, 1575
Foster, W.D., 2319.2, 2460, 2463.1, 2581.8
Fothergill, J., 1774, 4516–7, 5049, 5077
Fothergill, L.D., 4659.1
Fothergill, W.E., 6124
Foubeiran, E., 5649
Fourcroy, A.F., 1386.1, *2121*, 4439
Fourmestraux, J. de, 5807
Fourneau, E., 5288, 5690
Fournel, J., *1931.1*
Fournier, J.A., 2393, 2395, 4782, 4800
Foville, A.L.F., *4533*
Fowler, *6270*
Fowler, G.J., 1640
Fowler, G.R., 3179, 5623
Fowler, J., 2660.15
Fowler, *Sir* J.K., 4501.1
Fox, G.H., 3996, 4137
Fox, J., 3679, 3679.1
Fox, W.T., 4055, 4065, 4073, 4077–8
Fracastoro, G., 2364, 2528, 5371
Fraenkel, A., 3174
Fraenkel, B., 3281, 3285, 3296
Fraenkel, C., 5060.1
Fraenkel, E., 5210.1
Fraenkel-Conrat, H.L., 2527
Frame, J.D., 5546.4
Frampton, J., *1817*
France, L.C., *3047.12*
Frances-Chetti, A., 1757
Francis, E., 5176
Francis, T., 5498
Franco, P., 3573–4, 4279
Franco, R., 5460.1
François-Franck, C.E., 1417, 3022.1
Frania, M., *5447.1*
Frank, A.E., 3083, 3897
Frank, F., 6247
Frank, H.A., *4256*
Frank, J.P., 1599, 1965, *3809*, 3879, 4518
Frank, M., *427, 440*
Frank, O., 843
Frank, R., 3508, *3512*
Frank, R.G., Jr., 1588.17
Frankau, G., *4992.1*
Franke, H., 3978.1
Fränkel, F., 3865
Franken, F.H., 3666.7
Frankl-Hochwart, L. von, 4834
Franklin, B., *2094, 4992.2*, 5419, *6374.15*
Franklin, K.J., *757, 759, 1245*, 1583
Franks, *Sir* K., 3603
Franz, K., *5479*
Frapolli, F., 3751
Frappier, A., 2352
Fraser, F.W., 3215.7
Fraser, H., 3742
Fraser, *Sir* T.R., 1866.1, 1867, 1885, 2108
Frazer, *Sir* J.G., 184
Frazer, W.M., 1670

Halban, J. von, 6129, 6280
Halberstaedter, L., 5951
Halbertsma, T., 6244
Hald, J., 2091
Haldane, J.B.S., *253*, 254
Haldane, J.S., 891, 951, 951.1, 954, *957–8*, 961, 1977
Hale, C.W., *1947*
Hale, *Sir* M., 215
Hales, S., 765, *767*, 1596
Hall, M., 768.1, 1359, 2028.56, *4479*, 4812
Hall, M.C., 5368
Hall, R.J., 3568
Hall, R.W., *2160*
Hall, T.S., 143.1, *574*, 1588.6
Hallas-Moller, K., 3978
Haller, A. von, 54, 397, 438, 469.2, 534, 585, 587–8, *616*, 917, *985*, *1542*, 1833, 2732, 5789 *6746*, 6747
Haller, J.H., Jr., 6596.5
Hallervorden, J., 4724
Halley, E., 1687
Halliburton, W.D., 1295
Hallopeau, F.H., *4096.1*, 4101
Hallopeau, P., 3030
Hallpike, C.S., 3409
Halperin, B., *2660*
Halsted, W.S., 86.3, *2660*, 2966, 2969, 3488, *3568*, 3599, 3639.1, *3821*, 3860, 5640, 5679, *5683*, *5689*, *5756.3*, 5776–8
Haly Abbas, 42, *2193*
Ham, E.J. Ten., 1089
Ham, F.J., *5766.4*
Hamberg, M., 1931.7
Hamberg, U., *1155*
Hamberger, G.E., 918, 3424
Hambrecht, F.T., *5620.1*
Hamburger, C., 5970
Hamburger, F., 2591.1
Hamburger, H.J., 725
Hamby, W., *59*, *5790*
Hameed, H.A., *45*
Hamer, H.G., *4297*
Hamill, P., 1339
Hamilton, A., 2134
Hamilton, D.N.H., 6551.2
Hamilton, F.H., 1742, 4420, 5747
Hamilton, R., 5523
Hamilton, W.D., 257.1
Hammarsten, O., 877
Hammer, A., 2781
Hammon, W.M., 4672
Hammond, E.A., 6742.3
Hammond, J., *3666.5*
Hammond, W.A., 4542
Hammurabi, 1, 6471.90
Hampton, A.O., *4401*
Hamy, E.T.J., 203.2
Hanbury, D., 2032
Hancock, H., 3563

Hand, A., 6361, *6362*
Handerson, H.E., *6389*
Handley, W.S., 5782
Hanger, F.M., 3662
Hanot, V.C., 3624
Hanover, N.H., *1271.1*
Hansemann, D.P. von, 2626
Hansen, G.H.A., 2436, *2436.1*
Hansmann, G.H., 5541.2
Hanson, A.M., 1135
Hanson, F.R., 1945
Hanson, H.E., *2879*
Hanzal, F., *2719*
Hanzlik, P.J., 1914
Happold, F.C., *5072*
Hardaway, W.A., 4076
Hardisty, R.M., *3155.3*
Hardy, G.H., 243
Hardy, J., 4914.5
Hardy, J.D., 3047.19
Hardy, W.B., *1122*
Hare, E.S., *1328*, *5903*
Hare, R., 2578, 2068.15
Hare, W.K., 1446.2
Hargitay, B., *1246.1*, 1246.01
Hargrave, J., *57*
Hargraves, M.M., 2237.1
Harington, *Sir* C.R., 1137–8
Harington, *Sir* J., *51*, 1594
Harken, D.E., 3046.1
Harkins, H.N., 2261
Harkins, P.W., *4963.1*
Harkness, A.H., 2442.1
Harley, E.V.B., 717
Harley, G., 4171
Harley, G.W., 6466
Harley, J., 5344.5
Harms, H.P., *1086.1*
Harper, A.A., 1040.1
Harper, R.F., *1*, *6471.90*
Harrington, P.R., 4405.2
Harris, A., *2418*, 2418.1, *2419.2*
Harris, C.A., 3680
Harris, C.R.S., 1588.13
Harris, H., *3921*
Harris, H.F., 3756
Harris, L.J., 1078, 3708
Harris, P., *216.3*
Harris, S.A., 1088
Harris, S.H., 4275
Harris, W., 6321
Harris, W.R., 4435.6
Harrison, F., 3688
Harrison, J.H., *4257*
Harrison, R.G., 521, 558
Harrow, B., 1189
Hart, A.P., 3087.1
Hart, E.B., *1056*
Hart, P.C., *1186*
Hart, P.M d'A., 2359

Kimball, G., 6042
Kimmelsteiel, P., 4250
Kimpton, A.R., 2018.1
King, A.F.A., 5237
King, *Sir* E., 2014
King, E.J., *5225*
King, E.S.J., 3042
King, G., 1694
King, H., 5719
King, J., 6166–7
King, J.D., *5261*
King, L., *583*
King, T.W., 1126
Kinghorn, A., 5285.2
Kingsley, N.W., 3685.1
Kinmonth, J.B., 2700.1
Kinnersley, H.W., *1064*
Kinsell, L.W., 3908
Kircher, A., 580, 2528.1, 5118
Kirchheim, J. von, *363*
Kirkes, W.S., 2758
Kirkman, H., 1310
Kirkpatrick, J., 5416
Kirschner, M., *3012*, 3016, 4378, 5710
Kirstein, A., 3335
Kitai, R., *1207*
Kitasato, S., *Baron*, 2544, 5060, *5062*, 5149–50
Kite, C., 2028.54
Kite, J.H., 4403.1
Kjeldahl, J., 703
Klarenbeek, A., 5335, *5336*
Klasen, H.J., 5768.4
Klebs, A.C., *373*, 2050, *2192*, *5114*, 5140–1, 5436, 6776
Klebs, T.A.E., 549, 2173, 2327, 2392, 2535, 4212, 5031, 5055
Klein, E.E., 5080
Klein, G., 4405.02
Kleine, F.K., 5283.1
Klemperer, G., 3178
Klemperer, P., *2236*, 2237
Klencke, P.F.H., 2323
Klickstein, H., *2683*
Klieneberger, E., 2524.4
Kligfield, P., *2731*
Kligler, I.J., *5484.3*
Klimt, C.R., *4672*
Klinefelter, H.F., 3804
Kling, C., 4670.4
Klippel, M., 4131, 4362, 4386
Kloss, K., 3084
Klotz, O., 2918
Klupp, H., *5729*
Kluyskens, H., 6631.90
Knapp, A.H., 5964
Knapp, H., *5678*
Knapp, H.J., 5884, 5902
Knapp, R.E., 5320
Knapton, *399*
Knauer, C., *3659.2*

Knauer, E., 1178.1
Kneisel, F.C., 3679.8
Kneussel, C.F., 5181
Knickerbocker, G.G., *2883.4*
Knight, G.C., 4914.3
Knoefel, P.K., *1485*
Knoll, M., 269.3
Knoop, F., 728
Knotts, F.L., 1957
Know, R., *6623.01*
Knowles, R., 5301.1
Knox, R., 161, 415
Knutson, B., *5115*
Knutson, J.W., *3692.1*
Kobert, E.R., 2083
Kobert, R., *1788*
Koch, F.C., *1191*
Koch, M.B., *3150*
Koch, R., 86, 2331–3, 2544.1, 2457, 2488, 2495.1, 2503–4, *2533*, 2536, 2545, *3687*, 5040, *5106.1*, 108, 5167, 5636.1, 5923, *5930*
Koch, W.K., 3722
Kocher, E.T., 3473, 3600, 3826–7, 4425, 5619.1
Köcher, F., 6473.1
Koeberlé, E., 6051–3
Koebner, H., 4070.1
Koehn , C.J., 1076
Koelbing, H.M., *6467.2*
Koelsche, G.A., *1150*
Koetschet, P., *1931.1*
Kögl, F., 1071.1, 1089
Köhler, A., 269.1, 2182, 2817, 4377, 4387
Köhler, G.F., 2578.43
Köhler, W., 4991
Köhlmeier, W., *4154*
Kohn, M. *See* Kaposi, M.
Kolff, W.J., 4255
Kolisko, A., 6265
Kolle, F.S., 5756.5
Kolle, K., 5019
Kolle, W., 2517, 2562, 5111
Koller, *1880.1*
Koller, C., 5678, 5925
Koller, P.C., *2659.3*
Kölliker, R.A. von, 231, 487, 546, 618, 1219–20, 2078, *2683*
Kollmann, J.K.E., 427
Kolmer, J.A., 2413
Kolodny, A., 4394
Kolsky, M., *1931.1*
Kondo, K., 2578.41
König, F., 3069, 4350
Koniuszy, F.R., *1091*
Konjetzny, G.E., 3546
Kopech, G., 567.1
Kopetzky, S.J., 3411
Koplik, H., 5444
Köppen, W.P., 1782
Koprowski, H., 4672.1
Korányi, S, *Baron*, 4226

INDEX OF SUBJECTS

References are to entry numbers; page numbers are not used in the index.

actinomycin, carcinolytic action, 2660.8

actinomycosis, *Actinomyces bovis*, 5512

acumeter, 3364, 3387.1

acupressure, 5610

acupuncture, 6374.10–6374.16
    history, 6374.90, 6495.3

acute abdomen surgery, history, 5813.6

acute anterior poliomyelitis, 4664, 4665.1

acute ataxia, 4706.1

acute atrophy of bones, 4370

acute cystitis, conococcus, 6103

acute diseases, 1959.1

acute eczema, 3989

acute epididymitis operation, 4194

acute gastro-enteritis, 3481

acute glomerulonephritis, 4249

acute hallucinatory mania, 4849

acute hydrocephalus, 4635

acute infectious erythema, 5504

acute infective polyneuritis, 4639, 4647

acute intestinal obstruction, 3554

acute inversion, uterus, 6233

acute jaundice, separate from Leptospirosis
    icterohaemorrhagica, 5332

acute leukaemia, 3064.1
    vincristine, 3788.2

acute lymphocytic choriomeningitis, 4687

acute mastoiditis, 3369

acute middle-ear suppuration, paracentesis,
    3362

acute myeloblastic anaemia, cytosine
    orabinoside, 2660.3

acute nephritis, 4515

acute osteomyelitis, furuncle relationship,
    5619

acute otitis
    and abductor paralysis, 3398
    drainage treatment, 3371

acute pancreatitis, 3632

acute renal failure, parthogenesis, 4256.11

acute rheumatism, 4493
    childhood throat infections, 4507
    clinical history, 4492
    heart disease compared, 4494
    streptococci isolated, 4504.1
    throat infections, 4501.1

acute superior haemorrhagic
    polioencephalitis, 4641

Addison's disease, 3118, 3864
    eschatin treatment, 3874
    treatment, 3877
    (*see also* Biermer's disease)

adenocarcinomata of breast, 5778

adenoids, anaesthesia, 5709.1

adenoma sebaceum, 3989

adenoviruses discovery, 2526.2

adherent pericardium, 2800, 2805

Adie's syndrome, 5950

adiposis dolorosa, 3917

adrenal cortex, 1123

chemistry, 1152

extract, 3873

hormone, 1149, 3874, 3877

tumour removal, 3872

virilism, 3875

adrenal diseases, 3876

adrenal glands, 391
    immunity mechanism of body, 3793

adrenal insufficiency, 3873, 3877

adrenal medulla
    adrenaline content, 1141–1142
    tumours, 3866, 3871

adrenalectomy, carcinoma of prostate, 4276.1

adrenaline
    action, 1336
    in adrenal medulla, 1141–1142
    bronchial asthma, 3202.1
    isolated, 1146–1147
    pharmacological actions, 1928
    synthesis, 1147.1
    therapeutic uses, 1928

adrenals
    antitoxic to blood, 1140
    described, 1139

adrenocorticotrophic hormone
    isolation, 1174–1175
    rheumatoid arthritis treatment, 4508

adrenogenital syndrome, 3867

adrenotropic hormone isolation, 1170

adrenotropic receptors, sympathetic nervous
    system, 1929.4

adults, chronic arthritis, 4506

Aëdes aegypti
    dengue fever vector, 5472, 5474
    and yellow fever, 5460

Aëdes albopictus as dengue fever vector, 5475

aerial contamination, micro-organisms, 100

aerobic actinomycete described, 5512.1

aerobic carbohydrate metabolism, 751.1

aerobic glycolysis, 2651

aerobic organisms, anaerobic organisms
    compared, 2478

aerogenes bacillus, 2508

aerosporin antibiotic, 1937

Aesculapius
    disciples, 6721
    and musical sons, 6631.02

aesthetic plastic surgery, 5768.7

aesthetics, 149, 179

aetiology (*see* etiology)

Afar fossils, 214.3

afferent arterioles, 1231
    frog kidney, 1242

afferent nervous system, 1298

Africa
    Australopithecus (fossil man), 211.1,
    214.1
    camel history, 302
    lathyrism disease, 2077.1
    medicine, 6466

genetics, 254.3
history, 1588.10, 1588.18
micro-organisms, 1933.2
Paul Ehrlich, 86.4
biological antibodies, 2564.1
biological climatology, 2010
biological oxidation, 739
biological thought, 258.12
biological variations, statistical study, 233
biology, 258.11, 316
animal, 143.1
of death, 137
encyclopaedia, 290
German, 145.2
history, 141–142, 144–145, 534.3, 6661
mental defects, 4962.2
methodology handbook, 136
molecular, 254.1
nomenclature, 99.1
physical, 145.63
term coined, 105.1
Von Oken studies, 107
biomechanics
hand, 411.1
hip joint, 4400.5
motion, 604
biometric observations, genetics, 248
biopsy procedure, bone marrow, 3074, 3080, 3087–3088
biotin
deprivation, 3724
isolation, 1071.1
synthetic, 1088
biparental heredity, epigenesis relationship, 215.1
biparietal foetal cephalometry, ultrasound, 6235.1
Bipp, wounds treatment, 5644
birds
air sacs, 309
of America, 322
anatomy and physiology, 336
auditory and olfactory apparatus, 1453, 1458
bones compared to man, 283
German studies, 276.1
gill slits embryos, 480
haemocytozoa, 5249–5250
identified, 277
Leonardo da Vinci studies, 93–94
malaria parasites, 5238.1, 5246
natural history, 324
polyneuritis, 1047
sexual characteristics, 309
birth control, 1641.2, 1696.1
bismarsen, syphilis treatment, 2414
bismuth, syphilis treatment, 2394
bismuth meal
opaque to x-rays, 3519
roentgenology, 2687.1

bite-wing radiographs, 3692
Black Death (*see* pestilence; plague)
blacks
American medical history, 6594
health and diseases, 1601.1
and yellow fever, 5453.1
blackwater fever, 5235
history, 5264.1
bladder, 396, 2269
aeroscopic examination, 4187
bismuth subnitrate suspension, 4191.4
cancer, 2128.1
carcinoma radiotherapy, 4194.1
diverticula operation, 4189
exstrophy, 534.53, 4170, 6046
malignant diseases, 4194
muscle fibres, 4259.1
non-prostatic obstruction, 4165
rupture, 4169
stones history, 4289, 4297.1
stones removal, 4281
subtrigonal glands, 4185
surgery, 4175
transurethral fulguration, 4268
tumours, 4174, 4180, 4190
ureters catherization, 4187
Blalock–Taussig operation, 3043
blastodermic layers, 470–471
blastomeres, 505, 509
Blastomyces dermatitidis isolated from soil, 4154.7
blastomycetic dermatitis, 5530.1
blastomycosis
of skin, 5529.1
South American, 5532.1
bleeding
control after suprapubic prostatectomy, 4267
hereditary bleeding, 3087.2
blepharoplasty, 5738
blind
Helen Keller's works, 3399
Moon type, 5909
school, 5833
blindness, 4536
colour, 5911, 5916–5917
onchocerciasis, 5344.10
retinal artery embolism, 5882
Blocq's disease, 4573
blood, 2283
albumin, 3060
amino acids content, 730.1
analysis, 861, 3922
anatomy, 883
antibodies, 2601.1
antitoxic adrenals, 1140
bactericidal action, 2542
bank, 2026
calcium–bones relationship, 746
carbon dioxide dissociation, 958, 960

bowel
> hernia, 3584
> obstruction, 3479

brachial aneurysm, 2939

brachial artery
> aneurism treatment, 33
> traumatic aneurism, 2985

brachial plexus paralysis, 4553

Bracht–Wächter bodies, 2828

bradykinin discovered 1930

Brahma medicine, 8

braille described, 5851

brain
> abscess, 4638, 4853
> air in ventricles, 4884
> anatomy, 1254, 1378.1, 1379.1, 1406.01
> architectonics, 4942
> cephalins in tissue, 1415.1
> chemistry, 1380.1, 1386.1
> diseases, 2285.2, 4537, 4558, 4568
> disorders, 4511.02
> dissection, 373.1
> dropsy, 4634–4635
> electric currents, 1408.1
> electrodes location, 1435.1
> epilepsy, 4914.2
> fourth ventricle puncture, 3933
> functions, 1409
> galvanic current effects, 2003.2
> growth, 1425
> history, 1586, 1588.4, 1588.9
> injuries effects, 1446.1
> lesions, 4914.4
> life as a product, 115
> mammalian, 1396.01, 1420.1
> morbid anatomy, 2284
> myelins in tissue, 1415.1
> as organ of thought, 1378
> pathological studies, 2285.2
> phosphorus content, 1380.1
> physiology, 1382.2, 1574
> primates, 350
> pseudosclerosis, 4709
> pyogenic infective diseases, 4872
> radio-isotopes localization, 4615.2
> revascularization, 4914
> and sight defects, 4537
> simian, 1426
> speech centre, 1400, 4630
> stereotactic surgery, 4879.1, 4912.1
> structure, 401.2, 1379, 1403
> subprimate, 1426
> surgery, 4851.1, 4859, 4879, 5008
> *Treponema pallidum* and general paralysis, 4805
> wire gauze drain, 4886
> woodcuts, 368
> (*see also* cerebral entries)

brain atrophy

aphasia, 4707
> presenile dementia, 4707

brain stem
> primates, 350
> respiration regulation, 963
> syndrome, 5019.11

brain tumour, 4615.2, 4879–4879.01
> positional nystagmus, 4611.2
> retinal haemorrhage, 5870

Braxton Hicks's sign, 6189

Brazil
> crustacea, 221
> medicine, 6599, 6601
> yaws, 5293.1

breakbone fever (*see* dengue)

breast
> adenocarcinomata, 5778
> amputations, 36
> anatomy, 5769.1
> carcinoma metastasis, 2607
> diseases, 5769–5788
> plastic surgery, 5760, 5766
> reconstruction, 5766.6
> sero-cystic tumours, 5770
> surgery, 3195
> tumours, 5771, 5773, 5781, 5784

breast cancer, 2619, 2657, 5640, 5782–5782.1
> cure, 5776
> hypertrophy compared, 5553
> öophorectomy treatment, 5778.1

breathing through mouth, 3267

Breda's disease, 5293.1

Brenner tumour, 6109.1, 6118

Breslau Codex, 49

Breslau tables, 1687

Bright's disease, 2285, 4206, 4209, 4495
> and arteries, 4216
> chronic, 4215, 4253
> etiology, 2906.1
> kidney, 4250.1
> kidney operation, 4228
> pathological anatomy, 4217

Brill–Symmers disease, 3787

Brill's disease described, 5382, 5396.4

Briquet's ataxia, 4842

British anatomy, 461

British anti-lewisite, 1929

British Army
> medical service officers, 6723
> medical and surgical history, 2165

British botanicals, 2068.15

British cranial studies, 203

British glass, 2068.94

British herbals, 2068.15

British horticulture, 2068.15

British Isles
> bubonic plague history, 5145
> medicine, 6534–6551.4

British medicine, Vienna School, 6437

British pharmacopoeia, 1866

fingerprint identification, 186
medicine, 6491.9–6495.4
parasitic diseases, 2455
China root, therapeutic use, 1810.1
Chinese, pulse watch, 2670
chinocough (*see* whooping cough)
chironomia, 3346–3347
chiropody (*see* podiatry)
chirurgical observations, cataract, 2122
Chlamydia psittaci, agent of psittacosis, 5539
Chlamydia trachomatis, 5951, 5961
    isolated, 5991.1
Chlonorchis sinensis described, 5344.9
chloral discovered, 1852
chloral hydrate as hypnotic, 1869
chlorambucil, cancer chemotherapy, 2660.4
chlorambucil use in malignant lymphoma,
    3108.6
chloramine-T as antiseptic, 1903.2
chloramphenicol
    introduced, 1940
    production, 1938
    used in typhus, 5402
chloric ether
    as anaesthesia, 5648
    solutions, 1850
chloride of lime for antisepsis, 2219
chlorides distributed in nerve cells, 1300
chlorine disinfectant, 5633
chloroform
    as anaesthetic, 5654, 5657, 5666, 5673
    discovered, 1850–1852, 5648–5650
    and ether, 5730
    inhaler, 5663, 5668
    and morphine reaction, 5670
chloroma, 3055
chloroquine, *Plasmodium vivax* malaria
    treatment, 5261.1
chlorosis, 4301
    boarding schools, 3111
    described, 3109–3110, 3130
    haemoglobin change, 3120
    iron deficiency, 3114
    treatment, 3113
chlorotic anaemia, achylia gastrica as cause,
    3134
chlorpromazine, 1931.1
    psychosis treatment, 4962.3
chlortetracycline discovered, 1942
cholangiograms, 3650
cholecysto-intestinal anastomosis, 3507
cholecystography introduced, 3652
cholecystotomy
    gall stones removal, 3621
    Sim's operation, 3625
cholelithiasis, 3645
cholera, 2263, 2269, 5104–5112
    bacteriolysis, 2546
    described, 1815
    history, 5111.2, 5111.4, 5112

international sanitary code, 1610.1
    pathology, 2571.1
    pyocyanase as inhibitor, 1932.2
cholera vibrios, bacteriolysis, 5110
cholesteatomata effects on bone, 3385
cholesterol, 668.2
cholesterol-rich diet, arteriosclerosis, 2915
choline
    detection, 1338
    toxicity, 1897
cholinesterase inhibitors, 1344
chondrin isolated, 673
chondro-osteo-dystrophy, 4397.1
chondrodystrophic dwarfs in Denmark, 4404
chondrodystrophy inheritance, 4404
chorda tympani
    acetylcholine production, 1348
    described, 378.2
chorea
    chronic degenerative, 4699
    chronic hereditary, 4691
    electric, 4637
    hereditary, 4699
    minor, 4514
    post-paralytic, 4552
    speech defects, 4620
chorio-allantoic membrane, chick embryos,
    2524.1
choriocarcinoma, 6066.1
    histogenesis, 6097.1
    in North America, 6100
chorionepithelioma, 6097.1
chorionic neoplasms classified, 6094
chorionic tumours, 6031.1
choroid
    cauterization, 5980
    membrane description, 1501
    neoplasms radiation treatment, 5978
    plexus extirpation, 4888
    Sattler's layer, 1518
Christmas disease, 3108.1
chromaffin cell tumours described, 3871
chromatin, 122
chromidrosis, 4046
chromosomes
    in cell nucleus as inherited characteris-
    tics, 254.3
    development, 241.1
    genes relationship, 245.3–245.4
    heredity, 242.1
    individuality, 231.1
    meiosis, 242.1
    number in man, 256.5
    sex determination, 256.2, 518
chronaxia defined, 655
chronic abscesses, micrococci present 2494
chronic appendicitis, 3562
chronic arthritis
    adults, 4506
    childhood, 4499

gastroenterostomy, 3476, 3529, 3543
after-effects, 3538
gastrointestinal anastomosis, 3507, 3511
gastrointestinal motility, emotions effects,
1124
gastrointestinal tract, radioactive iron
absorption, 1040
gastrophotography, 3548
gastroptosis described, 3484
gastroscope, 3535.1
demonstration, 3558.3
flexible, 3553
Rosenheim's, 3516.1
gastroscopy, 3337, 3545
gastrostomy, 3451, 3457, 3463.1, 3468, 3486,
3512
oesophagus stricture, 3464, 3467
operation, 3523
tubo-valvular, 3549
valvular method, 3509
gastrosuccorrhoea described, 3478
gastrula, two-layered, 120
Gaucher's disease, anaemia, 3127
gauze face mask, 5641
Gee–Herter disease, 3528
Geisböck's disease, 3076
general paralysis, 4793, 4802
diagnosis with cerebrospinal fluid,
4804
and insanity, 4794, 4796–4797
mental disorders relationship, 4798
and paresis, 4799
Treponema pallidum in brain, 4805
generation, 534.2, 534.4
alteration, 217
Hippocratic treatise, 6485.61
history, 467.1–467.2
theory, 470
genes
artificial transmutation, 251.1
on chromosomes, 245.3–245.4, 246
cloning, 257.5
history, 258.5
linear series, 245.3–245.4
linkage, 242.3
recombination, 255.4
regulation, 256.9
theory, 251
transmutation, 251.1
X-chromosomes in mice, 256.7
genesis of animal cells, 112.1
genetic code, proteins, 256.8
genetics, 216.1, 222, 258.12, 2526.1
biochemical, 254.3
biometric observations, 248
chromatin mass, 255.5
control and biochemical reactions,
254.3
and DNA, 257.3
early study, 258.1–258.2

evolution of social behaviour, 257.1
history, 258.3–258.4
inherited defects, 253.2
intrauterine defects diagnosis, 6235.2
Mendelian, 248
mutation induction, 251.1
natural selection theory, 253
origin, 258.6–258.8
origin of species, 254.2
popular, 244
protein synthesis, 256.9
radiation effects, 251.1
recombination, 2526.1
textbook, 241
tissue transplantation, 2573.1
transduction effects, 256.1
transformations, 255.3
transplantation, 2578.30
variability, 242
Geneva Convention (1864), 2166
genital system, development in anterior
pituitary, 1167
genitals
abnormalities, 3876
hypoplasia in dogs, 1162
neoplasms, 2273
of rat, 296
genius, hereditary, 226
gentamicin isolated, 1947.5
gentian violet
burns treatment, 2258
staphylococci treatment, 1911
geographical distribution of plants, 145.55
geographical medicine, 1767, 1782.1
geographical pathology, 1776.1, 1778
geography
diseases, 1780
physical, 145.59
practical medicine, 1776
geriatrics, 1589.1, 1595, 1641.1
bibliography, 1671.11
history, 1605.1, 1671.61
study, 2222
Gerlach's stain histology, 548
Gerlach's valve, 994
German biology, 145.2
German flora, 1806
German measles (*see* rubella)
German medical school, 18.2
German medicinals, 1827
German medicine, 6558–6560
German Papyrus, 4, 6467.92
German people, physical characteristics, 176
German pharmacy, 2057
German physicians, bibliographies, 6768
German practical medicine, 1776
German surgery, 60.1, 5795
German universities, medical sciences,
1766.603
German war surgery history, 2182

germicides, mercurochrome, 1908
germinal epithelium, 492
germinal nuclei, genetic equivalents, 256.12
germinal vesicle, embryos, 476
germination, 519
germs
    in atmosphere, 2495
    diseases, 2475
    fermentation, 674
    layer classification, 485
    layer theory, 470, 479
    plasma continuity, 236
    putrefaction, 674
    theory, 2529
gerontology
    bibliography, 1671.11
    history, 1602.1
Gerson–Sauerbruch–Hermannsdorfer diet, 2345
Gerstmann's syndrome, 4605.3
Gestalt psychology, 4991
gestation, 6144.1
    tubo peritoneal ectopic, 6203
Ghon's primary focus, 3233
ghosts, 4916.2
giant lymph follicle hyperplasia, lymph nodes, 3786
giant urticaria, 4070
Gigli's saw
    craniotomy, 4874
    pubiotomy, 6204
gingivectomy, 3673.1
glanders, 2553, 5152
    bacteriology, 5154
    diagnosis, 5157–5158
    in horse transmitted to man, 5153
    infectious diseases, 5159
    Pfeifferella mallei as cause, 5156
glands
    Haversian, 387
    viscera differentiated, 1116
glandular fever (*see* infectious mononucleosis)
glandular nerves, paralytic secretions, 622
glass, British, 2068.94
glaucoma, 5820, 5871
    cyclodiathermy treatment, 5988
    filering cicatrix treatment, 5955
    intraocular pressure, 5842.1
    iridectomy treatment, 5881
    iridencleisis, 5952
    physostigmine treatment, 5913
    sclerectomy treatment, 5953
    sclero-corneal trephining, 5955
    small flap sclerotomy, 5958
    symptoms, 5842, 5848
glaucosan, 5970
glia cells discovered, 1271
glioma tumours, 4608

glomerular capillary pressures in frog kidney, 1242
glomerular circulation in frog kidney, 1238
glomerular filtration rate, 1241
glomerular urine composition, 1239
glomerulonephritis described, 4212, 4234
Glossina morsitans, 5269
Glossina palpalis, Trypanosoma transmission, 5283.1
glossitis, 3321
glossopharyngeal nerves, 1253, 1271.1
    frogs, 1266
glossopharyngeal neuralgia, 4896
glottis, oedema, 3262
glottiscope described, 3327
glucose
    in blood transfusions, 2019
    kidney action, 992.3
    in urine, 3931–3932
glucosides synthesis, 1903
glutathione isolated, 745
gluteal artery
    aneurysms, 2935, 2958
    ligation, 2926, 5581
glutin isolated, 673
glycaemia in diabetes, 3942
glycine
    isolated, 668.3
    myathenia gravis treatment, 4766
glycogens, 566.3
    catalytic transformation, 751.4
    discovered, 999.1
    hepatomegalic disease, 3656
glycosuria
    diabetes relationship, 3936, 3942
    from brain ventricle puncture, 3933
    islands of Langerhans relationship, 3962
    and retinitis, 3938
gnathodynamometer, 3689.2
goat's milk, undulant fever source, 5102
goitre
    burnt sponge remedy, 3808
    and cretinism, 3809
    deaf-mutism relationship, 3840.1
    described, 3806
    effects on eyelids, 3820
    endemic, 3805
    endemic cretinism, 3842
    exophthalmic, 2210, 3811, 3813
    iodine treatment, 3807, 3812
    operations, 3829
    pathogenesis, 3847
    seaweed treatment, 5551
    sporadic cretinism, 3842
    thyroidectomy, 3825–3826
gold
    chronic arthritis therapy, 4506.1
    tooth filling, 3666.84, 3689.1

deformities, 464, 6259
deformities classified, 6265
female, 6253–6254
fractures, 4416–4417
non-rachitic flat, 6259
osteomalacic, 6254
pus content, 6090
rachitic, 6259
spinosa, 6261
spondylolisthetic, 6262, 6264
various forms, 6260
pemphigus
chronic, 4152.1
erythematodes, 4151.2
foliaceus, 4037
gangrenosa, 4020
vegetans, 4087, 4101
penicilinase, 1933.3
penicillamine, 1934.2
penicillin
chemotherapeutic agent, 1934–1934.1
history, 2068.11
meningitis treatment, 4689.1
subacute bacterial endocarditis, 2880
syphilis treatment, 2418
used in gonorrheal infections, 5214.1
Penicillium, bacteria-inhibiting effect, 1932
Penicillium glaucum, antibacterial crystalline
produced, 1932.3, 1933
penis
plastic induration, 4163
reconstruction, 5766.2
pentaquine used in *Plasmodium vivax*
malaria, 5261.2
pentobarbitone sodium, intravenous use,
5712.1
pentosuria
chemical malformation, 3921
described, 3918
pepsin, 991
crystalline, 1038.1
peptic ulcer, 3454
gastritis relationship, 3546
hypothalamus relationship, 3552
jejunum, 3558.2
vagotomy, 3557
perception theory, 1529
percussor, 2675
percutaneous arterial catheterization, 2924.2
percutaneous transluminal, coronary
angioplasty, 2924.4
percutaneous tuberculosis reaction, 2339
perforated appendix, peritonitis, 3561, 3563,
3570
perfusion pump, 856.1
peri-uterine septic disease treatment, 6096
periarterial sympathectomy, 4885
periarteritis nodosa, 2906
hypersensitivity, 2924
pericardial effusion diagnosis, 2676

pericardial pseudocirrhosis in liver, 2803
pericardiectomy, constrictive pericarditis,
3030–3031
pericardiocentesis, 3021–3022
pericarditis
Avenzoar writings, 47
described, 2733
epistenocardiaca described, 2772
pericardium, stab wound/suture, 3022.2
peridontal diseases, 3666.82, 3676
peridural anaesthesia, 5702
perinaeum preserved in birth, 6156
perineal hernia, 3584
perineal prostatectomy, 4195, 4265–4265.1
modification, 4272
perineorrhaphy, 6078
periodicals
medical and scientific, 6774
scientific history, 6786.20
periodontia, clinical, 3690.1
periodontoclasia treatment, 3673.1
periosteum, osteogenetic layer, 420
Peripatetic School in Athens, 87.1
peripheral aneurysms bypass, 2915.1
peripheral circulation, 2236
peripheral ganglia paralysis, 1329.1
peripheral nerves, injury effects, 1299
peripheral neuritis, 4784
peripheral tabes, separated from medullary
tabes, 4785
peripheral vascular disease, 2919.1
perirenal insufflation of oxygen, kidney 4241
peritoneal dialysis in uraemia, 4242
peritoneal irrigation, renal failure treatment,
4256
peritoneum, 394
described, 1217
female, 4456
processus vaginalis, 77
peritonitis
described, 2279
from perforated appendix, 3561, 3563
suppurative, 3568
perityphlitis, 3565
pernicious anaemia
achylia gastrica relationship, 3134,
3143
bone marrow changes, 3125–3125.1,
3131.1
bone marrow pathology, 3142.1
described, 3112, 3116, 3118, 3124–
3125.3
desiccated stomach, 3144
hookworms in cats, 5359
injected liver extract, 3144.1, 3145.1
macrocytic anaemia, 3149
pregnancy, 3146
raw liver diet, 3140
vitamin B_{12}, 3154–3155
peroneal artery ligation, 2937

peroxidase systems function, 1059
perpetual arrhythmia, auricular fibrillation, 2830–2831, 2833
persecution mania, 4931
Persia
    manuscripts catalogue, 6786.30
    medicine, 6511–6515
    pharmacology, 1788
persistent dental capsule, 3681
personal hygiene, 1592, 1602
personalities, maladies, 4943
perspiration, body temperature, 590
pertussis immunization, 5087.2
Peru, medicine history, 6602
Peruvian bark, 1826, 5230.1
pestilence, 5114
    contagion, 5123
    and epidemics, 5113
    history, 5138
    history in France, 5137
    remedies, 5140
    (*see also* plague)
petechial typhus, typhoid compared, 5372.1
pethidine synthesis, 1927
Petri dish, 2505.1
Peyer's patches, 1100
peyote, 2086.1
    mescaline content, 1890.1
Pfannenstiel's incision, 6113
Pfeiffer phenomenon, 2546
Pfeifferella mallei, glanders cause, 5156
Pfeifferella whitmori isolated, 5159
Pfeiffer's phenomenon, 5110
pH in blood, 742
phaeochromocytoma described, 3865
phagocytes, 2538
phagocytosis, 2538
    of fat cells, 4151
phantastics, 2086
pharmaceutical pottery and porcelain, 2068.16
pharmaceutical trade literature, bibliography, 6786.32
pharmaceuticals dictionary, 1610
pharmacists, poetry, 6621
pharmacology
    anthology, 2068.4
    Arabia, 6508
    drugs, 1804, 1900, 2081
    early teaching, 1862.1
    experimental, 1909
    in Great Britain, 2035
    histamines, 1919
    history, 1906, 2036–2038, 2068.10, 2073
    hormones, 1125
    magnesium salts effects, 1894
    Persian, 1788
    pituitary gland, 1172
    textbook, 1881

    therapeutics, 1931.8
pharmacopoeia, 1810, 1816
    British, 1866
    first in United States, 1845
    London, 1821
    Paris, 1824
    unofficial drugs, 1874
pharmacy
    and the Bible, 2045
    chronicles, 2045
    development, 2067
    German, 2057
    history, 2040–2041, 2049, 2051–2052, 2055, 2058, 2064, 2068.5, 2068.7
    history in Great Britain, 2068.2
    and medicine, 2045, 6610.14
    and mythology, 2045
    and Shakespeare, 2045
pharyngeal paralysis, **Avenzoar** writings, 47
pharyngeal tonsil inflammation, 3283
pharyngotomy, 3265
pharynx
    carcinoma, 3196
    disease history, 3339
    treatment, 3280
phase contrast microscopy, 269.3
phenacetin introduced, 1883.3
phenformin, diabetes use, 3978.3
phenobarbitone, epilepsy treatment, 4823
phenolsulphonephthalein in renal function tests, 1896, 4236
phenoltetrachlorphthalein in hepatic function tests, 1896
phenylalanine, tyrosine metabolism, 3923.1
phenylhydrazine hydrochloride, polycythaemia treatment, 3084
phenylindanedione, 3107
phenylketonuria
    bacterial inhibition test, 3924.4
    described, 3924
    mental retardation, 3923.1
pheochromocytoma
    histamine test, 3869
Philadelphia
    relapsing fever epidemic, 5313
    yellow fever epidemic, 5451–5453.1, 5454.2
philately and medicine, 6639.2
Philippines medicine, 6604.39
philosophy, 88
    and medicine, 6645, 6647
phlebitis, post-operative, 3018
Phlebotomus
    Oroya fever vector, 5538.2
    and phlebotomus fever, 5477
Phlebotomus argentipes
    and India kala azar, 5302
    Leishmania donovani reproduction, 5301.1
phlebotomus fever from *Phlebotomus,* 5477

frog heart, 821
history, 2116
identified, 2080
industrial, 2134
on living body, 2075
microchemistry, 2080
minerals, 2069
muscular contractions, 2078
nerve endings reaction, 1893
submaxillary gland nerves, 1011
vegetables, 2069
Poitou colic
described, 2092
lead poisoning effects, 2095
polioencephalomyelitis, 4643, 4648
poliomyelitis, 4662, 4666
acute anterior, 4664, 4665.1
epidemic, 4667, 4670.4
history, 4672.5
immunization, 4672.1–4672.2
infectious, 4668
Lansing strain, 4671.1–4671.2
in monkeys, 4669
prophylactic agent, gamma globulin, 4672
virus strains, 4670.5–4670.6
polycentric knee arthroplasty, 4405.5
polycythaemia
hypertonica, 3076
phenylhydrazine hydrochloride, 3084
vera, 2991–2992, 3070, 3073
polygraph, 834, 2812
polymavirus
cell transformation, 2660.13
isolated, 2660.10
polymorphonuclear leucocytes, 3075
polymyxin
chemotherapeutic agent, 1941
discovered, 1937
polyneuritis, 4587
acute infective, 4639, 4647
in birds, 1047, 3744
polynucleotides, enzymatic synthesis, 752.3, 752.6
polype natural history, 306
polypetide protein molecule, 721
polyposis of colon, 3460
polypus, nose, 1609, 2122, 2607.1
polysaccharide antigens, 2573.2, 3198
polyuria and tuberculosis, 6361
polyvinyl sponge prosthesis, 2993.2
Ponceau fuchsin stain, 3875
pons
trigeminal nerve, 4896
varolii, 1377.2, 1478
poor, treatment of sick, 1657
popliteral aneurysm, 2925
popular medicine, 1794
population
behaviour, 253

classification, 171
ecology, 145.90
in England, 1694
evolution problems, 1713
geometrical proportional growth, 215
growth, 145.57–145.58
growth in United States, 1712
history, 1714
physical anomalies, 174
principles, 215.4, 1693
porokeratosis, 4068, 4114–4115
porphyrin, haematoporphyrin, 3914.1
portal venography, 2725.1
Porter's sign, 3254
portraits of doctors, 6610.10, 6621, 6711
portraiture, 154
Portugal medicine, 6577, 6579.1
positional nystagmus, brain tumour, 4611.2
post-mortem examinations, 2270, 2276
post-paralytic chorea, 4552
post-partum
haemorrhage, 3907.1
haemorrhage and abdominal ligature, 6214
necrosis and anterior pituitary, 3900
post-scarlatinal dropsy, 5074
posterior nerve roots, haemorrhagic inflammation, 4644
posterior parietal presentatin, 6263.1
posterior pituitary, oxytocic action, 1159
posterior rhizotomy, 4860.1, 4861.1
postsynaptic inhibition, ionic mechanism, 1310.2
posture, 661, 663.1
potash hydrate, 826
potassium bromide epilepsy treatment, 4813.1–4814
potassium chloride used in myathenia gravis, 4769
potassium compounds in heart tissue, 1337
potassium ferricyanide, oxygen in oxyhaemoglobin, 951
potassium iodide
roentgenography, 2692.2
syphilis treatment, 2379
potassium-argon dating, palaeoanthropology, 214.2
potters and lead poisoning, 2121
Pott's disease, 2320, 4303–4304, 4344
fracture treatment, 4359.1
tibia transplanted into spine, 4384.1
tuberculous, 4315
Pott's puffy tumour, 4850.5
practical anatomy, history, 442
practical hygiene, 1614
practical surgery, 5593, 5596
practice of medicine, 2215
praecordial leads, electrocardiography, 2868
praecypitine, 2556
pre-eclampsia, 6163.1